Molecular Biology of B-Cell and T-Cell Development

Contemporary Immunology

1. **Molecular Biology of B-Cell and T-Cell Development**
   Edited by John G. Monroe and Ellen V. Rothenberg, 1998
2. **Cytokine Knockouts**
   Edited by Scott K. Durum and Kathrin Muegge, 1998
3. **Immunosuppression and Human Malignancy**
   Edited by David Naor, 1990
4. **The Lymphokines**
   Edited by John W. Haddon, 1990
5. **Clinical Cellular Immunology**
   Edited by Howard H. Weetall, 1990

Molecular Biology of B-Cell and T-Cell Development

Edited by

John G. Monroe

University of Pennsylvania,
Philadelphia, PA

and

Ellen V. Rothenberg

California Institute of Technology,
Pasadena, CA

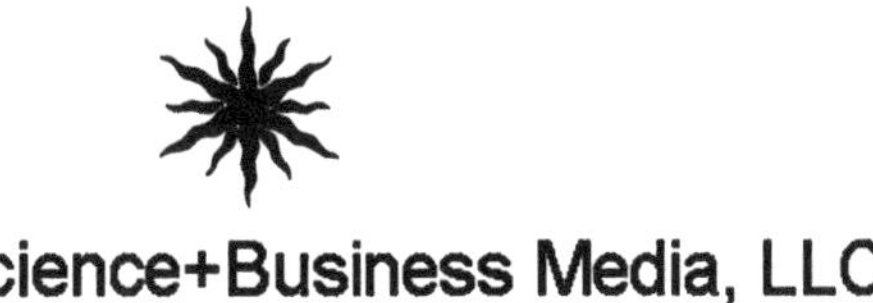

Springer Science+Business Media, LLC

Originally published by Humana Press Inc. in 1998
MyCopy version of the original edition 1998

This publication is printed on acid-free paper. ∞
ANSI Z39.48-1984 (American National Standards Institute) Permanence of Paper for Printed Library Materials.

Cover design by Patricia F. Cleary.

For additional copies, pricing for bulk purchases, and/or information about other Humana titles, contact Humana at the above address or at any of the following numbers: Tel.: 973-256-1699; Fax: 973-256-8341; E-mail: humana@humanapr.com or visit our Web site: http://humanapress.com

10 9 8 7 6 5 4 3 2 1
Library of Congress Cataloging in Publication Data

Molecular Biology of B-Cell and T-Cell Development / edited by
John G. Monroe and Ellen V. Rothenberg.
p. cm. — (Contemporary immunology)
Includes index.

DOI 10.1007/978-1-4757-2778-4
1. B cells. 2. T cells. 3. Hematopoietic stem cells.
I. Monroe, John Gordon, 1953- . II. Rothenberg, Ellen V. III. Series.

QR 185.8B15M64 1998
616.07' 97--dc21
DNLM/DLC
for Library of Congress 98-12613
CIP

www.springer.com/mycopy

Preface

Despite the tremendous diversity of the cells of the hematopoietic system, they are all derived from common precursor cells that are generated in the fetus and persist into adult life. In this regard, B and T lymphocytes, which comprise the two arms of the antigen-specific and inducible immune system, though functionally very different, are descendants of the same stem cell precursor. In the past several years, we have witnessed an explosion of information regarding the process by which differentiation of B- and T-cells from stem cells occurs. This information, like the answers to most important biological questions, has come from multiple and diverse directions.

Because all hematopoietic cells arise from common precursors, complex regulatory processes must be involved in determining commitment to various lineages. Understanding commitment to the B- or T-cell lineage remains incomplete; however, identification of transcription factors necessary for progression along specific B- and T-cell pathways suggests that we are on the verge of understanding the molecules involved in the initial fate-determining steps. Studies of this type previously could be accomplished only in nonmammalian systems that are more amenable to genetic approaches. However, new technologies allow increasingly elegant and informative studies in mammalian systems, particularly for cells of the hematopoietic system.

At the level of cell biology, significant progress has been made in the identification and characterization of hematopoietic stem cells and developmental stages associated with B- and T-cell development. Two advances have contributed to this progress. One is the ability to use constellations of cell-surface markers to provide extraordinary precision in the developmental characterization of individual cells. The other is the ability to culture and transfer hematopoietic cells in a variety of environments, and to define the responses of individual cells by cell-autonomous markers. As a result of these advances, cell transfer experiments with tightly defined precursor populations have even begun to dissect the process of commitment to B- and T-cell lineages, providing new evidence for a gradual, stepwise narrowing of developmental potential. T- and natural killer cells appear to be more closely related, by this measure, than T- and B-cells; whereas T- and most myeloerythroid cells appear much less closely related. These relationships provide a starting point for defining the target genes on which lineage-determining factors must work in driving commitment.

B- and T-cells are distinct from other hematopoietic cells in that the fully developed progeny are clonally unique. In order to avoid retention of nonfunctional or autoreactive clones, antigen receptor-mediated inducible selection events occur during defined stages in the development of these cells. These events, both positive and negative, are central to establishing the available immune system repertoire. Genetic, biochemical, and cellular approaches are each producing important insights into the molecular basis and cellular mechanisms underlying these selection events.

In the past, B- and T-cell malignancies have provided our only chance to study early stages of development of these cells. Cells "frozen" at particular stages of development by malignant transformation provided tools to study the phenotype and cell biology of developing B- and T-cells. Now, however, the ability to isolate normal cells at defined developmental stages affords us the ability to define the cell biology of these cells and thereby better understand the physiology of their transformed cell counterparts. The usefulness of this information lies in our ability to use it to alter the growth characteristics of specific B- and T-cell malignancies.

Finally, cells of the developing hematopoietic system are especially amenable to gene therapy approaches. Because they are now easily isolatable, capable of expansion, and relatively easy to maintain in culture, they provide convenient vehicles for the introduction of new genes.

Significant progress has been realized in all of the above areas over the past several years. This progress has yielded not only important insights into significant and fundamental areas of cell biology, but has influenced our thinking in terms of understanding human disease and new ways of therapeutic intervention into disease processes. The aim of *Molecular Biology of B-Cell and T-Cell Development* is to present an integrated and comprehensive presentation of these new advances in B and T lymphocyte development. Topics covered in this volume will be of interest to researchers and clinicians interested in hematopoiesis, immunology, cancer biology, and gene therapy.

John G. Monroe
Ellen V. Rothenberg

Contents

Contributors

KOICHI AKASHI • *Departments of Pathology and Developmental Biology, Stanford University School of Medicine, Stanford, CA*
NICOLE AVITAHL • *Cutaneous Biology Research Center, Massachussetts General Hospital, Harvard Medical School, Charlestown, MA*
BART BARLOGIE • *Departments of Medicine and Pathology, University of Arkansas for Medical Sciences and the Little Rock VAMC, Little Rock, AR*
LISA BORGHESI • *Department of Immunology, Oklahoma Medical Research Foundation, Oklahoma City, OK*
MEINRAD BUSSLINGER • *Research Institute of Molecular Pathology, Vienna, Austria*
JAN BUER • *Faculty of Medicine, Necker Institute, Paris, France*
MYRIAM CAPONE • *Department of Immunobiology, DNAX Research Institute, Palo Alto, CA*
SIMON R. CARDING • *Department of Microbiology, University of Pennsylvania, Philadelphia, PA*
KENNETH DORSHKIND • *Department of Pathology and Laboratory Medicine and The Jonsson Comprehensive Cancer Center, University of California Los Angeles School of Medicine, Los Angeles, CA*
ERASTUS C. DUDLEY • *Laboratory of Immunology, National Institutes of Health, Bethesda, MD*
ELAINE DZIERZAK • *Department of Cell Biology and Genetics, Erasmus University Medical Facility, Rotterdam, The Netherlands*
ANNE F. EDER • *Hospital of the University of Pennsylvania, Philadelphia, PA*
RICHARD FESTENSTEIN • *Division of Molecular Immunology, The National Institute for Medical Research, London, England*
KATIA GEORGOPOULOS • *Cutaneous Biology Research Center, Massachussetts General Hospital, Harvard Medical School, Charlestown, MA*
MICHAEL GIRARDI • *Department of Dermatology, Yale University School of Medicine, New Haven, CT*
RUDOLF GROSSCHEDL • *Department of Microbiology and Immunology, Howard Hughes Medical Institute, University of California, San Francisco, CA*

SUSAN C. GUBA • *Division of Hematology/Oncology, Department of Medicine,University of Arkansas for Medical Sciences, Little Rock, AR*
CYNTHIA J. GUIDOS • *Division of Immunology and Cancer, The Hospital for Sick Children, Toronto, Ontario, Canada*
ADRIAN HAYDAY • *Department of Biology, Section of Immunology, Yale University School of Medicine, New Haven, CT*
RICHARD R. HARDY • *Institute for Cancer Research, Fox Chase Cancer Center, Philadelphia, PA*
ERIC S. HOFFMAN • *Section of Immunology, Department of Biology, Yale University School of Medicine, New Haven, CT*
LISA J. JARVIS • *Department of Laboratory Medicine/Pathology, Centers for Immunology and Cancer, University of Minnesota Medical School, Minneapolis, MN*
BARBARA L. KEE • *Department of Biology, University of California, San Diego, La Jolla, CA*
PAUL W. KINCADE • *Immunobiology Program, Oklahoma Medical Research Foundation, Oklahoma City, OK*
LESLIE B. KING • *Department of Pathology and Laboratory Medicine, University of Pennsylvania, Philadelphia, PA*
DIMITRIS KIOUSSIS • *Division of Molecular Immunology, The National Institute for Medical Research, London, England*
MOTONARI KONDO • *Department of Pathology and Developmental Biology, Stanford University School of Medicine, Stanford, CA*
PETER LANSDORP • *Terry Fox Laboratory, British Columbia Cancer Agency, Department of Medicine, University of British Columbia, Vancouver, British Columbia, Canada*
TUCKER LEBIEN • *University of Minnesota Cancer Center, Minneapolis, MN*
CHRISTIAAN N. LEVELT • *Center for Cancer Research, Massachussetts Institute of Technology, Cambridge, MA*
YUE-SHENG LI • *Beijing Sai-Yin-Si Institute of Biotechnology, Beijing, People's Republic of China*
FERENC LIVAK • *Section of Immunobiology, Yale University School of Medicine, New Haven, CT*
KAY MEDINA • *Immunology Program, Oklahoma Medical Research Foundation, Oklahoma City, OK*
ALEXANDER MEDVINSKY • *Department of Cell Biology and Genetics, Erasmus University, Rotterdam, The Netherlands*
FRITZ MELCHERS • *Section of Immunology, Basel Institute for Immunology, Basel, Switzerland*
JOHN G. MONROE • *Department of Pathology and Laboratory Medicine, University of Pennsylvania, Philadelphia, PA*
ENCARNACION MONTECINO-RODRIGUEZ • *Department of Pathology and Laboratory Medicine and The Jonsson Comprehensive Cancer Center, University of California Los Angeles School of Medicine, Los Angeles, CA*

ALIKI NICHOGIANNOPOULOU • *Cutaneous Biology Research Center, Massachussetts General Hospital, Harvard Medical School, Charlestown, MA*
STEPHEN L. NUTT • *Research Institute of Molecular Pathology, Vienna, Austria*
STUART H. ORKIN • *Division of Hematology/Oncology, Children's Hospital and the Dana Farber Institute, Department of Pediatrics, Harvard Medical School, Howard Hughes Medical Insitute, Boston, MA*
KENJI ORITANI • *Immunobiology Program, Oklahoma Medical Research Foundation, Oklahoma City, OK*
CHRISTOPHER J. PAIGE • *The Wellesley Hospital Research Institute, Toronto, Ontario, Canada*
LORENA PASSONI • *Department of Molecular Cell and Developmental Biology and Section of Immunobiology, Yale University, New Haven, CT*
KIMBERLY PAYNE • *Immunobiology Program, Oklahoma Medical Research Facility, Oklahoma City, OK*
HOWARD T. PETRIE • *Memorial Sloan-Kettering Cancer Center, Cornell University Graduate School of Medical Sciences, New York, NY*
KAREN E. POLLOK • *Section of Pediatric Hematology/Oncology, Herman B. Wells Center for Pediatric Research, Riley Hospital for Children, Indiana University School of Medicine, Indianapolis, IN*
TANNISHTHA REYA • *Department of Microbiology and Immunology, Howard Hughes Medical Institute, University of California San Francisco, San Francisco, CA*
ELLEN V. ROTHENBERG • *Division of Biology, California Institute of Technology, Pasadena, CA*
PETER SANDEL • *Department of Pathology and Laboratory Medicine, University of Pennsylvania School of Medicine, Philadelphia, PA*
RICHARD A. SATER • *Department of Pathology and Laboratory Medicine, University of Pennsylvania School of Medicine, Philadelphia, PA*
ANNETTE M. SCHLAGETER • *Departments of Pathology and Developmental Biology, Stanford University School of Medicine, Stanford, CA*
EDWARD W. SCOTT • *Institute for Human Gene Therapy, University of Pennsylvania School of Medicine, Philadelphia, PA*
TAKAICHI SHIMOZATO • *Immunobiology Program, Oklahoma Medical Research Foundation, Oklahoma City, OK*
SUSAN SHINTON • *Institute for Cancer Research, Fox Chase Cancer Center, Philadelphia, PA*
MIKAEL SIGVARDSSON • *Howard Hughes Medical Institute and Departments of Microbiology and Biochemistry, University of California San Francisco, San Francisco, CA*
LESLIE E. SILBERSTEIN • *Department of Pathology and Laboratory Medicine, Hospital of the University of Pennsylvania, Philadelphia, PA*

GLENNDA SMITHSON • *Immunobiology Program, Oklahoma Medical Research Foundation, Oklahoma City, OK*
ALAIN P. VICARI • *DNAX Research Institute of Molecular and Cellular Biology, Palo Alto, CA*
HARALD VON BOEHMER • *Faculty of Medicine, Necker Institute, Paris, France*
ROBERT WASSERMAN • *Division of Oncology, Children's Hospital of Philadelphia and Department of Pediatrics, University of Pennsylvania School of Medicine, Philadelphia, PA*
IRVING L. WEISSMAN • *Departments of Pathology and Developmental Biology, Stanford University School of Medicine, Stanford, CA*
DAVID A. WILLIAMS • *Howard Hughes Medical Institute, Indiana University School of Medicine, Indianapolis, IN*
SUSAN WINANDY • *Cutaneous Biology Research Center, Massachussetts General Hospital, Harvard Medical School, Charlestown, MA*
THOMAS H. WINKLER • *Section of Immunology, Basel Institute for Immunology, Basel, Switzerland*
LI WU • *The Walter and Eliza Hall Institute of Medical Research, Melbourne, Victoria, Australia*
YOSHIO YAMASHITA • *Immunobiology Program, Oklahoma Medical Research Foundation, Oklahoma City, OK*
ZHONG ZHENG • *Immunobiology Program, Oklahoma Medical Research Foundation, Oklahoma City, OK*
ALBERT ZLOTNIK • *DNAX Research Institute of Molecular and Cellular Biology, Palo Alto, CA*

Part I

Stem Cells and Lineage Commitment Models

Chapter 1

Developmental Origins of Hematopoietic Stem Cells

Elaine Dzierzak and Alexander Medvinsky

1. Introduction

The hemato/lymphopoietic system is a dynamic continuum of differentiating cells leading to the production of numerous lineages of blood effector cells. In the adult, only a few immature undifferentiated hematopoietic stem cells are required to yield the enormous number of intermediate progenitors and effector cells produced daily. Although these founder cells of the adult mammalian blood system have been extensively studied, the developmental origins of definitive hematopoietic stem cells are controversial, and the subject of much current research. In this article, the authors review studies that explore the ontogeny of the hemato/lymphopoietic system and present current models of initiation, migration, lineage potential, and molecular programming of the cells involved in establishing the complex network in the adult. The combined results of studies on the origin and function suggest distinct embryonic and adult hierarchies on the cellular levels, whereas molecular studies suggest some, but not complete, overlap in the genetic programming of embryonic and adult hematopoietic cells.

2. Cellular Hierarchies in Mammalian Hematopoiesis

Throughout development, both the lineage complexity and the circulating nature of the mammalian hematopoietic system make it a difficult tissue to study. In vitro and in vivo assays to establish precursor-progeny associations in this rapidly differentiating system have made profound contributions to the understanding of the basis of blood production. The mouse has served as an excellent experimental model for adult mammalian hematopoiesis, and in agreement with many clinical observations in human hematology and transplantation, a hierarchical framework for the line of descent of all

From: *Molecular Biology of B-Cell and T-Cell Development*
Edited by: J. G. Monroe and E. V. Rothenberg

adult hemato/lymphopoietic effector cells has been long established in the authors' thinking. However, accumulating masses of data on mouse embryonic hematopoiesis strongly suggest a different and opposing hierarchical framework for hematopoiesis during ontogeny.

2.1. The Conventional Adult Hematopoietic Hierarchy

The textbook model of adult hematopoiesis reveals a branching network of cell intermediates between a small number of founder hematopoietic stem cells and numerous differentiated effector cells that vary in function *(1)*. The hematopoietic stem cell was established as the foundation of the hierarchy through in vivo transplantation studies, in which marked donor cells were adoptively transferred in lethally irradiated or hematopoietic deficient adult mouse recipients *(2,3)*. Clonal marking with retroviruses and limiting dilution transplantation studies further demonstrate that only a few hematopoietic stem cells in this cohort is contributing to the production of the extensive hematopoietic system at any point in time *(4–8)*. Thus, hematopoietic stem cells have the following properties;

1. Pluripotency for all hematopoietic lineages;
2. High proliferative potential;
3. Long-term maintenance and high level hematopoietic contribution; and
4. Self-renewal ability.

At this time, the long-term in vivo transplantation assay remains the only irrevocable method to identify functional hematopietic stem cells within a population. Other hematopoietic assays have provided evidence for the existence of many intermediate progenitors. The in vivo colony forming unit-spleen (CFU-S) assay that produces macroscopic colonies on the spleen of the irradiated recipient mice within 1–2 weeks of bone marrow injection, reveals a multipotent erythroid/myeloid progenitor that has high proliferative potential *(9)*. It is assumed that the CFU-S progenitor does not produce lymphoid cells. Some of these cells are self-renewing *(10)*, but they do not contribute long-term to hematopoiesis. In fact, CFU-S progenitors can be physically separated from hematopoietic stem cells *(11)*. More committed, as well as multipotent, erythroid-myeloid progenitors in adult bone marrow are revealed by the in vitro colony forming unit-culture (CFU-C) assay *(12)*. Multilineage and single lineage colonies containing erythroid, myeloid, and/or granulocytic cells appear shortly after plating in semisolid medium with addition of hematopoietic growth factors. CFU-C progenitors produce no lymphoid lineage cells nor are the CFU-Cs long-lived. Thus, both CFU-S and CFU-C progenitors can be placed downstream of the hematopoietic stem cell.

The analysis of progenitor cell lymphoid potential has relied on separate in vitro culture systems that provide a lymphoid-type microenvironment. Coculture systems utilizing B lymphoid-specific stromal cells and specific growth factors retrospectively demonstrate the B lymphoid potential of a progenitor *(13)*. Fetal thymic organ culture also reveals progenitor potential for the T lymphoid lineage *(14)*. Determining multipotency for the lymphoid lineages and the erythroid-myeloid lineages presents a problem with such in vitro assays, since growth factor/microenvironment requirements appear to be very different. Recently, a modification of the fetal thymic organ culture system has allowed for the in vitro production of all lineages erythro-myeloid, B lymphoid, and T lymphoid from single cells *(15)*. Although this in vitro assay detects no lymphoid committed B-T lineage progenitor, retrovirus clonal marking studies of bone marrow cells adoptively transferred suggest that there is a committed lymphoid progenitor *(16)*. Thus, branchpoints in the adult hierarchy between the separate lineages are still somewhat speculative, but the general adult hematopoietic hierarchical scheme, based on the progressive restriction of cellular differentiation potential, is well-established.

2.2. The Embryonic Hematopoietic Hierarchy

2.2.1. Sites of Embryonic Hematopoiesis

Until recently, it was thought that the yolk sac produced the first cells of the adult hematopoietic system *(17)*. Yolk sac hematopoietic cells were thought to migrate to the liver, which acted as the predominant site of hematopoiesis during fetal stages of development *(18)*. At neonatal stages, these cells were to migrate yet again to the bone marrow to reside throughout the adult stages of life. Such a model focused on the yolk sac and liver, as they are the most visually active hematopoietic sites undergoing extensive erythropoiesis. Although the preliver embryo body was also initially examined for CFU-C hematopoietic activity, little or no activity was found *(17)*. However, hematopoietic progenitor activity has been recently demonstrated in a preliver intraembryonic site containing no visually apparent hematopoietic foci *(19–21)*. This region, consisting of the dorsal aorta, gonads, and mesonephros (AGM), harbors potent hematopoietic progenitor/stem cell activity and is thought to generate the adult hematopoietic system. The temporal appearance of various hematopoietic activities in each of the three embryonic hematopoietic sites is described.

2.2.1.1. Yolk Sac

The most obvious early embryonic hematopoietic site is the yolk sac. The first differentiated hematopoietic cells, primitive erythrocytes, are found there at day 7.5 in mouse gestation (E7.5) *(22)*. Unlike the adult and fetal hematopoietic tissues, the yolk sac hematopoietic cells are formed intravascularly within structures known as blood islands. A close association of endothelial cells and hematopoietic cells in the blood islands has led to the proposal of a common progenitor cell, the hemangioblast, for these two distinct lineages of cells *(23)*. In vivo, the yolk sac produces predominantly erythroid cells. However, in vitro cultures of yolk sac cells demonstrate the presence of erythroid progenitors, as well as granulocyte-macrophage progenitors beginning at E7 *(17)*. Slightly later at E8.5, T lymphoid and B lymphoid progenitors are found in the yolk sac *(24–29)*. No definitive CFU-S progenitors are found in the yolk sac before mid-E9 *(20,30)*. Long-term repopulating hematopoietic stem cells in the yolk sac appear rather late in mouse gestation, at E11, when compared to the appearance of the more differentiated cells and CFU-C and CFU-S progenitors at this site *(17,21,31)*.

2.2.1.2. AGM

This intraembryonic region, which begins to form at E7 from the para-aortic splanchnopleural mesoderm, as well as closely associated tissue, has been examined by histologic sectioning for the presence of differentiating hematopoietic cells. No extravascular foci of hematopoietic cells are observed *(20)*. However, beginning at E7.5, multipotent hematopoietic progenitors are detected after organ culture and a two-step culture system that promotes the growth and differentiation of myeloid-erythroid, B lymphoid, and T lymphoid cells *(32)*. At E8.5, progenitors for B1a (CD5) B-cells are also detected when the para-aortic splanchnopleura is engrafted under the kidney capsule of SCID mice *(19)*. By E9, the first CFU-S progenitors appear in the AGM region *(20)*, and by late E10, the first long-term repopulating hematopoietic stem cells are detected *(21,31)*. The AGM region always produces definitive hematopoietic progenitors and stem cells to much higher levels of potency and probably at slightly earlier stages than the yolk sac.

2.2.1.3. Liver

At early E9, the evagination of the gut into the septum transversum forms the rudiment of the liver *(18)*. At this time in development, the liver is thought not to autonomously generate its own hematopoietic activity, but to be seeded by exogenous hematopoietic cells from other sites *(33)*. During late E9, the liver rudiment contains erythroblasts *(18,34)* and at E10, begins to produce differentiated erythroid cells. Committed myeloid progenitors appear at mid-E9, T-cell progenitors at E10 *(35)*, and granulocyte-macrophage and B lineage cells at E10–11 *(36,37)*. CFU-S progenitors, as well as hematopoietic stem cells, are detected in the liver beginning at E11, immediately after the increase of these activities in the AGM region *(20,38)*.

2.2.2. A Reversed Hierarchy in the Embryo

The extensive examination of differentiated hematopoietic cells, CFU-C, CFU-S, multipotent erythro-myelo-lymphoid progenitors, and long-term repopulating hematopoietic stem cells in the mouse embryo has revealed an ordered temporal appearance precisely opposite to what is expected from the conventional adult hematopoietic hierarchy *(39)* (Fig. 1). No hematopoietic stem cells are found before E10, yet primitive erythrocytes and myeloid progenitors are readily detected as early as E7.5. The late appearance of the long term repopulating hematopoietic stem cells that establish the entire adult hierarchy leads to two main hypotheses for the hematopoietic generation within the embryo (Fig. 1): 1) The rapidly differentiated hematopoietic cells in the early stage embryo are generated from a cohort of hematopoietic progenitors distinct and independent from those generating the adult hematopoietic hierarchy. 2) A pool of preadult hematopoietic stem cells may be generated early in the embryo; some cells of this cohort undergo rapid terminal differentiation (i.e., in the yolk sac), whereas others acquire more definitive progenitor- and stem cell-like characteristics in the AGM microenvironment. Thus, the lineage relationship of the cells generating the embryonic and adult hematopoietic hierarchies has yet to be established.

3. Determining the Embryonic Source of the Adult Hematopoietic System

3.1. Source Conservation Through Evolution

The earliest temporal appearance of each of the hematopoietic activities in distinct tissues in the mouse conceptus cannot convincingly indicate the generating source of the hematopoietic cells, since the hemato/lymphoid system is mobile. Beginning at E8.5, hematopoietic cells are disseminated via the vascular network throughout the mouse embryo *(32)*. Thus, because of the early establishment of the circulation, it is difficult to determine if independent hematopoietic generation occurs at multiple sites in the mouse embryo such as the yolk sac, AGM, and liver, or whether one tissue is the source of hematopoietic cells that colonize the other tissues.

Developmental studies typically rely on evolutionary comparisons for insight into cellular and genetic processes. Such evolutionary comparisons for early hematopoietic development are becoming increasingly important, and show a high degree of conservation between species. Although it was the widely held view for over 20 years that the originating source of the adult blood system in mammals was the yolk sac, studies on

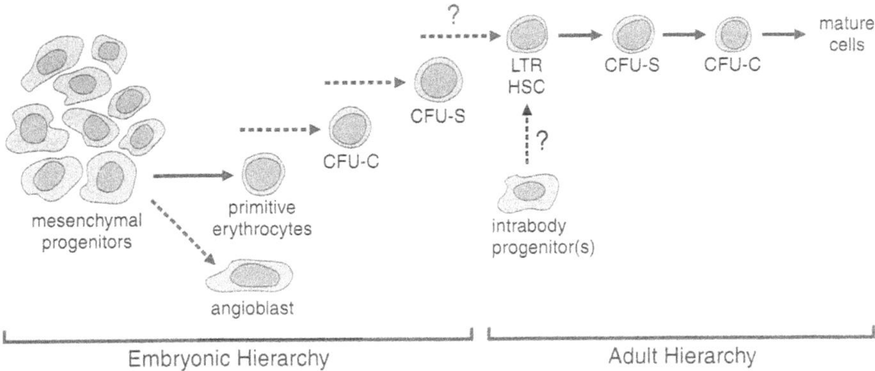

Fig. 1. Hematopoietic cell generation in the mouse embryo. The embryonic and the classical adult hematopoietic hierarchies appear in reverse orientation to each other. The embryonic hematopoietic hierarchy first contains primitive erythropoietic cells, CFU-C progenitors and then CFU-S progenitors. The lineage relationship between these hematopoietic cells of the embryonic hierarchy remains elusive (as indicated by dotted arrows). Yolk sac hematopoietic cells are derived from a population of mesenchymal progenitors which also produce cells of the endothelial lineage. As indicated by the dotted arrow, a common (hemangioblast) progenitor has been proposed.

The hematopoietic stem cell at the foundation of the adult hierarchy (leading to the production of CFU-S, CFU-C and mature, differentiated cells) may be generated by the same cohort of prestem cells as the embryonic hierarchy. Alternatively, the definitive hematopoietic stem cell may take its origin from independent intrabody progenitors. These two models for the origin of definitive hematopoiesis are indicated by the question marks.

nonmammalian vertebrates revealed two embryonic sources, an extraembryonic transient source (yolk sac) and an intraembryonic adult source (region containing the dorsal aorta and pro/mesonephros) *(39–48)*. Recent evidence on the initiation of adult hematopoietic stem cells in mammalian embryos shows strong analogies to nonmammalian vertebrate hematopoietic development and is consistent with the idea that the intraembryonic AGM region of mammals is the source of the definitive adult hematopoietic system.

3.1.1. An Intraembryonic Source of Definitive Hematopoiesis in Avian and Amphibian Embryos

Embryo chimera construction and grafting experiments performed before the establishment of vasculature from the yolk sac to the embryo body have shown that avian and amphibian embryos have two parallel, but independent sources of hemato/lymphopoietic activity *(42,43)*. In these experiments, species- or strain-specific or diploid-triploid marker differences were used to determine whether definitive hematopoietic cells are produced from the yolk sac or embryo body.

In avian embryos, the yolk sac generates only transient hematopoietic cell populations, whereas the embryo body is the exclusive contributing source of long-lived adult hematopoietic cells *(40,42,44)*. Within the ventral wall of the dorsal aorta, large hematopoietic foci were identified and contain high frequency CFU-C numbers supporting the idea that the area comprising the dorsal aorta gives rise to the definitive hematopoietic system *(45)*.

In amphibians, the yolk sac analogue, the ventral blood islands produce the first hematopoietic cells in the embryo *(46)*. Before the circulation is completed, the intraembryonic area containing the dorsal aorta and pro/mesonephros also produces hematopoietic activity. Both the ventral blood islands and the intraembryonic region contribute to different elements of the adult hematopoietic system. However, the intrabody region provides most of the cells of the adult blood *(47,48)*.

3.1.2. The AGM Region Autonomously and Exclusively Generates the First Definitive Hematopoietic Cells in the Mouse

Although two sites of hematopoiesis, the yolk sac and the AGM region, function in mouse ontogeny prior to the onset of liver hematopoiesis, cellular interchange between these two tissues obscures the specific site of hematopoietic stem cell generation. In nonmammalian vertebrates, the orthotopic embryo-grafting method has yielded conclusive results. However, the *in utero* development of the mouse embryo excludes such experimentation at the present time and requires alternative approaches. To examine the source of the definitive hematopoietic system in the mouse, an organ culture approach was taken in which isolated whole embryonic tissues are cultured separately from other tissues so that cells cannot be exchanged between hematopoietic sites *(31)*. These experiments demonstrate that isolated embryonic tissues can initiate and expand definitive CFU-S progenitors and hematopoietic stem cells in culture.

Beginning at early E10 and thereafter, the AGM region is able to expand the CFU-S progenitor pool when cultured as an intact tissue for 2–3 days. In contrast, cultures of E10 yolk sac only maintain CFU-S numbers at their initial level. When early E11 yolk sacs are explanted and cultured, large numbers of CFU-S progenitors are found, but they are not as abundant as those in the AGM region. The first long-term repopulating hematopoietic stem cells are found to be autonomously and exclusively generated and expanded (15-fold) by cultured E10 AGM regions. Hematopoietic stem cells are detected in yolk sac and liver at lower potency only beginning E11. Thus, as in nonmammalian vertebrates, the intraembryonic AGM region generates the potent adult hematopoietic system populating secondary hematopoietic tissues (liver and yolk sac), whereas the yolk sac itself, most likely contributes to low potency/transient hematopoiesis.

3.2. Migratory Nature of Hematopoietic Development

In the adult, the circulation serves as the most physiologic route for delivery of hematopoietic cells. Immature hemato/lymphopoietic progenitors and stem cells are associated with stromal cells in the extravascular space of the bone marrow and spleen. Cells undergoing differentiation quickly move intravascularly, through the circulation to other tissues and organs. Growth factor administration induces the efficient mobilization of hematopoietic precursors into blood *(49–50)*. Similarly, during development, the embryonic vasculature provides blood cells with migratory routes *(51)*, allowing mobilization and colonization to serve the immediate needs of the embryo. Accumulating evidence in amphibians, birds, and mice demonstrates that the sequential development of the hematopoietic system, leads to waves of colonization of secondary hemato/lymphopoietic territories *(38,39,52)* that occurs via circulation or through interstitial migration *(46)*.

3.2.1. Waves of Hematopoietic Colonization

3.2.1.1. Nonmammalian Vertebrates

Orthotopic grafting experiments with avian embryos have shown that the thymus is colonized by periodic waves of lymphoid precursors (Fig. 2) *(40,52)*. This colonization

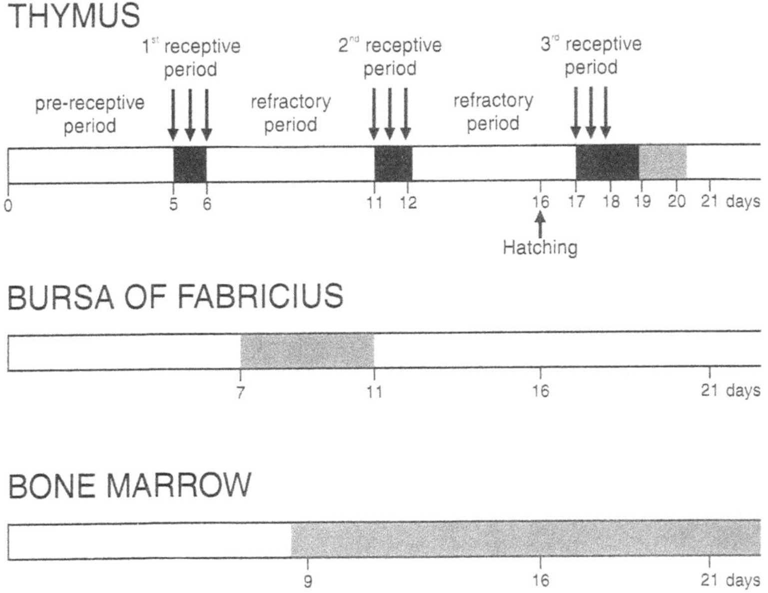

Fig. 2. Waves of colonization in quail hematopoietic tissues during development. Embryo grafting experiments in birds reveal cyclic receptive and refractory periods of thymus colonization. One wave of hematopoietic colonization is observed in the bursa of fabricius and the bone marrow. This figure is a composite of data from refs. *52,53*.

is punctuated with periods when the thymus is apparently not receptive *(53)*. The periods of receptivity of the thymus may reflect the recruitment of avian hematopoietic precursor cells by chemotactic peptides secreted by thymic epithelial cells. Labeled chick hematopoietic cells injected into the circulation traverse the perithymic basement membrane and intercalate with the thymic epithelium. The fibronectin receptor complex is at least partially involved in this process. In contrast, the bursa of Fabricius and the bone marrow are colonized during single, longer embryonic periods beginning at E7 and E9, respectively *(54)*. The colonization of these tissues is preferentially by intraembryonic-derived hematopoietic cells, with only a small transient contribution by yolk sac-derived cells *(55)*. Indeed, even the yolk sac blood islands were found to be seeded by cells from the intraembryonic region beginning at E5, indicating migration of these cells in various directions.

By similar embryo grafting approaches, amphibians demonstrate that the larval liver is initially populated by intrabody-derived hematopoietic cells *(56)*. However, such intrabody-derived cells are undetectable in the circulating blood, suggesting another means of migration. Slightly later and close to the time of metamorphosis, the clonal intrabody hematopoietic composition of the liver begins to fluctuate. This fluctuation continues throughout adulthood and represents waves of colonization by hematopoietic cells from both the ventral blood islands and the intrabody source. However, intrabody-derived cells are always the predominant adult blood cell type *(56,57)*.

In addition to the circulation, interstitial migration has been suggested as another means of transference of hematopoietic cells within the embryo. Interstitial migration within the amphibian embryo body has been shown to occur before the completion of vascular development *(46)* and has been suggested to be the means by which cells migrate in the early

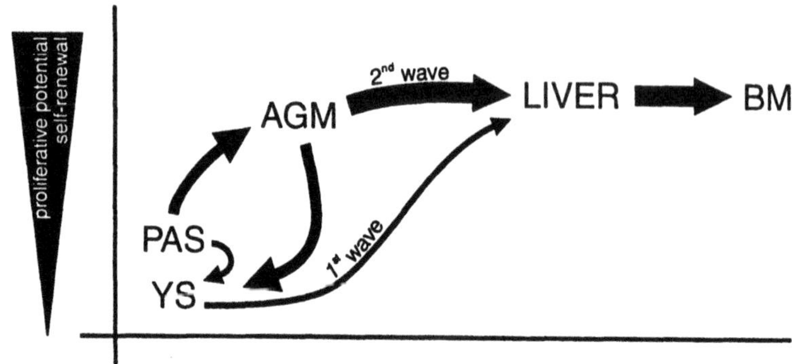

Fig. 3. Two waves of hematopoietic activity entering the fetal liver. The yolk sac and the AGM region are sources of hematopoietic progenitors/stem cells that colonize the fetal liver. At E9 the yolk sac contributes to the first wave containing primitive erythroid cells and CFU-C progenitors. Beginning at late E10, the AGM contributes CFU-S progenitors and hematopoietic stem cells to the second wave of liver colonization. An early wave of multipotent progenitor cells from the PAS is thought to colonize the yolk sac.

chick embryo *(55)*. In zebra fish embryos, the results of *in situ* analysis of GATA transcription factors *(58,59)* expression together with results of time-lapse microscopy of demonstrating the anterior migration of blood cells (M. Thompson and L. I. Zon, personal communication) suggests that before the onset of active circulation, cells located caudally in the intermediate cell mass of Oellacher migrate rostrally during development.

3.2.1.2. The Mouse

The liver rudiment contains hematopoietic cells beginning at the 28 somite pair stage in the E9 embryo *(34)*. The colonization of the mouse liver by exogenous hematopoietic cells has been demonstrated by explanting pre- and post-28 sp livers under the kidney capsule of adults *(33)*. Yolk sac hematopoietic cells are thought to be the source since organ cultures of E7 embryos without yolk sacs do not show any hematopoiesis, whereas those with yolk sacs are positive for CFU-Cs *(17)*. Also, after organ coculture of yolk sac and 25 sp liver rudiment (with a cell-permeable filter between), livers are found to contain yolk sac-derived erythropoietic cells *(60)*. Slightly later in development, the appearance of definitive CFU-S progenitors and long-term repopulating hematopoietic stem cells in organ cultures of AGM and liver support the hypothesis that a second wave of colonization begins at late E10/E11 *(31)*. Hence, it is generally accepted that two sequential waves of hematopoietic progenitors colonize the liver *(39)* (Fig. 3).

The first wave of colonization contains cells originating in the yolk sac, the initial hematopoietic source in the early embryo *(34)*. This wave consists of cells characteristic of the yolk sac at this developmental time and this cellular composition is well-reflected in the circulation. By the end of E9–E10, the liver rudiment contains primitive erythroid cells and committed progenitors *(17)*, but is deficient in CFU-S progenitors and hematopoietic stem cells *(20,21,31)*. By mid-late E10, the AGM region functions as the main generator of CFUS activity, and as the first tissue initiating hematopoietic stem cells *(20,21,31)*. These events precede by a half day the first detection of CFU-S and hematopoietic stem cells in the liver, strongly suggesting that the second wave of liver hematopoietic colonization at E11 is predominated by AGM-derived cells. This idea is supported by data on morphological similarity between spleen colonies produced by CFU-S progenitors from the AGM region and the liver *(38)*.

Recently, in the early stage mouse embryo (E7.5–E8.5), a preliver wave of colonization has been suggested to occur between the embryo body and the yolk sac *(32)*. Multipotential progenitors with erythroid-myeloid-lymphoid potential are present in the intraembryonic para-aortic splanchnopleura (PAS) beginning at E7.5. In contrast, in the E7.5 yolk sac, only progenitors with erythroid-myeloid potential are found. No multipotent progenitors with lymphoid potential are detected in the yolk sac until E8.5. Hence, the PAS cells may seed the yolk sac at E8.5 *(32)* in a similar manner that observed in the chick *(55)*.

3.3. Cell Surface Markers and the Relationship of AGM, Liver, and Bone Marrow Hematopoietic Stem Cells

The hematopoietic stem cells generated in the mouse AGM region possess functional repopulating ability equivalent to the hematopoietic stem cells found in the adult bone marrow and fetal liver. Taken together, the temporal appearance and spatial localization of definitive hematopoietic progenitors and the ability of the AGM region to expand the definitive hematopoietic progenitor/stem cell pool give strong support for fetal liver colonization by AGM-derived hematopoietic stem cells and hence, a direct lineage relationship between these cells. To further examine this lineage relationship, AGM cells have been recently characterized for cell surface phenotype. Previously, fetal liver and adult bone marrow hematopoietic stem cells have been extensively characterized for cell surface phenotype, and have been found to be c-kit+, CD34+, Sca-1+, and negative for lineage markers CD4, CD8, B220, and Gr-1 *(61,62)*. AGM hematopoietic stem cells share this pattern of surface marker expression *(63)* suggesting a direct relationship with fetal liver and bone marrow hematopoietic stem cells. Interestingly, a subset of AGM hematopoietic stem cells bear the mature lineage marker Mac-1 *(63)*, which is expressed on all hematopoietic stem cells in the fetal liver at E13 *(64)*, further supporting the lineage relationship between the cells in these tissues. Although positive for the AA4.1 fetal liver stem cell marker, E11 yolk sac cells lack the Sca-1 marker *(65)*, suggesting either separate hematopoietic differentiation pathways in embryonic and adult hematopoiesis which may depend on local microenvironment or independent hematopoietic hierarchies. The analysis of the AGM region for further markers will provide a better understanding of the hematopoietic lineage relationships within the embryo.

4. Lineage Potentials of Embryonic and Adult Hematopoietic Progenitors/Stem Cells

Previously, hematopoietic stem cells throughout mouse ontogeny were thought to be a homogeneous, self-renewing population with constant lineage potential that may vary depending upon microenvironment or assay conditions. However, the functional lineage potential of hematopoietic progenitors/stem cells varies during development. As a basis for further understanding the origins of the adult hematopoietic repertoire, a brief description of the differences in lineage potential of mouse embryonic, fetal, and adult hematopoietic progenitors and stem cells is provided.

4.1. Erythroid Lineage

During embryonic development, nucleated erythroid cells expressing embryonic globins are produced. In contrast, fetal and adult stage erythrocytes are enucleated and express adult globins *(22)*. It is now clear that individual erythroid progenitors from fetal liver can switch from a fetal to adult expression program *(66)*, and possibly result in adult erythroid cell morphology. However, the general populations of mature erythroid cells may be derived from developmentally separate stem cell populations *(67,68)*. Recently, it has been shown that fetal liver and adult bone marrow cells positive for c-kit differ in erythroid potential from c-kit negative yolk sac and fetal liver cells. In accordance with this, administration of anti-c-kit antibodies inhibit fetal liver hematopoiesis, but not yolk sac hematopoeisis *(69)*. Such results indicating differential regulation of primitive and definitive erythropoiesis may indicate the presence of at least two distinct progenitor/ stem cell populations.

4.2. Lymphoid Lineages

Differing lymphoid lineage potentials have been demonstrated in hematopoietic stem cells enriched from adult bone marrow and fetal liver populations. In the T lymphoid lineage, fetal liver hematopoietic stem cells are capable of producing Vγ3 and Vγ4 T cell subsets, whereas adult bone marrow stem cells are lacking in this potential and produce predominantly Vαβ T-cells *(70)*. In addition to fetal liver, E8.5 yolk sac cells produce Vγ3 and Vγ4 T-cells *(27,28)*. Similarly in the B lymphoid lineage, the B1a subset can be produced by the fetal liver *(71,72)*, splanchnopleural mesoderm *(19,73)*, and yolk sac *(24)*, but generally not by the adult bone marrow. Recently, it was found that the para-aortic splanchnopleura is the first tissue developing multipotent lymphoid-myeloid progenitors, and this occurs 1 day earlier than the appearance of such progenitors in the yolk sac *(32)*. Therefore, multipotent progenitors from the para-aortic splanchnopleura most likely colonize the yolk sac between E7.5 and E8.5. The para-aortic splanchnopleura remains as the single source of more committed B1a progenitors later in development. Thus, it is tempting to think that these intraembryonic progenitors produce the Vγ3 and Vγ4 subset of T-cells important for skin-related and mucosal immunity, and the B1a cell subset found predominantly in the peritoneum of the adult.

4.3. Macrophage Lineage

Two separate lineages of macrophages are thought to develop in ontogeny; primitive macrophages, and the monocytic lineage of macrophages *(73,74)*. The primitive macrophages are the first to appear in the yolk sac at E9. They most likely arise from a local hematopoietic progenitor and not a monocytic progenitor; promonocytic and monocytic cells are not found in the yolk sac at E9, whereas myeloid progenitors are found already at E7–8. The primitive macrophages colonize other embryonic tissues, including the fetal liver through the circulation. In contrast, adult macrophages do not migrate through the blood. These cells of the monocytic lineage begin to appear at E10 in the fetal liver as well as the yolk sac. It has been suggested that monocytic cells, which are part of the adult hematopoietic system, are derived from precursors in the AGM region, whereas the primitive macrophages are yolk sac derived *(75)*.

5. Molecular Hierarchies in Mammalian Hematopoiesis

The distinct functional subsets of cells within the individual lineages of the hematopoietic cells produced during embryonic or adult stages, along with the differing hematopoietic progenitors in the two pre-liver sites of hematopoiesis suggest differences in molecular genetic programs between embryonic and adult hematopoietic progenitors. Molecular changes have been found to occur at numerous levels. Changes have been

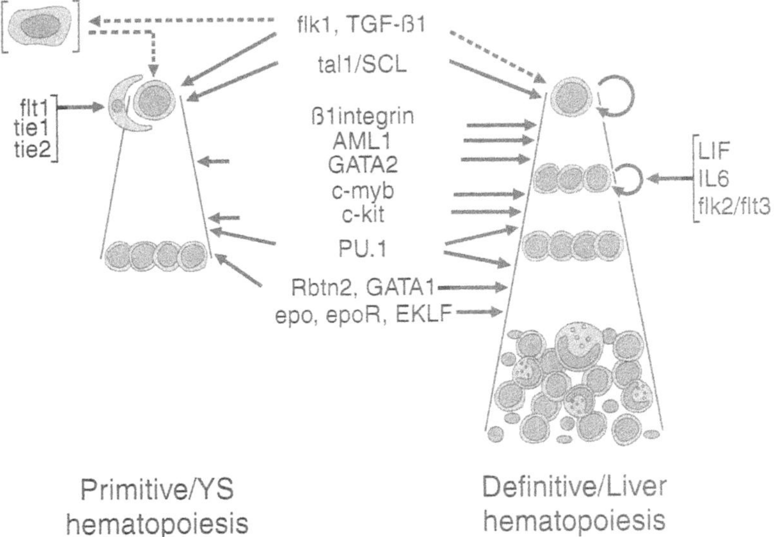

Fig. 4. Model of overlapping and differential genetic control in embryonic and adult hematopoiesis. Arrows indicate the part of the hematopoietic hierarchies affected by each gene as determined by analysis of mouse mutants. As the analysis of many of the mouse mutants is not yet experimentally conclusive, some genes may have other targets in the hematopoietic hierarchies not indicated here. Proposed effects are indicated by dotted arrows. The cell in the brackets in the upper left corner is the proposed hemangioblast.

found at the level of chromosome telomere length (reviewed by Landsdorp in Chapter 2), and at the level of single genes (for example, hematopoietic transcription factors reviewed by Orkin in Chapter 3). Gene targeting and the generation of mutant mice has revealed critical roles for numerous genes at early stages of hematopoietic development and suggest differential, but sometimes overlapping, genetic requirements in embryonic and adult hematopoiesis.

5.1. Mutant Mice as a Means of Examining Molecules Relevant in Development of the Hematopoietic System

The recent availability of mice mutant in genes affecting the hematopoietic system has been of great importance in the study of the origins and genetic progamming of the embryonic and adult hematopoietic system. Targeted germ line mutagenesis with embryonic stem (ES) cells has produced numerous lines of mice that are affected at early critical stages of hematopoiesis (Fig. 4). Generally, such germ-line gene mutations can be grouped by their effects and suggested roles in

1. Hematopoietic specification;
2. Progenitor/stem cell function;
3. Migration; or
4. Terminal hematopoietic differentiation.

These include gene products that function as transcription factors, growth factors, signaling molecules, and adhesion molecules. Several of these null mutations result in early embryonic lethality (E9–10), presumably affecting yolk sac hematopoiesis, whereas others are lethal at slightly later embryonic stages (E11–16), affecting definitive hematopoiesis. The generation of chimeric mice with homozygous mutant ES cells has enabled the additional analysis of roles for some of these genes at later developmental stages.

5.1.1. Genes Affecting Hematopoietic Specification

Specification to hematopoiesis occurs shortly after the onset of mesoderm formation in the mouse embryo. The inductive signals for commitment to the hematopoeitic lineage are unknown. However, mice mutant in the Flk-1 receptor tyrosine kinase gene *(76)* or the TGF-β1 (transforming growth factor-β1) gene *(77)* demonstrate that these gene products are involved in establishing hematopoietic and endothelial cells in the yolk sac. Flk-1 null embryos die *in utero* between E8.5 and E9.5. Their yolk sacs contain no blood islands or blood vessels. Only background levels of yolk sac hematopoietic progenitors and abortive development of endothelial precursors in some intraembryonic sites are found. TGF-β1 null embryos (only about 50%) die slightly later at E10.5. Similarly, yolk sac hematopoiesis is severely reduced. However, endothelial cells are produced in the absence of TGF-β1, but vessel formation and cellular adhesion is defective. Other receptor tyrosine kinase genes similar to Flk-1 such as Flt-1 *(78)*, tie-1 *(79,80)*, and tie-2/tek *(80)*, affect development of the endothelial network and angiogenesis but not yolk sac hematopoiesis. It will be important to study all of these gene mutations in chimeric mice, or conditional knockout mice so as to determine whether the same signals are required for specification of the adult hematopoietic system and to establish the relationship between the hematopoietic and endothelial cell lineages in later stage mouse embryos and adults. Such studies could also provide insight into the possible presence of the hypothetical hemangioblast *(23)* in the embryo.

In comparison, the tal1/SCL transcription factor is required for the generation of all hematopoietic cells, but not all endothethial cells *(81–84)*. Germline mutant embryos die early E9–10 and lack all yolk sac hematopoiesis *(83,84)*. Although yolk sac capillaries are initiated, vitelline vessel formation is blocked. Adult mutant ES cell chimeric mice with a high percentage of the donor cell type show no mutant ES cell contribution in the hematopoietic system *(81,82)*. Thus, tal1/SCL may be involved in the further specification of mesodermal cells to hematopoietic fate during the onset of both the embryonic and adult hematopoietic system.

5.1.2. Genes Affecting Progenitor/Stem Cell Function

In the yolk sac, hematopoiesis occurs multifocally. Such distribution of blood islands suggests that hematopoiesis may be initiated through numerous progenitors. These progenitors, of low proliferative potential, contribute to the relatively small pool of circulating embryonic erythrocytes. However in the adult, abundant hematopoiesis is the result of a few self-renewing definitive hematopoietic progenitors *(85)* with high proliferative potential, as shown by comparisons of yolk sac, fetal liver, and bone marrow in vitro colonies *(17)*. Thus, gene mutations differentially affecting yolk sac and fetal liver hematopoiesis may be involved in proliferative/clonogenic potential of hematopoietic progenitors and should be readily apparent. Alternatively, such genes may be involved in the generation, maintenance, or self-renewal of definitive progenitors/stem cells. Defects in these characteristics of progenitor/stem cells are more difficult to detect since in vivo, single hematopoietic progenitors/stem cells can generate a complete fully differentiated adult blood system *(8)*. Examples of some candidate genes leading to such proposed defects are found in mice mutant for the transcription factors GATA-2 *(86)*, core binding factor (CBF) *(87–90)*, GATA-3 *(91,92)*, myb *(93,94)* and PU.1 *(95–97)*, and for the receptor tyrosine kinase c-kit *(69,98,99)* and its ligand steel factor (SCF). More subtle examples are found in mice lacking growth factors interleukin-6 (IL-6) *(100)*, or leukemia inhibitory factor (LIF) *(101)*, or the receptor tyrosine kinase Flk-2/Flt-3 *(102)*. Brief descriptions of the effects of each mutation are given.

5.1.2.2. GATA-2

A germ line deficiency in the mouse GATA-2 transcription factor leads to embryonic lethality beginning at E10.5 *(86)*. Such embryos exhibit severe fetal liver anemia. Embryonic erythrocyte number in the yolk sac is slightly reduced, but in vitro clonogenic progenitors (CFU-Cs) are decreased 100-fold. In chimeric mice, no ES cell definitive hematopoietic contribution is observed in fetal liver or the adult. Embryonic progenitors are less affected, suggesting a defect at the level of the clonogenic potential of hematopoietic progenitors.

5.1.2.3. CBF

Mice lacking either *(87–89)* or both *(90)* subunits of the heterodimeric CBF transcriptional regulatory molecule present severe fetal liver anemia and embryonic lethality beginning at E12.5. Unlike GATA-2 mutants, yolk sac erythropoiesis is unaffected, whereas CFU-C progenitors in the yolk sac and fetal liver are absent. Hence, this gene may specifically act at the level of proliferation, generation, or maintenance of definitive hematopoietic progenitors/stem cells.

5.1.2.4. GATA-3

In mice null for GATA-3, embryonic lethality occurs beginning E11 *(91)*. Severe aberrations in fetal liver hematopoiesis are observed. At least a 10-fold decrease in fetal liver CFU-Cs is found, whereas yolk sac CFU-Cs are normal. In ES cell chimeric mice, the GATA-3 mutation does not prevent myeloid cell differentiation of ES derived cells, suggesting that GATA-3 affects only the T lymphoid lineage *(92)*. However, since contribution of GATA-3 null cells is always low, possible effects of this mutation on the proliferative potential of definitive hematopoietic progenitors cannot be excluded.

5.1.2.5. C-Myb

This proto-oncogene transcription factor is known to act on a variety of hematopoietic genes, and its downregulation is correlated with hematopoietic cell maturation. Lack of C-Myb results in the embryonic lethality of mice at E15 most likely because of fetal liver anemia that begins at E13 *(94)*. A decrease in multipotent granulocyte-macrophage progenitors and adult type erythrocytes suggest that a myeloid-erythroid progenitor is affected *(93)*, but other lineages and chimeric mice must be examined for further insight into the requirements for C-Myb.

5.1.2.6. c-kit

The genes for the receptor tyrosine kinase, c-kit and its ligand, SCF, have been found to be defective in W and Sl of strains of mice, respectively *(104,105)*. These mutant mice demonstrate deficiencies in hematopoiesis, primordial germ cell development, and pigmentation *(99)*. The most severe mutations result in lethality late in gestation (E16) or during neonatal periods. Although c-kit/SCF signaling does not appear to be involved in the embryonic development of hematopoietic stem cells, the hematopoietic system of the mutants is deficient in CFU-S progenitors and mast cells. Since SCF acts as an antiapoptotic *(106)* or proliferative agent *(69,98)* in hematopoietic progenitors including CFU-S, c-kit/SCF signaling may be required for clonogenicity/proliferation of CFU-S early in development, and/or may play a role in migration of early hematopoietic progenitors, as for primordial germ cells and melanocytes.

5.1.2.7. PU.1

Severe phenotype PU.1 knockout mice die of anemia at E18 *(97)*. In the yolk sac, erythroid and megakaryocyte differentiation are normal, but myeloid progenitors are reduced. In the fetal liver, erythrocyte numbers and CFU-Cs are reduced, and in vitro colony size much smaller. No lymphocyte development is detected. Using ES cell chimeras, the effects of the PU.1 mutation are cell autonomous *(96)* and independent of Ikaros, a pivotal transcription factor in lymphoid lineage specification *(103)*. Thus, PU.1 is probably involved in the proliferative potential of lymphoid-myeloid progenitors.

5.1.2.8. LIF

Viable adult animals do not require leukemia inhibitory factor (LIF). Hematopoiesis is visibly normal, but LIF null animals are dramatically decreased in several clonogenic progenitors including CFU-S *(101)*. Although bone marrow from such animals can promote survival of lethally irradiated recipient mice, limiting dilution or competitive repopulations must be performed to determine whether stem cell numbers are affected. It is suggested that LIF is required in the microenvironment as a progenitor/stem cell maintenance factor.

5.1.2.9. IL-6

Similar to LIF null mice, IL-6 deficient mice are decreased in CFU-S progenitors *(100)*. To examine the stem cell compartment, competitive repopulation experiments were performed and demonstrate a decrease in potency of hematopoietic stem cells. This, combined with a rapid transition of immature to committed progenitors, suggests that IL-6 plays a role in the maintenance of self-renewal.

5.1.2.10. Flk-2/Flt-3

These deficient mice also thrive as adults *(102)*. Although Flk-2/Flt-3 is expressed on a subset of hematopoietic stem cells, Flk-2/Flt-3 null mice are not decreased in CFU-S or pre-CFU-S numbers. Transplantation experiments reveal a deficiency in myeloid and lymphoid reconstitution by such cells and suggests effects on the proliferative potential rather than the self-renewal of immature hematopoietic progenitors.

5.1.3. Genes Affecting Hematopoietic Cell Migration

As described in previous sections, hematopoietic cell migration is important for the colonization of secondary hemtopoietic territories. Although many of the aforementioned listed genes are proposed to affect the proliferation/self-renewal of progenitor/stem cells, it cannot be ruled out that these genes play some role in the colonization process. However, there is convincing evidence for the role of integrins in cell migration. In vitro studies have suggested that integrins play a critical role in the differentiation and migration of hematopoietic cells. β1 intergrin is thought to play a role in the formation of CFU-S through adhesion to the spleen stroma *(107)*, and α4 integrin is thought to act at the level of adhesion of hematopoietic progenitors in the bone marrow *(108)*. Recently, the in vivo function of these genes has been examined in mutant mice.

Mutation of the β1 integrin gene results in preimplantation embryonic lethality *(109,110)*. Thus, the generation of chimeric mice with β1 integrin null ES cells was necessary to determine whether there is a requirement for β1 in hematopoiesis at any stages in development. Indeed, such a necessity was demonstrated, but it revealed that β1 is necessary for fetal liver, but not yolk sac hematopoiesis *(111)*. In vitro, β1 null yolk sac progenitors exhibit normal clonogenic and differentiation potential. Although β1 null cells are found in the circulation until E15, no such cells appear in the fetal liver, suggesting that they cannot colonize the fetal liver. This is further supported by the absence of β1 null cells in the adult bone marrow, thymus, and circulation.

Similar to β1 mutants, mice deficient in the α4 integrin also die in early embryonic stages *(108)*. Chimeric mouse studies reveal a role for α4 in the homing of B and T lymphocytes to adult hematopoietic tissues, but not fetal tissues. Not all hematopoietic lineages are affected, since monocytes and natural killer cells develop normally. Examination of earlier stage α4 mutant chimeric embryos may yield information on homing requirements for other progenitors and lineages in the yolk sac and AGM region of the developing mouse.

5.1.4. Genes Affecting Terminal Differentiation of Hematopoietic Cells

Several genes thought to be involved in the maturation of committed hematopoietic progenitors have been demonstrated in gene targeting experiments to differentially affect these cells during embryonic and definitive stages. A number of examples have been provided in the erythroid lineage. In mice deficient in the Rbtn-2 *(112)* or GATA-1 transcription factors *(113–115)*, there are no mature erythrocytes in the vessels of the embryo or yolk sac. Such mutant mice die of severe yolk sac anemia early in gestation at about E10.5. These factors are required for the differentiation of proerythroblasts to erythroid cells and are required for both embryonic and definitive erythropoiesis. However, mice lacking the EKLF transcription factor *(116,117)* and erythropoietin/erythropoietin receptor signaling molecules *(118,119)* are not affected in yolk sac erythropoiesis. Fatal anemia develops in early fetal life as erythropoiesis switches to the definitive program and null embryos die at about E16. Although the erythroid progenitor pool is normal, the lack of differentiation demonstrates that the molecular program for adult erythropoiesis requires additional factors that are not required for primitive erythropoiesis.

5.2. ES Cells as a Model of Embryonic Hematopoiesis?

The use of ES cells in the generation of mouse mutants has yielded great insight into the genes necessary for hematopoiesis during ontogeny and has revealed differences in the molecular requirements for yolk sac versus definitive hematopoiesis. In vitro hematopoietic differentiation of ES cells has also aided the study of early genetic events in the onset of blood cell development and has provided an accessible source for the analysis of hematopoietic progenitors for growth factor requirements and gene expression patterns *(120,121)*. However, ES cells appear to be limited in the production of adult hierarchy, despite the fact that some adult-type hematopoietic differentiation can be induced. Upon the removal of LIF, ES cells form embryoid bodies in which differentiation of many lineages of cells occurs, including hematopoietic cells *(122)*. In clonogenic assays, numerous hematopoietic growth factors added together with cells from such differentiating cultures induce erythroid, myeloid, and lymphoid colony formation *(123,124)*. Although low level, long-term multilineage progenitors have been found after in vivo transplantation of differentiating ES cells *(125,126)*, neither CFU-S progenitors nor true adult hematopoietic stem cells have been detected *(126)*. Thus, in vitro differentiating ES cells appear most similar in potential to those progenitors found in early stage yolk sac *(121)*. The lack of CFU-S progenitors and high level, long-term repopulating stem cells in the in vitro cultures, coupled with the recent in vivo evidence for the AGM region as the source of the adult definitive hematopoietic system, strongly suggests that ES cell cultures do not fully reflect all stages of hematopoietic development, particularly those leading to the establishment of the adult hierarchy. It is possible that a highly organized three-dimensional spatial microenvironment provided in vivo by the mouse AGM region, but not contained in embryoid bodies, is required to induce definitive progenitor/stem cell formation.

6. Human Developmental Hematopoiesis

The clinical use of fetal and cord blood cells in transplantation therapies has increased interest in the embryologic development of the human hematopoietic system *(127)*. Concerns about the molecular program, proliferative potential, lineage potential, expansion properties, and general cycling characteristics of early hematopoietic stem cells and progenitors have been raised in this context. Concerns focus mainly on the differences of embryonic hematopoietic stem cells compared to adult hematopoietic stem cells. Because of practical reasons and the lack of appropriate experimental systems, little is known about functional hematopoietic development and the early embryonic hierarchy in humans. Animal models have given insight into the embryonic and adult hierarchies and should provide insight into human developmental hematopoiesis and future therapeutic applications.

Information concerning human embryonic hematopoiesis comes mainly from descriptive studies. Yolk sac hematopoiesis begins in the middle of the third week of human gestation and decreases from week five until week eight, when it disappears. Although indirect, it is thought that yolk sac hematopoietic cells colonize the fetal liver. At week five, yolk sac burst forming units-erythroid (BFU-Es) decrease in frequency, while liver BFU-Es increase *(128)*. Further descriptive analyses suggest early thymus colonization at week seven *(129,130)* and bone marrow colonization at weeks 10–11 *(131)*. By 15–20 weeks in gestation, it is thought that both the bone marrow and fetal liver contain cells characteristically described as hematopoietic stem cells and such early fetal liver cells have been used successfully in clinical transplantations. Only recently have intrabody regions been examined for adult type hematopoietic progenitors/stem cells.

Clonogenic myeloid progenitors have been found in the yolk sac and body of 25–50 day gestational stage human embryos *(132)*. Erythroid and multipotent progenitors are also present in these tissues. And between 30 and 40 days into gestation, as many nonerythroid progenitors were found in the eviscerated embryo as in the liver. Descriptive immunohistochemical analyses have localized a cluster of cells adhering to the ventral endothethial wall of the dorsal aorta in five week preumbilical human embryos. These are phenotypically identical ($CD34^+CD38^-$) to adult hematopoietic progenitor/stem cells *(133)*. The presence of these cells corresponds well to findings in avian *(45)* and murine *(38,134)* embryos at equivalent developmental stages in which immature hematopoietic progenitors/stem cells are found on ventral wall of the dorsal aorta. Finally, $CD34^+$ cells from the human intraembryonic region yield large multilineage colonies after coculture on bone marrow stromal cells. Thus, like avian, amphibian, and murine embryos, the human embryo has potent hematopoietic activity within the intraembryo region containing the dorsal aorta. Further analyses should shed light on the potency of the human intraembryonic hematopoietic progenitor/stem cells compared to those in other embryonic and adult hematopoietic tissues.

7. Summary

The ontogeny of the hematopoietic system of mammals bears a striking resemblance to hematopoietic development in nonmammalian vertebrates. The appearance of the first long-term repopulating hematopoietic stem cells in the AGM region of the mouse embryo after the appearance of more differentiated hematopoietic progenitors and effector cells suggests that the AGM region gives birth to the long-lived adult blood system. The yolk sac appears to serve the immediate needs of the developing embryo. However, it remains to be elucidated whether the ancestors of the definitive hematopoietic stem cells originate from the AGM region, the yolk sac or some other embryonic tissue. Analyses at the level of lineage potential and phenotypic characterization of hematopoietic progenitors, as well as genetic hierarchies in the developing mouse embryo further suggest an important role for the AGM region in the generation of the adult hematopoietic hierarchy. Since the gradient of hematopoietic activities from the yolk sac to the intraembryonic regions appears to become progressively more complex, the relationship of the mesodermal cells giving rise to the embryonic and adult hematopoietic hierarchies both spatially and temporally should yield information on the induction of the adult hematopoietic stem cell, and provide novel signaling molecules potentially useful in clinical transplantation therapies.

References

1. Morrison, S. J., Uchida, N., and Weissman, I. L. (1995) The biology of hematopoietic stem cells. *Ann. Rev. Cell. Dev. Biol.* **11,** 35–71.
2. Abramson, S., Miller, R. G., and Phillips, R. A. (1977) The identification in adult bone marrow of pluripotent and restricted stem cells of the myeloid and lymphoid systems. *J. Exp. Med.* **145,** 1567–1579.
3. Micklem, H. S., Ford, C. E., Evans, E. P., and Gray, J. (1966) Interrelationships of myeloid and lymphoid cells: studies with chromosome-marked cells transfused into lethally irradiated mice. *Proc. R. Soc. Lond. B. Biol. Sci.* **165,** 78–102.
4. Capel, B., Hawley, R., Covarrubias, L., Hawley, T., and Mintz, B. (1989) Clonal contributions of small numbers of retrovirally marked hematopoietic stem cells engrafted in unirradiated neonatal W/Wv mice [published erratum appears in Proc Natl Acad Sci U S A 1989 Sep;86(18):7048]. *Proc. Natl. Acad. Sci. USA* **86,** 4564–4568.
5. Dick, J. E., Magli, M. C., Huszar, D., Phillips, R. A., and Bernstein, A. (1985) Introduction of a selectable gene into primitive stem cells capable of long-term reconstitution of the hemopoietic system of W/Wv mice. *Cell* **42,** 71–79.
6. Jordan, C. T., McKearn, J. P., and Lemischka, I. R. (1990) Cellular and developmental properties of fetal hematopoietic stem cells. *Cell* **61,** 953–963.
7. Keller, G., Paige, C., Gilboa, E., and Wagner, E. F. (1985) Expression of a foreign gene in myeloid and lymphoid cells derived from multipotent haematopoietic precursors. *Nature* **318,** 149–154.
8. Lemischka, I. R., Raulet, D. H., and Mulligan, R. C. (1986) Developmental potential and dynamic behavior of hematopoietic stem cells. *Cell* **45,** 917–927.
9. Till, J. and E. McCulloch. (1961) A direct measurement of the radiation sensitivity of normal mouse bone marrow cells. *Radiation Res.* **14,** 213–222.
10. Magli, M. C., Iscove, N. N., and Odartchenko, N. (1982) Transient nature of early haematopoietic spleen colonies. *Nature* **295,** 527–529.
11. Jones, R. J., Wagner, J. E., Celano, P., Zicha, M. S., and Sharkis, S. J. (1990) Separation of pluripotent haematopoietic stem cells from spleen colony-forming cells [see comments]. *Nature* **347,** 188–189.
12. Metcalf, D. (1984) The hemopoietic colony stimulating factors. Elsevier Science Publishers B. V., Amsterdam.
13. Whitlock, C. A. and Witte, O. N. (1982) Long-term culture of B lymphocytes and their precursors from murine bone marrow. *Proc. Natl. Acad. Sci. USA* **79,** 3608–3612.
14. Jenkinson, E. J., Franchi, L. L., Kingston, R., and Owen, J. J. (1982) Effect of deoxyguanosine on lymphopoiesis in the developing thymus rudiment in vitro: application in the production of chimeric thymus rudiments. *Eur. J. Immunol.* **12,** 583–587.
15. Kawamoto, H., Ohmura, K., and Katsura, Y. (1997) Direct evidence for the commitment of hematopoietic stem cells to T, B and myeloid lineages in murine fetal liver. *Int. Immunol.* **9,** 1011–1019.

16. Snodgrass, R. and Keller, G. (1987) Clonal fluctuation within the haematopoietic system of mice reconstituted with retrovirus-infected stem cells. *Embo. J.* **6,** 3955–3960.
17. Moore, M. A. and Metcalf, D. (1970) Ontogeny of the haemopoietic system: yolk sac origin of in vivo and in vitro colony forming cells in the developing mouse embryo. *Br. J. Haematol.* **18,** 279–296.
18. Johnson, G. R. and Jones, R. O. (1973) Differentiation of the mammalian hepatic primordium in vitro. I. Morphogenesis and the onset of haematopoiesis. *J. Embryol. Exp. Morphol.* **30,** 83–96.
19. Godin, I. E., Garcia-Porrero, J. A., Coutinho, A., Dieterlen-Lievre, F., and Marcos, M. A. (1993) Para-aortic splanchnopleura from early mouse embryos contains B1a cell progenitors. *Nature* **364,** 67–70.
20. Medvinsky, A. L., Samoylina, N. L., Muller, A. M., and Dzierzak, E. A. (1993) An early pre-liver intraembryonic source of CFU-S in the developing mouse. *Nature* **364,** 64–67.
21. Muller, A. M., Medvinsky, A., Strouboulis, J., Grosveld, F., and Dzierzak, E. (1994) Development of hematopoietic stem cell activity in the mouse embryo. *Immunity* **1,** 291–301.
22. Russell, E. S. and Bernstein, S. E. (1966) Blood and blood formation, p. 351–372. in *Biology of the Laboratory Mouse,* 2nd ed. (Green, E. L., ed.), McGraw-Hill, New York.
23. His, W. (1990) Lecithoblast und Angioblast der Wirbeltiere. *Abhandl. Math-Phys. Ges. Wiss.* **26,** 171–328.
24. Cumano, A., Furlonger, C., and Paige, C. J. (1993) Differentiation and characterization of B-cell precursors detected in the yolk sac and embryo body of embryos beginning at the 10- to 12-somite stage. *Proc. Natl. Acad. Sci. USA* **90,** 6429–6433.
25. Godin, I., Dieterlen-Lievre, F., and Cumano, A. (1995) B-lymphoid potential in pre-liver mouse embryo. *Semin. Immunol.* **7,** 131–141.
26. Huang, H., Zettergren, L. D., and Auerbach, R. (1994) In vitro differentiation of B cells and myeloid cells from the early mouse embryo and its extraembryonic yolk sac [see comments]. *Exp. Hematol.* **22,** 19–25.
27. Liu, C. P. and Auerbach, R. (1991) In vitro development of murine T cells from prethymic and preliver embryonic yolk sac hematopoietic stem cells. *Development* **113,** 1315–1323.
28. Liu, C. P. and Auerbach, R. (1991) Ontogeny of murine T cells: thymus-regulated development of T cell receptor-bearing cells derived from embryonic yolk sac. *Eur. J. Immunol.* **21,** 1849–1855.
29. Ogawa, M., Nishikawa, S., Ikuta, K., Yamamura, F., Naito, M., Takahashi, K., and Nishikawa, S. (1988) B cell ontogeny in murine embryo studied by a culture system with the monolayer of a stromal cell clone, ST2: B cell progenitor develops first in the embryonal body rather than in the yolk sac. *Embo. J.* **7,** 1337–1343.
30. Medvinsky, A. L. (1993) Ontogeny of the mouse hematopoietic system. *Sem. Dev. Biol.* **4,** 333–340.
31. Medvinsky, A. and Dzierzak, E. (1996) Definitive hematopoiesis is autonomously initiated by the AGM region. *Cell* **86,** 897–906.
32. Cumano, A., Dieterlen-Lievre, F., and Godin, I. (1996) Lymphoid potential, probed before circulation in mouse, is restricted to caudal intraembryonic splanchnopleura. *Cell* **86,** 907–916.
33. Johnson, G. R. and Moore, M. A. (1975) Role of stem cell migration in initiation of mouse foetal liver haemopoiesis. *Nature* **258,** 726–728.
34. Houssaint, E. (1981) Differentiation of the mouse hepatic primordium. II. Extrinsic origin of the haemopoietic cell line. *Cell Differ.* **10,** 243–252.
35. Eren, R., Zharhary, D., Abel, L., and Globerson, A. (1987) Ontogeny of T cells: development of pre-T cells from fetal liver and yolk sac in the thymus microenvironment. *Cell Immunol.* **108,** 76–84.
36. Morris, L., Crocker, P. R., Fraser, I., Hill, M., and Gordon, S. (1991) Expression of a divalent cation-dependent erythroblast adhesion receptor by stromal macrophages from murine bone marrow. *J. Cell. Sci.* **99,** 141–147.
37. Velardi, A. and Cooper, M. D. (1984) An immunofluorescence analysis of the ontogeny of myeloid, T, and B lineage cells in mouse hemopoietic tissues. *J. Immunol.* **133,** 672–677.
38. Medvinsky, A. L., Gan, O. I., Semenova, M. L., and Samoylina, N. L. (1996) Development of day-8 colony-forming unit-spleen hematopoietic progenitors during early murine embryogenesis: spatial and temporal mapping. *Blood* **87,** 557–566.
39. Dzierzak, E. and Medvinsky, A. (1995) Mouse embryonic hematopoiesis. *Trends Genet.* **11,** 359–366.
40. Dieterlen-Lievre, F. and Le Douarin, N. M. (1993) Developmental rules in the hematopoietic and immune systems of birds: how general are they? *Sem. Dev. Biol.* **4,** 325–332.
41. Zon, L. I. (1995) Developmental biology of hematopoiesis. *Blood* **86,** 2876–2891.

42. Dieterlen-Lievre, F. (1975) On the origin of haemopoietic stem cells in the avian embryo: an experimental approach. *J. Embryol. Exp. Morphol.* **33,** 607–619.
43. Turpen, J. B., Knudson, C. M., and Hoefen, P. S. (1981) The early ontogeny of hematopoietic cells studied by grafting cytogenetically labeled tissue anlagen: localization of a prospective stem cell compartment. *Dev. Biol.* **85,** 99–112.
44. Dieterlen-Lievre, F. and Martin, C. (1981) Diffuse intraembryonic hemopoiesis in normal and chimeric avian development. *Dev. Biol.* **88,** 180–191.
45. Cormier, F. and Dieterlen-Lievre, F. (1988) The wall of the chick embryo aorta harbours M-CFC, G-CFC, GM-CFC and BFU-E. *Development* **102,** 279–285.
46. Turpen, J. B., Knudson, C. M., and Hoefen, P. S. (1981) The early ontogeny of hematopoietic cells studied by grafting cytogenetically labeled tissue anlagen: localization of a prospective stem cell compartment. *Dev. Biol.* **85,** 99–112.
47. Kau, C. L. and Turpen, J. B. (1983) Dual contribution of embryonic ventral blood island and dorsal lateral plate mesoderm during ontogeny of hemopoietic cells in Xenopus laevis. *J Immunol* **131,** 2262–2266.
48. Maeno, M., Tochinai, S., and Katagiri, C. (1985) Differential participation of ventral and dorsolateral mesoderms in the hemopoiesis of Xenopus, as revealed in diploid-triploid or interspecific chimeras. *Dev. Biol.* **110,** 503–508.
49. Bodine, D. (1995) Mobilization of peripheral blood 'stem' cells: where there is smoke, is there fire? [editorial; comment]. *Exp. Hematol.* **23,** 293–295.
50. Cronkite, E. (1997) Response to "Mobilization of peripheral blood 'stem' cells: Where there is smoke, is there fire?" Yes, there have been many fires, leaving cold coals. *Experimen. Hematol.* **25,** 185–186.
51. Delassus, S. and Cumano, A. (1996) Circulation of hematopoietic progenitors in the mouse embryo. *Immunity* **4,** 97–106.
52. Le Douarin, N. M., Dieterlen-Lievre, F., and Oliver, P. D. (1984) Ontogeny of primary lymphoid organs and lymphoid stem cells. *Am. J. Anat.* **170,** 261–299.
53. Coltey, M., Jotereau, F. V., and Le Douarin, N. M. (1987) Evidence for a cyclic renewal of lymphocyte precursor cells in the embryonic chick thymus. *Cell Differ.* **22,** 71–82.
54. Le Douarin, N. M., Houssaint, E., Jotereau, F. V., and Belo, M. (1975) Origin of hemopoietic stem cells in embryonic bursa of Fabricius and bone marrow studied through interspecific chimeras. *Proc. Natl. Acad. Sci. USA* **72,** 2701–2705.
55. Martin, C., Beaupain, D., and Dieterlen-Lievre, F. (1978) Developmental relationships between vitelline and intra-embryonic haemopoiesis studied in avian 'yolk sac chimaeras'. *Cell. Differ.* **7,** 115–130.
56. Chen, X. D. and Turpen, J. B. (1995) Intraembryonic origin of hepatic hematopoiesis in Xenopus laevis. *J. Immunol.* **154,** 2557–2567.
57. Bechtold, T. E., Smith, P. B., and Turpen, J. B. (1992) Differential stem cell contributions to thymocyte succession during development of Xenopus laevis. *J. Immunol.* **148,** 2975–2982.
58. Detrich, H. W. R., Kieran, M. W., Chan, F. Y., Barone, L. M., Yee, K., Rundstadler, J. A., Pratt, S., Ransom, D., and Zon, L. I. (1995) Intraembryonic hematopoietic cell migration during vertebrate development. *Proc. Natl. Acad. Sci. USA* **92,** 10,713–10,717.
59. Neave, B., Rodaway, A., Wilson, S. W., Patient, R., and Holder, N. (1995) Expression of zebrafish GATA 3 (gta3) during gastrulation and neurulation suggests a role in the specification of cell fate. *Mech. Dev.* **51,** 169–182.
60. Cudennec, C. A., Thiery, J. P., and Le Douarin, N. M. (1981) In vitro induction of adult erythropoiesis in early mouse yolk sac. *Proc. Natl. Acad. Sci. USA* **78,** 2412–2416.
61. Spangrude, G. J., Heimfeld, S., and Weissman, I. L. (1988) Purification and characterization of mouse hematopoietic stem cells [published erratum appears in Science 1989 Jun 2;244(4908):1030]. *Science* **241,** 58–62.
62. Uchida, N. and Weissman, I. L. (1992) Searching for hematopoietic stem cells: evidence that Thy-1.1lo Lin- Sca-1+ cells are the only stem cells in C57BL/Ka-Thy-1.1 bone marrow. *J. Exp. Med.* **175,** 175–184.
63. Sanchez, M. J., Holmes, A., Miles, C., and Dzierzak, E. (1996) Characterization of the first definitive hematopoietic stem cells in the AGM and liver of the mouse embryo. *Immunity* **5,** 513–525.
64. Morrison, S. J., Hemmati, H. D., Wandycz, A. M., and Weissman, I. L. (1995) The purification and characterization of fetal liver hematopoietic stem cells. *Proc. Natl. Acad. Sci. USA* **92,** 10,302–10,306.

65. Huang, H. and Auerbach, R. (1993) Identification and characterization of hematopoietic stem cells from the yolk sac of the early mouse embryo. *Proc. Natl. Acad. Sci. USA* **90,** 10,110–10,114.
66. Wijgerde, M., Grosveld, F., and Fraser, P. (1995) Transcription complex stability and chromatin dynamics in vivo. *Nature* **377,** 209–213.
67. Ingram, V. M. (1972) Embryonic red blood cell formation. *Nature* **235,** 338–339.
68. Wong, P. M., Chung, S. W., Reicheld, S. M., and Chui, D. H. (1986) Hemoglobin switching during murine embryonic development: evidence for two populations of embryonic erythropoietic progenitor cells. *Blood* **67,** 716–721.
69. Ogawa, M., Nishikawa, S., Yoshinaga, K., Hayashi, S., Kunisada, T., Nakao, J., Kina, T., Sudo, T., Kodama, H., and Nishikawa, S. (1993) Expression and function of c-kit in fetal hemopoietic progenitor cells: transition from the early c-kit-independent to the late c-kit-dependent wave of hemopoiesis in the murine embryo. *Development* **117,** 1089–1098.
70. Ikuta, K., Kina, T., MacNeil, I., Uchida, N., Peault, B., Chien, Y. H., and Weissman, I. L. (1990) A developmental switch in thymic lymphocyte maturation potential occurs at the level of hematopoietic stem cells. *Cell* **62,** 863–874.
71. Hayakawa, K., Hardy, R. R., Herzenberg, L. A., and Herzenberg, L. A. (1985) Progenitors for Ly-1 B cells are distinct from progenitors for other B cells. *J. Exp. Med.* **161,** 1554–1568.
72. Herzenberg, L. A., Stall, A. M., Lalor, P. A., Sidman, C., Moore, W. A., Parks, D. R., and Herzenberg, L. A. (1986) The Ly-1 B cell lineage. *Immunol. Rev.* **93,** 81–102.
73. Naito, M. (1993) Macrophage heterogeneity in development and differentiation. *Arch. Histol. Cytol.* **56,** 331–351.
74. Naito, M., Umeda, S., Yamamoto, T., Moriyama, H., Umezu, H., Hasegawa, G., Usuda, H., Shultz, L. D., and Takahashi, K. (1996) Development, differentiation, and phenotypic heterogeneity of murine tissue macrophages. *J. Leukoc. Biol.* **59,** 133–138.
75. Bruijn, M. D. (1997) PhD. Thesis. Macrophage progenitor cells in mouse bone marrow. Erasmus University, Rotterdam.
76. Shalaby, F., Rossant, J., Yamaguchi, T. P., Gertsenstein, M., Wu, X. F., Breitman, M. L., and Schuh, A. C. (1995) Failure of blood-island formation and vasculogenesis in Flk-1–deficient mice. *Nature* **376,** 62–66.
77. Dickson, M. C., Martin, J. S., Cousins, F. M., Kulkarni, A. B., Karlsson, S., and Akhurst, R. J. (1995) Defective haematopoiesis and vasculogenesis in transforming growth factor-beta 1 knock out mice. *Development* **121,** 1845–1854.
78. Fong, G. H., Rossant, J., Gertsenstein, M., and Breitman, M. L. (1995) Role of the Flt-1 receptor tyrosine kinase in regulating the assembly of vascular endothelium. *Nature* **376,** 66–70.
79. Puri, M. C., Rossant, J., Alitalo, K., Bernstein, A., and Partanen, J. (1995) The receptor tyrosine kinase TIE is required for integrity and survival of vascular endothelial cells. *Embo. J.* **14,** 5884–5891.
80. Sato, T. N., Tozawa, Y., Deutsch, U., Wolburg-Buchholz, K., Fujiwara, Y., Gendron-Maguire, M., Gridley, T., Wolburg, H., Risau, W., and Qin, Y. (1995) Distinct roles of the receptor tyrosine kinases Tie-1 and Tie-2 in blood vessel formation. *Nature* **376,** 70–74.
81. Porcher, C., Swat, W., Rockwell, K., Fujiwara, Y., Alt, F. W., and Orkin, S. H. (1996) The T cell leukemia oncoprotein SCL/tal-1 is essential for development of all hematopoietic lineages. *Cell* **86,** 47–57.
82. Robb, L., Elwood, N. J., Elefanty, A. G., Kontgen, F., Li, R., Barnett, L. D., and Begley, C. G. (1996) The scl gene product is required for the generation of all hematopoietic lineages in the adult mouse. *Embo. J.* **15,** 4123–4129.
83. Robb, L., Lyons, I., Li, R., Hartley, L., Kontgen, F., Harvey, R. P., Metcalf, D., and Begley, C. G. (1995) Absence of yolk sac hematopoiesis from mice with a targeted disruption of the scl gene. *Proc. Natl. Acad. Sci. USA* **92,** 7075–7079.
84. Shivdasani, R. A., Mayer, E. L., and Orkin, S. H. (1995) Absence of blood formation in mice lacking the T-cell leukaemia oncoprotein tal-1/SCL. *Nature* **373,** 432–434.
85. Berger, C. N. and Sturm, K. S. (1996) Estimation of the number of hematopoietic precursor cells during fetal mouse development by covariance analysis. *Blood* **88,** 2502–2509.
86. Tsai, F. Y., Keller, G., Kuo, F. C., Weiss, M., Chen, J., Rosenblatt, M., Alt, F. W., and Orkin, S. H. (1994) An early haematopoietic defect in mice lacking the transcription factor GATA-2. *Nature* **371,** 221–226.

87. Okuda, T., van Deursen, J., Hiebert, S. W., Grosveld, G., and Downing, J. R. (1996) AML1, the target of multiple chromosomal translocations in human leukemia, is essential for normal fetal liver hematopoiesis. *Cell* **84,** 321–330.
88. Sasaki, K., Yagi, H., Bronson, R. T., Tominaga, K., Matsunashi, T., Deguchi, K., Tani, Y., Kishimoto, T., and Komori, T. (1996) Absence of fetal liver hematopoiesis in mice deficient in transcriptional coactivator core binding factor beta. *Proc. Natl. Acad. Sci. USA* **93,** 12,359–12,363.
89. Wang, Q., Stacy, T., Binder, M., Marin-Padilla, M., Sharpe, A. H., and Speck, N. A. (1996) Disruption of the Cbfa2 gene causes necrosis and hemorrhaging in the central nervous system and blocks definitive hematopoiesis. *Proc. Natl. Acad. Sci. USA* **93,** 3444–3449.
90. Wang, Q., Stacy, T., Miller, J. D., Lewis, A. F., Gu, T. L., Huang, X., Bushweller, J. H., Bories, J. C., Alt, F. W., Ryan, G., Liu, P. P., Wynshaw-Boris, A., Binder, M., Marin-Padilla, M., Sharpe, A. H., and Speck, N. A. (1996) The CBFbeta subunit is essential for CBFalpha2 (AML1) function in vivo. *Cell* **87,** 697–708.
91. Pandolfi, P. P., Roth, M. E., Karis, A., Leonard, M. W., Dzierzak, E., Grosveld, F. G., Engel, J. D., and Lindenbaum, M. H. (1995) Targeted disruption of the GATA3 gene causes severe abnormalities in the nervous system and in fetal liver haematopoiesis. *Nat. Genet.* **11,** 40–44.
92. Ting, C. N., Olson, M. C., Barton, K. P., and Leiden, J. M. (1996) Transcription factor GATA-3 is required for development of the T-cell lineage. *Nature* **384,** 474–478.
93. Lin, H. H., Sternfeld, D. C., Shinpock, S. G., Popp, R. A., and Mucenski, M. L. (1996) Functional analysis of the c-myb proto-oncogene. *Curr. Top. Microbiol. Immunol.* **211,** 79–87.
94. Mucenski, M. L., McLain, K., Kier, A. B., Swerdlow, S. H., Schreiner, C. M., Miller, T. A., Pietryga, D. W., Scott, W. J., Jr., and Potter, S. S. (1991) A functional c-myb gene is required for normal murine fetal hepatic hematopoiesis. *Cell* **65,** 677–689.
95. McKercher, S. R., Torbett, B. E., Anderson, K. L., Henkel, G. W., Vestal, D. J., Baribault, H., Klemsz, M., Feeney, A. J., Wu, G. E., Paige, C. J., and Maki, R. A. (1996) Targeted disruption of the PU.1 gene results in multiple hematopoietic abnormalities. *Embo. J.* **15,** 5647–5658.
96. Scott, E., Fisher, R., Olson, M., Kehrli, E., Simon, M., and Singh, H. (1997) PU.1 functions in a cell-autonomous manner to control the differentiation of multipotential lymphoid-myeloid progenitors. *Immunity* **6,** 437–448.
97. Scott, E. W., Simon, M. C., Anastasi, J., and Singh, H. (1994) Requirement of transcription factor PU.1 in the development of multiple hematopoietic lineages. *Science* **265,** 1573–1577.
98. Okada, S., Nakauchi, H., Nagayoshi, K., Nishikawa, S., Nishikawa, S., Miura, Y., and Suda, T. (1991) Enrichment and characterization of murine hematopoietic stem cells that express c-kit molecule. *Blood* **78,** 1706–1712.
99. Russell, E. S. (1979) Hereditary anemias of the mouse: a review for geneticists. *Adv. Genet.* **20,** 357–459.
100. Bernad, A., Kopf, M., Kulbacki, R., Weich, N., Koehler, G., and J. C. Gutierrez-Ramos. (1994) Interleukin-6 is required in vivo for the regulation of stem cells and committed progenitors of the hematopoietic system. *Immunity* **1,** 725–731.
101. Escary, J. L., Perreau, J., Dumenil, D., Ezine, S., and Brulet, P. (1993) Leukaemia inhibitory factor is necessary for maintenance of haematopoietic stem cells and thymocyte stimulation. *Nature* **363,** 361–364.
102. Mackarehtschian, K., Hardin, J. D., Moore, K. A., Boast, S., Goff, S. P., and Lemischka, I. R. (1995) Targeted disruption of the flk2/flt3 gene leads to deficiencies in primitive hematopoietic progenitors. *Immunity* **3,** 147–161.
103. Wang, J. H., Nichogiannopoulou, A., Wu, L., Sun, L., Sharpe, A. H., Bigby, M., and Georgopoulos, K. (1996) Selective defects in the development of the fetal and adult lymphoid system in mice with an Ikaros null mutation. *Immunity* **5,** 537–549.
104. Bernstein, A. (1993) Receptor tyrosine kinases and the control of hematopoiesis. *Sem. Dev. Biol.* **4,** 351–358.
105. Witte, O. N. (1990) Steel locus defines new multipotent growth factor. *Cell* **63,** 5–6.
106. Hassan, H. T. and Zander, A. (1996) Stem cell factor as a survival and growth factor in human normal and malignant hematopoiesis. *Acta. Haematol.* **95,** 257–262.
107. Williams, D. A., Rios, M., Stephens, C., and Patel, V. P. (1991) Fibronectin and VLA-4 in haematopoietic stem cell-microenvironment interactions. *Nature* **352,** 438–441.
108. Arroyo, A. G., Yang, J. T., Rayburn, H., and Hynes, R. O. (1996) Differential requirements for alpha4 integrins during fetal and adult hematopoiesis. *Cell* **85,** 997–1008.

109. Fassler, R. and Meyer, M. (1995) Consequences of lack of beta 1 integrin gene expression in mice. *Genes Dev.* **9,** 1896–1908.
110. Stephens, L. E., Sutherland, A. E., Klimanskaya, I. V., Andrieux, A., Meneses, J., Pedersen, R. A., and Damsky, C. H. (1995) Deletion of beta 1 integrins in mice results in inner cell mass failure and peri-implantation lethality. *Genes Dev.* **9,** 1883–1895.
111. Hirsch, E., Iglesias, A., Potocnik, A. J., Hartmann, U., and Fassler, R. (1996) Impaired migration but not differentiation of haematopoietic stem cells in the absence of beta1 integrins. *Nature* **380,** 171–175.
112. Warren, A. J., Colledge, W. H., Carlton, M. B., Evans, M. J., Smith, A. J., and Rabbitts, T. H. (1994) The oncogenic cysteine-rich LIM domain protein rbtn2 is essential for erythroid development. *Cell* **78,** 45–57.
113. Fujiwara, Y., Browne, C. P., Cunniff, K., Goff, S. C., and Orkin, S. H. (1996) Arrested development of embryonic red cell precursors in mouse embryos lacking transcription factor GATA-1. *Proc. Natl. Acad. Sci. USA* **93,** 12,355–12,358.
114. Pevny, L., Lin, C. S., D. A. V., Simon, M. C., Orkin, S. H., and Costantini, F. (1995) Development of hematopoietic cells lacking transcription factor GATA-1. *Development* **121,** 163–172.
115. Pevny, L., Simon, M. C., Robertson, E., Klein, W. H., Tsai, S. F., D. A. V., Orkin, S. H., and Costantini, F. (1991) Erythroid differentiation in chimaeric mice blocked by a targeted mutation in the gene for transcription factor GATA-1. *Nature* **349,** 257–260.
116. Nuez, B., Michalovich, D., Bygrave, A., Ploemacher, R., and Grosveld, F. (1995) Defective haematopoicsis in fetal liver resulting from inactivation of the EKLF gene. *Nature* **375,** 316–318.
117. Perkins, A. C., Sharpe, A. H., and Orkin, S. H. (1995) Lethal beta-thalassaemia in mice lacking the erythroid CACCC-transcription factor EKLF. *Nature* **375,** 318–322.
118. Lin, C. S., Lim, S. K., D'Agati, V., and Costantini, F. (1996) Differential effects of an erythropoietin receptor gene disruption on primitive and definitive erythropoiesis. *Genes Dev.* **10,** 154–164.
119. Wu, H., Liu, X., Jaenisch, R., and Lodish, H. F. (1995) Generation of committed erythroid BFU-E and CFU-E progenitors does not require erythropoietin or the erythropoietin receptor. *Cell* **83,** 59–67.
120. Keller, G. M. (1995) In vitro differentiation of embryonic stem cells. *Curr. Opin. Cell. Biol.* **7,** 862–869.
121. Muller, A., and Dzierzak, E. (1993) ES cells as a model of embryonic hematopoiesis? *Sem. Dev. Biol.* **4,** 341–350.
122. Doetschman, T. C., Eistetter, H., Katz, M., Schmidt, W., and Kemler, R. (1985) The in vitro development of blastocyst-derived embryonic stem cell lines: formation of visceral yolk sac, blood islands and myocardium. *J. Embryol. Exp. Morphol.* **87,** 27–45.
123. Nakano, T., Kodama, H., and Honjo, T. (1994) Generation of lymphohematopoietic cells from embryonic stem cells in culture. *Science* **265,** 1098–1101.
124. Kennedy, M., Firpo, M., Choi, K., Wall, C., Robertson, S., Kabrun, N., and Keller, G. (1997) A common precursor for primitive erythropoiesis and definitive haematopoiesis. *Nature* **386,** 488–493.
125. Hole, N., Graham, G. J., Menzel, U., and Ansell, J. D. (1996) A limited temporal window for the derivation of multilineage repopulating hematopoietic progenitors during embryonal stem cell differentiation in vitro. *Blood* **88,** 1266–1276.
126. Muller, A. M. and Dzierzak, E. A. (1993) ES cells have only a limited lymphopoietic potential after adoptive transfer into mouse recipients. *Development* **118,** 1343–1351.
127. Peault, B. (1996) Hematopoietic stem cell emergence in embryonic life: developmental hematology revisited. *J. Hematother.* **5,** 369–78.
128. Migliaccio, G., Migliaccio, A. R., Petti, S., Mavilio, F., Russo, G., Lazzaro, D., Testa, U., Marinucci, M., and Peschle, C. (1986) Human embryonic hemopoiesis. Kinetics of progenitors and precursors underlying the yolk sac—liver transition. *J. Clin. Invest.* **78,** 51–60.
129. Haynes, B. F., Martin, M. E., Kay, H. H., and Kurtzberg, J. (1988) Early events in human T cell ontogeny. Phenotypic characterization and immunohistologic localization of T cell precursors in early human fetal tissues [published erratum appears in J Exp Med 1989 Feb 1;169(2):603]. *J. Exp. Med.* **168,** 1061–1080.
130. Lobach, D. F., Hensley, L. L., Ho, W., and Haynes, B. F. (1985) Human T cell antigen expression during the early stages of fetal thymic maturation. *J. Immunol.* **135,** 1752–1759.

131. Charbord, P., Tavian, M., Humeau, L., and Peault, B. (1996) Early ontogeny of the human marrow from long bones: an immunohistochemical study of hematopoiesis and its microenvironment [see comments]. *Blood* **87,** 4109–4119.
132. Huyhn, A., Dommergues, M., Izac, B., Croisille, L., Katz, A., Vainchenker, W., and Coulombel, L. (1995) Characterization of hematopoietic progenitors from human yolk sacs and embryos. *Blood* **86,** 4474–4485.
133. Tavian, M., Coulombel, L., Luton, D., Clemente, H. S., F. Dieterlen-Lievre, and Peault, B. (1996) Aorta-associated CD34+ hematopoietic cells in the early human embryo. *Blood* **87,** 67–72.
134. Garcia-Porrero, J. A., Godin, I. E., and Dieterlen-Lievre, F. (1995) Potential intraembryonic hemogenic sites at pre-liver stages in the mouse. *Anat. Embryol. (Berl)* **192,** 425–435.

Chapter 2

Self-Renewal of Stem Cells

The Intrinsic Timetable Model

Peter M. Lansdorp

1. Introduction

Most blood cells have a limited life-span, and it is estimated that an adult human needs to produce between 10^{11} and 10^{12} mature blood cells per day to compensate for the daily loss of differentiated end cells. Ultimately, this enormous production of cells is derived from a population of hematopoietic stem cells that may need some form of self-renewal to sustain steady-state hematopoiesis and to reconstitute blood cell production following marrow injury.

The mechanisms that regulate the fate of hematopoietic stem cells are poorly understood. Hematopoietic growth factors and factors in the microenvironment are clearly essential to ensure the survival and differentiation of hematopoietic stem cells, but their role in the selection between self-renewal and lineage commitment options is unclear. Differences in the functional behavior of purified stem cells at different stages of development suggest that developmentally regulated intrinsic factors may play an important role in directing stem cell fate. Recent studies strongly implicate homeobox genes in these processes and have further emphasized the linkage between developmental and stem cell biology.

Changes in stem cell function during development correlate with measurable changes in telomere length, and loss of telomere repeats may limit the replicative potential of stem cells. A more detailed understanding of telomere length regulation in hematopoietic cells as well as insight into their actual divisional capacity are required to guide transplantation strategies involving limited numbers of stem cells (e.g., before ex vivo expansion and/or selection after gene transfer).

In this chapter, some issues related to the self-renewal and telomere biology of stem cells are discussed. For this purpose, definitions and assays of stem cells are introduced, and models that incorporate recent data are presented. No attempt is made to cover the

From: *Molecular Biology of B-Cell and T-Cell Development*
Edited by: J. G. Monroe and E. V. Rothenberg © Humana Press Inc., Totowa, NJ

extensive literature in these general areas. Instead, the author's personal view on these topics is presented in the hope to clarify concepts and stimulate further work.

2. Definition of Stem Cells

It could be argued that the life of dedicated experimental hematologists was easier in the 1960s and 1970s. Back then, a stem cell was a pluripotent cell with self-renewal potential that, in the mouse, could be found in various tissues, including fetal liver, bone marrow, and spleen. A convenient assay to detect and enumerate such "stem" cells was to inject cells from any such tissue into lethally irradiated recipients and score the number of macroscopic colonies in the colony forming unit-spleen (CFU-S) after a period of 9–14 days *(1)*. Although it was shown that only some and not all spleen colonies contained CFU-S that could be detected upon secondary transplantation, this heterogeneity in self-renewal was accepted and explained by components in their self-renewal that could be expressed as a specific self-renewal probability *(2)*. The situation became somewhat more complicated when it was shown that the colonies observed on day 9 were not the same or even related to those scored on day 14 *(3)*. This was probably the first example of a theme that has been repeated many times since in studies of stem cell biology, i.e., an underestimation of the functional heterogeneity within populations of cells with some form of "stem cell" properties. The climax of the CFU-S saga probably was the demonstration that precursors of CFU-S and not CFU-S themselves are responsible for long-term lympho-myeloid repopulation *(4)* as shown by the physical separation of pre-CFU-S from CFU-S d12 *(5)*.

Several assays have been proposed over the last decade that provide better estimates of cells with the potential to repopulate the lympho-myeloid lineages of marrow-ablated recipients. One particularly promising procedure is the competitive repopulation assay in which lethally irradiated recipients are transplanted with limiting numbers of syngeneic marked "test" cells, together with unmarked "helper" cells *(6,7)*. By scoring the fraction of recipients with lympho-myeloid repopulation by the test cells at various time points as a function of the number of transplanted cells, the number of individual "competitive repopulating units (CRU)" in a cell suspension can be determined by application of Poisson statistics. Two pieces of information indicate that even the CRU assay is not going to be the "ultimate" stem cell assay. As was previously found with purified human progenitor cells *(8)*, it now seems clear that the phenotype *(9)* and function *(10)* of CRU change quite dramatically during ontogeny. Second, both the detection of CRU and the behavior of CRU in vivo clearly are critically dependent on host factors, notably radiation dose *(11)*. Surprisingly, cells that are clearly capable of contributing to long-term hematopoiesis (exhibiting "stem cell" behavior) do not show such properties in recipients who have received low or very high radiation doses *(11)*. These observations indicate that the fate (and detection) of stem cells is not only influenced by largely unknown intrinsic factors (with a developmental component, *see* Subheading 3. below), but also by host factors that are poorly characterized. Taken together, these numerous observations have completely eroded the concept that "stem cells" represent a single type of immortal cell of which only the frequency and absolute numbers show variations in different tissues. Instead, it now appears that stem cells may accurately be defined as "pluripotent transplantable cells with variable replicative potential that are subject to developmental changes and unpredictable (stochastic) components in their behavior as well as poorly characterized interactions with the hematopoietic microenvironment from the host."

So what if experimental hematologists are having a rough time with stem cell assays and definitions of stem cells? The problem of course is that without a measure or a definition of what hematopoietic stem cells represent, it becomes very difficult to address questions such as "what are the molecular mechanisms controlling self-renewal" or, indeed, "do hematopoietic stem cells self-renew?"

3. Fate Determination in Stem Cells

Of fundamental interest to experimental hematologists and developmental biologists are the mechanisms that control the behavior of primitive hematopoietic cells. At any point in time, an individual "stem" cell has a choice to contribute either to the immediate future (by differentiating and producing committed progenitor cells) or to the more distant requirements for mature cells by undergoing a (functional) self-renewal division. It has been proposed that such decisions at the level of pluripotent stem cells can be depicted as stochastic processes that are intrinsic to the cells *(2,12)*. If this is true, the "stochastic" nature of stem cell decisions may have been at the root of the problems related to the assays and definition of stem cells that were discussed in Subheading 2. above. For example, if in order to detect a contribution to long-term hematopoiesis by a single stem cell, multiple self-renewal divisions each occurring with a certain probability are required, attempts to prospectively separate the cells that, only on retrospect, showed this type of behavior (i.e., by retroviral marking) from indistinguishable and functionally equivalent cells that, by chance, did not display this fate would simply be impossible. Alternatively, the fraction of stem cells with the capacity to produce sufficient stem cells (from early generations) could be very small relative to indistinguishable cells from later generations. The difficulties in purifying repopulating stem cells to homogeneity that have been encountered by many investigators would be in support of either model.

What are the factors that could be involved in stem cell fate decisions? The line of thinking during much of the past has been that cytokines and factors in the (micro-) environment of stem cells are the key regulators of stem cell fate *(13,14)*. The dramatic clinical effect of cytokines such as Erythropoietin, G-CSF, Stem Cell factor, Thrombopoietin, and others on various hematopoietic precursor cells have highlighted the important and critical role that cytokines play in the proliferation and differentiation of various hematopoietic progenitor cells. However, attempts to modulate cell fate decisions in the most primitive hematopoietic cells using cytokines have invariably been unsuccessful *(12,15,16)*. It now appears likely that the primary role of cytokines and the microenvironment in the biology of "stem" cells is to provide an essential, but primarily permissive environment required for their survival, proliferation, and differentiation. If factors in the microenvironment do not determine stem cell fate, what factors do? Important clues to this crucial question have been obtained by studies of the expression of homeobox genes in purified subpopulations of human hematopoietic cells *(17)*. It was shown that various members of the homeobox family of transcription factors are differentially expressed in functionally distinct subpopulations of $CD34^+$ bone marrow cells *(17)*, and that overexpression of HoxB4 in murine stem cells results in a remarkable expansion of cells with long-term lympho-myeloid repopulating potential *(18)*. Interestingly, all the recipients of HoxB4 transduced cells appeared hematologically normal and did not show signs of leukemic transformation *(18)*. Are the homeobox genes, the genes regulated by these genes, and/or the genes that are regulating the homeobox genes themselves the ultimate regulators of stem cell fate? What other transcription factors are involved? Is telomere shortening related in any way to developmental changes in gene expression, or is this measurable genetic change purely coincidental? Can models be derived that incorporate the essential components involved in transcriptional control of stem cell behavior, and can such information be used to manipulate stem cells ex vivo in a way that is clinically meaningful? The answer to these questions are eagerly awaited. However, given the complexity of transcriptional regulation in general and the problems related to the definition and assay of stem cells discussed in Subheading 2. above, a detailed understanding of the molecular control of stem cell fate may not be achieved in the short term.

4. Self-Renewal of Stem Cells?

Self-renewal is a word that is almost as vague and yet widely used as the word "stem cell." The weakest definition of self-renewal is the formation of secondary colonies by cells derived from a primary colony. Although the colony-forming cell in question may be a differentiated cell and known to be completely separate from transplantable stem cells, this type of replating is often referred to as self-renewal of the original colony-forming cell. The strongest experimental definition of self-renewal is probably the reconstitution of multiple mice with the progeny of the same marked stem cell *(19–21)*. This appears to represent stem cell self-renewal by the most stringent of criteria. Most use of the word "self-renewal" describes properties of hematopoietic cells somewhere in between these two extremes. If self-renewal is defined as the process in which a cell division results in two daughter cells that are identical to the parental cell in every way, self-renewal may in fact not exist. Indeed, the loss of telomeric DNA in hematopoietic cells (*see* Subheading 5. below) and the developmental changes in such cells (reviewed in ref. *22*) are difficult to reconcile with "true" self-renewal.

So what if self-renewal in absolute terms does not exist? Could "relative" self-renewal of hematopoietic stem cells satisfy the life-long requirements for blood cell production in normal individuals? What about the hematologic reconstitution in patients and experimental animals after myeloablation and transplantation? It was recently shown that an absolute increase in the number of CRU (*see* Subheading 2. above) can be found in irradiated recipients of limited numbers of CRU, indicative of at least some degree of functional self-renewal in vivo *(23)*. Interestingly, in these experiments fetal liver CRU showed a greater in vivo self-renewal capacity than adult bone marrow CRU and, irrespective of the source of cells, CRU numbers never regenerated to normal levels. Although these studies indicate that some degree of in vivo self-renewal of CRU is possible, the differences in repopulation potential between cells from different sources also indicate the existence of qualitative differences and a functional hierarchy even in the cells defined as CRU.

5. Loss of Telomeric DNA in Stem Cells

The correlation between telomere shortening and the replicative life-span of various somatic human cells (reviewed in ref. *24*), and studies demonstrating the expression of telomerase in cancer cells (reviewed in ref. *25*), have raised considerable interest in the structure and function of chromosome ends. Most information about the molecules and molecular mechanisms involved in the maintenance and function of telomeres has been obtained in studies of unicellular organisms *(26,27)*. Understanding the structure and function of telomeres in cells of multicellular organisms is complicated by questions

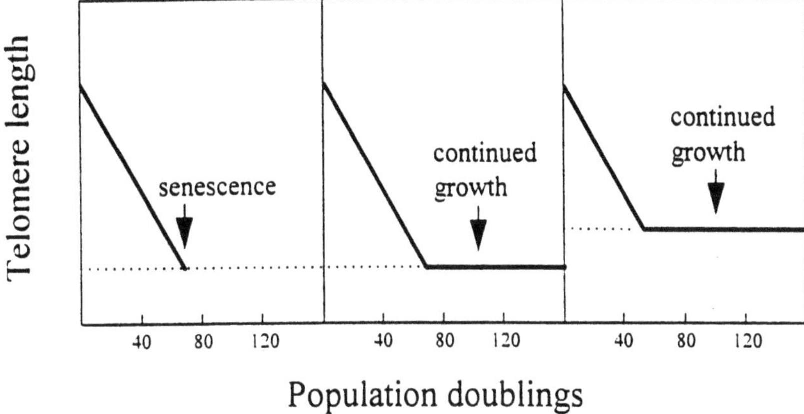

Fig. 1. Measurements of the telomere length in human cells do not necessarily indicate replicative history. In the three examples given, only telomerase negative cells (left panel) are expected to show a useful correlation between replicative life-span and average telomere length. The two panels on the right depict situations in which telomerase positive cells show differences in telomere length at which telomerase is activated to maintain telomeres. Such differences could be related to different levels in some of the molecules involved in telomere length regulation shown in Fig. 2.

about developmental biology, the organization of self-renewing tissues, replicative senescence and limitations of standard molecular techniques to address questions about telomere biology in heterogeneous cell suspensions, and rare cells such as stem cells.

The loss of telomere repeats in adult hematopoietic cells (including purified stem cell "candidates") relative to fetal hematopoietic cells *(28)* is in support of a finite and limited replicative potential of stem cells *(29)*. But what about the telomerase activity measured in stem cells *(30)*, and various models in which telomerase is postulated to extend the replicative life-span of stem cells *(31,32)*? A major problem in answering such questions is that the actual replicative life-span of stem cells is unresolved (*see* Subheading 7. below), consequently, the role of telomerase, if any in this parameter, is also in question. Telomerase is clearly expressed at very low levels in the most primitive, quiescent, $CD34^{+}CD38^{-}$ hematopoietic cells from adult bone marrow, and activity is markedly upregulated in $CD34^{+}CD38^{+}$ cells *(33,34)*. Recent studies also demonstrated telomerase activity in $CD34^{+}CD38^{-}$ cells from fetal liver *(35)*, arguably the best source of cycling stem cells from human tissue. Despite the presence of measurable telomerase, replicative telomere shortening has been observed in lymphocytes *(36)*, hematopoietic progenitor cells *(33)* and, in general, telomeres shorten in humans with age *(37,38)* and reviewed in ref. *24*). One possibility is that telomerase only acts on (very) short telomeres *(39)* and thereby increases the replicative life-span of telomerase positive cells to an unknown extent (Fig. 1). Alternatively, the measured telomerase activity in lymphocytes and hematopoietic cells may have no effect whatsoever on telomeres in vivo.

In order to address questions about the role of telomeres in mammalian cells, better tools to study the length of telomeres in single cells or limited numbers of cells are urgently needed. Recently, the use of quantitative fluorescence *in situ* hybridization (Q-FISH) for measurements of $(T_2AG_3)_n$ length of individual chromosomes was described *(39)*. With this technique, the replication-dependent shortening of human telomeres in metaphase chromosomes throughout the life-span of individual Epstein-Barr Virus

(EBV)-transformed B-cell clones from a male individual was analyzed *(40)*. Telomere fluorescence intensity values decreased at a calculated rate of ~60 bp/doubling and individual (sex) chromosomes showed the same rate of telomere loss. In agreement with published terminal restriction fragments (TRF) length measurements obtained from the same cells *(41)*, few telomere repeats were lost after more than 80 population doubling, suggestive of telomerase mediated telomere stabilization. A model that is compatible with these observations is shown in Fig. 1 (right panels). Could the telomerase activity measured in lymphocytes *(36)*, candidate human *(33–35)*, and murine *(30)* stem cells be capable of extending the replicative life-span in such cells in a similar manner as in these EBV-transformed B-cells (Fig. 1)? Furthermore, could variations in the threshold for telomerase activation vary between cells (e.g., as shown in the two right panels of Fig. 1)? In general, such considerations caution against the use of telomere length measurements as indicators of the replicative life-span or turnover of cells as in recent studies of lymphocytes *(42,43)*.

The amount of knowledge about the biology of telomeres has increased dramatically during the last few years, especially in unicellular organisms such as tetrahymena, oxytricha, yeast, and euplotes. A speculative model based on an interim report of the field (April 1997) is provided in Fig. 2 and its legend. Essential features of this hypothetical model are the potential contribution of many different telomere binding and/or capping proteins in telomere length regulation, and the exchange between an active elongating/telomerase complex and an inactive telomere cap, mediated by proteins binding to telomere repeats (sites 1–4 in Fig. 2). Most of the indicated molecules have not yet been cloned in humans and are proposed solely on the basis of expected homology with known molecules cloned in unicellular organisms. A major difference between the mortal somatic cells of vertebrates and the cells of immortal unicellular organisms is, of course, the replication-dependent loss of telomere repeats in somatic cells and their inevitable senescence. If anything, the regulation of telomere length in human cells is likely to be more complex than shown in Fig. 2. Oversimplifications related to the role of telomerase in cancer and immortality are difficult to fit into this complex picture.

6. The Intrinsic Timetable Model

In order to reconcile a finite replicative potential of stem cells with developmental changes in their function, telomere shortening and transplantation data, a simple model of stem cell biology, is proposed here (Fig. 3). This model, which is called the Intrinsic Timetable (IT) model, postulates that self-renewal is relative, under strict developmental control, and predictable for stem cells of the same generation, but unpredictable at the level of single cells. In the first version of the model (Fig. 3A), the self-renewal prob-

---

Fig. 2. Candidate molecules involved in the regulation of human telomere length. The speculative model shown is based on information from more well-characterized regulation of telomere length in unicellular organisms *(44,45)*. Most human homologs of the indicated proteins have not yet been cloned and the role of telomerase in somatic human cells is not clear. **(A)** Telomeric DNA showing 3' single strand overhand. **(B)** Putative regulators of telomere length in relation to telomeric DNA shown in A.

Proteins binding to double stranded telomere sequences *(46)*, (1 in the figure), are known to regulate human telomere length *(47)* possibly by anchoring telomeric DNA to specific sites in the nucleus *(48)*, at which other components of the macromolecular assembly (2–11

A

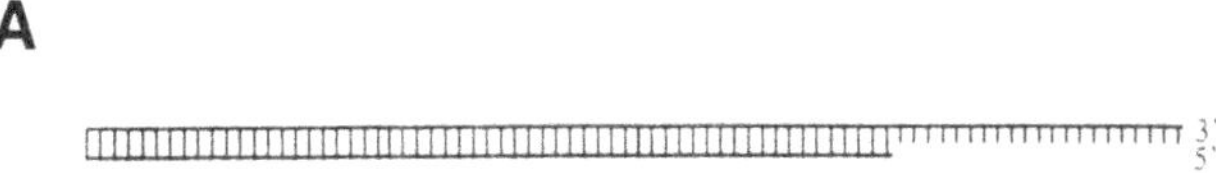

B

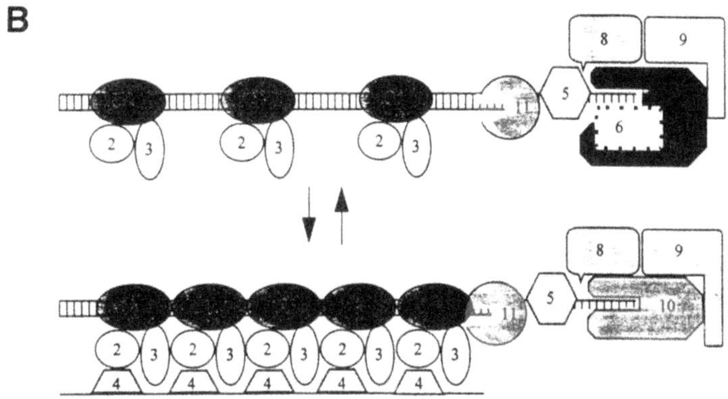

in the figure) are differentially concentrated. As telomeres shorten, insufficient TRF1 may be bound to direct chromosome ends to these nuclear matrix anchor sites which are postulated to be poorly accessible to the active telomerase complex (6–9 in figure). Upon exit from the nuclear matrix site, the inactive end cap complex (8–10 in the figure) is replaced by a macromolecular telomerase complex (6–9 in the figure) and telomeres are elongated or, in the absence of sufficient telomerase activity, cell cycle arrest and/or cells senescence is signaled. Upon elongation by telomerase, more TRF1 will be bound to the telomere, increasing the chance of telomere repositioning to the nuclear matrix. Putative human homologues (2,3 in the figure) of the yeast proteins Rif1p and Rif2p *(49)* will bind to TRF1 and may alter the chromatin structure near telomeres and thereby modulate telomere length in a similar manner as TRF-1. Alternatively, such homologs could mediate interaction with putative homologs of SIR3p and SIR4p *(50,51)* (4 in the figure). The size of the 3' single strand telomere overhang (shown more clearly in Fig. 3A) present at each human telomere *(52)* could be another important variable in telomere function and length regulation. In principle, the size of this single strand could be controlled by proteins binding to single strand repeats (5 in the figure) such as a putative homolog of yeast cdc 13 *(53)* or the β-subunit of Oxytricha telomere-binding protein either before or after folding of the 3' single strand into a higher order structure such as a G-quartet *(54)*; a putative 5'-3' exonuclease (11 in the figure) postulated to trim the 5' strand of telomeric DNA after replication *(52,55)*, and the macromolecular assembly at the very end of the 3' strand (7–10 in the figure). Several molecules are expected to be part of this end-capping assembly, which in the model exists either as an active telomerase complex capable of extending the 3' telomere end (top) or a passive cap (bottom). The active telomerase complex contains human telomerase RNA (6 in the figure, *[56]*) and a putative human homologue (7 in the figure) of Euplotes (p123) and yeast (Est2p) telomerase reverse transcriptase *(57)*, possibly together with the human homologs (8,9,10) of Tetrahymena p80 and p95 *(58)*, Euplotes p120 and p43 *(59)*, and/or ratTLP1 *(60)*. All of these molecules may also be part of the capping (catalytic inactive) complex and some of these proteins are expected to also interact with single strand binding proteins (5 in the figure). Regulation of telomere length may involve interactions of any of the indicated molecules 1–11, and differences in concentrations of these regulators between cells and possibly between specific chromosomes is expected to further complicate telomere length regulation in human cells.

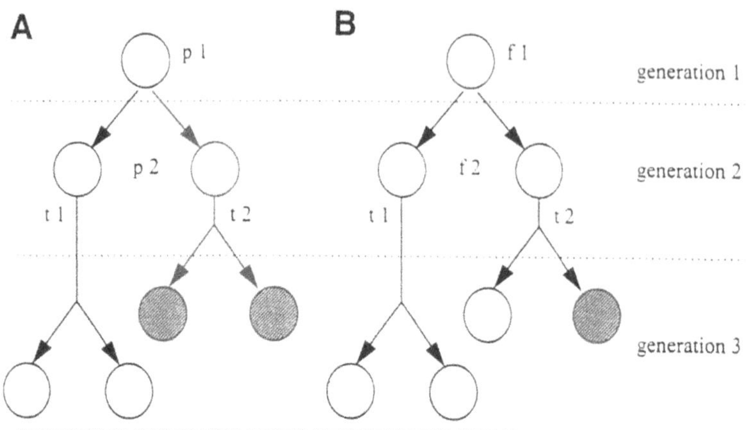

Fig. 3. The Intrinsic Timetable model of stem cell biology. In the two versions of the model shown, the probability of a "self-renewal" division (p) in a given stem cell (open circles) decreases from $1 > p > 0.5$ in fetal life to $p \geq 0.5$ in adult hematopoiesis (a) or, alternatively, the fraction of stem cells producing committed precursors (dashed circles) increases with each generation (b). In either case, the stem cell pool will increase during development and is maintained during steady state adult hematopoiesis. In principle, the size of the stem cell pool is given by either $(1+p)^n$ or $(1+f)^n$ with n being the number of stem cell divisions or generations. However, differences in turn-over (generation-time) between stem cells complicate application of this type of formula for the calculation of the stem cell pool at any particular age. The "self-renewal" of the stem cells in IT is "functional" and relative as the replicative potential of each stem cell decreases with each division and is ultimately limited by the number of telomeric repeats at chromosome ends. Finally, the time interval before daughter cells derived from an identical precursor enter mitosis is variable ($t1 \neq t2$), contributing to extensive heterogeneity in the replicative history of stem cells and consequently a functional hierarchy in different hematopoietic tissues.

ability (p) of stem cells is under developmental control, whereas in the alternative version (Fig. 3B) the fraction (f) of stem cells committed to differentiate increases with each subsequent generation. In both versions of the model, the size of the stem cell pool is regulated by changes in either p or f ($1 > p1 > p2 \geq 0.5$ or $0 < f1 < f2 \leq 1$) according to requirements at different stages of development and the replicative history of individual cells. The time interval before two daughter cells enter mitosis is postulated to vary ($t1 \neq t2$ in Fig. 3) as an important independent variable that is potentially subject to external control. Differences in turnover between stem cells from the same and from different generations result in a hierarchy of stem cells that differ in replicative history as well as p or f values corresponding to their generation.

The IT model is similar to the generation-age hypothesis proposed in the late 1970s *(61)*. In this hypothesis, the number of preceding cell divisions or generations increases the probability of individual stem cells to form two committed precursors. In IT, self-renewal and lineage commitment of stem cells are also intrinsic processes based on two alternative versions (Figs. 3A and B) of asymmetric cell divisions *(62–64)*. IT incorporates the observed loss of telomere DNA in candidate stem cells to indicate a timetable for stem cells in which self-renewal is relative and limited. In IT, the regulation of the cell cycle in stem cells is, furthermore, proposed to be subject to both intrinsic developmentally regulated control, as well as extrinsic regulation by factors of the host. Feed-

Table 1
A Limited Number of Cell Divisions May Generate a Large Number of Cells

Number of divisions	Number of cells produced	Comments
10	10^3	
20	10^6	
30	10^9	
40	10^{12}	Upper limit daily production blood cells in adults
50	10^{15}	
55	4×10^{16}	Upper limit life long production blood cells
60	10^{18}	
65	4×10^{19}	Enough blood cells for the life of a thousand individuals
75	4×10^{21}	Enough blood cells for the life of a million individuals

back from the latter results in the maintenance of most stem cells in a quiescent state during steady state adult hematopoiesis and stimulation of stem cell proliferation, following marrow injury. Finally, differences in the replicative history of stem cells are postulated to greatly contribute to the functional diversity and a functional hierarchy of stem cells in various hematopoietic tissues.

One of the most provocative predictions of IT is that life-long production of mature blood cells is derived from primordial stem cells with a limited replication potential. The observed loss of telomeric DNA in $CD34^+CD38^-$ cells from adult bone marrow relative to the DNA from fetal liver cells *(28)* is in support of this notion. In theory, only a limited number of cell divisions (< 100, Table 1) are needed to meet the life-long requirements for mature blood cells (estimated daily production 10^{12} cells/day in adults), if one assumes exponential cell production. According to this type of calculation, a replication potential of a hundred cell divisions indeed represents a large excess relative to maximum requirements for life-long steady-state hematopoiesis, and probably is also more than sufficient to explain regeneration and transplantation data. A limited replication potential of stem cells requires that few of such cells are wasted in the hematopoietic system (i.e., by apoptosis, selection or competition for limited stem cell "niches"). Economical use of a limited replication potential in stem cells is certainly compatible with the observation that most stem cells in adults (defined by almost any assay) are quiescent, noncycling cells.

Furthermore, IT predicts that the probability of a self-renewal division or the fraction of differentiating cells together with the overall turnover speed (generation time) of stem cells are linked in some way to their developmental stage and replicative history (generation). As a result, the organism ensures that the number of stem cells increases with the increase in cell mass, whereas also ensuring increased production of mature blood cells by increasing the numbers of stem cells that irreversibly commit to the various differentiation pathways. Several predictions based on IT can be tested, and IT cautions against prevalent notions about the self-renewal of hematopoietic stem cells. Some of the most urgent questions raised by the model are: how many times can stem cells divide, or what is the actual replicative potential of stem cells at various stages of development? What are the mechanisms behind the asymmetric cell divisions that result in either variable self-renewal or variable fractions of differentiating cells? To what extent are factors in the microenvironment (i.e., cytokines) capable of modulating self-renewal properties of stem cells? What are the mechanisms controlling the turnover time of stem cells in steady-state hematopoiesis and during hematopoietic regeneration? Are differences in the replicative history of stem cells reflected in their anatomical location and functional properties such as mobilization properties? Hopefully, the answers to some of these important questions will be available in the coming years.

7. Concluding Remarks

Stem cells remain elusive entities. As discussed above, simple questions such as "how many times can stem cells divide?" cannot be answered at this time with answers ranging from < 100 times (this paper) to > 5000 times *(65)*. The possibility that genetic differences in replicative potential are real and important seems increasingly likely. Such differences may ultimately favor the use of fetal liver or cord blood cells for certain clinical applications over autologous or allogeneic cells from adults. The major limitation related to the clinical use of fetal (and neonatal) stem cell sources appear to be related to the number of cells that can be obtained, and the (immunological) transplantation barriers that may become more significant as the number of cells in a transplant decreases. If ex vivo culture conditions could be developed that allow expansion of transplantable "stem" cells from fetal liver and/or cord blood, the use of such expanded cells may become a clinical option for transplantation in adult patients. The development of such culture conditions may not be straightforward *(66)*, but all the tools to make progress in this area appear to be available.

The role of telomeres in the biology of hematopoietic stem cells is currently largely unknown. Overall, telomeres shorten in hematopoietic cells with replication and with age, and the number of divisions that stem cells and lymphocytes can undergo may be limited as a result. However, low levels of telomerase in such cells may maintain the length of short telomeres and expand the replicative potential to an unknown extent. Q-FISH is a promising tool to analyze telomere length at the level of individual chromosomes. Application of Q-FISH and telomerase assays in studies of clonally expanded hematopoietic cells, and lymphocytes are expected to unravel some of the questions about the role of telomeres, telomerase, and telomere dynamics in the function and replication of hematopoietic cells.

What are the implications of the postulated finite replication potential of adult stem cells in transplantation? Taking into account the known genetic differences in telomere length *(67)* that may result in large differences in the actual proliferative potential in cells from different donors, the cautious approach would be not to transplant limited numbers of adult cells into (young) children as such cells may run out of replicative "steam" (telomere repeats) before the end of a normal life-span. Clearly, more data on the telomere length in hematopoietic cells of transplant recipients are needed to assess the degree to which such individuals are at risk. Limitations in replication potential may also complicate strategies aimed to "expand" limited numbers of adult stem cells "ex vivo." Without measures to prevent telomere shortening, increases in cell numbers are likely to coincide with a decreased replication potential of the expanded cells. This may especially be a problem in procedures such as gene marking in combination with selection of cells after gene transfer in which the recovery of the transfected cells of interest may be modest. Even if the right "stem" cells could be stimulated to proliferate into "self-renewal" divisions, such expansion would still be expected to coincide with loss of replication potential that eventually may limit their clinical usefulness. Increased knowledge of telomere biology in normal and malignant cells may point to ways in which telomere-related restriction in the replicative potential of somatic cells can be bypassed in the future. The obvious immediate solution to avoid problems related to such potential limitations of adult stem cell transplants is to use large numbers of cells and avoid manipulations that may result in significant losses of cells.

Acknowledgments

This work was supported by NIH grant AI29524 and by a grant from the National Cancer Institute of Canada with funds from the Terry Fox Run. Dr. G. Krystal is thanked for comments on the manuscript, which was typed by Colleen MacKinnon.

References

1. McCulloch, E. A. and Till, J. E. (1960) The radiation sensitivity of normal mouse bone marrow cells, determined by quantitative marrow transplantation into irradiated mice. *Radiat. Res.* **13,** 115–125.
2. Till, J. E., McCulloch, E. A., and Siminovitch, L. (1964) A stochastic model of stem cell proliferation, based on the growth of spleen colony-forming cells. *Proc. Natl. Acad. Sci. USA* **51,** 29–36.
3. Magli, M. C., Iscove, N. N., and Odartchenko, N. (1982) Transient nature of early haematopoietic spleen colonies. *Nature* **295,** 527–529.
4. Ploemacher, R. E. and Brons, R. H. C. (1989) Separation of CFU-S from primitive cells responsible for reconstitution of the bone marrow hemopoietic stem cell compartment following irradiation: Evidence for a pre-CFU-S cell. *Exp. Hematol.* **17,** 263–266.
5. Jones, R. J., Wagner, J. E., Celano, P., Zicha, M. S., and Sharkis, S. J. (1990) Separation of pluripotent haematopoietic stem cells from spleen colony-forming cells. *Nature* **347,** 188–189.
6. Szilvassy, S. J. and Cory, S. (1993) Phenotypic and functional characterization of competitive long-term repopulating hematopoietic stem cells enriched from 5-fluorouracil-treated murine marrow. *Blood* **81,** 2310–2320.
7. Szilvassy, S. J., Humphries, R. K., Lansdorp, P. M., Eaves, A. C., and Eaves, C. J. (1990) Quantitative assay for totipotent reconstituting hematopoietic stem cells by a competitive repopulation strategy. *Proc. Natl. Acad. Sci. USA* **87,** 8736–8740.
8. Lansdorp, P. M., Dragowska, W., and Mayani, H. (1993) Ontogeny-related changes in proliferative potential of human hematopoietic cells. *J. Exp. Med.* **178,** 787–791.
9. Rebel, V. I., Miller, C. L., Thornbury, G. R., Dragowska, W. H., Eaves, C. J., and Lansdorp, P. M. (1996) A comparison of long-term repopulating hematopoietic stem cells in fetal liver and adult bone marrow from the mouse. *Exp. Hematol.* **24,** 638–648.
10. Rebel, V. I., Miller, C. L., Eaves, C. J., and Lansdorp, P. M. (1996) The repopulation potential of fetal liver hematopoietic stem cells in mice exceeds that of their adult bone marrow counterparts. *Blood* **87,** 3500–3507.
11. Rebel, V. I., Miller, C. L., Spinelli, J. J., Thomas, T. E., Eaves, C. J., and Lansdorp, P. M. (1995) Nonlinear effects of radiation dose on donor-cell reconstitution by limited numbers of purified stem cells. *Biol. Blood Marrow Transplant.* **1,** 32–39.
12. Ogawa, M. (1993) Differentiation and proliferation of hematopoietic stem cells. *Blood* **81,** 2844–2853.
13. Dexter, T. M., Heyworth, C. M., Spooncer, E., and Ponting, I. L. O. (1990) The role of growth factors in self-renewal and differentiation of haemopoietic stem cells. *Philos. Trans. R. Soc. Lond. Biol.* **327,** 85–98.
14. Metcalf, D. (1991) Lineage commitment of hemopoietic progenitor cells in developing blast cell colonies: Influence of colony-stimulating factors. *Proc. Natl. Acad. Sci. USA* **88,** 11,310–11,314.
15. Fairbairn, L. J., Cowling, G. J., Reipert, B. M., and Dexter, T. M. (1993) Suppression of apoptosis allows differentiation and development of a multipotent hemopoietic cell line in the absence of added growth factors. *Cell* **74,** 823–832.
16. Mayani, H., Dragowska, W., and Lansdorp, P. M. (1993) Lineage commitment in human hemopoiesis involves asymmetric cell division of multipotent progenitors and does not appear to be influenced by cytokines. *J. Cell Physiol.* **157,** 579–586.
17. Sauvageau, G., Lansdorp, P. M., Eaves, C. J., Hogge, D. E., Dragowska, W. H., Reid, D. S., Largman, C., Lawrence, H. J., and Humphries, R. K. (1994) Differential expression of homeobox

genes in functionally distinct CD34+ subpopulations of human bone marrow cells. *Proc. Natl. Acad. Sci. USA* **91,** 12,223–12,227.

18. Sauvageau, G., Thorsteinsdottir, U., Eaves, C. J., Lawrence, H. J., Largman, C., Lansdorp, P. M., and Humphries, R. K. (1995) Overexpression of HOXB4 in hematopoietic cells causes the selective expansion of more primitive populations *in vitro* and *in vivo*. *Genes Dev.* **9,** 1753–1765.
19. Lemischka, I. R., Raulet, D. H., and Mulligan, R. C. (1986) Developmental potential and dynamic behavior of hematopoietic stem cells. *Cell* **45,** 917–927.
20. Fraser, C. C., Szilvassy, S. J., Eaves, C. J., and Humphries, R. K. (1992) Proliferation of totipotent hematopoietic stem cells in vitro with retention of long-term competitive in vivo reconstituting ability. *Proc. Natl. Acad. Sci. USA* **89,** 1968–1972.
21. Keller, G. and Snodgrass, R. (1990) Life span of multipotential hematopoietic stem cells in vivo. *J. Exp. Med.* **171,** 1407–1418.
22. Lansdorp, P. M. (1995) Developmental changes in the function of hematopoietic stem cells. *Exp. Hematol.* **23,** 187–191.
23. Pawliuk, R., Eaves, C., and Humphries, R. K. (1996) Evidence of both ontogeny and transplant dose-regulated expansion of hematopoietic stem cells in vivo. *Blood* **88,** 2852–2858.
24. Harley, C. B. (1995) Telomeres and Aging. in *Telomeres.* Blackburn, E. H. and Greider, C. W. (Eds.) Cold Spring Harbor Laboratory, Cold Spring Harbor, NY, pp. 247–265.
25. Harley, C. B., Kim, N. W., Prowse, K. R., Weinrich, S. L., Hirsch, K. S., West, M. D., Bacchetti, S., Hirte, H. W., Counter, C. M., Greider, C. W., Wright, W. E., and Shay, J. W. (1994) Telomerase, cell immortality, and cancer. Cold Spring Harbor Symp. Quant. Biol. 59, Cold Spring Harbor, NY, pp. 307–315.
26. Blackburn, E. H. (1994) Telomeres: no end in sight. *Cell* **77,** 621–623.
27. Zakian, V. A. (1995) Telomeres: Beginning to understand the end. *Science* **270,** 1601–1607.
28. Vaziri, H., Dragowska, W., Allsopp, R. C., Thomas, T. E., Harley, C. B., and Lansdorp, P. M. (1994) Evidence for a mitotic clock in human hematopoietic stem cells: loss of telomeric DNA with age. *Proc. Natl. Acad. Sci. USA* **91,** 9857–9860.
29. Lansdorp, P. M. (1995) Telomere length and proliferation potential of hematopoietic stem cells. *J. Cell Sci.* **108,** 1–6.
30. Morrison, S. J., Prowse, K. R., Ho, P., and Weissman, I. L. (1996) Telomerase activity in hematopoietic cells is associated with self-renewal potential. *Immunity* **5,** 207–216.
31. Holt, S. E., Shay, J. W., and Wright, W. E. (1996) Refining the telomere-telomerase hypothesis of aging and cancer. *Nature Biotechnol.* **14,** 834–837.
32. Autexier, C. and Greider, C. W. (1996) Telomerase and cancer: revisiting the telomere hypothesis. *Trends Biochem. Sci.* **21,** 387–391.
33. Hiyama, K., Hirai, Y., Kyoizumi, S., Akiyama, M., Hiyama, E., Piatyszek, M. A., Shay, J. W., Ishioka, S., and Yamakido, M. (1995) Activation of telomerase in human lymphocytes and hematopoietic progenitor cells. *J. Immunol.* **155,** 3711–3715.
34. Chiu, C-P., Dragowska, W., Kim, N. W., Vaziri, H., Yui, J., Thomas, T. E., Harley, C. B., and Lansdorp, P. M. (1996) Differential expression of telomerase activity in hematopoietic progenitors from adult human bone marrow. *Stem Cells* **14,** 239–248.
35. Yui, J., Chiu, C-P., and Lansdorp, P. M. (1998) Telomerase activity in candidate stem cells from fetal liver and adult bone marrow. *Blood,* in press.
36. Weng, N-P., Levine, B. L., June, C. H., and Hodes, R. J. (1996) Regulated expression of telomerase activity in human T lymphocyte development and activation. *J. Exp. Med.* **183,** 2471–2479.
37. Harley, C. B., Futcher, A. B., and Greider, C. W. (1990) Telomeres shorten during ageing of human fibroblasts. *Nature* **345,** 458–460.
38. Hastie, N. D., Dempster, M., Dunlop, M. G., Thompson, A. M., Green, D. K., and Allshire, R. C. (1990) Telomere reduction in human colorectal carcinoma and with ageing. *Nature* **346,** 866–868.
39. Lansdorp, P. M., Verwoerd, N. P., van de Rijke, F. M., Dragowska, V., Little, M-T., Dirks, R. W., Raap, A. K., and Tanke, H. J. (1996) Heterogeneity in telomere length of human chromosomes. *Hum. Mol. Genet.* **5,** 685–691.

40. Lansdorp, P. M., Poon, S., Chavez, E., Dragowska, V., Zijlmans, M., Bryan, T., Reddel, R., Egholm, M., Bacchetti, S., and Martens, U. (1997) Telomeres in the hematopoietic system. CIBA Foundation Symposium No. 211. Telomeres and Telomerase (in press).
41. Counter, C. M., Botelho, F. M., Wang, P., Harley, C. B., and Bacchetti, S. (1994) Stabilization of short telomeres and telomerase activity accompany immortalization of Epstein-Barr virus-transformed human B lymphocytes. *J. Virol.* **68,** 3410–3414.
42. Monteiro, J., Batliwalla, F., Ostrer, H., and Gregersen, P. K. (1996) Shortened telomeres in clonally expanded CD28$^-$CD8$^+$ T cells imply a replicative history that is distinct from their CD28$^+$CD8$^+$ counterparts. *J. Immunol.* **156,** 3587–3590.
43. Wolthers, K. C., Wisman, B. G., Otto, S. A., de Roda Husman, A. M., Schaft, N., de Wolf, F., Goudsmit, J., Coutinho, R. A., van der Zee, A. G., Meyaard, L., and Miedema, F. (1996) T cell telomere length in HIV-1 infection: no evidence for increased CD4$^+$ T cell turnover. *Science* **274,** 1543–1547.
44. Zakian, V. A. (1996) Structure, function, and replication of *Saccharomyces cerevisiae* telomeres. *Annu. Rev. Genet.* **30,** 141–172.
45. Greider, C. W. (1996) Telomere length regulation. *Annu. Rev. Biochem.* **65,** 337–365.
46. Chong, L., van Steensel, B., Broccoli, D., Erdjument-Bromage, H., Hanish, J., Tempst, P., and de Lange, T. (1995) A human telomeric protein. *Science* **270,** 1663–1667.
47. van Steensel, B. and de Lange, T. (1997) Control of telomere length by the human telomeric protein TRF1. *Nature* **385,** 740–743.
48. Mirabella, A. and Gartenberg, M. R. (1997) Yeast telomeric sequences function as chromosomal anchorage points in vivo. *EMBO J.* **16,** 523–533.
49. Wotton, D. and Shore, D. (1997) A novel Rap1p-interacting factor, Rif2p, cooperates with Rif1p to regulate telomere length in *Saccharomyces cerevisiae. Genes Dev.* **11,** 748–760.
50. Moretti, P., Freeman, K., Coodly, L., and Shore, D. (1994) Evidence that a complex of SIR proteins interacts with the silencer and telomere-binding protein RAP1. *Genes Dev.* **8,** 2257–2269.
51. Marcand, S., Buck, S. W., Moretti, P., Gilson, E., and Shore, D. (1996) Silencing of genes at nontelomeric sites in yeast is controlled by sequestration of silencing factors at telomeres by Rap1 protein. *Genes Dev.* **10,** 1297–1309.
52. Makarov, V. L., Hirose, Y., and Langmore, J. P. (1997) Long G tails at both ends of human chromosomes suggest a C strand degradation mechanism for telomere shortening. *Cell* **88,** 657–666.
53. Nugent, C. I., Hughes, T. R., Lue, N. F., and Lundblad, V. (1996) Cdc13p: a single-strand telomeric DNA-binding protein with a dual role in yeast telomere maintenance. *Science* **274,** 249–252.
54. Fang, G. and Cech, T. R. (1993) Characterization of a G-quartet formation reaction promoted by the β-subunit of the *Oxytricha* telomere-binding protein. *Biochemistry* **32,** 11,646–11,657.
55. Wellinger, R. J., Ethier, K., Labrecque, P., and Zakian, V. A. (1996) Evidence for a new step in telomere maintenance. *Cell* **85,** 423–433.
56. Feng, J., Funk, W. D., Wang, S-S., Weinrich, S. L., Avilion, A. A., Chiu, C-P., Adams, R. R., Chang, E., Allsopp, R. C., Yu, J., Le, S., West, M. D., Harley, C. B., Andrews, W. H., Greider, C. W., and Villeponteau, B. (1995) The RNA component of human telomerase. *Science* **269,** 1236–1241.
57. Lingner, J., Hughes, T. R., Shevchenko, A., Mann, M., Lundblad, V., and Cech, T. R. (1997) Reverse transcriptase motifs in the catalytic subunit of telomerase. *Science* **276,** 561–567.
58. Collins, K., Kobayashi, R., and Greider, C. W. (1995) Purification of tetrahymena telomerase and cloning of genes encoding the two protein components of the enzyme. *Cell* **81,** 677–686.
59. Lingner, J. and Cech, T. R. (1996) Purification of telomerase from Euplotes aediculatus: requirement of a primer 3' overhang. *Proc. Natl. Acad. Sci. USA* **93,** 10,712–10,717.
60. Nakayama, J., Saito, M., Nakamura, H., Matsuura, A., and Ishikawa, F. (1997) TLP1, A gene encoding a protein component of mammalian telomerase is a novel member of WD repeats family. *Cell* **88,** 1–20.
61. Rosendaal, M., Hodgson, G. S., and Bradley, T. R. (1979) Organization of haemopoietic stem cells: The generation-age hypothesis. *Cell Tissue Kinet.* **12,** 17–29.

62. Horvitz, H. R. and Herskowitz, I. (1992) Mechanisms of asymmetric cell division: two Bs or not two Bs, that is the question. *Cell* **68,** 237–255.
63. Amon, A. (1996) Mother and daughter are doing fine: asymmetric cell division in yeast. *Cell* **84,** 651–654.
64. Hirata, J., Nakagoshi, H., Nabeshima, Y., and Matsuzaki, F. (1995) Asymmetric segregation of the homeodomain protein Prospero during *Drosophila* development. *Nature* **377,** 627–630.
65. Potten, C. S. and Loeffler, M. (1990) Stem cells: attributes, cycles, spirals, pitfalls and uncertainties. Lessons for and from the crypt. *Development* **10,** 1001–1020.
66. Rebel, V. I. and Lansdorp, P. M. (1996) Culture of purified stem cells from fetal liver results in loss of in vivo repopulating potential. *J. Hematother.* **5,** 25–37.
67. Slagboom, P. E., Droog, S., and Boomsma, D. I. (1994) Genetic determination of telomere size in humans: A twin study of three age groups. *Am. J. Hum. Genet.* **55,** 876–882.

Chapter 3

Transcription Factors Regulating Early Hematopoietic Development and Lineage Commitment

Stuart H. Orkin

1. Introduction

The establishment of the hematopoietic system entails a series of developmental decisions, followed by expansion of immature progenitors or hematopoietic stem cells (HSCs) and the subsequent commitment of later progenitors to differentiation along selected lineages *(1)*. Within the early embryo, ventral (or posterior) mesoderm gives rise to presumptive hemangioblasts *(2)* that are further specified to embryonic erythroid precursors and vascular cells in the developing yolk sac blood islands (Fig. 1). Later, intraembryonic hematopoiesis occurs in the fetal liver, most likely seeded from progenitors or HSCs located in the aortic/gonad/mesonephros (AGM) region *(3–6)*. In addition to these important developmental decisions, amplification of hematopoietic progenitors within the yolk sac and embryonic compartments is necessary to provide the total number of cells required to meet increasing demands as the embryo grows. Various inductive events under the control of growth factors presumably lead to the origin of the hemangioblast, the specification of embryonic hematopoiesis, and the appearance of HSCs in the AGM region. The critical developmental decisions are thought to be executed by transcription factors, functioning in a combinatorial manner. These are the subject of this review. Genetic approaches have culminated in the identification of several transcription factors, or transcription factor associated proteins that are essential for various aspects of hematopoietic development. Examples are discussed below with the aim of defining some principles underlying hematopoietic development. The factors reviewed herein are summarized in Table 1 and are individually considered throughout the chapter.

From: *Molecular Biology of B-Cell and T-Cell Development*
Edited by: J. G. Monroe and E. V. Rothenberg © Humana Press Inc., Totowa, NJ

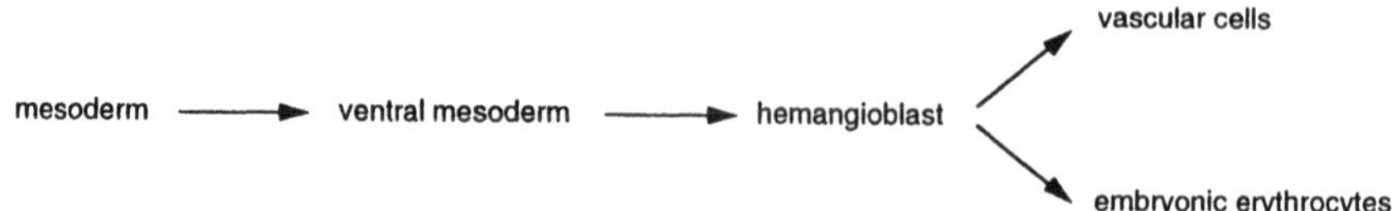

Fig. 1. Pathway of embryonic blood formation.

Table 1
Summary of Selected Transcriptional Factors and Their Roles in Hematopoiesis

Factor	Class	DNA-binding	Expression	Hematopoietic requirement
SCL/tal-1	b-HLH	+	hematopoietic: E, Meg, mast, prog., nonhemat.: vascular, CNS	all hematopoiesis
Rbtn2/ Lmo2	LIM	–	hematopoietic: E enriched, others nonhemat.: widespread (?)	embryonic RBCs (prob. all hematopoiesis)
GATA-1	GATA-zinc	+	hematopoietic: E, Meg, mast, prog., nonhemat.: Sertoli cells	E/Meg differentiation
GATA-2	GATA-zinc	+	hematopoietic: progenitors, Meg, mast, nonhemat.: widespread	proliferation/survival of hematopoietic prog.
GATA-3	GATA-zinc	+	hematopoietic: T-lymphoid nonhemat.: kidney, CNS	T-lymphoid cells
FOG	multitype-zinc	?	hematopoietic: E, Meg, progenitors, nonhemat.: (?)	E/Meg differentiation
AML1	runt	+	hematopoietic: not well defined nonhemat.: widespread (?)	definitive hematopoiesis

Abbreviations: b-HLH, basic-helix-loop-helix; E, erythroid; Meg, megakaryocytic; prog., progenitor; ?, unknown or uncertain from published work.

2. Genes Required for all Hematopoietic Lineages in a Cell-Autonomous Fashion

Those genes whose functions are essential for formation, expansion, or maintenance of HSCs would be expected to be required for development of all hematopoietic lineages. The clearest example of this class is the product of SCL/tal-1 (stem cell leukemia, T-ALL) gene *(7,8)*. The locus is frequently activated in acute lymphoblastic leukemia by chromosomal translocations and upstream interstitial deletions involving the *sil* locus *(9)* and encodes a basic helix-loop-helix (bHLH) family member that is expressed in limited sites in the developing embryo, particularly in extraembyonic mesoderm vascular cells, and the nervous system *(7,8,10–15)*. Expression of SCL/tal-1 transgenes targeted to T-cells is sufficient to induce lymphomas, demonstrating that under appropriate circumstances SCL/tal-1 is oncogenic *(16,17)*. Whether leukemogenesis induced by ectopic expression of SCL/tal-1 reflects the activation of an early hematopoietic program normally induced by SCL/tal-1 or interference with development through sequestration of heterodimeric partners, such as products of the E2A gene, is uncertain. Recent evidence has been interpreted to be consistent with the latter mechanism *(18)*.

Whichever proves to be the case, loss of SCL/tal-1 function through targeted mutation in murine embryonic stem (ES) cells prevents development of all hematopoietic lineages *(19–22)*. Embryos lacking SCL/tal-1 die by E10 with absent embryonic red blood cells in the yolk sac blood islands and the embryo proper. Of interest, endothelial cells are present in the yolk sac *(21,22)*, signifying proper specification of vascular cells from the presumptive hemangioblast. SCL/tal-1$^{-/-}$ ES cells do not generate any myeloerythroid precursors in vitro and also fail to contribute to hematopoiesis, including T- and B-lymphoid populations in the RAG-2 deficient blastocyst complementation assay *(19,23)*. These findings demonstrate that SCL/tal-1 is required in a nonredundant fashion at the very earliest stages of hematopoiesis, perhaps in the specification of a blood fate from the hemangioblast or thereafter, in the HSC to maintain itself, proliferate in response to growth factors, or to survive. At present, it is not possible to be more specific as to the stage of the block to hematopoietic development.

Current limitations in our understanding of SCL/tal-1's roles in development are the lack of identified target genes, and the absence of convenient assays of protein function. Of particular relevance to combinatorial models of regulation is the discovery that SCL/tal-1 associates with another leukemia oncoprotein, Rbtn2/Lmo2, a member of the zinc-finger LIM family *(24–26)*. Although Rbtn2/Lmo2 does not bind DNA on its own, it is believed to influence transcription through its physical interaction with SCL/tal-1, presumably mediated by the LIM domain of Rbtn2/Lmo2 and the bHLH domain of SCL/tal-1 *(25)*. Consistent with the notion that these proteins act in concert, at least in some circumstances, the loss of Rbtn2/Lmo2 function in the embryo also prevents embryonic erythropoiesis in the yolk sac blood islands *(26)*. Although the developmental potential of Rbtn2/Lmo2$^{-/-}$ ES cells needs to be more fully assessed, it seems probable that loss of Rbtn2/Lmo2 also blocks formation of other lineages. At first approximation; therefore, SCL/tal-1 and Rbtn2/Lmo2 are likely to function together within an essential protein complex to regulate critical target genes in the earliest hematopoietic compartment during embryogenesis. The block to development in their absence is envisioned to impair a precursor common to primitive erythropoiesis and definitive hematopoiesis, perhaps equivalent to the blast colony-forming cells detected in ES cells differentiated in vitro *(27)*.

Protein interactions of Rbtn2/Lmo2 may be more complex than suggested above and relate to its roles in early progenitors and/or erythroid precursors. Rbtn2/Lmo2 has been reported to interact, albeit weakly, with GATA-1 *(24)* (*see* Subheading 4.). Perhaps of greater potential relevance, Rbtn2/Lmo2 assembles in vitro on a bipartite DNA motif comprising an E-box (CAGGTG) followed 9 bp downstream by a GATA-site as part of a complex including SCL/tal-1, E47, GATA-1, and a LIM-interacting protein Ldb1/NL1 *(28–30)*. These in vitro findings provide additional evidence that Rbtn2/Lmo2 serves as a bridging molecule within larger transcriptional complexes. It will be important in the future to identify native gene regulatory elements in which this bipartite binding site resides. To date, target sites are unknown. Given the number of proteins already associated with the SCL/tal-1 and Rbtn2/Lmo2 complex and the recent identification of a highly specific GATA-interacting protein friend of GATA-1 (FOG) *(31)* (*see* Subheading 4.), it is likely that a variety of protein complexes exist in hematopoietic cells, perhaps changing their abundances as progenitors arise, commit to specific lineages, and mature along specific paths.

AML1 or CBFA2 provides another example of a gene discovered in the context of leukemia that serves an important role in hematopoietic development *(32–35)*. AML1 corresponds to the DNA-binding subunit of the heterodimeric core-binding factor (CBF). AML1, and its related genes CBFA1 and A3, bind DNA through a runt homology domain, named for the *Drosophila* pair-rule gene *runt*. Although AML1's expression is not restricted to the hematopoietic system throughout development, its loss, or that of its nonDNA-binding partner, leads to embryonic lethality, characterized by an intrinsic block to fetal liver hematopoiesis and intraembryonic hemorrhage *(32–35)*. Therefore,

AML1 appears to be required for some aspect of the formation, maintenance, or differentiation of adult progenitors or possibly the HSC itself.

3. Genes Influencing the Expansion of Immature Hematopoietic Progenitors

A functioning hematopoietic system depends on the proliferation of immature progenitor cells, both to provide sufficient cells during growth and development of the individual and to sustain blood cell production in the adult. The transcription factor GATA-2 plays a vital role in the proliferative capacity and/or survival of multipotential progenitors *(36–38)*. GATA-2, a member of the GATA-subfamily of zinc-finger proteins, is expressed at high level in immature progenitors and very likely in HSCs, as well. Expression is maintained in mast cells and megakaryocytes but repressed during erythroid maturation (*see* Subheading 4.) *(39)*. During embryonic development, GATA-2 expression is first seen in extraembryonic mesoderm in a region overlapping that for SCL/tal-1 and Rbtn2/Lmo2, implicating GATA-2 in formation of the first hematopoietic cells within the embryo *(40)*. Loss of GATA-2 function leads to embryonic lethality because of a quantitative defect in embryonic erythropoiesis *(37)*. In chimeric mice made by injection into wild-type blastocyts, GATA-$2^{-/-}$ ES cells fail to contribute appreciably to adult hematopoietic lineages. Contribution to B- and T-lymphocytes is exceedingly weak but detectable in some chimeras. In vitro differentiation of GATA-$2^{-/-}$ ES cells reveals a marked deficiency of multipotential progenitors *(41)*, particularly under conditions in which colony formation is dependent on stem cell factor (SCF, c-kit-ligand). Nonetheless, differentiation beyond the multipotential stage seems unaffected in erythroid, myeloid, megakaryocytic, and (presumably) lymphoid lineages. Mast cell formation appears blocked, most likely caused by an independent role for GATA-2 in the lineage *(41)*. Overall, findings are consistent with a critical function for GATA-2 in maintaining the proliferative capacity and/or viability of immature progenitor cells. Whether GATA-2 is required in a similar manner in HSCs is unknown, but plausible. The proposed role for GATA-2 at the progenitor level is independently supported by experiments of its enforced expression in immortalized chicken progenitor cells *(36)*. In this situation, erythroid maturation is blocked and cells remain in a proliferative state. The nature of the target genes regulated by GATA-2 in progenitors remain to be identified, although likely candidates are cytokine receptors, signaling molecules, or components of the cell-cycle machinery.

Homeodomain proteins figure very prominently in embryonic development *(42)* and, therefore, have long been entertained as regulators of hematopoiesis. Apart from the somewhat restricted expression of some *Hox* genes in hematopoietic cell lines, scant evidence existed until recently, linking specific Hox genes with any particular aspect of hematopoiesis. In a direct test of their potential involvement, a retrovirus containing *HOXB4* cDNA was transduced into murine bone marrow cells. Although no perturbation of specific lineages was observed, and leukemia was not induced, mice reconstituted with transduced marrow cells contained > 50-fold more HSCs *(43)*. This remarkable finding confirms the earlier observation implicating another *Hox* gene (*HOXB8*) in self-renewal of immature myeloid progenitors *(44)*. Thus, evidence is strengthening an association between *Hox* gene function and aspects of hematopoiesis. Given the number of Hox genes and their varying patterns of expression in hematopoietic progenitors and specific lineages, there is ample room for complex regulatory interactions and overlapping functions in vivo. The connection between *Hox* genes and hematopoietic development is underscored by two other situations. First, chromosomal translocations in myeloid leukemia have been described in which *HOXA9* is fused to nucleoporin *NUP98*, resulting in a chimeric protein that may block myeloid development in a dominant-negative manner *(45,46)*. Second, the *Drosophila trithorax*-related gene *Mll* (also known as HRX and ALL-1), which was discovered in chromosomal translocations associated with mixed-lineage leukemia, is a regulator of *HOX* genes in vivo *(47)*. Haploinsufficiency for *Mll* in mice leads to perturbed hematopoiesis, characterized principally by decreased numbers of red cells, platelets, and B-lymphocytes. A particular challenge for the future is relating *HOX* genes to specific downstream target genes or pathways. The complexity is daunting. Perhaps interbreeding of individual *HOX* knockout mice will eventually reveal dramatic effects of loss of function on hematopoietic progenitors or specific lineages.

Proteins of the homeobox family may also play important roles in the earliest steps in the patterning of mesoderm, ultimately to assume an hematopoietic fate. Through an expression cDNA screen in *Xenopus* the paired-class homeobox product known as *Mix.1* was identified as an inducer of ventral mesoderm *(48)*. Injection of its mRNA transforms dorsal mesoderm to a ventral fate and leads to excessive blood formation in embryos. Of particular interest, *Mix.1* expression is induced by BMP-4, a member of the transforming growth factor-β superfamily, which has been described as an inducer of hematopoietic activity in cultured ES cells *(49)*. Furthermore, a dominant inhibitory mutant of *Mix.1* blocks the ventralizing effects of BMP-4, placing *Mix.1* downstream in a BMP-4 signaling cascade *(48)*.

4. GATA-1: A Paradigm for an Hematopoietic-Specific Transcription Factor

The zinc-finger protein GATA-1, the founding member of the GATA-family, is perhaps the first "hematopoietic-specific" transcription factor to be studied in detail *(50,51)*. Except for Sertoli cells *(52)* of the testis where its function is uncertain, GATA-1's expression is restricted to the hematopoietic system within which it is highly expressed in erythroid, megakaryocytic, mast, and eosinophilic lineages and at lower level in multipotential progenitors *(53,54)*. Available evidence suggests that GATA-1 is not expressed in HSCs. However, during embryogenesis GATA-1 is expressed in extraembryonic mesoderm of the developing yolk sac blood islands and in embryonic erythroblasts *(40)*. The early appearance of GATA-1 during embryogenesis, taken together with lack of evidence for its expression in HSCs, may suggest that expression of GATA-1 is downregulated in HSCs and then upregulated in multipotential progenitors. In the immature hematopoietic compartment, GATA-1's expression is overlapping with that of GATA-2.

Among the hematopoietic transcription factors studied to date, GATA-1 is unique in its capacity to influence the phenotype of progenitor cells in which it is expressed. Forced expression of GATA-1 cDNA reprograms *myb-ets* transformed chicken progenitors along erythroid, eosinophilic, and thromboblastic (megakaryocytic) pathways concomitant with downregulation of myeloid markers *(55)*. Similarly, murine myeloid 416B cells are converted to megakaryocytes by expression of either GATA-1, GATA-2, or GATA-3, although induction of differentiation by GATA-2 and-3 correlates with activation of endogenous GATA-1 expression *(56,57)*. Again, megakaryocyte differentiation is accompanied by downregulation of myeloid markers. In chicken progenitors, GATA-1 induced lineage reprogramming appears to be dependent on the concentration of GATA-1 itself. These important observations suggest a competitive relationship between lineages modulated by the action of GATA-1.

Gene targeting experiments of the GATA-1 locus provide clear evidence that GATA-1 is essential for maturation of erythroid and megakaryocytic precursor cells. Loss of GATA-1 leads to a developmental arrest and apoptosis at the proerythroblast stage *(58–60)*. Thus, erythroid commitment takes place in the absence of GATA-1, presumably through the aegis of GATA-2, which remains elevated in the GATA-1⁻ cellular environment *(39)*. The failure to repress GATA-2 expression in GATA-1⁻ erythroid precursors underscores the dynamic relationship between these GATA-factors. Moreover, the switch from dependence on GATA-2 to GATA-1 accompanies the transition from proliferation to maturation and highlights the overlapping, but distinct, roles of these two transcription factors in hematopoietic development. GATA-1⁻ erythroid precursors also undergo apoptosis, establishing a link between GATA-1 and cell survival *(60)*. Although it is unclear as yet whether this relationship speaks to a direct role of GATA-1 in regulating apoptosis or an indirect consequence of other events in cellular maturation triggered by GATA-1, the observation that precursor cell survival relies on a critical transcription factor for the lineage makes biological sense. In the megakaryocytic lineage, the failure of cellular maturation is accompanied by unrestrained proliferation rather than apoptosis *(61)*. As a unifying model, it is suggested that GATA-1 is pivotal in controlling the balance between proliferative and maturation states of erythroid and megakaryocytic precursors and is required to drive terminal maturation. Apoptosis and proliferation can be viewed as alternative responses to impaired cellular differentiation. Despite GATA-1's ability to reprogram progenitor cell lines to specific lineage pathways, loss of expression is not accompanied by evident shifts in specific progenitors in hematopoietic colony assays from yolk sac cells of GATA-1⁻ embryos or GATA-1⁻ ES cells. This may reflect unique features of the progenitor cell lines used or compensatory mechanisms operating in non-transformed cells.

The available evidence indicates that GATA-1 is required quite late in the pathways of erythroid and megakaryocytic differentiation *(39,58,61)*, though it is expressed early in the hematopoietic hierarchy *(40,62)*. As GATA-1's function may be partially redundant with GATA-2 in immature cells, a role for GATA-1 prior to the stages at which it is required cannot be excluded. Analysis of the differentiation potential of ES cells with targeted mutations of both the GATA-1 and GATA-2 loci should clarify these possibilities.

Fundamental to understanding how GATA-1 acts is defining the mechanisms by which it participates in transcription. The prevailing view has been that GATA-1 binds its cognate recognition site in target *cis*-elements and activates transcription through interactions of its activation domains with components of the basal transcriptional machinery *(63,64)*. Indirect support for this scenario is provided by the demonstration that GATA-1 functions as a potent transactivator of reporters in fibroblastic cells and an "essential" amino-terminal region is transferable as an activation domain to an heterologous DNA-binding domain. More recent findings suggest an alternative manner in which GATA-1 is coupled to the transcriptional machinery.

The generation of a unique erythroid cell line derived from GATA-1⁻ ES cells affords the opportunity to examine GATA-1 function in erythroid differentiation, rather than in an artificial context *(65)*. Such experiments reveal that GATA-1's transactivation properties, as scored in conventional transfection settings, do not correlate with its capacity to program terminal erythroid maturation. Moreover, the amino-zinc finger of GATA-1, which is largely dispensable for DNA binding and transactivation in fibroblast assays *(64)*, is strictly required for erythroid differentiation. On the basis of these observations,

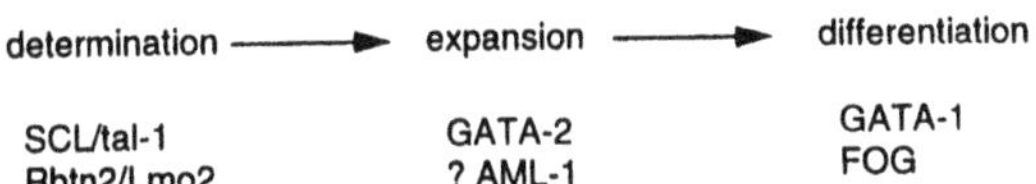

Fig. 2. Hypothesized requirements for specific transcriptional proteins in hematopoietic development. For purposes of discussion, the pathway is divided into phases of fate determination, expansion of progenitors (or HSCs), and lineage differentiation.

it has been proposed that the in vivo function of GATA-1 depends on a transcriptional cofactor *(65)*. The predicted cofactor, whose expression might be restricted among different cell types or lineages, would interact with the DNA-binding domain of GATA-1 and constitute a bridge to other proteins within a larger complex. In effect, GATA-1's primary function would be to identify sites within the chromatin and recruit a cell-specific complex to these regions.

Evidence in behalf of the cofactor model has recently been obtained through the isolation of a novel, multitype zinc-finger protein Friend of GATA-1 (FOG), which interacts specifically with the amino-finger of GATA-1 *(31)*. The expression of FOG parallels that of GATA-1 during murine hematopoietic development. Within hematopoietic lineages, the expression of GATA-1 and FOG is overlapping—both are expressed at high level in erythroid and megakaryocytic cells and at lower level in progenitors. However, mast cells express GATA-1, but not FOG. Most importantly, FOG synergizes with GATA-1 in transcription of a reporter containing an intact p45 NF-E2 gene hematopoietic-specific promoter and in cellular assays of both erythroid and megakaryocytic differentiation. These findings argue that FOG is, indeed, a cofactor for GATA-1 action in both erythroid and megakaryocytic lineages. Consistent with this general conclusion, mouse embryos lacking FOG are embryonic lethal at the yolk sac stage (A. Tsang, Y. Fujiwara, and S.H.O., unpublished data).

The possible roles for SCL/tal-1, Rbtn2/Lmo2, GATA-2, AML-1, GATA-1, and FOG discussed above are schematically summarized in Fig. 2. It is emphasized that this classification into genes involved in fate determination, progenitor expansion, and cellular differentiation should be considered tentative, as discussed more fully elsewhere *(66)*.

5. GATA-3: An Essential Factor for Development of the T-Cell Lineage

Soon after the cloning of GATA-1 cDNA, reduced stringency hybridization screening led to the isolation of a GATA-3, a member of the GATA-family whose expression among hematopoietic cells is highly restricted to T-lymphocytes and their precursors *(38,67,68)*. Functionally important GATA-motifs are present in promoters and enhancers of numerous T-cell expressed genes. Taken together with its prominent expression in developing thymus *(69)*, these data implied a role for GATA-3 in some aspects of T-cell development. These predictions have been borne out in recent genetic studies of GATA-3 function. Loss of GATA-3 leads to embryonic lethality in the mouse at midgestation because of myriad developmental abnormalities *(70)*. Analysis of the developmental potential of GATA-$3^{-/-}$ ES cells in chimeras demonstrates an essential function for production of T-cells, but not other hematopoietic lineages (including B-cells) *(71)*. Differentiation of GATA-$3^{-/-}$ T-cells is arrested at or prior to the earliest double-negative stage of thymocyte development. A later role for GATA-3 in directing cytokine gene expression in Th2 cells is indicated by experiments of Zheng and Flavell

(72). GATA-3 transcripts were noted to be selectively expressed in Th2, as compared with Th1, cells. GATA-3 activates an IL-4 promoter-reporter construct and is required for Th2 cytokine gene expression. Moreover, elevated GATA-3 in CD4 T-cells led to Th2 cytokine expression in Th1 cells. Thus, GATA-3 exerts critical effects at multiple levels within the T-cell lineage. The precise mechanisms by which GATA-3 affects transcription of its target genes is uncertain. Whether GATA-3 requires interacting cofactors, such as FOG, for in vivo function is unknown, but ripe for study.

6. Models of Lineage Commitment: Master Controls or Control by Committee?

"Commitment," as typically used in reference to hematopoiesis, implies a demonstrable, perhaps irreversible, fate decision. Models, naively fashioned after the simplest interpretation of early experiments of myogenesis induced by myoD *(73)*, posited unique roles of individual lineage-restricted regulators in commitment. Accordingly, one might anticipate the discovery of single transcription factors whose expression in multipotential progenitors (or HSCs) would lead to unilineage commitment and subsequent differentiation. Rigorous experimental tests of this simple model have not been possible, largely owing to the limited collection of HSC-like or progenitor cell lines available to serve recipients. The reprogramming of myeloid progenitors to megakaryocytic or erythroid/eosinophilic/megakaryocytic phenotypes *(55)* upon enforced GATA-1 comes the closest to this expectation. Nonetheless, under these circumstances, GATA-1 provokes differentiation along at least three different lineages in an apparently concentration-dependent manner. Besides the possible interplay of protein concentration, the nature of the recipient cell greatly influences the observed outcome. To complicate simple interpretation further, loss of GATA-1 function does not lead to a failure of lineage commitment in vivo.

Several recent observations taken together, suggest an alternative method by which lineages are selected. According to this model, lineage selection is not so much a matter of "commitment," but rather a somewhat unstable and progressive outcome of highly plastic and combinatorial regulatory interactions that are influenced by subtle effects operating at many different levels. One bit of indirect evidence supporting this view derives from consideration of the time at which lineage specificity is established during hematopoietic development. Prior to unilineage commitment and differentiation, hematopoietic progenitor cells express markers of both erythroid and myeloid lineages, including β-globin, myeloperoxidase, and lineage-affiliated cytokine receptors *(74)*, rather than only one set of lineage markers. These data support earlier observations of DNase I hypersensitivity that indicate activation of multilineage loci prior to unilineage commitment *(75)*. Selection of a particular lineage is then associated with extinction of DNase I hypersensitivity of specific loci and downregulation of gene expression. Thus, lineage specificity within the progenitor compartment may be considered a relative term. Consistent with this view, so-called lineage-restricted transcription factors, such as GATA-1, Pu.1, NF-E2, and FOG *(31,76–78)*, are expressed in multipotential progenitors prior to commitment to individual lineages.

If "promiscuity" exists with respect to lineage-restricted transcriptional regulators, how then might firm selection of a particular lineage be accomplished? Clues are beginning to emerge from recent findings which have defined protein-protein interactions that serve either to promote or inhibit transcription and progression along a particular lineage. An example of a partnership aimed at promoting lineage specific differentiation

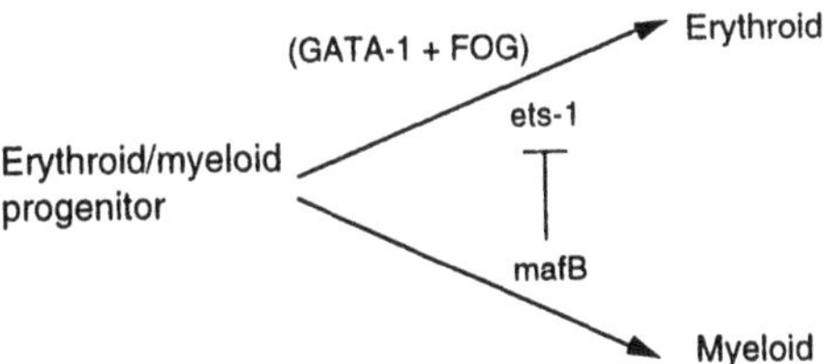

Fig. 3. Involvement of protein-protein interactions in erythroid and myeloid differentiation. GATA-1 and FOG are envisioned to act together in a positive fashion *(31)*, whereas mafB functions to repress the transcriptional activity of ets-1 in erythroid cells *(79)*.

is provided by the GATA-1/FOG interaction *(31)*. In this instance, FOG-dependence of GATA-1 function provides a combinatorial basis for erythroid and megakaryocytic development. Neither protein is sufficient to drive differentiation, but the combination exerts a potent stimulus. Protein interaction between mafB, a basic leucine-zipper polypeptide, and ets-1, a prototype of the ets-family of proteins, has been proposed to contribute to the choice between erythroid and myelomonocytic differentiation *(79)*. In this instance, expression of maf B, which is expressed specifically among myeloid cells within the hematopoietic system, blocks erythroid differentiation of chicken progenitor cells, presumably by interacting with the DNA-binding domain of ets-1 and inhibiting ets-1-mediated transactivation. Accordingly, maf B could serve complementary functions in hematopoietic development: maintenance of the myeloid phenotype and repression of erythroid development. Endowing single factors with dual actions reflects inherent cellular economy and allows for plasticity of hematopoietic lineages. The postulated positive and negative roles for the GATA-1/FOG and mafB/ets-1 interactions, respectively, are summarized in Fig. 3. The formation of larger protein complexes, such as those proposed to contain SCL/tal-1, Rbtn2, Lmo2, E47, Ldb1/NL1, GATA-1 *(30)*, may constitute a more elaborate mechanism by which specific transcriptional programs in hematopoietic cells are programmed.

If protein interactions that individually are of relatively low affinity form part of the combinatorial basis of lineage differentiation, changes in the abundance, rather than the "quality" or structure, of specific transcriptional components might exert important effects in vivo by altering the stoichiometry of critical, interacting proteins. Indeed, a ~fivefold reduction in the level of GATA-1 impairs erythroid cell maturation, but not erythroid precursor cell commitment *(80)*. The theme of modulating lineage selection or differentiation in part through subtle protein interactions can also easily accommodate positive or negative effects resulting from protein modifications. Moreover, signaling pathways downstream of cytokine receptors, which ultimately impinge on critical nuclear proteins, are readily integrated within these models.

If the proposal is to be accepted that fine-tuned combinatorial influences of protein concentration and protein-protein interactions participate in "commitment" of progenitors to specific pathways, how might unilineage differentiation become stabilized? Gene expression surveys suggest that following a phase of lineage "promiscuity" *(74)* appropriate lineage-specific transcription is evident *(81)*. "Fixation" of a lineage is also presumably associated with the shut-off or down-regulation of those products that promote development along other pathways. Crosstalk within a regulatory network is likely to be influenced by both positive and negative transcriptional effects exerted by some of the lineage-restricted transcription factors. As an example, the GATA-1-dependent re-

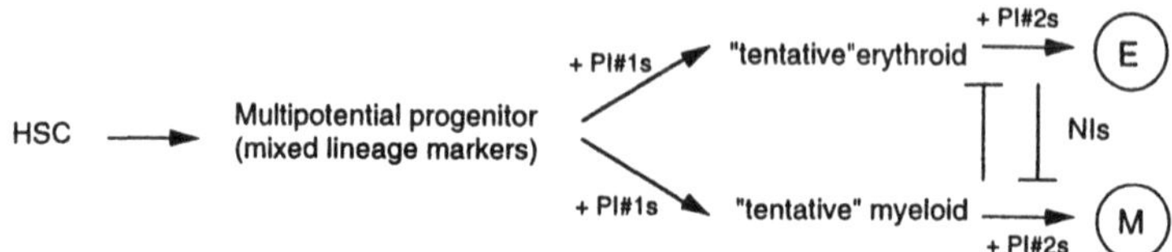

Fig. 4. Working model of lineage selection.

pression of GATA-2 expression observed during erythroid differentiation *(39)* may constitute part of the irreversible transition from a multipotential, proliferative progenitor to a single lineage, maturing erythroid precursor. The possibility that GATA-1 may inhibit expression of myeloid or lymphoid-restricted factors is worth exploring, as is the potential repression of GATA-1 expression by other lineage-restricted transcription factors.

A scheme for conceptualizing hematopoietic lineage commitment at the molecular level is summarized in Fig. 4. It is envisioned that multipotential progenitors express markers of diverse lineages. Positive influences (PI#1s) tend to initiate cells along one path or another in an unstable fashion. Such Pis might include the induction or repression of one or multiple proteins, a change in protein abundances or modifications, or effects of protein-protein interactions. Cells poised to proceed along a pathway are "tentatively" committed but require further positive influences (PI#2s), as well as negative influences (Nis) to stabilize a decision and drive single lineage differentiation. Again, Nis could influence transcriptional effects of large or small magnitude, protein modifications, or consequences of protein interactions.

The views espoused here, which extrapolate recent findings to the critical early decisions of HSCs or immature progenitors, are easily reconciled with contemporary models of combinatorial control of development in other tissues. The practical implications for further research in the field, however, are considerable if these concepts are further substantiated. First, the long-sought goal of identifying individual gene products that commit hematopoietic progenitors to single lineage fates may be elusive. The possibility remains open that such molecules will be demonstrated to exist, but current evidence does not give us confidence. Second, if these concepts are correct, the problem of lineage commitment, one of the cornerstones of hematopoiesis, will turn on defining intricate protein-protein interactions, transcriptional regulatory interactions, and quantitative features of expression, rather than the mere presence or absence of single components. Experimental validation of models will necessitate the development of sophisticated cellular systems suitable for investigating the postulated biochemical and genetic switches discussed here.

References

1. Orkin, S. H. (1996) Development of the hematopoietic system. *Curr. Opin. Genet. Devel.* **6,** 597–602.
2. Pardanaud, L., Yassine, F., and Dieterlen-Lievre, F. (1989) Relationship between vasculogenesis, angiogenesis, and haemopoiesis during avian ontogeny. *Development* **105,** 473–485.
3. Godin, I., Dieterlen-Lievre, F., and Cumano, A. (1995) Emergence of multipotent hemopoietic cells in the yolk sac and paraaortic splanchnopleura in mouse embryos, beginning at 8.5 days postcoitus. *Proc. Natl. Acad. Sci. USA* **92,** 773–777.
4. Godin, I. E., Garcia-Porrero, J. A., Coutinho, A., Dieterlen-Lievre, F., and Marcos, M. A. R. (1993) Para-aortic splanchnopleura from early mouse embryos contains B1a cell progenitors. *Nature* **364,** 67–70.

5. Medvinsky, A. and Dzierzak, E. (1996) Definitive hematopoiesis is autonomously initiated by the AGM region. *Cell* **86,** 897–906.
6. Medvinsky, A. L., Samoylina, N. L., Muller, A. M., and Dzierzak, E. A. (1993) An early pre-liver intraembryonic source of CFU-S in the developing mouse. *Nature* **364,** 64–66.
7. Begley, C. G., Aplan, P. D., Denning, S. M., Haynes, B. F., Waldmann, T. A., and Kirsch, I. R. (1989) The gene SCL is expressed during early hematopoiesis and encodes a differentiation-related DNA-binding motif. *Proc. Natl. Acad. Sci. USA* **86,** 10,128–10,132.
8. Chen, Q., Cheng, J.-T., Tsai, L.-H., Schneider, N., Buchanan, G., Carroll, A., Crist, W., Ozanne, B., Siciliano, M. J., and Baer, R. (1990) The tal gene undergoes chromosome translocation in T cell leukemia and potentially encodes a helix-loop-helix protein. *EMBO J.* **9,** 415–424.
9. Aplan, P. D., Lombardi, D. P., and Kirsch, I. R. (1991) Structural characterization of SIL, a gene frequently disrupted in T-cell acute lymphoblastic leukemia. *Mol. Cell. Biol.* **11,** 5462–5469.
10. Aplan, P. D., Begley, C. G., Bertness, V., Nussmeier, M., Ezquerra, A., Coligan, J., and Kirsch, I. R. (1990) The SCL gene is formed from a transcriptionally complex locus. *Mol. Cell. Biol.* **10,** 6426–6435.
11. Begley, C. G., Visvader, J., Green, A. R., Aplan, P. D., Metcalf, D., Kirsch, I. R., and Gough, N. (1991) Molecular cloning and chromosomal location of the mouse homolog of the human helix-loop-helix gene SCL. *Proc. Natl. Acad. Sci. USA* **88,** 869–873.
12. Green, A. R., Lints, T., Visvader, J., Harvey, R., and Begley, C. G. (1992) SCL is coexpressed with GATA-1 in hemopoietic cells but is also expressed in developing brain. *Oncogene* **6,** 475–479.
13. Kallianpur, A. R., Jordan, J. E., and Brandt, S. J. (1994) The SCL/TAL-1 gene is expressed in progenitors of both the hematopoietic and vascular systems during embryogenesis. *Blood* **83,** 1200–1208.
14. Mouthon, M.-A., Bernard, O., Mitjavila, M.-T., Romeo, P.-H., Vainchenker, W., and Mathieu-Mahul, D. (1993) Expression of tal-1 and GATA-binding proteins during human hematopoiesis. *Blood* **81,** 647–655.
15. Visvader, J., Begley, C. G., and Adams, J. M. (1991) Differential expression of the Lyl, SCL, and E2a helix-loop-helix genes within the hemopoietic system. *Oncogene* **6,** 187–194.
16. Condorelli, G. L., Facchiano, F., Valtieri, M., Proietti, E., Vitelli, L., Lulli, V., Huebner, K., Peschle, C., and Croce, C. M. (1996) T-cell-directed TAL-1 expression induces T-cell malignancies in transgenic mice. *Cancer Res.* **56,** 5113–5119.
17. Kelliner, M. A., Seldin, D. C., and Leder, P. (1996) Tal-1 induces T cell acute lymphoblastic leukemia accelerated by casein kinase IIa. *EMBO J.* **115,** 5160–5166.
18. Aplan, P. D., Jones, C. A., Chervinsky, D. S., Zhao, X. F., Ellsworth, M., Wu, C., McGuire, E. A., and Gross, K. W. (1997) An *scl* gene product lacking the transactivation domain induces bony abnormalities and cooperates with LMO1 to generate T-cell malignancies in transgenic mice. *EMBO J.* **16,** 2408–2419.
19. Porcher, C., Swat, W., Rockwell, K., Fujiwara, Y., Alt, F. W., and Orkin, S. H. (1996) The T-cell leukemia oncoprotein SCL/tal-1 is essential for development of all hematopoietic lineages. *Cell* **86,** 47–47.
20. Robb, L., Elwood, N. J., Elefanty, A. G., Kontgen, F., Li, R., Barnett, L. D., and Begley, C. G. (1996) The scl gene product is required for the generation of all hematopoietic lineages in the adult mouse. *EMBO J.* **15,** 4123–4129.
21. Robb, L., Lyons, I., Li, R., Hartley, L., Kontgen, F., Harvey, R. P., Metcalf, D., and Begley, C. G. (1995) Absence of yolk sac hematopoiesis from mice with a targeted disruption of the scl gene. *Proc. Natl. Acad. Sci. USA* **92,** 7075–7079.
22. Shivdasani, R., Mayer, E., and Orkin, S. H. (1995) Absence of blood formation in mice lacking the T-cell leukemia oncoprotein tal-1/SCL. *Nature* **373,** 432–434.
23. Chen, J., Lansford, R., Stewart, V., Young, F., and Alt, F. W. (1993) RAG-2-deficient blastocyst complementation: an assay of gene function in lymphocyte development. *Proc. Natl. Acad. Sci. USA* **90,** 4528–4532.
24. Osada, H., Grutz, G., Axelson, H., Forster, A., and Rabbitts, T. H. (1995) Association of erythroid transcription factors: complexes involving the LIM protein RBTN2 and the zinc-finger protein GATA1. *Proc. Natl. Acad. Sci. USA* **92,** 9585–9589.
25. Valge-Archer, V. E., Osada, H., Warren, A. J., Forster, A., Li, J., Baer, R., and Rabbitts, T. H. (1994) The LIM protein RBTN2 and the basic helix-loop-helix protein TAL1 are present in a complex in erythroid cells. *Proc. Natl. Acad. Sci. USA* **91,** 8617–8621.

26. Warren, A. J., Colledge, W. H., Carlton, M. B. L., Evans, M. J., Smith, A. J. H., and Rabbitts, T. H. (1994) The oncogenic cysteine-rich LIM domain protein Rbtn2 is essential for erythroid development. *Cell* **78,** 45–57.
27. Kennedy, M., Firpo, M., Choi, K., Wall, C., Robertson, S., Kabrun, N., and Keller, G. (1997) A common precursor for primitive erythropoiesis and definitive hematopoiesis. *Nature* **386,** 488–493.
28. Agulnick, A. D., Taira, M., Breen, J. J., Tanaka, T., Dawid, I. B., and Westphal, H. (1996) Functional and physical interaction of Ldb1, a novel LIM domain binding factor, with the LIM homeodomain protein Lhx1/Xlim-1. *Nature* **384,** 270–272.
29. Jurata, L. W., Kenny, D. A., and Gill, G. N. (1996) Nuclear LIM interactor, a rhombotin and LIM homeodomain interaction protein, is expressed in neuronal development. *Proc. Natl. Acad. Sci. USA* **93,** 11,693–11,698.
30. Wadman, I. S., Osada, H., Grutz, G. G., Agulnick, A. D., Westphal, H., Forster, A., and Rabbitts, T. H. (1997) The LIM-only protein Lmo2 is a bridging molecule assembling an erythroid, DNA-binding complex which include TAL1, E47, GATA-1, and Ldb1/NL1 proteins. *EMBO J.* **16,** 3145–3157.
31. Tsang, A. P., Visvader, J. E., Turner, C. A., Fujiwara, Y., Yu, C., Weiss, M. J., Crossley, M., and Orkin, S. H. (1997) FOG, a multitype zinc finger protein, acts as a cofactor for transcription factor GATA-1 in erythroid and megakaryocytic differentiation. *Cell* **90,** 109–119.
32. Okuda, T., Deursen, J. v., Hiebert, S. W., Grosveld, G., and Downing, J. R. (1996) AML1, the target of multiple chromosomal translocations in human leukemia, is essential for normal fetal liver hematopoiesis. *Cell* **84,** 321–330.
33. Sasaki, K., Yagi, H., Bronson, R. T., Tominaga, K., Matsunashi, T., Deguchi, K., Tani, Y., Kishimoto, T., and Komori, T. (1996) Absence of fetal liver hematopoiesis in mice deficient in transcriptional coactivator core binding factor b. *Proc. Natl. Acad. Sci. USA* **93,** 12,359–12,363.
34. Wang, Q., Stacy, T., Binder, M., Marin-Padilla, M., Sharpe, A. H., and Speck, N. A. (1996) Disruption of the *Cbfa2* gene causes necrosis and hemorrhaging in the central nervous system and blocks definitive hematopoiesis. *Proc. Natl. Acad. Sci. USA* **93,** 3444–3449.
35. Wang, Q., Stacy, T., Miller, J. D., Lewis, A. F., Gu, T.-L., Huang, X., Bushweller, J. H., Bories, J.-C., Alt, F. W., Ryan, G., Liu, P. P., Wynshaw-Boris, A., Binder, M., Marin-Padilla, M., Sharpe, A. H., and Speck, N. A. (1996) The CBFb subunit is essential for CBFa2(AML1) function in vivo. *Cell* **87,** 697–708.
36. Briegel, K., Lim, K.-C., Plank, C., Beug, H., Engel, J., and Zenke, M. (1993) Ectopic expression of a conditional GATA-2/estrogen receptor chimera arrests erythroid differentiation in a hormone-dependent manner. *Genes Dev.* **7,** 1097–1109.
37. Tsai, F.-Y., Keller, G., Kuo, F. C., Weiss, M. J., Chen, J.-Z., Rosenblatt, M., Alt, F., and Orkin, S. H. (1994) An early haematopoietic defect in mice lacking the transcription factor GATA-2. *Nature* **371,** 221–226.
38. Yamamoto, M., Ko, L. J., Leonard, M. W., Beug, H., Orkin, S. H., and Engel, J. D. (1990) Activity and tissue-specific expression of the transcription factor NF-E1 multigene family. *Genes Dev.* **4,** 1650–1662.
39. Weiss, M. J., Keller, G., and Orkin, S. H. (1994) Novel insights into erythroid development revealed through *in vitro* differentiation of GATA-1-embryonic stem cells. *Genes Dev.* **8,** 1184–1197.
40. Silver, L. and Palis, J. (1997) Initiation of murine embryonic erythropoiesis: a spatial analysis. *Blood* **89,** 1154–1164.
41. Tsai, F.-Y. and Orkin, S. H. (1997) Transcription factor GATA-2 is required for proliferation/survival of early hematopoietic cells and mast cell formation, but not for erythroid and myeloid terminal differentiation. *Blood* **89,** 3636–3643.
42. Krumlauf, R. (1994) *Hox* genes in vertebrate development. *Cell* **78,** 191–201.
43. Sauvageau, G., Thorsteinsdottir, U., Eaves, C. J., Lawrence, H. J., Largman, C., Landsorp, P. M., and Humphries, R. K. (1995) Overexpression of HOXB4 in hematopoietic cells causes the selective expansion of more primitive populations in vitro and in vivo. *Genes Dev.* **9,** 1753–1765.
44. Perkins, A. C. and Cory, S. (1993) Conditional immortalization of mouse myelomonocytic, megakaryocytic and mast cell progenitors by the Hox-2.4 homeobox gene. *EMBO J.* **12,** 3835–3846.
45. Borrow, J., Shearman, A. M., Stanton, J. V. P., Becher, R., Collins, T., Williams, A. J., Dube, I., Katz, F., Kwong, Y. L., Morris, C., Ohyashiki, K., Toyama, K., Rowley, J., and Housman,

D. E. (1996) The t translocation in acute myeloid leukemia fuses the genes for nucleoporin NUP98 and class I homeoprotein HOXA9. *Nat. Genet.* **12,** 159–167.
46. Nakamura, T., Largaespada, D. A., Lee, M. P., Johnson, L. A., Ohyashiki, K., Toyama, K., Chen, S. J., Willman, C. L., Chen, I.-M., Feinberg, A. P., Jenkins, N. A., Copeland, N. G., and Shaughnessy, J. D. J. (1996) Fusion of the nucleoporin gene NUP98 to HOXA9 by the chromosome translocation t(7;11)(p15;p15) in human myeloid leukemia. *Nat. Genet.* **12,** 154–158.
47. Yu, B. D., Hess, J. L., Horning, S. E., Brown, G. A. J., and Korsmeyer, S. J. (1995) Altered Hox expression and segmental identity in Mll-mutant mice. *Nature* **378,** 505–508.
48. Mead, P. E., Brinvanlou, I. H., Kelley, C. M., and Zon, L. I. (1996) BMP-4 responsive regulation of dorsoventral patterning by the homeobox protein Mix.1. *Nature* **382,** 357–360.
49. Johnasson, B. M. and Wiles, M. V. (1995) Evidence for involvement of activin A and bone mrophogenetic protein 4 in mammalian mesoderm and hematopoietic development. *Mol. Cell. Biol.* **15,** 141–151.
50. Evans, T. and Felsenfeld, G. (1989) The erythroid-specific transcription factor eryf1: a new finger protein. *Cell* **58,** 877–885.
51. Tsai, S. F., Martin, D. I., Zon, L. I., D'Andrea, A. D., Wong, G. G., and Orkin, S. H. (1989) Cloning of cDNA for the major DNA-binding protein of the erythroid lineage through expression in mammalian cells. *Nature* **339,** 446–451.
52. Yomogida, K., Ohtani, H., Harigae, H., Ito, E., Nishimune, Y., Engel, J. D., and Yamamoto, M. (1994) Developmental stage- and spermatogenic cycle-specific expression of transcription factor GATA-1 in mouse Sertoli cells. *Development* **120,** 1759–1766.
53. Martin, D. I. K., Zon, L. I., Mutter, G., and Orkin, S. H. (1990) Expression of an erythroid transcription factor in megakaryocytic and mast cell lineages. *Nature* **344,** 444–446.
54. Zon, L. I., Yamaguchi, Y., Yee, K., Albee, E. A., Kimura, A., Bennett, J. C., Orkin, S. H., and Ackerman, S. J. (1993) Espression of mRNA for the GATA-binding proteins in human eosinophils and basophils: potential role in gene transcription. *Blood* **81,** 3234–3241.
55. Kulessa, H., Frampton, J., and Graf, T. (1995) GATA-1 reprograms avian myelomonocytic cells into eosinophils, thromboblasts and erythroblasts. *Genes Dev.* **9,** 1250–1262.
56. Visvader, J. and Adams, J. M. (1993) Megakaryocytic differentiation induced in 416B myeloid cells by GATA-2 and GATA-3 transgenes or 5-azacytidine is tightly coupled to GATA-1 expression. *Blood* **82,** 1493–1501.
57. Visvader, J. E., Elefanty, A. G., Strasser, A., and Adams, J. M. (1992) GATA-1 but not SCL induces megakaryocytic differentiation in an early myeloid line. *EMBO J.* **11,** 4557–4564.
58. Fujiwara, Y., Browne, C. P., Cunniff, K., Goff, S. C., and Orkin, S. H. (1996) Arrested development of embryonic red cell precursors in mouse embryos lacking transcription factor GATA-1. *Proc. Natl. Acad. Sci. USA* **93,** 12,355–12,358.
59. Pevny, L., Simon, M. C., Robertson, E., Klein, W. H., Tsai, S.-F., D'Agati, V., Orkin, S. H., and Costantini, F. (1991) Erythroid differentiation in chimeric mice blocked by a targeted mutation in the gene for transcription factor GATA-1. *Nature* **349,** 257–260.
60. Weiss, M. J. and Orkin, S. H. (1995) Transcription factor GATA-1 permits survival and maturation of erythroid precursors by preventing apoptosis. *Proc. Natl. Acad. Sci. USA* **92,** 9623–9627.
61. Shivadasani, R. A., Fujiwara, Y., McDevitt, M. A., and Orkin, S. H. (1997) A lineage-selective knockout establishes the critical role of transcription factor GATA-1 in megakaryocyte growth and platelet development. *EMBO J.* **16,** 3965–3973.
62. Leonard, M., Brice, M., Engel, J. D., and Papayannopoulou, T. (1993) Dynamics of GATA transcription factor expression during erythroid differentiation. *Blood* **82,** 1071–1079.
63. Evans, T. and Felsenfeld, G. (1991) Trans-activation of a globin promoter in non-erythroid cells. *Mol. Cell. Biol.* **11,** 843–853.
64. Martin, D. I. K. and Orkin, S. H. (1990) Transcriptional activation and DNA-binding by the erythroid factor GF-1/NF-E1/Eryf 1. *Genes Dev.* **4,** 1886–1898.
65. Weiss, M. J., Yu, C., and Orkin, S. H. (1997) Erythroid-cell-specific properties of transcription factor GATA-1 revealed by phenotypic rescue of a gene-targeted cell line. *Mol. Cell. Biol.* **17,** 1642–1651.
66. Orkin, S. H. and Zon, L. I. (1997) Genetics of erythropoiesis: induced mutations in mice and zebrafish. *Ann. Rev. Genet.* **31,** 33–60.
67. Ho, I.-C., Vorhees, P., Marin, N., Oakley, B. K., Tsai, S.-F., Orkin, S. H., and Leiden, J. M. (1991) Human GATA-3: a lineage-restricted transcription factor that regulates the expression of the T cell receptor a gene. *EMBO* **10,** 1187–1192.

68. Ko, L. J., Yamamoto, M., Leonard, M. W., George, K. M., Ting, P., and Engel, J. D. (1991) Murine and human T-lymphocyte GATA-3 factors mediate transcription through a cis-regulatory element within the human T-cell receptor d gene enhancer. *Mol. Cell. Biol.* **11,** 2778–2784.
69. Oosterwegel, M., Timmerman, J., Leiden, J., and Clevers, H. (1992) Expression of GATA-3 during lymphocyte differentiation and mouse embryogenesis. *Dev. Immunol.* **3,** 1–11.
70. Pandolfi, P. P., Roth, M. E., Karis, A., Leonard, M. W., Dzierzak, E., Grosveld, F. G., Engel, J. D., and Lindenbaum, M. H. (1995) Targeted disruption of the GATA3 gene causes severe abnormalities in the nervous system and in fetal liver haematopoiesis. *Nat. Genet.* **11,** 40–44.
71. Ting, C.-N., Olson, M. C., Barton, K. P., and Leiden, J. M. (1996) Transcription factor GATA-3 is required for development of the T-cell lineage. *Nature* **384,** 474–478.
72. Zheng, W. and Flavell, R. A. (1997) The transcription factor GATA-3 is necessary and sufficient for Th2 cytokine gene expression in CD4 T cells. *Cell* **89,** 587–596.
73. Weintraub, H., Davis, R., Tapscott, S., Thayer, M., Krause, M., Benezra, R., Blackwell, T. K., Turner, D., Rupp, R., Hollenberg, S., Zhuang, Y., and Lassar, A. (1991) The myoD gene family: nodal point during specification of the muscle cell lineage. *Science* **251,** 761–766.
74. Hu, M., Kruase, D., Greaves, M., Sharkis, S., Dexter, M., Heyworth, C., and Enver, T. (1997) Multilineage gene expression precedes commitment in the hemopoietic system. *Genes Dev.* **11,** 774–785.
75. Jimenez, G., Griffiths, S. D., Ford, A. M., Greaves, M. F., and Enver, T. (1992) Activation of the β-globin locus control region precedes commitment to the erythroid lineage. *Proc. Natl. Acad. Sci. USA* **89,** 10,618–10,622.
76. Andrews, N. C., Erjument-Bromage, H., Davidson, M. B., Tempst, P., and Orkin, S. H. (1993) Erythroid transcription factor (NF-E2) is a haematopoietic-specific basic-leucine zipper protein. *Nature* **362,** 722–728.
77. Scott, E. W., Simon, M. C., Anastasi, J., and Singh, H. (1994) Requirement of transcription factor PU.1 in the development of multiple hematopoietic lineages. *Science* **265,** 1573–1577.
78. Sposi, N. M., Zon, L. I., Care, A., Valtieri, M., Testa, U., Gabbianelli, M., Mariani, G., Bottero, L., Mather, C., Orkin, S. H., and Peschle, C. (1992) Cycle-dependent initiation and lineage-dependent abrogation of GATA-1 expression in pure differentiating hematopoietic progenitors. *Proc. Natl. Acad. Sci. USA* **89,** 6353–6357.
79. Sieweke, M. H., Tekotte, H., Frampton, J., and Graf, T. (1996) MafB is an interaction partner and repressor of Ets-1 that inhibits erythroid differentiation. *Cell* **84,** 49–60.
80. McDevitt, M. A., Shivdasani, R. A., Fujiwara, Y., Yang, H., and Orkin, S. H. (1997) A "knock-down" mutation created by *cis*-element gene targeting reveals the dependence of red blood cell maturation on the level of transcrption factor GATA-1. *Proc. Natl. Acad. Sci. USA* **94,** 6781–6785.
81. Brady, G., Billia, F., Knox, J., Hoang, T., Kirsch, I. R., Voura, E. B., Hawley, R. B., Cumming, R., Buchwald, M., Siminovitch, K., Miyamoto, N., Boehmelt, G., and Iscove, N. N. (1995) Analysis of gene expression in a complex differentiation hierarchy by global amplification of cDNA from single cells. *Curr. Biol.* **5,** 909–922.

Part II

Intrinsic Factors Regulating B and T Lymphopoiesis

Chapter 4

The Ikaros Gene Family in Hemopoietic Differentiation

Nicole Avitahl, Aliki Nichogiannopoulou, Katia Georgopoulos, and Susan Winandy

1. Introduction

The molecular events that enable the progeny of a hemopoietic stem cell (HSC) to become committed to the erythroid, myeloid, or lymphoid lineages are still to be defined. Differentiated hemopoietic lineages originate from common multipotent progenitor cells that undergo a series of divisions and commitment steps, giving rise to precursor cells with increasingly restricted differentiation potentials. The functional and phenotypic changes that occur as a cell differentiates are determined by changes in gene expression. These changes are directed by cell signaling events, which induce a cascade of regulatory factors that ultimately affect the transcriptional program of the cell. Therefore, an important key to understanding hemopoiesis is identifying the transcription factors that regulate the transition through stages of differentiation. The *Ikaros* family of transcription factors has been shown to play an integral role in the determination and differentiation of the lymphoid lineage. This chapter will discuss the founder of this family of transcription factors, *Ikaros*, as well as its more lymphoid-restricted homolog, *Aiolos*, and what is known to date about the roles of these proteins in hemopoiesis and lymphocyte differentiation.

2. The Role of Zinc-Finger Domains in Ikaros Activity

The *Ikaros* gene encodes, by means of alternative splicing, a family of zinc-finger proteins that are expressed in the developing hemopoietic systems of mice and humans *(1–3)*. To date, six Ikaros isoforms have been identified, which are expressed from the hemopoietic stem cell to mature lymphocytes (Ik-1 through Ik-6). These proteins belong to the family of Krüppel-like zinc-finger DNA-binding proteins, yet they display some

From: *Molecular Biology of B-Cell and T-Cell Development*
Edited by: J. G. Monroe and E. V. Rothenberg © Humana Press Inc., Totowa, NJ

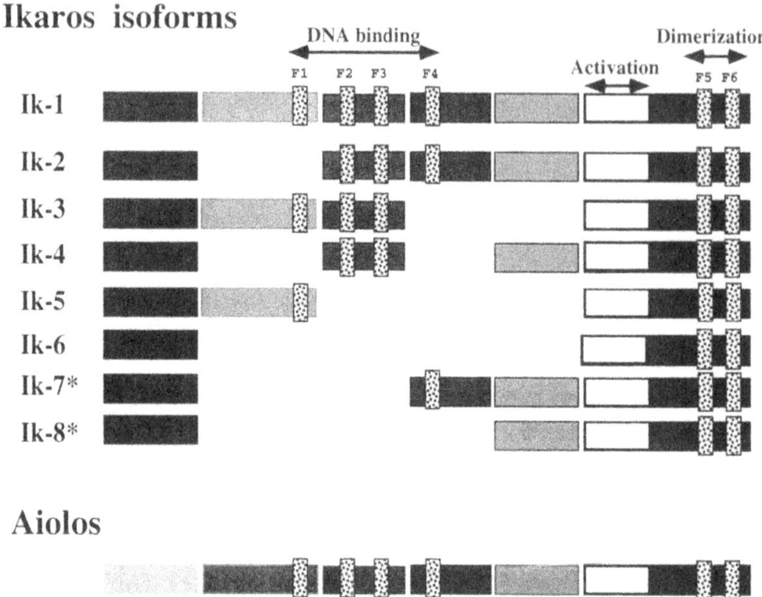

Fig. 1. Schematic representation of Ikaros isoforms and Aiolos protein. Zinc-finger domains involved in DNA binding and dimerization are indicated by horizontal arrows. The location of a conserved activation domain between Ikaros and Aiolos proteins is shown as a white rectangle. Stars by Ikaros isoforms indicate their exclusive production from the mutant dominant negative (DN) locus.

unique features. The Krüppel-like zinc-finger modules present in these proteins are spatially arranged in two domains that are functionally distinct (Fig. 1). All of the Ikaros proteins share a common C-terminus with two zinc fingers, which constitutes a dimerization domain, whereas their N-terminal domains can contain from one to four finger motifs, which are essential for mediating DNA binding. High-affinity DNA-binding activity on a single binding site requires a minimum of three N-terminal zinc finger domains *(2)*. Therefore, only three of the Ikaros proteins, Ik-1, Ik-2 and Ik-3, meet this requirement, and one of the Ikaros proteins, Ik-4, with two N-terminal zinc fingers, can only bind to tandem recognition sites. Although these isoforms share a common core consensus (GGGA) in their selected DNA-binding sites, each isoform displays a preference for different flanking nucleotide sequences as well as differing binding affinities. Ikaros proteins with less than two N-terminal zinc fingers (Ik-5 and Ik-6) cannot bind DNA *(2)*. These isoforms do not activate transcription from consensus Ikaros binding sites when ectopically expressed in fibroblasts, whereas the DNA-binding isoforms that are able to enter the nucleus (Ik-1 and Ik-2) do *(2)*.

The C-terminal zinc-finger domain, shared by all isoforms, mediates homo- and heterodimeric protein interactions that are pivotal for the activity of Ikaros proteins as transcription factors *(4)*. When dimerization of transcriptionally competent Ikaros isoforms is prevented by mutation of one or both of the C-terminal zinc fingers, DNA binding affinity and transcriptional activity of these proteins is severely compromised *(4)*. Therefore, formation of dimers between isoforms with an N-terminal domain capable of binding DNA (Ik-1, Ik-2 and Ik-3) dramatically increases their affinities for DNA and activities in transcription *(4)*. Furthermore, heterodimers formed between isoforms with a DNA-binding domain (Ik-1, Ik-2, and Ik-3) and those which lack a DNA-binding domain (Ik-5 and Ik-6) cannot bind DNA or function as transcriptional activators *(4)*. Ikaros proteins without a DNA-binding domain can play a dominant-negative role in transcription by interfering with the activity of isoforms that can bind DNA. This observation suggests the possibility of a regulatory role for these isoforms in attenuation of Ikaros activity in hemopoietic cells and their progenitors.

The N- and C-terminal zinc-finger domains of the Ikaros proteins may also be essential for directing their correct subcellular localization. In lymphocytes, Ikaros proteins are nuclear with no detectable cytoplasmic localization *(4)*. Visualization of Ikaros proteins within the cell by immunohistochemistry reveals an intense punctate staining within the nucleus *(4)*. This staining pattern suggests that Ikaros proteins participate in the formation of large protein or protein–DNA complexes. However, when Ikaros proteins with less than three N-terminal zinc fingers (Ik-5 and Ik-6) are expressed ectopically in the absence of proteins with three or more N-terminal zinc fingers (Ik-1, Ik-2, Ik-3 and Ik-4), the former are retained in the cytoplasm *(2)*. In contrast, Ikaros proteins with a deletion of the C-terminal zinc-finger domain enter the nucleus, indicating that dimerization itself is not necessary for nuclear localization.

3. The Transcriptional Activation Domain of Ikaros

Studies in which the Ikaros isoforms Ik-1, Ik-2, and Ik-3 were ectopically expressed in fibroblasts have established the role of Ikaros proteins as potential transcriptional activators *(2)*. The transcriptional activation domain of Ikaros lies upstream of the C-terminal zinc fingers within exon 7 (Fig. 1). This activation domain is bipartite, consisting of an acidic and a hydrophobic stretch of amino acids that are functionally distinct. The stretch of acidic amino acids can independently activate transcription when tethered to a heterologous DNA binding domain, whereas the hydrophobic residues cannot *(4)*. However, the presence of the hydrophobic residues greatly enhances the level of transcriptional activity provided by the acidic amino acids. The role of the hydrophobic region may be to stabilize interactions that take place between the acidic region and the basal transcription machinery. Alternatively, the hydrophobic region may control accessibility of the acidic region by influencing local secondary and/or tertiary protein structure. Interestingly, when the full-length Ikaros protein is tethered to a heterologous DNA-binding domain, it is a weaker transcriptional activator than the bipartite activation domain alone *(4)*. A change in Ikaros protein conformation brought about after binding to its cognate recognition sequences, which does not occur when Ikaros binds via the heterologous DNA-binding domain, may be essential for an optimal interaction between its activation domain and the basal transcription machinery. The accessibility of the Ikaros activation domain may also be regulated by protein interactions that take place through the C-terminal zinc fingers and through additional interaction domains on the Ikaros proteins (J. Koipally and K. Georgopoulos, unpublished results). Such intra- and intermolecular protein interactions may provide a pivotal mechanism for modulating the role of the Ikaros proteins in transcription during lymphocyte maturation.

4. Expression of the *Ikaros* Gene

Ikaros was first identified as a protein capable of binding to the enhancer of the CD3-δ and to the promoter of the terminal deoxynucleotide transferase (TdT) gene, both of which are expressed at early stages of T-cell differentiation *(1,5)*. However, *Ikaros*

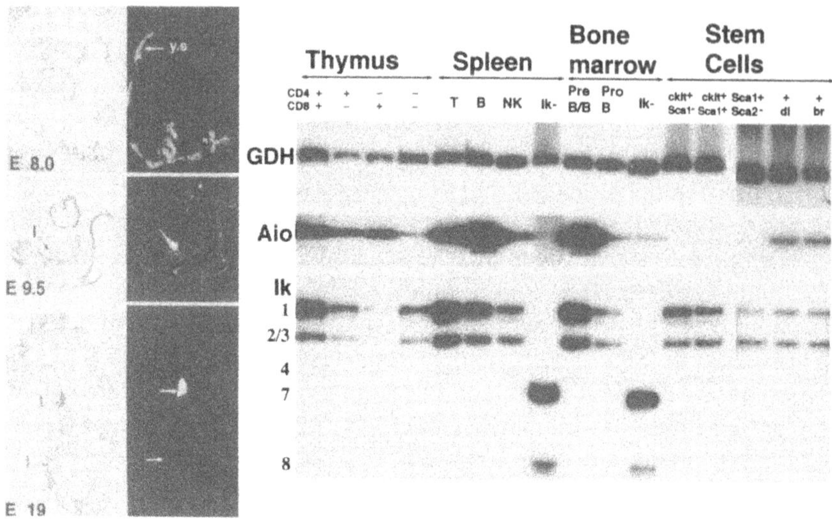

Fig. 2. Expression of *Ikaros* and *Aiolos* during fetal and adult lymphopoiesis. *Left—In situ* hybridization studies showing *Ikaros* expression in fetal lymphopoietic sites. *Ikaros* antisense riboprobe was hybridized to E8–E19 embryonic sections. Arrows point to hybridizing tissues. y.s. = yolk sac, l = liver, t = thymus. *Right*—RT-PCR experiments showing expression of *Ikaros* and *Aiolos* in adult hemopoietic cells. cDNAs were prepared from sorted populations isolated from the thymus, spleen and bone marrow of wild-type and $DN^{-/-}$ mutant (indicated by Ik-) mice. Populations enriched for hemopoietic stem cells were sorted based on the cell surface markers c-kit, Sca-1 and Sca-2. dl = dull, br = bright. *Ikaros* cDNA was amplified using primers derived from exons 2 and 7, which generate multiple bands corresponding to the alternatively spliced products of the *Ikaros* pre-mRNA transcript (*see* Fig. 1). The isoforms represented by each band are indicated at the side. Bands corresponding to isoforms 7 and 8 are generated from the mutant *Ikaros* locus, as described in Fig. 1. *Aiolos* cDNA was amplified using primers derived from exons 3 and 7 which generate a single band corresponding to the cDNA shown in Fig. 1. The glyceraldehyde 3-phosphate dehydrogenase gene was used as a reference. GDH = glyceraldehyde 3-phosphate dehydrogenase, Ik = Ikaros, Aio = Aiolos.

expression is not restricted to the T lineage; rather, it is expressed at varying levels in nearly all hemopoietic cells. The only exception to the hemopoietic-specific expression of *Ikaros* is during embryogenesis, when it is also expressed in the corpus striatum of the developing brain. *In situ* hybridization studies show that *Ikaros* is first expressed at embryonic day 7.5–8 (E7.5–E8) in distinct cells of the splanchnopleura region (T. Ikeda and K. Georgopoulos, unpublished results) and at E8 in the yolk sac. Subsequently, it is expressed at E9.5 in the fetal liver primordium, as it becomes the major site of hemopoiesis in the embryo proper *(1)*. *Ikaros* is first detected in the fetal thymus at E12. By E16 it is detected at high levels in the thymus and at lower levels in the fetal liver, correlating with the first wave of expansion of T-cell precursors in the thymus and with a shift from primitive to more committed erythroid and myeloid precursors in the fetal liver. Analyses of sorted populations from fetal liver and adult bone marrow show that *Ikaros* is expressed in the population of cells that are positive for the cell surface markers c-kit and Sca-1 *(6)*, (Fig. 2), a population highly enriched for HSCs *(7,8)*. This suggests that *Ikaros* may play a role in the earliest stages of hemopoiesis. Indeed, this is borne out by the phenotype of mice that are homozygous for a dominant-negative mutation in *Ikaros*. These mice, which will be described in detail in another section, are severely immunodeficient and manifest problems in all branches of hemopoietic cell development.

Ikaros is expressed at all stages of lymphoid development, from the HSC through to mature B- and T-cells (Fig. 2). Within the T-cell lineage, it is expressed in all γδ T-cells, albeit at lower levels than in αβ T-cells, as well as in natural killer (NK) and thymic dendritic antigen presenting cells (APCs). *Ikaros* expression is higher in maturing and terminally differentiated B- and T-cells than in their progenitors and in HSCs. The fact that *Ikaros* is expressed at all stages of lymphoid development suggests that it not only has a role in early lymphopoiesis, but also at later stages of this process.

As mentioned in the previous section, the *Ikaros* gene encodes for a family of proteins by means of alternate splicing of the mRNA. Since non-DNA-binding isoforms of Ikaros (Ik-5 and Ik-6) can interfere with the activities of DNA-binding isoforms (Ik-1, Ik-2 and Ik-3), one mechanism by which Ikaros activity could be regulated is through modulation of relative expression levels of the different isoforms. However, the results of reverse transcription-polymerase chain reaction (RT-PCR) experiments show that at the RNA level, the relative levels of the different isoforms remain comparable from the HSC stage throughout hemopoiesis and lymphoid development. Ikaros isoforms 1 and 2 are expressed at much higher levels than isoforms 3, 4, and 5 *(2)*. Therefore, the expression of the various Ikaros isoforms does not appear to be regulated during hemopoiesis.

5. *Ikaros* Function In Vivo

5.1. A C-Terminal Deletion Results in an Ikaros-Null Mutation

Two mutant mouse strains have been generated in which different functional domains of the Ikaros protein were targeted. These mutations give rise to mice with distinct hemopoietic defects. To determine the direct effect of loss of Ikaros activity in the development of the hemopoietic system, a mutation was targeted that resulted in deletion of most of the coding region of exon 7 including its 5' splice donor site *(9)*. The deleted domain, shared by all of the Ikaros proteins (Fig. 1), contains the C-terminal dimerization zinc fingers that are required for protein–protein interactions, the bipartite transcriptional activation domain, and a further domain with a potential regulatory role *(4)* (J. Koipally and K. Georgopoulos, unpublished results). The mutant *Ikaros* locus produces unstable proteins so that mice homozygous for this mutation are functionally null for Ikaros activity.

Ikaros-null mice have selective defects in hemopoiesis *(9)*. They display an early and complete block in B-cell development during both fetal and adult life. This complete block is manifested by the absence, from both the fetal liver and the adult bone marrow, of cells committed to the B- and B-1 cell lineages *(10–12)*. NK cells and thymic dendritic APCs, which arise from the earliest described T-cell progenitor *(13–15)*, are either absent or significantly reduced in these mice. *Ikaros*-null mice also lack peripheral lymphatic centers. Inguinal, axial, cervical, and mesenteric lymph nodes, as well as Peyer's patches and lymphoid follicles in the gastrointestinal tract, are absent because of a developmental block, rather than to the absence of circulating lymphocytes. Transplantation of these mice with wild-type bone marrow repopulates the lymphoid compartment but fails to reconstitute lymph nodes, suggesting a developmental block in lymph node generation that cannot be overcome in the adult (A. Nichogiannopoulou and K. Georgopoulos, unpublished results).

Lack of Ikaros activity has distinct effects on fetal and adult waves of T-cell differentiation. The fetal waves are completely absent in *Ikaros*-null mice. The thymus is devoid of all identifiable lymphoid progenitors throughout fetal development, and for the first days postnatally *(9)*. However, between days 3 and 5 postpartum, small numbers of thymocytes are detected in the thymic rudiment that expand and differentiate within the next few weeks to become mature $CD4^+$ and $CD8^+$ progeny. A reduction in $CD4^-$ $CD8^-$ T-cell receptor (TCR) negative immature thymocytes is evident; the authors hypothesize that this is caused by a reduced input from the prothymocyte compartment in the bone marrow (J-H. Wang and K. Georgopoulos, unpublished results).

The absence of fetal thymocyte development is further manifested by the absence of dendritic epidermal Vγ3 T-cells in the skin of *Ikaros*-null mice *(9)*. Development of these specialized T-cells is restricted to fetal stages of development and it has been shown that both the fetal origin of HSCs, as well as the fetal thymic microenvironment are indispensable for their generation *(16,17)*. Mucosal epithelial Vγ4 T-cells, however, which are known to originate from a second wave of fetal thymocyte development *(18,19)*, are present in a normal distribution and density *(9)*. This apparent discrepancy can be explained by the reported residual potential of adult HSCs to generate Vγ4 T-cells *(17)*. Extrathymically derived intestinal intraepithelial γδ T-cells and adult-derived γδ thymocytes and splenocytes are also absent or significantly reduced in *Ikaros*-null mice.

Postnatal αβ T-cell development proceeds abnormally in the absence of Ikaros. Thymocyte profiles are skewed towards $CD4^+CD8^-$ cells and precursors in transition to this phenotype *(9)*. This suggests a deregulation of the CD4 versus CD8 lineage commitment decision in the absence of Ikaros. In addition, $CD4^+$ and $CD8^+$ single positive thymocytes from *Ikaros*-null mice hyperproliferate in response to TCR stimulation *(9)*, and from the onset of T-cell development, oligoclonal T-cell expansions are observed in the mutant thymus. As mutant mice get older, one or a few transformed T-cell clones predominate in the thymus and are eventually exported to the periphery. The hyperproliferative phenotype and the oligo/monoclonal expansion of T-cells in *Ikaros*-null mice suggest a role for *Ikaros* as a tumor suppressor during T-cell differentiation.

In contrast to the severe lymphoid defects seen in the *Ikaros*-null mice, erythroid and myeloid differentiation appear unaffected, and these populations comprise the majority of the bone marrow and spleen in mutant mice.

5.2. Deletion of the DNA-Binding Domain Results in a Dominant-Negative Ikaros Mutation

A second *Ikaros* mutation was constructed, in which the high-affinity DNA-binding domain contained within exons 3 and 4 of the *Ikaros* gene was deleted *(20)*. Proteins generated by this mutated locus cannot bind DNA. However, these mutant isoforms have an intact C-terminal zinc-finger dimerization domain and can therefore interfere in a dominant-negative fashion with wild-type Ikaros proteins. In lymphocytes heterozygous for this mutation, mutant Ikaros proteins colocalize to the nucleus with the DNA-binding isoforms made by the intact wild-type allele *(4)*. Within the nucleus, they can sequester the wild-type Ikaros proteins into transcriptionally inactive heterodimers. In addition, the dominant-negative effect may be manifested against other proteins, which interact with Ikaros, such as the lymphoid-restricted *Ikaros* family member, Aiolos *(6)*. In mice homozygous for the dominant-negative *Ikaros* mutation, mutant isoforms might interfere with the activity of factors that dimerize and work in concert with Ikaros during the earliest stages of hemopoiesis. In this way, the mutant proteins would have detrimental effects on the fate determination of various hemopoietic lineages.

The severity of the phenotype of mice bearing this *Ikaros* mutation, hereafter termed dominant-negative (DN), confirms this hypothesis. *Ikaros* $DN^{-/-}$ mice display an early and complete block in the development of both fetal and adult lymphoid lineages *(20)*. An impairment of normal granulocyte development is also evident by the lack of cells expressing the granulocyte maturation marker Gr-1. This may be the cause of the inability of $DN^{-/-}$ mice to fight off the opportunistic infections to which they eventually succumb. These animals are also characterized by a 10-fold decrease in bone marrow cellularity, concomitant with a dramatic increase in extramedullary erythro- and myelopoiesis in the spleen. Blood smears and differential counts reveal developmental abnormalities that cannot be attributed solely to the ongoing infection. *Ikaros* $DN^{-/-}$ bone marrow and spleen cells perform poorly in all the commonly employed assays of hemopoietic stem and progenitor cell activity. For example, wild-type bone marrow cells completely populate unconditioned *Ikaros* $DN^{-/-}$ mice, replacing even those lineages that appear unaffected by the mutation, (i.e., erythroid and myeloid). These results strongly indicate a severe competitive disadvantage of *Ikaros* $DN^{-/-}$ stem cells compared to their wild-type counterparts. In addition to the competitive disadvantage, the numbers of stem cells are dramatically reduced, as is demonstrated by transplantation experiments. The reduction in stem cell numbers is also evidenced by the fact that the bone marrow Lin^{-}/c-kit^{+}/Sca-1^{+} population that is enriched for HSCs is virtually absent in *Ikaros* $DN^{-/-}$ bone marrow.

These findings reveal a redundant role for *Ikaros* in the earliest hemopoietic commitment events. This role appears to be shared with other transcription factors which can substitute for Ikaros function in *Ikaros*-null, but not in $DN^{-/-}$ mice.

6. The Role of *Ikaros* in T-Cell Homeostasis

6.1. Lymphocyte Development in Ikaros $DN^{+/-}$ Mice

The authors' studies with mice heterozygous for the dominant-negative *Ikaros* DNA-binding mutation ($DN^{+/-}$) further establish the *Ikaros* gene as an essential regulator of proliferation and homeostasis in the lymphocyte lineage *(21)*. Within developing T lymphocytes, distinct thresholds of Ikaros activity are required to regulate lineage specification and maturation. Low levels of Ikaros are required for lymphocyte specification, whereas higher levels are required within the T-cell lineage for proper maturation and antigen-mediated proliferative responses (Fig. 3).

Initially, *Ikaros* $DN^{+/-}$ mice have normal lymphoid populations, as determined by flow cytometry. However, "phenotypically normal" $DN^{+/-}$ thymocytes and splenocytes display augmented proliferative responses when triggered via the B- or T-cell receptor in vitro *(21)* (S. Winandy and K. Georgopoulos, unpublished results). This phenotype is most dramatic in $DN^{+/-}$ thymocyte populations, which, in wild-type animals, proliferate very poorly in response to TCR activation signals. When phenotyping experiments were performed with $DN^{+/-}$ thymocyte populations after TCR stimulation, it was discovered that the cells primarily responsible for this hyperproliferation are the mature $CD4^{+}CD8^{-}$ and $CD4^{-}CD8^{+}$ cells (S. Winandy and K. Georgopoulos, unpublished results).

In vivo, changes in the lymphocyte compartments are first detected in the thymuses of older $DN^{+/-}$ mice between two and three months of age *(21)*. Expansion in the intermediate double positive ($CD4^{+}/CD8^{int}/TCR^{int}$ and $CD4^{int}/CD8^{+}/TCR^{int}$) and in single positive ($CD4^{+}/TCR^{hi}$ and $CD8^{+}/TCR^{hi}$) thymocyte compartments is detected.

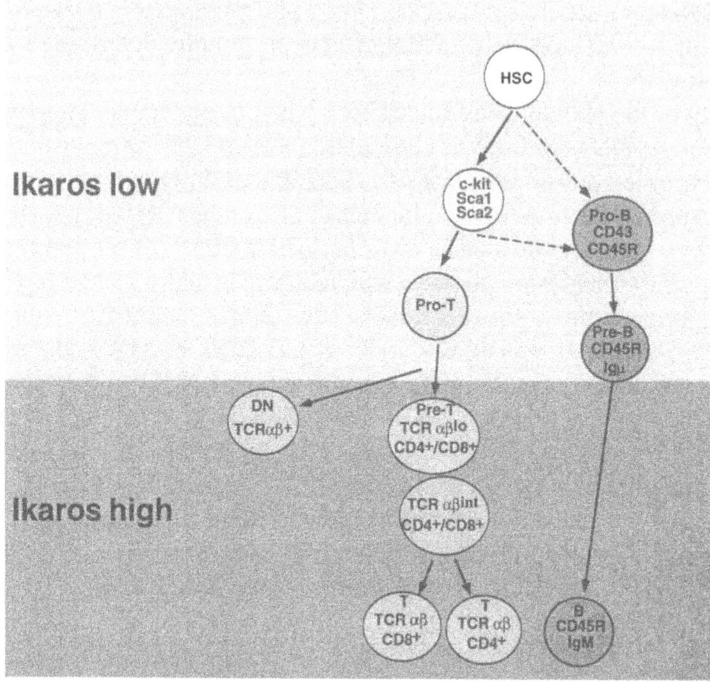

Fig. 3. Lymphocyte differentiation pathways showing the different thresholds of Ikaros activity necessary for specification vs maturation and proliferation.

Intermediate double positive thymocytes are cells in transition to the single positive stage and are in the process of being positively and negatively selected *(22)*. During these selection events, triggering through TCR should lead to either maturation in the absence of proliferation (positive selection) or apoptosis (negative selection) *(22–27)*. Impairment of the selection process that regulates the transition from an early double positive ($CD4^+/CD8^{int}/TCR^{lo}$) to an intermediate ($CD4^+/CD8^{int}/TCR^{int}$ and $CD4^{int}/CD8^+/TCR^{int}$) to a single positive ($CD4^+/TCR^{hi}$ and $CD8^+/TCR^{hi}$) thymocyte may result in the accumulation of these transitional stage intermediates and an increase in the number of single positive cells in the thymus. This phenotype may be a direct result of the hyperproliferative response of thymocytes to activation stimuli observed in vitro.

6.2. Transformation of T-Cells in Ikaros $DN^{+/-}$ Mice

Ikaros $DN^{+/-}$ mice develop highly malignant T-cell leukemias and lymphomas with 100% penetrance between 3 and 6 months of age *(21)*. The disease is characterized by complete takeover of the hemopoietic organs with clonal lymphoblastic T-cells and extensive infiltration by these cells of nonlymphoid organs such as lung, liver, and kidney. In all cases, the malignant cells express the CD3/T-cell receptor αβ (TCR αβ) complex. However, coreceptor phenotype of the accumulating T-cell population differs between mice. $CD8^+$ populations arise with the highest frequency, but $CD4^+$, $CD4^+CD8^+$ and $CD4^-CD8^-$ populations are also detected. Within a given animal, a percentage of these lymphoblastic T-cells express the CD25 (interleukin-2 receptor) activation marker. This percentage varies between animals and is highest at later stages of the disease. In addition, most of the cell lines established from these mice express CD25, strongly suggesting that expression of CD25 correlates with a high degree of malignancy. Interestingly, however, the authors have found no evidence of production of interleukin-2 (IL-2) by these transformed cells.

Outgrowth of clonal T-cell populations is first detected in the thymus, defining this organ as the point of origin of these malignant T-cells. This observation, together with the augmented proliferative response of $DN^{+/-}$ thymocytes to triggering through the TCR and the phenotype of accumulating thymocytes in the two- to three-month $DN^{+/-}$ thymuses, led the authors to hypothesize that the targets for transformation are developing thymocytes undergoing inappropriate proliferative responses during their transition from the double to the single positive stage. The expression of CD25 on these abnormal cells may indicate an aberrant response to positive and/or negative selection signals that results in their activation.

Genetic analysis of the malignant T-cells in the *Ikaros* $DN^{+/-}$ mice revealed loss of *Ikaros* heterozygosity. However, these malignant cells contained a normal number of chromosomes, indicating that the loss of the wild-type allele was caused by either aberrant mitotic segregation of the two mutant alleles, a gene conversion event or a deletion of the wild-type *Ikaros* gene. Loss of the wild-type *Ikaros* allele may be directly linked to the malignant transformation of $DN^{+/-}$ thymocytes. Alternatively, loss of *Ikaros* heterozygosity may confer a growth advantage to these cells that may undergo additional genetic events before they transform. Loss of heterozygosity has been well-documented in the tumor progression of cells heterozygous for mutations in tumor suppressor genes such as p53, retinoblastoma and APC *(28–30)*.

The dominant-negative nature of the transformation phenotype has been confirmed by generation of transgenic mice using a CD2 minigene construct to express a mutant Ikaros protein lacking exons 3 and 4. This minigene is expressed in all thymocytes and mature T-cells. The appearance and time course of development of leukemias and lymphomas, which are phenotypically identical to those observed in the $DN^{+/-}$ mice, is inversely correlated to the number of integrated transgenes (S. Winandy and K. Georgopoulos, unpublished results). However, in transformed cells, expression from the wild-type *Ikaros* allele is retained, demonstrating that the transformation phenotype is caused by a gain of function effect from the mutant Ikaros proteins.

6.3. Staging the Transformation Event

In order to identify the target thymocyte population(s) for transformation, the *Ikaros* $DN^{+/-}$ genotype has been bred onto genetic backgrounds that arrest T-cell development at different stages within the thymus. Mice homozygous for a mutation in the recombination activating gene 1 ($RAG1^{-/-}$) cannot recombine their TCR genes. Therefore, thymocytes do not express either pre-TCR (TCRβ chain in conjunction with the surrogate TCRα chain gp33 and the CD3 complex) or TCR and are blocked at the double negative ($CD4^-CD8^-$) stage of development *(31)*. $DN^{+/-}$ × $RAG1^{-/-}$ mice do not develop leukemias and lymphomas, suggesting that cells at this early stage of differentiation are refractory to transformation (S. Winandy and K. Georgopoulos, unpublished results). However, when a TCR αβ transgene was bred into the $DN^{+/-}$ × $RAG1^{-/-}$ background, the transformation phenotype was restored (S. Winandy and K. Georgopoulos, unpublished results). This suggests that TCR signaling pathways may have to be intact for thymocytes to transform under the influence of the *Ikaros* mutation. This hypothesis is strengthened by the result of breeding the $DN^{+/-}$ phenotype onto a TCRα $chain^{-/-}$ background. In these mice, differentiation of thymocytes does not progress beyond the $CD4^+CD8^+TCR^-$ stage because of the inability of the cells to express their TCRα chain gene *(32)*. However, thymocytes do express the pre-TCR; therefore, pre-TCR signaling pathways are operational. $DN^{+/-}$ × $TCR\alpha^{-/-}$ thymocytes do transform with kinetics equal to or greater than those observed in $DN^{+/-}$ mice (S. Winandy and K. Georgopoulos, unpublished results). This suggests that the TCR$\alpha^{-/-}$ background promotes accumulation of cells at a stage vulnerable to transformation—the CD4$^+$CD8$^+$ double positive, pre-TCR$^+$ stage. Therefore, immature thymocytes deficient in Ikaros activity can be targets for transformation only in the presence of intact TCR or pre-TCR signaling pathways.

6.4. Transformation in Ikaros-Null Mice

A dominant-negative mutation in one *Ikaros* allele promotes transformation in immature thymocytes. This may be caused by the functional inactivation of wild-type Ikaros proteins or to a dominant-negative effect on other proteins with which Ikaros interacts.

The central and independent role of *Ikaros* in maintenance of T-cell growth control and homeostasis is observed by the phenotype of the *Ikaros*-null mice. Lack of all Ikaros activity at the earliest stages of T-cell development in these mice results in deregulated maturation, hyperproliferation in response to TCR activation signals, and eventually, transformation of thymocytes. The transformation event occurs with reproducibly faster kinetics than that of the DN$^{+/-}$ thymocytes. Clonal expansions are detected within the *Ikaros*-null postnatal thymus as early as 10 days after the appearance of T-cell precursors. By as soon as 1 month of age, a single thymocyte clone predominates. The stage in thymocyte development during which these clones begin to expand has been defined as at or before the CD4$^+$CD8$^+$ stage, the same developmental window vulnerable to transformation in the DN$^{+/-}$ mice. This phenotype proves that loss of Ikaros activity alone, in the absence of dominant-negative interfering isoforms, can lead to transformation of immature thymocytes.

However, the *Ikaros*-null transformation is not phenotypically identical to that observed in the DN$^{+/-}$ mice. After loss of heterozygosity, DN$^{-/-}$ clones are highly aggressive in their growth properties. These clones can grow indefinitely in vitro in the absence of added cytokines, whereas very few of the *Ikaros*-null clones display this property. Furthermore, whereas the DN$^{-/-}$ clones easily and quickly form solid tumors in adoptive transfer experiments in nude mice, very few of the *Ikaros*-null clones do, and the kinetics of tumor outgrowth is significantly slower. The more aggressive phenotype of the DN$^{-/-}$ malignancies suggests a dual molecular event. It is hypothesized that a decrease of Ikaros activity, either by the absence of the protein (*Ikaros*-null mice) or by its retention in nonfunctional complexes (DN$^{+/-}$ mice) leads to deregulated growth of immature thymocytes. However, development of a highly aggressive malignancy requires functional loss of another protein, one which interacts with Ikaros. One good candidate is the Aiolos protein, whose expression is dramatically upregulated during the transition from the pro-T CD4$^-$CD8$^-$ to the pre-T CD4$^+$CD8$^+$ stage. This increase in Aiolos protein expression implicates an important role for Aiolos at this developmental stage, the same stage targeted for transformation in both the *Ikaros*-null and DN$^{+/-}$ mice. Moreover, Aiolos, as well as wild-type Ikaros protein, can be coimmunoprecipitated with the dominant-negative Ikaros protein, confirming that Aiolos is a target of dominant-negative interference by the mutant Ikaros proteins (J. Koipally and K. Georgopoulos, unpublished results).

7. *Aiolos*—A Gene Related to *Ikaros*

The fact that the dominant-negative *Ikaros* mutation gave rise to a more severe phenotype in mice than the null mutation suggested that Ikaros proteins interact not only with each other, but with non-Ikaros proteins as well. According to this hypothesis, the phenotype of the *Ikaros*-null mice would be caused by loss of functional Ikaros proteins, whereas the more severe phenotype of the DN$^{-/-}$ mice would be a result of the combined loss of functional Ikaros proteins in addition to interference with the activity of proteins that interact with Ikaros. Therefore, experiments were undertaken to identify proteins that interact with Ikaros proteins. Since *Ikaros* is homologous in the zinc-finger regions to the *Drosophila* gene *Hunchback*, it seemed likely that this was a motif that was conserved and duplicated in the murine genome, so that it might exist in several murine genes. Therefore, one strategy used to identify proteins that interact with Ikaros was to screen for genes that are homologous to *Ikaros* in the C-terminal zinc-finger dimerization region, as the products of such putative genes would be likely to be capable of dimerizing with Ikaros proteins. Such a screen resulted in the identification of the gene *Aiolos (6)*, which is the first extensively characterized homolog of *Ikaros*.

Like Ikaros, the Aiolos protein is encoded by seven exons and contains six zinc fingers, with the four amino-terminal fingers mediating DNA binding and the two carboxy-terminal fingers mediating dimerization (Fig. 1). Also like Ikaros, Aiolos binds DNA and is an activator of transcription. Aiolos and Ik-1, the largest of the Ikaros isoforms, share extensive regions of homology, with the highest degrees of homology occurring in the zinc-finger regions, which constitute the dimerization and the DNA-binding domains. Thus, Ikaros and Aiolos proteins form hetero- and homodimers with equal efficiency, and Ikaros and Aiolos homodimers have comparable DNA-binding specificities and affinities *(6)*. Given their similar properties, homo- and heterodimers of these proteins are likely to regulate the expression of the same set of target genes. However, differences in the expression patterns and functional properties of Ikaros and Aiolos proteins may modulate the activity of a complex which forms over a specific DNA binding site during development. Ikaros and Aiolos proteins also contain regions of nonhomology. These regions may play a role in the distinct functional roles of these proteins in hemopoiesis (J. Koipally and K. Georgopoulos, unpublished results).

Unlike the *Ikaros* mRNA, the *Aiolos* mRNA is not alternatively spliced; thus, the *Aiolos* gene does not generate any non-DNA-binding isoforms. Furthermore, the *Ikaros* and *Aiolos* genes differ in their expression patterns. Although *Ikaros* is expressed very early in hemopoiesis and its expression levels do not vary greatly, the expression of *Aiolos* is more restricted and varied. In the developing embryo, *Aiolos* is first expressed at day E16 in the fetal thymus, i.e., at a stage when committed T-cell precursors are differentiating and expanding from the CD4$^-$CD8$^-$ to the CD4$^+$CD8$^+$ stage. This is in contrast to *Ikaros,* which is expressed in fetal hemopoietic progenitor cells within the yolk sac and fetal liver, as well as in the earliest T-cell precursors in the E12–E14 fetal thymus. In the adult, *Ikaros* is expressed in populations that are enriched for the more primitive erythroid and myeloid progenitors (c-kit$^+$/Sca-1$^-$) and in populations which are enriched for pluripotent HSCs (c-kit$^+$/Sca-1$^+$) (Fig. 2) *(6)*. *Aiolos* is not expressed in either of these populations. However, it is expressed at low levels in the c-kit$^+$/Sca-1$^+$/Sca-2$^+$ cells that have increased potential for lymphoid differentiation *(33)*. Therefore, *Aiolos* expression seems to correlate with the earliest step in lymphoid commitment and may play a redundant role in this commitment step.

Aiolos is expressed at low levels in B220$^+$IgM$^-$CD43$^+$ pro-B cells and in CD4$^-$CD8$^-$ pro-T-cells, but becomes dramatically upregulated at the later B220$^+$IgM$^-$CD43$^-$pre-B-cell and CD4$^+$CD8$^+$ pre-T-cell stages. In mature lymphoid cells, *Aiolos* is expressed at higher levels in B- than in T-cells, with the highest levels being expressed in mature naive B-cells and terminally differentiated plasma cells in the periphery.

The function of *Aiolos* is presently being elucidated. Ongoing studies suggest an essential role at later stages of B- and T-cell differentiation, i.e., during maturation rather than specification. However, this does not preclude a redundant role during B- and T-cell specification.

8. Conclusion

Ikaros and *Aiolos* were the first two genes to be identified in what is turning out to be a family of genes encoding homologous zinc-finger DNA-binding proteins. Although *Ikaros* and *Aiolos* are highly homologous, they clearly have different essential roles in lymphoid differentiation and maturation. These different roles are likely to be a result of the different expression patterns, as well as inherent functional differences between the two proteins. The expression pattern of *Ikaros* and the phenotypes of the *Ikaros*-mutant mice demonstrate that this gene is an essential determinant of lymphoid cell fate in fetal and adult hemopoiesis. The related gene *Aiolos* does not share this specification property. Consistent with its different expression pattern, it appears to play a specialized role at later stages in the B- and T-cell lineages, playing a role in maturation rather than specification. At later stages, e.g., after lineage commitment, both *Ikaros* and *Aiolos* function to regulate differentiation and/or homeostasis of B and T lymphocytes. The authors' current model proposes that Ikaros proteins are the central factors of a complex network directing lymphocyte development and homeostasis. Since both Ikaros and Aiolos are transcription factors, it is most likely that these proteins drive lymphopoiesis by coordinating programs of stage-specific gene expression. This idea is supported by the fact that there are Ikaros/Aiolos consensus sites in the regulatory regions of several hemopoietic- and lymphoid-specific genes, e.g., TdT, RAG1, λ_5, V_{preB}, CD3-δ, -ε -γ, TCR-δ, -β, -α, Igα , the IgH and IgL loci, IL2R-α, SHP-1, and c-kit.

The hyperproliferative phenotype of $DN^{+/-}$ and *Ikaros*-null lymphocytes indicates that Ikaros proteins also function as regulators of lymphoid proliferation. Ikaros may regulate the expression of factors involved in signal transduction or cell cycle control. Alternatively, it may participate directly in modulating the activity of cell cycle control proteins, such as cyclins. The authors propose that Ikaros proteins carry out such a complex array of varied functions by interactions with different functional partners. One such partner is the related protein Aiolos, but current experiments indicate that Ikaros proteins also interact with several unrelated proteins. Identification of these proteins and disruption of the genes encoding them will provide further clues to the mechanism by which *Ikaros* regulates lymphocyte development and homeostasis. Independent studies on gene expression in lymphocyte populations of *Ikaros*-mutant mice should also reveal target genes whose expression is regulated by *Ikaros*, as well as provide insight into how these genes are controlled.

Since *Ikaros* appears to function so widely throughout lymphopoiesis, understanding the mechanisms of *Ikaros* function should aid greatly in elucidating the steps involved in lymphocyte differentiation and how the transition through each step of this complex pathway is regulated.

Acknowledgments

The authors wish to thank J. Koipally for communicating unpublished data, P. Wu for general support and P. Foran for secretarial help. N. Avitahl is a junior fellow of the Leukemia Society of America, K. Georgopoulos is a Scholar of the Leukemia Society of America and S. Winandy is a Cancer Research Institute Fellow. This work was supported by National

Institutes of Health grants RO1-AI38342AO2 and RO1-AI33062-04 to K. Georgopoulos and a core grant from the Cutaneous Biology Research Center (Shiseido Co. Ltd.).

References

1. Georgopoulos, K., Moore, D. D., and Derfler, B. (1992) Ikaros, an early lymphoid-specific transcription factor and a putative mediator for T cell commitment. *Science* **258,** 808–812.
2. Molnár, Á. and Georgopoulos, K. (1994) The Ikaros gene encodes a family of functionally diverse zinc finger DNA-binding proteins. *Mol. Cell. Biol.* **14,** 8292–8303.
3. Molnár, Á., Wu , P., Largespada, D. A., Vortkamp, A., Scherer, S., Copeland, N. G., Jenkins, N. A., Bruns, G., and Georgopoulos, K. (1996) The Ikaros gene encodes a family of lymphocyte-restricted zinc finger DNA-binding proteins, highly conserved in human and mouse. *J. Immunol.* **156,** 585–592.
4. Sun, L., Liu, A., and Georgopoulos, K. (1996) Zinc finger-mediated protein interactions modulate Ikaros activity, a molecular control of lymphocyte development. *EMBO J.* **15,** 5358–5369.
5. Hahm, K., Ernst, P., Lo, K., Kim, G. S., Turck, C., and Smale, S. T. (1994) The lymphoid transcription factor LyF-1 is encoded by specific, alternatively spliced mRNAs derived from the *Ikaros* gene. *Mol. Cell. Biol.* **14,** 7111–7123.
6. Morgan, B., Sun, L., Avitahl, N., Andrikopoulos, K., Ikeda, T., Gonzales, E., Wu, P., Neben, S., and Georgopoulos, K. (1997) Aiolos: a lymphoid restricted transcription factor that interacts with Ikaros to regulate lymphocyte differentiation. *EMBO J.* **16,** 2004–2013.
7. Okada, S., Nakauchi, H., Nagayoshi, K., Nishikawa, S., Nishikawa, S., Miura, Y., and Suda, T. (1991) Enrichment and characterization of murine hematopoietic stem cells that express the c-kit molecule. *Blood* **78,** 1706–1712.
8. Spangrude, G. J., Heimfeld, S., and Weissman, I. L. (1988) Purification and characterization of mouse hematopoietic stem cells. *Science.* **241,** 58–62.
9. Wang, J.-H., Nichogiannopoulou, A., Wu, L., Sun, L., Sharpe, A. H., Bigby, M., and Georgopoulos, K. (1996) Selective defects in the development of the fetal and adult lymphoid system in mice with an *Ikaros*-null mutation. *Immunity* **5,** 537–549.
10. Hardy, R. R., Carmack, C. E., Li, Y. S., and Hayakawa, K. (1994) Distinctive developmental origins and specificities of murine $CD5^+$ B cells. *Immunol. Rev.* **137,** 91–118.
11. Hardy, R. R. and Hayakawa, K. (1991) A developmental switch in B lymphopoiesis. *Proc. Natl. Acad. Sci. USA* **88,** 11550–11554.
12. Melchers, F., Strasser, A., Bauer, S. R., Kudo, A., Thalmann, P., and Rolink, A. (1991) B cell development in fetal liver. *Adv. Exp. Med. Biol.* **292,** 201–205.
13. Ardavin, C., Wu, L., Li, C., and Shortman, K. (1993) Thymic dendritic cells and T cells develop simultaneously in the thymus from a common precursor population. *Nature* **362,** 761–763.
14. Shortman, K. and Wu, L. (1996) Early T lymphocyte progenitors. *Annu. Rev. Immunol.* **14,** 29–47.
15. Wu, L., Vremec, D., Ardavin, K., Winkel, G., Süss, I. L., Maraskovsky, E., Cook, W., and Shortman, K. (1995) Mouse thymus dendritic cells: kinetics of development and changes in surface markers during maturation. *Eur. J. Immunol.* **25,** 418–425.
16. Ikuta, K., Kina, T., MacNeil, I., Uchida, N., Peault, B., Chien, Y. H., and Weissman, I. L. (1990) A developmental switch in thymic lymphocyte maturation potential occurs at the level of hematopoietic stem cells. *Cell.* **62,** 863–874.
17. Ikuta, K. and Weissman, I. L. (1991) The junctional modifications of a T cell receptor γ chain are determined at the level of thymic precursors. *J. Exp. Med.* **174,** 1279–1282.
18. Ito, K., Bonneville, M., Takagaki, Y., Nakanishi, N., Kanagawa, O., Krecko, E. G., and Tonegawa, S. (1989) Different γδ T-cell receptors are expressed on thymocytes at different stages of development. *Proc. Natl. Acad. Sci. USA* **86,** 631–635.
19. Itohara, S., Farr, A. G., Lafaille, J. J., Bonneville, M., Takagaki, Y., Haas, W., and Tonegawa, S. (1990) Homing of a γδ thymocyte subset with homogeneous T-cell receptors to mucosal epithelia. *Nature* **343,** 754–757.
20. Georgopoulos, K., Bigby, M., Wang, J.-H., Molnár, Á., Wu, P., Winandy, S., and Sharpe, A. (1994) The Ikaros gene is required for the development of all lymphoid lineages. *Cell* **79,** 143–156.
21. Winandy, S., Wu, P., and Georgopoulos, K. (1995) A dominant mutation in the *Ikaros* gene leads to rapid development of leukemia and lymphoma. *Cell* **83,** 289–299.

22. Chan, S. H., Cosgrove, D., Waltzinger, C., Benoist, C., and Mathis, D. (1993) Another view of the selective model of thymocyte selection. *Cell* **73,** 225–236.
23. Ashton-Rickardt, P. G., van Kaer, L., Schumacher, T. N. P., Ploegh, H. L., and Tonegawa, S. (1993) Peptide contributes to the specificity of positive selection of $CD8^+$ T cells in the thymus. *Cell* **73,** 1041–1049.
24. Hogquist, K., Jameson, S., Heath, W., Howard, J., Bevan, M., and Carbone, F. (1994) T cell receptor antagonist peptides induce positive selection. *Cell* **76,** 17–27.
25. Janeway, C. A., Jr. (1994) Thymic selection: two pathways to life and two to death. *Immunity* **1,** 3–6.
26. Takahama, Y., Suzuki, H., Katz, K. S., Grusby, M. J., and Singer, A. (1994) Positive selection of $CD4^+$ T cells by TCR ligation without aggregation even in the absence of MHC. *Nature* **371,** 67–70.
27. Vasquez, N. J., Kane, L. P., and Hedrick, S. M. (1994) Intracellular signals that mediate thymic negative selection. *Immunity* **1,** 45–56.
28. Cavenee, W. K., Dryja, T. P., Phillips, R. A., Benedict, W. F., Godbout, R., Gallie, B. L., Murphree, A. L., Strong, L. C., and White, R. L. (1983) Expression of recessive alleles by chromosomal mechanisms in retinoblastoma. *Nature* **305,** 779–784.
29. Ichii, S., Horii, A., Nakatsuru, S., Furayama, J., Utsunomiya, S., and Nakamura, Y. (1992) Inactivation of both APC alleles in an early stage of colon adenomas in a patient with familial adenomatous polyposis (FAP). *Hum. Mol. Gen.* **1,** 387–390.
30. Meltzer, S. J., Yin, J., Huang, Y., McDaniel, T. K., Newkirk, C., Iseri, O., Vogelstein, B., and Resau, J. H. (1991) Reduction to homozygosity involving p53 in esophageal cancers demonstrated by the polymerase chain reaction. *Proc. Natl. Acad. Sci. USA* **88,** 4976–4980.
31. Mombaerts, P., Iacomini, J., Johnson, R. S., Herrup, K., Tonegawa, S., and Papaioannou, V. E. (1992) RAG-1-deficient mice have no mature B and T lymphocytes. *Cell* **68,** 869–877.
32. Mombaerts, P., Clarke, A. R., Rudnicki, M. A., Iacomini, J., Itohara, S., Lafaille, J. J., Wang, L., Ichikawa, Y., Jaenisch, R., Hooper, M. L., and Tonegawa, S. (1992) Mutations in T-cell antigen receptor genes α and β block thymocyte development at different stages. *Nature* **360,** 225–231.
33. Antica, M., Wu, L., Shortman, K., and Scollay, R. (1994) Thymic stem cells in the mouse bone marrow. *Blood* **84,** 111–117.

Chapter 5

Transcriptional Control of B-Cell Differentiation by EBF and E2A

Mikael Sigvardsson and Rudolf Grosschedl

1. Introduction

B-cell differentiation is a complex developmental process that ultimately generates antibody-secreting plasma cells. The B-cell lineage involves multiple stages of differentiation that have been characterized by the expression of cell surface markers and the rearrangement status of the immunoglobulin (Ig) loci (Fig. 1). The earliest characterized cells that are committed to the B-cell lineage express the surface markers B220, CD43, AA4.1 and have the Ig heavy chain locus in germline configuration *(1,2)*. Pro-B and pre-B-cells express genes that are involved in the rearrangement of the Ig gene loci and signal transduction through the pre-B-cell receptor (reviewed in 3,4). In particular, these cells express the recombinase-activating genes (Rag1 and Rag2), the terminal deoxytransferase gene (TdT), the λ5 and VpreB genes encoding the Ig surrogate light chains, and the mb-1 and B29 genes encoding the Igα and Igβ proteins that mediate signaling. The pro-B- and pre-B-cells can be subdivided into populations that express different combinations of cell surface markers and may represent distinct stages of differentiation (Fig. 1) *(1,5)*. Further differentiation generates immature B-cells that have rearranged their Ig light chain locus and have downregulated the expression of the λ5 and VpreB surrogate light genes (reviewed in ref. *6*). Taken together, these early stages of B-cell differentiation represent the antigen-independent phase that occurs predominantly in the adult bone marrow. The late stages of B-cell differentiation that occur in peripheral lymphoid organs involve activation of B-cells by antigen and/or T helper cells and the generation of antibody-secreting plasma cells. These late stages of differentiation also result in somatic hypermutation of the Ig genes and antibody class switching (reviewed in ref. *7*).

The complex differentiation program of the B-cell lineage is dependent on the function of multiple transcription factors (reviewed in refs. *8–10*). Many transcription factors have been identified that are expressed predominantly in cells of the lymphoid lineages

From: *Molecular Biology of B-Cell and T-Cell Development*
Edited by: J. G. Monroe and E. V. Rothenberg © Humana Press Inc., Totowa, NJ

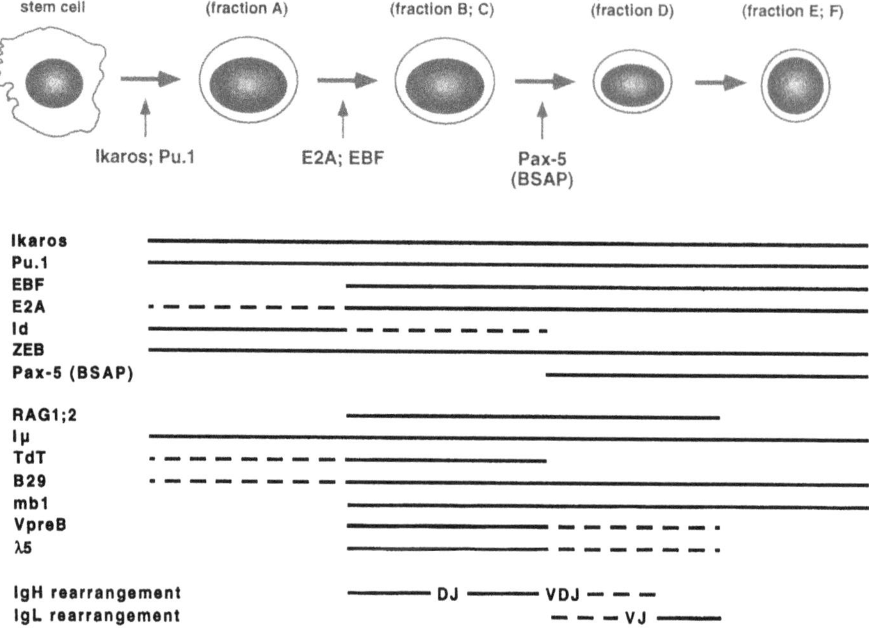

Fig. 1. Schematic diagram of early B-cell differentiation and the expression patterns of transcription factors and cell surface markers. The stages of B-cell differentiation representing the early, antigen-independent phase are indicated on the top. Transcriptional control points are indicated by arrows. Targeted inactivations of transcription factors result in an arrest of B-cell differentiation. Expression patterns of transcription factors discussed in the text are shown in the middle. The expression of cell surface markers and the rearrangement of immunoglobulin loci are indicated on the bottom. Dotted lines indicate low levels of expression or gene rearrangement.

and/or at specific stages of B-cell differentiation. The biological role of these transcription factors has been examined by targeted gene inactivations. These experiments have shown that these cell type-specific transcription factors contribute to the regulation of the B-cell lineage. The transcription factor Ikaros *(11,12)* is important for the generation of all lymphoid cell types *(13)*, whereas Pu.1 *(14,15)* regulates the generation of B lymphoid and myeloid cells *(16)*. Targeted inactivation of the genes encoding early B-cell factor (EBF) *(17)*, and E2A protein *(18)* both result in a complete arrest of B-cell differentiation prior to Ig gene rearrangement *(19–21)*. Finally, the Pax5 gene encoding the B-cell specific activator protein (BSAP) (*1*; reviewed in ref. *22*), controls B-cell differentiation at a subsequent stage that is defined by the completion of gene rearrangement of the Ig heavy chain locus *(23,24)*.

In this review, the authors discuss the current knowledge concerning the expression patterns, the biochemical and functional properties of the EBF and E2A proteins, which both regulate early B-cell differentiation.

2. Expression, Biochemical, and Functional Properties of EBF

2.1. Expression of EBF

EBF was identified as a protein that interacts with a functionally important site in the promoter of the mb-1 gene *(25,26)*. EBF is expressed in pro-B-, pre-B-, and B-cells, but

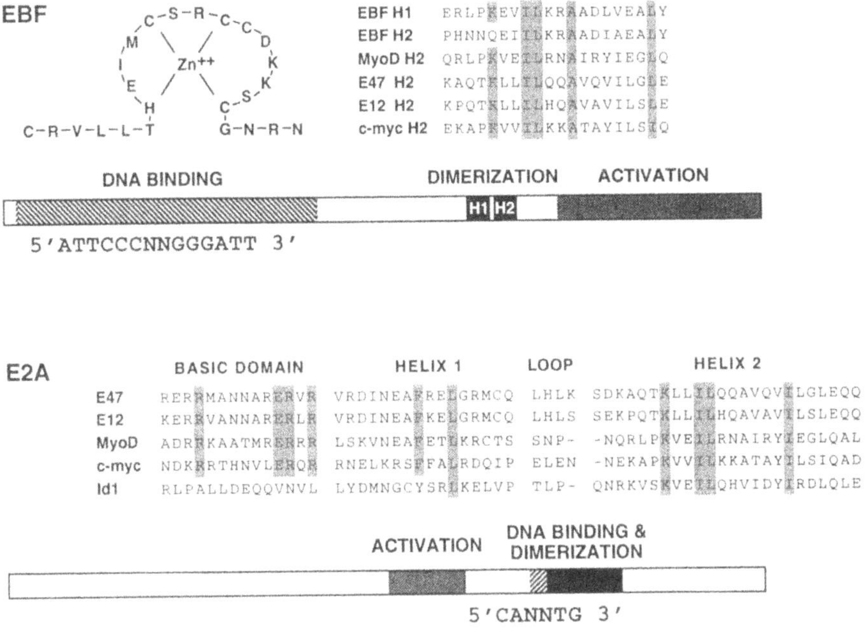

Fig. 2. Schematic representation of the functional domains of EBF and E47. The DNA-binding domains are indicated by a striped box and the dimerization domains are shown as black boxes. The transcriptional activation domains are shown as gray boxes. Above the schematic diagram of the polypeptides, the amino acids important for DNA-binding and protein dimerization are shown. Residues that are conserved between EBF and/or HLH proteins are indicated by shaded boxes. Below the graphic representation of the polypeptides, the consensus target sites for the EBF and E2A proteins are shown.

not at the plasma cell stage *(17,25)*. However, this transcription factor is also expressed in several nonlymphoid tissues that include adipose tissue and brain *(17)*. In olfactory neurons, the same transcription factor has also been identified as Olf-1 *(27,28)*. Purification and subsequent cloning of EBF has indicated that this protein is unrelated to other classes of transcription factors *(17,29)*. Recently, a *Drosophila* homolog of EBF, termed collier, has been identified *(30)*.

2.2. DNA Binding by EBF

EBF forms a homodimer independent of DNA binding *(17,29)*. The dimerization of EBF is dependent on a protein domain encompassing two α-helices that are related to helix 2 of the dimerization domain of helix-loop-helix (HLH) transcription factors (Fig. 2) *(17,31)*. The DNA-binding domain of EBF spans approx 200 amino acids that contain several cysteine and histidine residues. Although the DNA-binding domain of EBF cannot be aligned to any known DNA-binding motif, it contains an unusual arrangement of histidines and cysteines ($H\text{-}X_3\text{-}C\text{-}X_2\text{-}C\text{-}X_5\text{-}C$) that are important for DNA binding (Fig. 2). This motif appears to represent a metal-coordination motif because zinc is essential for DNA binding by EBF *(31)*.

EBF binds to variants of the palindromic sequence 5'ATTCCCNNGGGAAT *(29)*. In naturally occuring binding sites for EBF, a significant degeneracy of this consensus sequence has been observed *(25,28,32,33)*. On optimized and correctly spaced binding sites, the DNA-binding domain of EBF can form homodimers, whereas binding of EBF to degenerate sites also requires the dimerization domain *(31)*. Many binding sites for EBF overlap with the core binding site, 5'TGGGAAT, for the transcription factor, Ikaros *(34)*, and its close relative, Aiolos *(35)*. Ikaros can bind DNA as a monomer but has also been shown to form homodimers and heterodimers with Aiolos *(35,36)*. Although EBF and Ikaros are both expressed during B-cell differentiation, no evidence has yet been provided, suggesting that these transcription factors collaborate or compete with each other.

2.3. Functional Properties of EBF

Functional analysis of EBF has revealed two transcriptional activation domains *(31)*. A serine/threonine-rich domain resides in the carboxy terminus of EBF (Fig. 2). This activation domain can stimulate transcription when fused to a GAL4 DNA-binding domain. In addition, the DNA-binding domain alone can increase transcription from optimized binding sites but does not function in the context of a GAL4 fusion protein. EBF was initially shown to activate the promoter of the mb-1 gene *(25)*. This promoter includes binding sites for the transcription factors Sp1, Ets proteins, and BSAP *(25,37,38)*. Unlike typical transcriptional activators, EBF does not significantly stimulate transcription from multimerized binding sites. However, EBF can function in the context of the natural mb-1 promoter, suggesting that EBF may collaborate with other transcription factors *(25)*. Although the mb-1 promoter is a biochemical target for EBF, the endogenous mb-1 gene can be expressed in cells lacking both EBF and BSAP *(33)*. Likewise, an EBF-binding site has been identified in the κ light chain promoter, which is active in plasma cells that do not express EBF *(32)*. Thus, the mb-1 and κ genes may not represent genetic targets for EBF.

The understanding of the role of a transcription factor in cell differentiation depends on the knowledge of potential genetic targets. Recently, the Ig surrogate light chain genes were identified as direct genetic targets for EBF *(33)*. Transient or stable transfection of EBF in an immature hematopoietic cell line, Ba/F3, induced expression of the endogenous λ5 and VpreB genes (*see* also Subheading 5). Although EBF appears to act as a transcriptional activator in the regulation of these genes, EBF may also be involved in negative regulation. Ectopic expression of EBF in plasma cells has been found to downregulate the expression of a co-transfected Ig reporter gene *(32)*. A dual functional role for a transcription factor has been shown for several proteins, including BSAP, (reviewed in ref. *22*). BSAP is expressed in pro-B-, pre-B-, and mature B-cells, but not in plasma cells and activates transcription from the mb-1, CD19 and blk promoters *(38–40)*. In contrast, BSAP acts as a repressor in the regulation of the joining chain gene *(41)* and in the function of the IgH 3'α enhancer *(42–44)*.

3. Expression, Biochemical, and Functional Properties of E2A Proteins

3.1. Expression of E2A Proteins

The E2A gene encodes the transcription factors E12 and E47/E2-5 that are generated from alternatively spliced mRNAs *(18,45,46)*. The alternatively used exons encode distinct basic helix-loop-helix (bHLH) domains that differ in dimerization- and DNA-binding properties (Fig. 2). The E12 and E47 gene products have been detected in all cells examined. Likewise, two other related bHLH genes, E2-2 and HEB, are expressed ubiquitously *(45,47)*. Together with the *Drosophila* daughterless protein, these bHLH proteins represent one class of the family of bHLH transcription factors (reviewed in ref. *48*). Another class is represented by cell type-specific proteins such MyoD, Myogenin, Myf-5, and the *Drosophila* achaete-scute protein. Other bHLH proteins, which are characterized by an additional leucine zipper dimerization motif, include TFE3, TFE-B, and Myc, as well as the Myc-interacting proteins Mad and Max *(49)*. A final class of HLH proteins includes the Id proteins and Emc, which contain an HLH dimerization domain, but cannot bind DNA because of the absence of a basic domain (*see* Fig. 2). Id proteins appear to modulate bHLH protein function by the formation of DNA-nonbinding heterodimeric complexes *(36,50,51)*.

In B lymphoid cells, a specific DNA-binding activity that contains E2A proteins has been identified as B-cell factor 1 (BCF1) *(52,53)*. In contrast to the formation of cell type-specific heterodimeric proteins that contain both E47 and a myogenic protein of the MyoD family *(54–56)*, BCF1 is composed of an E47 homodimer *(57)*. The formation of the E47 homodimer has been suggested to involve the formation of a disulfide bond between two E47 molecules *(58)* and the activity of a phosphatase that mediates B-cell specific modification of E47 *(59)*. In addition, the formation of BCF1 may be influenced by the relative levels of Id proteins during B-cell differentiation. Pro-B- and pre-B-cells contain abundant levels of Id protein and low levels of E2A and E2–2 proteins *(2,48)*. In mature B-cells, the expression of E2A proteins increases whereas the expression of Id decreases *(60,61)*.

3.2. Biochemical Features of E2A Proteins

Proteins of the bHLH family of transcription factors bind a core nucleotide sequence initially identified by in vivo footprinting of the Ig heavy chain enhancer *(62)*. This sequence motif, 5'CANNTG, has been referred to as an E-box. The two central basepairs and the nucleotides immediately adjacent to the core determine the affinity for a particular bHLH dimer *(63,64)*. DNA-binding by bHLH proteins involves both a HLH dimerization domain and basic amino acids that are located immediately adjacent to the HLH domain (Fig. 2) *(65)*. Crystallography of the E47 bHLH dimer bound to DNA has revealed that each E47 subunit contacts one half site of the binding site, with the basic region interacting with the major groove, and helix two of the HLH domain interacting with the phosphate backbone on the opposite side of the DNA *(66)*.

3.3. Functional Properties of E2A Proteins

E47 contains a transcriptional activation domain that is located in the amino-terminal part of the protein and consists of a loop and an adjacent amphipathic helix (Fig. 2) *(45,67)*. This transactivation domain can stimulate transcription when fused to a Gal4 DNA-binding domain. E2A proteins are thought to play a role in the development of multiple cell lineages. Specifically, in association with the myogenic proteins MyoD, Myogenin, and Myf-5, E2A proteins participate in the induction of muscle cell differentiation (reviewed in refs. *68,69*). E47 has also been shown to play an important role in cell cycle regulation because induced expression of E47 in stably transfected NIH/3T3 cells results in a cell cycle arrest *(70)*. The function of E47 can be altered by association with Id proteins because ectopic expression of Id in B-cells directly affects the function of transfected Ig enhancers *(51)* and the differentiation of B-cells *(71)*. Finally, other bHLH proteins have also been implicated in B-cell specific gene expression and differentiation. TFE3, TFE-B, USF, and E2–2 participate in the regulation of the Ig heavy chain enhancer (reviewed in ref. *72*), and Myc and Myn may act in the differentiation and proliferation of B-cells *(73,74)*. Thus, HLH proteins play multiple roles in B-cell differentiation, and understanding of the interplay between these proteins will provide important information about the B-cell developmental pathway.

Several genetic target genes for E47 have been identified by ectopic overexpression of this protein in pre-T-cells and fibroblastic cells *(75,76)*. These experiments have shown that the lymphoid specific genes, Oct2, Rag1 and TdT, are upregulated in E47-overexpressing cells. In addition to an increase in the frequency of D-J rearrangements in the Ig heavy chain locus in pre-T-cells, overexpression of E47 has been found to upregulate Iμ sterile transcripts, which initiate immediately downstream of the IgH enhancer *(77,78)*. Iμ transcription has been correlated with IgH enhancer activity and gene rearrangement (reviewed in ref. *79*).

The function of E2A proteins has been studied extensively in the regulation of the IgH enhancer which contains multiple E-boxes. Three of the four E-boxes were found to bind members of the bHLH family of proteins that mediate enhancer function in collaboration with other transcription factors that bind to the enhancer *(72,80–85)*. DNA binding and transcriptional activation of bHLH proteins at the IgH enhancer appears also to be regulated by association with Id proteins *(51,86)*, and by competition with the repressor, ZEB *(87–89)*. ZEB binds the μE4 and μE5 sites in non-B-cells, and this repressor is physically displaced by the binding of E47 homodimers in B-cells.

4. Roles of EBF and E2A Proteins in B-Cell Differentiation

4.1. Arrest of B-Cell Differentiation in EBF- and E2A-Deficient Mice

Targeted gene inactivation provides a powerful strategy with which protein function can be studied. Gene knockout experiments in mice have shown that many transcription factors are important for the differentiation of specific cell lineages and for mouse development in general. Homologous inactivation of the EBF and E2A genes have shown that both transcription factors are essential for B-cell differentiation *(19–21)*. EBF-deficient mice have normal T-cell populations, but lack B-cells. Specifically, the mutant mice lack B-cells that express the surface markers HSA, BP1, and IgM, and that transcribe the λ5, VpreB, and mb-1 genes *(21)*. In addition, no rearrangements of the Ig heavy or light chain loci could be detected in the EBF-deficient mice, although these mice contain some B220-positive cells that express Il-7-receptor and Iμ transcripts. Thus, targeted inactivation of EBF results in a block of differentiation of the earliest pro-B-cells, representing fraction A, according to Hardy et al *(1)*.

A similar block in B-cell differentiation has been observed in mice lacking the E2A transcription factors although the specific phenotype depends on the targeted mutation *(19,20)*. In one case, the targeting construct was designed to mutate specifically the E12 bHLH domain; however, neither E12 nor E47 transcripts were detected in the knockout mice, and B-cell differentiation was blocked at essentially the same stage as in EBF deficient mice *(19)*. In contrast, deletion of both E12 and E47 bHLH domains by a targeted mutation resulted in a block of B-cell differentiation preceding the expression of any B-cell marker *(20)*. The molecular basis for the difference of these mutant phenotypes is unknown, but it may be related to the expression of a mutant form of E2A proteins in the mice carrying a deletion of both E12 and E47 bHLH domains.

4.2. Functional Redundancy of bHLH Proteins in B-Cell Development

The individual roles of E12 and E47 proteins in B-cell differentiation have been studied further in E47 knockout mice that express either an E12 or an E47 transgenic construct *(90)*. In E47 deficient mice that have also a reduced number of E12 transcripts,

B-cell differentiation is significantly impaired, and the B-cell phenotype is similar to that of the E2A mutant mice. Expression of an E12 transgene in the E47 deficient mice was found to allow for early B-cell differentiation, although the expression levels of the λ5 and mb-1 genes and the frequency of V-D-J recombination were low, and no IgM-expressing B-cells were detected. E2A knockout mice expressing an E47 transgene generate IgM-positive cells, albeit at a very low level. In E2A knockout mice expressing both E47 and E12, the number of B-cells was increased relative to the mice expressing either transgene alone. Thus, E12 appears to enhance the ability of E47 to promote B-cell differentiation, and both transcription factors may act in a partially redundant manner.

A functional interplay between HLH proteins in the control of B-cell differentiation has also been demonstrated by the analysis of mice that are trans-heterozygous for E2A proteins and the bHLH proteins HEB and/or E2–2 *(91)*. Mice homozygous for a targeted mutation in the E2–2 or HEB genes, have a twofold decrease in the number of pro-B-cells in fetal liver as compared to wild type animals *(91)*. A similar modest B-cell phenotype has been observed in mice lacking one allele of E47, whereas no sigificant reduction in the number of B-cell numbers has been detected in fetal livers from mice heterozygous for a mutation in the HEB or E2-2 genes. However, mice that are trans-heterozygous for either E2A/E2-2 or E2A/HEB display a four-fold reduced number of B-cells in the fetal liver. These data were interpreted to suggest that E2-2 and HEB proteins can collaborate with E2A proteins in the control of B lymphocyte differentiation. The mechanism underlying the dose dependence of bHLH proteins is unclear, but the phenotypes of the trans-heterozygous mice may be explained by the ability of HEB and E2-2 proteins to titrate out Id the negative regulator, thereby increasing the available pool of E2A activator proteins. A similar decrease in the number of pre-B-cells was also observed in mice heterozygous for the mutation in the EBF gene *(21)*. Thus, the expression levels of both EBF and E2A proteins may be tightly regulated in vivo.

5. Collaboration Between EBF and E47 in the Activation of B-Cell Specific Genes

The similarity of the B-cell deficiency in EBF- and E2A-deficient mice raises the possibility that these transcription factors act in concert to regulate genes important for B-cell differentiation. This possibility has been addressed recently by ectopic expression of EBF and E47 in the immature hematopoietic cell line Ba/F3, which lacks EBF and BCF1 *(33)*. Stable or transient overexpression of EBF in Ba/F3 cells induces low levels of expression of the endogenous surrogate light chain genes, λ5 and VpreB. Expression of E47, or an E47 forced dimer alone, did not induce expression of the surrogate light chain genes, but in collaboration with EBF E47 induced λ5 and VpreB expression to levels that were similar to those observed in pre-B-cells. This functional cooperation between EBF and E47 was further supported by transient transfections of a λ5 promoter/enhancer reporter construct. EBF or E47 alone induced modest reporter activity, whereas coexpression of both transcriptional factors resulted in a marked upregulation of reporter activity *(33)*.

The λ5 and VpreB genes appear to be direct targets for EBF and E47 because both transcription factors interact directly with the enhancer/promoter region of these genes. The promoter/enhancer of the λ5 gene was shown to contain three functionally important EBF sites and four E-boxes *(33,92,93)*. The mechanism underlying the functional synergy between EBF and E2A is still unknown.

6. Concluding Remarks

In summary, the transcription factors EBF and E2A are essential for B-cell differentiation. Although several genetic targets for E2A and EBF proteins have been identified recently, the known targets are unlikely to account for the phenotype of the mice carrying targeted mutations in the EBF or E2A genes. Additional target genes may have to be identified to understand the regulatory role of these proteins in B-cell differentiation. The functional synergy between EBF and E2A proteins is reminiscent of the collaborations between regulatory proteins that have been observed in the control of several other cell differentiation systems. One aspect of the collaboration between EBF and E2A proteins might be the enhancement of the accuracy of B-cell-specific gene control in the mouse.

Acknowledgments

The authors thank Mary O'Riordan for critically reading the manuscript, Ross Okamura for his help with the preparation of the figures, and Jacqueline Bruszewski-Walters for preparation of the manuscript.

References

1. Hardy, R., Carmack, C., Shinton, S., Kemp, J., and Hayakawa, K. (1991) Resolution and characterization of pro-B and pre-pro-B cell stages in normal mouse bone marrow. *J. Exp. Med.* **173,** 1213–1225.
2. Li, Y.-S., Wasserman, R., Hayakawa, K., and Hardy, R. (1996) Identification of the earliest B lineage stage in mouse bone marrow. *Immunity* **5,** 572–535.
3. Alt, F., Oltz, E., Young, F., Gorman, J., Taccioli, G., and Chen, J. (1992) V-D-J recombination. *Immunol. Today* **13,** 306–314.
4. Melchers, F., Karasuyama, H., Haasner, D., Bauer, S., Kudo, A., Sakaguchi, N., Jameson, B., and Rolink, A. (1993) The surrogate light chain in B-cell development. *Immunol. Today* **14,** 60–68.
5. Rolink, A., Grawunder, U., Winkler, T. H., Karasuyama, H., and Melchers, F. (1994) IL-2 receptor a chain (CD25, TAC) expression defines a crucial stage in pre-B cell development. *Int. Immunol.* **6,** 1257–1264.
6. Borst, J., Jacobs, H., and Brouns, G. (1996) Composition and function of T cell receptor and B cell receptor complexes on precursor lymphocytes. *Curr. Opin. Immunol.* **8,** 181–190.
7. Berek, C. and Ziegner, M. (1993) The maturation of the immune response. *Immunol. Today* **14,** 400–404.
8. Hagman, J. and Grosschedl, R. (1994) Regulation of gene expression at early stages of B cell differentiation. *Curr. Opin. Immunol.* **6,** 222–230.
9. Singh, H. (1996) Gene targeting reveals a hierarchy of transcription factors regulating specification of lymphoid cell fates. *Curr. Opin. Immunol.* **8,** 160–165.
10. Fitzsimmons, D. and Hagman, J. (1996) Regulation of gene expression at early stages of B cell and T cell differentiation. *Curr. Opin. Immunol.* **8,** 166–174.
11. Georgopoulos, K., Moore, D., and Derfler, B. (1992) Ikaros, an early lymphoid specific transcription factor and a putative mediator for T cell commitment. *Science* **258,** 808–812.
12. Hahm, K., Ernst, P., Lo, K., Kim, G. S., Turck, C., and Smale, S. T. (1994) The lymphoid transcription factor LyF-1 is encoded by specific, alternatively spliced mRNAs derived from the Ikaros gene. *Mol. Cell Biol.* **14,** 7111–7123.
13. Georgopoulos, K., Bigby, M., Wang, J., Molnar, A., Wu, P., Winandy, S., and Sharpe, A. (1994) The IKAROS gene is required for the development of all lymphoid lineages. *Cell* **79,** 143–156.
14. Klemsz, M. J., McKercher,S. R. , Celada, A., Van Beveren, C., and Maki, R. A. (1990) The macrophage and B cell-specific transcription factor PU.1 is related to the *ets* oncogene. *Cell* **61,** 113–124.
15. Moreau-Gachelin, F. Spi-1/Pu.1 an oncogene of the ets family. (1994) *Biochim. Biophys. Acta* **1198,** 149–163.
16. Scott, E., Simon, M., Anastasi, J., and Singh, H. (1994) Requirement of transcription factor PU.1 in the development of multiple hematopoietic lineages. *Science* **265,** 1573–1577.

17. Hagman, J., Belanger, C., Travis, A., Turck, C., and Grosschedl, R. (1993) Cloning and functional characterization of early B-cell factor, a regulator of lymphocyte-specific gene expression. *Genes Dev.* **7,** 760–773.
18. Murre, C., Schonleber Mc-Caw, P., and Baltimore, D. (1989a) A new DNA binding and dimerization motif in immunoglobulin enhancer binding, daughterless, MyoD, and myc proteins. *Cell* **56,** 777–783.
19. Bain G., Robanus Maandag, E., Izon, D., Amsen, D., Kruisbeek, A., Weintraub, B., Krop, I., Schlissel, M., Feeney, A., van Roon, M., van der Valk, M., te Riele, H., Berns, A., and Murre, C. (1994) E2A proteins are required for proper B cell development and initiation of immunoglobulin gene rearrangements. *Cell* **79,** 885–892.
20. Zhuang, Y., Soriano, P., and Weintraub, H. (1994) The helix-loop-helix gene E2A is required for B cell formation. *Cell* **79,** 875–884.
21. Lin, H. and Grosschedl, R. (1995) Failure of B-cell differentiation in mice lacking the transcription factor EBF. *Nature* **376,** 263–267.
22. Busslinger, M. and Urbanek, P. (1995) The role of BSAP (Pax-5) in B cell development. *Curr. Opin. Genet. Dev.* **5,** 595–601.
23. Urbanek, P., Wang, Z.-Q., Fetka, I., Wagner, E., and Busslinger, M. (1994) Complete block of early B cell differentiation and altered patterning of the posterior midbrain in mice lacking Pax5/BSAP. *Cell* **79,** 901–912.
24. Nutt, S., Urbanek, P., Rolink, A., and Busslinger, M. (1997) Essential functions of Pax-5 (BSAP) in pro-B cell development: difference between fetal and adult B lymphopoesis and reduced V- to DJ recombination in the IgH locus. *Genes Dev.* **11,** 476–491.
25. Hagman, J., Travis, A., and Grosschedl, R. (1991) A novel lineage-specific nuclear factor regulates mb-1 gene transcription at the early stages of B cell differentiation. *EMBO J.* **10,** 3409–3417.
26. Feldhaus, A., Mbangkollo, D., Arvin, K., Klug, C. H. S., and Singh, H. (1992) BlyF, a novel cell-type- and stage-specific regulator of the B-lymphocyte gene *mb-1*. *Mol. Cell Biol.* **12,** 1126–1133.
27. Kudrycki, K., Stein-Izsak, C., Behn, C., Grillo, M., Akeson, R., and Margolis, F. (1993) Olf-1 binding site: Characterisation of an olfactory neuron specific promoter motif. *Mol. Cell. Biol.* **13,** 3002–3014.
28. Wang, M. and Reed, R. (1993) Molecular cloning of the olfactory neuronal transcription factor Olf-1 by genetic selection in yeast. *Nature* **364,** 121–126.
29. Travis, A., Hagman, J., Hwang, L., and Grosschedl, R. (1993) Purification of early-B-cell factor and characterization of its DNA-binding specificity. *Mol. Cell. Biol.* **13,** 3392–3400.
30. Crozatier, M., Valle, D., Dubois, L., Ibnsouda, S., and Vincent, A. (1996) Collier, a novel regulator of Drosophila head development, is expressed in a single mitotic domain. *Curr. Biol.* **6,** 707–718.
31. Hagman, J., Gutch, M., Lin, H., and Grosschedl, R. (1995) EBF contains a novel zinc coordination motif and multiple dimerization and transcriptional activation domains. *EMBO J.* **14,** 2907–2916.
32. Sigvardsson, M., Åkerblad, P., and Leanderson, T. (1996) Early B cell Factor interacts with a subset of κ promoters. *J. Immunol.* **156,** 3788–3796.
33. Sigvardsson, M., O'Riordan, M., and Grosschedl, R. (1997) EBF and E47 collaborate to induce expression of the endogenous immunoglobulin surrogate light chain genes. *Immunity*, **7,** 25–36.
34. Molnar, A. and Georgopoulos, K. (1994) The IKAROS gene encodes a family of functionally diverse zinc finger DNA-binding proteins. *Mol. Cell. Biol.* **14,** 8292–8303.
35. Morgan, B., Sun, L., Avitahl, N., Andrikopolous, K., Ikeda, T., Gonzales, E., Wu, P., Neben, S., and Georgopolous, K. (1997) Aiolos, a lymphoid restricted transcription factor that interacts with Ikaros to regulate lymphocyte differentiation. *EMBO J.* **16,** 2004–2013.
36. Sun, L., Aiping, L., and Georgopoulos, K. (1996) Zinc finger-mediated protein interactions modulate Ikaros activity, a molecular control of lymphocyte development. *EMBO J.* **15,** 5358–5369.
37. Travis, A., Hagman, J., and Grosschedl, R. (1991) Heterogeneously initiated transcription from the Pre-B- and B-cell-specific *mb-1* promoter: Analysis of the requirement for upstream factor-binding sites and initiation site sequences. *Mol. Cell Biol.* **11,** 5756–5766.
38. Fitzsimmons, D., Hodsdon, W., Wheat, W., Maira, S.-M., Wasylyk, B., and Hagman, J. (1996) Pax-5 (BSAP) recruits Ets proto-oncogene family proteins to form functional ternary complexes on a B-cell-specific promoter. *Genes Dev.* **10,** 2198–2211.
39. Kozmik, Z., Wang, S., Dorfler, P., Adams, B., and Busslinger, M. (1992) The promoter of the CD19 gene is a target for the B cell specific transcription factor BSAP. *Mol. Cell. Biol.* **12,** 2662–2672.

40. Zwollo, P. and Desiderio, S. (1994) Specific recognition of the blk promoter by the B lymphoid transcription factor B-cell-specific activator protein. *J. Biol. Chem.* **269,** 15310–15317.
41. Rinkenberger, J., Wallin, J., Johnson, K., and Koshland, M. (1996) An interleukin-2 signal relieves the BSAP (Pax5)-mediated repression of the immunoglobulin J chain gene. *Immunity* **5,** 377–386.
42. Singh, M. and Birshtein, B. K. (1993) NF-HB (BSAP) is a repressor of the murine immunoglobulin heavy-chain 3'α enhancer at early stages of B-cell differentiation. *Mol. Cell Biol.* **13,** 3611–3622.
43. Neurath, M., Stuber, E., and Wakatsuki, Y. (1994) The murine Ig 3' α enhancer is a target site with repressor function for the B cell lineage-specific transcription factor BSAP. *J. Immunol.* **153,** 730–742.
44. Neurath, M. F., Max, E. E., and Strober, W. (1995) Pax5 (BSAP) regulates the murine immunoglobulin 3'α enhancer by suppressing binding of NF-αP, a protein that controls heavy chain transcription. *Proc. Natl. Acad. Sci. USA* **92,** 5336–5340.
45. Henthorn, P., Kiledjian, M., and Kadesch, T. (1990) Two distinct transcription factors that bind the immunoglobulin enhancer μE5/κE2 motif. *Science* **247,** 467–470.
46. Nelson, C., Shen, L.-P., Meister, A., Fodor, E., and Rutter, W. J. (1990) Pan: a transcriptional regulator that binds chymotrypsin, insulin, and AP-4 enhancer motifs. *Genes Dev.* **4,** 1035–1043.
47. Hu, J.-S., Olson, E. N., and Kingston, R. E. (1992) HEB, a helix-loop-helix protein related to E2A and ITF2 that can modulate the DNA-binding ability of myogenia regulatory factors. *Mol. Cell. Biol.* **12,** 1031–1042.
48. Murre, C., Bain, G., van Dijk, M., Engel, I., Furnari, B., Massari, M., Matthews, J., Quong, M., Rivera, R., and Stuiver, M. (1994) Structure and function of helix-loop-helix proteins. *Bioch. et Bioph. Acta* 1**218,** 129–135.
49. Lüscher, B. and Eisenman, R. (1990) New light on myc and myb. Part 1 myc. *Genes Dev.* **4,** 2025–2035.
50. Benezra, R., Davis, R., Lockshon, D., Turner, D., and Weintraub, H. (1990) The protein Id: a negative regulator of helix-loop-helix DNA binding proteins. *Cell* **61,** 49–59.
51. Wilson, R., Kiledjian, M., Shen, C.-P., Benezra, R., Zwollo, P., Dymecki, S., Desiderio, S., and Kadesch, T. (1991) Repression of immunoglobulin enhancers by the helix-loop-helix protein Id: implications for B-lymphoid-cell development. *Mol. Cell. Biol.* **11,** 6185–6191.
52. Bain G., Gruenwald, S., and Murre, C. (1993) E2A and E2-2 are subunits of B-cell-specific E2-box DNA-binding proteins. *Mol. Cell. Biol.* **13,** 3522–3529.
53. Jacobs, Y., Xin, X.-Q., Dorshkind, K., and Nelson, C. (1994) Pan/E2A expression precedes immunoglobulin heavy-chain expression during B lymphopoiesis in nontransformed cells, and Pan/E2A proteins are not detected in myeloid cells. *Mol. Cell Biol.* **14,** 4087–4096.
54. Murre, C., Schonleber Mc-Caw, P., Vaessin, H., Caudy, M., Jan, L., Jan, Y., Cabrera, C., Buskin, J., Hauschka, S., Lassar, A., Weintraub, H., and Baltimore, D. (1989b) Interactions between heterologous helix-loop-helix proteins generate complexes that bind specifically to a common DNA sequence. *Cell* **58,** 537–544.
55. Brennan, T. and Olson, E. (1990) Myogenin resides in the nucleus and acquires high affinity for a conserved enhancer element upon heterodimerization. *Genes Dev.* **4,** 582–595.
56. Lassar, A., Davis, R., Wright, W., Kadesch, W. T., Murre, C., Vovonova, A., Baltimore, D., and Weintraub, H. (1991) Functional activity of myogenic bHLH proteins requires hetero-oligomerization with E12/E47-like proteins in vivo. *Cell* **66,** 305–315.
57. Shen, C.-P. and Kadesch, T. (1995) B cell specififc DNA binding by an E47 homodimer. *Mol. Cell. Biol.* **15,** 4518–4524.
58. Benezra, R. (1995) An intermolecular disulfide bond stabilizes E2A homodimers and is required for DNA binding at physiological temperatures. *Cell* **79,** 1057–1067.
59. Sloan, S., Shen, C.-P., McGarrick-Walmsley, R., and Kadesch, T. (1996) Phosphorylation of E47 as a potential determinant of B cell specific activity. *Mol. Cell. Biol.* **16,** 6900–6908.
60. Murre, C., Voronova, A., and Baltimore, D. (1991) B-cell- and myocyte-specific E2-box-binding factors contain E12/E47-like subunits. *Mol. Cell. Biol.* **11,** 1156–1160.
61. Saisanit, S. and Sun, X.-H. (1995) A novel enhancer, the pro-B enhancer, regulates Id1 gene expression in progenitor B cells. *Mol. Cell Biol.* **15,** 1513–1521.
62. Ephrussi, A., Church, G., Tonegawa, S., and Gilbert, W. (1985) B-lineage-specific interactions of a immunoglobulin enhancer with cellular factors in vivo. *Science* **227,** 134–140.

63. Alex, R., Sozeri, O., Meyer, S., and Dildrop, R. (1992) Determination of the DNA sequence recognized by the bHLH domain of the N-myc protein. *Nucleic Acids Res.* **20,** 2257–2263.
64. Blackwell, T., Huang, J., Ma, A., Kretzner, L., Alt, F., Eisenman, R., and Weintraub, H. (1993) Binding of myc proteins to canonical and noncanonical DNA sequences. *Mol. Cell. Biol.* **13,** 5216–5224.
65. Davis, R., Cheng, P., Lassar, A., and Weintraub, H. (1990) The MyoD DNA binding domain contains a recognition code for muscle specific gene activation. *Cell* **60,** 733–746.
66. Ellenberger, T., Fass, D., Arnaud, M., and Harrison, S. (1994) Crystal structure of transcription factor E47: E-box recognition by a basic region helix-loop-helix dimer. *Genes Dev.* **8,** 970–980.
67. Quong, M., Massari, M., Zwart, R., and Murre, C. (1993) A new transcriptional activation motif restricted to a class of Helix-loop-helix proteins is functionally conserved in both yeast and mammalian cells. *Mol. Cell. Biol.* **13,** 792–800.
68. Olsen, E. (1990) MyoD family: a paradigm for development? *Genes Dev.* **4,** 1454–1461.
69. Wright, W. (1992) Muscle basic helix-loop-helix proteins and the regulation of myogenisis. *Curr. Opin. Genet. Dev.* **2,** 243–248.
70. Peverali, F., Ramqvist, T., Saffrich, R., Pepperkok, R., Barone, M., and Philipson, L. (1994) Regulation of G1 progression by E2A and Id helix-loop-helix proteins. *EMBO J.* **13,** 4291–4301.
71. Sun, X.-H. (1994) Constitutive expression of the Id1 gene impairs mouse B cell development. *Cell* **79,** 893–900.
72. Ernst, P. and Smale, S. (1995) Combinatorial regulation of transcription II: the immunoglobulin μ heavy chain gene. *Immunity* **2,** 427–438.
73. Adams, J., Harris, A., Pinkert, C., Corcoran, L., Alexander, W., Cory, S., Palmiter, R., and Brinster, R. (1985) The c-myc oncogene driven by immunoglobulin enhancers induces lymphoid malignancy in transgenic mice. *Nature* **318,** 533–538.
74. Stanton, L., Watt, R., and Marcu, K. (1983) Translocation, breakage and truncated transcripts of c-myc oncogene in murine plasma-cytomas. *Nature* **303,** 401–406.
75. Schlissel, M., Voronova, A., and Baltimore, D. (1991) Helix-loop-helix transcription factor E47 activates germ-line immunoglobulin heavy-chain gene transcription and rearrangement in a pre-T-cell line. *Genes Dev.* **5,** 1367–1376.
76. Choi, J., Shen, C.-P., Radomska, H., Eckhardt, L., and Kadesch, T. (1996) E47 activates the Ig-heavy chain and TdT loci in non-B cells. *EMBO J.* **15,** 5014–5021.
77. Lennon, G. and Perry, R. (1985) C μ-containing transcripts initiate heterogeneously within the IgH enhancer region and contain a novel 5'-nontranslatable exon. *Nature* **318,** 475–478.
78. Su, L. and Kadesch, T. (1990) The immunoglobulin heavy chain enhancer functions as the promoter for Iμ sterile transcription. *Mol. Cell. Biol.* **10,** 2619–2624.
79. Alt, F., Blackwell, T., and Yancopoulos, G. (1987) Development of the primary antibody repertoire. *Science* **238,** 1079–1087.
80. Lenardo, M., Pierce, J., and Baltimore, D. (1987) Protein binding sites in Ig gene enhancers determine transcriptional activity and inducibility. *Science* **236,** 1573–1577.
81. Park, K. and Atchison, M. L. (1991) Isolation of a candidate repressor/activator, NF-E1 (YY-1, δ), that binds to the immunoglobulin κ 3' enhancer and the immunoglobulin heavy-chain μ E1 site. *Proc. Natl. Acad. Sci. USA* **88,** 9804–9808.
82. Nelsen, B., Tian, G., Erman, B., Gregoire, J., Maki, R., Graves, B., and Sen, R. (1993) Regulation of lymphoid specific Immunoglobulin m heavy chain gene enhancer by ets-domain proteins. *Science* **261,** 82–86.
83. Rivera, R. S., Stuiver, M. H., Steenbergen, R., and Murre, C. (1993) Ets proteins: New factors that regulate immunoglobulin heavy-chain gene expression. *Mol. Cell Biol.* **13,** 7163–7169.
84. Erman, B. and Sen, R. (1996) Context-dependent transactivation domains activate the immunoglobulin-μ heavy-chain gene enhancer. *EMBO J.* **15,** 4665–4675.
85. Kadesch, T. (1992) Helix-loop-helix proteins in the regulation of immunoglobulin gene transcription. *Immunol. Today* **13,** 31–36.
86. Sun, X.-H., Copeland, N. A., Jenkins, N. A., and Baltimore, D. (1991) Id proteins Id1 and Id2 selectively inhibit DNA binding by one class of helix-loop-helix proteins. *Mol. Cell Biol.* **11,** 5603–5611.
87. Ruezinsky, D., Beckmann, H., and Kadesch, T. (1991) Modulation of the IgH enhancer's cell type specificity through a genetic switch. *Genes Dev.* **5,** 29–37.
88. Williams, T. W., Moolten, D., Burlien, J., Romano, J., Bhaerman, R., Godillot, A., Mellon, M., Rauscher, F. J., III, and Kant, J. A. (1991) Identification of a zinc finger protein that inhibits IL-2 gene expression. *Science* **254,** 1791–1794.

89. Genetta, T., Ruezinsky, D., and Kadesch, T. (1994) Displacement of an E-box-binding repressor by basic helix-loop-helix proteins: implications for B-cell specificity of the immunoglobulin heavy-chain enhancer. *Mol. Cell. Biol.* **14,** 6153–6163.
90. Bain G., Robanus Maandag, E., te Riele, H., Feeney, A., Sheeny, A., Schlissel, M., Shinton, A., Hardy, R., and Murre, C. (1997) Both E12 and E47 allow commitment to the B cell lineage. *Immunity* **6,** 145–154.
91. Zhuang, Y., Cheng, P., and Weintraub, H. (1996) B-lymphocyte development is regulated by the combined dosage of three basic helix-loop-helix genes, E2A, E2-2, and HEB. *Mol. Cell. Biol.* **16,** 2898–2905.
92. Kudo, A., Sakaguchi, N., and Melchers, F. (1987) Organization of the murine Ig-related λ5 gene transcribed selectively in pre-B lymphocytes. *EMBO J.* **6,** 103–107.
93. Yang, J., Glozak, M., and Blomberg, B. (1995) Identification and localization of a developmental stage-specific promoter activity from the murine λ5 gene. *J. Immunol.* **155,** 2498–2514.

Chapter 6

Role of the Transcription Factor BSAP (Pax-5) in B-Cell Development

Meinrad Busslinger and Stephen L. Nutt

1. Introduction

The development of B-lymphocytes from hematopoietic stem cells is a highly ordered and coordinated process that results in antigen-responsive B-cells with individual immunoglobulin receptors. This developmental pathway can be dissected into several stages according to the differential expression of specific cell surface markers, the distinctive growth factor requirements, and the sequential rearrangement of immunoglobulin heavy *(IgH)* and light *(IgL)* chain genes (reviewed in ref. *1*). To date, two different classification schemes are in use that rely on the analysis of different sets of cell surface markers (Fig. 1). Hardy et al. *(2,3)* have employed the differential expression of CD43, heat stable antigen (HSA), BP-1, IgM, and IgD to divide B-cell development into seven distinct stages (A–F) (Fig. 1, bottom). Instead, Rolink et al. *(4)* have ordered the different B-lymphocyte subpopulations in the bone marrow by cell size and expression of c-*kit,* CD25, and the surrogate light chains VpreB and λ5 (Fig. 1, top). These analyses demonstrated that the earliest B-cell progenitors are large cycling cells and are in the process of D_H-to-J_H rearrangement of the *IgH* locus and can be cloned in vitro on stromal cells in the presence of IL-7. An important checkpoint in early B-cell development ensures the positive selection of those late pro-B- (pre-BII-) cells that have completed a productive V_H-to-D_HJ_H rearrangement, and thus transiently express the μ protein as part of the pre-B-cell receptor complex (Fig. 1). Signaling through this pre-B-cell receptor promotes allelic exclusion at the *IgH* locus, triggers proliferative cell expansion and induces differentiation to small pre-B-cells, which undergo *IgL* (κ or λ) gene rearrangements. Immature B-cells subsequently emerge that synthesize the IgM form of the B-cell receptor and become subjected to selection by antigen. The expression of homing receptors enables these cells to populate peripheral lymphoid organs where they participate as mature B-cells in immunological reactions and undergo terminal differentiation to immunoglobulin-secreting plasma cells (reviewed in ref. *5*).

From: *Molecular Biology of B-Cell and T-Cell Development*
Edited by: J. G. Monroe and E. V. Rothenberg © Humana Press Inc., Totowa, NJ

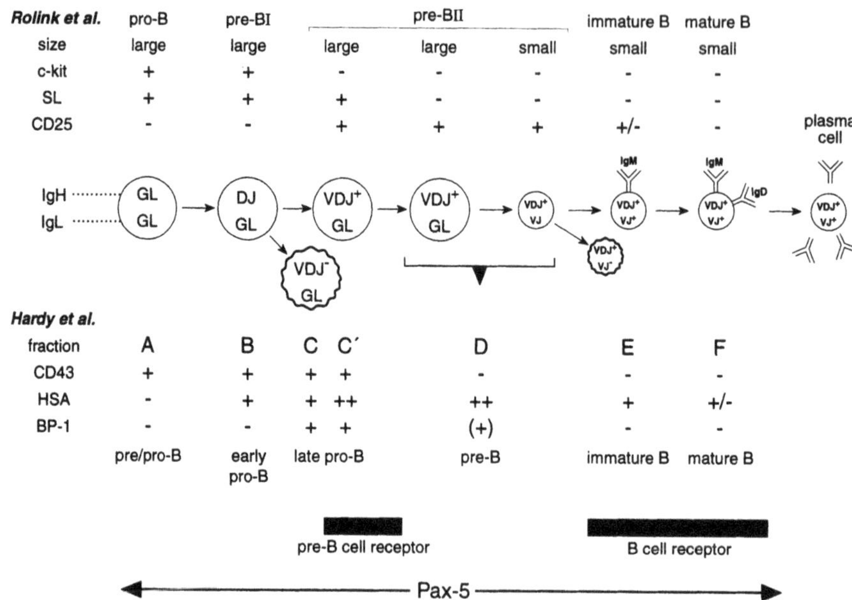

Fig. 1. Schematic diagram of murine B-cell development. The different developmental stages of B-lymphopoiesis are shown together with their characteristic cell surfacer markers which are used for the classification according to Rolink et al. *(4)* (top) or Hardy et al. *(2)* (bottom). Large and small circles represent proliferating and resting cells, respectively. Cells destined to die are indicated by wavy outlines. Gray shading highlights the early pro-B-cell stage at which B-cell development is arrested in the Pax-5-deficient bone marrow *(40)*. GL, germline; SL, surrogate light chain; HSA, heat-stable antigen.

The differential gene regulation underlying B-cell development occurs primarily at the transcriptional level. A number of B-lymphoid and stage-specific transcription factor have been identified as critical determinants of B-cell-specific gene expression by detailed analysis of *cis*-regulatory regions of B-lymphoid effector genes (reviewed in ref. *6*). Targeted inactivation of the corresponding transcription factor genes in the mouse germline demonstrated that these regulators fulfill important functions in the control of different aspects of B-cell development. Among these transcription factors is the B-cell-specific activator protein (BSAP), which is encoded by the *Pax-5* gene. The hierarchy of transcriptional control in B-lymphopoiesis has been the focus of several recent reviews *(7–9)*. In this chapter, the authors will therefore discuss only the literature dealing with the role of BSAP (Pax-5) in B-cell development and in the regulation of B-lymphoid gene expression.

2. Discovery of the Transcription Factor BSAP

2.1. Identification of BSAP as the Product of the Pax-5 *Gene*

The B-cell-specific activator protein BSAP was initially discovered as a DNA-binding activity displaying the same DNA sequence recognition as the sea urchin transcription factor (TSAP) that is involved in the developmental regulation of two pairs of histone H2A and H2B genes *(10,11)*. The DNA-binding activity of BSAP was detected in cell lines corresponding to the pro-B-, pre-B-, and mature B-cell stages, but not in cell lines

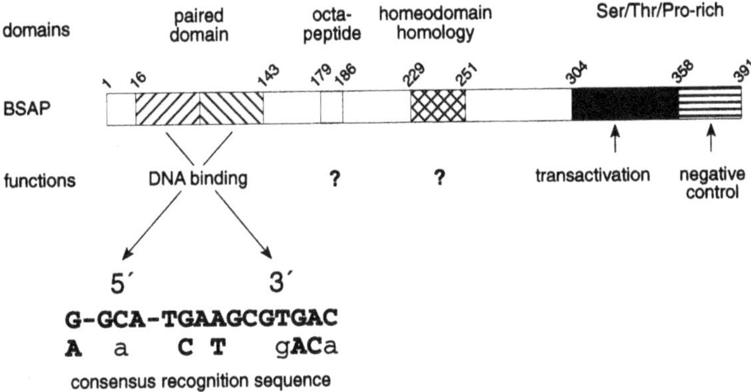

Fig. 2. Structure of BSAP and its consensus recognition sequence. A schematic diagram of the different domains of BSAP is shown together with the corresponding amino acid positions *(12)* and an up-dated consensus recognition sequence of the paired domain *(128)*.

derived from terminally differentiated plasma cells or other hematopoietic lineages *(11)*. The biochemical characterization of this DNA-binding activity revealed that BSAP consists of a single glycosylated polypeptide with an apparent molecular weight of 50 kD *(11,12)*. Protein purification and cDNA cloning identified BSAP as the protein product of *Pax-5 (12)*. The mammalian *Pax* genes code for a small family of nine developmental regulators that are defined by the presence of a highly conserved DNA-binding motif of 128 amino acids, the so-called paired domain *(13,14)*. BSAP (Pax-5) shares high sequence similarity with Pax-2 and Pax-8, which constitute together a subclass of Pax proteins *(12)*. Members of the *Pax-2/5/8* gene family have since been isolated from the sea urchin, *C. elegans* and *Drosophila* genomes, thus pointing to an ancient evolutionary origin of these genes *(15)*. Interestingly, the paired domains of these evolutionarily distant members are almost identical in sequence and consequently recognize DNA in a similar manner, thus explaining why BSAP (Pax-5) could be identified as a mammalian homologue of the sea urchin TSAP protein by DNA-binding assays.

2.2. Identity of other DNA-Binding Activities with BSAP

DNA-binding activities with a similar sequence specificity and B-lymphoid expression pattern as BSAP were independently found by several groups in their search for B-cell-specific proteins that are involved in different aspects of *IgH* and *IgL* gene regulation (*see* Subheading 6.2., 8.1., 9.1., and 9.2.). These DNA-binding activities have been referred to as KLP *(16)*, Sα-BP *(17)*, HF-HB *(18)*, NFSμ-B_1 *(19)*, and EBB-1 *(20)*. In the meantime, all of these DNA-binding proteins have been shown to be identical with BSAP as they recognize genuine BSAP-binding sites and react with BSAP-specific antibodies *(21–23)*.

3. DNA-Binding and Transactivation Properties of BSAP

Like other transcription factors, BSAP possesses also a modular structure (Fig. 2). It contains a paired domain at the N-terminus, an evolutionary conserved octapeptide, a central region homologous to the first half of the paired-type homeodomain of other Pax proteins, and a serine/threonine/proline-rich region at the C-terminus *(12)*. Mutational analysis localized the DNA-binding and transactivation functions within the N- and C-terminal sequences of BSAP, respectively *(12,24)*. No function has yet been assigned to the conserved octapeptide and the homeodomain homology region. However, it is conceivable that these motifs are involved in the interaction of BSAP with other transcription factors or components of the basal transcription machinery.

The DNA-binding function of the conserved paired domain was first discovered by in vitro mutagenesis of the *Drosophila* Paired *(14)* and mammalian Pax-1 *(25)* proteins. However, the sequence recognition by the paired domain was considered at the time to be highly degenerate, as no reasonable consensus sequence could be deduced from several known Pax-binding sites. This paradoxical situation could be resolved by detailed mutational analysis of BSAP, which uncovered the bipartite nature of the paired domain and its recognition sequence and which resulted in the definition of a consensus sequence *(21)*. According to this model, the paired domain is composed of two subdomains that bind to two distinct half-sites in adjacent major grooves of the DNA helix (Fig. 2). The recognition sequence for BSAP spans 17 nucleotides and is thus exceptionally long compared to other DNA-binding proteins *(21)*. Moreover, both half-sites contribute to the overall affinity of a given BSAP-binding site according to their match with the consensus sequence *(21)*. However, none of the naturally occurring binding sites completely conforms to the consensus sequence. Instead, they contain compensatory base changes in one of the two half-sites, thus explaining the seemingly degenerate DNA sequence recognition of Pax proteins *(21)*. X-ray crystallographic analysis of the paired domain-DNA complex has subsequently confirmed the bipartite model of the paired domain by demonstrating that each of the two subdomains consists of a helix-turn-helix motif resembling the structure of the homeodomain *(26)*.

A potent transactivation domain of 55 amino acids was identified within the C-terminal sequences of BSAP by in vitro mutagenesis and transient transfection experiments *(24)*. The function of this transactivation domain is negatively regulated by adjacent sequences from the extreme C-terminus (Fig. 2). Moreover, the C-terminal regulatory module consisting of activating and inhibitory sequence is functional in many different cell types and has been conserved in all vertebrate members of the Pax-2/5/8 family *(24)*. Negatively regulated transactivation domains are usually a characteristic feature of inducible transcription factors that are activated in response to intracellular signaling. Hence, the presence of a regulated transactivation function in BSAP suggests that this transcription factor may also be at the receiving end of signal transduction in the nucleus. However, no direct link between signaling in B-lymphocytes and transcriptional activation of BSAP could so far be demonstrated *(24)*.

4. B-Lymphoid Expression Pattern of *Pax-5*

4.1. Pax-5 *Expression During B-Cell Development*

The expression of *Pax-5* was initially studied in transformed cell lines of murine and human origin, which represent different developmental stages of B-lymphopoiesis *(11,12)*. These analyses indicated that the *Pax-5* mRNA and the BSAP protein are expressed in these established cell lines at a constant level from the pro-B to the mature B-cell stage. BSAP expression was, however, neither detected in plasmacytoma and myeloma cells nor in cell lines of other hematopoietic lineages. The strict lineage fidelity of BSAP expression within a large panel of transformed cell lines suggested at the time that Pax-5 may play an essential role in defining the B-cell phenotype *(11)*. This hypothesis has subsequently been confirmed by gene inactivation experiments (*see* Subheading 5.).

Some aspects of the *Pax-5* expression pattern have also been analyzed in primary B-lymphocytes. Recent advances in cell sorting and the availability of an anti-CD19 antibody made it possible to isolate and characterize the earliest B-lineage progenitor cells from the bone marrow of the mouse *(28,29)*. These analyses revealed that the earliest cell fraction A, as defined by Hardy et al. *(2)* (Fig. 1), is heterogeneous, containing precursors of natural killer cells and B-lymphocytes. Based on differences in the cell surface phentoype, the earliest B-lymphoid progenitors could be further subdivided into an earlier fraction A1, and a later fraction A2. BSAP transcripts could already be detected in cells of fraction A1, indicating that *Pax-5* expression is initiated during the commitment phase of B-lymphopoiesis *(29)*. Moreover, a recent analysis of large pro-B- and small pre-B-cells suggests that the DNA-binding activity of BSAP may be down-modulated upon signaling through the pre-B-cell receptor *(30)*. In addition, mitogenic activation of resting splenic B-cells was shown to moderately increase the DNA-binding activity of BSAP *(31)*. Hence, *Pax-5* expression appears to be fine-tuned in primary B-lymphocytes in response to signal transduction, which contrasts with the constitutive expression observed in established B-cell lines.

4.2. The Regulation of Pax-5 Expression During Terminal B-Cell Differentiation

The shut-off of *Pax-5* transcription during terminal differentiation is still a controversial issue, as the absence of *Pax-5* expression in plasmacytoma and myeloma cell lines is difficult to verify in primary plasma cells for two principal reasons. First, plasma cells are short-lived and not very abundant in B-lymphoid tissues. Second, plasma cells cannot be unequivocally enriched or even isolated by immunological methods, as no cell surface marker specific for plasma cells is known to date. In the absence of such a marker, two group have isolated cells with a plasma cell-like morphology by sorting human bone marrow for cells with high CD38 expression levels *(32,33)*. However, it is important to note that CD38 is also present on activated B-cells and cells of other hematopoietic lineages. Human "plasma" cells defined by this criterion transcribe *PAX-5* and its target gene *CD19*, whereas primary myeloma cells lack *PAX-5* and *CD19* expression altogether *(34)*. This finding is in apparent contradiction with observations made with in vitro differentiation of mouse splenic B-cells. In this case, *Pax-5* expression is repressed upon stimulation of mature B-cells to undergo terminal plasma cell differentiation *(35,36)*. Hence, it remains to be seen whether the observed discrepancy reflects a difference between human and murine plasma cells or, more likely, results from the different experimental definitions of plasma cells.

4.3. Transcription of the Pax-5 Gene from Two Distinct Promoters

The *Pax-5* gene is transcribed from two differentially regulated promoters, resulting in the splicing of two alternative 5' exons (1A and 1B) to the common coding sequences of exons 2–10 *(37)* (Fig. 3). The upstream promoter is almost exclusively used in B-lymphoid tissues, whereas the downstream promoter is not only active in B-lymphocytes, but also in the developing CNS and adult testis. Using a transgenic approach, the authors have recently searched for regulatory elements within the 5' region of the *Pax-5* gene. However, twenty-five kb of DNA sequences upstream of exon 2 were unable to elicit B-cell-specific expression of a *lacZ* gene in transgenic mice, whereas a midbrain-specific enhancer could be localized to a 600-bp fragment within this 5' region (P. Pfeffer and M. Busslinger, unpublished data). Interestingly, however, 12 kb of 5' flanking

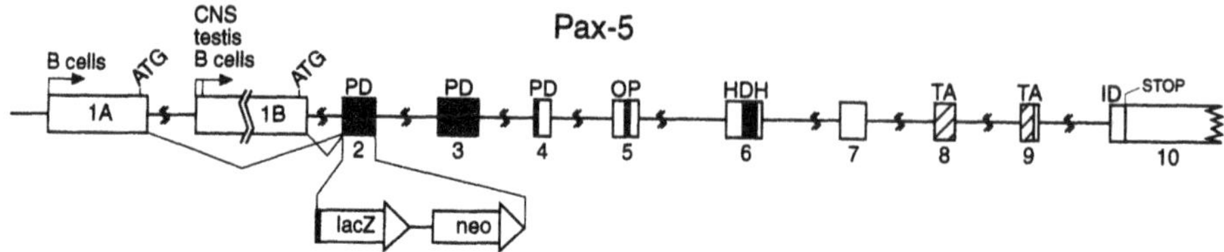

Fig. 3. Structure of the *Pax-5* gene. The exon-intron structure of the entire *Pax-5* gene is shown together with the tissue specificity of its two promoters. The translation start codon is provided by the alternatively used exons 1A and 1B, which are spliced onto the common coding sequences of exons 2–10. The exons coding for the paired domain (PD), conserved octapeptide (OP), homeodomain homology region (HDH), transactivation domain (TA), and inhibitory domain (ID) are shown. For details *see* ref. *37*. As indicated, the mouse *Pax-5* gene was inactivated by an in-frame insertion of *lacZ* coding sequences at the 5' end of exon 2 *(38)*.

sequences (upstream of exon 1A) were sufficient to promote transcription of a reporter gene in stably transfected B-cell lines to the same high level as the endogenous *Pax-5* gene (S. Vambrie and M. Busslinger, unpublished data). Hence, at least two control regions are required for B-cell-specific transcription of *Pax-5,* i.e., the immediate 5' flanking sequences and a currently unidentified regulatory element within the locus that renders the *Pax-5* gene accessible to the transcription machinery in primary B-lymphocytes.

5. Essential Functions of *Pax-5* in Early B-Cell Development

5.1. Pax-5 *is Essential for Progression of Adult B-Lymphopoiesis Beyond the Early Pro-B-Cell Stage*

The expression pattern of *Pax-5* suggests a role for this transcription factor in neural development, B-lymphopoiesis, and spermatogenesis. To study the in vivo function of *Pax-5*, the authors have inactivated this gene in the mouse germline by replacing exon 2 with *lacZ* coding sequences in embryonic stem (ES) cells (Fig. 3). The phenotypic analysis of Pax-5 (–/–) mutant mice revealed an essential role for Pax-5 in midbrain patterning and B-cell development, whereas spermatogenesis was unaffected *(38)*. However, the midbrain phenotype of Pax-5-deficient embryos is relatively mild, suggesting that the loss of Pax-5 function in the developing midbrain is partially compensated for by expression of the closely related *Pax-2* gene. Indeed, the midbrain and cerebellum entirely fails to develop in *Pax-2*, *Pax-5* double mutant embryos *(39)*. In contrast to the situation in the developing CNS, *Pax-5* is the only member of the *Pax* gene family that is expressed in the B-lymphoid lineage *(12)*.

Pax-5 mutant mice fail to produce small pre-B-, B-, and plasma cells and lack immunoglobulins in their serum because of a complete arrest of B-cell development at an early stage *(38)*. The conventional $CD5^-$ B-lymphocytes (B-2 cells) and the $CD5^+$ B-1 cells are equally affected in these mice, indicating that *Pax-5* is required for the differentiation of both B-cell subpopulations. However, the bone marrow of Pax-5-deficient mice generates large $CD43^+$ pro-B-cells *(38)*. The precise developmental stage of the differentiation block was investigated by detailed expression analysis of cell surface proteins and by the growth factor requirement of Pax-5-deficient pro-B-cells *(40)*. Flow cytometric analyses indicated that B-cell development in the bone marrow is arrested at the early pro-B- (pre-BI-) cell stage (Figs. 1 and 4). Moreover, these Pax-5-deficient pro-B-cells

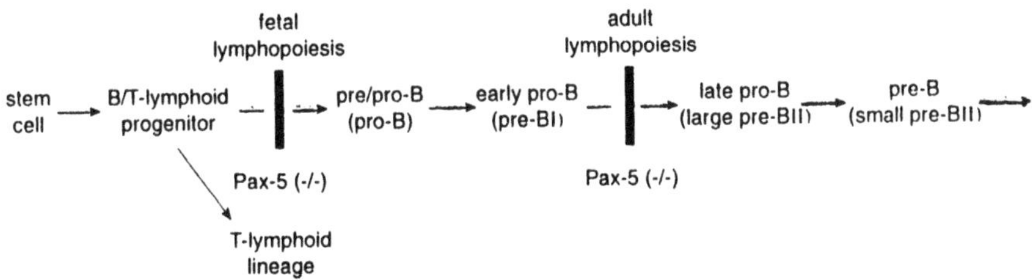

Fig. 4. Differential dependency of fetal and adult pro-B-cell development on Pax-5. A schematic diagram of early B-cell development is shown together with the developmental block observed in fetal and adult B-lymphopoiesis of *Pax-5* mutant mice. The different developmental stages are referred to in the nomenclature of Hardy et al. *(2)* and Rolink et al. *(4)* (in brackets)

are capable of long-term proliferation in vitro in the presence of stromal cells and IL-7. Furthermore, bone marrow transplantation experiments demonstrated that the developmental block in adult B-lymphopoiesis results from a direct, B-cell autonomous effect of the *Pax-5* mutation instead of being the indirect consequence of an interference with stromal cell differentiation *(40)*.

5.2. Pax-5 *is Required for B-Lineage Commitment in the Fetal Liver*

B-cell development is arrested at an earlier stage in the fetal liver of *Pax-5* mutant embryos than in adult bone marrow (Fig. 4). B-lymphoid progenitors could neither be detected by flow cytometry nor analysis of B-cell-specific transcripts in the Pax-5-deficient fetal liver *(40)*. Moreover, no pro-B-cell cultures could be established in vitro, thus confirming that the absence of Pax-5 leads to the loss of the earliest B-lineage-committed precursor cells in the fetal liver *(40)*. However, Pax-5-deficient fetal liver cells could give rise to the development of early pro-B-cells in the bone marrow upon transplantation into lethally irradiated mice *(40)*. Hence, Pax-5 is required at two distinct developmental stages in the different microenvironments of fetal and adult B-lymphopoiesis. In the fetal liver, *Pax-5* is required right from the onset of its transcription for B lineage commitment (Fig. 4). In contrast, Pax-5 expression in the bone marrow does not appear to fulfill a critical function early in pro-B-cell development, as it is essential only for progression beyond the early pro-B- (pre-BI-) cell stage (Fig. 4). For this reason, it is difficult to position *Pax-5* within the regulatory hierarchy of B-lymphopoiesis, which has recently been deduced from the phenotypic analysis of mice lacking different transcription factor genes (reviewed in ref. *8,9*). In adult bone marrow, Pax-5 would appear to function downstream of the transcription factors encoded by the *Ikaros (41)*, *E2A (42,43)*, and *EBF (44)* genes, whereas in the fetal liver Pax-5 may act at the same level or even upstream of these transcription factors.

5.3. Pax-5 *and the Proliferation Control of B-Lymphocytes*

Pax-5 has been implicated in the control of B-cell proliferation, as antisense oligonucleotide-mediated inhibition of BSAP synthesis prevented the activation of resting splenic B-cells upon mitogenic stimulation *(31)*. Moreover, the proliferative capacity of established B-cell lines was also severely reduced by treatment with BSAP-specific antisense oligonucleotides, whereas no effect was observed with randomized oligonucleotides *(31)*. In contrast, cell cycle analysis of the early pro-B-cell compartment revealed that these cells proliferate equally well in vivo in the presence or absence of

Pax-5 *(40)*. In addition, pro-B-cells from Pax-5-deficient or wild-type bone marrow also grow with similar kinetics ex vivo in the presence of stromal cells and IL-7. Therefore, it appears that the proliferation of B-lymphocytes in the bone marrow does not require Pax-5 early in the lineage but may become dependent on this transcription factor at later stages of B-cell differentiation (*see* also Section 10).

6. *Pax-5* and the V(D)J Rearrangements of Immunoglobulin Genes

6.1. Reduced V-to-DJ Recombination at the IgH Locus in Pax-5-Deficient Pro-B-Cells

The rearrangement of immunoglobulin genes is temporally regulated during early B-cell development, as the D_H-to-J_H joining usually precedes the V_H-to-D_HJ_H rearrangement at the *IgH* locus followed by recombination of the *IgL* genes (Fig. 1). The status of immunoglobulin gene rearrangement in Pax-5-deficient pro-B-cells was analyzed by single cell and quantitative PCR assays *(40)*. These experiments revealed that the *Pax-5* (–/–) pro-B-cells undergo D_H-to-J_H rearrangements of the *IgH* locus at normal frequency. In contrast, the V_H-to-D_HJ_H rearrangements were ~50-fold reduced compared to wild-type pro-B-cells. These data, therefore, indicate a role for Pax-5 in the developmental pathway controlling V-to-DJ recombination *(40)*. Gain- and loss-of-function experiments have previously implicated the ubiquitiously expressed transcription factors of the *E2A* gene in the control of D_H-to-J_H rearrangements *(42,45)*. D_HJ_H rearrangements at the *IgH* locus are known to occur promiscuously in T-lymphocytes, whereas the V_H-to-D_HJ_H rearrangements take place only in the B-lymphoid lineage. Therefore, these data suggest that *Pax-5* is involved in the control of the B-cell-specific step of V(D)J recombination.

The transition from the pro-B- to the pre-B-cell stage is an important checkpoint in B-cell development (Fig. 1). Productive rearrangement of the *IgH* gene initiates this transition by signaling through the pre-B-cell receptor complex, which is composed of the rearranged μ chain, the surrogate light chain proteins λ5 and VpreB and the signal-transducing proteins Igα and Igβ *(27)*. The pro-B- to pre-B-cell transition is abrogated by targeted inactivation of genes, which code for components of the pre-B-cell receptor (μ, λ5, Igβ) *(46–49)* or which are essential for immunogobulin gene recombination (RAG-1 and RAG-2) *(50,51)*. Expression of a functionally rearranged μ transgene can complement the recombination defect of RAG-deficient mice, thus resulting in expression of the pre-B-cell receptor and in progression to the pre-B-cell stage *(52–54)*. The *Pax-5* gene mutation interferes with the efficient synthesis of two components of the pre-B-cell receptor, i.e., the μ chain and Igα (mb-1) protein (Table 1) (*see* Subheading 7.3.). It is therefore possible that the inability to form a functional pre-B-cell receptor could be the cause for the developmental arrest in Pax-5-deficient bone marrow. This hypothesis was tested by introducing functional immunoglobulin transgenes into Pax-5-deficient mice and examined their effect on B-cell development by analyzing the expression pattern of cell surface proteins (Fig. 1) and the ex vivo clonability of bone marrow cells, which is usually lost upon transition to the pre-B-cell stage. By both criteria, neither expression of a functionally rearranged μ transgene *(55)* nor expression of a μ-Igβ fusion gene *(52)* were able to advance B-cell development to the pre-B-cell stage in *Pax-5* mutant mice (C. Thévenin and M. Busslinger, unpublished data). Interestingly, the μ-Igβ fusion protein can signal the transition from the pro-B- to pre-B-cell stage, even in the absence of μ, Igα, and Igβ proteins *(52,56)*. The inability of the μ-Igβ transgene to

Table 1
Expression of BSAP target genes at the pro-B-cell stage.

gene	pro-B cells +/+	pro-B cells -/-
CD19	++++	-
mb-1	+++	+
N-myc	++	+
λ5	+++	+++
VpreB	++++	++++
blk	++	++
XBP-1	++	++

The expression of putative BSAP target genes was determined by RNase protection analysis in pro-B- (pre-BI-) cells established from wild-type (+/+) and Pax-5 (–/–) bone marrow. The relative mRNA levels in the presence and absence of Pax-5 are schematically shown for those genes that were previously suggested to be regulated by BSAP. For details *see* ref. *40* and *68*.

complement the *Pax-5* defect demonstrates furthermore that neither the absence of V_H-to-D_HJ_H rearrangement nor the reduced Igα expression can be responsible for the developmental block in *Pax-5* mutant mice (C. Thévenin and M. Busslinger, unpublished data). It is concluded, therefore, that mutation of the *Pax-5* gene arrests pro-B-cell development at an early stage, which is not yet responsive to pre-B-cell receptor signaling.

6.2. A Possible Role for Pax-5 in Igκ Gene Rearrangements

The chromatin accessability of the immunoglobulin recombination substrates appears to be a key factor in the control of the V(D)J recombination process, as the transcription of germline gene segments usually precedes their DNA rearrangement *(57,58)*. Transcriptional activation is thought to open up the local chromatin structure and thus to target immunoglobulin gene regions for V(D)J recombination. Two germline κ^o transcripts are synthesized in mouse pre-B-cells prior to V-J rearrangement of the *Igκ* locus. One of these transcripts is initiated 3.5 kb 5' of the J_κ gene cluster *(59)* and is processed to a sterile 1.1-kb RNA lacking any coding potential *(60)*. Transcription of a second 0.8-kb κ^o RNA is initiated immediately upstream of the mouse $J_\kappa 1$ segment *(60,61)* within a region that contains two binding sites (KI and KII) for the κ locus protein (KLP) (ref. *16*; Fig. 7A). A sequence closely resembling the KI site was found at a similar position relative to the nonamer-heptamer recombination signal sequence in the chicken Igλ locus *(62)*. This sequence element proved to be essential for efficient DNA rearrangement of the chicken Igλ gene in transgenic mice *(62)*. Importantly, specific mutation of only the KI and KII sites by gene targeting also affected the V-J rearrangement process at the mouse κ locus *(63)*. These elegant experiments clearly demonstrated that the KI and KII sequences function as *cis*-acting recombination-enhancing elements *(63)*. Interestingly, the KLP protein *(16)* is expressed during B-cell development in a manner that is highly reminiscent of BSAP *(11)*. Indeed, the KI and KII sites have recently been shown to correspond to genuine BSAP recognition sequences, thus demonstrating that KLP and BSAP are one and the same protein *(23)*. Hence, these data implicate BSAP in the control of κ gene rearrangements.

7. BSAP-Dependent Gene Regulation in Early B-Lymphopoiesis

7.1. Genetic Identification of BSAP Target Genes

Insight into the regulatory function of BSAP critically depends on the identification of genes that are controlled by this transcription factor. The most commonly used approach for identifying target genes relies on the characterization of gene regulatory regions, whereby a factor-binding site is identified by protein–DNA binding assay, followed by functional analysis in transiently transfected cells. In this manner, BSAP has been implicated in different aspects of immunoglobulin gene regulation (*see* Subheadings 8. and 9.) and in the control of the genes coding for the cell surface protein CD19 *(64)*, the membrane protein Igα (mb-1) *(65)*, the tyrosine kinase Blk *(66)*, the transcription factor XBP-1 *(67)*, and the surrogate light chains λ5 and VpreB1 *(20)*. However, the identification of target genes by promoter analyses assumes that a functional BSAP-binding site identified by transient transfection experiments is also important for the regulation of the endogenous gene. In contrast, loss-of-function experiments, combined with a selective induction system, allow the direct identification of endogenous target genes. The in vitro clonability of Pax-5-deficient pro-B-cells thus provides an important tool for the search of BSAP-regulated genes. Comparative expression analysis of ~50 known B-cell-specific genes in wild-type and Pax-5-deficient pro-B-cells resulted in the identification of three genes, *CD19*, *mb-1(Igα)*, and *N-myc*, which are down-regulated in the absence of BSAP at the early pro-B-cell stage *(40,68)* (Table 1). The expression of all three genes can be rapidly induced by estrogen in Pax-5-deficient pro-B-cells expressing a BSAP-estrogen receptor fusion protein, thus identifying these genes as direct targets for BSAP regulation *(68)*. The expression of *blk*, *XBP-1*, *λ5*, and *VpreB1* was, however, unaffected by the absence of BSAP *(40)* (Table 1). Hence, this genetic evidence strongly argues against a critical role of BSAP in the regulation of these four genes in clear contradiction to the published data *(20,66,67)*. In this context, it is also interesting to note that BSAP does not regulate the expression of the transcription factor genes *PU.1*, *Ikaros*, *EBF*, *E2A*, *Sox-4*, *Oct-2*, and *OBF-1*, which have been implicated at different levels in the developmental control of B-lymphopoiesis *(40)*. Hence, Pax-5 does not exert its effect on B-cell development by controlling the expression of other known transcription factors.

7.2. Complete Loss of CD19 Transcription in the Absence of BSAP

CD19 was suggested to be a BSAP target gene based on promoter analysis, which identified a high-affinity BSAP-binding site instead of a TATA-box in the –30 region of this gene *(64)*. Moreover, in vivo footprinting experiments demonstrated that this site is fully occupied by BSAP only in CD19-expressing B-cells *(64)* (Fig. 5). Other transcription factors, in addition to BSAP, are likely to contribute to the regulation of the *CD19* gene. However, these regulators have not yet been identified, as the B-cell-specific activity of the CD19 promoter could not be reproduced in transiently transfected cells *(64)*. Importantly, Pax-5-deficient pro-B-cells do neither express the CD19 protein nor mRNA, thus indicating a central role for BSAP in the transcriptional regulation of the *CD19* gene *(40)* (Table 1). The complete loss of *CD19* transcription in these cells strongly suggests that the interaction of BSAP with the –30 region is critical for recruiting the basal transcription machinery to the *CD19* promoter.

The CD19 protein forms a complex with the complement receptor CD21, CD81, and Leu-13 on the surface of mature B-cells (reviewed in ref. *69*). This complex associates with surface immunoglobulin receptors, whereby CD19 acts as a costimulatory molecule to lower the threshold for antigen-dependent signaling *(70)*. In agreement with this function, the processes of B-cell activation, selection, and maturation are severely impaired in mice lacking *CD19 (71,72)*. However, B-lymphoid development up to the mature B-cell stage was unperturbed in the bone marrow of these mice *(71,72)*, thus demonstrating that *CD19* cannot be one of the critical target genes responsible for the differentiation block in *Pax-5* mutant mice.

7.3. Recruitment of Ets Proteins to the mb-1 (Igα) *Promoter by BSAP*

Pax-5-deficient pro-B-cells express the *mb-1* gene at a 5–10-fold lower level compared with pro-B-cells from wild-type mice *(68)*. Hence, in contrast to *CD19* transcription, BSAP contributes to, but it is not absolutely required, for *mb-1* promoter activity. Transient transfection and protein-DNA binding analyses revealed a relatively complex structure of the *mb-1* promoter that is controlled by at least four different transcriptional regulators *(65,73–75)* (Fig. 5A). The ubiquitious transcription factor Sp1 binds to the –40 region, where it may be involved in the selection of transcription start sites *(75)*. Members of the *Ets* proto-oncogene family can regulate the *mb-1* promoter by binding to the –50 region *(73)*, whereas the B-cell-specific transcription factors EBF and BSAP both contribute to the B-lymphoid expression of *mb-1* by interacting with upstream elements at –170 and –80, respectively *(65,74)*. In the context of the *mb-1* promoter, BSAP has been shown to function as a docking protein that efficiently recruits Ets transcription factors to a suboptimal binding site at position –70 *(65)*. Mutation of the BSAP-binding site not only interferes with binding of Ets proteins to the adjacent site, but also reduces the activity of the *mb-1* promoter fivefold in transfected cells *(65)*, which compares favorably with a 5–10-fold lower expression level of the endogenous *mb-1* gene in Pax-5-deficient pro-B-cells *(68)*. In in vitro binding assays, the paired domain of BSAP is already sufficient to recruit Ets proteins into ternary complexes with DNA *(65)*. Consistent with this finding, retrovirus-mediated expression of a BSAP paired domain peptide is able to restore wild-type *mb-1* expression levels in Pax-5-deficient pro-B-cells, thus indicating that the C-terminal transactivation function of BSAP is dispensable for *mb-1* gene regulation *(68)*.

The role of the Igα (mb-1) signaling protein in B-lymphopoiesis has so far been analyzed in a mouse mutant containing a deletion of the cytoplasmic tail of Igα. Early B-cell development is only mildly impaired in this mouse, most likely because the introduced mutation does not generate an *mb-1* null phenotype *(76)*. However, the failure of the μ-Igβ transgene to partially rescue the B-lymphoid defect of *Pax-5* mutant mice (*see* section 6.1) strongly argues that the reduced *mb-1* expression cannot be responsible for the early developmental arrest in Pax-5-deficient bone marrow.

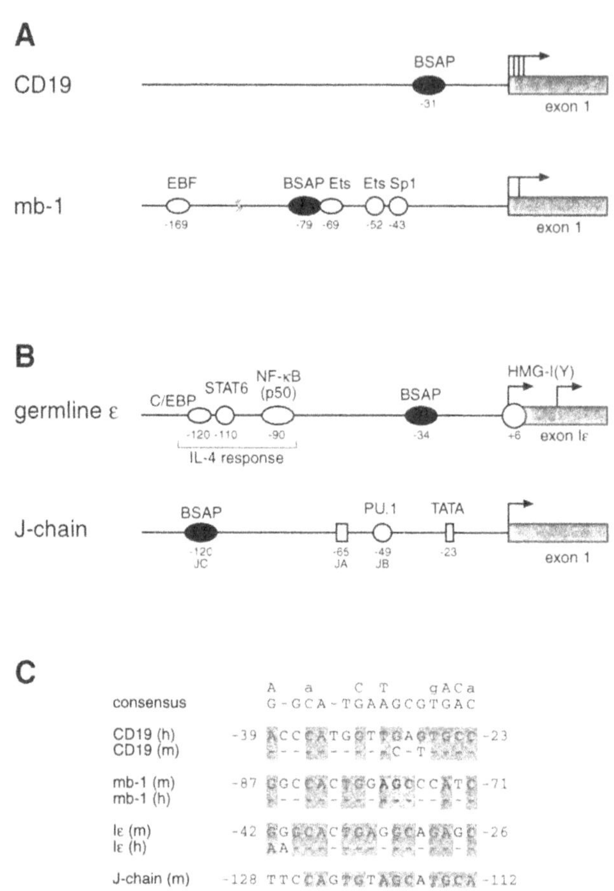

Fig. 5. Functional BSAP-binding sites in the proximal promoter of B-cell-specific genes. **(A)** Genuine BSAP target genes whose expression is affected by the absence of Pax-5 at the pro-B-cell stage. The *CD19* gene contains a functional BSAP-binding site in the –30 promoter region *(64)*. Multiple binding sites for ubiquitous and B-cell-specific transcription factors are present in the promoter of the *mb-1* (*Igα*) gene *(65,74,75)*. **(B)** BSAP target genes which are expressed at later stages of B-cell differentiation. BSAP-dependent regulation of the *IgH* germline ε promoter *(22,81,84)* and the J-chain gene *(89)* was inferred from protein-DNA binding, in vitro mutagenesis and transient cell transfection experiments. **(C)** Alignment of functional BSAP-binding sites with the consensus recognition sequence of the paired domain *(128)*. Base pairs matching the consensus sequence are indicated by grey overlay, and nucleotide positions are shown relative to the first prominent transcription start site. m, mouse; h, human.

7.4. BSAP is Essential for IL-7 Induction of the N-myc *Gene*

The N-*myc* gene is expressed in different tissues during mouse ontogeny *(77)*. Within the B-lymphoid lineage, the N-*myc* gene is transcribed only in pro-B- and pre-B-cells, but not at more mature stages of B-cell differentiation (B-cells and plasma cells) *(77)*. Moreover, N-*myc* expression is rapidly induced by IL-7 in these B-lymphoid precursor cells, indicating that N-*myc*, like c-*myc*, is an early response gene in these cells *(78)*. The IL-7-induced synthesis of N-*myc* mRNA results both from an increased rate of transcription initiation as well as from a release of a transcription attenuation block *(78)*. Interestingly, Pax-5-deficient pro-B-cells, which are cultured in the presence of IL-7, express a 5–10-fold lower steady-state level of N-*myc* mRNA *(68)*. A similarly low basal level of N-*myc* expression is seen in wild-type pro-B-cells after IL-7 withdrawal *(68,78)*. Furthermore, the response of the N-*myc* gene to IL-7 stimulation is delayed and reduced in Pax-5-deficient pro-B-cells, suggesting that BSAP is essential for mediating the IL-7 effect. To date, the transcriptional control region of the N-*myc* gene has not yet been characterized, and hence, no information is available about regulatory sequences that confer BSAP-dependent regulation to the N-*myc* gene. However, recent gene targeting experiments have demonstrated that B-cell development proceeds normally in the absence of N-*myc* function *(79)*. In summary, the authors have identified three genes, *CD19*, *mb-1* and N-*myc* that depend on BSAP for their expression at the pro-B-cell stage. However, the down-regulation of none of these genes appears to be causally involved in the early developmental bock observed in Pax-5-deficient bone marrow.

8. BSAP-Dependent Gene Regulation in Activated B-Cells

8.1. The Activation of the IgH *Germline* ε *Promoter Depends on BSAP*

Following antigen stimulation, mature IgM^+IgD^+ B-cells often switch to the expression of a different *IgH* constant region (C_H) gene, which results in a change of the effector function, but not the antigen specificity of an antibody molecule. This process, known as immunoglobulin class switching, leads to deletional DNA recombination between repetitive switch (S) regions, which are located upstream of each of seven C_H genes (except for Cδ) (reviewed in ref. *80*). The selection of a particular C_H gene for class switching is governed by distinct classes of cytokines (IL-4, IFN-γ, TGFβ) and B-cell mitogens (LPS, CD40L). The recombination process is normally preceded by transcription of the selected switch region that is thus made accessible to the recombination machinery. These germline C_H transcripts are initiated at a cytokine-inducible promoter, which is located upstream of a noncoding exon (know as exon I_H) and the switch region (reviewed in ref. *80*). A search for B-cell-specific DNA-binding activities involved in switching recombination led to the identification of several BSAP-binding sites within or upstream of switch regions *(17–19,81)*. However, only the BSAP recognition sequence located in the germline ε promoter was shown to be functionally relevant for the regulation of class switching (Fig. 5B).

B-cells activate germline ε transcription, and subsequently switch to the IgE isotype upon activation by IL-4 plus LPS or CD40 signaling. In agreement with this observation, the germline ε promoter contains an IL-4-responsive region which consists of recognition sequences for the transcription factors Stat6 (NF-IL4), C/EBPβ (NF-IL6) and NF-κB (p50) *(82)* (Fig. 5B). Moreover, the nonhistone chromosomal protein HMG-I(Y) interacts with the initiation region where it apparently represses basal transcription from the Iε promoter in the absence of IL-4 signaling *(83)*. Both the mouse *(22,81)* and human *(84)* germline ε promoters also contain a BSAP-binding site instead of a TATA box in the –30 region. Hence, BSAP interacts with both the Iε and CD19 promoters in a very similar manner (Fig. 5A). The functional significance of the BSAP-binding site for Iε transcription is, however, still controversial, as three groups obtained different results by in vitro mutagenesis and transient transfection experiments. The BSAP-binding site in the –30 region was essential for only basal *(82)*, only induced *(84)*, or basal and induced activity *(22,81)* of the germline ε promoter. As the Pax-5-deficient mouse could not be used to resolve this controversy (because of its early developmental block), a transdominant paired domain polypeptide was used for analysis in stable transfectants of the mature B-cell line M12.4.1. An excess of this peptide, which consists only of the DNA-binding domain of BSAP, interfered with LPS plus IL-4 induction of endogenous germline ε transcripts, possibly by competing endogenous BSAP away from its binding site (A. Morrison and M. Busslinger, unpublished data). This evidence together with the transient transfection data thus implicates BSAP in the regulation of germline ε transcription and consequently in switching to the IgE isotype.

8.2. BSAP-Mediated Repression of the J-Chain Gene

The J-chain gene codes for an immunoglobulin joining (J) protein that is essential for the assembly and secretion of pentamer IgM antibodies *(85)*. Consistent with this function, the J-chain gene is tightly regulated at the transcriptional level and is induced only in antigen-activated B-cells in response to the T-cell lymphokines IL-2 and IL-5 *(86)*. Transcriptional activation of the mouse J-chain gene is preceded by the formation of a nuclease-hypersensitive region, which extends up to position –170 in the promoter. Three major control elements have been defined with this region by deletion analyses (Fig. 5B). Two adjacent sequences, JA and JB, are positive regulatory elements, which are responsible for high promoter activity in J-chain-expressing plasmacytoma cell lines *(87)*. The B-cell- and macrophage-specific Ets protein PU.1 is known to activate the J-chain promoter in plasma cells by binding to the JB element *(88)* (Fig. 5B). In contrast, BSAP has recently been shown to silence the J-chain promoter at earlier stages of B-cell development by interacting with the negative regulatory element JC *(89)* (Fig. 5B). Consistent with this finding, the expression of the endogenous J-chain gene was reduced ~ fivefold by ectopic expression of BSAP in plasma cell lines *(89)*. Therefore, it was suggested that the down-regulation of *Pax-5* expression during terminal plasma cell differentiation relieves the mouse J-chain gene from negative regulation by BSAP. The analysis of the bovine J-chain gene revealed high conservation of the proximal promoter sequences (including the JA and JB elements) between rodents and cattle *(90)*. However, a BSAP-binding site is absent at the equivalent position in the bovine J-chain gene because of the lack of sequence conservation in the upstream promoter region *(90)*, suggesting that BSAP may repress this gene through a different mechanism, if at all. In summary, it is interesting to note that BSAP appear to have a dual regulatory role during the activation phase of a primary immune response, as it can function as an activator of the *I*ε promoter and as a repressor of the murine J-chain gene.

9. The Role of BSAP in the Regulation of Immunoglobulin 3' Enhancers

9.1. Negative Regulation of the IgH 3' Enhancer by BSAP

The expression of the immunoglobulin heavy-chain gene is under the control of the intronic Eμ enhancer and a complex regulatory region, which is located 3' of the Cα gene (Fig. 6). These downstream regulatory sequences contain four tissue- and cell stage-specific DNase I hypersensitive sites (HS), which function together as a locus control region (LCR) in plasma cells *(91)*. Of these regulatory elements, the 3'α enhancer (3'αE) encompassing the hypersensitive sites 1 and 2 has been analyzed in greatest detail. This enhancer is located ~16 kb downstream of the mouse Cα gene *(92)*, and its activity is largely restricted to activated B-cells and plasma cells where it contributes to maximal expression of secreted

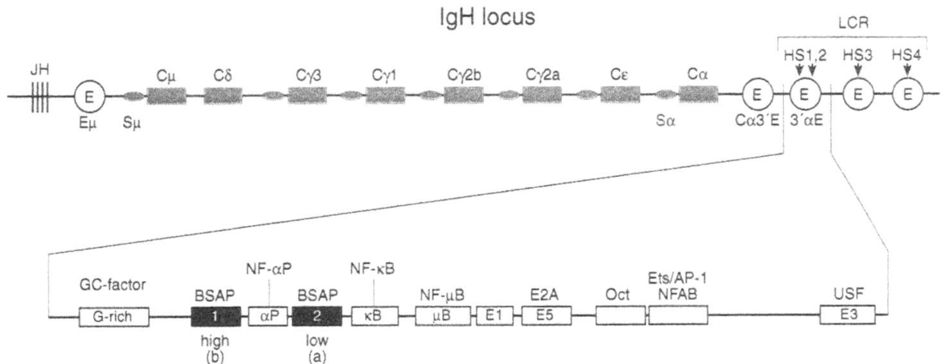

Fig. 6. Structure of the 3'α enhancer of the mouse *IgH* locus. Schematic diagram of the *IgH* locus and the regulatory region of the 3'α enhancer. The high- and low-affinity BSAP-binding sites 1 and 2 *(98)* are also referred to as sites b and a *(99)*, respectively. Note that the BSAP site 1 and NF-κB site have not been conserved in the rat 3'α enhancer *(92)*. See text for further explanation.

immunoglobulins *(91–93)*. Targeted deletion of the 3'αE region revealed an essential function of this enhancer not only in immunoglobulin gene transcription *(94)*, but also in class switching *(95)*. The 3'α enhancer consists of a complex array of recognition sequences for different transcription factors, which mediate enhancer activation in response to signaling in stimulated B-cells (Fig. 6). Among these transcription factors is BSAP whose expression pattern appears to be inversely correlated with 3'α enhancer activity in mature B-cell and plasma cell lines, respectively. Hence, BSAP has been implicated as a repressor of the 3'α enhancer. However, a rather complex picture about this repressive function of BSAP has emerged in the literature, as the data contributed by three different laboratories are contradictory in certain aspects and thus appear controversial at present. The role of BSAP in the regulation of the 3'α enhancer activity has also been the focus of two recent reviews that may be consulted for different views on this topic *(96,97)*.

BSAP interacts in vitro with two sites in the mouse 3'α enhancer *(98,99)*. The high-affinity binding site 1 (also referred to as site b) conforms well with the BSAP consensus recognition sequence in contrast to the low-affinity site 2 (a) *(98,99)* (Fig. 6). Curiously, however, the high-affinity site 1 has been deleted in the rat *(35)* despite the fact that the 3'α enhancer sequences have otherwise been highly conserved in rodents *(92,100)*. In vivo footprint analyses indicated that BSAP binds to site 1 in the mouse enhancer *(101)* but to site 2 in the rat enhancer *(35)*. As shown by transient cell transfection experiments, BSAP is able to repress the mouse 3'α enhancer through both the high- and low-affinity binding sites in B-cell lines *(98,99,102)*. In agreement with this finding, ectopic expression of BSAP down-regulates the activity of the 3'α enhancer three-to-fivefold in plasma cell lines. Moreover, inhibition of endogenous BSAP synthesis by antisense oligonucleotide treatment *(98)*, or blockage of the endogenous BSAP site 1 by hybridization with a specific triple helix-forming oligonucleotide *(101)*, led to increased 3'α enhancer activity in mature B-cells. On the basis of these data, it has been postulated that BSAP represses the 3'α enhancer in early development up to the mature B-cell stage, and that the 3'α enhancer is activated upon down-regulation of *Pax-5* expression during terminal plasma cell differentiation *(98,99)*. However, a detailed time-course analysis of enhancer activation and BSAP down-regulation revealed that the rapid physiological stimulation of the 3'α enhancer in splenic B-cells cannot be blocked by the presence of BSAP, which is lost only later in activated blast cells *(35)*. Hence, the regulation of the 3'α enhancer by BSAP may be more complex than advertised.

Two models have to date been put forward to explain BSAP-mediated repression of the 3'α enhancer. In their in vivo footprint studies, Neurath et al. *(101)* observed an inverse binding pattern at the BSAP site 1 and the adjacent NF-αP site in B-cells and plasma cells despite the fact that the Ets-like protein NF-αP is expressed in both cell types. Hence, these authors hypothesized that BSAP blocks activation in B-cells by preventing the positive regulator NF-αP from binding to the 3'α enhancer. Birshtein's group discovered in their mutagenesis analysis that three transcription factors, a G-rich DNA-binding protein, NF-κB, and Oct factors, are essential for full activation of the 3'α enhancer in plasma cells *(102,103)*. Binding of the same three factors is, however, required in B-cells for negative regulation by BSAP, suggesting that the 3'α enhancer is subject to concerted repression by a multiprotein complex *(102,103)*. In summary, BSAP appears to exert a negative effect on immunogloblin synthesis and secretion by repressing the *IgH* 3'α enhancer in B-lymphocytes prior to terminal plasma cell differentiation. Several aspects of this BSAP-mediated inhibition require, however, further experimental clarification.

9.2. BSAP Modulates the Chromatin Structure and Activity of the κ 3' Enhancer

The rearrangement and expression of the immunoglobulin κ gene is regulated by two enhancers that are located in the intron (iEκ) and 8.5 kb downstream of the Cκ gene (3'Eκ) *(104)* (Fig. 7A). Contrary to the situation in the *IgH* locus, both κ enhancers are activated at the same stage in B-cell development. Hence, the activity of the 3' κ enhancer can be induced by LPS treatment in pre-B-cell lines and then remains high in mature B-cells and plasma cells *(104–106)*. Transgenic studies have implicated the 3' κ enhancer as a critical element for hypermutation and high level expression of rearranged κ transgenes in activated B-cells *(105,107)*. Moreover, the use of transgenic recombination substrates revealed that the 3' κ enhancer determines both the correct temporal regulation and B-lymphoid specificity of the V-to-J rearrangement at the κ locus *(108)*. Targeted deletion of the 3' κ enhancer in the mouse germline confirmed a critical role of this regulatory element in rearrangement as well as expression of the κ gene in resting B-cells *(109)*. Interestingly however, the expression of the κ gene was unaffected in activated and antibody-secreting B-lymphocytes of 3'EκΔ mutant mice, suggesting that so far unknown regulatory elements in the κ locus can compensate for the loss of the 3' κ enhancer at these terminal stages of B-cell differentiation *(109)*. The activity of the 3' κ enhancer depends on several different transcription factors, some of which are the same proteins involved in the regulation of the *IgH* 3'α enhancer (compare Figs. 6 and 7A). BSAP is one of these proteins, although the evidence available to date would suggest different functions for BSAP in the context of the two enhancers.

Functional analyses of the mouse and human 3' κ enhancer revealed that the transcription factors PU.1 and Pip (NF-EM3) *(110–112)*, HLH proteins encoded by the *E2A* gene *(106,111)*, members of the ATF/CREM family *(113)*, and NF-E1 (YY-1) *(114)* are involved in determining the activity of the 3' κ enhancer (Fig. 7A). BSAP was identified as a DNA-binding activity of the mouse 3' κ enhancer by in vivo footprint and chromatin analyses, using established cell lines that represent different stages of B-cell development *(115)*. An early type of chromatin structure is seen in pre-B- and

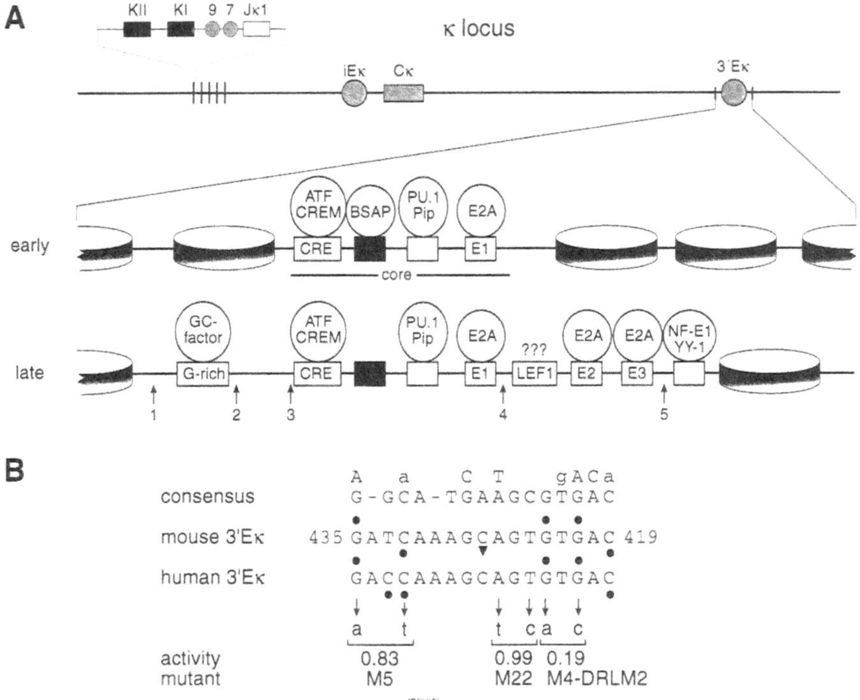

Fig. 7. BSAP and the chromatin structure of the κ 3' enhancer. **(A)** Schematic diagram of the immunoglobulin κ locus. The 'early' and 'late' chromatin structures of the κ 3' enhancer are indicated together with the occupancy of the different factor-binding sites and the positions of five DNase I hypersensitive sites. Adapted from Roque et al. *(115)*. See text for further description of the κ 3' enhancer. The KI and KII sequences located upstream of the Jκ1 element are recognized by the KLP protein *(16)*, which was recently shown to be identical with BSAP *(23)*. The nonamer and heptamer recombination signal sequences are indicated by 9 and 7, respectively. **(B)** In vivo footprint pattern and functional analysis of the BSAP-binding site present in the κ 3' enhancer. The BSAP-binding sites of the mouse *(104)* and human *(116)* κ 3' enhancer were aligned with the consensus recognition sequence of the paired domain *(128)*. Nucleotides are numbered according to the published mouse 3'Eκ DNA sequence *(104)*. Filled circles denote G-residues in the upper or lower DNA strand which are protected from methylation by dimethyl sulfate in vivo in murine *(115)* and human *(111)* B-cell lines. A hypersensitive G-residue is indicated by an arrowhead. Linker scan mutations of the human BSAP-site are shown together with their activity relative to the wild-type κ 3' enhancer which was determined by transient transfection assay in a human B-cell line *(111)*.

B-cells where the DNase I-hypersensitive region encompasses the core enhancer (Fig. 7A). Genomic footprint experiments revealed binding of ATF/CREM, BSAP, PU.1/Pip, and E2A proteins within this open chromatin region. The 3' κ enhancer is, however, embedded in a different chromatin structure in plasma cells (late type), where the DNase I-sensitive sequences extend beyond the core region. Furthermore, the appearance of five hypersensitive sites underscores the drastic change in chromatin structure that correlates with binding of additional proteins on both sides of the core enhancer (Fig. 7A). As BSAP is absent in plasma cells and in the chromatin of the late type, it is tempting to speculate that the down-regulation of BSAP expression may be causally linked to the chromatin reorganization in plasma cells *(115)*. A different picture has recently emerged from investigating the in vivo occupancy of the 3' κ enhancer in primary pro-B- and pre-B-cells *(30)*. In this case, a footprint characteristic of BSAP was only observed in pro-B-cells, whereas binding of the ATF/CREM and PU.1/Pip proteins was predominantly seen in pre-B-cells. Contrary to the analysis of established cell lines, BSAP may interfere with binding of the ATF/CREM and PU.1/Pip proteins in primary pro-B-cells, thus preventing activation of the 3' κ enhancer prior to the pre-B-cell stage *(30)*. However, this model of κ gene activation is unlikely to hold true in its simple form, as the absence of BSAP does not lead to premature κ gene expression in Pax-5-deficient pro-B-cells (S. Nutt and M. Busslinger, unpublished data).

The sequence and function of the 3' κ enhancer have been highly conserved between human and mouse *(111,116)*. Importantly, the BSAP-binding sites of both enhancers are not only identical in sequence (except for one nucleotide position), but also show a similar in vivo footprint in human and murine B-cell lines *(111,115)* (Fig. 7B). The observed pattern of methylation protection is typical of BSAP *(21)*, and is lost in plasma cell lines *(115)*, thus positively identifying BSAP as the in vivo DNA-binding activity. The human 3' κ enhancer has been subjected to extensive linker scan mutagenesis and functional analysis in transiently transfected B-cells *(111)*. Although the binding sites for the E2A and PU.1 proteins were identified in this manner, a third functionally important region could not be interpreted at the time in terms of a DNA-binding activity. Interestingly, three mutations in this region were generated within the BSAP recognition sequence. Two of them (M5 and M22) did neither decrease the match with the BSAP consensus sequence nor significantly affect the activity of the 3' κ enhancer *(111)* (Fig. 7B). In contrast, a third mutation (M4-DRLM2) not only altered two critical residues in the BSAP-binding site (Fig. 7B), but also resulted in a fivefold reduction of enhancer activity *(111)* (Fig. 7B). Hence, the reinterpretation of these data suggests that BSAP acts as a positive regulator of the 3' κ enhancer in mature B-cells in contrast to its function as a repressor of the *IgH* 3'α enhancer at the same developmental stage.

10. Oncogenic Activation of *PAX-5* by Chromosomal Translocations in Non-Hodgkin Lymphomas

10.1. Activation by Enhancer Insertion

An oncogenic role has been proposed for *PAX* genes primarily on the basis of a consistent involvement of *PAX-3* and *PAX-7* in the genesis of alveolar rhabdomyosarcoma. In this pediatric muscle tumor, a specific translocation between one of the two *PAX* loci and the fork head domain gene *FKHR* generates a novel fusion gene that codes for a potent chimaeric transcription factor *(117,118)*. *PAX-5* has so far been implicated in the formation of medulloblastoma, as its expression is frequently deregulated in this tumor *(119)*. The localization of the human *PAX-5* gene to chromosome 9p13 *(120)* has recently led to the discovery that *PAX-5* is involved in a specific translocation, t(9;14)(p13;q32), recurring in a small subset of nonHodgkin lymphomas. These tumors are referred to as small lymphocytic lymphomas of the plasmacytoid subtype and can give rise to more aggressive large-cell lymphomas *(121)*. The initial characterization of a t(9;14) breakpoint from a diffuse large-cell lymphoma (KIS-1) demonstrated that the *IgH* locus on 14q32 was juxtaposed to chromosome 9p13 sequences of unknown function *(122)*. Subsequently, *PAX-5* was identified as the second translocation partner by localizing the KIS-1 breakpoint 1807 bp upstream of exon 1A of *PAX-5* *(37)*. As a

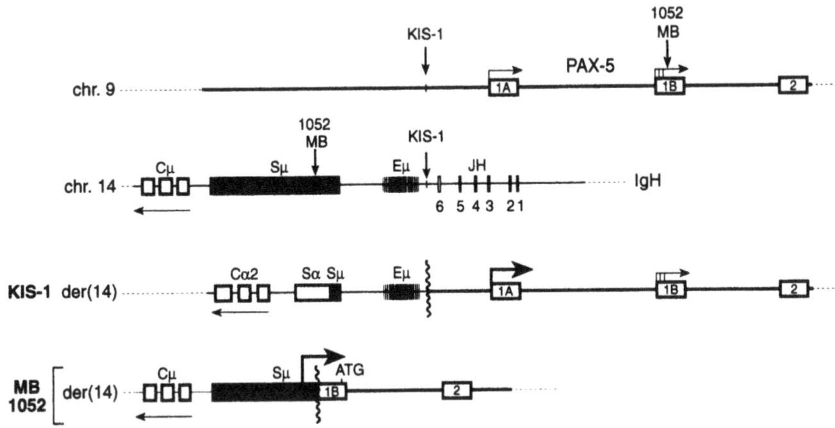

Fig. 8. Chromosomal translocations between the *PAX-5* and *IgH* loci in three patients with non-Hodgkin lymphoma. The 5' region of the *PAX-5* gene, the J_H-to -Cμ region of the *IgH* locus and the corresponding translocation breakpoints present on the derivative chromosome 14 in the lymphomas of the patients KIS-1 *(37)*, 1052 *(123)* and MB *(124)* are schematically diagrammed.

consequence, the potent Eμ enhancer of the *IgH* gene was brought into close proximity of the *PAX-5* promoters in the KIS-1 lymphoma (Fig. 8). Importantly, this translocation did not affect the coding region of *PAX-5* and therefore must be regarded as a regulatory mutation, which results in deregulation of *PAX-5* expression. Indeed, the transcription of *PAX-5* is increased about 10-fold in KIS-1 cells compared with normal B-cell lines *(123,124)*.

10.2. Activation by Promoter Replacement

A novel translocation breakpoint between the *PAX-5* and *IgH* loci has recently been characterized in a patient (case 1052) diagnosed with lymphoplasmacytoid lymphoma *(123)*. Subsequently, the authors have identified a third patient (MB) with an almost identical translocation by screening $CD5^{low}$ non-Hodgkin lymphomas *(124)*. In both cases, the translocation occurred within exon 1B of *PAX-5* and the Sμ switch region of the *IgH* locus, which dissociated the *PAX-5* gene from its own control region (Fig. 8). As a result, *PAX-5* was brought under the control of a new promoter that is located in the Sμ switch sequences *(124)*. However, the Eμ enhancer is absent from the der(14) chromosome (Fig. 8), suggesting that the Sμ switch promoter is activated by the downstream 3' enhancers of the *IgH* locus. In agreement with this interpretation, the expression of *PAX-5* mRNA and protein was drastically increased in the malignant B-lymphocytes of patient MB *(124)*.

Both the enhancer and promoter insertions of the t(9;14) translocation may activate *PAX-5* as an oncogene in two different ways. The increase in *PAX-5* expression could per se result in deregulation of the BSAP function, as the activity of Pax transcription factors often shows a narrow concentration dependence, which is also reflected by the haploinsufficient nature of most *PAX* gene mutations (reviewed in ref. *125*). Apart from such quantitative effects, the insertion of regulatory elements of the *IgH* locus is likely to force the *PAX-5* gene to remain active during the terminal phase of B-cell differentiation when the endogenous *PAX-5* gene is usually switched off. In this context, it is interesting to note that *PAX-5* has been implicated in the proliferation control of mature

B-cells by antisense oligonucleotide inhibition experiments *(31)*. Hence, the forced expression of *PAX-5* may prevent activated B-cells from exiting the cell cycle and could thus block the completion of the plasma cell differentiation program. This notion is supported by the plasmacytoid nature of the malignant B-lymphocytes containing the t(9;14) translocation.

11. Monoallelic Expression of *Pax-5* and the Haploinsufficiency of Mammalian *Pax* Genes

The most unusual and characteristic feature of mammalian *Pax* genes is their haploinsufficiency, which results in the frequent association of heterozygous *Pax* gene mutations with human disease syndromes and mouse developmental mutants (reviewed in ref. *125*). The function of these transcription factors is therefore thought to be particularly sensitive to gene dosage, as mutation of one allele already results in developmental abnormalities. One possible model to account for the haploinsufficiency of *Pax* genes is the so-called monoallelic expression theory. According to this hypothesis, a given *Pax* gene is transcribed from only one of its two alleles, and hence the cells of an expressing tissue can be subdivided into two populations that transcribe either allele 1 or 2. Both cell populations can participate in normal development and differentiation, as long as the two alleles contain wild-type sequences. However, if one allele is mutated, one subpopulation of cells lacks the function of the respective *Pax* gene and may therefore not contribute to tissue formation, which could lead to phenotypic abnormalities.

A direct test of the monoallelic expression hypothesis depends on the possibility to follow the transcription of individual *Pax* gene alleles in vivo. Such a possibility was provided by the analysis of B-lymphocytes from heterozygous *Pax-5* (+/–) mice for the following reasons. First, as the expression of CD19 is strictly dependent on the presence of BSAP (*see* Subheading 7.2.), only cells expressing the wild-type *Pax-5* allele can be stained with an anti-CD19 antibody, and are subsequently detected as $CD19^+$ cells by flow cytometric analysis (Fig. 9A). Second, the inactivated *Pax-5* allele contains an in-frame *lacZ* gene insertion; hence, its transcription leads to the synthesis of β-galactosidase, the activity of which can also be monitored by flow cytometric analysis using a fluorogenic substrate (Fig. 9A). Analysis of the B-cell compartments of heterozygous *Pax-5* (+/–) fetal liver and bone marrow demonstrated that the majority of the B-lymphocytes express the CD19 protein, yet display no β-galactosidase activity *(126)* (Fig. 9B). Hence, most heterozygous B-lymphocytes express exclusively the wild-type *Pax-5* allele in vivo, thus supporting the hypothesis of allele-specific regulation of the *Pax-5* gene. Interestingly, this monoallelic expression pattern of *Pax-5* was independent of the parental orgin of the two *Pax-5* alleles *(126)*.

The phenomenon of monoallelic *Pax-5* expression was further investigated by establishing pro-B-cell lines from heterozygous mice in vitro. Single cell cloning experiments and time course analyses demonstrated that individual cell colonies were able to switch expression between alleles within two weeks *(126)*. Moreover, replication timing analyses by fluorescence *in situ* hybridization (FISH) demonstrated that both *Pax-5* alleles are synchronously replicated during S-phase in B-cells of heterozygous mice *(125)*. In summary, the allele-specific regulation of *Pax-5* is stochastic, reversible, independent of parental origin, and does not correlate with asynchronous replication in contrast to the monoallelic expression of genomically imprinted genes. As predicted, the monoallelic expression of *Pax-5* generates a haploinsufficient phenotype at the cellular level in heterozygous *Pax-5* (+/–) mice. Cells that express only the mutant (*lacZ*) allele are

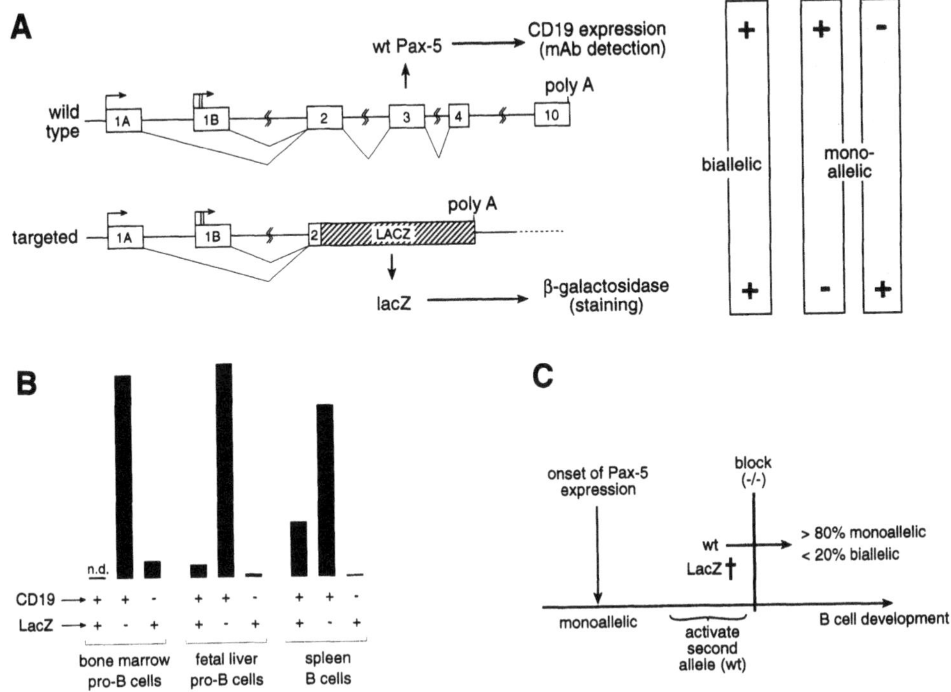

Fig. 9. Monoallelic expression of *Pax-5* in B-lymphocytes of heterozygous *Pax-5* (+/–) mice. **(A)** Schematic diagram of the wild-type and disrupted *Pax-5* alleles. **(B)** Percentages of bi- and mono-allelically expressing B-lymphocytes in fetal liver, bone marrow, and spleen. The bar graph indicates the different percentages of CD19 and/or lacZ expressing cells, which were determined by flow cytometric analysis of the respective B-cell compartment *(126)*. **(C)** Model to account for mono- and bi-allelically expressing B-lymphocytes.

absent in the B-lymphoid lineage past the developmental block of the *Pax-5* mutation (Fig. 9B, C). Hence, heterozygous pro-B-cells, which initially switch on the mutant *Pax-5* allele, can only participate in later development if they also activate the wild-type allele early on. These B-lymphocytes may account for the small percentage of biallelically expressing cells (Fig. 9B, C). Interestingly, the Pax-5 (+/–) mouse has been ideal to prove the monoallelic expression theory, although it is phenotypically normal and does not provide a model for a human inherited disease. The main reasons for this apparent discrepancy are the functional redundancy of Pax-2 and Pax-5 in the developing midbrain *(39)*, and the fact that a twofold reduction in B-cells is without phenotypic consequence. Hence, the human *PAX-5* gene could not be linked to a primary immunodeficiency syndrome *(127)*.

12. Concluding Remarks

Several different experimental approaches have implicated BSAP (Pax-5) as a key regulator at all stages of B-cell development. However, there is still little known about direct target genes, which mediate the different effects of BSAP in B-lymphopoiesis. A systematic search for such genes may be greatly facilitated by the availability of Pax-5-deficient pro-B-cell lines and a BSAP-specific induction system. Moreover, the plethora of functions that have been ascribed to BSAP at late stages of B-cell differentiation will have to be scrutinized in genetic tests by using the Cre-loxP system for conditional inactivation of *Pax-5* in late B-cell development. Transgenic experiments will be required to define the B-cell-specific control region of *Pax-5,* and thus to identify the upstream regulators of this gene in the genetic hierarchy of hematopoiesis. In addition, overexpression studies in transgenic mice may help to clarify the oncogenic role of *Pax-5* in B-lymphocytes, whereas elucidation of the molecular mechanism underlying the monoallelic expression of *Pax-5* will be a challenging task for the future.

Acknowledgments

The authors are grateful to P. Pfeffer for critical reading of this manuscript. This work was supported by the IMP and, in part, by the Austrian Industrial Research Promotion Fund.

References

1. Rolink, A. and Melchers, F. (1991) Molecular and cellular origins of B lymphocyte diversity. *Cell* **66,** 1081–1094.
2. Hardy, R. R., Carmack, C. E., Shinton, S. A., Kemp, J. D., and Kayakawa, K. (1991) Resolution and characterization of pro-B and pre-pro-B cell stages in normal mouse bone marrow. *J. Exp. Med.* **173,** 1213–1225.
3. Li, Y.-S., Hayakawa, K., and Hardy, R. R. (1993) The regulated expression of B lineage associated genes during B cell differentiation in bone marrow and fetal liver. *J. Exp. Med.* **178,** 951–960.
4. Rolink, A., Grawunder, U., Winkler, T. H., Karasuyama, H., and Melchers, F. (1994) IL-2 receptor α chain (CD25,TAC) expression defines a crucial stage in pre-B cell development. *Int. Immunol.* **6,** 1257–1264.
5. Melchers, F., Rolink, A., Grawunder, U., Winkler, T. H., Karasuyama, H., Ghia, P., and Andersson, J. (1995) Positive and negative selection events during B lymphopoiesis. *Curr. Opin. Immunol.* **7,** 214–227.
6. Hagman, J. and Grosschedl, R. (1994) Regulation of gene expression at early stages of B-cell differentiation. *Curr. Opin. Immunol.* **6,** 222–230.
7. Busslinger, M. and Urbánek, P. (1995) The role of BSAP (Pax-5) in B cell development. *Curr. Opin. Genet. Dev.* **5,** 595–601.
8. Clevers, H. C. and Grosschedl, R. (1996) Transcriptional control of lymphoid development: lessons from gene targeting. *Immunol. Today* **17,** 336–343.
9. Singh, H. (1996) Gene targeting reveals a hierarchy of transcription factors regulating specification of lymphoid cell fates. *Curr. Opin. Immunol.* **8,** 160–165.
10. Barberis, A., Superti-Furga, G., Vitelli, L., Kemler, I., and Busslinger, M. (1989) Developmental and tissue-specific regulation of a novel transcription factor of the sea urchin. *Genes Dev.* **3,** 663–675.
11. Barberis, A., Widenhorn, K., Vitelli, L., and Busslinger, M. (1990) A novel B-cell lineage-specific transcription factor present at early but not late stages of differentiation. *Genes Dev.* **4,** 849–859.
12. Adams, B., Dörfler, P., Aguzzi, A., Kozmik, Z., Urbánek, P., Maurer-Fogy. I., and Busslinger, M. (1992) *Pax-5* encodes the transcription factor BSAP and is expressed in B lymphocytes, the developing CNS, and adult testis. *Genes Dev.* **6,** 1589–1607.
13. Bopp, D., Burri, M., Baumgartner, S., Frigerio, G., and Noll, M. (1986) Conservation of a large protein domain in the segmentation gene *paired* and in functionally related genes of *Drosophila. Cell* **47,** 1033–1040.
14. Treisman, J., Harris, E., and Desplan, C. (1991) The paired box encodes a second DNA-binding domain in the Paired homeo domain protein. *Genes Dev.* **5,** 594–604.
15. Czerny, T., Bouchard, M., Kozmik, Z., and Busslinger, M. (1997) The characterization of novel *Pax* genes of the sea urchin and *Drosophila* reveal an ancient evolutionary origin of the *Pax2/5/8* family. *Mech. Dev.* **67,** 179–192.

16. Weaver, D. and Baltimore, D. (1987) B lymphocyte-specific protein binding near an immunoglobulin κ-chain gene *J* segment. *Proc. Natl. Acad. Sci. USA* **84,** 1516–1520.
17. Waters, S. J., Saikh, K. U., and Stavnezer, J. (1989) A B-cell-specific nuclear protein that binds to DNA sites 5' to immunoglobulin Sα tandem repeats is regulated during differentiation. *Mol. Cell. Biol.* **9,** 5594–5601.
18. Liao, F., Giannini, S. L., and Birshtein, B. K. (1992) A nuclear DNA-binding protein expressed during early stages of B-cell differentiation interacts with diverse segments within and 3' of the IgH chain gene cluster. *J. Immunol.* **148,** 2909–2917.
19. Xu, L., Kim, M. G., and Marcu, K. B. (1992) Properties of B cell stage specific and ubiquitous nuclear factors binding to immunoglobulin heavy chain gene switch regions. *Int. Immunol.* **4,** 875–887.
20. Okabe, T., Watanabe, T., and Kudo, A. (1992) A pre-B- and B cell-specific DNA-binding protein, EBB-1, which binds to the promoter of the V_{preB1} gene. *Eur. J. Immunol.* **22,** 37–43.
21. Czerny, T., Schaffner, G., and Busslinger, M. (1993) DNA sequence recognition by Pax proteins: bipartite structure of the paired domain and its binding site. *Genes Dev.* **7,** 2048–2061.
22. Liao, F., Birshtein, B. K., Busslinger, M., and Rothman, P. (1994) The transcription factor BSAP (NF-HB) is essential for immunoglobulin germ-line ε transcription. *J. Immunol.* **152,** 2904–2911.
23. Tian, J., Okabe, T., Miyazaki, T., Takeshita, S., and Kudo, A. (1997) Pax-5 is identical to EBB-1/KLP and binds to the VpreB and λ5 promoters as well as the KI and KII sites upstream of the Jκ genes. *Eur. J. Immunol.* **27,** 750–755.
24. Dörfler, P. and Busslinger, M. (1996) C-terminal activating and inhibitory domains determine the transactivation potential of BSAP (Pax-5), Pax-2 and Pax-8. *EMBO J.* **15,** 1971–1982.
25. Chalepakis, G., Fritsch, R., Fickenscher, H., Deutsch, U., Goulding, M., and Gruss, P. (1991) The molecular basis of the *undulated/Pax-1* mutation. *Cell* **66,** 873–884.
26. Xu, W., Rould, M. A., Jun, S., Desplan, C., and Pabo, C. O. (1995) Crystal structure of the paired domain-DNA complex at 2.5 Å resolution reveals structural basis for Pax developmental mutations. *Cell* **80,** 639–650.
27. Borst, J., Jacobs, H., and Brouns, G. (1996) Composition and function of T-cell receptor and B-cell receptor complexes on precursor lymphocytes. *Curr. Opin. Immunol.* **8,** 181–190.
28. Rolink, A., ten Boekel, E., Melchers, F., Fearon, D. T., Krop, I., and Andersson, J. (1996) A subpopulation of $B220^+$ cells in murine bone marrow does not express CD19 and contains natural killer cell progenitors. *J. Exp. Med.* **183,** 187–194.
29. Li, Y.-S., Wasserman, R., Hayakawa, K., and Hardy, R. R. (1996) Identification of the earliest B lineage stage in mouse bone marrow. *Immunity* **5,** 527–535.
30. Shaffer, A. L., Peng, A., and Schlissel, M. S. (1997) In vivo occupancy of the κ light chain enhancers in primary pro- and pre-B cells: a model of κ locus activation. *Immunity* **6,** 131–143.
31. Wakatsuki, Y. W., Neurath, M. F., Max, E. E., and Strober, W. (1994) The B cell-specific transcription factor BSAP regulates B cell proliferation. *J. Exp. Med.* **179,** 1099–1108.
32. Harada, H., Kawano, M. M., Huang, N., Harada, Y., Iwato, K., Tanabe, O., Tanaka, H., Sakai, A., Asaoku, H., and Kuramoto, A. (1993) Phenotypic difference of normal plasma cells from mature myeloma cells. *Blood* **81,** 2658–2663.
33. Pellat-Deceunynck, C., Bataille, R., Robillard, N., Harousseau, J.-L., Rapp, M.-J., Juge-Morineau, N., Wijdenes, J., and Amiot, M. (1994) Expression of CD28 and CD40 in human myeloma cells: a comparative study wit normal plasma cells. *Blood* **84,** 2597–2603.
34. Mahmoud, M. S., Huang, N., Nobuyoshi, M., Lisukov, I. A., Tanaka, H., and Kawano, M. M. (1996) Altered expression of Pax-5 gene in human myeloma cells. *Blood* **87,** 4311–4315.
35. Andersson, T., Neurath, M. F., Grant, P. A., and Pettersson, S. (1996) Physiological activation of the IgH 3' enhancer in B lineage cells is not blocked by Pax-5. *Eur. J. Immunol.* **26,** 2499–2507.
36. Stüber, E., Neurath, M., Calderhead, D., Fell, H. P., and Strober, W. (1995) Cross-linking of OX40 ligand, a member of the TNF/NGF cytokine family, induces proliferation and differentiation in murine splenic B cells. *Immunity* **2,** 507–521.
37. Busslinger, M., Klix, N., Pfeffer, P., Graninger, P. G., and Kozmik, Z. (1996) Deregulation of *PAX-5* by translocation of the Eμ enhancer of the *IgH* locus adjacent to two alternative *PAX-5* promoters in a diffuse large-cell lymphoma. *Proc. Natl. Acad. Sci. USA* **93,** 6129–6134.
38. Urbánek, P., Wang, Z.-Q., Fetka, I., Wagner, E. F., and Busslinger, M. (1994) Complete block of early B cell differentiation and altered patterning of the posterior midbrain in mice lacking Pax5/BSAP. *Cell* **79,** 901–912.

39. Urbánek, P., Fetka, I., Meisler, M. H., and Busslinger, M. (1997) Cooperation of *Pax2* and *Pax5* in midbrain and cerebellum development. *Proc. Natl. Acad. Sci. USA* **94,** 5703–5708.
40. Nutt, S. L., Urbánek, P., Rolink, A., and Busslinger, M. (1997) Essential functions of Pax5 (BSAP) in pro-B cell development: difference between fetal and adult B lymphopoiesis and reduced *V*-to-*DJ* recombination at the *IgH* locus. *Genes Dev.* **11,** 476–491.
41. Wang, J.-H., Nichogiannopoulou, A., Wu, L., Sun, L., Sharpe, A. H., Bigby, M., and Georgopoulos, K. (1996) Selective defects in the development of the fetal and adult lymphoid system in mice with an Ikaros null mutation. *Immunity* **5,** 537–549.
42. Bain, G., Maandag, E. C. R., Izon, D. J., Amsen, D., Kruisbeek, A. M., Weintraub, B. C., Krop, I., Schlissel, M. S., Feeney, A. J., van Roon, M., van der Valk. M., te Riele, H. P. J., Berns, A., and Murre, C. (1994) E2A proteins are required for proper B cell development and initiation of immunoglobulin gene rearrangements. *Cell* **79,** 885–892.
43. Zhuang, Y., Soriano, P., and Weintraub, H. (1994) The helix-loop-helix gene E2A is required for B cell formation. *Cell* **79,** 875–884.
44. Lin, H. and Grosschedl, R. (1995) Failure of B-cell differentiation in mice lacking the transcription factor EBF. *Nature* **376,** 263–267.
45. Schlissel, M., Voronova, A., and Baltimore, D. (1991) Helix-loop-helix transcription factor E47 activates germ-line immunoglobulin heavy-chain gene transcription and rearrangement in a pre-T cell line. *Genes Dev.* **5,** 1367–1376.
46. Ehlich, A., Schaal, S., Gu, H., Kitamura, D., Müller, W., and Rajewsky, K. (1993) Immunoglobulin heavy and light chain genes rearrange independently at early stages of B cell development. *Cell* **72,** 695–704.
47. Gong, S. and Nussenzweig, M. C. 1996. Regulation of an early developmental checkpoint in the B cell pathway by Igβ. *Science* **272,** 411–414.
48. Kitamura, D., Kudo, A., Schaal, S., Müller, W., Melchers, F., and Rajewsky, K. (1992) A critical role of λ5 protein in B cell development. *Cell* **69,** 823–831.
49. Kitamura, D., Roes, J., Kühn, R., and Rajewsky, K. (1991) A B cell-deficient mouse by targeted disruption of the membrane exon of the immunoglobulin μ chain gene. *Nature* **350,** 423–426.
50. Mombaerts, P., Iacomini, J., Johnson, R. S., Herrup, K., Tonegawa, S., and Papaioannou, V. E. (1992) RAG-1-deficient mice have no mature B and T lymphocytes. *Cell* **68,** 869–877.
51. Shinkai, Y., Rathbun, G., Lam, K.-P., Oltz, E. M., Stewart, V., Mendelsohn, M., Charron, J., Datta, M., Young, F., Stall, A. M., and Alt, F. W. (1992) RAG-2-deficient mice lack mature lymphocytes owing to inability to initiate V(D)J rearrangement. *Cell* **68,** 855–867.
52. Papavasiliou, F., Misulovin, Z., Suh, H., and Nussenzweig, M. C. (1995) The role of Igβ in precursor B cell transition and allelic exclusion. *Science* **268,** 408–411.
53. Spanopoulou, E., Roman, C. A. J., Corcoran, L. M., Schlissel, M. S., Silver, D. P., Nemazee, D., Nussenzweig, M. C., Shinton, S. A., Hardy, R. R., and Baltimore, D. (1994) Functional immunoglobulin transgenes guide ordered B-cell differentiation in Rag-1-deficient mice. *Genes Dev.* **8,** 1030–1042.
54. Young, F., Ardman, B., Shinkai, Y., Landford, R., Blackwell, T. K., Mendelsohn, M., Rolink, A., Melchers, F., and Alt, F. W. (1994) Influence of immunoglobulin heavy- and light-chain expression on B-cell differentiation. *Genes Dev.* **8,** 1043–1057.
55. Grosschedl, R., Weaver, D., Baltimore, D., and Costantini, F. (1984) Introduction of a μ immunoglobulin gene into the mouse germ line: specific expression in lymphoid cells and synthesis of functional antibodies. *Cell* **38,** 647–658.
56. Sanchez, M., Misulovin, Z., Burkhardt, A. L., Mahajan, S., Costa, T., Franke, R., Bolen, J. B., and Nussenzweig, M. (1993) Signal transduction by immunoglobulin is mediated through Igα and Igβ. *J. Exp. Med.* **178,** 1049–1055.
57. Schlissel, M. S. and Baltimore, D. (1989) Activation of immunoglobulin kappa gene rearrangement correlates with induction of germline kappa gene transcription. *Cell* **58,** 1001–1007.
58. Yancopoulos, G. D. and Alt, F. W. (1985) Developmentally controlled and tissue-specific expression of unrearranged V_H gene segments. *Cell* **40,** 271–281.
59. Van Ness, B. G., Weigert, M., Coleclough, C., Mather, E. L., Kelley, D. E., and Perry, R. P. (1981) Transcription of the unrearranged mouse C_κ locus: sequence of the initation region and comparison of activity with a rearranged V_κ-C_κ gene. *Cell* **27,** 593–602.
60. Martin, D. J. and Van Ness, B. G. (1990) Initiation and processing of two kappa immunoglobulin germ line transcripts in mouse B cells. *Mol. Cell. Biol.* **10,** 1950–1958.

61. Leclercq, L., Butkeraitis, P., and Reth, M. (1989) A novel germ-line J_κ transcript starting immediately upstream of $J_\kappa1$. *Nucleic Acids Res.* **17,** 6809–6819.
62. Lauster, R., Reynaud, C.-A., Mårtensson, I.-L., Peter, A., Bucchini, D., Jami, J., and Weill, J.-C. (1993) Promoter, enhancer and silencer elements regulate rearrangement of an immunoglobulin transgene. *EMBO J.* **12,** 4615–4623.
63. Ferradini, L., Gu, H., De Smet, A., Rajewsky, K., Reynaud, C.-A., and Weill, J.-C. (1996) Rearrangement-enhancing element upstream of the mouse immunoglobulin kappa chain J cluster. *Science* **271,** 1416–1420.
64. Kozmik, Z., Wang, S., Dörfler, P., Adams, B., and Busslinger, M. (1992) The promoter of the CD19 gene is a target for the B-cell-specific transcription factor BSAP. *Mol. Cell. Biol.* **12,** 2662–2672.
65. Fitzsimmons, D., Hodsdon, W., Wheat, W., Maira, S.-M., Wasylyk, B., and Hagman, J. (1996) Pax-5 (BSAP) recruits Ets proto-oncogene family proteins to form functional ternary complexes on a B-cell-specific promoter. *Genes Dev.* **10,** 2198–2211.
66. Zwollo, P. and Desiderio, S. (1994) Specific recognition of the *blk* promoter by the B-lymphoid transcription factor B-cell-specific activator protein. *J. Biol. Chem.* **269,** 15,310–15,317.
67. Reimold, A. M., Ronath, P. D., Li, Y.-S., Hardy, R. R., David, C. S., Strominger, J. L., and Glimcher, L. H. (1996) Transcription factor B cell lineage-specific activator protein regulates the gene for human X-box binding protein 1. *J. Exp. Med.* **183,** 393–401.
68. Nutt, S. L., Morrison, A., Dörfler, P., Rolink, A., and Busslinger, M. (1998) Identification of BSAP (Pax-5) target genes in early B-cell development by loss- and gain-of-function experiments. *EMBO J.,* in press.
69. Tedder, T. F., Inaoki, M., and Sato, S. (1997) The CD19–CD21 complex regulates signal transduction thresholds governing humoral immunity and autoimmunity. *Immunity* **6,** 107–118.
70. Carter, R. H. and Fearon, D. T. (1992) CD19, Lowering the threshold for antigen receptor stimulation of B lymphocytes. *Science* **256,** 105–107.
71. Engel, P., Zhou, L.-J., Ord, D. C., Sato, S., Koller, B., and Tedder, T. F. (1995) Abnormal B lymphocyte development, activation, and differentiation in mice that lack or overexpress the CD19 signal transduction molecule. *Immunity* **3,** 39–50.
72. Rickert, R. C., Rajewsky, K., and Roes, J. (1995) Impairment of T-cell-dependent B-cell responses and B-1 cell development in CD19–deficient mice. *Nature* **376,** 352–355.
73. Hagman, J. and Grosschedl, R. (1992) An inhibitory carboxyl-terminal domain of Ets-1 and Ets-2 mediates differential binding of ETS family factors to promoter sequences of the *mb-1* gene. *Proc. Natl. Acad. Sci. USA* **89,** 8889–8893.
74. Hagman, J., Travis, A., and Grosschedl, R. (1991) A novel lineage-specific nuclear factor regulates *mb-1* gene transcription at the early stages of B cell differentiation. *EMBO J.* **10,** 3409–3417.
75. Travis, A., Hagman, J., and Grosschedl, R. (1991) Heterogeneously initiated transcription from the pre-B- and B-cell-specific *mb-1* promoter: analysis of the requirement for upstream factor-binding sites and initiation site sequences. *Mol. Cell. Biol.* **11,** 5756–5766.
76. Torres, P. M., Flaswinkel, H., Reth, M., and Rajewsky, K. (1996) Aberrant B cell development and immune response in mice with a compromised BCR complex. *Science* **272,** 1804–1808.
77. Zimmerman, K. A., Yancopoulos, G. D., Collum, R. G., Smith, R. K., Kohl, N. E., Denis, K. A., Nau, M. M., Witte, O. N., Toran-Allerand, D., Gee, C. E., Minna, J. D., and Alt, F. W. (1986) Differential expression of *myc* family genes during murine development. *Nature* **319,** 780–783.
78. Morrow, M. A., Lee, G., Gillis, S., Yancopoulos, G. D., and Alt, F. W. (1992) Interleukin-7 induces N-*myc* and c-*myc* expression in normal precursor B lymphocytes. *Genes Dev.* **6,** 61–70.
79. Malynn, B. A., Demengeot, J., Stewart, W., Charron, J., and Alt, F. W. (1995) Generation of normal lymphocytes dereived from N-*myc*-deficient embryonic stem cells. *Int. Immunol.* **7,** 1637–1647.
80. Stavnezer, J. (1996) Immunoglobulin class switching. *Curr. Opin. Immunol.* **8,** 199–205.
81. Rothman, P., Li, S. C., Gorham, B., Glimcher, L., Alt, F., and Boothby, M. (1991) Identification of a conserved lipopolysaccharide-plus-interleukin-4-responsive element located at the promoter of the germ line ε transcript. *Mol. Cell. Biol.* **11,** 5551–5561.
82. Delphin, S. and Stavnezer, J. (1995) Characterization of an interleukin 4 (IL-4) responsive region in the immunoglobulin heavy chain germline ε promoter: regulation by NF-IL-4, a C/EBP family member and NF-κB/p50. *J. Exp. Med.* **181,** 181–192.

83. Kim, J., Reeves, R., Rothman, P., and Boothby, M. (1995) The non-histone chromosomal protein HMG-I(Y) contributes to the repression of the immunoglobulin heavy chain germ-line ε RNA promoter. *Eur. J. Immunol.* **25,** 798–808.
84. Thienes, C., De Monte, L., Monticelli, S., Busslinger, M., Gould, H. J., and Vercelli, D. (1997) The transcription factor B cell-specific activator protein (BSAP) enhances both IL-4- and CD40-mediated activation of the human ε germline promoter. *J. Immunol.*, **158,** 5874–5882.
85. Niles, M. J., Matsuuchi, L., and Koshland, M. E. (1995) Polymer IgM assembly and secretion in lymphoid and nonlymphoid cell lines: Evidence that J chain is required for pentamer IgM synthesis. *Proc. Natl. Acad. Sci. USA* **92,** 2884–2888.
86. Blackman, M. A., Tigges, M. A., Minie, M. E., and Koshland, M. E. (1986) A model system for peptide hormone action in differentiation: interleukin 2 induces a B lymphoma to transcribe the J chain gene. *Cell* **47,** 609–617.
87. Lansford, R. D., McFadden, H. J., Siu, S. T., Cox, J. S., Cann, G. M., and Koshland, M. E. (1992) A promoter element that exerts positive and negative control of the interleukin 2-responsive J-chain gene. *Proc. Natl. Acad. Sci. USA* **89,** 5966–5970.
88. Shin, M. K. and Koshland, M. E. (1993) Ets-related protein PU.1 regulates expression of the immunoglobulin J-chain gene through a novel Ets-binding element. *Genes Dev.* **7,** 2006–2015.
89. Rinkenberger, J. L.,Wallin, J. J., Johnson, K. W., and Koshland, M. E. (1996) An interleukin-2 signal relieves BSAP (Pax5)-mediated repression of the immunoglobulin J chain gene. *Immunity* **5,** 377–386.
90. Kulseth, M. A. and Rogne, S. (1994) Cloning and characterization of the bovine immunoglobulin J chain cDNA and its promoter region. *DNA Cell Biol.* **13,** 37–42.
91. Madisen, L. and Groudine, M. (1994) Identification of a locus control region in the immunoglobulin heavy-chain locus that deregulates c-*myc* expression in plasmacytoma and Burkitt's lymphoma cells. *Genes Dev.* **8,** 2212–2226.
92. Dariavach, P., Williams, G. T., Campbell, K., Pettersson, S., and Neuberger, M. S. (1991) The mouse IgH 3'-enhancer. *Eur. J. Immunol.* **21,** 1499–1504.
93. Arulampalam, V., Grant, P. A., Samuelsson, A., Lendahl, U., and Pettersson, S. (1994) Lipopolysaccharide-dependent transactivation of the temporally regulated immunoglobulin heavy chain 3' enhancer. *Eur. J. Immunol.* **24,** 1671–1677.
94. Lieberson, R., Ong, J., Shi, X., and Eckhardt, L. A. (1995) Immunoglobulin gene transcription ceases upon deletion of a distant enhancer. *EMBO J.* **14,** 6229–6238.
95. Cogné, M., Lansford, R., Bottaro, A., Zhang, J., Gorman, J., Young, F., Cheng, H.-L., and Alt, F. W. (1994) A class switch control region at the 3' end of the immunoglobulin heavy chain locus. *Cell* **77,** 737–747.
96. Michaelson, J. S., Singh, M., and Birshtein, B. K. (1996) B cell lineage-specific activator protein (BSAP): a player at multiple stages of B cell development. *J. Immunol.* **156,** 2349–2351.
97. Neurath, M. F., Stüber, E. R., and Strober, W. (1995) BSAP: a key regulator of B-cell development and differentiation. *Immunol. Today* **16,** 564–569.
98. Neurath, M. F., Strober, W., and Wakatsuki, Y. (1994) The murine Ig 3'α enhancer is a target site with repressor function for the B cell lineage-specific transcription factor BSAP (HF-HB, Sα-BP). *J. Immunol.* **153,** 730–742.
99. Singh, M. and Birshtein, B. K. (1993) NF-HB (BSAP) is a repressor of the murine immunoglobulin heavy-chain 3'α enhancer at early stages of B cell differentiation. *Mol. Cell. Biol.* **13,** 3611–3622.
100. Pettersson, S., Cook, G. P., Brüggemann, M., Williams, G. T., and Neuberger, M. S. (1990) A second B cell-specific enhancer 3' of the immunoglobulin heavy-chain locus. *Nature* **344,** 165–168.
101. Neurath, M. F., Max, E. E., and Strober, W. (1995) Pax5 regulates the murine immunoglobulin 3'α enhancer by affecting binding of NF-αP, a protein that controls heavy chain transcription. *Proc. Natl. Acad. Sci. USA* **92,** 5336–5340.
102. Singh, M. and Birshtein, B. K. (1996) Concerted repression of an immunoglobulin heavy-chain enhancer, 3'αE(hs1,2). *Proc. Natl. Acad. Sci. USA* **93,** 4392–4397.
103. Michaelson, J. S., Singh, M., Snapper, C. M., Sha, W. C., Baltimore, D., and Birshtein, B. K. (1996) Regulation of 3' IgH enhancers by a common set of factors including κB-binding proteins. *J. Immunol.* **156,** 2828–2839.
104. Meyer, K. B., and Neuberger, M. S. (1989) The immunoglobulin κ locus contains a second, stronger B-cell-specific enhancer which is located downstream of the constant region. *EMBO J.* **8,** 1959–1964.

105. Meyer, K. B., Sharpe, M. J., Surani, M. A., and Neuberger, M. S. (1990) The importance of the 3'-enhancer in immunoglobulin κ gene expression. *Nucleic Acids Res.* **18,** 5609–5615.
106. Pongubala, J. M. R. and Atchison, M. L. (1991) Functional characterization of the developmentally controlled immunoglobulin kappa 3' enhancer: regulation by Id, a repressor of helix-loop-helix transcription factors. *Mol. Cell. Biol.* **11,** 1040–1047.
107. Betz, A. G., Milstein, C., González-Fernández, A., Pannell, R., Larson, T., and Neuberger, M. S. (1994) Elements regulating somatic hypermutation of an immunoglobulin κ gene: a critical role for the enhancer/matrix attachment region. *Cell* **77,** 239–248.
108. Hiramatsu, R., Akagi, K., Matsuoka, M., Sakumi, K., Nakamura, H., Kingsbury, L., David, C., R.Hardy, R., Yamamura, H.-I., and Sakano, H. (1995) The 3' enhancer region determines the B/T specificity and pro-B/pre-B specificity of immunoglobulin V_κ-J_κ joining. *Cell* **83,** 1113–1123.
109. Gorman, J. R., van der Stoep, N., Monroe, R., Cogne, M., Davidson, L., and Alt, F. W. (1996) The Igκ 3' enhancer influences the ratio of Igκ versus Igλ B lymphocytes. *Immunity* **5,** 241–252.
110. Eisenbeis, C. F., Singh, H., and Storb, U. (1995) Pip, a novel IRF family member, is a lymphoid-specific, PU.1–dependent transcriptional activator. *Genes Dev.* **9,** 1377–1387.
111. Judde, J.-G. and E.Max, E. (1992) Characterization of the human immunoglobulin kappa gene 3' enhancer: functional importance of three motifs that demonstrate B-cell-specific in vivo footprints. *Mol. Cell. Biol.* **12,** 5206–5216.
112. Pongubala, J. M.R., Nagulapalli, S., Klemsz, M. J., McKercher, S. R., Maki, R. A., and Atchison, M. L. (1992) PU.1 recruits a second nuclear factor to a site important for immunoglobulin κ 3' enhancer activity. *Mol. Cell. Biol.* **12,** 368–378.
113. Pongubala, J. M. R. and M.Atchison, L. (1995) Activating transcription factor 1 and cyclic AMP response element modulator can modulate the activity of the immunoglobulin κ 3' enhancer. *J. Biol. Chem.* **270,** 10304–10313.
114. Park, K. and Atchison, M. L. (1991) Isolation of a candidate repressor/activator, NF-E1 (YY-1, δ), that binds to the immunoglobulin κ 3' enhancer and the immunoglobulin heavy-chain μE1 site. *Proc. Natl. Acad. Sci. USA* **88,** 9804–9808.
115. Roque, M. C., Smith, P. A., and Blasquez, V. C. (1996) A developmentally modulated chromatin structure at the mouse immunoglobulin k 3' enhancer. *Mol. Cell. Biol.* **16,** 3138–3155.
116. Müller, B., Stappert, H., and Reth, M. (1990) A physical map and analysis of the murine Cκ-RS region show the presence of a conserved element. *Eur. J. Immunol.* **20,** 1409–1411.
117. Davis, R. J., D'Cruz, C. M., Lovell, M. A., Biegel, J. A., and Barr, F. G. (1994) Fusion of *PAX7* to *FKHR* by the variant t(1;13)(p36;q14) translocation in alveolar rhabdomyosarcoma. *Cancer Res.* **54,** 2869–2872.
118. Galili, N., Davis, R. J., Fredericks, W. J., Mukhopadhyay, S., Rauscher III, F. J., Emanuel, B. S., Rovera, G., and Barr, F. G. (1993) Fusion of a fork head domain gene to *PAX3* in the solid tumour alveolar rhabdomyosarcoma. *Nature Genet.* **5,** 230–235.
119. Kozmik, Z., Sure, U., Rüedi, D., Busslinger, M., and Aguzzi, A. (1995) Deregulated expression of *PAX-5* in medulloblastoma. *Proc. Natl. Acad. Sci. USA* **92,** 5709–5713.
120. Stapleton, P., Weith, A., Urbánek, P., Kozmik, Z., and Busslinger, M. (1993) Chromosomal localization of seven *PAX* genes and cloning of a novel family member, *PAX-9*. *Nature Genet.* **3,** 292–298.
121. Offit, K., Parsa, N. Z., Filippa, D., Jhanwar, S. C., and Chaganti, R. S. K. (1992) t(9;14)(p13;q32) denotes a subset of low-grade non-Hodgkin's lymphoma with plasmacytoid differentiation. *Blood* **80,** 2594–2599.
122. Ohno, H., Furukawa, T., Fukuhara, S., Zong, S. Q., Kamesaki, H., Shows, T. B., Le Beau, M. M., McKeithan, T. W., Kawakami, T., and Honjo, T. (1990) Molecular analysis of a chromosomal translocation, t(9;14)(p13;q32), in a diffuse large-cell lymphoma cell line expressing the Ki-1 antigen. *Proc. Natl. Acad. Sci. USA* **87,** 628–632.
123. Iida, S., Rao, P. H., Nallasivam, P., Hibshoosh, H., Butler, M., Louie, D. C., Dyomin, V., Ohno, H., Chaganti, R. S. K., and Dalla-Favera, R. (1996) The t(9;14)(p13;q32) chromosomal translocation associated with lymphoplasmacytoid lymphoma involves the *PAX-5* gene. *Blood* **88,** 4110–4117.
124. Morrison, A., Jäger, U., Chott, A., and Busslinger, M. (1998) Deregulated *PAX-5* transcription from a translocated *IgH* promotes in marginal zone lymphoma. *Mol. Cell. Biol.,* submitted.
125. Strachan, T. and Read, A. P. (1994) PAX genes. *Curr. Opin. Genet. Dev.* **4,** 427–438.
126. Nutt, S. L., Vambrie, S., Steinlein, P., Weith, A., and Busslinger, M. (1997) Monoallelic expression of *Pax-5* (BSAP) is responsible for the haploinsufficient phenotype of heterozygous *Pax-5* mutant mice. *Nature,* submitted.

127. Vorechovsky, I., Koskinen, S., Paganelli, R., Smith, E. C. I., Busslinger, M., and Hammarström, L. (1995) The *PAX5* gene: a linkage and mutation analysis in candidate human primary immunodeficiencies. *Immunogenet.* **42,** 149–152.
128. Czerny, T. and Busslinger, M. (1995) DNA-binding and transactivation properties of Pax-6, three amino acids in the paired domain are responsible for the different sequence recognition of Pax-6 and BSAP (Pax-5). *Mol. Cell. Biol.* **15,** 2858–2871.

Chapter 7

The Role of PU.1 in the Regulation of Lymphoid and Myeloid Hematopoietic Progenitors

Edward W. Scott

1. The Big Picture of Hematopoiesis

Mammalian development begins with a single totipotent cell that undergoes an ordered process of differentiation to form a complex multicellular organism. The hematopoietic system is an accessible model system with which to study differentiation into distinct lineages. The hematopoietic stem cell (HSC) retains its pluripotent differentiative capacity throughout the lifespan of an organism. Homeostasis is maintained by a constant, ordered, and tightly regulated developmental cascade. Hematopoietic stem cells differentiate through a hierarchical array of multipotent and monopotent progenitor cells to form all cell types of the blood and lymph, including lymphocytes, granulocytes, monocytes, erythrocytes, and megakaryocytes. The regulatory pathways that control hematopoiesis consist of several interconnected mechanisms. One level of regulation is the transcriptional control of hematopoietic specific gene expression. Other mechanisms that regulate homeostasis involve the interaction of soluble hematopoietic growth factors with their cognate cell-surface receptors, and cell/cell interactions within the hematopoietic microenvironment.

Given that the HSC can develop into at least eight distinct lineages, how is the end-point determined? An ideal solution would be a master commitment switch for each lineage that functions in a manner similar to myoD in muscle differentiation *(1)*. This switch would program (or reprogram) a cell to differentiate along a given hematopoietic lineage. To date, no such switch has been identified for any hematopoietic lineage. Commitment to any given lineage is likely to require a combination of transcription factors induced in response to cell/cell interactions and a growth factor milieu. Specific combinations trigger the transcriptional activation of lineage specific genes. The com-

From: *Molecular Biology of B-Cell and T-Cell Development*
Edited by: J. G. Monroe and E. V. Rothenberg © Humana Press Inc., Totowa, NJ

mitment and subsequent lineage development of individual progenitors reflects the overall environment of the cell: transcription factors, growth factors, and cell/cell contacts. This "combinatorial" model of lineage commitment appears to be the most likely, since very few transcription factors are expressed in only a single cell lineage, and none are capable of initiating an entire program of lineage development *(2)*. Investigation of this morass of events is hampered by the biological equivalent of the Heisenberg uncertainty principle. The simple act of holding one parameter constant for study has untoward effects on the other factors involved. Put another way, your results are only as good as your assay.

The B- and T-lymphocyte lineages are a case in point. Committed lymphoid progenitors have been well-characterized *(3,4)*; however, the relationship of the lymphoid lineages to other multipotential intermediates remains unclear. Progenitors for the lymphoid lineages are very difficult to assay in vitro and require specialized culture conditions that do not support the growth of other hematopoietic lineages. Conversely, commonly used methylcellulose or spleen colony forming assays are incapable of measuring lymphoid potential *(5,6)*. Therefore, lymphoid progenitors are often depicted as being derived from a separate multipotent progenitor than the myeloid and erythroid lineages *(7)*. Cumano and colleagues have recently described assays that detect a multipotential lymphoid/myeloid progenitor cell from the fetal liver *(8–10)*. The initial assay consisted of plating single fetal liver derived hematopoietic progenitors ($AA4.1^+$, Lin^-) on a S17 stromal cell layer in the presence of IL-7. These conditions supported the outgrowth of both B-cells and macrophages, and the authors were able to demonstrate that a single progenitor could give rise to both cell lineages. This is a prime example of using a novel assay to define heretofore unknown potentialities during hematopoietic development.

The recent spate of knockout animals that effect hematopoiesis have merely confirmed the complexity of commitment decisions during hematopoietic development. Hematopoietic stem cells are thought to develop from the mesoderm in the aorta-gonad-mesonephros (AGM) region during embryogenesis *(11)*. This represents the first of many commitment events during hematopoiesis. The receptor tyrosine kinase Flk-1 is required for this event *(12)*, as is the transcription factor SCL/tal-1 *(13,14)*. Growth factors and growth factor receptors such as kit-ligand and c-kit receptor *(15)*, GM-CSF, and GM-CSFR *(16)* are also required for proper hematopoietic development. The importance of cell adhesion molecules cannot be overlooked. The $\alpha4$ integrin is required for lymphocyte development in the bone marrow *(17)*. These and other knockouts have provided genetic confirmation for what was already suspected. Every aspect of hematopoiesis is interrelated and required for proper development.

2. The Role of Transcription Factors in Hematopoiesis

One key to unraveling these complex regulatory pathways has been the identification of *cis*-regulatory elements required for the expression of lineage-restricted genes. Once identified, a *cis*-element can be used to clone the nuclear factors (usually transcription factors) that bind to the element. These transcription factors can often be shown to regulate the expression of multiple genes within a given lineage. The GATA family of proteins is a case in point. GATA-1 is the founding member of this family and was originally cloned on the basis of its ability to bind a GATA consensus motif. GATA-1, GATA-2, and GATA-3 have all been knocked out, and all have effects on hematopoiesis. Deletion of GATA-1 blocks erythroid maturation at the proerythroblast stage *(18)*. GATA-2 knockouts have a more profound hematopoietic defect characterized by severe anemia, and an almost total block to hematopoiesis *(19)*. GATA-3$^{-/-}$ mice die from anemia and exhibit hemorrhaging as well as brain and spinal cord defects *(20)*. Gene targeting of other transcription factors such as C-Myb, SCL/TAL-1, and AML-1 has also resulted in severe defects to hematopoiesis *(13,14, 21,22)*. The C/EBP family of transcription factors may play a more restricted role in hematopoietic development. C/EBP proteins are expressed in multiple tissues but appear restricted to the myeloid lineage during hematopoiesis. C/EBPα knockouts have a significant defect in granulocyte production as well as a variety of nonhematopoietic defects *(23)*. Additional details can be found in several recent reviews on the role of transcription factors in hematopoiesis *(24–26)*.

The leukemogenic nature of transcription factors was initially realized from studies utilizing animal models of leukemia. Many of the most studied systems utilize avian retroviruses capable of consistently and efficiently inducing leukemias in chickens *(27)*. One such retrovirus, E26, transforms myeloblasts and early multipotential progenitors. E26 contains a fusion protein between C-Myb and a then novel transcription factor. The novel factor was named *E*- *T*wenty *S*ix-1, or Ets-1. Both C-Myb and Ets-1 are transcription factors that normally function during hematopoietic development. As noted above, C-Myb plays a critical role in the earliest stages of hematopoietic development and appears to be required for the development of all hematopoietic lineages with the possible exception of megakaryocytes *(21)*. *Ets*-1 is primarily expressed in T-cells and appears to be required for proper T-cell maturation and function.

Ets-1 was the founding member of a large family of transcription factors, the *Ets* family. *Ets*-proteins are thought to regulate gene expression during a number of biological processes including developmental programs, lymphocyte activation, growth control, and transformation (for a review *see* refs. *28,29)*. Proteins are grouped into the *Ets* family on the basis of a common DNA binding motif, the "*ets* domain." The *Ets* family is conserved throughout a broad range of divergent species from metazoan nematodes to man *(30–32)*. All *ets* family members bind to a common DNA sequence motif C/A GGA A/T. As with other transcription factors, *ets* proteins have been demonstrated to contain multiple functional domains, including transcriptional activation and protein interaction domains. *Ets* proteins can be further divided into subfamilies based upon similarities outside the *ets* domain *(29)*. Three highly unrelated *Ets* family members, *PU.1*, *Fli-1*, and *v-ets*, nevertheless, can all induce erythroleukemias, suggesting convergent function despite divergent structure *(33–35)*.

3. The Role of PU.1 in Hematopoiesis: In Vitro Evidence

The *Ets*-family transcription factor PU.1 has been suggested to be a regulator of hematopoiesis based on two lines of evidence. *PU.1* was initially isolated as the product of the *Spi-1* proto-oncogene *(36)*. The *Spi-1/PU.1* locus is the site of integration of the spleen focus-forming provirus (SFFV) in 95% of murine erythroleukemias induced by Friend virus complexes *(37)*. SFFV proviral insertion leads to overexpression of PU.1 in erythroblasts, which has been shown to be sufficient for their immortalization *(38)*. Subsequent chemically induced differentiation of these erythroleukemic lines leads to a down regulation of PU.1 expression *(39,40)*. Therefore, PU.1 may play a role in regulating the proliferation and differentiation of normal erythroid progenitors during hematopoiesis.

The *PU.1* locus is also a common site of viral integration in the murine-AIDS (MAIDS) model. Infection of mice with the defective MAIDS virus induces a polyclonal expan-

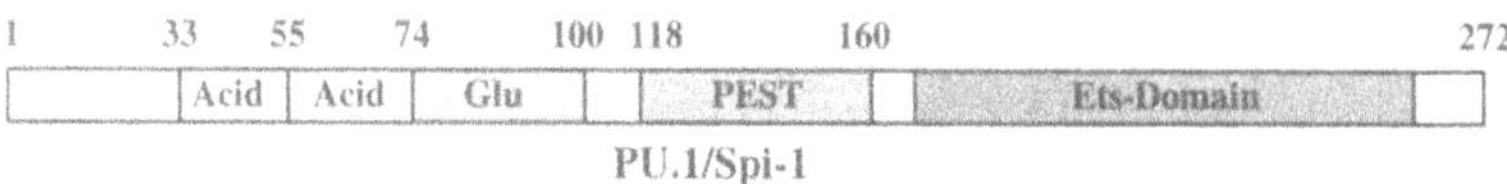

Fig. 1. Structure of the PU.1 Protein.

sion of infected B-cells *(41)*. Additional genetic changes result in the expansion becoming oligoclonal. One such change is MAIDS integration into the *PU.1* locus that can lead to B- and T-cell disfunction associated with the immunodeficiency syndrome. A similar series of events have been observed in the acquired immunodeficiency syndrome-related lymphoproliferative disorder in HIV infected individuals *(42)*, and the posttransplant lyphoproliferative disorder in immunosuppressed organ recipients *(43)*. Both lymphoproliferative disorders are closely associated with polyclonal expansion of EBV-infected B-cells that can progress into monoclonal malignant B-cell lymphomas. Several latent gene products of EBV, LMP-1, and EBNA-2, for example, are either known oncogenes or are required for growth transformation of the B-cells *(44,45)*. Recently, several groups have shown that PU.1 is an essential component that interacts with EBNA-2 to transactivate the LMP-1 oncogene *(46,47)*. This suggests that PU.1 is required for the induction of the EBV associated B-cell lymphoproliferative disorders in humans. Given the fact that *PU.1* plays an important role in several transformation processes for multiple blood cell types, understanding the normal function of this gene during hematopoietic development may provide insight into the transformation process.

PU.1 was independently cloned on the basis of its binding to a purine rich sequence, GAGGAA (PU box), in an MHC class II gene promoter *(48)*. *PU.1* is expressed specifically in hematopoietic tissues with high levels of expression in the monocytic, granulocytic, and B-lymphoid lineages *(49–51)*. It is expressed at lower levels in immature erythroid cells but not in their mature counterparts. PU.1 is expressed at low levels in human $CD34^+$, $CD38^-$ cells and is upregulated upon their differentiation along the myeloid lineage *(52)*. In mice, PU.1 is expressed in fetal HSC (Sca-1^+, Thy-1.1^+, CD$11b^+$, Lin^-) but not in adult HSC (Sca-1^+, Thy 1.1^+, Lin^-, CD $11b^-$) (C. Klug and I. Weissman, personal communication). The role that PU.1 plays in the commitment decisions of these early hematopoietic progenitors remains to be fully elucidated.

PU.1 is a 272 amino acid protein consisting of multiple functional domains, (Fig. 1) *(48,53–55)*. The *Ets*-family DNA binding domain is located at the carboxy terminus of the protein and is encoded by exon five *(48,56)*. The structure of the PU.1 DNA binding domain has recently been determined to be a winged helix-turn-helix motif *(57)*. The amino terminus of the protein contains multiple transcriptional activation domains, including two acid-rich regions and a glutamine-rich region *(48,58)*. It should be noted that PU.1 is not a particularly strong transcriptional activator by itself in transient transfection type assays. This has necessitated the use of reporter constructs containing multimerized PU.1 binding sites to map the activation domains of PU.1. The activation and DNA-binding domains are separated by a proline, glutamic acid, serine, and threonine-rich (PEST) region, which is often associated with protein degradation *(59)*. Through protein-protein interactions within the PEST domain, PU.1 recruits a second transcription factor, NF-EM5/PIP, to bind to the Ig kappa 3' and Ig lambda 2–4 enhancers *(55,58,60,61)*. Phosphorylation of PU.1 at serine 148 is required for this interaction *(60,63)*.

PU.1 is highly related (43% overall identity) to another *Ets*-protein termed Spi-B *(63)*. These two proteins have nearly identical DNA-binding specificities *(64)*, and overlapping patterns of expression within the B-lymphoid lineage *(49)*. Spi-B is also capable of binding to the kappa 3' enhancer, recruiting NF-EM5/PIP and transactivating Igκ-enhancer dependent reporter constructs (Abe Brass, personal communication). Moreau-Gachelin and colleagues have recently demonstrated the ability of both PU.1 and Spi-B to bind to the *c-fes* promoter in vitro *(64)*. They noted, however, that only PU.1 bound the site from extracts prepared from the Raji B-cell lymphoma line that expresses both proteins. This may reflect differences in protein modification resulting in altered DNA binding activity for PU.1 and Spi-B within the Raji B-cell line.

PU.1 has been demonstrated to interact with several additional proteins. Through the transactivation domain, PU.1 binds to both the TATAA box binding protein, TBP, and the retinoblastoma or Rb protein *(53,65)*. The interaction with TBP is particularly compelling for myeloid-specific genes. Most myeloid-specific promoters lack TATAA boxes but have PU.1 binding sites proximal to their transcriptional initiation sites (*see* ref. *26* for a review). PU.1 may activate transcription of these genes in part via the recruitment of TBP binding. This interaction may begin the assembly of the basic transcriptional machinery at the site of initiation. The interaction of PU.1 and Rb may also have functional relevance. Weintraub et al. recently demonstrated that Rb can block the transactivation ability of PU.1. *(65)*. This study, however, employed an artificial promoter construct and inhibitory effects of the PU.1:: Rb interaction on a native promoter remains to be demonstrated.

Nagulapilli et al. used a Far Western blot technique to assay for additional proteins that physically interact with PU.1 *(66)*. NF-IL6β (C/EBPδ), a leucine zipper transcription factor, was shown to interact with the carboxyl-terminal 28 amino acids of PU.1. This interaction required the leucine zipper motif of NF-IL6β, and the two proteins synergistically activated transcription of an artificial promoter construct. Once again, the functional role of this interaction in vivo remains unclear, although C/EBP proteins clearly play a role in myeloid gene expression. This same study demonstrated interactions between PU.1 and two HMG domain proteins, HMG I/Y, and SSRP. The functional role of these interactions was not addressed.

4. The Role Of PU.1 in the Lymphoid and Myeloid Lineages

For all their similarities, *Ets*-family members still play very individualized roles within a broad range of tissues. Defining how subtle differences in protein expression and structure establish these unique functions is a key step in understanding the process of lineage commitment. In the B-lymphoid lineage, PU.1 is implicated in regulating transcription of the immunoglobulin (Ig) heavy (μ) *(55)* and light chain genes (κ and λ) *(55,60,61)*, the *mb-1* gene *(68,69)*, and the J-chain gene *(70)*. The PU.1 binding site in the κ 3' enhancer (kE3') is required for the proper regulation of V_{κ}-J_{κ} DNA rearrangements *(71)*. Mutation of this site permitted V_{κ}-J_{κ} rearrangements to occur in T-cells. Therefore, in the B-cell lineage, PU.1 can transactivate transcription over large distances by contributing to enhancer function. The Igκ3' enhancer is the most thoroughly studied of the B-cell specific, PU.1–dependent regulatory elements. PU.1 binds to kE3' along with many other proteins such as PIP, ATF1, CREM, c-Fos, c-Jun, and E2A. Pongubala and Atchison have recently shown that these proteins form a higher-order complex on kE3', and that each protein is required for complex formation *(72)*. Furthermore, they demonstrated that the combination of PU.1, PIP, c-Fos, and c-Jun can activate kE3' in NIH-3T3 fibroblasts. A most interesting finding was that the transactivation domain of PU.1 was not required for the combinatorial activation of kE3'. PU.1 mutants lacking amino acids 33–100, combined with the other proteins, activated kE3' 75% as well as wild type PU.1. However, in the absence of PU.1 only minimal enhancer activity was observed.

In monocytes, PU.1 appears to regulate the transcription of a large proportion of myeloid-specific genes including: colony-stimulating factor receptor genes (G-CSFR, GM-CSFR, and M-CSFR), the myeloid integrins CD11b and CD18, FcγR I and FcγR IIIA, the scavenger receptor, and many others (reviewed in ref. *26*). Inhibition of PU.1 function via antisense oligonucleotides has been shown to inhibit the ability of human CD34$^+$ cells to differentiate along the myeloid lineage in vitro *(52)*. In the myeloid lineage, PU.1 regulates transcription through sites located immediately proximal to the site of transcriptional initiation. The majority of myeloid-specific genes lack a TATAA box. PU.1 is postulated to recruit TBP, thereby initiating the formation of the basic transcriptional machinery and the start of transcription. Many of these myeloid promoters also contain binding sites for C/EBP family members. The observation that PU.1 interacts with NF-IL6β (C/EBPδ) may indicate the potential of PU.1 to bind to other C/EBP family members. Therefore, PU.1 appears to function in a fundamentally different way in the lymphoid and myeloid lineages. Whether B-cell or myeloid-specific genes are expressed may reflect PU.1 interacting with different transactivation partners within the distinct lineages.

5. Genetic Analysis of PU.1 Function

The previous studies utilized a wide array of molecular biological techniques to infer PU.1 function in vivo. To definitively prove the function of PU.1 during hematopoiesis, the author used a genetic approach based on gene targeting of the *PU.1* loci in embryonic stem (ES) cells *(73)*. Since PU.1 must bind DNA to function, the author deleted the ets-DNA binding domain of *PU.1,* replacing it with the *neo* selectable marker. Therefore, even if a truncated protein were made, it could not function. Disruption of *PU.1* resulted in prenatal lethality, as *PU.1*$^{-/-}$ embryos die around day 17 out of 21 days of gestation *(74)*. It should be noted that the exact time of death is variable with a few *PU.1*$^{-/-}$ pups being stillborn (<10%). Mutant embryos produced normal numbers of megakaryocytes and erythroid progenitors, however, enucleated erythrocytes were reduced in number in some embryos. Subsequent backcrossing of the mutation onto a C57BL/6 background has severely reduced the incidence of anemic *PU.1*$^{-/-}$ embryos (E. Scott, unpublished result). Histological staining for lysozyme and myeloperoxidase, coupled with flow cytometric staining (FACS) for the myeloid specific cell surface markers CD11b/CD18 and Gr-1, indicated that myelopoiesis was blocked at a very early stage in *PU.1*$^{-/-}$ fetal livers. FACS analysis for the B-lymphoid marker B220 and the T-lymphoid markers Thy1/CD2 and CD4/CD8 demonstrated that no lymphoid precursors were produced in the mutant embryos. Reverse transcriptase-PCR (RT-PCR) for Ig gene rearrangements and the expression of early B- and T-cell genes confirmed the early nature of the block to lymphoid differentiation.

Subsequent CFU or Colony Forming Unit assays on day 16 fetal liver cells confirmed the complete lack of myeloid progenitors (CFU-G, CFU-M, CFU-GM, CFU-GEMM), but normal numbers of erythroid (CFU-E) and megakaryoid (CFU-EMeg, CFU-Meg) progenitors *(75)*. In addition, analysis of progenitors present in day 8.5 and 10.5 yolk sacs indicated that the defect in myeloid differentiation is also observed during yolk sac hematopoiesis *(76)*. Thus, PU.1 is different from other transcription factors such as EKLF (erythroid Kruppel-like factor), C-Myb, and GATA-3 *(20,77,78)*, which are only essential for fetal liver hematopoiesis. These results suggested that *PU.1* may be required for commitment to the lymphoid and myeloid lineages during hematopoietic differentiation. They also provide genetic support for the existence of a *PU.1*-dependent multipotent progenitor that gives rise to lymphocytes, monocytes, and granulocytes. Progenitors with both myeloid and B-lymphoid potential have been found in the fetal liver through the use of in vitro clonogenic assays *(10,79,80)*. Although the lineage defects induced by the *PU.1* mutation are most simply interpreted as the loss of a common multipotent *PU.1*-dependent progenitor, separate requirements for *PU.1* in committed progenitors of each lineage cannot be ruled out.

Several aspects of the *PU.1*$^{-/-}$ animals were unexpected. The very early nature of the defect would not have been predicted based on the known expression pattern of *PU.1*. Given that *PU.1* is only expressed at high levels in the myeloid and B-lymphoid lineages, defects would have been predicted to manifest *after* commitment to these lineages. Furthermore, given the complete lack of *PU.1* expression in the T-cell lineage, no defect would have been predicted. More recently, a second targeted disruption of the *PU.1* locus has been reported *(81)*. The second approach generated a different targeted allele and slightly different results. The targeting construct used by McKercher et al. *(81)* inserted the *neo* selectable marker 35 amino acids downstream of the author's deletion site. Their construct was also designed to retain the remainder of the exon encoding the DNA binding domain, thereby deleting no portion of the *PU.1* locus. In addition, slightly different versions of the *neo* selectable marker were employed in opposite orientations. McKercher et al. *(81)* observed *PU.1*$^{-/-}$ pups being born, but dying within 48 hrs because of septicemia. Analysis of these pups yielded a phenotype very similar to the author's mutation, namely, no mature B- or T-cells and no myeloid cells. However, by treating the *PU.1*$^{-/-}$ pups with antibiotics, they were able to extend their survival one to two weeks. These older pups exhibited a delayed and reduced maturation of thymocytes with the production of both CD4$^+$ and CD8$^+$ cells in the thymus. B-cell development also progressed further with this mutation. In contrast with the author's mutation, B220$^+$ cells were clearly present in the fetal liver and bone marrow. The surface phenotype of the B220$^+$ cells does not correspond to any previously recognized B-cell progenitor, and the cells fail to rearrange the immunoglobulin loci. Partial myeloid maturation also appears in these animals when treated with antibiotics. Subsequent examination of the bone marrow of these animals demonstrated that they suffer from ostopetrosis because of a lack of osteoclast formation *(82)*.

One intriguing possibility to explain these differences in observed phenotype between the two *PU.1* knockouts would be the partial retention of PU.1 function in the McKercher knockout *(81)*. If partial PU.1 function is retained, it could explain the T-cell phenotype observed in the McKercher mutant *(81)*. Since PU.1 is expressed at low levels in multipotent progenitors, there may be a lower threshold of PU.1 activity required to initiate the subsequent steps in their differentiation. The higher levels of PU.1 expressed in the B-cell and myeloid lineages may reflect a high threshold of PU.1 activity required for their maturation. Since known T-cell progenitors do not express PU.1, a low level of PU.1 activity may be sufficient to allow commitment to the T-cell lineage. Once a commitment decision to the T-cell lineage was made, *PU.1* would not be required for maturation. This is almost exactly what is seen in the mutation of McKercher et al *(81)*. The delay in T-cell development observed could reflect the expansion of a few committed T-cell progenitors that escaped the block imposed by partial PU.1 function. The production of B220$^+$ cells expressing low levels of certain B-cell specific genes and limited myeloid development would also be explained by this hypothesis. Since a higher threshold level of PU.1 function would be required for progression down the B-cell or myeloid differentiation pathway, these cells would be prevented from maturing.

6. Secondary Genetic Experiments

The generation and initial characterization of a knockout mouse does not provide definitive proof of gene function in and of itself. Are the phenotypes observed a direct result of the engineered mutation? Were other mutations introduced that are contributing to the phenotype? Hematopoietic defects like those observed in the *PU.1*$^{-/-}$ animals can arise from intrinsic defects in the development of hematopoietic progenitors, or from the lack of extrinsic factors supplied by the hematopoietic microenvironment. The *Rb* knockout is a very good example of the later phenomenon. *Rb*$^{-/-}$ embryos die by E16 and have apparent defects in enucleated erythrocyte production *(83,84)*. *Rb*$^{-/-}$ fetal livers exhibit a profoundly disturbed architecture with very few hepatocytes present. *RB*$^{-/-}$ ES cells were used to generate chimeric animals in order to test whether the hematopoietic defect observed in *Rb*$^{-/-}$ animals was cell intrinsic in nature *(85)*. The *Rb*$^{-/-}$ ES cells fully contributed to the production of mature enucleated erythrocytes in the chimeric animals. This indicated that the defect seen in the homozygous mutant animals was caused by a failure of the hematopoietic microenvironment, rather than Rb playing a direct role in erythropoiesis.

We tested the cell intrinsic nature of the *PU.1* mutation in two ways. First, by a chimeric animal analysis using *PU.1*$^{-/-}$ ES cells. Second, by adoptively transferring *PU.1*$^{-/-}$ fetal liver progenitors into lethally irradiated adult recipients. Wild-type and *PU.1*$^{-/-}$ ES cells were used to generate chimeric animals with 50–70% ES cell contribution based on coat color analysis. The mutant ES cells contributed equally to nonhematopoietic tissues when compared with wild-type ES cells. However, *PU.1*$^{-/-}$ ES cells did not contribute to any hematopoietic lineage in the adult chimeras. Even adult chimeras of greater then 90% *PU.1*$^{-/-}$ ES cell contribution showed no contribution to the lymphoid, myeloid, or erythroid lineages. The lack of erythroid contribution in the adult chimeras was puzzling because of the normal numbers of erythroid progenitors observed in *PU.1*$^{-/-}$ fetal livers. Therefore, contribution of *PU.1*$^{-/-}$ ES cells to E16 chimeras was analyzed and the expected degree of contribution to erythropoiesis was observed. When *PU.1*$^{-/-}$ fetal liver progenitors were adoptively transferred to lethally irradiated hosts a similar phenomenon was observed. *PU.1*$^{-/-}$ progenitors are unable to provide long-term radioprotection to the recipient animals with death ensuing two to three weeks after irradiation. *PU.1*$^{-/-}$ progenitors were unable to contribute to the myeloid or lymphoid lineages. Contributions to these lineages were observed in control transfers of wild-type progenitors. However, at three weeks post transfer contribution of the *PU.1*$^{-/-}$ fetal progenitors to bone marrow erythropoiesis was observed. Subsequent competitive reconstitution assays have demonstrated that *PU.1*$^{-/-}$ progenitors are able to contribute to bone marrow erythropoiesis for one month. After one month, either the fetal *PU.1*$^{-/-}$ progenitors fail to thrive in the bone marrow, or they are simply out competed by wild-type progenitors (J. Lovelock and E. Scott, unpublished results). When the fetal liver multipotential progenitor population (AA4.1^{+}, Lin^{-}) was characterized in more detail, a significant reduction in cell number was observed by flow cytometry *(75)*. It has also been shown that the adoptive transfer of wild-type HSC to *PU.1*$^{-/-}$ embryos in utero rescues the animal. Rescued *PU.1*$^{-/-}$ animals are indistinguishable from wild-type littermates at six weeks of age. The hematopoietic system of the rescued mutants is composed entirely of wild-type donor derived cells (E. Scott, unpublished results). Tondravi *(82)* and McKercher et al. *(81)*, reported a similar rescue via HSC transfer into newborn *PU.1*$^{-/-}$ mutants. These data collectively prove that the hematopoietic defect observed in *PU.1*$^{-/-}$ mice is cell intrinsic in nature and cannot be complemented by any factors supplied in trans by a wild-type microenvironment. The lack of contribution to erythropoiesis in adult chimeras, and the failure of fetal liver derived *PU.1*$^{-/-}$ progenitors to either reconstitute or radioprotect adult animals suggest that there may be differing requirements for PU.1 in fetal vs adult hematopoiesis.

7. An Alternative Approach

Given the complexity of continuing analysis of PU.1 function in animals, we wanted to utilize the capability of ES cells to differentiate in vitro to provide a simplified system to study hematopoiesis. This in vitro differentiation (IVD) system is capable of producing multiple hematopoietic lineages including; macrophages, neutrophils, megakaryocytes, and erythrocytes *(86)*. *PU.1*$^{-/-}$ ES cells were generated by sequential gene targeting. Southern blot analysis was used to confirm that both alleles of *PU.1* had been disrupted *(76)*.

During in vitro differentiation, ES cells form three-dimensional structures known as embryoid bodies (Ebs), containing a variety of embryonic cells *(86,87)*. When differentiated Ebs produce primitive erythrocytes, macrophages, early megakaryocytes, and rare neutrophils *(86)*. *PU.1*$^{+/+}$, *PU.1*$^{+/-}$, and *PU.1*$^{-/-}$ ES cells were differentiated for 11 days and examined both morphologically and immunochemically for macrophage production. May-Grunwald-Giemsa staining of cytospins prepared from *PU.1*$^{-/-}$ Ebs failed to detect monocytes, macrophages, or neutrophils. Immunocytochemical staining for the macrophage cell surface markers CD11b (immature, mature) and F4/80 (mature) was performed on adherent cell populations isolated from Ebs. *PU.1*$^{+/+}$ and *PU.1*$^{+/-}$ Ebs clearly produced macrophages that stained for both CD11b and F4/80. *PU.1*$^{-/-}$ Ebs did not produce macrophages. Myeloid gene expression was examined by RT-PCR, using RNA harvested from whole embryoid bodies. *PU.1*$^{-/-}$ Ebs expressed a variety of early myeloid/multipotential progenitor genes such as CD34, GATA-2, G-CSFR, GM-CSFR, and low levels of MPO. The analysis was extended to examine the expression of genes expressed later in myeloid development (CD11b, CD18, CD64, M-CSFR). The expression of these genes was ablated or reduced below detection by the *PU.*1 mutation. Henkel et al confirmed these data with an independent line of *PU.1*$^{-/-}$ ES cells *(88)*. The lack of myeloid maturation in the *PU.1*$^{-/-}$ Ebs recapitulates the myeloid defect seen in *PU.1*$^{-/-}$ animals, thus providing a simplified system with which to analyze myelopoiesis.

The ES cell differentiation system has also been used to examine the development of early B-cell progenitors in vitro. Wild-type and *PU.1*$^{-/-}$ ES cells were differentiated in the presence of IL-11 and IL-7 for 18 days prior to harvesting RNA. RT-PCR analysis was used to examine the expression of early B-cell markers. Wild-type ES cells differentiated to the point of expressing the IL 7 receptor and *B29* but were still negative for *Rag* and *TdT* expression. Therefore, the IVD system is only able to detect very early events in B-cell development. *PU.1*$^{-/-}$ ES cells, however, never expressed *IL-7R*, and B29 expression was greatly reduced (E. W. Scott, unpublished results). The residual expression of *B29* may reflect the presence of multipotential progenitors in the *PU.1*$^{-/-}$ Ebs. The IVD results, taken together, strongly suggest that the block to both B-lymphoid and myeloid development induced by the *PU.1* mutation occurs prior to lineage commitment at the level of a multipotential progenitor.

8. Genetic Analysis of Hematopoiesis in a Tissue-Culture Dish

The final genetic proof of the function of PU.1 requires the complementation of the *PU.1*$^{-/-}$ phenotype by reintroducing the gene. To address this requirement, a transgene carrying the *PU.1* cDNA under the control of the native promoter was transfected into *PU.1*$^{-/-}$ ES cells. The PU.1 transgene rescued the ability of the *PU.1*$^{-/-}$ ES cells to differentiate into mature macrophages *(76)*. The presence of macrophages was confirmed by immunochemical staining for the macrophage-specific markers CD11b and F4/80. RT-PCR analysis also confirmed the re-expression of the M-CSFR and CD64. The rescue of myeloid differentiation proved that the *PU.1* mutation caused the observed phenotype and not untoward effects on a second locus. The culmination of a four-year proof of function in a mammal that would have taken two weeks in yeast.

The ability to rescue the *PU.1* mutation with a transgene provides a very powerful genetic tool to examine the functional significance of the structural components of PU.1. The readout of the in vitro differentiation system is the production of normal, functional, mature macrophages. No artificial reporter constructs in transient transfection assays with transformed cell lines. No inferences about in vivo function-based biochemical analysis. Simply a means to genetically test mutant versions of PU.1 during myeloid development. The PU.1 transgene was engineered to allow the easy introduction of mutant PU.1 cDNAs into *PU.1*$^{-/-}$ ES cells. All mutations selected for assay have been previously characterized for their effects on PU.1 function in vitro. Each mutant has been stably expressed both by in vitro translation and in transformed cell lines. Acidic activation domain mutants were fully capable of promoting mature macrophage development during IVD. This is in stark contrast to the absolute requirement for this domain in transactivation assays with reporter constructs. However, the glutamine rich domain was absolutely required for macrophage development even though its mutation had only minor effects in vitro. Deletion of the PEST domain appears to stabilize the PU.1 protein during transient transfection assays. Indeed, this prompted the activation domain mapping studies to be performed in the absence of the PEST domain *(58)*. Once again, the PEST domain proved to be essential for the development of macrophages. Deletion of the carboxy terminal 24 amino acids of PU.1 blocks NF-IL6β (C/EBPδ) binding in solution, and its ability to bind DNA in electrophoretic mobility shift assays. This deletion had no effect on myeloid differentiation during IVD. Larger deletions of the *ets*-DNA binding domain did, however, prevent the rescue of myelopoiesis (Robert Fisher and E. W. Scott, unpublished results).

The conclusions that can be drawn from this type of analysis have potentially wide ranging implications. The acidic activation domain of PU.1 had the greatest transactivating potential in transient assays, yet deletion of the domain has no effect on myelopoiesis. Weiss et al. have recently demonstrated that the transactivation domain of the GATA-1 protein is not required for the terminal erythroid maturation of a transformed erythroblastic cell line, G1E *(89)*. Another example of a differentiation assay yielding unexpected results with regards to transactivation. The acidic activation domain of PU.1 may still be required for B-cell development. Future experiments with chimeric animals will address this question. Since PU.1 acts proximally in myeloid cells and distally in B-cells to the site of transcriptional initiation, different domains of the protein may well be required. Such findings would suggest some very interesting knock-in experiments for future studies.

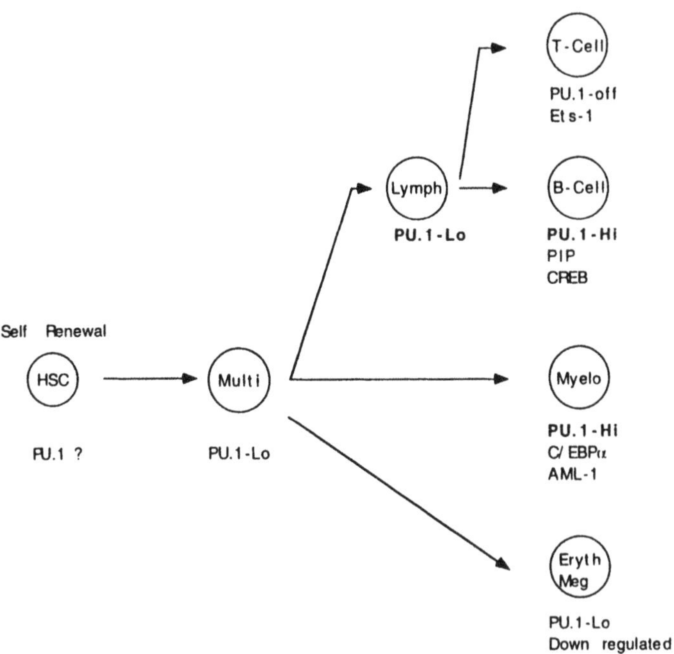

Fig. 2. Role of PU.1 in Hematopoiesis. Bold lettering indicates progenitors that require PU.1 during hematopoiesis.

9. PU.1 and Hematopoietic Lineage Commitment

What is the role of PU.1 in commitment to the lymphoid and myeloid lineages? The accumulated evidence makes two things clear. First, PU.1 is not sufficient to commit cells along the lymphoid or myeloid lineage. The expression of PU.1 in fetal HSC and erythroid progenitors is sufficient to rule that possibility out. Second, the author's data strongly suggested that PU.1 is required for lymphoid or myeloid commitment to take place. At the very least, PU.1 is required for B-cell and myeloid maturation beyond the very early progenitor stage. Figure 2 presents a model of PU.1 function during hematopoietic development. The expression of PU.1 in long-term self-renewing hematopoietic stem cell is difficult to determine because of the limited ability to isolate these cells. PU.1 is expressed at low levels in multipotential progenitor cells. Erythrocyte development requires that this low level expression of PU.1 be downregulated for progression past the erythroblast stage.

In the myeloid lineage, PU.1 is essential for maturation and perhaps commitment. PU.1 expression is upregulated in myeloid cells where it is necessary for the expression of a wide variety of myeloid-specific genes. PU.1 is not sufficient for myeloid gene expression. Rather, PU.1 acts in conjunction with other transcription factors such as AML-1 and C/EBPα to direct myeloid-specific expression. A similar situation exists in the B lymphoid lineage. PU.1 is *required* for the expression of B-cell specific genes such as Ig kappa, but it is not *sufficient.* In the B-cell lineage PU.1 appears to interact with a different group of transcription factors (PIP, CREM, ATF, E2A) than in the myeloid lineage.

One model of lineage commitment hypothesizes that the combination of transcription factors expressed by a multipotential progenitor cell determines its ultimate fate. Hu et al. examined gene expression in early multipotent progenitor cells *(90).* They demonstrated multilineage gene expression (a mix of lineage specific genes) within single cells. This could represent fluctuations in transcription factor expression prior to lineage commitment. Stochastic or environmental factors may determine the eventual transcription factor balance within any given cell. In this model, small alterations in transcription factor combinations would be sufficient to explain the large phenotypic differences seen among hematopoietic lineages. In addition, one transcription factor such as PU.1 could easily play different roles in separate lineages by interacting with different partners. Alternatively, lineage-specific coactivators may still function as "master switches" to induce lineage commitment. Until all transcription factors have been identified and tested within the hematopoietic system, or specific combinations of factors are shown to reprogram cell fate, this question will remain unresolved.

References

1. Olson, E. N., Brennan, T. J., Chakraborty, T., Cheng, T. C., Cserjesi, P., Edmondson, D., James, G., and Li, L. (1991) Molecular control of myogenesis: antagonism between growth and differentiation. *Mol. Cell. Biochem.* **104,** 7–13.
2. Orkin, S. (1996) Development of the Hematopoietic system. *Curr. Opinion Genet. Dev.* **6,** 597–602.
3. Hardy, R. R., Carmack, C. E., Shinton, S. A., Kemp, J. D., and Hayakawa, K. (1991) Resolution and characterization of pro-B and pre-pro-B cell stages in normal mouse bone marrow. *J. Exp. Med.* **173,** 1213–1225.
4. Rothenberg, E. V. (1992) The development of functionally responsive T cells. *Adv. Immunol.* **51,** 85–214.
5. Harrison, D. E. (1992) Evaluating functional abilities of primitive hematopoietic stem cell populations. *Curr. Topics Microbiol. Immunol.* **177,** 13–30.
6. Spangrude, G. J. (1992) The pre-spleen colony-forming unit assay: measurement of spleen colony-forming unit regeneration. *Curr. Topics Microbiol. Immunol.* **177,** 31–39.
7. Dexter, T. M. and Spooncer, E. (1987) Growth and differentiation in the hematopoietic system. *Ann. Rev. Cell Biol.* **3,** 423–441.
8. Cumano, A., Kee, B. L., Ramsden, D. A., Marshall, A., Paige, C. J., and Wu, G. E. (1994) Development of B lymphocytes from lymphoid committed and uncommitted progenitors. *Immunol. Rev.* **137,** 5–33.
9. Cumano, A. and Paige, C. J. (1992) Enrichment and characterization of uncommitted B-cell precursors from fetal liver at day 12 of gestation. *EMBO J.* **11,** 593–601.
10. Cumano, A., Paige, C. J., Iscove, N. N., and Brady, G. (1992) Bipotential precursors of B cells and macrophages in murine fetal liver. *Nature* **356,** 612–615.
11. Muller, A. M., Medvinsky, A., Strouboulis, J., Grosveld, F., and Dzierzak, E. (1994) Development of hematopoietic stem cell activity in the mouse embryo. *Immunity* **1,** 291–301.
12. Shalaby, F., Rossant, J., Yamaguchi, T. P., Gertsenstein, M., Wu, X. F., Breitman, M. L., and Schuh, A. C. (1995) Failure of blood-island formation and vasculogenesis in Flk-1–deficient mice. *Nature* **376,** 62–66.
13. Porcher, C., Swat, W., Rockwell, K., Fujiwara, Y., Alt, F. W., and Orkin, S. H. (1996) The T cell leukemia oncoprotein SCL/tal-1 is essential for development of all hematopoietic lineages. *Cell* **86,** 47–57.
14. Robb, L., Lyons, I., Li, R., Hartley, L., Kontgen, F., Harvey, R. P., Metcalf, D., and Begley, C. G. (1995) Absence of yolk sac hematopoiesis from mice with a targeted disruption of the scl gene. *Proc. Natl. Acad. Sci. USA* **92,** 7075–7079.

15. Morrison-Graham, K. and Takahashi, Y. (1993) Steel factor and c-kit receptor: from mutants to a growth factor system. *Bioessays* **15,** 77.
16. Lieschke, G. J. (1997) CSF-deficient mice: what have they taught us? Ciba Foundation Symposium **204,** 60–74; discussion 74–7.
17. Arroyo, A., Wang, J., Rayburn, H., and Hynes, R. (1996) Differential requirements for alpha-4 integrins during fetal and adult hematopoiesis. *Cell* **85,** 997–1008.
18. Pevny, L., Simon, M. C., Robertson, E. J., Klien, W. H., Tsai, S. F., D'Agati, V., Orkin, S. H., and Costantini, F. (1991) Erythroid differentiation in chimeric mice blocked by a targeted mutation in the gene for transcription factor GATA-1. *Nature* **349,** 257–260.
19. Tsai, F. Y., Keller, G., Kuo, F. C., Weiss, M., Chen, J., Rosenblatt, M., Alt, F. W., and Orkin, S. H. (1994) An early haematopoietic defect in mice lacking the transcription factor GATA-2. *Nature* **371,** 221–226.
20. Pandolfi, P. P., Roth, M. E., Karis, A., Leonard, M. W., Dzierzak, E., Grosveld, F. G., Engel, J. D., and Lindenbaum, M. H. (1995) Targeted disruption of the GATA3 gene causes severe abnormalities in the nervous system and in fetal liver haematopoiesis [see comments]. *Nature Genetics* **11,** 40–44.
21. Mucenski, M. L., Mclain, K., Kier, A. B., Swerdlow, S. H., Schreiner, C. M., Miller, T. A., Pietryga, D. W., Scott, W. J., and Potter, S. S. (1991) A functional c-myb gene is required for normal murine fetal hepatic hematopoiesis. *Cell* **65,** 677–689.
22. Okuda, T., van Deursen, J., Hiebert, S. W., Grosveld, G., and Downing, J. R. (1996) AML1, the target of multiple chromosomal translocations in human leukemia, is essential for normal fetal liver hematopoiesis. *Cell* **84,** 321–330.
23. Zhang, D., Zhang, P., Wang, N., Hetherington, C., Darlington, G., and Tenen, D. (1997) Absence of colony-stimulating factor singnaling and neutrophil development in CCAAT enhancer binding protein α-deficient mice. *Proc. Natl. Acad. Sci USA* **94,** 569–574.
24. Orkin, S. (1995) Transcription factors and hematopoietic development. *J. Biol. Chem.* **270,** 4955–4958.
25. Shivdasani, R. A. and Orkin, S. H. (1996) The transcriptional control of hematopoiesis. *Blood* **87,** 4025–4039.
26. Tenen, D., Hromas, R., Licht, J., and Zhang, D. (1997) Transcription factors, normal myeloid development, and leukemia. *Blood* **90,** 489–519.
27. McNagny, K. M. and Graf, T. (1996) Acute avian leukemia viruses as tools to study hematopoietic cell differentiation. *Current Topics Microbiol. Immunol.* **212,** 143–162.
28. Macleod, K., Leprince, D., and Stehelin, D. (1992) The ets gene family. *Trends Biochem. Sci.* **17,** 251–256.
29. Wasylyk, B., Hahn, S. L., and Giovane, A. (1993) The Ets family of transcription factors [published erratum appears in Eur J Biochem 1993 Aug 1;215(3):907]. *Eur. J. Biochem.* **211,** 7–18.
30. Degnan, B. M., Degnan, S. M., Naganuma, T., and Morse, D. E. (1993) The ets multigene family is conserved throughout the Metazoa. *Nucleic Acids Res.* **21,** 3479–3484.
31. Reddy, E. S. and Rao, V. N. (1988) Structure, expression and alternative splicing of the human c-ets-1 proto-oncogene. *Oncogene Res.* **3,** 239–246.
32. Watson, D. K., McWilliams, M. J., Lapis, P., Lautenberger, J. A., Schweinfest, C. W., and Papas, T. S. (1988) Mammalian ets-1 and ets-2 genes encode highly conserved proteins. *Proc. Natl. Acad. Sci. USA* **85,** 7862–7866.
33. Ben-David, Y. and Bernstein, A. (1991) Friend virus-induced erythroleukemia and the multistage nature of cancer. *Cell* **66,** 831–834.
34. Ben-David, Y., Giddens, E. B., Letwin, K., and Bernstein, A. (1991) Erythroleukemia induction by Friend murine leukemia virus: insertional activation of a new member of the ets gene family, Fli-1, closely linked to c-ets-1. *Genes Dev.* **5,** 908–918.
35. Metz, T. and Graf, T. (1991) Fusion of the nuclar oncoproteins v-*Myb* and v-*Ets* is required for the leukemogenicity of E26 virus. *Cell* **66,** 95–105.
36. Goebl, M. G. (1990) The PU.1 transcription factor is the product of the putative oncogene Spi-1. *Cell* **61,** 1165–1166.
37. Moreau-Gachelin, F., Tavitian, A., and Tambourin, P. (1988) Spi-1 is a putative oncogene in virally induced murine erythroleukemias. *Nature* **331,** 277–280.
38. Schuetze, S., Stenberg, P. E., and Kabat, D. (1993) The Ets-related transcription factor PU.1 immortalizes erythroblasts. *Mol. Cell. Biol.* **13,** 5670–5678.

39. Delgado, M. D., Hallier, M., Meneceur, P., Tavitian, A., and Moreau-Gachelin, F. (1994) Inhibition of Friend cells proliferation by spi-1 antisense oligodeoxynucleotides. *Oncogene* **9,** 1723–1727.
40. Schuetze, S., Paul, R., Gliniak, B. C., and Kabat, D. (1992) Role of the PU.1 transcription factor in controlling differentiation of Friend erythroleukemia cells. *Mol. Cell. Biol.* **12,** 2967–2975.
41. Huang, M., Takac, M., Kozak, C. A., and Jolicoeur, P. (1995) The murine AIDS defective provirus acts as an insertional mutagen in its infected target B cells. *J. Virol.* **69,** 4069–4078.
42. Dolcetti, R., Gloghini, A., De Vita, S., Vaccher, E., De Re, V., Tirelli, U., Carbone, A., and Boiocchi, M. (1995) Characteristics of EBV-infected cells in HIV-related lymphadenopathy: implications for the pathogenesis of EBV-associated and EBV-unrelated lymphomas of HIV-seropositive individuals. *Int. J. Cancer* **63,** 652–659.
43. Leblond, V., Sutton, L., Dorent, R., Davi, F., Bitker, M. O., Gabarre, J., Charlotte, F., Ghoussoub, J. J., Fourcade, C., Fischer, A., and et al. (1995) Lymphoproliferative disorders after organ transplantation: a report of 24 cases observed in a single center. *J. Clin. Oncol.* **13,** 961–968.
44. Hanto, D. W. (1995) Classification of Epstein-Barr virus-associated posttransplant lymphoproliferative diseases: implications for understanding their pathogenesis and developing rational treatment strategies. *Ann. Rev. Med.* **46,** 381–394.
45. Vousden, K. H. and Farrell, P. J. (1994) Viruses and human cancer. *Bri. Medi. Bull.* **50,** 560–581.
46. Johannsen, E., Koh, E., Mosialos, G., Tong, X., Kieff, E., and Grossman, S. R. (1995) Epstein-Barr virus nuclear protein 2 transactivation of the latent membrane protein 1 promoter is mediated by J kappa and PU.1. *J. Virol.* **69,** 253–262.
47. Laux, G., Adam, B., Strobl, L. J., and Moreau-Gachelin, F. (1994) The Spi-1/PU.1 and Spi-B ets family transcription factors and the recombination signal binding protein RBP-J kappa interact with an Epstein-Barr virus nuclear antigen 2 responsive cis-element. *EMBO J.* **13,** 5624–5632.
48. Klemsz, M. J., McKercher, S. J., Celada, A., Van Beveren, C., and Maki, R. A. (1990) The macrophage and B cell-specific transcription factor PU.1 is related to the ets oncogene. *Cell* **61,** 113–124.
49. Chen, H. M., Zhang, P., Voso, M. T., Hohaus, S., Gonzalez, D. A., Glass, C. K., Zhang, D. E., and Tenen, D. G. (1995) Neutrophils and monocytes express high levels of PU.1 (Spi-1) but not Spi-B. *Blood* **85,** 2918–2928.
50. Galson, D. L., Hensold, J. O., Bishop, T. R., Schalling, M., D'Andrea, A. D., Jones, C., Auron, P. E., and Housman, D. E. (1993) Mouse beta-globin DNA-binding protein B1 is identical to a proto-oncogene, the transcription factor Spi-1/PU.1, and is restricted in expression to hematopoietic cells and the testis. *Mol. Cell. Biol.* **13,** 2929–2941.
51. Hromas, R., Orazi, A., Neiman, R. S., Maki, R., Van Beveran, C., Moore, J., and Klemsz, M. (1993) Hematopoietic lineage- and stage-restricted expression of the ETS oncogene family member PU. 1. *Blood* **82,** 2998–3004.
52. Voso, M. T., Burn, T. C., Wulf, G., Lim, B., Leone, G., and Tenen, D. G. (1994) Inhibition of hematopoiesis by competitive binding of transcription factor PU. 1. *Proc. Natl. Acad. Sci. USA* **91,** 7932–7936.
53. Hagemeier, C., Bannister, A. J., Cook, A., and Kouzarides, T. (1993) The activation domain of transcription factor PU.1 binds the retinoblastoma (RB) protein and the transcription factor TFIID in vitro: RB shows sequence similarity to TFIID and TFIIB. *Proc. Natl. Acad. Sci. USA* **90,** 1580–1584.
54. Nagulapalli, S., Pongubala, J., and Atchison, M. (1995) Multiple proteins physically interact with PU.1. *J. Immunol.* **155,** 4330–4338.
55. Pongubala, J. M., Nagulapalli, S., Klemsz, M. J., McKercher, S. R., Maki, R. A., and Atchison, M. L. (1992) PU.1 recruits a second nuclear factor to a site important for immunoglobulin kappa 3' enhancer activity. *Mol. Cell. Biol.* **12,** 368–378.
56. Moreau-Gachelin, F., Ray, D., Mattei, M., Tambourin, P., and Tavitian, A. (1989) The putative oncogene Spi-1: murine chromosomal localization and transcriptional activation in murine acute erythroleukemias. *Oncogene* **4,** 1449–1456.
57. Kodandapani, R., Pio, F., NI, C., Piccialli, G., Klemsz, M., McKercher, S., Maki, R., and Ely, K. (1996) A new pattern for helix-turn-helix recognition revealed by the PU.1 ets-domain-DNA complex. *Nature* **380,** 456–459.
58. Klemsz, M. and Maki, R. (1996) Activation of transcription by PU.1 requires both acidic and glutamine domains. *MCB* **16,** 390–397.

59. Rodgers, S., Wells, R., and Rechsteiner, M. (1986) Amino acid sequences common to rapidly degraded proteins: the PEST hypothesis. *Science* **234,** 364–368.
60. Eisenbeis, C. F., Singh, H., and Storb, U. (1995) Pip, a novel IRF family member, is a lymphoid-specific, PU.1–dependent transcriptional activator. *Genes Dev.* **9,** 1377–1387.
61. Eisenbeis, C. F., Singh, H., and Storb, U. (1993) PU.1 is a component of a multiprotein complex which binds an essential site in the murine immunoglobulin lambda 2-4 enhancer. *Mol. Cell. Biol.* **13,** 6452–6461.
62. Pongubala, J. M., Van Beveren, C., Nagulapalli, S., Klemsz, M. J., McKercher, S. R., Maki, R. A., and Atchison, M. L. (1993) Effect of PU.1 phosphorylation on interaction with NF-EM5 and transcriptional activation. *Science* **259,** 1622–1625.
63. Ray, D., Bosselut, R., Ghysdael, J., Mattei, M. G., Tavitian, A., and Moreau-Gachelin, F. (1992) Characterization of Spi-B, a transcription factor related to the putative oncoprotein Spi-1/PU. 1. *Mol. Cell. Biol.* **12,** 4297–4304.
64. Ray-Gallet, D., Mao, C., Tavitian, A., and Moreau-Gachelin, F. (1995) DNA binding specificities of Spi-1/PU.1 and Spi-B transcription factors and identification of a Spi-1/Spi-B binding site in the c-fes/c-fps promoter. *Oncogene* **11,** 303–313.
65. Weintraub, S., Chow, K., Luo, R., Zhang, S., He, S., and Dean, D. (1995) Mechanism of active transcriptional repression by the retinoblastoma protein. *Nature* **375,** 812–815.
66. Nagulapalli, S., Pongubala, J. M. R., and Atchison, M. L. (1995) Multiple proteins physically interact with PU. 1. *JI* **155,** 4330.
67. Nelsen, B., Tian, G., Erman, B., Gregoire, J., Maki, R., Graves, B., and Sen, R. (1993) Regulation of lymphoid-specific immunoglobulin mu heavy chain gene enhancer by ETS-domain proteins. *Science* **261,** 82–86.
68. Feldhaus, A. L., Mbangkollo, D., Arvin, K. L., Klug, C. A., and Singh, H. (1992) BLyF, a novel cell-type and stage-specific regulator of the B-lymphocyte gene mb-1. *Mol. Cell. Biol.* **12,** 1126–1133.
69. Hagman, J. and Grosschedl, R. (1992) An inhibitory carboxyl-terminal domain in Ets-1 and Ets-2 mediates differential binding of Ets family factors to promoter sequences of the mb-1 gene. *Proc. Natl. Acad. Sci. USA* **89,** 8889–8893.
70. Shin, M. K. and Koshland, M. E. (1993) Ets-related protein PU.1 regulates expression of the immunoglobulin J-chain gene through a novel Ets-binding element. *Genes Dev.* **7,** 2006–2015.
71. Hiramatsu, R., Akagi, K., Matsuoka, M., Kingsbury, L., David, C., Hardy, R. R., Yamamura, K., and Sakano, H. (1995) The 3' Enhancer Region Determines the B/T Specificity and Pro-B/Pre-B Specificity of Immunoglobulin V_κ-J_κ Joining. *Cell* 83, 1113–1123.
72. Pongubala, J. and Atchison, M. (1997) PU.1 can participate in an active enhancer complex without its transcriptional activation domain. *Proc. Natl. Acad. Sci. USA* **94,** 127–132.
73. Robertson, E. J. (1987) Teratocarcinomas and embryonic stem cells a practical approach. IRL Press, Oxford.
74. Scott, E. W., Simon, M. C., Anastasi, J., and Singh, H. (1994) Requirement of transcription factor PU.1 in the development of multiple hematopoietic lineages. *Science* **265,** 1573–1577.
75. Scott, E., Fisher, R., Olson, M., Kehrli, E., Simon, M., and Singh, H. (1997) PU.1 functions in a cell-autonomous manner to control the differentiation of multipotential lymphoid-myeloid progenitors. *Immunity* **6,** 437–447.
76. Olson, M. C., Scott, E. W., Hack, A. A., Su, G. H., Tenen, D. G., Singh, H., and Simon, M. C. (1995) PU.1 is not essential for early myeloid gene expression but is required for terminal myeloid differentiation. *Immunity* **3,** 703–714.
77. Nuez, B., Michalovich, D., Bygrave, A., Ploemacher, R., and Grosveld, F. (1995) Defective haematopoiesis in fetal liver resulting from inactivation of the EKLF gene. *Nature* **375,** 316–318.
78. Perkins, A., Sharpe, A., and Orkin, S. (1995) Lethal β-thalassaemia in mice lacking the erythroid CACCC-transcription factor EKLF. *Nature* **375,** 318–322.
79. Hirayama, F., Shih, J. P., Awgulewitsch, A., Warr, G. W., Clark, S. C., and Ogawa, M. (1992) Clonal proliferation of murine lymphohemopoietic progenators in culture. *Proc. Natl. Acad. Sci. USA* **89,** 5907–5911.
80. Kee, B. L., Cumano, A., Iscove, N. N., and Paige, C. J. (1994) Stromal cell independent growth of bipotent B cell—macrophage precursors from murine fetal liver. *Intl. Immunol.* **6,** 401–407.
81. McKercher, S., Torbett, B., Anderson, K., Henkel, G., Vestal, D., Baribault, H., Klemsz, M., Feeney, A., Wu, G., Paige, C., and Maki, R. (1996) Targeted disruption of the PU.1 gene results in multiple hematopoietic abnormalities. *EMBO* **15,** 5647–5658.

82. Tondravi, M., McKercher, S., Anderson, K., Erdmann, J., Quiroz, M., Maki, R., and Teitelbaum, S. (1997) Osteopetrosis in mice lacking haematopoietic transcription factor PU.1. *Nature* **386,** 81–84.
83. Jacks, T., Fazeli, A., Schmitt, E. M., Bronson, R. T., Goodell, M. A., and Weinberg, R. A. (1992) Effects of an Rb mutation in the mouse. *Nature* **359,** 295–300.
84. Lee, E. Y., Chang, C. Y., Hu, N., Wang, Y. J., Lai, C. C., Herrup, K., Lee, W. H., and Bradley, A. (1992) Mice deficient for Rb are nonviable and show defects in neurogenesis and haematopoiesis. *Nature* **359,** 288–294.
85. Williams, B. O., Schmitt, E. M., Remington, L., Bronson, R. T., Albert, D. M., Weinberg, R. A., and Jacks, T. (1994) Extensive contribution of Rb-deficient cells to adult chimeric mice with limited histopathological consequences. *EMBO J.* **13,** 4251–4259.
86. Keller, G., Kennedy, M., Papayannopoulou, T., and Wiles, M. V. (1993) Hematopoietic commitment during embryonic stem cell differentiation in culture. *Mol. Cell. Biol.* **13,** 473–486.
87. Doetschman, T., Eistetter, H., Katz, M., Schmidt, W., and Kemler, R. (1985) The *in vitro* development of blastocyst-derived embryonic stem cell lines: formation of visceral yolk sac, blood islands, and myocardium. *J. Embryol. Exp. Morphol.* **87,** 27–45.
88. Henkel, G., McKercher, S., Yamamoto, H., Anderson, K., Oshima, R., and Maki, R. (1996) PU.1 but not Ets-2 is essential for macrophage development from embryonic stem cells. *Blood* **88,** 2917–2926.
89. Weiss, M., YU, C., and Orkin, S. (1997) Erythroid-specific properties of transcription factr GATA-1 revealed by phenotypic rescue of a gene targeted cell line. *Mol. Cell. Biol.* **17,** 1642–1651.
90. Hu, M., Krause, D., Greaves, M., Sharkis, S., Dexter, M., Heyworth, C., and Enver, T. (1997) Multilineage gene expression precedes commitment in the hematopoietic system. *Genes Dev.* **11,** 774–785.

Chapter 8

Chromatin Structure and Lineage Determination

Dimitris Kioussis and Richard Festenstein

1. Introduction

It is commonplace nowadays to state that the identity of a cell is determined by the expression of a subset of genes present in its nucleus. Many of these genes are necessary for the survival of the cell and are, by and large, expressed in all types of cells, regardless of lineage. They have come to be known as housekeeping genes. In addition, cells belonging to a particular tissue express a set of genes which is characteristic of the lineage to which they belong. Such genes are called tissue-specific genes, and their regulated expression defines the characteristic function and hence, the identity of the cell. An example of such tissue-specific genes are those that encode for surface molecules; antibodies recognizing these structures have made the analysis and identification of cells of particular lineage feasible.

Understanding the regulation of the tissue-specific expression of certain genes provides a tool to examine the processes underlying decisions made during cell differentiation. For instance, elucidating the mechanism that determines that the CD3 genes are kept silent in B-cells but are expressed in T-cells, or, conversely, why immunoglobulin genes are expressed in B-cells but are silent in T-cells, would greatly enhance our insight into lineage formation.

This chapter focuses on the function of a T-cell specific regulatory element that has provided a model system for assessing fundamental aspects of mammalian gene regulation—namely, processes by which a cell may "decide" whether or not to express a particular gene; conditions that may influence this decision, and mechanisms whereby a cell may "remember" to express or silence particular genes and, hence, "lock" into a specific phenotype.

From: *Molecular Biology of B-Cell and T-Cell Development*
Edited by: J. G. Monroe and E. V. Rothenberg © Humana Press Inc., Totowa, NJ

2. Regulation of Gene Expression

2.1. Elements Necessary for Gene Expression

DNA regions within or around the genes control their tissue-specific expression to a large extent. Chief among such *cis* regulatory elements are promoters and enhancers that mediate their function through interactions with proteins of the transcriptional machinery that can have a tissue specific distribution.

2.1.1. Promoters

These elements that are found 5' of most functional genes play an essential role in defining the start site for transcription. In many instances, this function is mediated via an AT rich sequence known as the TATA box *(1)* or, in the absence of this element, by an alternative sequence known as the "Initiator" (Inr) which is not so well defined *(2)*.

2.1.2. Enhancers

Originally identified in viruses, enhancers were shown in cell transfection assays to increase the level of transcription, regardless of their orientation or position with respect to the gene *(3,4)*. Enhancers are associated with many eukaryotic genes and are capable of functioning at considerable distances from them (reviewed in ref. *5*). In many cases, their action is restricted to specific cell types, and this correlates with the existence of nuclear proteins that act as tissue-specific transcription factors. Mutational studies have identified additional so-called Upstream Activating Sequences (UAS), which often lie within a 100 bp region upstream of the start site *(6)*. As with enhancers, UAS have been shown to define both the tissue specificity and efficiency of transcription.

2.1.3. Silencers

Like enhancers, silencers also exhibit tissue specificity, although only a few have been identified. Notably, the recent identification of a silencer within the T-cell specific CD4 gene indicates a potential role for such elements in defining cell lineage specific gene expression *(7–9)*.

2.2. Chromatin Configuration

In addition to the aforementioned elements that determine transcription of a gene, in recent years, it has become apparent that expressed genes acquire a different configuration within the nucleus in comparison with those that are not expressed. Several assays have been devised to detect such conformational differences, and one of them examines the methylation state of the gene. It is widely accepted that the majority of expressed genes within mammalian cells are unmethylated at the CpG dinucleotide sequence, whereas silent genes are methylated at this position. This has been attributed to the differential three-dimensional configuration of the DNA/protein complexes, which either prohibits methyltransferases from acting on it or encourages specific methylases to remove already existing methyl groups *(10)*.

An alternative way to look at the conformational state of the gene is to study its accessibility to certain macromolecules such as nucleases. One of them, DNase I, has been extremely useful in this respect. When nuclei of cells are incubated with increasing amounts of DNase I, the expressed genes are preferentially degraded, whereas silent genes appear to be resistant to the action of the enzyme. In fact, the degradation by DNase I is such that particular regions are specifically digested, allowing the identification of DNase I hypersensitive regions within the expressed genes. Such hypersensitive sites can be mapped within a 50–200 bp accuracy, following restriction enzyme digestion and Southern blot analysis of the gene locus. Numerous studies have shown that there is very good correlation between DNase I hypersensitivity and the presence of regulatory elements *(11)*.

The different behavior of the DNA in these assays is thought to reflect its differential packaging within the nucleus of the examined cells. In the nucleus, DNA is assembled in macromolecular nucleic acid/protein complexes, giving rise to a structure that is collectively known as chromatin. It is generally accepted that chromatin can be divided into two types depending on its microscopic appearance in interphase nuclei when stained with Giemsa; the barely visible variety is known as "euchromatin," and the densely staining type is known as "heterochromatin." Most of the expressing genes in a nucleus appear to be associated with euchromatic regions, whereas silent genes are thought to exist within the densely packed heterochromatin. Examples of regions within a nucleus that are heterochromatic throughout the cell cycle are the centromeric or telomeric portions of the chromosomes and are known as "constitutively heterochromatic." However, along the chromosome and interspersed within euchromatic regions containing expressed genes are additional stretches of DNA containing silenced genes that are assembled in a form known as "facultative heterochromatin." It is thought that the distribution of euchromatin and "facultative" heterochromatin along the chromosomes is different between cells from different lineages *(12)*. This hypothesis also stipulates that cells of the same lineage have similar distribution patterns of euchromatin and heterochromatin along their chromosomes. It is very likely that this is accomplished by differential interactions of the DNA with tissue-specific as well as ubiquitous nuclear proteins. It follows that this pattern is decided at some point during differentiation, and that the latter is stably maintained by the cells belonging to a certain lineage.

2.3. Transgenic Mice and Position Effects

Recent years have seen intense activity in the search of DNA regions that regulate gene expression and the molecular mechanisms that underlie their function. With the introduction of transgenic technology, it became possible to study gene regulation in mammals in vivo (for review *see* ref. *13*). In this approach, the transgene integrates directly into the mouse genome and is then packaged into chromatin and higher order structures. Moreover, the transgene is now subject to both tissue-specific and developmentally regulated expression. Early attempts established that there was a large variability in gene expression between different transgenic lines carrying identical DNA constructs *(14)*. Each trangenic line carried its transgene array at a different chromosomal site, and in most cases, the expression level was greatly reduced and bore no relationship to the number of transgene copies integrated. Moreover, tissue-specific expression of the transgene was frequently lost. It was suggested that this aberrant transcriptional activity was determined by the site of integration of the transgene. This implied that most chromosomal locations imposed a negative effect on transcription and/or that the *cis*-acting elements included in the transgene constructs (promoters and enhancers); although capable of sustaining high level transcription in other assays, these were not sufficient to activate transcription irrespective of chromosomal integration site in vivo *(15,16)*.

The possibility that the positioning of genes to abnormal locations could dramatically impair gene expression had been raised by geneticists studying chromosomal translocations in the early part of this century *(17–19)*. These effects were termed "chromosomal

Position Effects" (PE). These observations suggested the possibility that for correct regulation, a given gene would have to be located in regions "permissive" for transcription. Thus, the position effects that were now being observed in transgenic animals could potentially provide essential additional information regarding the mechanism of action of *cis*-acting regulatory elements.

2.4. Locus Control Regions

Transgenic research on gene expression led to the discovery of a new class of regulatory element, locus control regions (LCRs), which can overcome these repressive position effects in transgenic mice *(20)*. There are many similarities between enhancers and LCRs. Both contain multiple binding sites for transcription factors, can exhibit tissue specificity, interact with their cognate promoters to activate transcription, and can function in an orientation independent fashion and at considerable distances from their associated genes. However, in contrast to enhancers, it was found that LCRs could direct tissue-specific transgene-copy number dependent physiological expression, regardless of the chromosomal site of integration. This discovery was an essential step toward bringing classical genetic observations and direct gene expression studies to a scientifically fruitful juxtaposition.

One of the earliest observations concerning LCRs was that a DNA fragment containing the human β-globin gene linked to a cluster of DNase I hypersensitive regions far upstream in the locus could direct a high level, tissue specific, and gene copy number dependent expression of the gene in transgenic mice *(20)*. Shortly after this discovery, a cluster of DNase I hypersensitive regions defining a T-cell specific LCR was identified downstream of the human CD2 gene *(21)*. Subsequently, a number of other sequences have been nominated for LCR function, complying to a varying degree to the criteria of position independent, copy number dependent, tissue-specific, and physiological levels (per transgene copy) of expression *(22–31)*.

Although the precise mechanism for achieving position independent expression has not been defined, it is likely that cooperation among the individual regulatory sites (which corresponded to DNase I hypersensitivity regions) results in establishing and/or maintaining a transcriptionally competent chromatin domain *(20)*. In order to unravel the mechanisms governing position effects, we sought to identify the nature/composition of the site of transgene integration in the host genome that apparently imposes negative position effects, the type of effect that such integration has on the expression of the transgene, and the sequences within an LCR that are necessary to overcome these position effects.

3. An Experimental System to Study Chromatin Structure and Gene Regulation in Mammalian T-Cells

3.1. T-Cell Development

T-cells are derived from hematopoietic stem cells that originate in the bone marrow or fetal liver but go through much of their development in the thymus *(32)*. It is during their differentiation in that organ that self-reactive T-cells are eliminated through a process known as negative selection. At the same time, positive selection of T-cells with a wide range of antigen specificities takes place. The majority of T-cells are not subject to selection and die by, so called, 'neglect' *(33–35)*.

Specific stages of T-cell maturation are identified by the presence or absence of cell surface markers (cluster differentiation [CD] markers). Many of these markers are coded for by genes that are members of the immunoglobulin supergene family and are glycoproteins. CD44 and Thy 1 are some of the first markers detectable on the surface of progenitor T-cells and are present on cells found in the subcapsular region of the thymus. This prothymocyte then loses expression of CD44, but transiently gains expression of heat stable antigen (HSA) and the IL-2 receptor. CD2, CD5, CD8, CD1, CD3, and CD4 are then expressed in a temporal order (for summary, *see* ref. *36*). The emerging mature T-cell population can be further subdivided on the basis of whether they express the coreceptor molecules CD4 or CD8 on their surface. The expression of the latter molecules is mutually exclusive in mature T-cells.

It is obvious from the dramatic changes in the surface phenotype of the developing thymocyte that the expression of specific genes at different stages in development is strictly regulated. Such precise control mechanisms underlying the decision whether to express key genes are also likely to apply at crossroads during early stages of fetal development, or during the differentiation of pluripotent haemopoietic stem cells into the various blood cell types, thus orchestrating organogenesis and tissue-specific lineage formation.

We decided to examine gene expression during thymocyte development and develop a model of tissue-specific gene regulation by examining the elements that control the expression and affect the chromatin structure of a T-cell specific gene, namely the human CD2 gene (hCD2).

3.2. The Human CD2 Gene

The human CD2 molecule, a member of the immunoglobulin supergene family, is a 55 kDa glycoprotein that appears on T-cells early in their differentiation and remains on their surface throughout their life *(37)*. The relevance of CD2 function in T-cell development has been called into question recently, as neither disruption of the CD2 gene, nor anti-CD2 antibody treatment of fetal thymic organ cultures in mouse, were shown to have any detectable effect *(38)*.

The genomic structure of human CD2 has been determined, and it was found that it consists of five exons and intervening sequences spanning a region of approx 15 kb. A 28.5 kb genomic fragment including 4.5 kb of upstream sequence and 9 kb of downstream flanking sequence, as well as the coding region of the human CD2 gene, has been introduced into the germline of mice to generate transgenic animals *(39)*. These mice have been shown to express the transgene at high levels, and this expression is position independent, copy number dependent, and tissue specific, indicating the presence of an LCR *(21)*. Furthermore, thymus specific DNase I hypersensitive sites were found within the 5' and 3' flanking regions of the hCD2 gene in nuclei obtained from these animals. One such site has been mapped to a position immediately 5' of the first exon within the promoter of the gene. Two further sites were found approx 0.5 kb and 1.0–1.5 kb 3' of the polyadenylation signal of the gene.

Deletional analysis of the 3' flanking region has localized the minimum region required to confer LCR function on the human CD2 minigene within a 2 kb sequence immediately downstream of the gene *(40)*. To enable the functional dissection of the LCR, the DNase I hypersensitive sites (HSS) were localized at high resolution within the hCD2 3' 2 kb flanking region shown to be sufficient for LCR function. Such analysis revealed three clusters of sites (HSS 1–3) (Fig. 1). The upstream HSS cluster (HSS 1) of strong hypersensitive sites coincides with the region known to function as a classical enhancer, whereas the weak HSS region 2 and the stronger HSS region 3 appear to have no enhancer

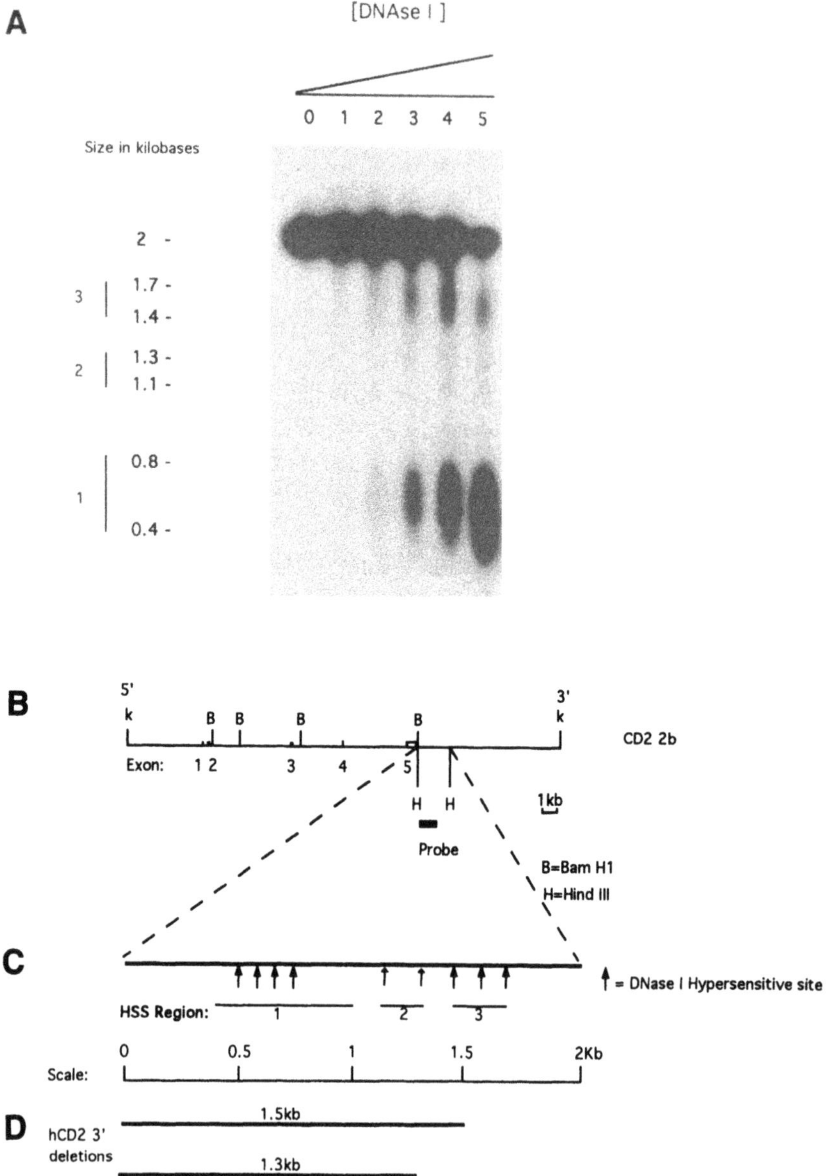

Fig. 1. High-resolution DNAse I hypersensitive site analysis of the hCD2 Locus Control Region. **(A)** Southern blot analysis of DNA from DNAse I treated nuclei from hCD2 transgenic mice (CD2 2b). **(B)** The full hCD2 genomic transgene construct carried by CD2 2b mice. The 2kb *Hind*III fragment with full LCR function is indicated together with the probe used to visualize it. **(C)** Map showing the DNAse I hypersensitive sites identified in lanes 3–5 arranged in three regions. **(D)** 3' deletions of the 2 kb *Hind*III fragment which were linked to the hCD2 minigene to generate transgenic lines in which HSS 3 was either partially deleted (1.5 kb) or omitted (1.3 kb).

activity in transient transfection assays *(41)*. Since it is possible that HSS without an enhancer function are nevertheless important for LCR function, we investigated the function of the downstream HSS cluster (HSS region 3) by generating transgenic mouse lines in which these sites were deleted. These transgenic mouse lines were analyzed at the DNA, RNA, and most importantly, at the protein level. Using hCD2 monoclonal antibodies and flow cytometry, the latter analysis provided us with a measure of the quantity of hCD2 protein expressed on the cell surface of individual thymocytes and T-cells.

3.3. Position Effect Variegation in Mice Transgenic for a hCD2 Gene Lacking Region HSS3 of its LCR

The frequency distribution of thymocytes expressing hCD2 derived from the hCD2 transgenic mouse lines carrying sequential 3' → 5' deletions of the 3' flanking DNA, was compared with thymocytes obtained from a nontransgenic mouse. All transgenic lines carrying transgenes with the full LCR (which contains all 3 HSSs) express hCD2 protein in a characteristic unimodal distribution on all thymocytes and T-cells. However, thymocytes from a proportion of transgenic mouse lines carrying the hCD2 minigene linked to either 1.5 or 1.3 kb of immediate 3' flanking DNA (i.e., in which downstream DNase I HSS region 3 has been partially deleted or omitted) show a disrupted distribution of expression. Thus, in the case of the CD2 1.5 kb transgenics, five out of seven lines show the expected unimodal distribution of expression, but the remaining two show a bimodal distribution indicated by a population of thymocytes positive for hCD2 and a population with either low or undetectable hCD2 expression. Furthermore, out of 6 CD2 1.3 kb transgenic lines, three show a similar bimodal distribution of hCD2 expression.

This effect is apparently transgene copy number and orientation independent since two out of four additional transgenic lines carrying the 1.3 kb in the reverse orientation (CD2 1.3 kb B) also have bimodal distributions of hCD2 expression on thymocytes and peripheral T-cells. The authors, therefore, conclude that transgenes without the HSS3 sometimes result in a mosaic expression pattern. This type of position effect bears a striking similarity to position effect variegation (PEV) as described in *Drosophila,* and recently yeast (for reviews *see* refs. *42–44*). PEV occurs when a euchromatic gene is translocated to a region of heterochromatin with the result that expression of the gene is then silenced in a proportion of cells. This is thought to be caused by spreading of heterochromatin, which varies from cell to cell, thus sometimes including the translocated gene in a proportion of cells, thereby silencing it. The characteristic red and white patches visible in the compound eyes of *Drosophila* is the phenotype associated with such a translocation of the white gene (which codes for red eye) to a region of centromeric heterochromatin (for review and references therein *see* refs. *45,46*). These patches are thought to represent the clonal expansion of a progenitor cell, in which the expression of the white gene is determined and maintained through successive cell divisions.

In pursuit of the analogy with PEV in *Drosophila,* immunostaining frozen sections of thymuses of mice with a mosaic expression revealed the arrangement of thymocytes in clusters, which are either positive or negative for hCD2 expression. In contrast, a uniform staining of all thymocytes was seen in a thymus of a transgenic mouse carrying the full LCR *(47).*

In conclusion, mouse lines carrying the hCD2 minigene under the control of only 1.3 kb of 3' LCR sequences in which the downstream HSS region 3 has been omitted, can exhibit a variegated phenotype within the thymus. This phenotype is inherited and is evident in all the mice of the same line. In addition, flow cytometric analysis confirmed that the extent of variegation in these mice is similar within all subsets of thymocyte populations indicating that this pattern of expression is established early in thymocyte development and maintained in subsequent differentiation steps.

3.4. Variegation is Associated with a Centromeric Chromosomal Location of the hCD2 Transgene and an Altered Chromatin Configuaration

As mentioned in Subheading 2.3., the site of integration can influence the expression of the hCD2 transgene; therefore, we sought to define better its chromosomal location using fluorescence *in situ* hybridization (FISH). The results confirmed that the truncated LCR transgenes are subjected to PEV when located within centromeric heterochromatin. In contrast, when an identical transgene is located in the long arm of the chromosome, the expression pattern is unimodal. These results confirm that the variegation observed in hCD2 transgenics appears to be induced by centromeric heterochromatin as described for classical PEV in *Drosophila.* In order to assess whether an intact LCR could overcome the position effects imposed by centromeric heterochromatin, we examined the integration site in mice carrying a hCD2 transgene linked to a full LCR including HSS region 3, and found that when such a transgene is integrated at the centromere, the mice show no variegated expression. This data (summarized in Fig. 2) indicate that sequences within HSS region 3 of the hCD2 LCR are essential for overcoming the highly unfavorable heterochromatic environment associated with the centromere. It is of interest that DNase I hypersensitivity of the transgenic locus was found to be different in expressing cells when compared to the nonexpressing population. Thus, no hypersensitive site formation was detected in the hCD2$^-$ population of thymocytes, whereas the expressing cells had reconstructed a chromatin configuration, which allows access to the DNase I *(47)*.

3.5. Enhancer Function is Intact in the Expressing Cells of Variegating Mice

As mentioned in Subheading 3.3., a proportion of the transgenic lines that carry 1.3 or 1.5 kb of 3' flanking DNA show a variegated expression pattern. The transgene constructs in these mice contain the classically defined transcriptional enhancer sequences (associated with HSS region 1), but they have either a partial deletion of HSS 3 (CD2 1.5 kb) or complete omission of this region (CD2 1.3 kb). We have determined hCD2 expression levels, using flow cytometry, on the group of thymocytes expressing hCD2 within four of these variegating transgenic lines and found that the expressing cells obtained from the variegating lines are expressing hCD2 in a transgene copy dependent manner (R.F., unpublished). The copy-dependent expression in these cells indicates that the hCD2 enhancer is functioning at the predicted level, provided the transgene in these thymocytes is in an active chromatin configuration (*see* Subheading 3.4.); the partial deletion or complete omission of HSS region 3 has no effect on the level of expression within such cells. This result is in agreement with the lack of classical enhancer function of this region as shown by transient transfection assays *(41)*.

3.6. The Decision to Express hCD2 or Not in a Variegating Line is Stochastic and Stable

Further examination of variegating mice indicated that the decision to open and maintain the expression of the hCD2 transgene in homozygote transgenic mice was taken by the two allelic chromosomes independently from each other and in a manner that appears random or stochastic. Thus, in a homozygous variegating mouse thymus, there were three cell populations regarding the level of hCD2 expression (negative, intermediate, or high) and these populations were consistent with having none, one, or both alleles expressed, respectively. The presence of cells that express only one allele sug-

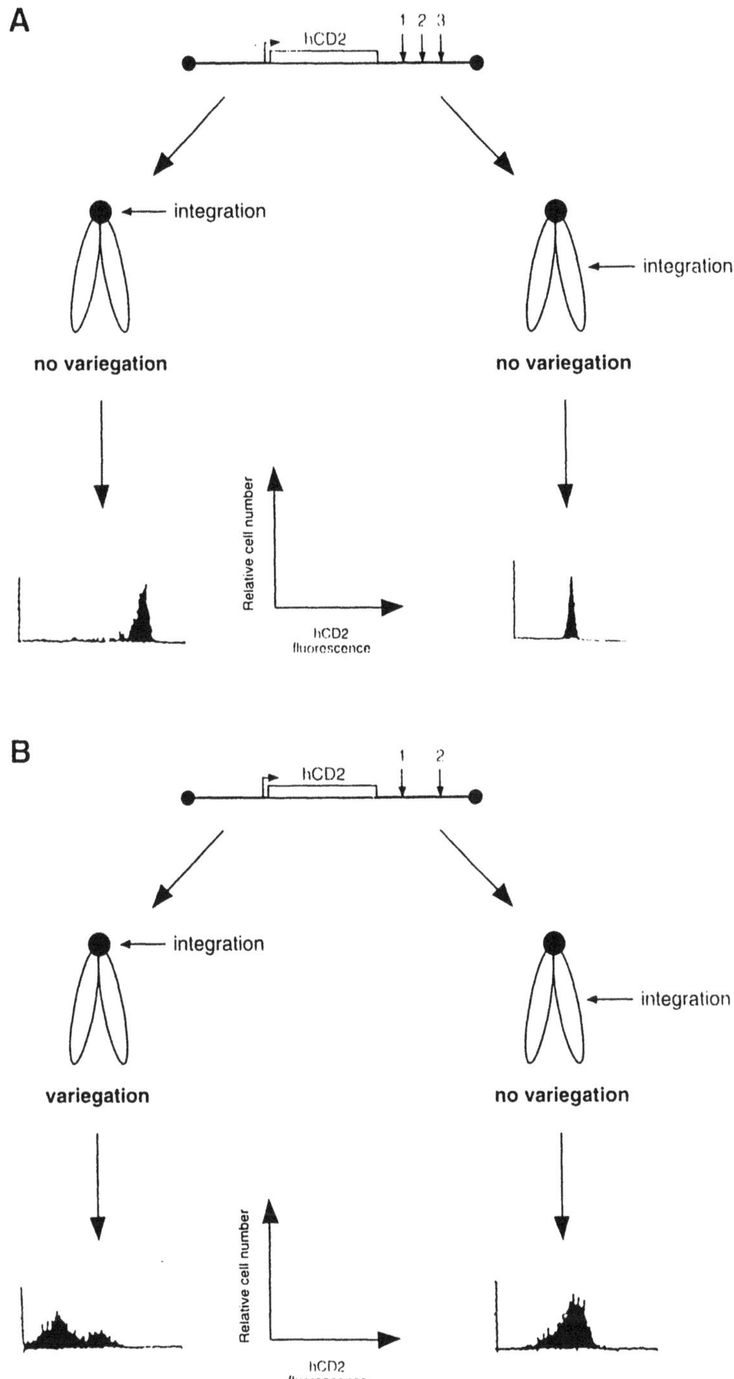

Fig. 2. Chromosomal localisation influences the pattern of expression of genes with an incomplete set of regulatory elements. **(A)** hCD2 transgenes with full Locus Control Region elements (HSS 1, 2, and 3) express in all T-cells regardless of whether they are integrated in the centromere or the long arm of the chromosome. **(B)** hCD2 transgenes with a deletion in the Locus Control Region (HSS 1 and HSS 2) exhibit a mosaic expression pattern, if they integrate at the centromere, whereas integration in the long arm of the chromosome results in a unimodal pattern of expression.

gests that the decision to open the chromatin is taken by each chromosome independently (Fig. 3). This situation appears to be similar to the one seen in mice transgenic for a hCD2 gene linked to the immunoglobulin heavy chain enhancer *(48)*.

A key question arising from the phenomenon of PEV addresses the question of lineage commitment. It has been observed that the expression pattern in a variegating *Drosophila* eye follows a patchy distribution with sectors either expressing the gene and others where the gene is expressed at a low level or is completely silenced. Since in eye development these patches corresponded to a lineage of cells generated from a single progenitor, it was important to show that the decision to express the hCD2 transgene was inherited by the daughter cells. The significance of this finding would relate to the nature of cellular "memory," with respect to lineage-specific gene expression and would provide a biological system for investigating the molecular basis of such phenomena.

Using the hCD2 transgenic mice, we addressed this question by culturing T-cells derived from variegating strains in vitro. The T-cells were obtained from the lymph nodes of variegating transgenic lines, stained with Thy 1 (to identify T-cells) and hCD2 monoclonal antibodies. Following sorting by means of a fluorescence activated cell sorter (FACS), into $hCD2^+$ and $hCD2^-$ populations, the cells were cultured for two days in the presence of pdbU and ionomycin. The inclusion of BrdU in the culture medium allowed the authors to subsequently assess which cells had undergone division. The cells were then harvested and restained for hCD2 and BrdU.

The results using cells from one of the variegating mouse lines are shown in Fig. 4. Panel A shows the expression pattern for hCD2 on the unsorted population of cells. Panel B i) and C i) shows the cells after sorting into $hCD2^-$ and $hCD2^+$ populations, respectively, before culture in vitro. As seen, the purity of the populations was in excess of 80%. The right histogram plot in panels B ii) and C ii) shows the result of concomitant staining for BrdU incorporation for both populations, and it indicates that over 85% of cells have divided in both populations during this period. The left histogram plot in Panel B ii) and C ii) shows the pattern of expression on the same populations after this period in culture, indicating that despite cell division, these cells retain their phenotype. These results show that the information as to the expression status of this gene is passed on by a cell with a given phenotype to its progeny. Since it is possible in this system to separate cells according to their phenotype, it is now possible to investigate the nature of this putative "epigenetic imprint."

4. Discussion and Hypothesis

4.1. Making and Maintaining the Decision to Express or Not at the Chromatin Level

Previous studies using transient transfection assays showed that the impairment of expression related to mutating an SV40 enhancer was associated with a decrease in the number of cells expressing, rather than a decrease in the level of expression per cell *(49)*. Additional studies appear to confirm this result *(4,50,51)*.

The model that begins to emerge is one in which the individual HSS within an LCR act together to increase the probability of establishing an active transcriptional unit in the expressing cells. Thus, early in the development of a cell lineage, the individual HSS would act together to establish a stable transcriptional unit in competition with heterochromatin forming proteins. The stability of this complex is impaired by locating a transgene (in which an LCR element has been deleted) in a heterochromatic environment

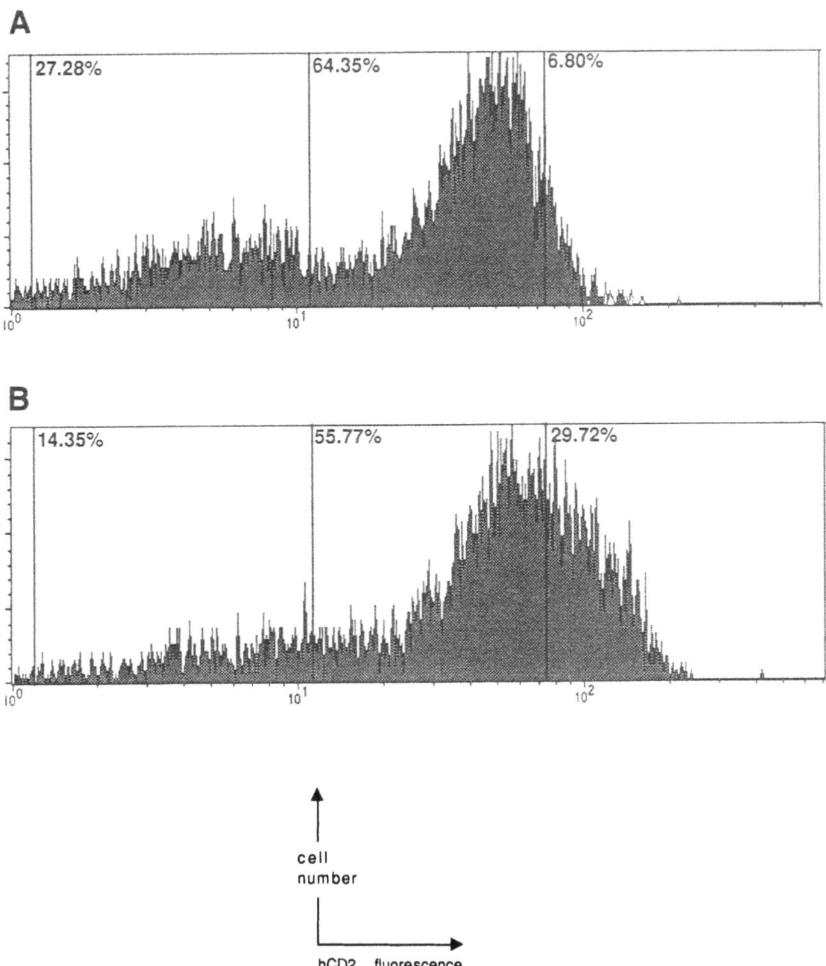

Fig. 3. The decision to express hCD2 in a variegating transgenic line is stochastic. **(A)** A histogram plot of human CD2 expression on peripheral T-cells from a mouse (CD2 1.3B), which is hemizygote for the transgene. The plot is divided into three regions with the proportion of cells falling into these categories indicated. The result indicates essentially a bimodal expression pattern either $hCD2^+$ (65%) or $hCD2^-$ (27%). **(B)** Identical analysis to that shown in panel A done on a mouse homozygote for the same transgene (CD2 1.3B). The results now indicate three levels of hCD2 expression. A reduction in the proportion of hCD2– (14%) T-cells, a decrease in the intermediate population of hCD2 expressing T-cells (56%) and a significant number of T-cells expressing hCD2 at a high level (30%) from both transgene alleles. Thus, it appears from this analysis that the decision to express from each allele is independent; the relative proportions suggest that the decision to express is random.

(e.g., the centromere), thus decreasing the probability of establishing an open and active chromatin domain at the transgene locus. Such a correlation between stability and probability has already been suggested to explain how the β-globin LCR may function. In this case, a flip-flop model for LCR function has been proposed in which an LCR-holocomplex appears to interact alternately with embryonic and adult genes within the

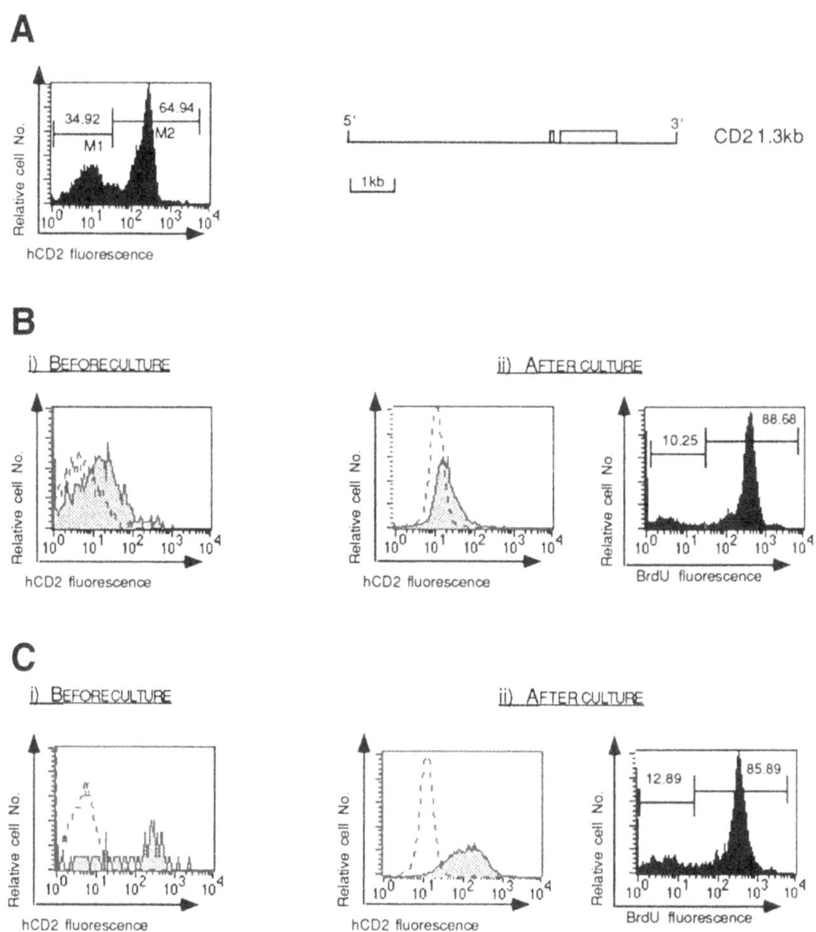

Fig. 4. hCD2+ and hCD2- transgenic T-cell populations retain their phenotype after proliferation in vitro. **(A)** A histogram plot showing a bimodal pattern of hCD2 expression on T-cells obtained from a mouse carrying the CD2 1.3 kb B transgene. The percentages of cells in gates M1 and M2 are shown. **(B i)** and **(C i)** Histogram plots obtained after sorting the populations shown in (A) into hCD2$^-$ and hCD2$^+$ populations. These cells were put into culture with PDBU and Ionomycin to stimulate proliferation. **(B ii)** and **(C ii)** The reassessment of the hCD2 phenotype after two days in culture, is presented as the left histogram plot indicating that the majority of cells retain their hCD2 phenotype. BrdU was included in the culture medium, thus the histogram plot shown on the right of this panel indicates that over 85% of the cells in these cultures have divided.

locus. The LCR can apparently only interact with one gene at a time. During development, the stability of this interaction decreases in the case of the embryonic genes and increases in the case of the adult gene. This process is presumably regulated by factors that influence the stability of this interaction, thus enabling a developmental switch in expression *(52)*.

Taken together, the data discussed so far indicate that the position of a gene within the chromosome in transgenic mice can have dramatic effects on its expression, and that the components of heterochromatin and the mechanisms underlying the maintenance of gene repression or activation are likely to be conserved from yeast through *Drosophila* to mammals.

It is logical, therefore, to review some of the recent advances in the study of PEV in *Drosophila* and the related phenomenon of Telomere Position Effect (TPE), which has recently been described in yeast, and in which a variegating phenomenon is induced when a gene is placed in close proximity to the telomeric sequences of the chromosome *(53)*.

4.2. Models for Regulation of Gene Expression in PEV

A number of models have been put forward to explain the loss of gene expression associated with PEV including DNA elimination *(43,54)*, and nuclear compartmentalization *(55)*. The fact that mutations in single genes can modify the extent of variegation has led to models for chromatin structure and function. The most widely accepted explanation is one that relies on the laws of mass action *(56)*. In such a model within a particular genetic locus, an activating or repressing multimeric protein complex is formed that is dependent on the presence of many different proteins; the equilibrium of this reaction being exquisitely sensitive to the concentration of the individual constituents. Thus, in the absence of PEV, an identical complex is formed in all the relevant loci. In cases of PEV, however, some chromosomes establish activating complexes at the relevant locus, whereas others establish repressive ones, depending on the availability of the different components. These models fit well with the observed ability to modify the extent of variegation in TPE in yeast and PEV in *Drosophila* (e.g., by overexpressing proteins that are components of these complexes) *(53,57–60)*.

Up to 120 genes, which can act as modifiers of PEV, have been identified in *Drosophila* by genetic studies (for a comprehensive analysis of 43 of these mutations, *see* ref. *61*). These are known as suppressors or enhancers of PEV. In some cases, the genes have been cloned and their associated proteins characterized. Some of these are known ubiquitous components of chromatin, such as histones, or proteins with a more restricted distribution along the chromosome (for review, *see* ref. *62*).

4.3. HP1, Polycomb, Trithorax Proteins

4.3.1. HP1

Probably the most studied example of a PEV modifier is Heterochromatin Protein 1 (HP1), which is encoded by Su(var)205 (**Su**ppresser of **Var**iegation 205) and has been shown to associate with heterochromatic regions such as the chromocenter by antibody staining of polytene chromosomes. HP1 binds to chromatin rather than directly to DNA and induces silencing of the relevant genes. Point mutations in HP1 gene result in suppression of variegation, thus restoring the wild-type phenotype. Moreover, this effect can be reversed by the introduction of the wild-type HP1 as a transgene. In addition, HP1 overexpression enhances variegation. These effects have also been shown to be dosage dependent *(59)*. Homologs of HP1 have been cloned from a diverse range of species, including mammals, implying possible conservation of function *(63–65)*.

4.3.2. Polycomb

Another mechanism for the maintenance of gene repression came to light with the discovery of a *Drosophila* protein known as Polycomb, which binds to chromatin rather than a specific DNA sequence. Immunoprecipitation experiments demonstrated Polycomb Group members (Pc-G) to be part of a repressive macromolecular complex of proteins similar to the one postulated in heterochromatin mediated silencing. There are a number of other parallels between this form of silencing and that described in PEV. The centromere associated protein HP1 shares homology with Polycomb significantly within a 37 amino acid stretch known as the "chromodomain" *(66)*. This domain is essential for the silencing function of both HP1 and Polycomb *(67)*. It is not known how Polycomb is targeted to specific loci. As yet, none of the members of the Pc-G have been shown to demonstrate sequence-specific binding. However, *cis*-acting sequences that can direct Pc-G-mediated gene repression have been described within the ultrabithorax complex, and are known as polycomb response elements (PRE) *(68)*. When linked to a reporter gene, these elements have the property of rendering a transgene susceptible to variegation even when located at euchromatic sites in the *Drosophila* genome *(69)*.

Interestingly, mutations in the polycomb group proteins alter the extent of this variegation in a fashion analogous to PEV. The similarities between polycomb and HP1 were further investigated in transgenic *Drosophila* using transgenes coding for chimeric molecules *(70)*. In these experiments, it was possible to redirect silencing proteins normally associated with centromeric heterochromatin to the ultrabithorax complex and vice versa. One model invoked to explain the mechanism of Pc-G-mediated gene repression is the chromatin accessibility model, in which multiple, cooperating Pc-G complexes form a heterochromatin like structure that prevents activators and/or basal transcription factors from contacting the DNA *(71)*. Recently a number of mammalian homologs of the Pc-G genes have been investigated in mice and *Drosophila* by transgenesis *(72)*.

4.3.3. Trithorax

On the other end of the spectrum, Trithorax proteins are required for the maintenance of homeotic gene expression patterns established by the transient expression of segmentation genes during *Drosophila* embryogenesis. There are twenty members of the *Drosophila* trithorax group (trx-G) of transcriptional activators that are thought to act, at least in part, as antagonists of the Pc-G and function, by maintaining an active transcriptional state at particular loci (for review *see* ref. *73*). Antibody staining of polytene chromosomes reveals 63 specific sites for trithorax, which colocalizes with Polycomb at their known targets *(74)*. Some mammalian genes have been identified which contain sequences sharing homology with the *Drosophila* trithorax genes *(75–78)*.

4.4. Acetylation of Histone Tails

In recent years, studies have indicated that histones may play a more rigorous role in specific gene regulation than their ubiquitous presence would imply. Thus, in *S. cerevesiae*, deletional studies of the histone tails have identified protein domains with specialized functions in regulating both the activation and repression of gene expression *(79)*. Amino acid substitutions have further localized these functions to specific lysine residues. These lysines are subject to posttranslational acetylation that in some studies appear to correlate with the transcriptional activity of the genes with which those histone molecules are associated.

Using antibodies against hyperacetylated histone tails, it was possible to immunoprecipitate chromatin containing DNA sequences from the transcriptionally active β-globin locus *(80)*. Complementary DNase I sensitivity mapping identified a region of general sensitivity that also coincided with the active locus. The flanking chromatin was found to lack both of these features. These findings support the concept of a transcriptionally competent chromatin domain associated with hyperacetylation of histones.

Further evidence for a correlation between transcription and histone acetylation comes from studies using cytogenetic staining for hyperactylated histone H4 tails *(81)*. It was shown that the inactive X chromosome in humans and mice is hypoacetylated. From this and other data, it has been suggested that the hyperacetylation of the histone tails may provide a means whereby the transcriptionally active state for a specific gene within a given cell is maintained or alternatively, provide an access point for transcription factors.

Although little is known about the processes involved in maintaining histone acetylation and deacetylation, histone acetyltransferases (HATs) *(82–84)*, and deacetylases have been identified and are likely to play an essential role in this process *(85,86)*. Furthermore, inhibition of the deacetylases has already provided evidence that this modification is functionally important for gene regulation *(85)*.

The recent discovery that a yeast adapter protein (GCN5p) that had already been shown to play an essential role in gene regulation, also has HAT activity has also provided a potentially important link between these two processes *(83)*. Such proteins, by acetylating the histone tails of specific nucleosomes, may facilitate the access of nonhistone DNA binding proteins to their recognition sequences, thereby enabling transcriptional activation (*83*; for review *see* ref. *87*).

On the other hand, a genetic modifier (RPD3) of PEV and TPE in *Drosophila* and yeast was shown to be part of a complex with deacetylase activity; recently a series of experiments indicated that such regulatory mechanisms also operate in mammalian cells *(88–93)*.

4.5. Heterochromatin Formation and Cell Lineage Determination

In *Drosophila* PEV, modification of the extent of variegation can be induced by heat shocking embryos, which have not yet turned on transcription of the variegating gene. This implies the existence of a "determinative event" at the chromatin level that takes place during a developmental window of opportunity prior to expression *(94)*. The nature of this event is unknown; however, it is tempting to draw analogies with the mammalian phenomenon of genomic imprinting in which a gene is marked, probably by methylation during germ cell formation *(95,96)*. This so-called imprint determines whether that particular allele will be expressed. It may be that in PEV the decision whether to express or not is likewise recorded by such an epigenetic modification.

The similarities between the physiological maintenance of gene repression in the homeotic locus by the Polycomb system and the identification of sequences that recruit this heterochromatin-like silencing apparatus indicate that *cis*-acting sequences can act as nucleation sites for heterochromatinization. It may be that the repetitive sequences associated with centromeres or telomeres (e.g., α-satellite DNA) act as heterochromatin nucleation sites, e.g., in the case of TPE, a DNA-binding sequence for the heterochromatin recruiting factor RAP 1 has been identified, and the molecular basis for "heterochromatinization" is relatively well-characterized.

The conservation of these regulatory phenomena among diverse organisms such as mice, *Drosophila,* and yeast is very encouraging, and the hCD2 system described in the first part of this chapter can be used to investigate the function of other potentially important mammalian homologs of modifiers of PEV.

The independent regulation of expression of allelic loci as revealed in the experimental system described in Subheading 3. has additional repercussions in interpreting cases of haploinsufficiency. In this genetic phenomenon, one allele is apparently silenced in a random fashion, whereas the other is active and expressing. However, if one of the alleles is mutated, and the normal allele is silenced, a loss of function can occur with the subsequent death of the affected cell. Recent research has associated disease with haploinsufficiency (for review, *see* ref. *97*). The apparent randomness in activation or inactivation of the different alleles within a cell may also have implications in situations where stochastic elements seem to control a developmental process: for instance, in the upstream decisions taken by the developing thymocyte to commit to the CD4 or CD8 lineage *(98–102)*.

5. Concluding Remarks

It is possible that biological mechanisms similar to those underlying PEV determine cell fate by regulating tissue specific gene expression at key branch points during differentiation (e.g., the development of the T and B lymphocyte lineages during hematopoeisis). Thus, in addition to identifying a *cis*-acting element essential for preventing PEV, we have developed a mammalian system enabling the study of the mechanism of chromatin or DNA modifications, which determine and maintain the fate of specific cells with respect to the expression of a lineage specific gene. The ability to separate sufficient numbers of such cells according to their expression status will enable further studies on the *cis*- and *trans*-acting factors, as well as the epigenetic modifications, which are required for the commitment to and persistence of tissue specific gene expression in mammals.

References

1. Benoist, C. and Chambon, P. (1981) In vivo sequence requirements of the SV40 early promoter region. *Nature* **290,** 304–310.
2. Lo, K. and Smale, S. T. (1996) Generality of a functional initiator consensus sequence. *Gene* **182,** 13–22.
3. Banerji, J., Rusconi, S., and Schaffner, W. (1981) Expression of a beta-globin gene is enhanced by remote SV40 DNA sequences. *Cell* **27,** 299–308.
4. Moreau, P., Hen, B., Waslylyk, R., Everett, M., Gaub, M. P., and Chambon, P. (1981) The SV40 72-bp repeat has a striking effect on gene expression both in SV40 and other chimeric recombinants. *Nucleic Acids Res.* **9,** 6047–6068.
5. Kennison, J. A. (1993) Transcriptional activation of Drosophila homeotic genes from distant regulatory elements. *Trends Genet.* **9,** 75–79.
6. Serfling, E., Jasin, M., and Schaffner, W. (1985) Enhancers and eukaryotic gene transcription. *Trends Genet.* **1,** 224–230.
7. Donda, A., Schulz, M., Burki, K., De Libero, G., and Uematsu, Y. (1996) Identification and characterization of a human CD4 silencer. *Eur. J. Immunol.* **26,** 493–500.
8. Sawada, S., Scarborough, J. D., Killeen, N., and Littman, D. R. (1994) A lineage-specific transcriptional silencer regulates CD4 gene expression during T lymphocyte development. *Cell* **77,** 917–929.
9. Siu, G., Wurster, A. L., Duncan, D. D., Soliman, T. M., and Hedrick, S. M. (1994) A transcriptional silencer controls the developmental expression of the CD4 gene. *EMBO J.* **13,** 3570–3579.
10. Eden, S. and Cedar, H. (1994) Role of DNA methylation in the regulation of transcription. *Curr. Opin. Genet. Dev.* **4,** 255–259.
11. Gross, D. S. and Garrard, W. T. (1988) Nuclease hypersensitive sites in chromatin. *Ann. Rev. Biochem.* **57,** 159–197.
12. Cook, P. R. (1973) Hypothesis on differentiation and the inheritance of gene superstructure. *Nature* **245,** 23–25.
13. Grosveld, F. and Kollias, G. (1992) Transgenic Animals. (London, Academic Press).
14. Palmiter, R. D. and Brinster, R. L. (1986) Germline transformation of mice. *Ann. Rev. Genet.* **20,** 465–499.
15. Dobie, K., Mehtali, M., McClenaghan, M., and Lathe, R. (1997) Variegated gene expression in mice. *Trends Genet.* **13,** 127–130.
16. Milot, E., Fraser, P., and Grosveld, F. (1996) Position effects and genetic disease. *Trends Genet.* **12,** 123–126.
17. Dobzhansky, T. (1936) Position effects on genes. *Biol. Rev.* **11,** 364–434.
18. Lewis, E. B. (1950) The phenomenon of position effect. *Adv. Genet.* **3,** 73–115.
19. Sturtevant, A. H. (1925) The effects of unequal cross-over at the Bar-locus in Drosophila. *Genetics* **10,** 117–147.
20. Grosveld, F., van Assendelft, G. B., Greaves, D. R., and Kollias, G. (1987) Position-independent, high-level expression of the human beta-globin gene in transgenic mice. *Cell* **51,** 975–985.
21. Greaves, D. R., Wilson, F., Lang, G., and Kioussis, D. (1989) Human CD2 3'-flanking sequences confer high-level T-cell specific position independent gene expression in transgenic mice. *Cell* **56,** 979.

22. Bonifer, C., Vidal, M., Grosveld, F., and Sippel, A. S. (1990) Tissue specific and position independent expression of complete gene domain for chicken lysozyme in transgenic mice. *EMBO J.* **9,** 2843–2848.
23. Carson, S., and Wiles, M. V. (1993) Far upstream regions of class II MHC Ea are necessary for position-independent, copy-dependent expression of Ea transgene. *Nucleic Acids Res.* **21,** 2065–2072.
24. Dale, T. C., Krnacik, M. J., Schmidhauser, C., Yang, C. L., Bissell, M. J., and Rosen, J. M. (1992) High-level expression of the rat whey acidic protein gene is mediated by elements in the promoter and 3' untranslated region. *Mol. Cell Biol.* **12,** 905–914.
25. Diaz, P., Cado, D., and Winoto, A. (1994) A Locus Control Region in the T cell receptor alpha/ delta locus. *Immunity* **1,** 207–217.
26. Palmiter, R. D., Sandgren, E. P., Koeller, D. M., and Brinster, R. L. (1993) Distal regulatory elements from the mouse metallothionein locus stimulate gene expression in transgenic mice. *Mol. Cell. Biol.* **13,** 5266–5275.
27. Reitman, M., Lee, E., Westphal, H., and Felsenfeld, G. (1990) Site-independent expression of the chicken beta A-globin gene in transgenic mice. *Nature* **348,** 749–752.
28. Schedl, A., Montoliu, L., Kelsey, G., and Schutz, G. (1993) A yeast artificial chromosome covering the tyrosinase gene confers copy number-dependent expression in transgenic mice. *Nature* **362,** 258–261.
29. Strauss, W. M., Dausman, J., Beard, C., Johnson, C., Lawrence, J. B., and Jaenisch, R. (1993) Germ line transmission of a yeast artificial chromosome spanning the murine alpha 1(I) collagen locus. *Science* **259,** 1904–1907.
30. Talbot, D., Descombes, P., and Schibler, U. (1994) The 5' flanking region of the rat LAP (C/EBP beta) gene can direct high-level, position-independent, copy number-dependent expression in multiple tissues in transgenic mice. *Nucleic Acids Res.* **22,** 756–766.
31. Whitelaw, C. B., Harris, S., McClenaghan, M., Simons, J. P., and Clark, A. J. (1992) Position-independent expression of the ovine beta-lactoglobulin gene in transgenic mice. *Biochem. J.* **286,** 31–39.
32. Davis, M. M. and Bjorkman, P. J. (1988) T-cell antigen receptor genes and T-cell recognition. *Nature* **334,** 395–401.
33 Adkins, B., Mueller, C., Okada, C. Y., Reichert, R., Weissman, I. L., and Spangrude, G. J. (1987) Early events in T-cell maturation. *Ann. Rev. Immunol.* **5,** 325–365.
34. Blackman, M., Kappler, J., and Marrack, P. (1990) The role of the T cell receptor in positive and negative selection of developing T cells. *Science* **248,** 1335–1341.
35. Kappler, J. W., Roehm, N., and Marrack, P. C. (1987) T cell tolerance by clonal elimination in the thymus. *Cell* **149,** 273–280.
36. Ritter, M. A. and Crispe, I. N. (1992) The thymus in focus. *Book IRL Press* 34–36.
37. Driscoll, P. C., Cyster, J. G., Campbell, I. D., and Williams, A. (1991) Structure of domain 1 of rat T lymphocyte CD2 antigen. *Nature* **353,** 762–765.
38. Killeen, N., Stuart, S. G., and Littman, D. R. (1992) Development and function of T cells in mice with a disrupted CD2 gene. *EMBO J.* **11,** 4329–4336.
39. Lang, G., Wotton, D., Owen, M. J., Sewell, W. A., Brown, M. H., Mason, D. Y., Crumpton, M. J., and Kioussis, D. (1988) The structure of the human CD2 gene and its expression in transgenic mice. *EMBO J.* **7,** 1675–1682.
40. Lang, G., Mamalaki, C., Greenberg, D., Yannoutsos, N., and Kioussis, D. (1991) Deletion analysis of the human CD2 gene locus control region in transgenic mice. *Nucleic Acids Res.* **19,** 5851–5856.
41. Lake, R. A. and Wotton, D. (1990) A 3' transcriptional enhancer regulates tissue-specific expression of the human CD2 gene. *EMBO J.* **9,** 3129–3136.
42. Allshire, R. C., Javerzat, J.-P., Redhead, N. J., and Cranston, G. (1994) Position Effect Variegation at fission yeast centromeres. *Cell* **76,** 157–169.
43. Karpen, G. H. (1994) Position-effect variegation and the new biology of heterochromatin. *Curr. Opin. Genet. Dev.* **4,** 281–291.
44. Singh, P. B., Miller, J. R., Pearce, J., Kothary, R., Burton, R. D., Paro, R., James, T. C., and Gaunt, S. J. (1991) A sequence motif found in a Drosophila heterochromatin protein is conserved in animals and plants. *Nucleic Acids Res.* **19,** 789–794.
45. Henikoff, S. (1992) Position effect and related phenomena. *Curr. Opin. Genet. Dev.* **2,** 907–912.
46. Henikoff, S. (1990) Position-effect variegation after 60 years. *Trends Genet.* **12,** 422–426.

47. Festenstein, R., Tolaini, M., Corbella, P., Mamalaki, C., Parrington, J., Fox, M., Miliou, A., Jones, M., and Kioussis, D. (1996) Locus control region function and heterochromatin-induced position effect variegation. *Science* **271,** 1123–1125.
48. Elliott, J., Festenstein, R., Tolaini, M., and Kioussis, D. (1995) Random activation of a transgene under the control of a hybrid hCD2 locus control region/Ig enhancer regulatory element. *EMBO J.* **14,** 575–584.
49. Weintraub, H. (1988) Formation of stable transcription complexes as assayed by analysis of individual templates. *Proc. Natl. Acad. Sci. USA* **85,** 5819–5823.
50. Moon, A. M. and Ley, T. J. (1991) Functional properties of the beta-globin locus control region in K562 erythroleukemia cells. *Blood* **77,** 2272–2284.
51. Walters, M. C., Fiering, S., Eidemiller, J., Magis, W., Groudine, M., and Martin, D. I. K. (1995) Enhancers increase the probability but not the level of gene expression. *Proc. Natl. Acad. Sci. USA* **92,** 7125–7129.
52. Wijgerde, M., Grosveld, F., and Fraser, P. (1995) Transcription complex stability and chromatin dynamics *in vivo*. *Nature* **377,** 209–213.
53. Gottschling, D. E., Aparicio, O. M., Billington, B. L., and Zakian, V. A. (1990) Position effect at S. cerevisiae telomeres, reversible repression of Pol II transcription. *Cell* **63,** 751–762.
54. Karpen, G. H. and Spradling, A. C. (1990) Reduced DNA polytenization of a minichromosome region undergoing position-effect variegation in Drosophila. *Cell* **63,** 97–107.
55. Wakimoto, B. T. and Hearn, M. G. (1990) The effects of chromosome rearrangement on the expression of heterochromosomal genes in Chromosome 2L in melanogaster, D. *Genetics* **125,** 141–154.
56. Locke, J., Kotarski, M. A., and Tartof, K. D. (1988) Dosage-dependent modifiers of positional effect variegation in Drosophila and a mass action model that explains their effect. *Genetics* **120,** 181–198.
57. Aparicio, O. M., Billington, B. L., and Gottschling, D. E. (1991) Modifiers of position effect are shared between telomeric and silent mating-type loci in S. cerevisiae. *Cell* **66,** 1279–1287.
58. Aparicio, O. M. and Gottschling, D. E. (1994) Overcoming telomeric silencing: a trans-activator competes to establish gene expression in a cell cycle-dependent way. *Genes Dev.* **8,** 1133–1146.
59. Eissenberg, J. C., Morris, G. D., Reuter, G., and Hartnett, T. (1992) The heterochromatin-associated protein HP-1 is an essential protein in Drosophila with dosage-dependent effects on position-effect variegation. *Genetics* **131,** 345–352.
60. Renauld, H., Aparicio, O. M., Zierath, P. D., Billington, B. L., Chhablani, S. K., and Gottschling, D. E. (1993) Silent domains are assembled continuously from the telomere and are defined by promoter distance and strength, and by SIR3 dosage. *Genes Dev.* **7,** 1133–1145.
61. Wustmann, G., Szidonya, J., Taubert, H., and Reuter, G. (1989) The genetics of position-effect variegation modifying loci in Drosophila melanogaster. *Mol. Gen. Genet.* **217,** 520–527.
62. Reuter, G. and Spierer, P. (1992) Position effect variegation and chromatin proteins. *Bioessays* **14,** 605–612.
63. Epstein, H., James, T. C., and Singh, P. B. (1992) Cloning and expression of Drosophila HP1 homologs from a mealybug, Planococcus citri. *J. Cell. Sci.* **101,** 463–474.
64. Hamvas, R. M., Reik, W., Gaunt, S. J., Brown, S. D., and Singh, P. B. (1992) Mapping of a mouse homolog of a heterochromatin protein gene the X chromosome. *Mamm. Genome* **2,** 72–75.
65. Saunders, W. S., Chue, C., Goebl, M., Craig, C., Clark, R. F., Powers, J. A., Eissenberg, J. C., Elgin, S. C., Rothfield, N. F., and Earnshaw, W. C. (1993) Molecular cloning of a human homologue of Drosophila heterochromatin protein HP1 using anti-centromere autoantibodies with anti-chromo specificity. *J. Cell. Sci.* **104,** 573–582.
66. Paro, R. and Hogness, D. S. (1991) The Polycomb protein shares a homologous domain with a heterochromatin-associated protein of Drosophila. *Proc. Natl. Acad. Sci. USA* **88,** 263–267.
67. Chang, Y. L., King, B. O., M. O'Connor, Mazo, A., and Huang, D. H. (1995) Functional reconstruction of trans regulation of the Ultrabithorax promoter by the products of two antagonistic genes, trithorax and Polycomb. *Mol. Cell. Biol.* **15,** 6601–6612.
68. Simon, J., Chiang, A., Bender, W., Shimell, M. J., and O'Connor, M. (1993) Elements of the Drosophila bithorax complex that mediate repression by Polycomb group products. *Dev. Biol.* **158,** 131–144.
69. Chan, C. S., Rastelli, L., and Pirrotta, V. (1994) A Polycomb response element in the Ubx gene that determines an epigenetically inherited state of repression. *EMBO J.* **13,** 2553–2564.
70. Platero, J. S., Hartnett, T., and Eissenberg, J. C. (1995) Functional analysis of the chromo domain of HP1. *EMBO J.* **14,** 3977–3986.

71. Paro, R. (1990) Imprinting a determined state into the chromatin of Drosophila. *Trends Genet.* **6,** 416–421.
72. Muller, J., Gaunt, S., and Lawrence, P. A. (1995) Function of the Polycomb protein is conserved in mice and flies. *Development* **121,** 2847–2852.
73. Simon, J. (1995) Locking in stable states of gene expression: transcriptional control during Drosophila development. *Curr. Opin. Cell. Biol.* **7,** 376–385.
74. Chinwalla, V., Jane, E. P., and Harte, P. J. (1995) The Drosophila trithorax protein binds to specific chromosomal sites and is co-localized with Polycomb at many sites. *EMBO J.* **14,** 2056–2065.
75. Khavari, P. A., Peterson, C. L., Tamkun, J. W., Mendel, D. B., and Crabtree, G. R. (1993) BRG1 contains a conserved domain of the SWI2/SNF2 family necessary for normal mitotic growth and transcription. *Nature* **366,** 170–174.
76. Mbangkollo, D., Burnett, R., McCabe, N., Thirman, M., Gill, H., Yu, H., Rowley, J. D., and Diaz, M. O. (1995) The human MLL gene: nucleotide sequence, homology to the Drosophila trx zinc-finger domain, and alternative splicing. *DNA Cell. Biol.* **14,** 475–483.
77. Randazzo, F. M., Khavari, P., Crabtree, G., Tamkun, J., and Rossant, J. (1994) Brg1: a putative murine homologue of the Drosophila brahma gene, a homeotic gene regulator. *Dev. Biol.* **161,** 229–242.
78. Yu, B. D., Hess, J. L., Horning, S. E., Brown, G. A., and Korsmeyer, S. J. (1995) Altered Hox expression and segmental identity in Mll-mutant mice. *Nature* **378,** 505–508.
79. Kayne, P., Ung-Jin, K., Mullen, J. R., Yoshizaki, F., and Grunstein, M. (1988) Extremely conserved histone H4 N terminus is dispensable for growth but essential for repressing the silent mating loci in yeast. *Cell* **55,** 27–39.
80. Hebbes, T. R., Thorne, A. W., and Crane-Robinson, C. (1994) A direct link between core histone acetylation and transcriptionally active chromatin. *EMBO J.* **7,** 1395–1402.
81. Jeppesen, P. and Turner, B. M. (1993) The inactive X chromosome in female mammals is distinguished by a lack of histone H4 acetylation, a cytogenetic marker for gene expression. *Cell* **74,** 281–289.
82. Brownell, J. E. and Allis, C. D. (1995) An activity gel assay detects a single, catalytically active histone acetyltransferase subunit in Tetrahymena macronuclei. *Proc. Natl. Acad. Sci. USA* **92,** 6364–6368.
83. Brownell, J. E., Zhou, J., Ranalli, T., Kobayashi, R., Edmondson, D. G., Roth, S. Y., and Allis, C. D. (1996) Tetrahymena histone acetyltransferase A: a homologue to yeast Gcn5p linking histone acetylation to gene activation. *Cell* **84,** 843–851.
84. Kleff, S., Andrulis, E. D., Anderson, C. W., and Sternglanz, R. (1995) Identification of a gene encoding a yeast histone H4 acetyltransferase. *J. Biol. Chem.* **270,** 24,674–24,677.
85. Fanti, L., Berloco, M., and Pimpinelli, S. (1994) Carnitine suppression of position-effect variegation in Drosophila melanogaster. *Mol. Gen. Genet.* **244,** 588–595.
86. Taunton, J., Hassig, C. A., and Schreiber, S. L. (1996) A mammalian histone deacetylase related to the yeast transcriptional regulator Rpd3p. *Science* **272,** 408–411.
87. Wolffe, A. P. and Pruss, D. (1996) Targeting chromatin disruption: transcription regulators that acetylate histones. *Cell* **84,** 817–819.
88. Alland, L., Muhle, R., Hou Jr, H., Potes, J., Chin, L., Schreiber-Agus, N., and DePinho, R. A. (1997) Role for N-CoR and histone deacetylase in Sin3-mediated transcriptional repression. *Nature* **387,** 49–55.
89. Hassig, C. A., Fleischer, T. C., Billin, A. N., Schreiber, S. L., and Ayer, D. E. (1997) Histone deacetylase activity is required for full transcriptional repression by mSin3A. *Cell* **89,** 341–347.
90. Heinzel, T., Lavinsky, R. M., M. T-M., Soderstrom, M., Laherty, C. D., Torchia, J., Yang, W.-M., Brard, G., Ngo, S. D., Davie, J. R., Seto, E., Eisenman, R. N., Rose, D. W., Glass, C. K., and Rosenfeld, M. G. (1997) A complex containing N-CoR, mSin3 and histone deacetylase mediates transcriptional repression. *Nature* **387,** 43–48.
91. Kadosh, D. and Struhl, K. (1997) Repression by Ume6 involves recruitment of a complex containing Sin3 corepressor and Rpd3 histone deacetylase to target promoters. *Cell* **89,** 365–371.
92. Laherty, C. D., Yang, W.-M., Sun, J.-M., Davie, J. R., Seto, E., and Eisenman, R. N. (1997) Histone deacetylases associated with mSin3 corepressor mediate mad transcriptional repression. *Cell* **89,** 349–356.
93. Nagy, L., Kao, H.-Y., Chakravarti, D., Lin, R. J., Hassig, C. A., Ayer, D. E., Schreiber, S. L., and Evans, R. M. (1997) Nuclear receptor repression mediated by a complex containing SMRT, mSin3A, and histone deacetylase. *Cell* **89,** 373–380.

94. Singh, P. B. (1994) Molecular mechanisms of cellular determination: their relation to chromatin structure. *J. Cell. Sci.* **107,** 2653–2668.
95. Bartolomei, M. S., Webber, A. L., Brunkow, M. E., and Tilghman, S. M. (1993) Epigenetic mechanisms underlying the imprinting of the mouse H19 gene. *Genes Dev.* **7,** 1663–1673.
96. John, R. M. and Surani, M. A. (1996) Imprinted genes and regulation of gene expression by epigenetic inheritance. *Curr. Opin. Cell. Biol.* **8,** 348–353.
97. Engelkamp, D. and van Heyningen, V. (1996) Transcription factors in disease. *Curr. Opin. Genet. Dev.* **6,** 334–342.
98. Chan, S. H., Cosgrove, D., Waltzinger, C., Benoist, C., and Mathis, D. (1993) Another view of the selective model of thymocyte selection. *Cell* **73,** 225–236.
99. Corbella, P., Moskophidis, D., Spanopoulou, E., Mamalaki, C., Tolaini, M., Itano, A., Lans, D., Baltimore, D., Robey, E., and Kioussis, D. (1994) Functional commitment to helper T cell lineage precedes positive selection and is independent of T cell receptor MHC specificity. *Immunity* **1,** 269–276.
100. Davis, C. B., Killeen, N., Crooks, M. E. C., Raulet, D., and Littman, D. R. (1993) Evidence for a stochastic mechanism in the differentiation of mature subsets of T lymphocytes. *Cell* **73,** 237–247.
101. Itano, A., Kioussis, D., and Robey, E. (1994) Stochastic component to development of class I major histocompatibility complex-specific T cells. *Proc. Natl. Acad. Sci. USA* **91,** 220–224.
102. Robey, E., Chang, D., Itano, A., Cado, D., Alexander, H., Lans, D., Weinmaster, G., and Salmon, P. (1996) An activated form of Notch influences the choice between CD4 and CD8 T cell lineages. *Cell* **87,** 483–492.

Part III

Extrinsic Factors Regulating B and T Lymphopoiesis

Chapter 9

The Role of Cytokines in Hematolymphoid Development

Tannishtha Reya and Simon R. Carding

1. The Hematopoietic Microenvironment: An Overview

For an uncommitted mesodermally derived stem cell to develop into a functionally mature blood cell, it must be capable of proliferation, commitment, differentiation, survival, and homing. These complex processes are tightly regulated by signals derived from the cells that make up the microenvironment in which hematopoiesis takes place. These include a variety of cell types, both nonhematopoietic fixed-tissue cells such as fibroblasts and epithelial cells (collectively referred to as "stromal cells"), and hematopoietic cells themselves. These cells influence hematopoiesis in three major ways: by providing signals through direct cell–cell contact, by secreting components of the extracellular matrix (ECM), and, by secreting soluble factors. Together, these signals comprise the hematopoietic inductive microenvironment or HIM *(1)*. Microenvironments within different hematopoietic tissues are distinct and specialized in supporting the development of specific hematopoietic cell populations. For example, the thymus that almost exclusively supports T-cell development consists of a separate class of epithelial cells, bone marrow-derived cells, and cytokines that are different from that in the bone marrow, which supports the development of myeloid, erythroid, and B-cells. The intriguing observation that precursor cells from the thymus, when injected into recipient mice *(2)*, or cultured in vitro with bone marrow stromal cells *(3)*, can give rise to B-cells and/or macrophages, exemplifies the inductive nature of hematopoietic microenvironments and demonstrates the ability of different sites to support the generation of distinct hematopoietic cell lineages.

2. Cytokines: Properties and Function

Cytokines are soluble proteins that act through specific cell surface receptors and participate in diverse biological events. They act on both hematopoietic and nonhematopoietic cells,

From: *Molecular Biology of B-Cell and T-Cell Development*
Edited by: J. G. Monroe and E. V. Rothenberg © Humana Press Inc., Totowa, NJ

regulating processes ranging from the immune response and inflammation *(4)*, to osteopoiesis and the endometrial cycle *(5,6)*. The ability of soluble factors to control the growth and differentiation of hematopoietic cells was initially demonstrated using in vitro cell culture systems *(7,8)* from which factors that influence the survival, proliferation, and differentiation of immature hematopoietic cells could be purified and biochemically identified.

The behavior and action of cytokines are complex. They are pleiotropic and exert a diverse array of effects on a variety of cell types. For example, Interleukin-2 (IL-2) affects a variety of cell types including B-cells, T-cells, natural killer (NK) cells, and monocytes/macrophages *(9)*. Cytokines are also frequently redundant, for instance both tumor necrosis factor α (TNFα) and tumor necrosis factor β (TNFβ) potentiate antigen presentation, bactericidal and, tumoricidal functions of macrophages, and promote differentiation of monocytes *(10–12)*. Not only do cytokines have diverse effects on a variety of cell types, but they also have the capacity to regulate one another's production and activity. For example, IL-2 can promote the production of IL-1, IL-5, IL-6, interferon gamma (IFNγ), and granulocyte macrophage-colony stimulating factor (GM-CSF) (reviewed in ref. *13*), whereas transforming growth factor β (TGFβ) can inhibit the production of IL-1, IL-6, IL-7, and TNF *(14,15)*. Cytokines can act synergistically to enhance a particular cellular response (e.g., IL-3, GMCSF, IL-1, and erythropoietin act together to promote the growth of colony forming unit-megakaryocyte (CFU-Meg and the production of megakaryocytes in vitro *[16]*), or antagonistically to inhibit responses to one another (e.g., IL-4 antagonizes the effects of IL-2 on B-cell proliferation *[17]*, and reduces the number of myeloid colonies in IL-3–stimulated bone marrow cultures *[18]*). Finally, an important characteristic of cytokines is that in contrast to hormones, they mainly act locally as paracrine and autocrine factors. The release of cytokines into the circulatory system at high levels can cause a series of pathological reactions including fever and eosinophilia *(19)*. Because of their varied and potent influences, cytokines are finely regulated in vivo. Their production and usage are tightly controlled and compartmentalized, for example, by interaction with ECM *(20–23)*, to ensure that their biological effects are focused on the appropriate targets at the right time *(24,25)*.

3. Cytokines in Development

Evidence for the influence of cytokines on the development of hematopoietic progenitor cells comes mainly from various in vitro assay systems in which growth and differentiation is dependent on the addition of various cytokines. Experiments utilizing cytokine neutralizing antibodies, and mutant mice that lack genes encoding particular cytokines or cytokine receptors, have demonstrated the importance of such factors for the development of hematopoietic cells in vivo. These experiments have shown that cytokines made by both nonhematopoietic stromal cells, as well as by hematopoietic cells, are powerful modulators of hematopoiesis.

3.1. Cytokines Produced by Hematopoietic Cells

Hematopoietic cells can influence one another's development through the production of cytokines. For instance, IL-4 produced by mast cells, basophils, and T-cells synergizes with monocyte-derived granulocyte-colony stimulating factor (G-CSF) *(18)* to have stimulatory effects on bone marrow cells. G-CSF and macrophage-colony stimulating factor (M-CSF) *(26,27)* produced by activated monocytes, macrophages, and B-cells *(26–31)*, stimulate formation of granulocyte and macrophage colonies, respectively, in vitro, and act synergistically with other factors to stimulate formation of colonies of other lineages. Interleukin-3, produced primarily by T-cells, supports the growth of multiple lineages (e.g., colony forming units-granulocyte erythroid macrophage megakaryocytic [CFU-GEMM], CFU-GM, blast forming units-erythroid [BFU-E], and colony forming units-eosinophil/basophil [CFU-Eo/Ba] and sustains the survival of colony forming units-granulocyte [CFU-G] *(32–34)*. GM-CSF, produced by monocytes and T-cells, has activities similar to IL-3, although it is less effective in sustaining multilineage progenitor cells *(33)*.

As in the bone marrow, intrathymic production of cytokines such as IL-4 and IL-2 *(35–37)*, IFNγ *(35)*, TNFα *(38)*, IL-7 *(39)*, and Stem Cell Factor (SCF) *(39)* by thymocytes suggests that they may be required for normal thymic development. Numerous in vitro studies utilizing these cytokines have provided evidence for effects on proliferation or differentiation of bulk populations as well as specific subsets of thymocytes. For example, IL-1 *(40)* and IFNγ *(41)* have been implicated in the growth of immature, $CD4^{-}CD8^{-}$, thymocytes, and γδ cells, as well as being able to regulate expression of major histocompatability (MHC) molecules in the thymus *(42)*. On the other hand, IL-4 has been shown to induce proliferation of various thymocyte subsets *(35,43)*. The use of anti-cytokine or cytokine receptor antibodies in fetal thymic organ culture (FTOC) has also proven useful in identifying growth promoting cytokines and the cells that use them. For example, a role for SCF in immature growth and development has been suggested from studies demonstrating that antibodies against its receptor, c-kit, exert a strong inhibitory influence on T-cell development in FTOC *(44)*. The observation that IL-1, IL-4 and IFNγ made by thymocytes can induce human thymic epithelial cell lines to produce cytokines, such as SCF *(45)*, suggests that thymocytes are not the only source of cytokines in the thymus and that stromal cells can directly influence thymocyte development through the production and release of various cytokines.

3.2. Growth Factors Produced by Nonhematopoietic Cells

An important way in which stromal cells can influence the growth and development of hematopoietic cells is through the production of cytokines. Some of these cytokines, such as M-CSF and TGFβ *(46–49)*, are produced constitutively, whereas others, such as IL-1, TNF, IL-6, IL-7, G-CSF, and GM-CSF *(49–53)* are made in response to stimulation. In either case, these cytokines act in much the same way as those produced by hematopoietic cells; by regulating the survival, growth, and differentiation of cells of GM-CSF various hematopoietic lineages directly or indirectly.

Stromal cell-derived cytokines have been shown to play an important role in the development of the myeloid lineage. For example, fibroblasts and bone marrow stromal cells can produce GM-CSF *(54,55)*, G-CSF *(50,54,55)*, and M-CSF *(54)*, that are important in stimulating and sustaining early myeloid progenitor cell expansion and development. In vitro studies have shown that IL-6 produced by fibroblasts and bone marrow stromal cells synergizes with M-CSF to promote formation of macrophage colonies *(56)* and with G-CSF or IL-3 to promote formation of granulocytic colonies *(57)*. IL-1, also produced by fibroblasts, has been shown to function as an inducer of CSF production by endothelial cells *(54,58)* and T-cells *(59)* and may thereby influence myelopoiesis indirectly.

Interestingly, few of these cytokines have been detected in long-term bone marrow cultures that support hematopoiesis *(60)*, which has called into question the physiologic relevance of the growth factors used in in vitro colony assays. One explanation for this apparent paradox is that undetectable levels of these cytokines may be physiologically active, particularly if they are concentrated in the appropriate microenvironment by association with stromal cells or ECM in long-term cultures *(20)*. Alternatively, stromal cells in such cultures may be capable of supporting hematopoiesis in the absence of these cytokines, or there may be as yet undefined growth factors that influence this process.

Stromal cell-derived factors influence lymphocyte development as well. In the B-cell compartment, one of the most important regulators of development is IL-7. Produced by bone marrow stromal cells *(61)*, IL-7 influences B-cell development by promoting proliferation of B-cell progenitors *(62)*. The importance of this effect has been demonstrated in studies showing that mice treated with antibodies against IL-7 *(61)* display impaired B lymphocyte development. Similarly, mutant mice lacking IL-7 or IL-7R *(63,64)* have been shown to have severely reduced numbers of developing B-cells.

Although IL-7 is the most intensively studied cytokine that influences B-cell development, other cytokines like c-kit and its ligand *(65)* and insulin-like growth factor-1 *(66)* have also been implicated in the proliferation and differentiation of immature B-cells. In the thymus, a number of different cytokines produced by epithelial cells have been implicated in T-cell development. Many epithelial cells in culture have been shown to constitutively produce IL-1 *(67)*, IL-7 *(68)*, M-CSF *(69)* and IL-6 *(70)*, that have the capacity to influence thymocyte growth and development *(71–73)*. In vitro experiments suggest that IL-7 produced by thymic epithelial cells can induce proliferation of thymocytes *(68)*. Studies showing that IL-7–transgenic mice have two to three times as many thymocytes as wild-type mice *(74)*, that mice treated with antibodies against IL-7 *(61)* have impaired T lymphocyte development, and that adult IL-7-deficient (IL-$7^{-/-}$) *(64)* and IL-$7R^{-/-}$ *(63)* mice have severely reduced numbers of developing T-cells all corroborate these findings. The temporally regulated production of IL-1α, IL-1β, IL-3, and IL-6 by murine fetal thymic stromal cells *(75)* and the production of IL-1 and G-CSF by human fetal thymic epithelial cells *in situ* *(76)*, also implicates the involvement of these cytokines in thymic development.

Although many of the aforementioned cytokines stimulate hematopoietic cell growth and development, there are also cytokines that are inhibitory for progenitor cells. These include the interferons *(77–79)*, TNFα *(77,80–83)*, and macrophage inflammatory protein-1α (MIP-1α) *(84–87)*. Experiments demonstrating that neutralizing antibodies to TGFβ and antisense-TGFβ can enhance the proliferation of primitive progenitor cells *(88,89)* suggest that at least some of these negative regulatory factors are important in vivo to control the number of hematopoietic progenitors and the fate of their descendants.

Of the cytokines that influence hematopoietic cells, IL-2 is one of the most extensively studied and characterized and has a wide range of influences on hematopoietic cells. Since the involvement of IL-2 in hematolymphoid development is a major focus of the authors' own research, they will use this cytokine to explore in detail the variety of ways in which a soluble growth factor can exert its influence on developing hematopoietic cells, and how its mechanism of action is different on cells at different stages of their development and in different hematopoietic tissues. Its pleiotropism and specificity forms the basis of many questions about the fascinating nature of cytokine action. Moreover, it is important that the requirement for IL-2 in hematolymphoid cell development and hematopoiesis in general be understood from a clinical point of view, since IL-2 and antibodies capable of preventing its interaction with IL-2 receptor (IL-2R) bearing cells have and continue to be used as immunotherapeutic agents for patients with a variety of hematopoietic disorders and malignancies.

4. Interleukin-2 (IL-2)

Discovered in 1976 as a growth factor capable of maintaining the proliferation of bone marrow T-cells *(90)*, IL-2 was originally designated T-cell growth factor. It was later cloned in 1983 *(91)* and renamed IL-2.

Since its discovery, receptors for this cytokine have been shown to be expressed on cells in almost every hematopoietic compartment and lineage, including mature T, B, NK cells, and monocyte/macrophages *(9)*, developing thymocytes *(92)*, developing B-cells *(93,94)* and myeloid cells *(95)*. IL-2 has been found to influence the activity of these cells by inducing proliferation and differentiation, and under different circumstances, by preventing these same activities, or by promoting cell death.

4.1. The IL-2 Receptor Complex and Signaling

IL-2 is a 15.5 kDa protein that acts as a monomer. To date, the IL-2R complex (Fig. 1) has been shown to consist of three chains, α (p55), β (p75) and γ (p64) (reviewed in ref. *96*). The β chain has been shown to be a component of the receptor complex for the cytokine IL-15 *(97)*, and γ is also part of the receptor for IL-4 *(98,99)*, IL-7 *(100,101)*, IL-9 *(102)* and IL-15 *(103)*.

The characteristics of IL-2 receptors and signaling pathways that are triggered in response to IL-2 binding have been most widely studied in mature T-cell clones, and in lymphoid and fibroblast cell lines transfected with various combinations of the genes encoding the IL-2R chains. These studies have suggested that the α chain is essential for high affinity binding of IL-2, but on its own is not capable of transducing any signals *(104,105)*. In contrast, the β and γ chains of the receptor mediate only intermediate affinity binding of IL-2 but have been shown to be important in signaling *(104–110)* and internalization of IL-2 *(111,112)*. It should be mentioned that since signal transduction was commonly assayed by measuring proliferation *(113,114)*, it is possible that various receptor chain combinations such as αβ or αγ, while unable to transduce signals sufficient for induction of proliferation, are still capable of initiating signaling pathways important for other biological functions *(115)*. In many cell types the structure, and as a result, the activity of the IL-2R complex is regulated by cellular activation. For example, resting T-cells constitutively express IL-2Rβ and γ *(112,116)* and antigen receptor-mediated activation results in production of IL-2, which binds to the intermediate affinity βγ receptor and induces expression of the α chain, upregulation of the β receptor chain, and IL-2 production *(117)*. This in turn allows formation of the receptor complex that is capable of binding IL-2 with high affinity and transducing a mitotic signal.

4.2. Evidence for IL-2's Importance in Hematopoiesis

A number of studies suggest that the IL-2/IL-2R signaling pathway may play a role in hematopoietic development. Although the primary focus of these studies has been on intrathymic T-cell development, a substantial amount of recent evidence implicates IL-2 in the regulation of developing cells of the NK and myeloid lineages also.

Figure 2 summarizes the distribution of IL-2–production and IL-2R expression (the β-chain signifies expression of functional receptors) by developing hematopoietic cells that has been obtained from the results of the authors' own studies and those of others.

4.2.1. IL-2 as a Regulator of T-Cell Differentiation

In spite of the numerous studies that have been undertaken during the past 12 years to evaluate the role of IL-2 in T-cell development, its precise role remains controversial

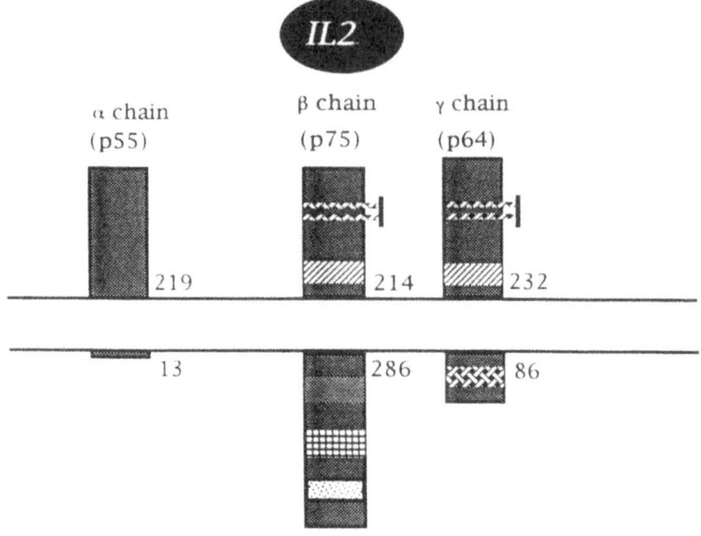

KEY:
Disulfide bonds
WSXWS motif
Ser rich region
Acidic region
Pro rich region
SH2-like domain

Subunits	IL-2 binding (Kd)
α	10^{-6} M
β	10^{-7} M
γ	Not detectable
αβ	10^{-10} M
αγ	10^{-6} M
βγ	10^{-9} M
αβγ	10^{-11} M

Fig. 1. A schematic representation of the IL-2R structure and binding affinities for IL-2.

(reviewed in ref. *75*). The observation that a major subset of both mouse and human $CD4^-CD8^-$ thymocytes expresses IL-2Rα *(118–120)* suggests that cells may require IL-2 at this stage of development. This was supported by the more recent findings that IL-2Rα is expressed in a temporally regulated manner in the fetal thymus, and that its expression is paralleled by the production of IL-2 *(36,92)*. The recent development of reagents to detect the other IL-2 receptor chains have shown that they are also expressed on thymocytes. Using antibodies to the β chain of the IL-2R, it was shown that 6–10% of thymocytes also express IL-2Rβ *(121)*. Moreover, IL-2Rγ detected by PCR and Southern analysis has been shown to be expressed throughout thymic development *(98)*.

Although studies of IL-2R expression suggest that IL-2 may regulate T-cell development, experiments to analyze its functional relevance have yielded contradictory results. In some in vitro studies, IL-2 has been shown to promote thymocyte proliferation *(37)*, whereas in others, IL-2 has been found to abrogate thymocyte proliferation and differentiation *(122–124)*, or not have any effect at all *(119,125,126)*. Apparently contradictory observations have also been made in studies in which anti–IL-2R anti-

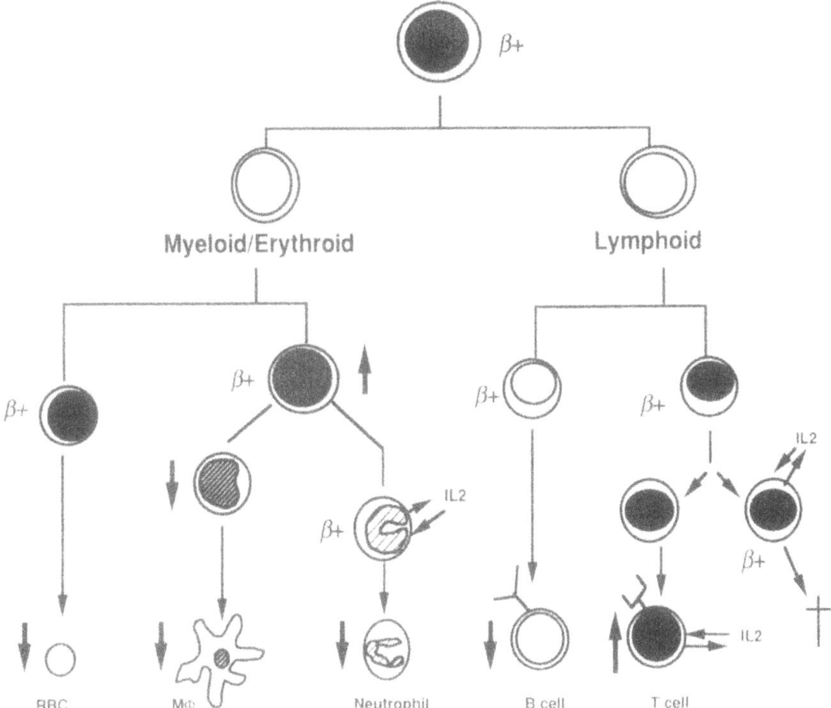

Fig. 2. Expression of IL-2 and IL-2Rs by hematopoietic cells. The production of IL-2 and expression of the β-chain of the IL-2R complex are shown for the lymphoid, myeloid and erthyroid cell lineages as determined by analyses of hematopoietic cells in the murine fetal liver and adult bone marrow. The thick arrows indicate the effects of IL-2-deficiency on the distribution and number of cells present in IL-$2^{-/-}$ mice. Upward pointing arrows indicate an increase and downward pointing arrows a decrease in cell number. For a more detailed explanation *see* Subheading 4.2.

bodies were added to FTOC; in some case such treatment abrogated T-cell development *(127)* whereas in others it had no effect *(128)*.

Analysis of the function of IL-2 in vivo has yielded somewhat more consistent results. For example, administration of anti–IL-2Rα antibodies to pregnant mice has been shown to block the proliferation and differentiation of double negative cells in the thymi of their offspring *(129)*. Although using antibodies to the β chain of the IL-2R to block IL-2 utilization *in utero* did not result in any apparent defect in αβ T-cell development, it did cause a loss of a subset of γδ cells *(121)*, suggesting that IL-2 is required for normal development of this lineage. Similar to its effects *in utero,* the presence of anti–IL-2Rα antibodies in sublethally irradiated adult mice retarded reconstitution by radioresistant intrathymic stem cells *(130)*. In mice expressing a human IL-2Rα transgene, in which thymocytes express a nonfunctional murine IL-2Rβ-human IL-2Rα heterodimer, T-cell development was blocked *(131)*. Finally, in mice expressing a human IL-2Rβ transgene, in which thymocytes express high affinity (α and β) IL-2Rs, thymocyte development proceeded normally *(132)*. Based on these studies, it seems likely that IL-2 functions to promote or regulate the proliferation and differentiation of thymocytes.

Some of the variability in the influence seen on immature T-cells may reflect the complexity in its activity; similar experiments carried out at a slightly different gestational stages or in adult vs fetal mice (circumstances under which the milieu of other cytokines and the expression of surface receptors on thymocytes may differ), may result in apparently contradictory results. Moreover, because a number of functional studies used antibodies, differences in the efficiency of antibody treatment, and differences in the blocking ability of antibodies to IL-2 vs antibodies to its receptors may also yield different results.

These and many other past studies of thymocytes (reviewed in ref. *75*) are consistent with a direct requirement for IL-2 during T-cell development. Although initial studies of lymphocyte development in IL-$2^{-/-}$ mice failed to identify any overt affect of IL-2 deficiency on T-cell development *(133)*, subsequent studies identifying abnormalities in thymic development *(95)* now support the findings of previous studies, that IL-2 does play a role in T-cell development. IL-$2^{-/-}$ mice develop a fatal autoimmune disorder characterized by hyperactivation of peripheral T-cells, lymphadenopathy, splenomegaly, hemolytic anemia, and colitis *(134,135)*. The analyses of IL-$2^{-/-}$ mice bred onto the athymic *nu/nu* background and RAG-$2^{-/-}$ mice reconstituted with IL-$2^{-/-}$ bone marrow have shown that the immunopathology in these mice depends upon the intrathymic differentiation of T-cells carrying the IL-2^{-}–mutation *(136)*. Other studies identifying phenotypic changes in subsets of thymocytes *(137,138)*, or abnormal cytokine production *(138)* by IL-$2^{-/-}$ thymocytes also implicate defects in thymic development as the underlying basis of disease pathology in these mice. The authors' own analysis of these animals has shown that they develop a thymic disorder resulting in the disruption of T-cell development *(95)*. Interestingly, this disorder was shown to be a result of abnormalities in thymic stromal cell populations, rather than any intrinsic defect in T-cell progenitors. Within the stroma, there was a progressive loss of cortical epithelial cells and bone marrow-derived monocytes/macrophages. This loss of macrophages is apparent within the first week of birth in germ-free IL-$2^{-/-}$ mice, prior to the export of functionally mature thymocytes into the periphery, excluding the possibility that this defect is caused by dysfunctional T-cells. Instead, the authors' findings suggest that IL-2 is required for the generation and perhaps maintenance of thymic monocytes/macrophages, some of which are known to express functional IL-2R *(139)*. Consistent with this interpretation are the results obtained from additional studies in which the authors have obtained compelling evidence for the direct involvement of IL-2 in myeloid cell development (discussed in section 4.2.3, below).

Although the evidence in favor of IL-2 being involved and required for T-cell development is now very compelling, the generation of T-cells in the absence of IL-2 in IL-$2^{-/-}$ mice is inconsistent with many of the studies carried out previously, and the direct dependency on IL-2 by $CD4^-CD8^-$ thymocytes for their growth and/or differentiation. However, the presence of self-reactive T-cells and autoimmunity in IL-$2^{-/-}$ mice suggest that IL-2 may influence later stages of T-cell development and perhaps thymocyte selection. The presence of lymphoid hyperplasia and autoimmunity in gnotobiotic IL-$2^{-/-}$ mice is consistent with a defect in central and/or peripheral tolerance as being responsible for disease rather than an uncontrolled peripheral T-cell response to environmental antigens *(140)*. If and how IL-2 influences these processes is currently not known and relies, at least in part, in determining what the underlying basis of abnormal thymocyte development in IL-$2^{-/-}$ mice is.

One clue as to its mechanism of action has been obtained from the authors' analyses of thymocyte death and selection in normal wild-type mice, TCR-transgenic mice and IL-$2^{-/-}$ mice. They have shown that IL-2/IL-2R interactions are required for mediating susceptibility to apoptosis in thymocytes that have undergone TCR-mediated activation (H. Bassiri, P. Egan, and S. R. Carding, unpublished observations). Using monoclonal anti-CD3 antibodies to experimentally induce cortical thymocyte apoptosis, dying thymocytes were shown to produce IL-2 and upregulate high affinity IL-2Rs *in situ*. Similar results were obtained using the MHC class II-restricted ovalbumin-specific TCR transgenic mice, DO11.10, *(141)*. On sections of thymus from ovalbumin-treated transgenic mice, IL-2 protein was detected within a large number of clusters of apoptotic cells situated in the cortex and medulla. Intracellular staining and flow cytometric analyses of cells recovered from DO11.10 mice injected with ovalbumin identified IL-2–producing cells as $CD4^{lo}8^{lo}$, small (low FSC) and transgene-$TCR^{int/hi}$, consistent with an apoptotic phenotype. The ability of anti–IL-2R antibodies at least partially to prevent the deletion of TCR-transgene positive, $CD4^+CD8^+$ thymocytes in mice-administered antigen demonstrates that IL-2/IL-2R interactions are directly involved in antigen-mediated deletion of at least some MHC class II restricted thymocytes. The hypothesis that IL-2 is involved in thymocyte apoptosis was tested directly by determining the consequences of IL-2–deficiency on activation-induced cell (AICD) death of thymocytes in IL-$2^{-/-}$ mice. In the absence of IL-2, thymocytes were refractory to anti-CD3 induced apoptosis. This insensitivity to anti-CD3–induced apoptosis could, however, be overcome by providing an exogenous source of IL-2 at the time of administering anti-CD3. The induction of apoptosis was dependent upon both IL-2 and anti-CD3, since IL-2 given alone did not result in an increase in the number of apoptotic cells detected in sections of thymus from anti-CD3-treated IL-$2^{-/-}$ mice. Together with the impaired deletion of antigen-activated peripheral IL-$2^{-/-}$ T-cells *(142)*, these results provide an explanation for the presence of self-reactive $CD4^+$ T-cells and autoimmunity in IL-$2^{-/-}$ *(134,143)*, IL-$2R\alpha^{-/-}$ *(144)*, and IL-$2R\beta^{-/-}$ *(145)* mice. They also provide direct evidence for a requirement for the IL-2/IL-2R signaling pathway in the induction of thymocyte apoptosis and the elimination of self-reactive thymocytes, particularly those reactive with self antigens presented by MHC class II molecules. Finally, the authors' results may also provide an explanation for some of the contrasting effects of IL-2 or anti-IL-2/IL-2R antibodies on thymocyte growth, survival, and development both in vitro and in vivo.

These novel findings raise an interesting question. Does the elimination of self-reactive MHC class I-restricted thymocytes require or involve IL-2/IL-2R interactions? The inability to detect any effect of IL-2–deficiency on the deletion of self-reactive thymocytes in MHC class I-restricted TCR transgenic mice crossed onto the IL-$2^{-/-}$ background *(146)*, and the authors' inability to detect IL-2 production by apoptotic class I-restricted thymocytes during coculture with antigen (Bassiri and Carding, unpublished observations) suggest that there may be alternative pathways of thymocyte apoptosis. The elimination of MHC class II-restricted T-cells may, therefore, be mechanistically distinct from class I-restricted T-cells, which appears to be IL-2-independent. This possibility is currently under investigation in the authors' laboratory.

Although most previous experiments have focused on the influence of IL-2 on $\alpha\beta$ T-cell development, there is also some evidence that IL-2 is required for $\gamma\delta$ T-cell development. The observation of IL-$2R\beta$ expression on developing $\gamma\delta$ cells in the thymus, and the demonstration that in utero anti–IL-$2R\beta$ antibody treatment results in a loss of $V\gamma5^+$ cells in the thymus and dendritic epithelial cells from the skin *(121)*, suggest that IL-2 may be necessary for the development of some $\gamma\delta$ cell populations. More recent studies, of mice deficient in syk (a kinase implicated in IL-2R signaling *(147)*, support this idea since these mice show a striking loss of dendritic epidermal T-cells *(147)*. Interestingly, IL-2Rγ-deficient mice show a complete absence of γδ T-cells in the thymus and the periphery *(148,149)*, suggesting that IL-2 may have an even broader role in γδ T-cell development. Although some of the defects in IL-2Rγ mice may reflect a requirement for other cytokines whose receptors utilize this chain (e.g., IL-4, IL-7, IL-9, or IL-15), the authors' laboratory has recently obtained more direct evidence for a requirement for IL-2 in the development of $\gamma\delta^+$ intestinal intraepithelial lymphocytes (IEL) *(140)*. In contrast to wild-type littermates, the number of $\gamma\delta^+$ IELs in the small intestine of germfree IL-$2^{-/-}$ mice were dramatically reduced, and bone marrow from IL-$2^{-/-}$ mice could not regenerate $\gamma\delta^+$ IEL upon transfer to lethally irradiated wild-type congenic mice. Together with the observation that $\gamma\delta^+$ IEL are also reduced in IL-2R$\beta^{-/-}$ mice *(150)*, the authors' findings identify an essential role for the IL-2/IL-2R signaling pathway in the development of γδ IELs.

It is apparent from all of these studies of IL-2 and T-cell development that IL-2's influence is not restricted to one particular cell type or stage of development. One attractive possibility, therefore, is that IL-2 has multiple effects during T-cell development and that the nature of its influence is dictated by the developmental stage of IL-2R-bearing cells.

4.2.2. IL-2 in the Regulation of B- and NK Cell Development

Although far fewer studies have examined the effects of IL-2 on development of non-T-cells, there is some evidence that it has a role to play in these processes as well. Since the IL-2 receptors expressed on mature B-cells can mediate a proliferative response to IL-2 *(151–154)*, it is possible the recent reports of IL-2Rα expression by pre-B-cells, *(94,155)* indicate a role for the cytokines in proliferation and differentiation of these cells as well. The authors' observation of IL-2Rβ expression on $B220^+$ cells in the fetal liver and bone marrow, and that these cells can proliferate in response to IL-2 *(156)* also suggest that there may be a requirement for this cytokine in developing B-cells. However, it should be noted that the $B220^+$ pro B-cells may also contain some NK precursors, and the expression of IL-2Rβ may actually reflect its expression in this lineage of cells. An influence of IL-2 on NK cell development is suggested by the finding that their development in neonatal mice can be blocked by administering anti-IL-2R antibodies *(121)* and is severely compromised in IL-2R$\beta^{-/-}$ mice *(150)*.

4.2.3. IL-2 in the Regulation of Myeloid Cell Development

Secreted proteins with structural and functional similarities to IL-2 have been identified in invertebrates (the protozoan pheromone, Er-1) that rely on phagocytic cells to eliminate invading pathogens (discussed in ref. *157*). Although it is not known if this invertebrate IL-2 homolog influences or regulates phagocytic cell activity, it is interesting to speculate that IL-2 may have evolved from a factor whose original function was to regulate cellular defense mechanisms (phagocytes) other than lymphocytes. It perhaps not surprising, therefore, that IL-2 can influence the development and activity of mammalian myeloid cells.

Evidence for the involvement of IL-2 in myelopoiesis comes from patient studies, animal studies using normal and genetically engineered mice, as well as in vitro experiments using isolated cells. Administration of IL-2 to cancer patients has been shown to result in an increase in the number of circulating erythroid (BFU-E), myeloid (CFU-GM), and/or multi-lineage (CFU-GEMM) progenitor cells *(158–160)*. The ability of recombinant IL-2 to promote the growth and development of hematopoietic progenitors *(161)* and myeloid precursors *(162)* in in vitro culture is also consistent with a direct role for IL-2 in regulating hematopoietic cell activity. The authors' observation that IL-2 can promote the growth and development of highly purified immature myeloid cells in vitro, and that its absence in IL-$2^{-/-}$ mice results in impaired granulocyte and macrophage development, provide more direct evidence for the ability of IL-2 to regulate myelopoiesis *(163)*.

The accumulation of immature myeloid cells and the absence of blood neutrophils and populations of tissue-specific macrophages in IL-$2^{-/-}$ mice suggest that the absence of IL-2 results in an inability of immature cells to progress to more mature fully differentiated cells. The occurrence of a similar granulocytic abnormality in IL-2R$\beta^{-/-}$ mice *(145)* is also consistent with the involvement of the IL-2/IL-2R signaling pathway in regualting myelomonocytic cell generation. Based upon the inability of IL-$2^{-/-}$ bone marrow cells to sustain myelopoiesis in lethally irradiated mice and in long-term bone marrow cultures, this defective hematopoietic disorder is most likely a result of an intrinsic proliferative and/or developmental defect in a hematopoietic stem or myeloid progenitor cell population. Since IL-$2^{-/-}$ bone marrow cells can contribute to the long-term reconstitution of lymphocyte lineages in bone marrow chimeras, this would argue against a stem cell defect since this would prevent multilineage reconstitution. These observations are consistent with the hypothesis that the myeloid progenitor cell defect in IL-$2^{-/-}$ mice is caused by a direct requirement for IL-2 for their growth, and possibly development. However, it is possible that IL-2 may influence myeloid cell development in other ways: for example, by functioning as a competence factor enabling developing myeloid cells to acquire responsiveness to other growth and differentiation factors. The loss of mature granulocytes and macrophages may also result from an inability of immature cells to progress to the more mature stages. Finally, the finding that in vitro exposure to IL-2 prevents apoptosis in mature neutrophils *(164)* suggest that if IL-2 acts in a similar way in vivo, its absence may contribute to the loss of mature granulocytes in IL-$2^{-/-}$ mice. Further studies are required in order to determine if these mechanisms contribute to the myeloid cell defects seen in IL-$2^{-/-}$ mice.

The increase in the number of circulating erythroid (BFU-E), myeloid (CFU-GM), and/or multi-lineage (CFU-GEMM) progenitor cells in cancer patients after immunotherapy with IL-2 *(158–160)* suggests that IL-2 may regulate progenitor activity in humans. Moreover, the finding that addition of recombinant IL-2 to cultures of T-cell–depleted, enriched populations of human bone marrow hematopoietic progenitors *(161)* and murine myeloid precursors *(162)* can promote their growth and development is consistent with a direct role for IL-2 in regulating hematopoietic cell activity. These observations are also supported by the finding that human immunodeficiency as a result of defective IL-2 production *(165)* is associated with deficient hematopoiesis in the bone marrow (K. Weinberg, personal communication).

4.3. Requirement for IL-2 in the Generation and Maintenance of HIMs

The microenvironment for any developing hematopoietic cell includes other hematopoietic and nonhematopoietic cells, as well as the growth factors, adhesion molecules, and extracellular matrix components they produce. Even subtle alterations in this microenvironment can dramatically influence hematopoietic development and activity. Therefore, it may be useful to consider the ways in which IL-2 may affect hematopoietic cells and nonhematopoietic stromal cells to create a microenvironment capable of supporting hematopoiesis.

4.3.1. Influences of Lymphoid and Myeloid Cells

The pleiotropic effects of IL-2 on T-cells can clearly have important repercussions for development of other hematopoietic lineages. The effects of T-cells on hematopoiesis may be mediated by cytokines such as IFNγ *(166)*, TNF, IL-4, and GM-CSF *(13)*. Since T-cell production of these cytokines can be regulated by IL-2, the loss of IL-2 in mutant mice could result in a loss of growth factors necessary for the development of hematopoietic cells. This notion is supported by experiments demonstrating that removal of marrow T-cells results in a reduction of BFU-E activity by 50% *(167)* because of the loss of burst promoting-activity, which is normally produced by T-cells in response to IL-2 *(168)*. Effects such as these may explain why the removal of T-cells from donor bone marrow samples adversely effects the efficiency of engraftment in bone marrow transplant patients (discussed in ref. *169*). However, the significance of these studies are unclear in light of the fact that T-cell-deficient mice such as SCID and athymic *nu/nu* mice do not exhibit defects in hematopoiesis. Moreover, in vitro long-term bone marrow cultures from nude mice, and T-cell-depleted cultures from normal mice *(170)*, can be maintained successfully for many months. Therefore, it is possible that IL-2 is required to maintain normal T-cell function and that its absence leads to aberrant T-cell mediated inhibition of hematopoiesis. There are many examples of such inhibition. For instance, IL-2–stimulated T-cells have been shown, under some circumstances, to inhibit in vitro granulocyte-macrophage and erythroid colony formation *(171–173)* as well as uncommitted progenitor cell colony formation *(79)*. In patients with aplastic anemia, it has been shown that T-cells suppress colony formation *(174)* that appears to be a result of the production of IFNγ since anti-IFNγ antibodies could restore hematopoietic cell colony forming activity in bone marrow cells from these patients *(175)*.

Cytokine-mediated inhibition of hematopoietic cell development may be of particular relevance for B-cell development since TNFα and IL-4 have both been shown to have potent inhibitory effects on immature B-cells. For example, IL-4 has been found to inhibit stromal cell-dependent growth of pre-B-cells and proliferation of early hematopoietic progenitor cells *(176)*. Similarly, exogenously added TNFα can inhibit IL-7-induced growth of early B lineage cells in culture *(177)*, and inhibition of in vitro bone marrow colony formation *(178)*. This mechanism of inhibition of hematopoiesis has been shown to be physiologically relevant in experiments demonstrating that bone marrow failure and suppression of hematopoietic colony formation in HIV infected patients *(179)* is mediated by TNFα.

The hematopoietic failure, and in particular the anemia and defective B-cell development, that occurs in IL-$2^{-/-}$ *(134,143)* and IL-2Rβ$^{-/-}$ *(145)* mice has been attributed to the presence of dysfunctional T-cells. The authors' preliminary finding that the bone marrow of IL-$2^{-/-}$ mice contains elevated numbers of TNFα- and IL-4- (but not IFNγ) producing T-cells (T. Reya and S. R. Carding, unpublished observations) and that the transfer of splenic T-cells from IL-$2^{-/-}$ mice to normal C57BL.6 mice causes a reduction in the number of B220$^+$ cells in the host bone marrow, suggests that T-cells that have developed in the absence of IL-2 have deleterious effects on hematopoiesis. However, since the presence of IL-$2^{-/-}$ T-cells does not interfere with the development of normal myeloid cells in vivo or in vitro *(163)* it is unlikely that these cells are responsible for the defective myelopoiesis seen in IL-$2^{-/-}$ mice (*see* Subheading 4.2.3., above). In contrast, the colitis observed in IL-$2^{-/-}$ mice is likely to be caused by T-cells, since IL-$2^{-/-}$ T-cells can transfer disease to otherwise healthy wild-type mice and, IL-$2^{-/-}$ mice lacking both T- and B-cells do not show symptoms of colitis, whereas mice that lack only B-cells do *(180)*.

4.3.2. Stromal Cell and Bone Influences

Stromal cells form a critical part of the hematopoietic microenvironment providing important cell-cell contacts, producing cytokines and secreting extracellular matrix components necessary for the growth of hematopoietic cells. Surprisingly, the authors have found that both thymic *(95)* and bone marrow (T. Reya and S. R. Carding, unpublished observations) stromal cells from IL-$2^{-/-}$ mice are deficient in their ability to support hematopoiesis. In the thymus, this is because of the loss or absence of myeloid (macrophages) and MHC class II-expressing epithelial cells. In the bone marrow, the alkaline phosphatase-positive presumptive stromal cell precursor *(181)* population is almost completely absent from primary cultures of IL-$2^{-/-}$ cells. The addition of exogenous IL-2 to these cultures partially restored fibroblast-like cells, suggesting that IL-2 may act directly on certain stromal cell populations to promote or regulate their growth and development. There is some additional evidence that nonhematopoietic cells such as fibroblasts may utilize IL-2 for their growth and function *(115,182)*. Since stromal cells contribute significantly to the hematopoietic microenvironment, the loss of precursor and mature stromal cells in the bone marrow of IL-$2^{-/-}$ mice could contribute to many of the hematopoietic defects observed.

Besides interacting with classical stroma, developing hematopoietic cells are likely to interact with bone cells as well. The fact that greater numbers of stem cells can be found near the surface of the bone compared to central regions *(183,184)* raises the possibility that progenitors may require interactions with cells at the bone surface, or utilize extracellular matrix or soluble factors secreted by these cells. In fact, bone cells have been documented to produce cytokines that support multipotent progenitor cell growth *(185–189)*. Osteoblasts, in particular, have been shown to constitutively produce M-CSF, IL-6 *(190)* and GM-CSF *(191)*. In addition, these cells produce components of the stromal matrix such as collagen and proteoglycans, and have been demonstrated to support hematopoietic progenitor cell growth in in vitro cultures *(192)*. The deficiency of alkaline-phosphatase–positive stromal cells in bone marrow cultures from IL-$2^{-/-}$ mice suggests that osteoblasts, which also express this enzyme, may indeed be targets of IL-2. Thus, the fact that IL-$2^{-/-}$ mice have fragile bones with increased fibrosis may reflect a loss of the normal microenvironment necessary for hematopoiesis.

Just as hematopoietic cells may rely on nonhematopoietic elements (stroma and bone cells) for their development, stroma and bone cells may require hematopoietic cells as well. For instance, much evidence points to the growth of bone cells from marrow stroma; in experiments in which marrow cells were implanted into a host animal in a diffusion chamber, these cells generated bone and cartilage *(193–195)*. Thus, a defect in hematopoiesis could in turn cause loss of both bone cells and stroma. Osteoclasts are also believed to originate from hematopoietic progenitors in the bone marrow *(196,197)*. In fact, most studies suggest that they derived from the monocyte/macrophage lineage *(198)*. Since cells of this lineage have IL-2 receptors and myelopoiesis is compromised in IL-$2^{-/-}$ mice, a loss of IL-2 may directly affect the development or function of osteoclasts as well.

5. Differential Requirement for IL-2 During Ontogeny

In the authors' attempt to understand IL-2's role in hematopoiesis, they have examined the evidence for its influence at both the fetal and adult stages of ontogeny. The fact that cells expressing IL-2R and producing IL-2 are present in fetal liver and thymus, as well as adult bone marrow and thymus, implies that cells at these stages of an animals development may utilize this cytokine in hematopoiesis. Thus, it is intriguing that the hematopoietic defect in IL-2 mutant mice does not become apparent until well after birth.

One explanation for this late onset of disease is a differential requirement for IL-2 during the fetal and adult phases of hematopoiesis. A number of studies have demonstrated differences between fetal and adult progenitor cells. These include differences in developmental potential *(199,200)*, T-cell receptor repertoire *(199)*, B-cell repertoire (B1 and B2 cells) *(201)*, tissue-specific macrophages *(202,203)*, erythrocyte hemoglobin gene expression *(204)*, and B-cell class II expression *(205,206)*. Moreover, fetal and adult hematopoietic cells appear to differ functionally. In studies examining colony-forming ability, it was demonstrated that the number of CFU-S per spleen colony decreased during ontogeny *(207,208)*. Fetal stem cells have also been documented to have higher turnover rates *(209)* compared to adult stem cells. Some of these changes may occur as a result of the shift in hematopoiesis from fetal liver to bone marrow, whereas others may reflect an age-related changes in growth and differentiation requirements and age-related changes in the structure, composition, and function of HIM. Adult hematopoietic stem and progenitor cells, as well as stromal cell populations, which comprise the microenvironments in which they develop might, therefore, be more dependent upon IL-2 than their fetal counterparts.

It is also possible that the defects in IL-2$^{-/-}$ mice occur only in the adult because of the appearance during adulthood of a mature hematopoietic population (e.g., T-cells) that can influence hematopoiesis. In the absence of IL-2, this regulatory cell may be absent or may exhibit an abnormal function that is capable of disrupting hematopoiesis. Compensatory mechanisms (such as cytokines with functions similar to IL-2) that are present primarily in fetal life may help explain the late onset of disease in IL-2$^{-/-}$ mice. The possibility that the hematopoietic defect is apparent during fetal development but is rescued by maternal transfer of IL-2 seems unlikely since in IL-2$^{-/-}$ mice born to homozygous, IL-2$^{-/-}$ mothers the disease is also late onset *(140)*.

6. Redundant Functions of IL-2 in Hematopoiesis

In reviewing the evidence supporting a role for IL-2 in hematopoietic development and function, it is clear that although many of the phenotypes of IL-2 and IL-2R mutant mice are similar, there are also differences. For example, IL-2$^{-/-}$ *(135)* and IL-2R$\alpha^{-/-}$ *(144)* mice develop T-cell–mediated colitis, whereas the IL-2R$\gamma^{-/-}$ *(148,149)* and the IL-2R$\beta^{-/-}$ mice *(145)* do not, and IL-2R$\gamma^{-/-}$ mice have defects that occur earlier than those in the other three mutants. Although these inconsistencies may reflect the incorporation of the β and γ chains as being part of other cytokine receptors and the inability to respond to cytokines other than IL-2, some of them may result from the fact that mice lacking a particular receptor chain may still be able to respond to IL-2 with partial signals transduced through the remaining components of the receptor.

Based on the fact that IL-2R are expressed on numerous hematopoietic progenitor cells (*see* Fig. 2), it would be predicted that the defects specifically affect a number of progenitors directly. Although this is a possibility that needs to be investigated, if such defects are not present, this would imply that IL-2's function is effectively compensated by other cytokines. Compensation has been documented in multiple systems where a single gene mutation did not show the expected defects; however, upon crossing the mice to other mice with separate mutations, various defects became apparent. For example, although fyn, and src mutant mice had nonoverlapping phenotypes, and mice mutant for yes showed no phenotypic changes, src/fyn and src/yes double mutants die perinatally, whereas the fyn/yes double mutants develop degenerative renal disease *(210)*, defects not evident in mice mutant for either fyn or yes. Candidates for compensatory cytokines include those whose receptors share one of the IL-2 receptor chains. For instance, since the γ chain can be utilized by IL-4, IL-7, IL-9, and IL-15 *(99–103,211)* it is possible that in the absence of IL-2 one of these cytokines can substitute for its functions. In the case of the IL-$2^{-/-}$ mice, they have been bred to mice lacking IL-4 *(212)* and analysis of lymphoid development did not reveal any developmental defects of immature or mature lymphoid cells *(213)*. However, the antiviral CTL responses of mice lacking both IL-2 and IL-4 was significantly impaired compared to mice lacking either IL-2 or IL-4. This identifies IL-4 as a cytokine that can compensate for the function of IL-2 either during T-cell activation or during development of the T-cells responsible for mounting an immune response *(212)*. Such compensatory pathways could occur in the IL-2Rβ- and α-deficient mice also, whereas in the absence of γ itself, none of the cytokines would be able to compensate and the mutation would result in multiple defects. In light of the severe defects in the lymphoid compartments in IL-2R$\gamma^{-/-}$ mice, it seems likely that this reflects a requirement for cytokines other than IL-2 that act through it; the similarity in defects in lymphocyte development of these mice and the IL-$7^{-/-}$ *(64)* and IL-$7R^{-/-}$ *(63)* mice suggest that IL-7 is the most important cytokine.

The fact that functional receptors are expressed on hematopoietic progenitor cells that are localized at sites of hematopoiesis in which IL-2 is also produced, makes it highly likely that these cells do respond in some manner to IL-2. Therefore, the absence of defects that arise from direct dependence on IL-2 is more indicative of redundant cytokine pathways than the possibility that IL-2 does not influence the cells that express its receptors. Designing experiments that distinguish the effects of compensatory cytokines, partial signals through receptor components and requirements for other cytokines that act through shared receptors would help clarify the specific role of IL-2 in hematopoiesis.

7. A Model and Future Studies

It is clear from the above discussion (Subheadings 4.2.–4.3.) that there are many possible mechanisms by which IL-2 exerts its influence on hematopoietic and nonhematopoietic cells. Here, the authors propose one model that may help guide future experiments (Fig. 3). Based on previous findings about IL-2's influences on various hematopoietic cells, and their own studies, they propose that IL-2 regulates hematopoiesis in three distinct ways. It acts directly on immature hematopoietic cells that express its receptor promoting their survival, growth, and differentiation into mature cells. It regulates the production of other cytokines, which in turn control the growth and differentiation of hematopoietic cells. Finally, it acts to maintain the development and function of the stromal cells that make up the hematopoietic microenvironment.

The authors' data suggest that among the most critical targets of IL-2 are cells of the myeloid lineage. They propose that IL-2 is required for myeloid cell development, directly acting to promote the growth and development of IL-$2R^{+}$ progenitor cells. Thus, in the absence of IL-2, myeloid development is disrupted, and there is an accumulation of immature myeloid cells, and a relative absence of mature cells of this lineage. The authors also hypothesize that IL-2 regulates cytokine secretion by cells of the myeloid and T lineages. Based on this notion they propose that the absence of IL-2 causes dysregulated production of cytokines such as TNFα and IL-4, by myeloid cells, and this in turn disrupts hematopoietic progenitor growth and B-cell development. IL-2 controls a similar cytokine pathway in T-cells as well,

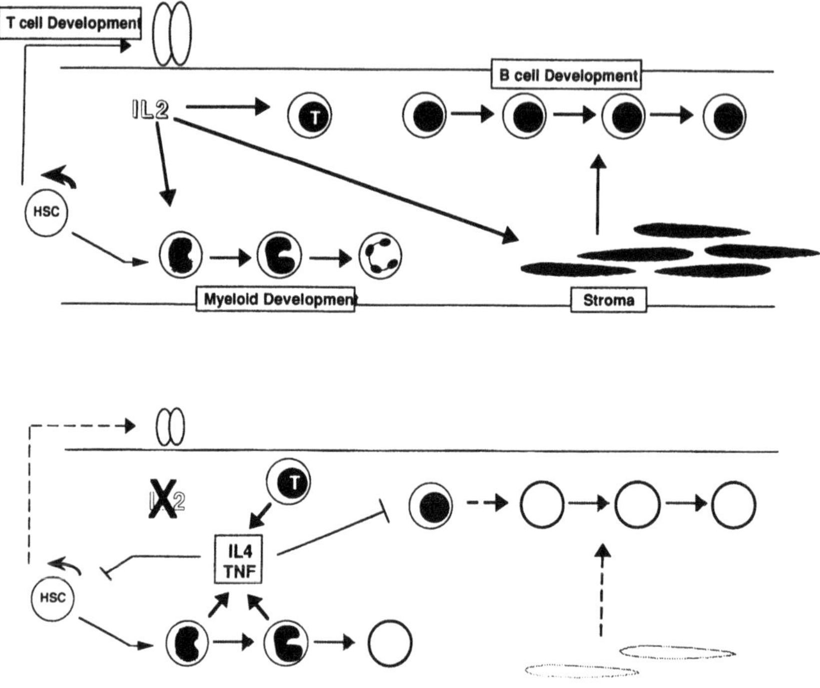

Fig. 3. The role of IL-2 in hematopoiesis: a model. The figure depicts the ways in which IL-2 normally regulates bone marrow hematopoiesis (upper) and the consequences of its abscence (lower). Through its ability to interact directly with IL-2R–expressing progenitor cells, by regulating the production of cytokines by immature and mature cells, and through its interaction with stromal cells, IL-2 can influence the survival, growth and differentiation of immature hematopoietic cells into mature cells. For more detailed explanation *see* Subheading 7. HSC, hematopoietic stem cell.

and in its absence T-cells overproduce IL-4 and TNFα. Finally, IL-2 also affects stromal cells directly by regulating the expression of adhesion molecules that are important in normal stromal development and function. The loss of IL-2 results in the decrease in stromal cell development, which directly or indirectly results in abnormal bone formation.

Further experiments can be designed to test the model proposed above (Fig. 3), and to investigate other possible mechanisms by which IL-2 regulates hematolymphoid cell development. Various types of genetically engineered mice could be used for these studies. Utilization of mutants in which IL-2R can be eliminated in specific cell types (e.g., myeloid cells or T-cells), would provide insight into the role of IL-2 in these cells. In a complex system such as hematopoiesis, analysis of tissue-specific mutant mice may be the only way to determine the dependence of each hematopoietic compartment on IL-2, as well as the dependence of other hematopoietic components on the targeted cells. The role of IL-2 in fetal and adult life may also be clarified by generating inducible IL-2 deficient mice, for example using the thymidine kinase/gancyclovir cell ablation system to eliminate IL-2-producing cells *(214)*, which would allow its role at particular stages of development of the hematopoietic systems to be investigated. To identify requirements for IL-2 that may be masked by compensatory pathways, mice in which both IL-2 and the IL-2R are inactivated would be useful, since this approach would prevent partial signals and eliminate compensation that may occur through particular chains of the IL-2 receptor complex. Mice that express mutant receptors lacking signaling domains may provide another way to approach the same issue. Moreover, crossing IL-$2^{-/-}$ mice with mice deficient for other cytokines that could potentially compensate for its function, might also reveal novel roles for IL-2. Comparison of IL-$2^{-/-}$ mice to mutants lacking other cytokines that act through common receptor chains (such as IL-7 or IL-15) may distinguish requirements for IL-2 from requirements for other growth factors. To identify the defects that occur in the various hematopoietic lineages, it would also be useful to generate an in vitro system in which the aberrant cells of interest could be analyzed in the absence of the other defects. Cell lines from IL-$2^{-/-}$ mice should provide a useful system for such detailed analyses. For example, this would prove to be of enormous value in further elucidating the nature of the interaction between developing T-cells and stromal cells in the thymus that determines the fate of thymocytes and how IL-2 influences this outcome. It would also enable studies of the intracellular signaling pathways induced by antigenic stimuli during lymphocyte development to be carried out, providing insights into the downstream effectors of IL-2.

Acknowledgments

The authors would like to thank all of the members of the Carding laboratory for their assistance in the preparation of this review. The studies performed in the authors laboratory were supported in part by grants from the W.W. Smith Charitable Trust, The American Cancer Society (JFRA-399, RPG-97-027), the NIH (AI-31972, HL-51749) and the University of Pennsylvania Research Foundation and Cancer Center.

References

1. Trentin, J. J. (1970) Influence of hematopoietic organ stroma (hemopoietic microenvironment) on stem cell differentiation, in *Regulation of Hematopoiesis* (Gordon, A. S., ed.), Meredith, New York, pp. 161–186.
2. Wu, L., Antica, M., Johnson, G., Scollay, R., and Shortman, K. (1991) Developmental potential of the earliest precursor cells from the the adult mouse thymus. *J. Exp. Med.* **174,** 1617–1627.
3. Watson, J. D., Morrissey, P. J., Namen, A. E., Conlon, P. J., and Widmer, M. B. (1989) Effect of IL-7 on the growth of fetal thymocytes in culture. *J. Immunol.* **143,** 1215–1222.
4. Miller, M. D. and Krangel, M. S. (1992) Biology and biochemistry of the chemokines: A family of chemotactic and inflammatory cytokines. *Crit. Rev. Immunol.* **12,** 17–46.
5. Lorenzo, J. A. (1991) The role of cytokines in the regulation of local bone resorption. *Crit. Rev. Immunol.* **11,** 195–213.
6. Tabibzadeh, S. (1991) Human endometrium: an active site of cytokine production and action. *Endocrine Rev.* **12,** 272–290.
7. Bradley, T. R. and Metcalf, D. (1966) The growth of mouse bone marrow cells in vitro. *Aust. J. Exp. Biol. Med. Sci.* **44,** 287–299.
8. Ichikawa, Y., Pluznik, D. H., and Sachs, L. (1966) In vitro control of the development of macrophage and granulocyte colonies. *Proc. Natl. Acad. Sci. USA* **56,** 488–495.
9. Smith, K. (1988) Interleukin **2,** Inception, Impact, and implications. *Science* **240,** 1169–1176.
10. Chen, B. D.-M. and Najor, F. (1987) Macrophage activation by interferon alpha and beta is associated with a loss of proliferative capacity: role of interferon alpha and beta in the regulation of macrophage proliferation and function. *Cell. Immunol.* **106,** 343–354.
11. Moore, R. N., Larsen, H. S., Horohov, D. W., and Rouse, B. T. (1984) Endogenous regulation of macrophage proliferative expansion by colony stimulating factor-induced interferon. *Science* **223,** 178–181.
12. Schultz, R. M. and Chirigos, M. A. (1978) Similarities among factors that render macrophages tumoricidal in lymphokine and interferon preparations. *Cancer. Res.* **38,** 1003–1007.

13. Kroemer, G., Andreu-Sanchex, J. L., Gonzalo, J. A., Gutierrez-Ramos, J. C., and Martinez-A, C. (1991) Interleukin-2, autotolerance, and autoimmunity. *Adv. Immunol.* **50,** 147–235.
14. Schluesener, H. J. and Lider, O. (1989) Transforming growth factors β1 and β2: cytokines with identical immunosuppressive effects and a potential role in the regulation of autoimmune T cell function. *J. Neuroimmunol.* **24,** 249–258.
15. Wahl, S. M., Allen, J. B., Wong, H. L., Dougherty, S. F., and Ellingsworth, L. R. (1990) Antagonistic and agonistic effects of transforming growth factor-β and IL-1 in rheumatoid synovium. *J. Immunol.* **145,** 2514–2519.
16. Hoffman, R. (1989) Regulation of megakaryocytopoiesis. *Blood* **74,** 1196–1212.
17. Karray, S., deFrance, T., Merle-Béral, H., Banchereau, J., Debré, P., and Galanaud, P. (1988) Interleukin 4 counteracts the interleukin 2-induced proliferation of monoclonal B cells. *J. Exp. Med.* **168,** 85–94.
18. Vellenga, E., de Wolfe, J. T. M., Beentjes, J. A. M., Esselink, M. T., Smit, J. W., and Halie, M. R. (1990) Divergent effects of interleukin-4 (IL-4) on the granulocyte colony-stimulating factor and IL-3-supported myeloid colony formation from normal and leukemic bone marrow cells. *Blood* **75,** 633–637.
19. Alegre, M.-L., Vandenabeele, P., Depierreuz, M., Florquin, S., Deschodt-Lanckman, M., Flamand, V., Moser, M., Leo, O., Urbain, J., Fiers, W., and Goldman, M. (1991) Cytokine release syndrome induced by the 145-2C11 anti-CD3 monoclonal antibody in mice: prevention by high doses of methylprednisone. *J. Immunol.* **146,** 1184–1191.
20. Gordon, M. Y., Riley, G. P., Watt, S. M., and Greaves, M. F. (1987) Compartmentalization of a haematopoietic growth factor (GM-CSF) by glycosaminoglycans in the bone marrow microenvironment. *Nature* **326,** 403–405.
21. Li, Y.-S., Milner, P. G., Chauhan, A. K., Watson, M. A., Hoffman, R. M., Kodner, C. M., Milbrandt, J., and Deuel, T. F. (1990) Cloning and expression of a developmentally regulated protein that induces mitogenic and neurite outgrowth activity. *Science* **250,** 1690–1692.
22. Merenmies, J. and Rauvala, H. (1990) Molecular cloning of the 18-kDa growth-associated protein of developing brain. *J. Biol. Chem.* **265,** 16,721–16,728.
23. Roberts, R., Gallagher, J., Spooncer, E., Allen, T. D., Bloomfield, F., and Dexter, T. M. (1988) Heparan sulfate bound growth factors: a mechanism for stromal cell mediated haemopoiesis. *Nature* **332,** 376–378.
24. Kroemer, G., Cuende, E., and Martinez-A, C. (1993) Compartmentalization of the peripheral immune system. *Adv. Immunol.* **53,** 157–216.
25. Kroemer, G., Toribio, M. L., and Martinez-A, C. (1991) Interleukin-2: counteracting pleiotropism by compartmentalization. *New Biologist* **3,** 219–229.
26. Oster, W., Lindemann, A., Mertelsmann, R., and Herrmann, F. (1989) Granulocyte-macrophage colony-stimulating factor (CSF) and multilineage CSF recruit human monocytes to express granulocyte CSF. *Blood* **73,** 64–67.
27. Wieser, M., Bonifer, R., Oster, W., Lindemann, A., Mertelsmann, R., and Herrmann, F. (1989) Interleukin-4 induces secretion of CSF for granulocytes and CSF for macrophages by peripheral blood monocytes. *Blood* **73,** 1105–1108.
28. Horiguchi, J., Warren, M. K., and Kufe, D. (1987) Expression of the macrophage-specific colony-stimulating factor in human monocytes treated with granulocyte-macrophage colony-stimulating factor. *Blood* **69,** 1259–1261.
29. Pistoia, V., Ghio, R., Roncella, S., Cozzolino, F., Zupo, S., and Ferrarini, M. (1987) Production of colony-stimulating activity by normal and neoplastic human B lymphocytes. *Blood* **69,** 1340–1347.
30. Rambaldi, A., Young, D. C., and Griffin, J. D. (1987) Expression of the M-CSF (CSF-1) gene by human monocytes. *Blood* **69,** 1409–1413.
31. Vellenga, E., Rambaldi, A., Ernst, T. J., Ostapovicz, D., and Griffin, J. D. (1988) Independent regulation of M-CSF and G-CSF gene expression in human monocytes. *Blood* **71,** 1529–1532.
32. Bot, F. J., v. Eijk, L., Schipper, P., and Lowenberg, B. (1989) Effects of human interleukin-3 on granulocytic colony-forming cells in human bone marrow. *Blood* **73,** 1157–1160.
33. Leary, A. G., Yang, Y.-C., Clark, S. C., Gasson, J. C., Golde, D. W., and Ogawa, M. (1987) Recombinant gibbon interleukin-3 supports formation of human multilineage colonies and blast cell colonies in culture: Comparison with recombinant human granulocyte-macrophage colony stimulating factor. *Blood* **70,** 1343–1348.
34. Valent, P., Schmidt, G., Besemer, J., Mayer, P., Zenke, G., Liehl, E., Hinterberger, W., Lechner, K., Maurer, D., and Bettelheim, P. (1989) Interleukin-3 is a differentiation factor for human basophils. *Blood* **73,** 1763–1769.

35. Carding, S. R., Jenkinson, E. J., Kingston, R., Hayday, A. C., Bottomly, K., and Owen, J. J. T. (1989) Developmental control of lymphokine gene expression in fetal thymocytes during T cell ontogeny. *Proc. Natl. Acad. Sci. USA* **86,** 3342–3345.
36. Yang-Snyder, J. A. and Rothenberg, E. V. (1993) Developmental and anatomical patterns of IL-2 gene expression in vivo in the murine thymus. *Dev. Immunol.* **3,** 85–102.
37. Zúñiga-Pflücker, J. C., Smith, K. A., Tentori, L., Pardoll, D. M., Longo, D. L., and Kruisbeek, A. M. (1990) Are the IL-2 receptors expressed in the murine fetal thymus functional? *Dev. Immunol.* **1,** 59–66.
38. Deman, J., Martin, M.-T., Delvenne, P., Humblet, C., Boniver, J., and Defresne, M. P. (1992) Analysis by *in situ* hybridization of cells expressing mRNA for tumor-necrosis factor in the developing thymus of mice. *Dev. Immunol.* **2,** 103–109.
39. Wiles, M. V., Ruiz, P., and Imhof, B. A. (1992) Interleukin-7 expression during mouse thymus development. *Eur. J. Immunol.* **22,** 1037–1042.
40. Lynch, F. and Shevach, E. M. (1992) Activation requirements of newborn thymic gamma delta T cells. *J. Immunol.* **149,** 2307–2314.
41. Ransom, J., Fischer, M., Mosmann, T., Yokota, T., DeLuca, D., Schumacher, J., and Zlotnik, A. (1987) Interferon-gamma is produced by activated immature mouse thymocytes and inhibits the interleukin 4-induced proliferation of immature thymocytes. *J. Immunol* **139,** 4102–4108.
42. Zlotnik, A. and Kelner, G. S. (1994) Cytokines in the adult thymus, in *Intrathymic T-Cell Development* (Nikolic-Zugic, J., R.G. Landes, Austin, TX, p. 64–75.
43. Zlotnik, A., Ransom, J., Frank, G., Fischer, M., and Howard, M. (1987) Interleukin 4 is a growth factor for activated thymocytes: possible role in T-cell ontogeny. *Proc. Natl. Acad. Sci. USA* **84,** 3856–3860.
44. Godfrey, D. I., Zlotnik, A., and Suda, T. (1992) Phenotypic and functional characterization of c-kit expression during intrathymic T cell development. *J. Immunol.* **149,** 2281–2285.
45. Galy, A. H. and Spits, H. (1991) IL-1, IL-4, and IFN-gamma differentially regulate cytokine production and cell surface molecule expression in cultured human thymic epithelial cells. *J. Immunol.* **147,** 3823–3830.
46. Gimble, J. M., Pietrangeli, C., Henley, A., Dorheim, M. A., Silver, J., Namen, A., Takeichi, M., Goridis, C., and Kincade, P. W. (1989) Characterization of murine bone marrow and spleen-derived stromal cells: analysis of leukocyte marker and growth factor mRNA transcript levels. *Blood* **74,** 303–311.
47. Harigaya, K., Cronkite, E. P., Miller, M. E., and Shadduck, R. K. (1981) Murine bone marrow cell line producing colony-stimulating factor. *Proc. Natl. Acad. Sci. USA* **78,** 6963–6966.
48. Hunt, P., Robertson, D., Weiss, D., Rennick, D., Lee, F., and Witte, O. N. (1987) A single bone marrow-derived stromal cell type supports the in vitro growth of early lymphoid and myeloid cells. *Cell* **48,** 997–1007.
49. Akashi, M., Loussararian, A. H., Adelman, D. C., Saito, M., and Koeffler, H. P. (1990) Role of lymphotoxin in expression of interleukin 6 in human fibroblasts. Stimulation and regulation. *J. Clin Invest.* **85,** 121–129.
50. Fibbe, W. E., Van Damme, J., Billiau, A., Duinkerken, N., Lurvink, E., Ralph, P., Altrock, B. W., Kaushansky, K., Willemze, R., and Falkenburg, J. H. (1988) Human fibroblasts produce granulocyte-CSF, macrophage-CSF, and granulocyte-macrophage-CSF following stimulation by interleukin-1 and poly(rI).poly(rC). *Blood* **72,** 860–866.
51. Fibbe, W. E., van Damme, J., Billiau, A., Goselink, H. M., Voogt, P. J., van Eeden, G., Ralph, P., Altrock, B. W., and Falkenburg, J. H. (1988) Interleukin 1 induces human marrow stromal cells in long-term culture to produce granulocyte colony-stimulating factor and macrophage colony-stimulating factor. *Blood* **71,** 430–435.
52. Nemunaitis, J., Andrews, D. F., Crittenden, C., Kaushansky, K., and Singer, J. W. (1989) Response of simian virus 40 (SV40)-transformed, cultured human marrow stromal cells to hematopoietic growth factors. *J. Clin. Invest.* **83,** 593–601.
53. Slack, J. L., Nemunaitis, J., Andrews, D. F., and Singer, J. W. (1990) Regulation of cytokine and growth factor gene expression in human bone marrow stromal cells transformed with simian virus 40. *Blood* **75,** 2319–2327.
54. Kaushansky, K., Lin, N., and Adamson, J. W. (1988) Interleukin 1 stimulates fibroblasts to synthesize granulocyte-macrophage and granulocyte colony-stimulating factors: mechanism for the hematopoietic response to inflammation. *J. Clin. Invest.* **81,** 92–97.

55. Yamato, K., El-Hajjaoui, Z., Kuo, J. F., and Koeffler, H. P. (1989) Granulocyte-macrophage colony-stimulating factor: signals for its mRNA accumulation. *Blood* **74,** 1314–1320.
56. Bot, F., van Eijk, L., Broeders, L., Aarden, L., and Lowenberg, B. (1989) Interleukin-6 synergizes with M-CSF in the formation of macrophage colonies from purified human marrow progenitor cells. *Blood* **73,** 435–437.
57. Caracciolo, D., Clark, S. C., and Rovera, G. (1989) Human interleukin-6 supports granulocytic differentiation of hematopoietic progenitor cells and acts synergistically with GM-CSF. *Blood* **73,** 666–670.
58. Zsebo, K. M., Yuschenkoff, V. N., Schiffer, S., Chang, D., McCall, E., Dinarello, C. A., Brown, M. A., Altrock, B., and Bagby, G. C. (1988) Vascular endothelial cells and granulopoiesis: interleukin-1 stimulates release of G-CSF and GM-CSF. *Blood* **71,** 99–103.
59. Herrmann, F., Oster, W., Meuer, S. C., Lindemann, A., and Mertelsmann, R. H. (1988) Interleukin 1 stimulates T lymphocytes to produce granulocyte-monocyte colony-stimulating factor. *J. Clin. Invest.* **81,** 1415–1418.
60. Allen, T. D., Dexter, T. M., and Simmons, P. J. (1990) Marrow biology and stem cells, in *Colony Stimulating Factors: Molecular and Cellular Biology,* (Dexter, T. M., Garland, J. M., and Testa, N. G., eds.), Marcel Dekker, New York, pp. 1–38.
61. Grabstein, K. H., Waldschmidt, T. J., Finkelman, F. D., Hess, B. W., Alpert, A. R., Boiani, N. E., Namen, A. E., and Morrissey, P. J. (1993) Inhibition of murine B and T lymphopoiesis in vivo by an anti-interleukin 7 monoclonal antibody. *J. Exp. Med.* **178,** 257–264.
62. Namen, A. E., Lupton, S., Hjerrild, K., Wignall, J., Mochizuki, D. Y., Schmeirer, A., Mosley, B., March, C. J., Urdal, D., and Gillis, S. (1988) Stimulation of B cell progenitors by cloned murine interleukin-7. *Nature* **333,** 571.
63. Peschon, J. J., Morrissey, P. J., Grabstein, K. H., Ramsdell, F. J., Maraskovsky, E., Gliniak, B. C., Park, L. S., Ziegler, S. F., Williams, D. E., Ware, C. B., Meyer, J. D., and Davison, B. L. (1994) Early lymphocyte expansion is severely impaired in interleukin 7 receptor-deficient mice. *J. Exp. Med.* **180,** 1955–1960.
64. von Freeden-Jeffry, U., Vieira, P., Lucian, L. A., McNeil, T., Burdach, S. E., and Murray, R. (1995) Lymphopenia in interleukin (IL)-7 gene-deleted mice identifies IL-7 as a nonredundant cytokine. *J. Exp. Med.* **181,** 1519–1526.
65. Rolink, A., Streb, M., Nishikawa, S.-I., and Melchers, F. (1991) The c-kit encoded tyrosine kinase regulates the proliferation of early pre-B cells. *Eur. J. Immunol.* **21,** 2609–2613.
66. Landreth, K. S., Narayanan, R., and Dorshkind, K. (1992) Insulin-like growth factor-1 regulates B cell differentiation. *Blood* **80,** 1207–1210.
67. Le, P. T., Tuck, D. T., Dinarello, C. A., Haynes, B. F., and Singer, K. H. (1987) Human thymic epithelial cells produce interleukin 1. *J. Immunol.* **138,** 2520–2526.
68. Murray, R., Suda, T., Wrighton, N., Lee, F., and Zlotnik, A. (1989) IL-7 is a growth and maintenance factor for mature and immature thymocyte subsets. *Int. Immunol.* **1,** 526–531.
69. Galy, A. H., Spits, H., and Hamilton, J. A. (1993) Regulation of M-CSF production by cultured human thymic epithelial cells. *Lymphokine Cytokine Res.* **12,** 265–270.
70. Le, P. T., Lazorick, S., Whichard, L. P., Yang, Y. C., Clark, S. C., Haynes, B. F., and Singer, K. H. (1990) Human thymic epithelial cells produce IL-6, granulocyte-monocyte-CSF, and leukemia inhibitory factor. *J. Immunol.* **145,** 3310–3315.
71. DeLuca, D. and Mizel, S. B. (1986) I-A-positive nonlymphoid cells and T cell development in murine fetal thymus organ cultures: interleukin 1 circumvents the block in T cell differentiation induced by monoclonal anti-I-A antibodies. *J. Immunol.* **137,** 1435–1441.
72. Nakano, N., Kikutani, H., and Kishimoto, T. (1990) Differential effects of IL-2 and IL-6 on the development of three distinct precursor T-cell populations in the thymus. *Dev. Immunol.* **1,** 77–84.
73. Peault, B., Khazaal, I., and Weissman, I. L. (1994) In vitro development of B cells and macrophages from early mouse fetal thymocytes. *Eur. J. Immunol.* **24,** 781–784.
74. Samaridis, J., Casorati, G., Traunecker, A., Iglesias, A., Gutierrez, J. C., Muller, U., and Palacios, R. (1991) Development of lymphocytes in interleukin 7-transgenic mice. *Eur. J. Immunol.* **21,** 453–460.
75. Carding, S. R., and Tannishtha. (1994) Cytokines in the fetal thymus, in *Intrathymic T-Cell Development,* (Nikolić-Žugić, J., ed.), R. G. Landes Company, Austin, TX, p. 46–63.
76. Haynes, B. F. (1990) Human thymic epithelium and T cell development: current issues and future directions. *Thymus* **16,** 143–157.
77. Broxmeyer, H. E., Williams, D. E., Lu, L., Cooper, S., Anderson, S. L., Beyer, G. S., Hoffman, R., and Rubin, B. Y. (1986) The suppressive influences of human tumor necrosis factors on bone

marrow hematopoietic progenitor cells from normal donors and patients with leukemia: synergism of tumor necrosis factor and interferon-gamma. *J. Immunol.* **136,** 4487–4495.
78. Rigby, W. F. C., Ball, E. D., Guyre, P. M., and Fanger, M. W. (1985) The effects of recombinant DNA-derived interferons on the growth of myeloid progenitor cells. *Blood* **65,** 858–861.
79. Zoumbos, N. C., Djeu, J. Y., and Young, N. S. (1984) Interferon is the suppressor of hematopoiesis generated by stimulated lymphocytes in vitro. *J. Immunol.* **133,** 769–774.
80. Jacobsen, S. E., Ruscetti, F. W., Dubois, C. M., and Keller, J. R. (1992) Tumor necrosis factor alpha directly and indirectly regulates hematopoietic progenitor cell proliferation: role of colony-stimulating factor receptor modulation. *J. Exp. Med.* **175,** 1759–1772.
81. Murphy, M., Perussia, B., and Trinchieri, G. (1988) Effects of recombinant tumor necrosis factor, lymphotoxin, and immune interferon on proliferation and differentiation of enriched hematopoietic precursor cells. *Exp. Hematol.* **16,** 131–138.
82. Peetre, C., Gullberg, U., Nilsson, E., and Olsson, I. (1986) Effects of recombinant tumor necrosis factor on proliferation and differentiation of leukemic and normal hemopoietic cells in vitro: Relationship to cell surface receptor. *J. Clin. Invest.* **78,** 1694–1700.
83. Roodman, G. D., Bird, A., Hutzler, D., and Montgomery, W. (1987) Tumor necrosis factor-alpha and hematopoietic progenitors: Effects of tumor necrosis factor on the growth of erythroid progenitors CFU-E and BFU-E and the hematopoietic cell lines K562, HL60 and HEL cells. *Exp. Hematol.* **15,** 928–935.
84. Broxmeyer, H. E., Sherry, B., Lu, L., Cooper, S., Carow, C., Wolpe, S. D., and Cerami, A. (1989) Myelopoietic enhancing effects of murine macrophage inflammatory proteins 1 and 2 on colony formation in vitro by murine and human bone marrow granulocyte/macrophage progenitor cells. *J. Exp. Med.* **170,** 1583–1594.
85. Broxmeyer, H. E., Sherry, B., Lu, L., Cooper, S., Oh, K.-O., Tekamp-Olson, P., Kwon, B. S., and Cerami, A. (1990) Enhancing and suppressing effects of recombinant murine macrophage inflammatory proteins on colony formation in vitro by bone marrow myeloid progenitor cells. *Blood* **76,** 1110–1116.
86. Graham, G. J., Wright, E. G., Hewick, R., Wolpe, S. D., Wilkie, N. M., Donaldson, D., Lorimore, S., and Pragnell, I. B. (1990) Identification and characterization of an inhibitor of haemopoietic stem cell proliferation. *Nature* **344,** 442–444.
87. Maze, R., Sherry, B., Kwon, B. S., Cerami, A., and Broxmeyer, H. E. (1992) Myelosuppressive effects in vivo of purified recombinant murine macrophage inflammatory protein-1 alpha. *J. Immunol.* **149,** 1004–1009.
88. Eaves, C. J., Cashman, J. D., Kay, R. J., Dougherty, G. J., Otsuka, T., Gaboury, L. A., Hogge, D. E., Lansdorp, P. M., Eaves, A. C., and Humphries, R. K. (1991) Mechanisms that regulate the cell cycle status of very primitive hematopoietic cells in long-term human marrow cultures. II. Analysis of positive and negative regulators produced by stromal cells within the adherent layer. *Blood* **78,** 110–117.
89. Hatzfeld, J., Li, M. L., Brown, E. L., Sookdeo, H., Levesque, J. P., O'Toole, T., Gurney, C., Clark, S. C., and Hatzfeld, A. (1991) Release of early human hematopoietic progenitors from quiescence by antisense transforming growth factor beta 1 or Rb oligonucleotides. *J. Exp. Med* **174,** 925–929.
90. Morgan, D. A., Ruscetti, F. W., and Gallo, R. (1976) Selective in vitro growth of T lymphocytes from normal human bone marrows. *Science* **193,** 1007–1008.
91. Taniguchi, T., Matsui, H., Fujita, T., Takaoka, C., Kashima, N., Yoshimoto, R., and J. Hamuro. (1983) Structure and expression of a cloned cDNA for human interleukin-2. *Nature* **302,** 305–310.
92. Carding, S. R., Hayday, A. C., and Bottomly, K. (1991) Cytokines in T cell development. *Immunol. Today* **12,** 239–245.
93. Chen, J., Ma, A., Young, F., and Alt, F. (1994) IL2 receptor alpha chain expression during early B lymphocyte differentiation. *Int. Immunol.* **6,** 1265–1268.
94. Rolink, A., Grawunder, U., Winkler, T. H., Karasuyama, H., and Melchers, F. (1994) IL-2 receptor α chain (CD25, TAC) expression defines a crucial stage in pre-B cell development. *Int. Immunol.* **6,** 1257–1264.
95. Reya, T., Bassiri, H., Biancaniello, R., and Carding, S. R. (1998) Thymic stromal cell abnormalities and dysregulated T cell development in IL2-deficient mice. *Dev. Immunol.* in press.
96. Nakamura, M., Asao, H., Takeshita, T., and Sugamura, K. (1993) Interleukin-2 receptor heterotrimer complex and intracellular signaling. *Sem. Immunol.* **17,** 309–317.
97. Grabstein, K. H., Eisenman, J., Shanebeck, K., Rauch, C., Srinivasan, S., Fung, V., Beers, C., Richardson, J., Schoenborn, M. A., Ahdieh, M., Johnson, L., Alderson, M. R., Watson, J. D.,

Anderson, D. M., and Giri, J. G. (1994) Cloning of a T cell growth factor that interacts with the β chain of the interleukin-2 receptor. *Science* **264,** 965–968.

98. Kondo, M., Ohashi, Y., Tada, K., Nakamura, M., and Sugamura, K. (1994) Expression of the mouse interleukin-2 receptor γ chain in various populations of the thymus and spleen. *Eur. J. Immunol.* **24,** 2026–2030.
99. Russell, S. M., Keegan, A. D., Harada, N., Nakamura, Y., Noguchi, M., Leland, P., Friedmann, M. C., Miyajima, A., Puri, R. K., Paul, W. E., and Leonard, W. J. (1993) Interleukin-2 receptor γ chain: A functional component of the interleukin-4 receptor. *Science* **262,** 1880–1883.
100. Kondo, M., Takeshita, T., Higuchi, M., Nakamura, M., Sudo, T., Nishikawa, S., and Sugamura, K. (1994) Functional participation of the IL-2 receptor gamma chain in IL-7 receptor complexes. *Science* **263,** 1453–1454.
101. Noguchi, M., Nakamura, Y., Russell, S. M., Ziegler, S. F., Tsang, M., Cao, X., and Leonard, W. J. (1993) Interleukin-2 receptor γ chain: a functional component of the interleukin-7 receptor. *Science* **262,** 1877–1880.
102. Russell, S. M., Johnston, J. A., Noguchi, M., Kawamura, M., Bacon, C. M., Friedmann, M., Berg, M., McVicar, D. W., Witthuhn, B. A., Silvennoinen, O., Goldman, A. S., Schmalstieg, F. C., Ihle, J. N., O'Shea, J. J., and Leonard, W. J. (1994) Interaction of IL-2Rβ and γc chains with Jak1 and Jak3: implications for XSCID and XCID. *Science* **266,** 1042–1045.
103. Giri, J. G., Ahdieh, M., Eisenman, J., Shanebeck, K., Grabstein, K., Kumaki, S., Namen, A., Park, L. S., Cosman, D., and Anderson, D. (1994) Utilization of the β and γ chains of the IL-2 receptor by the novel cytokine IL-15. *EMBO J.* **13,** 2822–2830.
104. Siegel, J. P., Sharon, M., Smith, P. L., and Leonard, W. L. (1987) The IL-2 receptor β chain (p70): role in mediating signals for LAK, NK, and proliferative activities. *Science* **238,** 75–78.
105. Tsudo, M., Goldman, C. K., Bongiovanni, K. F., Chan, W. C., Winton, E. F., Yagita, M., Grimm, E. A., and Waldmann, T. A. (1987) The p75 peptide is the receptor for interleukin 2 expressed on large granular lymphocytes and is responsible for interleukin 2 activation of these cells. *Proc. Natl. Acad. Sci. USA* **84,** 5394–5398.
106. Arima, N., Kamio, M., Imada, K., Hori, T., Hattori, T., Tsudo, M., Okuma, M., and Uchiyama, T. (1992) Pseudo-high affinity interleukin 2 (IL-2) receptor lacks the third component that is essential for functional IL-2 binding and signaling. *J. Exp. Med.* **176,** 1265–1272.
107. Asao, H., Takeshita, T., Ishii, N., Kumaki, S., Nakamura, M., and Sugamura, K. (1993) Reconstitution of functional interleukin 2 receptor complexes on fibroblastoid cells: involvement of the cytoplasmic domain of the gamma chain in two distinct signaling pathways. *Proc. Natl. Acad. Sci. USA* **90,** 4127–4131.
108. Taniguchi, T. and Minami, Y. (1993) The IL-2/IL-2 receptor system: a current overview. *Cell* **73,** 5–8.
109. Voss, S. D., Leary, T. P., Sondel, P. M., and Robb, R. J. (1993) Identification of a direct interaction between interleukin 2 and the p64 interleukin 2 receptor gamma chain. *Proc. Natl. Acad. Sci. USA* **90,** 2428–2432.
110. Zurawski, S. M., Imler, J.-L., and Zurawski, G. (1990) Partial agonist/antagonist mouse interleukin-2 proteins indicate that a third component of the receptor complex functions in signal transduction. *EMBO J.* **9,** 3899–3905
111. Imler, J.-L. and Zurawski, G. (1992) Receptor binding and internaliation of mouse interleukin-2 derivatives that are partial agonists. *J. Biol. Chem.* **267,** 13,185–13,190.
112. Takeshita, T., Asao, H., Ohtani, K., Ishii, N., Kumaki, S., Tanaka, N., Munakata, H., Nakamura, M., and Sugamura, K. (1992) Cloning of the γ chain of the human IL-2 receptor. *Science* **257,** 379–382.
113. Nakamura, Y., Russell, S. M., Mess, S. A., Friedmann, M., Erdos, M., Francois, C., Jacques, Y., Adelstein, S., and Leonard, W. J. (1994) Heterodimerization of the IL2 receptor β- and γ-chain cytoplasmic domains is required for signalling. *Nature* **369,** 330–333.
114. Nelson, B. H., Lord, J. D., and Greenberg, P. D. (1994) Cytoplasmic domains of the of interleukin 2 receptor β and γ chains mediate the signal for T-cell proliferation. *Nature* **369,** 333–336.
115. Plaisance, S., Rubenstein, E., Alileche, A., Benoit, P., Jasmin, C., and Azzarone, B. (1993) The IL2 receptor present on human embryonic fibroblasts is functional in the absence of P64/IL2Rγ chain. *Int. Immunol.* **5,** 843–848.
116. Hatakeyama, M., Kono, T., Kobayashi, N., Kawahara, A., Levin, S. D., Perlmutter, R. M., and Taniguchi, T. (1991) Interaction of the IL-2 receptor with the *src*-family kinase $p56^{lck}$: identification of novel intermolecular association. *Science* **252,** 1523–1528.
117. Greene, W. C. and Leonard, W. J. (1986) The human interleukin-2 receptor. *Ann. Rev. Immunol.* **4,** 69–95.

118. De la Hera, A., Toribio, M. L., Marquez, C., Marcos, M. A., Cabrero, E., and Martinez-A, C. (1986) Differentiation of human mature thymocytes: existence of a T3+4-8– intermediate stage. *Eur. J. Immunol.* **16,** 653–658.
119. Raulet, D. H. (1985) Expression and function of interleukin-2 receptors on immature thymocytes. *Nature* **314,** 101–103.
120. Toribio, M. L., De la Hera, A., Marcos, M. A., Marquez, C., and Martinez-A, C. (1989) Activation of the interleukin 2 pathway precedes CD3-T cell receptor expression in thymic development. Differential growth requirements of early and mature intrathymic subpopulations. *Eur. J. Immunol.* **19,** 9–15.
121. Tanaka, T., Takeuchi, Y., Shiohara, T., Kitamura, F., Nagasaka, Y., Hamamura, K., Yagita, H., and Miyasaka, M. (1992) *In utero* treatment with monoclonal antibody to IL-2 receptor β-chain completely abrogates development of Thy-1+ dendritic epidermal cells. *Int. Immunol.* **4,** 487–491.
122. Skinner, M., Le Gros, G., Marbrook, J., and Watson, J. D. (1987) Development of fetal thymocytes in organ cultures: Effect of interleukin 2. *J. Exp. Med.* **165,** 1481–1493.
123. Waanders, G. A. and Boyd, R. L. (1990) The effects of interleukin 2 on early and late thymocyte differentiation in foetal thymus organ culture. *Int. Immunol.* **2,** 461–468.
124. Waanders, G. A., Godfrey, D. I., and Boyd, R. L. (1989) Modulation of T-cell differentiation in murine fetal thymus organ cultures. *Thymus* **13,** 73–82.
125. Habu, S., Okumura, K., Diamantstein, T., and Shevach, E. (1985) Expression of interleukin 2 receptor on murine fetal thymocytes. *Eur. J. Immunol.* **15,** 456–460.
126. von Boehmer, H., Crisanti, A., Kisielow, P., and Haas, W. (1985) Absence of growth by most receptor-expressing fetal thymocytes in the presence of interleukin-2. *Nature* **314,** 539–540.
127. Jenkinson, E. J., Kingston, R., and Owen, J. J. T. (1987) Importance of IL-2 receptors in intrathymic generation of cells expressing T-cell receptors. *Nature* **329,** 160–162.
128. Plum, J., and de Smedt, M. (1988) Differentiation of thymocytes in fetal organ culture: lack of evidence for the functional role of the interleukin 2 receptor expressed by prothymocytes. *Eur. J. Immunol.* **18,** 795–799.
129. Tentori, L., Longo, D. L., Zúñiga-Pflücker, J. C., Wing, C., and Kruisbeek, A. M. (1988) Essential role of the interleukin 2- interleukin 2 receptor pathway in thymocyte maturation in vivo. *J. Exp. Med.* **168,** 1741–1747.
130. Zúñiga-Pflücker, J. C. and Kruisbeek, A. M. (1990) Intrathymic radioresistant stem cells follow an IL-2/IL-2R pathway during thymic regeneration after sublethal irradiation. *J. Immunol.* **144,** 3736–3740.
131. Gutierrez-Ramos, J. C., Martinez, A. C., and Kohler, G. (1990) Analysis of T cell subpopulation in human IL-2R-alpha transgenic mice: expansion of Thy.1.2- thymocytes and depletion of double-positive T cell precursors. *Immunol. Res.* **140,** 661–674.
132. Nishi, M., Ishida, Y., and Honjo, T. (1988) Expression of functional interleukin-2 receptors in human light chain/Tac transgenic mice. *Nature* **331,** 267–269.
133. Schorle, H., Holtschke, T., Hunig, T., Schimpl, A., and Horak, I. (1991) Development and function of T cells in mice rendered interleukin-2 deficient by gene targeting. *Nature* **352,** 621–624.
134. Horak, I., Löhler, J., Ma, A., and Smith, K. A. (1995) Interleukin-2 deficient mice: a new model to study autoimmunity and self-tolerance. *Immunol. Rev.* **148,** 35–43.
135. Sadlack, B., Merz, H., Schorle, H., Schimpl, A., Feller, A. C., and Horak, I. (1993) Ulcerative colitis-like disease in mice with a disrupted interleukin-2 gene. *Cell* **75,** 253–261.
136. Krämer, S., Schimpl, A., and Hunig, T. (1995) Immunopathology of interleukin (IL) 2-deficient mice: thymus dependence and supression by thymus-depedent cells with and intact IL-2 gene. *J. Exp. Med.* **182,** 1769–1776.
137. Hanke, T., Mitnacht, R., Boyd, R., and Hünig, T. (1994) Induction of interleukin-2 receptor β-chain expression by self-recognition in the thymus. *J. Exp. Med.* **180,** 1629–1636.
138. Lúdvíksson, B. R., Gray, B., Strober, W., and Ehrhardt, R. O. (1997) Dysregulated intrathymic development in the IL2-deficient mouse leads to colitis-inducing thymocytes. *J. Immunol.* **158,** 104–111.
139. Rocha, B., Lehuen, A., and Papiernik, M. (1988) IL2–dependent proliferation of thymic accessory cells. *J. Immunol.* **140,** 1076–1080.
140. Contractor, N. V., Bassiri, H., Reya, T., Park, A. Y., Baumgart, D. C., Wasik, M., Emerson, S. G., and Carding, S. R. (1998) Lymphoid hyperplasia, autoimmunity and compromised intestinal intraepithelial lymphocyte development in colitis-free gnotobiotic Interleukin 2-deficient mice. *J. Immunol.* **160,** 385–394.

141. Murphy, K., Heimberger, A., and Loh, D. (1990) Induction by antigen of intrathymic apoptosis of CD4+CD8+TCRlo thymocytes in vivo. *Science* **250,** 1720–1723.
142. Kneitz, B., Herrmann, T., Yonehara, S., and Schimpl, A. (1995) Normal clonal expansion but impaired Fas-mediated cell death and anergy induction in interleukin-2-deficient mice. *Eur. J. Immunol.* **25,** 2572–2577.
143. Sadlack, B., Löhler, J., Schorle, H., Klebb, G., Haber, H., Sickel, E., Noelle, R. J., and Horak, I. (1995) Generalized autoimmune disease in interleukin-2-deficient mice is triggered by an uncontrolled activation and proliferation of CD4+ T cells. *Eur. J. Immunol.* **25,** 3053–3059.
144. Willerford, D. M., Chen, J., Ferry, J. A., Davidson, L., Ma, A., and Alt, F. W. (1995) Interleukin-2 receptor α chain regulates the size and content of the peripheral lymphoid compartment. *Immunity* **3,** 521–530.
145. Suzuki, H., Kundig, T. M., Furlonger, C., Wakeman, A., Timms, E., Matsuyama, T., Schmits, R., Simard, J. J. L., Ohashi, P., Griesser, H., Taniguchi, T., Paige, C. J., and Mak, T. W. (1995) Deregulated T cell activation and autoimmunity in mice lacking interleukin-2 receptor β. *Science* **268,** 1472–1476.
146. Krämer, S., Mamalaki, C., Horak, I., Schimpl, A., Kioussis, D., and Hünig, T. (1994) Thymic selection and peptide-induced activation of T cell receptor-transgenic CD8 T cells in interleukin-2-deficient mice. *Eur. J. Immunol.* **24,** 2317–2322.
147. Turner, M., Mee, P. J., Costello, P. S., Williams, O., Price, A. A., Duddy, L. P., Furlong, M. T., Geahlen, R. L., and Tybulewicz, V. L. (1995) Perinatal lethality and blocked B-cell development in mice lacking the tyrosine kinase Syk. *Nature* **378,** 298–302.
148. Cao, X., Shores, E. W., Hu-Li, J., Anver, M. R., Kelsall, B. L., Russell, S. M., Drago, J., Noguchi, M., Grinberg, A., Bloom, E. T., Paul, W. E., Katz, S. I., Love, P. E., and Leonard, W. J. (1995) Defective lymphoid development in mice lacking expression of the common cytokine receptor γ chain. *Immunity* **2,** 223–238.
149. DiSanto, J. P., Müller, W., D. Guy-Grand, Fischer, A., and Rajewsky, K. (1995) Lymphoid development in mice with a targeted deletion of the interleukin 2 receptor γ chain. *Proc. Natl. Acad. Sci. USA* **92,** 377–381.
150. Suzuki, H., Duncan, G., Takimoto, H., and Mak, T. W. (1997) Abnormal development of intestinal intraepithelial lymphocytes and peripheral natural killer cells in mice lacking the IL2-receptor β chain. *J. Exp. Med.* **185,** 499–505.
151. Jung, L. K. L., Hara, T., and Fu, S. M. (1984) Detection and functional studies of p60–65 (Tac antigen) on activated human B cells. *J. Exp. Med.* **160,** 1597–1565.
152. Longo, D., L., Gelman, E., P., Cossman, J., Young, R., A., Gallo, R. C., O'Brien, S., and Matis, L. A. (1984) Isolation of HTLV-transformed B-lymphocyte clone from a patient with HTLV-associated adult T cell leukemia. *Nature* **310,** 505–506.
153. Muraguchi, A., Kehri, J. H., Longo, D. L., Volkman, D. J., Smith, K. A., and Fauci, A. S. (1985) Interleukin 2 receptors on human B cells: implications for the role of interleukin 2 in human B cell function. *J. Exp. Med.* **161,** 181–197.
154. Robb, R. J. (1984) Interleukin-2: The molecule and its function. *Immunology Today* **5,** 203–206.
155. Jianzhu, C., Ma, A., Young, F., and Alt, F. (1994) IL-2 receptor α chain expression during early B lymphocyte differentiation. *Int. Immunol.* **6,** 1265–1268.
156. Reya, T., Yang-Snyder, J. A., Rothenberg, E. V., and Carding, S. R. (1996) Regulated expression and function of CD122 (Interleukin-2/Interleukin-15R-β) during lymphoid development. *Blood* **87,** 190–201.
157. Horton, J. and Ratcliffe, N. (1996) Evolution of immunity, in *Immunology,* (Roitt, I., Brostoff, J., and Male, D., eds.), Mosby, London, p. 15.1–15.22.
158. Gambacorti-Passerini, C., Hank, J. A., Borchert, A., Moore, K., Malkovska, V., and Sondel, P. (1991) In vivo effects of multiple cycles of recombinant interleukin-2 (IL2) on peripheral granulocyte-macrophage hematopoietic progenitors circulating in the blood of cancer patients. *Tumori* **77,** 420–422.
159. Schaafsma, M. R., Fibbe, W. E., Van Der Harst, D., Duinkerken, N., Brand, A., Osanto, S., Franks, C. R., Willemze, R., and Falkenberg, J. H. F. (1990) Increased numbers of circulating haematopoietic progenitor cells after treatment with high-dose interleukin-2 in cancer patients. *Brit. J. Haematol.* **76,** 180–185.
160. Tritarelli, E., Rocca, E., Testa, U., Boccoli, G., Camagna, A., Calabresi, F., and Peschle, C. (1991) Adoptive immunotherapy with high-dose interleukin-2: kinetics of circulating progenitors correlates with interleukin-6, granulocyte colony stimulating factor level. *Blood* **77,** 741–749.

161. Michalevicz, R., Campana, D., Katz, F. E., Janossy, G., and Hoffbrand, A. V. (1988) Recombinant interleukin 2 and anti-Tac influence the growth of enriched multipotent hemopoietic progenitors: proposed hypothesis for different responses in early and late progenitors. *Leukemia Res.* **12,** 113–121.
162. Baccarini, M., Schwinger, M., and Lohmann-Matthes, M.-L. (1989) Effect of human recombinant IL2 on murine macrophage precursors. *J. Immunol* **142,** 118–125.
163. Reya, T., Contractor, N. V., Couzens, M. C., Wasik, M. A., Emerson, S. G., and Carding, S. R. (1998) Abnormal myelocytic cell development in interleukin-2 (IL2) deficient mice: evidence for the involvement of IL2 in myelopoiesis. *Blood* **91,** 1–14.
164. Pericle, F., Liu, J. H., Diaz, J. I., Blanchard, D. K., Wei, S., Forni, G., and Djeu, J. Y. (1994) Interleukin-2 prevention of apoptosis in human neutrophils. *Eur. J. Immunol.* **24,** 440–444.
165. Weinberg, K. P. R. (1990) Severe combined immunodeficiency due to a specific defect in the production of interleukin-2. *N. Engl. J. Med.* **322,** 1718–1723.
166. Ye, J., Ortaldo, J. R., Conlon, K., R. Winkler-Pickett, and Young, H. A. (1995) Cellular and molecular mechanisms of IFN-gamma production induced by IL-2 and IL-12 in a human NK cell line. *J. Leuk. Biol.* **58,** 225–233.
167. Estrov, Z., Roifman, C., Wang, Y. P., Grunberger, T., Gelfand, E. W., and Freedman, M. H. (1986) The regulatory role of interleukin 2-responsive T lymphocytes on early and mature erythroid progenitor proliferation. *Blood* **67,** 1607–1610.
168. Skettino, S., Phillips, J., Camer, L., Nagler, A., and Greenberg, P. (1988) Selective generation of erythroid burst-promoting activity by recombinant human interleukin 2-stimulated human T lymphocytes. *Blood* **71,** 907–914.
169. Quinones, R. R. (1993) Hematopoietic engraftment and graft failure after bone marrow transplantation. *Am. J. Pediat. Hematol-Oncol.* **15,** 3–17.
170. Garland, J. M. and Dexter, T. M. (1982) Expression of 20-alpha hydroxysteroid dehydrogenase in murine long-term bone marrow cultures. *Eur. J. Immunol.* **12,** 998–1001.
171. Burdach, S. and Levitt, L. (1987) Receptor-specific inhibition of bone marrow erythropoiesis by reconbinant DNA-derived interleukin-2. *Blood* **69,** 1368–1375.
172. Frassoni, F., Bacigalupo, A., Podesta, M., van Lint, M. T., Piaggio, G., and Marmont, A. (1982) Generation of CFU-C suppressor T cells in vitro. III. Failure of mitogen-primed T cells from patients with chronic granulocytic leukemia to inhibit the growth of normal CFU-C. *Blood* **60,** 1447–1452.
173. Kerndrup, G. and Hokland, P. (1988) Natural killer cell-mediated inhibition of bone marrow colony formation (CFU-GM) in refractory anaemia (preleukaemia): evidence for patient-specific cell populations. *Br. J. Haematol.* **69,** 457–462.
174. Bacigalupo, A., Podesta, M., Mingari, M., Moretta, L., Van Lint, M., and Marmont, A. (1980) Immune suppression of hematopoiesis in aplastic anemia: activity of T-gamma lymphocytes. *J. Immunol.* **125,** 1449–1453.
175. Zoumbos, N. C., Gascon, P., Djeu, J. Y., and Young, N. S. (1985) Interferon is a mediator of hematopoietic suppression in aplastic anemia in vitro and possibly in vivo. *Proc. Natl. Acad. Sci. USA* **82,** 188–192.
176. Rennick, D., Yang, G., Muller-Sieburg, C., Smith, C., Arai, N., Takabe, Y., and l. Gemmel, L. (1987) Interleukin 4 (B-cell stimulatory factor 1) can enhance or antagonize the factor-dependent growth of hemopoietic progenitor cells. *Proc. Natl. Acad. Sci. USA* **84,** 6889–6893.
177. Wang, J., Lin, Q., Langston, H., and Cooper, M. (1995) Resident bone marrow macrophages produce Type 1 interferons that can selectively inhibit interleukin-7-driven growth of B lineage cells. *Immunity* **3,** 475–484.
178. Selleri, C., Sato, T., Anderson, S., Young, N. S., and Maciejewski, J. P. (1995) Interferon-gamma and tumor necrosis factor-alpha suppress both early and late stages of hematopoiesis and induce programmed cell death. *J. Cell. Physiol.* **165,** 538–546.
179. Maciejewski, J. P., Weichold, F. F., and Young, N. S. (1994) HIV-1 suppression of hematopoiesis in vitro mediated by envelope glycoprotein and TNF-alpha. *J. Immunol.* **153,** 4303–4310.
180. Ma, A., Datta, M., Margosian, E., Chen, J., and Horak, I. (1995) T cell, but not B cells are required for bowel inflammation in interleukin-2 deficient mice. *J. Exp. Med.* **182,** 1567–1572.
181. Westen, H. and Bainton, D. F. (1979) Association of alkaline-phosphatase-positive reticulum cells in bone marrow with granulocytic precursors. *J. Exp. Med.* **150,** 919–937.
182. Plaisance, S., Rubenstein, E., Alileche, A., Krief, P., Augery-Bourget, Y., Sahraoui, Y., Jasmin, C., Suarez, C., and Azzarone, B. (1992) Expression of interleukin-2 receptor on human fibroblasts and its biological significance. *Int. Immunol.* **4,** 739–746.

183. Gong, J. K. (1978) Endostial marrow: a rich source of hematopoietic stem cells. *Science* **199,** 1443–1445.
184. Lord, B. I. and Hendry, H. H. (1972) The distribution of haemopoietic colony-forming units in the mouse femur and its modification by X-rays. *Br. J. Radiol.* **45,** 110–115.
185. Chan, S. H. and Metcalf, D. (1972) Local production of colony-stimulating factor within the bone marrow: role of nonhematopoietic cells. *Blood* **40,** 646–649.
186. Feyen, J. H., Elford, P., Di Padova, F. E., and Trechsel, U. (1989) Interleukin-6 is produced by bone and modulated by parathyroid hormone. *J. Bone Min. Res.* **4,** 633–638.
187. Horowitz, M. C., Coleman, D. L., Flood, P. M., Kupper, T. S., and Jilka, R. L. (1989) Parathyroid hormone and lipopolysaccharide induce murine osteoblast-like cells to secrete a cytokine indistinguishable from granulocyte-macrophage colony-stimulating factor. *J. Clin. Invest.* **83,** 149–157.
188. Horowitz, M. C., Coleman, D. L., Ryaby, J. T., and Einhorn, T. A. (1989) Osteotropic agents induce the differential secretion of granulocyte-macrophage colony-stimulating factor by the osteoblast cell line MC3T3-E1. *J. Bone Min. Res.* **4,** 911–921.
189. Lowik, C. W., van der Pluijm, G., Bloys, H., Hoekman, K., Bijvoet, O. L., Aarden, L. A., and Papapoulos, S. E. (1989) Parathyroid hormone (PTH) and PTH-like protein (PLP) stimulate interleukin-6 production by osteogenic cells: a possible role of interleukin-6 in osteoclastogenesis. *Biochem. Biophys. Res. Comm.* **162,** 1546–1552.
190. Benayahu, D., Horowitz, M., Zipori, D., and Wientroub, S. (1992) Hemopoietic functions of marrow-derived osteogenic cells. *Calcified Tissue Int.* **51,** 195–201.
191. Taichman, R. S. and Emerson, S. G. (1994) Human osteoblasts support hematopoiesis through the production of granulocyte colony-stimulating factor. *J. Exp. Med.* **179,** 1677–1682.
192. Taichman, R. S., Reilly, M. J., and Emerson, S. G. (1996) Human osteoblasts support human hematopoietic progenitor cells in in vitro bone marrow cultures. *Blood* **87,** 518–524.
193. Friedenstein, A. J., Chailakhjan, R. K., and Lalykina, K. S. (1970) The development of fibroblast colonies in monolayer cultures of guinea-pig bone marrow and spleen cells. *Cell Tissue Kinet.* **3,** 393–403.
194. Friedenstein, A. J., Deriglasova, U. F., Kulagina, N. N., Panasuk, A. F., Rudakowa, S. F., Luria, E. A., and Ruadkow, I. A. (1974) Precursors for fibroblasts in different populations of hematopoietic cells as detected by the in vitro colony assay method. *Exp. Hematol.* **2,** 83–92.
195. Friedenstein, A. J. (1976) Precursor cells of mechanocytes. *Int. Rev. Cytol.* **47,** 327–359.
196. Hagenaars, C. E., van der Kraan, A. A., Kawliarang-de Hass, E. W., Visser, J. W., and Nijweide, P. J. (1989) Osteoclast formation from cloned pluripotent hemopoietic stem cells. *Bone Miner.* **6,** 179–189.
197. Scheven, B. A. A., Visser, J. W. M., and Nijweide, P. J. (1986) In vitro osteoclast generation from different bone marrow fractions, including a highly enriched haemapoietic stem cell population. *Nature* **321,** 79–81.
198. Jee, W. S. S. and Nolan, P. D. (1963) Origin of osteoclasts from fusion of phagocytes. *Nature* **200,** 225–226.
199. Ikuta, K., Kina, T., MacNeil, I., Uchida, N., Peault, B., Chien, Y. H., and Weissman, I. L. (1990) A developmental switch in thymic lymphocyte maturation potential occurs at the level of hematopoietic stem cells. *Cell* **62,** 863–874.
200. Ikuta, K., Uchida, N., Friedman, J., and Weissman, I. L. (1992) Lymphocyte development from stem cells. *Ann. Rev. Immunol.* **10,** 759–783.
201. Hardy, R. R. and Hayakawa, K. (1991) A developmental switch in B lymphopoiesis. *Proc. Natl. Acad. Sci. USA* **88,** 11,550–11,554.
202. Naito, M. (1993) Macrophage heterogeniety in development and differentiation. *Arch. Histol. Cytol.* **56,** 331–351.
203. Naito, M., Umeda, S., Yamamoto, T., Moriyama, H., Umezu, H., Hasegawa, G., Usuda, H., Shultz, L. D. and Takahashi, K. (1996) Development, differentiation and phenotypic heterogeneity of murine tissue macrophages. *J. Leuk. Biol.* **59,** 133–138.
204. Stamatoyannopoulos, G. and Nienhuis, A. W. (1987) Human hemoglobin switching, in *Molecular Basis of Blood Disease* (Stamatoyannopoulos, G., ed.), Saunders, Philadelphia, p. 66–84.
205. Hayakawa, K., Tarlinton, D., and Hardy, R. R. (1994) Absence of MHC class II expression distinguishes fetal from adult B lymphopoiesis in mice. *J. Immunol.* **152,** 4801–4807.
206. Lam, K.-P., and Stall, A. M. (1994) Major histocompatibility complex class II expression distinguishes two distinct B cell developmental pathways during ontogeny. *J. Exp. Med.* **180,** 507–516.

207. Lansdorp, P. M., Dragowska, W., and Mayani, H. (1993) Ontogeny-related changes in proliferative potential of human hematopoietic cells. *J. Exp. Med.* **178,** 787–791.
208. Moore, M. A. S. and Metcalf, D. (1970) Ontogeny of the haemopoietic system: Yolk sac origin of in vivo and in vitro colony forming cells in the developing mouse embryo. *Br. J. Haematol.* **18,** 279–296.
209. Christensen, R. D. (1988) Developmental changes in pluripotent hematopoietic progenitors. *Early Hum. Dev.* **16,** 195–205.
210. Stein, P. L., Vogel, H., and Soriano, P. (1994) Combined deficiencies of Src, Fyn, and Yes tyrosine kinases in mutant mice. *Genes Dev.* **8,** 1999–2007.
211. Kondo, M., Takeshita, T., Naoto, I., Nakamura, M., Watanabe, S., Arai, K.-I., and Sugamura, K. (1993) Sharing of the interleukin-2 (IL-2) receptor γ chain between receptors for IL-2 and IL-4. *Science* **262,** 1874–1876.
212. Bachmann, M. F., Schorle, H., Kuhn, R., Muller, W., Hengartner, H., Zinkernagel, R. M., and Horak, I. (1995) Antiviral immune responses in mice deficient for both interleukin-2 and interleukin-4. *J. Virol.* **69,** 4842–4846.
213. Sadlack, B., Kuhn, R., Schorle, H., Rajewsky, K., Muller, W., and Horak, I. (1994) Development and proliferation of lymphocytes in mice deficient for both interleukins-2 and -4. *Eur. J. Immunol.* **24,** 281–284.
214. Minasi, L.-A., Kamogawa, Y., Carding, S. R., Bottomly, K., and Flavell, R. A. (1993) Ablation of interleukin-2–producing cells isolated from transgenic mice. *J. Exp. Med.* **177,** 2205–2210.

Chapter 10

Life/Death Decisions in B Lymphocyte Precursors

A Role for Cytokines, Cell Interaction Molecules, and Hormones

Paul W. Kincade, Kay Medina, Glennda Smithson, Zhong Zheng, Kenji Oritani, Lisa Borghesi, Yoshio Yamashita, Kimberly Payne, and Takaichi Shimozato

1. Introduction

The bone marrow and thymus are remarkable factories for blood cells. Although impressively large numbers of cells of various types are produced, the output is carefully controlled. Lymphocytes that emerge from these organs are essential to life, but some are potentially capable of inducing autoimmune disease or malignancy. For that reason, intricate mechanisms have evolved for checking the maturing cells for quality and functional capability. Blood cells of most types can be made in other organs, as is particularly obvious during embryonic life, or when the marrow is ablated. However, this is not the case during normal adult circumstances, and it has long been a goal to determine what is special about central lymphoid tissues. Extraordinary progress has been made in discovering cytokines and cell interaction molecules produced in those sites, and we are beginning to understand how each delivers positive and negative signals for lymphocyte formation. However, additional interesting molecules are still being found, and new roles are being ascribed to previously known ones. The focus of this chapter will be on several classes of molecules expressed within the bone marrow environment. Their study may reveal mechanisms that control the movement of lymphocyte precursors within and from bone marrow, the rate of lymphocyte production, and how defective or potentially harmful cells are eliminated.

2. Cell Surface Correlates of Key Differentiation Events

A wealth of information has accumulated about cell surface markers that can be used to identify and subdivide B lineage populations. These will be extensively discussed

From: *Molecular Biology of B-Cell and T-Cell Development*
Edited by: J. G. Monroe and E. V. Rothenberg © Humana Press Inc., Totowa, NJ

elsewhere in this volume and need only be briefly considered here as a background to the current studies of the marrow microenvironment. Although there is no internationally accepted nomenclature for B-cell precursors, tradition dictates that only cells that express μ heavy chains of immunoglobulin (Ig) without conventional immunoglobulin light chains should be referred to as "pre-B" cells. Less mature cells that are presumably committed to this lineage can be appropriately designated "pro-B." Both categories of cells can be subdivided on the basis of size and/or mitotic activity, as well as expression of surface markers.

Murine B lineage lymphoid cells were originally identified and separated on the basis of CD45R/B220 expression *(1,2)*. Greater resolution of differentiation steps was obtained by staining for the nuclear antigen TdT or cytoplasmic μ chains and, although fixation of the cells was required, this approach had considerable analytical value *(3,4)*. Hardy and colleagues found that subpopulations of viable B-cell precursors could be discriminated by flow cytometry on the basis of surface CD24 density and the expression of CD43 and BP-1 (*5*; also *see* Chapter 14). This extremely important innovation has been widely adopted, but a direct comparison with the intracellular staining classification developed by Osmond has only recently been performed (Lu, Smithson, Kincade, and Osmond, submitted). The authors sorted bone marrow subpopulations according to the Hardy classification and determined that, although the "fractions" generally represent a progression in differentiation, none are homogeneous with respect to either TdT or cytoplasmic μ expression. The most uniform category of cells (fraction "D") is discriminated by small size and lack of surface CD43. A number of investigators have shown that these are virtually all $c\mu^+$ pre-B-cells, but even this population is heterogeneous with respect to the extent to which cells have rearranged immunoglobulin light chain genes (*6–8*; Lu, et al. submitted). Indeed, B-cell precursors can also be subdivided based on Ig gene rearrangement status, expression of pre-B-cell receptors and other markers *(9,10)*.

It has been known for some time that no isoforms of CD45 are completely restricted to cells of the B lineage *(2,11)*. Therefore, development of antibodies to the murine homolog of CD19 was a welcome advance *(12,13)*. This marker appears to be acquired by pro-B-cells at a stage partly corresponding to Hardy's fraction "B" and to be B lymphocyte lineage specific *(14,15)*. CD25 (the IL-2Rα chain) display has been used as one characteristic of pre-B-cells and is not expressed on the surface of B lymphocyte precursors in RAG gene targeted mice *(8,16)*. In the authors' experience, although some B lineage precursors that express CD25 have cytoplasmic μ, not all $c\mu^+$ cells express CD25. Therefore, one must be cautious in using CD25 expression as the sole criterion for enumerating $c\mu^+$ pre-B-cells. CD25 display may be a more useful indicator of rearrangement status/capability than for determining the degree of lineage progression in pro-B populations.

The receptor for stem cell factor, c-kit, can be used to discriminate cells at two stages of differentiation *(17)*. Multipotential stem cells in bone marrow express c-kit at high levels *(18,19)*. The authors have recently found that this receptor is subsequently downregulated in B-cell progenitor populations. A c-kit$^-$ to c-kit^{low} bone marrow population seems to represent an intermediate between stem cells and CD45R$^+$ pro-B-cells. The receptor is expressed at low levels on a minority pro-B-cells and then lost before entry at a stage corresponding to Hardy's fraction "D" (K. Payne manuscript in preparation). In culture, and perhaps also in vivo, stem cell factor can augment B lymphopoiesis (*see* below). B lineage cells that have the c-kit receptor have the highest cloning efficiency on stromal cells *(20)*. However, the authors find that c-kit$^-$ pro-B-cells clone only slightly less efficiently (K. Payne, manuscript in preparation).

There are precursors of NK cells, as well as B-cells, within the CD45R$^+$, CD19$^-$ (Hardy's fraction "A") population, and this category is heterogeneous with respect to AA4.1 antigen expression *(14,15)*. AA4.1 has also been extensively used to enrich stem cells and bi-potential precursors from fetal liver *(21)*. Low level expression of the CD4 antigen has been identified as a characteristic of early precursors with the potential to form B and T lymphocytes, as well as dendritic cells *(22)*. Hardy has recently proposed that the combination of CD4, AA4.1, and CD45R can be used to discriminate the earliest B lineage precursors, and it will be important to learn if any pattern of surface antigen expression correlates with loss of options to generate cells of other types *(14)*.

To summarize, an impressive array of surface markers are available for resolving and sorting murine B lineage precursors. They have been extremely useful for characterizing gene targeted, transgenic, and experimentally manipulated mice. This is especially the case when requirements for growth and differentiation in culture are shown to be distinct for cells with different markers *(5,14,23,24)*. Furthermore, many laboratories have extensively used PCR and direct staining approaches to determine how intracellular events correlate with changes in cell surface phenotype. The resulting information has provided insight into critical checkpoints in differentiation, and the authors' objective is to learn how those events are regulated by signals from the microenvironment in bone marrow.

3. Cytokines and Ectoenzymes that Promote B Lymphocyte Formation

The discovery of interleukin 7 (IL-7) represented a significant advance in understanding B lymphocyte formation, and there is substantial information to suggest that it also has an important role in the thymus. B lineage differentiation is abruptly shut down in mice injected with a neutralizing antibody to IL-7, and development of humoral immunity is blocked by targeting of genes that encode either the α or γ chains of the IL-7 receptor *(25–27)*. The point of arrest in all of these circumstances is at a relatively early pro-B-cell stage (precedes Hardy's fraction "C"). The authors developed a clonal assay for cells that can proliferate solely in the presence of recombinant IL-7 and determined that they were exclusively large in size *(28)*. Cells that developed within the colonies were almost exclusively cytoplasmic μ positive pre-B-cells. More recently, it was found that most of the clonable cells have surface characteristics of fractions "B and C" and lack CD25 (*29*; also *see* Smithson, manuscript in preparation). CD25 display normally corresponds to successful rearrangement of μ heavy chains *(8,16)*. Therefore, precursors that are poised to expand primarily under the influence of this cytokine may not yet have initiated CD25 synthesis. A much larger number of cells can thrive in the presence of IL-7 if stromal cells and their products are also available *(5,30)*. The authors recently modified their cloning assay by inclusion of an adherent stromal cell underlayer, with an additional agar spacer layer to block direct stromal cell-lymphocyte interactions (G. Smithson, manuscript in preparation). Diffusible products from the stromal layer increased the cloning efficiency of lymphocyte precursors as much as ninefold. Interestingly, B-cell precursors from mutant SCID mice were IL-7 responsive in this circumstance, but marrow cells from RAG or λ5 gene targeted mice were not. Although IL-7 is clearly a survival and proliferation factor, recent mutation studies indicate that it may have an additional distinct role in promoting early differentiation events *(31)*.

It is interesting that B lineage differentiation proceeds to a later stage (Hardy's fraction "C") and is less compromised in mice whose IL-7 gene has been targeted than in IL-7R knock out mice *(25,27,32)*. One explanation might be that there is compensatory expression of a cytokine with overlapping functions that shares the same receptor. Farr and colleagues described a product of a unique thymic stromal cell line, which was subsequently cloned and designated thymic stromal-derived lymphopoietin (TSLP) *(33,34)*. The available information suggests that normal murine B lineage precursors are responsive to TSLP in culture, and it will be important to learn if this is an essential stimulus. Another cytokine must also be invoked to explain the expansion of human B lymphocyte precursors. Human, as compared to murine, pre-B-cells are poorly responsive to recombinant IL-7 in culture *(35)*. In addition, formation of pre-B-cells is not impaired in patients that lack the common chain of the IL-7 receptor *(36)*. While it is not a potent growth factor, IL-7 does augment the maturation of early human precursors and induce some differentiation events in culture *(37,38)*.

Though flt ligand (FL) and stem cell factor (SCF) are better known for their effects on hematopoietic progenitors, it appears they may also function as cofactors with other cytokines in promoting differentiation and expansion of pro-B-cells. Each of these cytokines can be produced by stromal cells in either soluble or transmembrane forms and both signal through receptor tyrosine kinases. Interactions between the cytokine/receptor pairs FL/Flk-3 *(39)* and SCF/c-kit *(18,40)* are not absolutely required for production of B-cells. However, both have been shown to synergize with IL-7 in supporting B lymphopoiesis *(41)*. Interactions involving FL/Flk-3 seem to be more critical than those with SCF/c-kit. Disrupting the gene for the Flk-3 receptor resulted in a reduction of pro- and pre-B-cells, however, numbers of more mature B lineage cells was normal *(39)*. Flk-3 is expressed in Hardy's fractions "A" and "B," but is absent from fraction "C" *(42)*. This pattern of expression at an early pro-B stage is consistent with a reported role for a combined IL-7 and FL signal in promoting B-cell commitment and differentiation *(43)*.

Mutations at either the W (encodes c-kit) or Sl (encodes SCF) loci result in macrocytic anemia and abnormalities relating to stem cell expansion *(44)*. These mutations can be simulated by injections of blocking antibodies to c-kit that result in loss of erythroid and myeloid, but not B lineage cells in the bone marrow *(18)*. Consistent with this, fetal liver cells from W/W mutant mice generated B-cells when transferred to RAG targeted mice *(40)*. Much more drastic reductions in pro- and pre-B-cells were seen when Flk-3 deficient mice were crossed with c-kit deficient mice *(39)*. Given the transient expression of c-kit in Hardy's fraction "C" (K. Payne manuscript in preparation), these data suggest that SCF/c-kit interactions, although not essential for B-cell differentiation, can play a role in expansion of cells late in the pro-B compartment. Thus, it appears that FL and SCF have complementary functions and expression patterns. FL and IL-7 function during an early pro-B stage to promote lineage commitment and differentiation, whereas SCF and IL-7 promote expansion of the late pro-B compartment. This is consistent with the dual role for IL-7 in proliferation and differentiation noted above *(31)*.

A number of other substances have been found to augment the growth of murine pre-B-cells, but more study is required to determine their relative importance. There is a single report describing a widely expressed cytokine, pre-B enhancing factor (PBEF), that synergizes with IL-7 plus SCF *(45)*. A unique signal sequence trap strategy was used to discover a cDNA fragment of a stromal cell product that was initially designated SDF-1 *(46)*. The same molecule was isolated in full length form on the basis of its ability to enhance the growth of a stromal cell dependent pre-B-cell clone and renamed PBSF *(47)*. Mice whose pre-B-cell growth stimulatory factor (PBSF) gene has been disrupted die of cardiac defects, but there are also striking abnormalities in lymphohematopoiesis *(48)*. It was speculated that PBSF might be required for migration of hemopoietic cells, and indeed, it is chemotactic for stem cells *(49)*. This chemokine is also the natural ligand for the fusin coreceptor for HIV infection *(50)*.

At least three ecto-enzymes influence the growth of pre-B-cells. BST-1 was initially cloned from human stromal cell lines that significantly supported the growth of the DW34 pre–B-cell clone *(51)*. This ADP-ribosyl cyclase enzyme is attached to the cell membrane via a glycosylphosphatidylinositol linkage. The distribution of BST-1 (also known as BP-3) is different in the mouse, where it is expressed on maturing B lineage precursors, but not stromal cells. Its distribution differs from CD38, another ecto-enzyme with similar activity *(52)*. Aminopeptidase A (BP-1) is expressed on pre-B-cells and some stromal cells in marrow *(53)*. There is evidence to suggest it favors B lymphopoiesis by degrading small peptides derived from nonlymphoid cells *(54)*. Although neutral endopeptidase (CD10) is expressed on both stromal cells and pre-B-cells in humans, it is present on stromal cells and absent from pre-B-cells of mice *(55)*. A role for CD10 in marrow is less clear, but it can degrade peptide hormones, such as the neuropeptide VIP. As discussed below, vasoactive intestinal peptide (VIP) can inhibit B lymphopoiesis *(56)*. Therefore, an appropriate balance of positive and negative regulators may be maintained in the vicinity of B-cell precursors by such ecto-enzymes.

The leptin receptor has recently been shown to be expressed on lympho-hematopoietic cells and may participate in lymphopoiesis *(57,58)*. Reduced numbers of peripheral lymphocytes and B-cell precursors were found in *db/db* mice, which have defective leptin receptors *(57)*. Leptin was shown to synergize with stem cell factor and several other cytokines, including IL-7, in production of lymphocytes in culture. It is produced by stromal cell lines obtained from fetal liver and presumably also by marrow adipocytes.

Interleukin 11 is a stromal cell product that probably promotes survival and expansion of early precursors and stem cells *(59,60)*. It has been effectively used to increase production of B lymphocyte lineage cells in culture from bipotential fetal cells. Interleukin 6 is also capable of interacting in a positive way with stem cells *(60)*. IL-10 has been described as both a stimulus and as an inhibitor for B lymphopoiesis, but it appeared not to have either activity in our culture systems (*61,62* and G. Smithson, unpublished).

4. Cell Interaction Molecules and the Extracellular Matrix

Physical interactions between cells in bone marrow are as critical as those that occur in lymphoid tissues during immune responses. Rare multipotential stem cells are held in protected niches throughout life, and these sites are most likely located in the subendosteal area. A network of venous sinuses runs through the center of bone marrow and represents the point of egress of newly formed cells into the blood stream. Maturing and proliferating precursors migrate between these two extremes, making physical contact with various cell types en route. In the case of B lineage precursors, interactions with one or more types of stromal cells provides access to the critical growth and differentiation factors discussed in Subheading 3. Although macrophages and other phagocytic cells recognize and quickly eliminate apoptotic lymphocytes, they may also release substances that influence lymphopoiesis. Some of these are negative regulators, which will be discussed in Subheading 6. The term "cell adhesion molecules" is commonly used to describe ones that mediate physical attachment, but most of them have additional roles, such as transmission of signals. Several that have been studied with respect to B lymphopoiesis will be discussed here in a larger context as "cell interaction molecules." These not only facilitate communication between cells in bone marrow, but between lympho-hematopoietic cells and a rich extracellular matrix.

It was exciting to find that antibodies to CD44 prevented formation of lymphoid and myeloid cells in long-term bone marrow cultures *(63)*. This was followed soon after by the description of a new cell adhesion mechanism involving CD44 and hyaluronan (HA) *(64)*. Although a wealth of information subsequently accumulated about this receptor/ligand pair, their precise roles in bone marrow remain speculative. The function of many cell interaction molecules, including CD44, is controlled to a remarkable degree following their display on cell surfaces. While a majority of cells in bone marrow and elsewhere express this molecule, very few constitutively use it as a hyaluronan receptor (reviewed in ref. *65*). However, there are circumstances where B lymphocytes become hyaluronan binding cells, and considerable progress has been made in understanding how they differ from other lymphocytes.

Ten of the exons in the CD44 gene can be alternatively spliced, yielding an extraordinary potential for molecular diversity *(65)*. Although it initially appeared that variable mRNA splicing would solely account for whether the molecule could recognize hyaluronan *(66)*, this was found not to be the case. The authors found that multiple CD44 variants have HA binding capability, provided they are expressed in a permissive cell type *(67)*. Also, lymphocytes can convert from a nonbinding to a hyaluronan binding state, without changing the pattern of CD44 mRNA expression *(65)*. The cytoplasmic tail of many cell interaction molecules, including CD44, can have a dramatic influence on the ability of extracellular domains to mediate adhesive functions *(68)*. This opens the possibility that association with cytoskeletal, other intracellular, or transmembrane proteins can reversibly modulate CD44 functions, and there is evidence to support each of these ideas. However, there are also conflicting findings and remaining uncertainty about how intracellular events control extracellular function (commonly termed "inside out signaling") *(69)*.

Hodes and colleagues first noticed that the CD44 expressed on activated B-cells was slightly smaller in size than that on resting cells and attributed this difference to glycosylation *(70)*. Two other labs simultaneously and independently demonstrated that subclones of the same cell line could express CD44 that was functionally and structurally different *(71,72)*. For example, the authors prepared soluble CD44–Ig fusion proteins from CHO cells that do not constitutively recognize hyaluronan. This lack of function (no HA recognition) also characterized the soluble molecule but was restored by treatment with a sialidase *(71)*. More recently, it was found that the degree of terminal sialylation of CD44 expressed by a pair of CHO cell clones differed in correspondence to their ability to recognize hyaluronan *(73)*. In addition, a reduction in glucose concentrations in the tissue culture medium to 25% of the normal level caused nonhyaluronan binding CHO cells to acquire this binding function. The same transformation occurred when the cells were grown as a solid tumor, where it is known that glucose concentrations can be quite low. Thus, the function of this molecule can be modulated to a remarkable degree by the cellular environment, with glucose concentrations being one important variable. These examples primarily involve attachment of carbohydrate to CD44 via asparagine linkages and demonstrate that glycosylation can negatively regulate CD44 function. However, there have also been convincing reports that a minimal degree of glycosylation can be required for proper folding of the molecule and posttranslational modifications involving O-linkages can also influence CD44 function *(73a,74)*.

CD44 is related to a number of molecules that are collectively referred to as hyaladherins, and a structure for one member of this family has recently been solved by molecular modeling and NMR *(75)*. In addition, a number of epitopes recognized by monoclonal antibodies have been localized on the molecule, including ones that enhance or block ligand recognition *(76)*. This information will be very helpful for understanding how particular glycoforms modify binding site conformation. For example, an epitope corresponding to a blocking antibody is located within the predicted binding site for HA, is situated next to a motif for N-linked carbohydrate and is itself influenced by glycosylation. Antibodies are powerful tools for discovering and manipulating the functions of cell interaction molecules. They may also mimic substances encountered in the natural environment.

Although CD44 and other hyaladherins have no primary sequence homology to C-type lectins such as the selectins, strong homology was revealed in terms of the overall structure *(75)*. This important discovery places CD44 within an even broader context of recognition molecules. Gene targeting studies now underway in a number of laboratories should reveal the degree of functional redundancy that exists between them in vivo.

The function of a second pair of molecules in bone marrow is more straightforward. Murine pre-B-cells adhere to stromal cells in culture and it was found that this was primarily mediated by VLA-4 on the former and VCAM-1 on the latter *(77,78)*. Others found that this pair of recognition molecules has an even broader utilization and is also important in human bone marrow *(79,80)*. Although VCAM-1 was originally described as an inducible molecule on inflamed endothelial cells, the authors found that it was constitutively expressed on a subpopulation of stromal cells and endothelial cells within bone marrow *(77,81)*. If these molecules tether lympho-hematopoietic cells in marrow, disruption by antibody treatment might be expected to dislodge them and even mobilize immature cells into the blood stream. Treatment of mice with anti–VCAM-1 weakened the association of stromal cell clusters in marrow, and others reported that treatment with anti–VLA-4 resulted in egress of stem cells in primates *(82,83)*. Additionally, it was reported that short-term migration of transplanted stem cells into bone marrow was diminished by treatment of mice with antibodies to either VLA-4 or VCAM-1 *(84)*. These findings have obvious and important implications for therapy relating to bone marrow. It should also be noted that a variety of inflammatory conditions and transplant rejection have been manipulated by antibodies to VLA-4 or VCAM-1 *(85–88)*. This demonstrates not only the degree to which individual molecules can participate in disparate functions, but also the unexpected nature of applications that can result from basic studies.

One surprising finding has resulted from gene targeting studies and merits comment. Disruption of genes for either the α_4 or β_1 chains of the VLA-4 integrin, or VCAM-1 interferes with implantation and subsequent development of murine embryos *(89–91)*. This is consistent with observations suggesting that recognition between this pair of molecules is critical for multiple embryonic events. However, although the vast majority of these artificial mutations are embryonic lethal, there is a small incidence of survivors in one strain of VCAM-1 targeted mice *(92)*. Such animals appear normal in all respects, but they can transmit the mutant phenotype and abnormalities to offspring. If the conclusion is correct that there is no residual VCAM-1 expression in these exceptional animals, this report raises the important question of compensatory expression of molecules with overlapping function.

The authors developed a new approach to discovery of cell interaction molecules in bone marrow *(93)*. A cDNA library was first prepared from stromal cells and then enriched for sequences containing signal peptides. The logic was that this would facilitate isolation of transcripts corresponding to transmembrane and secreted molecules. A second step then involved expression of pools from the library, as soluble Ig-fusion proteins and individual clones were selected that encoded molecules capable of binding to a stromal cell dependent pre-B-cell clone. Seven molecules were thus identified as stromal cell products that might have counter-receptors on lymphocyte precursors. Most of them would be classified as matrix associated, or matrix interaction molecules, and none of them had previously attracted the authors' attention for other reasons. Biglycan, matrix glycoprotein SC-1, and a novel molecule that the authors' designated stromal interaction molecule (originally SIM1, renamed STIM1) all potentiated the IL-7 dependent proliferation of pre-B-cells when present as soluble Ig-fusion proteins.

One of the stromal cell molecules, syndecan 4, inspired detailed study for other reasons. Monoclonal antibodies to syndecan 4 were prepared with the objective of localizing stromal cells that express it in bone marrow or disrupting some stromal cell functions. However, it was learned that the molecule is also a differentiation marker for B lineage cells and the authors' antibodies preferentially recognize them in marrow cell suspensions. Thus, it is present on two types of cells whose close physical interaction is essential for B-cell formation. The function of this heparan sulfated proteoglycan (HSPG) remains highly speculative, but one possibility is that it serves as a docking site for essential growth and differentiation factors. Interesting candidates include chemokines such as PBSF, hepatocyte growth factor, platelet-derived growth factor, fibroblast growth factor, TGF-β, IL-3, G/M-CSF, γIFN, and IL-7. All of these molecules have been shown to bind to HSPGs, and there would be important implications to their presentation within the vicinity of B-cell precursor expansion. The recognition of pre–B-cells by stromal cell derived STIM1 or syndecan 4-Ig fusion proteins was blocked by heparin *(93)*, and manuscript in preparation. Furthermore, addition of heparin to long term bone marrow cultures blocked formation of lymphoid, but not myeloid cells (Borghesi, Yamashita, and Kincade, manuscript in preparation). It will be interesting to determine if this resulted from interference with cell-cell, cell-matrix, or cell-cytokine interactions, which are normally dependent on HSPG. Similar issues are raised by the discovery that biglycan is a stromal cell product. This matrix component can bind and neutralize TGF-β, a known negative regulator of lympho-hematopoiesis *(28,94,95)*.

5. Hormones as Negative Regulators of Lymphopoiesis

The authors were fortunate to discover that B lymphopoiesis is markedly suppressed during pregnancy in mice *(96)*. This observation was followed by the finding that artificial elevation of sex steroids resulted in preferential reduction in B lymphocyte precursors *(97)*. It is important to note that multiple hormonal and other changes occur during pregnancy, and this situation is not perfectly reproduced by manipulation of estrogen. For example, the distal skeleton of mice undergoes an osteosclerotic reaction in response to estrogen treatment with a resulting decrease in marrow volume. In contrast, numbers of total nucleated cells in marrow are not obviously influenced by pregnancy. It is possible that the rise of estrogen during pregnancy is compensated by changes in other hormones, but the authors have studied only one combination of two sex steroids. Although treatment with progesterone alone was without obvious influence, it made pre-B-cells numbers more sensitive to estrogen. Mechanisms through which the two hormones synergize in this situation need to be explored. The authors will note below an additional difference between responses of B-cell precursors to pregnancy and estrogen treatment. However, subsequent studies directed at understanding mechanisms through which sex steroids influence bone marrow have focused on estrogens and androgen.

This phenomenon would be important within the context of pregnancy alone, but it acquired much greater significance with observations relating to hormonal deficiencies. Hypogonadal (hpg/hpg) mice are defective with respect to sex steroid synthesis and have greatly elevated numbers of B-cell precursors in bone marrow *(98)*. These values were brought within the normal range by estrogen replacement. Castrated male mice also have elevated numbers of pre-B-cells, and additional experiments were performed to assess the relative contribution of male and female sex steroids (*98,99* and Smithson, Couse, Korach, and Kincade, submitted). Male testicular feminization (*tfm/tfm*) mice lack a functional androgen receptor and have similar abnormalities to those in hypogonadal animals. In each of these examples, the populations of B-cell precursors that undergo the greatest change (small $CD43^-$ pre-B-cells) are the same ones that dramatically decline during pregnancy. These results strongly suggest that both androgens and estrogens contribute to normal rates of B lymphocyte formation. The androgen receptor is known to control enzymes important in estrogen synthesis; thus, it is formally possible that this class of hormone works indirectly via estrogen. However, treatment with a nonmetabolizable form of testosterone (DHT) suppressed IL-7 responding B-cell precursors in bone marrow and DHT reduced B-cell precursor expansion in stromal cell cocultures *(29* and unpublished observations). Consequently, testosterone may be sufficient to regulate B-cell production.

Numbers of splenic B-cells were found to be increased approximately twofold in both *hpg/hpg* and *tfm/tfm* mice. This could result from greater output of newly formed lymphocytes from the marrow, but the authors cannot exclude the possibility that sex steroids also influence survival and/or proliferation of mature lymphocytes. It is interesting that the numbers of splenic B-cells do not fall below normal either during pregnancy or when IL-7 is depleted with a neutralizing antibody *(26,96)*. As might be expected, B-cells with immature characteristics ($sIgM^{hi}$,$sIgD^{lo}$,$CD24^{hi}$) disappear from the marrow, peripheral blood, and spleen during pregnancy or following estrogen treatment (unpublished observations).

The authors predicted that B lymphopoiesis would be markedly dysregulated and expanded in mice whose estrogen receptor (ERα) had been targeted. However, no abnormalities were observed in male $ER\alpha^{-/-}$ mice and female $ER\alpha^{-/-}$ mice had slightly reduced numbers of pre-B-cells (Smithson, Couse, Korach, and Kincade, submitted). This initially puzzling result might have several interesting explanations. For example, estrogen might regulate B lymphopoiesis via an estrogen receptor independent mechanism. However, a drug that blocks ER specific functions also interferes with estrogen mediated suppression in vitro *(100* and Smithson, Couse, Lorach, and Kincade, submitted). Another possibility is that there is a compensatory regulation of B lymphopoiesis by androgens in $ER\alpha^{-/-}$ mice. Androgen levels are normal in male, but elevated in female $ER\alpha^{-/-}$ mice *(101)*. However, it was found that stromal cell clones isolated from $ER\alpha^{-/-}$ are responsive to estrogen in culture, an observation that is most interesting within the context of a second, recently discovered, estrogen receptor (ERβ) *(102–105)*. The ligand and DNA binding domains of this receptor are very similar to those of ERα and blocked by many of the same drugs *(102,105)*. The authors found transcripts for ERβ in $ER\alpha^{-/-}$ mice and in stromal cell clones derived from them. Furthermore, levels of estrogen are very high in female $ER\alpha^{-/-}$ mice, presumably as a result of inadequate feedback regulation of the pituitary *(101)*. The authors tentatively conclude that there are at least two estrogen receptors in bone marrow stromal cells and ablation of both might be required to disregulate B lymphopoiesis in female mice. Androgens and the androgen receptor may play the same role in males.

Stromal cells are known to have functional estrogen receptors, and the authors' observations are consistent with them being one target of sex steroids in bone marrow *(29,106)*. Exposure of normal or transformed B-cell precursors to estrogen in the absence of stromal cells had no obvious effect and did not induce the characteristic phenotypic changes that occur during pregnancy or in hormone-treated mice. However, estrogen reduced the expansion of precursors in culture when stromal cells were also present *(29)*. Medium conditioned by stromal cells that had been briefly treated with estrogen was also suppressive. These findings suggest that estrogen may trigger the release of a negative regulator, whose nature remains unknown.

A number of candidate molecules have been eliminated or deemed to be unlikely mediators of the hormonal influence on marrow. The expression of several substances can be upregulated by estrogen: TGFβ and IGF-1 in osteoblastic cells *(107–109)*, TNF in the uterus *(110)*, and IL-1 and NO in macrophages *(111,112)*, and cathepsin D in breast cancer cells *(113)*. Some of these (TGFβ, TNF, and IL-1) have also been reported to suppress B-cell precursor growth *(28,114–116)*. However, the authors found that neutralizing antibodies to TGFβ, IFNβ (*117*; also *see* L. Borghesi, submitted), or IL-4 *(118)* did not prevent estrogen from suppressing B-cell precursor expansion in cocultures with OP42 stromal cells. Other factors such as IGF-1 and cathepsin D had no detrimental effects of precursor growth (*29,119,120*; also *see* G. Smithson, unpublished observations). Furthermore, estrogen did not induce NO production in our estrogen responsive stromal cell line, eliminating it as a potential estrogen-induced inhibitor.

With respect to cell numbers, the greatest degree of hormone-related change occurs at the small pre–B-cell stage. However, a number of observations indicate that sex steroids influence earlier events. Stromal cell cocultures initiated with stem cells are more affected by estrogen than those that utilize more differentiated (fraction "A") precursors (*29*; also *see* Medina, manuscript in preparation). Furthermore, an important change was documented in residual fraction "B" pro-B-cells in estrogen-treated mice. Although transcripts for a number of B lineage genes were detectable, RAG-1 was usually absent in these animals. This finding may be key to understanding why there is a marked depression in numbers of cytoplasmic μ heavy chain positive cells with estrogen treatment (Medina, manuscript in preparation).

In contrast to the effects of estrogen on B lymphopoiesis in normal mice, no changes were documented in animals that express a strong human Bcl-2 transgene. This might indicate that the fate of precursors during pregnancy or after estrogen treatment involves apoptosis. Therefore, it was a surprise to learn that treatment of either normal or RAG gene targeted mice with estrogen leads to the survival of cells that appear to be defective. As discussed in Subheading 2., successful immunoglobulin gene rearrangement and expression of cytoplasmic μ heavy chains is a feature of nearly all small $CD43^-$ pre-B-cells in normal mice. However, there is a conspicuous population of small, $CD43^-$, μ^- cells in marrow of animals that have been estrogen treated (Medina, manuscript in preparation). Several B lineage markers including CD19 are expressed by these "pseudo pre-B-cells," and they have nuclear TdT. The TdT enzyme is normally extinguished when cytoplasmic μ chains appear *(8,121)*. The cells also differ from normal small pre-B-cells in lacking CD25. As discussed in Subheading 2., CD25 expression normally correlates with successful heavy chain gene rearrangement *(8,16)*. Further study concerning the origin and fate of "pseudo pre-B" cells may be informative about life/death decisions in B-cell precursors in more normal circumstances.

A substantial percentage of B lineage lymphocytes in normal animals fail to successfully rearrange either μ heavy chain allele, and these defective cells probably undergo apoptosis. Their selective death might result in part from intrinsic signals. However, a variety of evidence suggests that some type of quality control mechanism is built into precursors such that they are not allowed to proceed beyond a certain check point (large pro-B, fraction "C") without display of specific surface receptors. Gene targeting and transgene replacement experiments indicate that a "pre-B receptor complex," containing transmembrane μ and the associated Ig-α/Ig-β signaling molecules, along with V_{pre-B} and λ_5, surrogate light chains, is normally required for progression to the small pre-B-cell stage *(7,122,123)*. This transition is preceded at the large pre–B-cell stage by several rounds of unusually rapid replication *(5,8)*. Thus, large pre–B-cells may require interaction with some unknown ligand in the environment via their primitive receptors to signal their proliferation, subsequent exit from the cell cycle, survival, and initiation of light chain gene rearrangement. However, the authors' observations with estrogen-treated mice demonstrate that loss of surface CD43 and progression to a small resting state is not absolutely linked to μ chain expression. It has also been proposed that macrophage-like cells in the bone marrow provide signals that preferentially encourage death of defective lymphocytes *(117)*, and macrophage products that induce apoptosis will be discussed in Subheading 6. Regardless of what intrinsic and extrinsic signals initiate defective lymphocyte death, their fate is to be ingested by phagocytic cells *(124)*.

There are several possible explanations for the appearance of "pseudo pre-B" cells in estrogen treated mice. For example, an estrogen induced mediator may act on early precursors and bypass the requirement for signal delivery via the pre-B-cell receptor complex. The authors have found that "pseudo pre-B" cells, like normal small pre-B-cells, express Bcl-X_L, and it will be important to learn how this survival gene is regulated. As a second possibility, death signals that are normally provided by macrophage-like cells and/or phagocytic processes could be hormone sensitive. Thus, defective cells would be allowed to survive for an abnormally long time. However, this explanation is likely to be incomplete, because estrogen reduced expansion of B lineage cells in cultures containing only lymphocytes and stromal cells *(29)*. RAG-1 expression at the early pro–B-cell (fraction "B") stage is the earliest estrogen-sensitive event that the authors have clearly documented. Definition of the molecular mediators of that response could be key to understanding how sex steroids control the numbers of B-cells that are produced, as well as the fate of defective cells that are normally destined to die.

6. Other Negative Regulators

There is increasing realization that the output of bone marrow is controlled by a balance between positive and negative signals from the microenvironment. In addition to estrogen, a number of substances have the potential to limit B lymphopoiesis. Transforming growth factor β (TGF-β) was the first cytokine shown to inhibit the IL-7 dependent expansion of pre-B-cells *(28,95)*. However, the authors subsequently found that myelopoiesis was more sensitive to TGF-β than B lymphocyte formation in culture *(125)*. This is consistent with a variety of studies that suggest this molecule may be an important regulator at the stem cell stage. B lineage lymphocyte formation can be inhibited in culture, as well as in vivo by IL-1α *(126,127)*. Similarly, apoptosis can be induced in normal and transformed pre-B-cells by prostaglandin E2 *(128* and manuscript in preparation). Type II interferons are particularly interesting because genetic manipulations that result in over-expression or hypersensitivity cause pre-B-cell deficiency *(129,130)*. Wang and Cooper found that IL-7 responsive pre-B-cells undergo apoptosis when exposed to IFN-α/β and suggested that defective lymphocytes might be particularly sensitive *(117)*. Their analyses also indicated that IFN-β might be constitutively present in the bone marrow. As discussed below, life/death decisions in pre-B-cells probably depend on their integration of multiple signals from the environment.

The authors recently discovered an interesting pathway through which type II IFN might be produced. The marrow has a nerve supply, and neuropeptides have been identified in that site *(131)*. Addition of vasoactive intestinal peptide (VIP) to bone marrow cultures suppressed pre-B-cell growth, but only when macrophages were present *(56)*. VIP induced production of IFN-α by adherent marrow cells and the cytokine suppressed clonal expansion of pre-B-cells. There are reports that pre-B-cells may be directly responsive in culture to another neuropeptide, CGRP *(132)*. Further study might reveal if neuronal/neuropeptide influence actually occurs in vivo and whether it is operable under steady-state or stress-induced conditions.

Pre-B-cells spontaneously die by apoptosis when removed from bone marrow and placed in culture, but the rate of their disappearance decreases substantially when they are allowed to contact stromal cells *(133)*. Conversely, apoptosis is markedly increased when pre-B-cells are exposed to glucocorticoids, PGE-2, IL-1α, or type II interferons. It is interesting that, although stromal cell contact delays the rate of apoptosis induced by most of these agents, it has no effect on that elicited by type II IFN. Stromal cell conditioned medium provides only partial protection from spontaneous and induced apoptosis, so it will be important to learn what transmembrane or matrix associated molecules are involved. Antibodies to a number of stromal cell interaction molecules did not influence pre–B-cell survival in these cultures. Maturing lymphocyte precursors clearly integrate multiple signals from their environment, and the particular combination may determine if they are allowed to proceed beyond discrete check points in differentiation.

7. Conclusion

Although it may now be possible to make B lymphocyte precursors from stem cells in vitro *(43,133)*, it remains a challenge to do so in a situation where all components of the medium are defined and to efficiently take the cells to a mature, functional state. This would indicate that although we know a great deal about the composition of bone marrow, all components have probably not been identified. Furthermore, we have not learned how to present regulatory molecules to maturing blood cells in a natural way. Clearly, there is a great need to understand more about the microanatomy of bone marrow, and particularly with respect to the placement of molecules discussed in this chapter. Culture studies have revealed that an impressive number of substances can potentially be made by stromal cells (Fig. 1). However, a great deal more work is required to learn what combinations are made by individual stromal cells within marrow *(134,135)*. Certain cytokines, including IL-1, IL-3, IL-4, and IL-10 can positively regulate some stages of lympho-hematopoiesis and have the opposite effect at other stages or in other circumstances *(61,62,114,125,126,133,136)*. This indicates that B lymphopoiesis must be considered within the context of cell movement. Maturing cells probably enter, and are affected by, discrete physical compartments as they make their way towards the point of departure into the bloodstream.

The negative regulatory role of sex steroids discussed here must be studied and considered within a larger endocrine context. Hormones of the hypothalamic-pituitary-thyroid axis are particularly interesting, and there is evidence that both IGF-1 and thyroxine contribute in a positive way to B lymphopoiesis (*120,137,138 see* also Chapter 11). Furthermore, there are probably more similarities than differences in the way lymphocytes are made in the thymus and bone marrow. As just one example, lymphopoie-

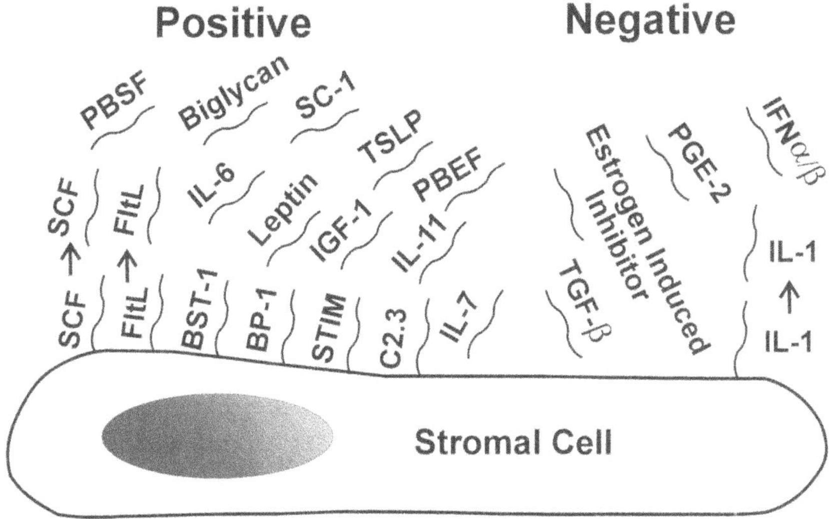

Fig. 1. Stromal cells produce many substances that can influence B lymphopoiesis in a positive or negative way. This conclusion is derived largely from studies of stromal cell clones, and it is unlikely that all of these molecules are simultaneously produced by individual stromal cells *in situ*. The proximity of B lineage precursors to these substances is governed by cell adhesion molecules such as VCAM-1 (not shown). Some of the cytokines are produced in both transmembrane and soluble forms as indicated. Also, many of the factors (IL-7, PBSF, TGF-β) may be docked on heparan sulfated proteoglycans such as syndecan-4 (not illustrated).

sis in both sites is negatively influenced by estrogen (reviewed in ref. *140*). Although both of these organs produce lymphocytes from stem cells or uncommitted progenitors, it must be remembered that lymphocytes can also be generated in another way. That is, B-cells are made via clonal expansion during immune responses. Interesting similarities are being found between lymphocytes in germinal centers and pre-B-cells within bone marrow *(141)*. Therefore, it will be important to learn if hormones or the other components of the marrow microenvironment discussed here regulate peripheral lymphocyte expansion.

Acknowledgments

The authors research is supported by grants AI 20069 and AI 19884 from the National Institutes of Health.

References

1. Coffman, R. L. and Weissman, I. L. (1981) A monoclonal antibody that recognizes B cells and B cell precursors in mice. *J. Exp. Med.* **153,** 269–279.
2. Kincade, P. W., Lee, G., Watanabe, T., Sun, L., and Scheid, M. P. (1981) Antigens displayed on murine B lymphocyte precursors. *J. Immunol.* **127,** 2262–2268.
3. Landreth, K. S., Kincade, P. W., Lee, G., and Medlock, E. S. (1983) Phenotypic and functional characterization of murine B lymphocyte precursors isolated from fetal and adult tissues. *J. Immunol.* **131,** 572–580.
4. Osmond, D. G. (1990) B cell development in the bone marrow. *Semin. Immunol.* **2,** 173–180.
5. Hardy, R. R., Carmack, C. E., Shinton, S. A., Kemp, J. D., and Hayakawa, K. (1991) Resolution and characterization of pro-B and pre-pro-B cell stages in normal mouse bone marrow. *J. Exp. Med.* **173,** 1213–1225.

6. Ehlich, A., Martin, V., Muller, W., and Rajewsky, K. (1994) Analysis of the B-cell progenitor compartment at the level of single cells. *Curr. Biol.* **4,** 573–583.
7. Rajewsky, K. (1996) Clonal selection and learning in the antibody system. *Nature* **381,** 751–758.
8. Rolink, A., Grawunder, U., Winkler, T. H., Karasuyama, H., and Melchers, F. (1994) IL-2 receptor α chain (CD25, TAC) expression defines a crucial stage in pre-B cell development. *Intl. Immunol.* **6,** 1257–1264.
9. Melchers, F., Rolink, A., Grawunder, U., Winkler, T. H., Karasuyama, H., Ghia, P., and Andersson, J. (1995) Positive and negative selection events during B lymphopoiesis. *Current Opinion Immunol.* **7,** 214–227.
10. Rolink, A. and Melchers, F. (1993) Generation and regeneration of cells of the B-lymphocyte lineage. *Curr. Opin. Immunol.* **5,** 207–217.
11. Scheid, M. P., Landreth, K. S., Tung, J. S., and Kincade, P. W. (1982) Preferential but nonexclusive expression of macromolecular antigens on B-lineage cells. *Immunol. Rev.* **69,** 141–159.
12. Krop, I., de Fougerolles,A. R., Hardy, R. R., Allison, M., Schlissel, M. S., and Fearon, D. T. (1996) Self-renewal of B-1 lymphocytes is dependent on CD19. *Eur. J. Immunol.* **26,** 238–242.
13. Sato, S., Ono, N., Steeber, D. A., Pisetsky, D. S., and Tedder, T. F. (1996) CD19 regulates B lymphocyte signaling thresholds critical for the development of B-1 lineage cells and autoimmunity. *J. Immunol.* **157,** 4371–4378.
14. Li, Y.-S., Wasserman, R., Hayakawa, K., and Hardy, R. R. (1996) Identification of the earliest B lineage stage in mouse bone marrow. *Immunity* **5,** 527–535.
15. Rolink, A., Ten Boekel, E., Melchers, F., Fearon, D. T., Krop, I., and Andersson, J. (1996) A subpopulation of B220+ cells in murine bone marrow does not express CD19 and contains natural killer cell progenitors. *J. Exp. Med.* **183,** 187–194.
16. Chen, J., Ma, A., Young, F., and Alt, F. (1994) IL-2 receptor α chain expression during early B lymphocyte differentiation. *Int. Immunol.* **6,** 1265–1268.
17. Era, T., Nishikawa, S., Sudo, T., Wang, F. H., Ogawa, M., Kunisada, T., and Hayashi, S. (1994) How B-precursor cells are driven to cycle. *Immunol. Rev.* **137,** 35–51.
18. Ogawa, M., Matsuzaki, Y., Nishikawa, S., Hayashi, S., Kunisada, T., Sudo, T., Kina, T., Nakauchi, H., and Nishikawa, S. (1991) Expression and function of c-kit in hemopoietic progenitor cells. *J. Exp. Med.* **174,** 63–71.
19. Okada, S., Nakauchi, H., Nagayoshi, K., Nishikawa, S., Miura, Y., and Suda, T. (1991) Enrichment and characterization of murine hematopoietic stem cells that express c-*kit* molecule. *Blood* **78,** 1706–1712.
20. Rolink, A., Haasner, D., Nishikawa, S.-I., and Melchers, F. (1993) Changes in frequencies of clonable pre B cells during life in different lymphoid organs of mice. *Blood* **81,** 2290–2300.
21. Kee, B. L. and Paige, C. J. (1996) In vitro tracking of IL-7 responsiveness and gene expression during commitment of bipotent B-cell/macrophage progenitors. *Curr. Biol.* **6,** 1159–1169.
22. Shortman, K. and Wu, L. (1996) Early T lymphocyte progenitors. *Annu. Rev. Immunol.* **14,** 29–47.
23. Hayashi, S., Kunisada, T., Ogawa, M., Sudo, T., Kodama, H., Suda, T., Nishikawa, S., and Nishikawa, S. (1990) Stepwise progression of B lineage differentiation supported by Interleukin 7 and other stromal cell molecules. *J. Exp. Med.* **171,** 1683–1695.
24. Sudo, T., Ito, M., Ogawa, Y., Iizuka, M., Kodama, H., Kunisada, T., Hayashi, S.-I., Ogawa, M., Sakai, K., Nishikawa, S., and Nishikawa, S.-I. (1989) Interleukin 7 production and function in stromal cell-dependent B cell development. *J. Exp. Med.* **170,** 333–338.
25. DiSanto, J. P., Müller, W., Guy-Grand, D., Fischer, A., and Rajewsky, K. (1995) Lymphoid development in mice with a targeted deletion of the interleukin 2 receptor gamma chain. *Proc. Natl. Acad. Sci. USA* **92,** 377–381.
26. Grabstein, K. H., Waldschmidt, T. J., Finkelman, F. D., Hess, B. W., Alpert, A. R., Boiani, N. E., Namen, A. E., and Morrissey, P. J. (1993) Inhibition of murine B and T lymphopoiesis in vivo by an anti-interleukin 7 monoclonal antibody. *J. Exp. Med.* **178,** 257–264.
27. Peschon, J. J., Morrissey, P. J., Grabstein, K. H., Ramsdell, F. J., Maraskovsky, E., Gliniak, B. C., Park, L. S., Ziegler, S. F., Williams, D. E., Ware, C. B., Meyer, J. D., and Davison, B. L. (1994) Early lymphocyte expansion is severely impaired in interleukin 7 receptor-deficient mice. *J. Exp. Med.* **180,** 1955–1960.
28. Lee, G., Namen, A. E., Gillis, S., Ellingsworth, L. R., and Kincade, P. W. (1989) Normal B cell precursors responsive to recombinant murine IL-7 and inhibition of IL-7 activity by transforming growth factor-β. *J. Immunol.* **142,** 3875–3883.

29. Smithson, G., Medina, K., Ponting, I., and Kincade, P. W. (1995) Estrogen suppresses stromal cell-dependent lymphopoiesis in culture. *J. Immunol.* **155,** 3409–3417.
30. Hayashi, C., Kunisada, T., Ogawa, M., Sudo, T., Kodama, H., Suda, T., Nishikawa, S., and Nishikawa, S. I. (1990) Stepwise progression of a B lineage differentiation supported by interleukin 7 and other stromal cell molecules. *J. Exp. Med.* **171,** 1683–1695.
31. Corcoran, A. E., Smart, F. M., Cowling, R. J., Crompton, T., Owen, M. J., and Venkitaraman, A. R. (1996) The interleukin-7 receptor chain transmits distinct signals for proliferation and differentiation during B lymphopoiesis. *EMBO Journal* **15,** 1924–1932.
32. Von Freeden-Jeffry, U., Vieira, P., Lucian, L. A., McNeil, T., Burdach, S. E. G., and Murray, R. (1995) Lymphopenia in interleukin (IL)-7 gene-deleted mice identifies IL-7 as a nonredundant cytokine. *J. Exp. Med.* **181,** 1519–1526.
33. Friend, S. L., Hosier, S., Nelson, A., Foxworthe, D., Williams, D. E., and Farr, A. (1994) A thymic stromal cell line supports in vitro development of surface IgM^+ B cells and produces a novel growth factor affecting B and T lineage cells. *Exp. Hematol.* **22,** 321–328.
34. Ray, R. J., Furlonger, C., Williams, D. E., and Paige, C. J. (1996) Characterization of thymic stromal-derived lymphopoietin (TSLP) in murine B cell development in vitro. *Eur. J. Immunol.* **26,** 10–16.
35. Pribyl, J. A. R. and Lebien, T. W. (1996) Interleukin 7 independent development of human B cells. *Proc. Natl. Acad. Sci. USA* **93,** 10,348–10,353.
36. Leonard, W. J. (1994) The defective gene in X-linked severe combined immunodeficiency encodes a shared interleukin receptor subunit: implications for cytokine pleiotropy and redundancy. *Curr. Opin. Immunol.* **6,** 631–635.
37. Dittel, B. N. and Lebien, T. W. (1995) The growth response to IL-7 during normal human B cell ontogeny is restricted to B-lineage cells expressing CD34. *J. Immunol.* **154,** 58–67.
38. Ryan, D. H., Nuccie, B. L., Ritterman, I., Liesveld, J. L., Abboud, C. N., and Insel, R. A. (1997) Expression of interleukin-7 receptor by lineage-negative human bone marrow progenitors with enhanced lymphoid proliferative potential and B-lineage differentiation capacity. *Blood* **89,** 929–940.
39. Mackarehtschian, K., Hardin, J. D., Moore, K., Boast, S., Goff, S. P., and Lemischka, I. (1995) Targeted disruption of the *flk2/flt3* gene leads to deficiencies in primitive hematopoietic progenitors. *Immunity* **3,** 147–161.
40. Takeda, S., Shimizu, T., and Rodewald, H. R. (1997) Interactions between c-kit and stem cell factor are not required for B-cell development in vivo. *Blood* **89,** 518–525.
41. Hirayama, F., Lyman, S. D., Clark, S. C., and Ogawa, M. (1995) The *flt3* ligand supports proliferation of lymphohematopoietic progenitors and early B-lymphoid progenitors. *Blood* **85,** 1762–1768.
42. Wasserman, R., Li, Y.-S., and Hardy, R. R. (1995) Differential expression of the Blk and Ret tyrosine kinases during B lineage development is dependent on Ig rearrangement. *J. Immunol.* **155,** 644–651.
43. Veiby, O. P., Lyman, S. D., and Jacobsen, S. E. W. (1996) Combined signaling through interleukin-7 receptors and flt3 but not c-*kit* potently and selectively promotes B-cell commitment and differentiation from uncommitted murine bone marrow progenitor cells. *Blood* **88,** 1256–1265.
44. Witte, O. N. (1990) Steel locus defines new multipotent growth factor. *Cell* **63,** 5–6.
45. Samal, B., Sun, Y., Stearns, G., Xie, C., Suggs, S., and McNiece, I. (1994) Cloning and characterization of the cDNA encoding a novel human pre-B-cell colony enhancing factor. *Mol. Cell Biol.* **14,** 1431–1437.
46. Tashiro, K., Tada, H., Heilker, R., Shirozu, M., Nakano, T., and Honjo, T. (1993) Signal sequence trap: A cloning strategy for secreted proteins and type I membrane proteins. *Science* **261,** 600–603.
47. Nagasawa, T., Kikutani, H., and Kishimoto, T. (1994) Molecular cloning and structure of a novel pre-B cell growth stimulating factor (PBSF). *Proc. Natl. Acad. Sci. USA* **91,** 2305–2309.
48. Nagasawa, T., Hirota, S., Tachibana, K., Takakura, N., Nishikawa, S., Kitamura, Y., Yoshida, N., Kikutani, H., and Kishimoto, T. (1996) Defects of B-cell lymphopoiesis and bone-marrow myelopoiesis in mice lacking the CXC chemokine PBSF/SDF-1. *Nature* **382,** 635–638.
49. Aiuti, A., Webb, I. J., Bleul, C., Springer, T., and Gutierrez-Ramos, J. C. (1997) The chemokine SDF-1 is a chemoattractant for human $CD34^+$ hematopoietic progenitor cells and provides a new mechanism to explain the mobilization of $CD34^+$ progenitors to peripheral blood. *J. Exp. Med.* **185,** 111–120.

50. Nagasawa, T., Nakajima, T., Tachibana, K., Iizasa, H., Bleul, C. C., Yoshie, O., Matsushima, K., Yoshida, N., Springer, T. A., and Kishimoto, T. (1996) Molecular cloning and characterization of a murine pre-B-cell growth-stimulating factor stromal cell-derived factor 1 receptor, a murine homolog of the human immunodeficiency virus 1 entry coreceptor fusin. *Proc. Natl. Acad. Sci. USA* **93,** 14726–14729.
51. Kaisho, T., Ishikawa, J., Oritani, K., Inazawa, J., Tomizawa, H., Muraoka, O., Ochi, T., and Hirano, T. (1994) BST-1, a surface molecule of bone marrow stromal cell lines that facilitates pre-B cell growth. *Proc. Natl. Acad. Sci. USA* **91,** 5325–5329.
52. Ishihara, K., Kobune, Y., Okuyama, Y., Itoh, M., Lee, B. O. K., Muraoka, O., and Hirano, T. (1996) Stage-specific expression of mouse BST-1/BP-3 on the early B and T cell progenitors prior to gene rearrangement of antigen receptor. *Int. Immunol.* **8,** 1395–1404.
53. Wu, Q., Lahti, J. M., Air, G. M., Burrows, P. D., and Cooper, M. D. (1990) Molecular cloning of the murine BP-1/6C3 antigen: A member of the zinc-dependent metallopeptidase family. *Proc. Natl. Acad. Sci. USA* **87,** 993–997.
54. Welch, P. A. (1995) Regulation of B cell precursor proliferation by aminopeptidase A. *Int. Immunol.* **7,** 737–746.
55. Kee, B. L., Paige, C. J., and Letarte, M. (1992) Characterization of murine CD10, an endopeptidase expressed on bone marrow adherent cells. *Int. Immunol.* **4,** 1041–1047.
56. Shimozato, T. and Kincade, P. W. (1997) Indirect suppression of IL-7-responsive B cell precursors by vasoactive intestinal peptide. *J. Immunol.* **158,** 5178–5184.
57. Bennett, B. D., Solar, G. P., Yuan, J. Q., Mathias, J., Thomas, G. R., and Matthews, W. (1996) A role for leptin and its cognate receptor in hematopoiesis. *Curr. Biol.* **6,** 1170–1180.
58. Gainsford, T., Willson, T. A., Metcalf, D., Handman, E., McFarlane, C., Ng, A., Nicola, N. A., Alexander, W. S., and Hilton, D. J. (1996) Leptin can induce proliferation, differentiation, and functional activation of hemopoietic cells. *Proc. Natl. Acad. Sci. USA* **93,** 14564–14568.
59. Hirayama, F., Shih, J. P., Awgulewitsch, A., Warr, G. W., Clark, S. C., and Ogawa, M. (1992) Clonal proliferation of murine lymphohemopoietic progenitors in culture. *Proc. Natl. Acad. Sci. USA* **89,** 5907–5911.
60. Kee, B. L., Cumano, A., Iscove, N. N., and Paige, C. J. (1994) Stromal cell independent growth of bipotent B cell/macrophage precursors from murine fetal liver. *Int. Immunol.* **6,** 401–407.
61. Elia, J. M., Hamilton, B. L., and Riley, R. L. (1995) IL-10 inhibits IL-7-mediated murine pre-B cell growth in vitro. *Exp. Hematol.* **23,** 323–327.
62. Fine, J. S., Macosko, H. D., Grace, M. J., and Narula, S. K. (1994) Influence of IL-10 on murine CFU-pre-B formation. *Exp. Hematol.* **22,** 1188–1196.
63. Miyake, K., Medina, K., Hayashi, S.-I., Ono, S., Hamaoka, T., and Kincade, P. W. (1990) Monoclonal antibodies to Pgp-1/CD44 block lympho-hemopoiesis in long-term bone marrow cultures. *J. Exp. Med.* **171,** 477–488.
64. Miyake, K., Underhill, C. B., Lesley, J., and Kincade, P. W. (1990) Hyaluronate can function as a cell adhesion molecule and CD44 participates in hyaluronate recognition. *J. Exp. Med.* **172,** 69–75.
65. Lesley, J., Hyman, R., and Kincade, P. W. (1993) CD44 and its interaction with the extracellular matrix. *Adv. Immunol.* **54,** 271–335.
66. Stamenkovic, I., Aruffo, A., Amiot, M., and Seed, B. (1991) The hematopoietic and epithelial forms of CD44 are distinct polypeptides with different adhesion potentials for hyaluronate-bearing cells. *EMBO J.* **10,** 343–348.
67. He, Q., Lesley, J., Hyman, R., Ishihara, K., and Kincade, P. W. (1992) Molecular isoforms of murine CD44 and evidence that the membrane proximal domain is not critical for hyaluronate recognition. *J. Cell Biol.* **119,** 1711–1719.
68. Lesley, J., He, Q., Miyake, K., Hamann, A., Hyman, R., and Kincade, P. W. (1992) Requirements for hyaluronic acid binding by CD44: a role for the cytoplasmic domain and activation by antibody. *J. Exp. Med.* **175,** 257–266.
69. Isacke, C. M. (1994) The role of the cytoplasmic domain in regulating CD44 function. *J. Cell Sci.* **107,** 2353–2359.
70. Hathcock, K. S., Hirano, H., Murakami, S., and Hodes, R. J. (1993) CD44 expression on activated B cells: Differential capacity for CD44-dependent binding to hyaluronic acid. *J. Immunol.* **151,** 6712–6722.
71. Katoh, S., Zheng, Z., Oritani, K., Shimozato, T., and Kincade, P. W. (1995) Glycosylation of CD44 negatively regulates its recognition of hyaluronan. *J. Exp. Med.* **182,** 419–429.

72. Lesley, J., English, N., Perschl, A., Gregoroff, J., and Hyman, R. (1995) Variant cell lines selected for alterations in the function of the hyaluronan receptor CD44 show differences in glycosylation. *J. Exp. Med.* **182,** 431–437.
73. Zheng, Z., Cummings, R. D., Pummill, P. E., and Kincade, P. W. (1997) Growth as a solid tumor or reduced glucose concentration in culture reversibly induce CD44 mediated hyaluronan recognition by Chinese hamster ovary cells. *J. Clin. Invest.* **100,** 1217–1229.
73a. Bartolazzi, A., Nocks, A., Aruffo, A., Spring, F., and Stamenkovic, I. (1996) Glycosylation of CD44 is implicated in CD44–mediated cell adhesion to hyaluronan. *J. Cell Biol.* **132,** 1199–1208.
74. Bennett, K. L., Modrell, B., Greenfield, B., Bartolazzi, A., Stamenkovic, I., Peach, R., Jackson, D. G., Spring, F., and Aruffo, A. (1995) Regulation of CD44 binding to hyaluronan by glycosylation of variably spliced exons. *J. Cell Biol.* **131,** 1623–1633.
75. Kohda, D., Morton, C. J., Parkar, A. A., Hatanaka, H., Inagaki, F. M., Campbell, I. D., and Day, A. J. (1996) Solution structure of the link module: A hyaluronan-binding domain involved in extracellular matrix stability and cell migration. *Cell* **86,** 767–775.
76. Zheng, Z., Katoh, S., He, Q., Oritani, K., Miyake, K., Lesley, J., Hyman, R., Hamik, A., Parkhouse, R. M. E., Farr, A. G., and Kincade, P. W. (1995) Monoclonal antibodies to CD44 and their influence on hyaluronan recognition. *J. Cell Biol.* **130,** 485–495.
77. Miyake, K., Medina, K., Ishihara, K., Kimoto, M., Auerbach, R., and Kincade, P. W. (1991) A VCAM-like adhesion molecule on murine bone marrow stromal cells mediates binding of lymphocyte precursors in culture. *J. Cell Biol.* **114,** 557–565.
78. Miyake, K., Weissman, I. L., Greenberger, J. S., and Kincade, P. W. (1991) Evidence for a role of the integrin VLA-4 in lympho-hemopoiesis. *J. Exp. Med.* **173,** 599–607.
79. Ryan, D. H., Nuccie, B. L., Abboud, C. N., and Winslow, J. M. (1991) Vascular cell adhesion molecule-1 and the integrin VLA-4 mediate adhesion of human B cell precursors to cultured bone marrow adherent cells. *J. Clin. Invest.* **88,** 995–1004.
80. Simmons, P. J., Masinovsky, B., Longenecker, B. M., Berenson, R., B. Torok-Storb, and Gallatin, W. M. (1992) Vascular cell adhesion molecule-1 expressed by bone marrow stromal cells mediates the binding of hematopoietic progenitor cells. *Blood* **80,** 388–395.
81. Jacobsen, K., Kravitz, J., Kincade, P. W., and Osmond, D. G. (1996) Adhesion receptors on bone marrow stromal cells: In vivo expression of vascular cell adhesion molecule-1 by reticular cells and sinusoidal endothelium in normal and gamma-irradiated mice. *Blood* **87,** 73–82.
82. Funk, P. E., Kincade, P. W., and Witte, P. L. (1994) Native associations of early hemopoietic stem cells and stromal cells isolated in bone marrow cell aggregates. *Blood* **83,** 361–369.
83. Papayannopoulou, T. and Nakamoto, B. (1993) Peripheralization of hemopoietic progenitors in primates treated with anti-VLA_4 integrin. *Proc. Natl. Acad. Sci. USA* **90,** 9374–9378.
84. Papayannopoulou, T., Craddock, C., Nakamoto, B., Priestley, G. V., and Wolf, N. S. (1995) The VLA4/VCAM-1 adhesion pathway defines contrasting mechanisms of lodgement of transplanted murine hemopoietic progenitors between bone marrow and spleen. *Proc. Natl. Acad. Sci. USA* **92,** 9647–9651.
85. Baron, J. L., Reich, E.-P., Visintin, I., and Janeway, C. A., Jr. (1994) The pathogenesis of adoptive murine autoimmune diabetes requires an interaction between α4–integrins and vascular cell adhesion molecule-1. *J. Clin. Invest.* **93,** 1700–1708.
86. Isobe, M., Suzuki, J., Yagita, H., Okumura, K., and Sekiguchi, M. (1994) Effect of anti-VCAM-1 and anti-VLA-4 monoclonal antibodies on cardiac allograft survival and response to soluble antigens in mice. *Transplant. Proc.* **26,** 867–868.
87. Orosz, C. G., Ohye, R. G., Pelletier, R. P., Van Buskirk, A. M., Huang, E., Morgan, C., Kincade, P. W., and Ferguson, R. M. (1993) Treatment with anti-vascular cell adhesion molecule 1 monoclonal antibody induces long-term murine cardiac allograft acceptance. *Transplantation* **56,** 453–460.
88. Steffen, B. J., Butcher, E. C., and Engelhardt, B. (1994) Evidence for involvement of ICAM-1 and VCAM-1 in lymphocyte interaction with endothelium in experimental autoimmune encephalomyelitis in the central nervous system in the SJL/J mouse. *Am.J.Pathol.* **145,** 189–201.
89. Gurtner, G. C., Davis, V., Li, H., McCoy, M. J., Sharpe, A., and Cybulsky, M. I. (1995) Targeted disruption of the murine *VCAM1* gene: essential role of VCAM-1 in chorioallantoic fusion and placentation. *Genes Dev.* **9,** 1–14.
90. Kwee, L., Baldwin, H. S., Shen, H. M., Stewart, C. L., Buck, C., Buck, C. A., and Labow, M. A. (1995) Defective development of the embryonic and extraembryonic circulatory systems in vascular cell adhesion molecule (VCAM-1) deficient mice. *Development* **121,** 489–503.

91. Yang, J. T., Rayburn, H., and Hynes, R. O. (1995) Cell adhesion events mediated by α_4 integrins are essential in placental and cardiac development. *Development* **121,** 549–560.
92. Friedrich, C., Cybulsky, M. I., and Gutierrez-Ramos, J. C. (1996) Vascular cell adhesion molecule-1 expression by hematopoiesis-supporting stromal cells is not essential for lymphoid or myeloid differentiation in vivo or in vitro. *Eur. J. Immunol.* **26,** 2773–2780.
93. Oritani, K. and Kincade, P. W. (1996) Identification of stromal cell products which interact with Pre-B cells. *J. Cell. Biol.* **134,** 771–782.
94. Hildebrand, A., Romarís, M., Rasmussen, L. M., Heinegård, D., Twardzik, D. R., Border, W. A., and Ruoslahti, E. (1994) Interaction of the small interstitial proteoglycans biglycan, decorin and fibromodulin with transforming growth factor β. *Biochem. J.* **302,** 527–534.
95. Lee, G., Ellingsworth, L. R., Gillis, S., Wall, R., and Kincade, P. W. (1987) B transforming growth factors are potential regulators of B lymphopoiesis. *J. Exp. Med.* **166,** 1290–1299.
96. Medina, K. L., Smithson, G., and Kincade, P. W. (1993) Suppression of B lymphopoeisis during normal pregnancy. *J. Exp. Med.* **178,** 1507–1515.
97. Medina, K. L. and Kincade, P. W. (1994) Pregnancy related steroids are potential negative regulators of B lymphopoiesis. *Proc. Natl. Acad. Sci. USA* **91,** 5382–5386.
98. Smithson, G., Beamer, W. G., Shultz, K. L., Christianson, S. W., Shultz, L. D., and Kincade, P. W. (1994) Increased B lymphopoiesis in genetically sex steroid-deficient Hypogonadal (hpg) mice. *J. Exp. Med.* **180,** 717–720.
99. Wilson, C. A., Mrose, S. A., and Thomas, D. W. (1995) Enhanced production of B lymphocytes after castration. *Blood* **85,** 1535–1539.
100. Wakeling, A. E., Dukes, M., and Bowler, J. (1991) A potent specific pure antiestrogen with clinical potential. *Cancer Res.* **51,** 3867–3873.
101. Couse, J. F., Curtis, S. W., Washburn, T. F., Lindzey, J., Golding, T. S., Lubahn, D. B., Smithies, O., and Korach, K. S. (1995) Analysis of transcription and estrogen insensitivity in the female mouse after targeted disruption of the estrogen receptor gene. *Mol. Endocrinology* **9,** 1441–1454.
102. Kuiper, G. G. J. M., Carlsson, B., Grandien, K., Enmark, E., Haggblad, J., Nilsson, S., and Gustafsson, J. (1997) Comparison of the ligand binding specificity and transcript tissue distribution of estrogen receptors α and β. *Endocrinology* **138,** 863–870.
103. Kuiper, G. G. J. M., Enmark, E., Pelto-Huikko, M., Nilsson, S., and Gustafsson, J. (1996) Cloning of a novel estrogen receptor expressed in rat prostate and ovary. *Proc. Natl. Acad. Sci. USA* **93,** 5925–5930.
104. Mosselman, S., Polman, J., and Dijkema, R. (1996) ERβ: identification and characterization of a novel human estrogen receptor. *FEBS Let.* **392,** 49–53.
105. Tremblay, G. B., Tremblay, A., Copeland, N. G., Gilbert, D. J., Jenkins, N. A., Labrie, F., and Giguere, V. (1997) Cloning, chromosonal localization, and functional analysis of the murine estrogen receptor β. *Mol. Endocrinology* **11,** 353–365.
106. Bellido, T., Girasole, G., Passeri, G., Yu, X.-P., Mocharla, H., Jilka, R. L., Notides, A., and Manolagas, S. C. (1993) Demonstration of estrogen and vitamin D receptors in bone marrow-derived stromal cells: Up-regulation of the estrogen receptor by 1,25–dihydroxyvitamin-D_3. *Endocrinology* **133,** 553–562.
107. Finkelman, R. D., Bell, N. H., Strong, D. D., Demers, L. M., and Baylink, D. J. (1992) Ovariectomy selectively reduces the concentration of transforming growth factor β in rat bone: Implications for estrogen deficiency-associated bone loss. *Proc. Natl. Acad. Sci. USA* **89,** 12,190–12,193.
108. Gray, T. K., Mohan, S., Linkhart, T. A., and Baylink, D. J. (1989) Estradiol stimulates in vitro the secretion of insulin-like growth factors by the clonal osteoblastic cell line, UMR106. *Biochem. Biophys. Res. Commun.* **158,** 407–412.
109. Komm, B. S., Terpening, C. M., Benz, D. J., Graeme, K. A., Gallegos, A., Korc, M., Greene, G. L., O'Malley, B. W., and Haussler, M. R. (1988) Estrogen binding, receptor mRNA, and biologic response in osteoblast-like osteosarcoma cells. *Science* **241,** 81–83.
110. De, M., Sanford, T. R., and Wood, G. W. (1992) Interleukin-1, interleukin-6, and tumor necrosis factor alpha are produced in the mouse uterus during the estrous cycle and are induced by estrogen and progesterone. *Dev. Biol.* **151,** 297–305.
111. Hu, S.-K., Mitcho, Y. L., and Rath, N. C. (1988) Effect of estradiol on interleukin 1 synthesis by macrophages. *Int. J. Immunopharmac.* **10,** 247–252.
112. Shami, P. J. and Weinberg, J. B. (1996) Differential effects of nitric oxide on erythroid and myeloid colony growth from $CD34^+$ human bone marrow cells. *Blood* **87,** 977–982.

113. Westley, B. and May, F. E. B. (1991) Estrogen-regulated messenger RNA's in human breast cancer cells, in *Regulatory Mechanisms in Breast Cancer* (Lippman, M. and Dickson, R., eds.), Kluwer Academic, Boston, pp. 259–271.
114. Billips, L. G., Petitte, D., and Landreth, K. S. (1990) Bone marrow stromal cell regulation of B lymphopoiesis: Interleukin-1 (IL-1) and IL-4 regulate stromal cell support of pre-B cell production in vitro. *Blood* **75,** 611–619.
115. Hirayama, F., Clark, S. C., and Ogawa, M. (1994) Negative regulation of early B lymphopoiesis by interleukin 3 and interleukin 1α. *Proc. Natl. Acad. Sci. USA* **91,** 469–473.
116. Ryan, D. H., Nuccie, B. L., Ritterman, I., Liesveld, J. L., and Abboud, C. N. (1994) Cytokine regulation of early human lymphopoiesis. *J. Immunol.* **152,** 5250–5258.
117. Wang, J., Qun, L., Langston, H., and Cooper, M. D. (1995) Resident bone marrow macrophages produce type 1 interferons that can selectively inhibit interleukin-7-driven growth of B lineage cells. *Immunity.* **3,** 475–484.
118. Rennick, D., Yang, G., Muller-Sieburg, C., Smith, C., Arai, N., Takabe, Y., and Gemmell, L. (1987) Interleukin 4 (B-cell stimulatory factor 1) can enhance or antagonize the factor-dependent growth of hemopoietic progenitor cells. *Proc. Natl. Acad. Sci. USA* **84,** 6889–6893.
119. Gibson, L. F., Piktel, D., and Landreth, K. S. (1993) Insulin-like growth factor-1 potentiates expansion of interleukin-7 dependent pro-B cells. *Blood* **82,** 3005–3011.
120. Landreth, K. S., Narayanan, R., and Dorshkind, K. (1992) Insulin-like growth factor-I regulates pro-B cell differentiation. *Blood* **80,** 1207–1212.
121. Wasserman, R., Li, Y.-S., and Hardy, R. R. (1997) Down-regulation of terminal deoxynucleotidyl transferase by Ig heavy chain in B lineage cells. *J. Immunol.* **158,** 1133–1138.
122. Lassoued, K., Nuñez, C. A., Billips, L., Kubagawa, H., Monteiro, R. C., Lebien, T. W., and Cooper, M. D. (1993) Expression of surrogate light chain receptors is restricted to a late stage in pre-B cell differentiation. *Cell* **73,** 73–86.
123. Winkler, T. H., Rolink, A., Melchers, F., and Karasuyama, H. (1995) Precursor B cells of mouse bone marrow express two different complexes with the surrogate light chain on the surface. *Eur. J. Immunol.* **25,** 446–450.
124. Jacobsen, K. A., Prasad, V. S., Sidman, C. L., and Osmond, D. G. (1994) Apoptosis and macrophage-mediated deletion of precursor B cells in the bone marrow of *Eμ-myc* transgenic mice. *Blood* **84,** 2784–2794.
125. Dorshkind, K. (1988) IL-1 inhibits B cell differentiation in long term bone marrow cultures. *J. Immunol.* **141,** 531–538.
126. Hayashi, S., Gimble, J. M., Henley, A., Ellingsworth, L. R., and Kincade, P. W. (1989) Differential effects of TGF beta on lymphohemopoiesis in long-term bone marrow cultures. *Blood* **74,** 1711–1717.
127. Fauteux, L. J. and Osmond, D. G. (1996) IL-1 as a systemic modifier of B lymphopoiesis-Recombinant IL-1α binds to stromal cells and sinusoid endothelium in bone marrow and perturbs precursor B cell dynamics. *J. Immunol.* **156,** 2376–2383.
128. Brown, D. M., Warner, G. L., Ales-Martinez, J. E., Scott, D. W., and Phipps, R. P. (1992) Prostaglandin E_2 induces apoptosis in immature normal and malignant B lymphocytes. *Clin. Immunol. Immunopathol.* **63,** 221–229.
129. Matsuyama, T., Kimura, T., Kitagawa, M., Pfeffer, K., Kawakami, R., Watanabe, N., Kundig, T., Amakawa, R., Kishihara, K., Wakeham, A., Potter, J., Furlonger, C. L., Narendran, A., Suzuki, H., Ohashi, P. S., Paige, C. J., Taniguchi, T., and Mak, T. W. (1993) Targeted disruption of IRF-1 or IRF-2 results in abnormal type I IFN gene induction and aberrant lymphocyte development. *Cell* **75,** 83–97.
130. Yamada, G., Ogawa, M., Akagi, K., Miyamoto, H., Nakano, N., Itoh, S., Miyazaki, J., Nishikawa, S., Yamamura, K., and Taniguchi, T. (1991) Specific depletion of the B-cell population induced by aberrant expression of human interferon regulatory factor 1 gene in transgenic mice. *Proc. Natl. Acad. Sci. USA* **88,** 532–536.
131. Felten, D. L., Felten, S. Y., Carlson, S. L., Olschowka, J. A., and Livnat, S. (1985) Noradrenergic and peptidergic innervation of lymphoid tissue. *J. Immunol.* **135,** 755s-765s.
132. McGillis, J. P., Humphreys, S., Rangnekar, V., and Ciallella, J. (1993) Modulation of B lymphocyte differentiation by calcitonin gene-related peptide (CGRP). II. Inhibition of LPS-induced kappa light chain expression by CGRP. *Cell. Immunol.* **150,** 405–416.
133. Borghesi, L. A., Smithson, G., and Kincade, P. W. (1997) Stromal cell modulation of negative regulatory signals that influence apoptosis and proliferation of B-lineage lymphocytes. *J. Immunol.* **159,** 4171–4179.

134. Ball, T. C., Hirayama, F., and Ogawa, M. (1995) Lymphohematopoietic progenitors of normal mice. *Blood* **85,** 3086–3092.
135. Deryugina, E. I., Ratnikov, B. I., Bourdon, M. A., and Müller-Sieburg, C. E. (1994) Clonal analysis of primary marrow stroma: functional homogeneity in support of lymphoid and myeloid cell lines and identification of positive and negative regulators. *Exp. Hematol.* **22,** 910–918.
136. Funk, P. E., Stephan, R. P., and Witte, P. L. (1995) Vascular cell adhesion molecule 1-positive reticular cells express interleukin-7 and stem cell factor in the bone marrow. *Blood* **86,** 2661–2671.
137. King, A. G., Wierda, D., and Landreth, K. S. (1988) Bone marrow stromal cell regulation of B-lymphopoiesis: 1. The role of macrophages, interleukin-1, and interleukin-4 in pre-B cell maturation. *J. Immunol.* **141,** 2016–2026.
138. Jardieu, P., Clark, R., Mortensen, D., and Dorshkind, K. (1994) In vivo administration of insulin-like growth factor-I stimulates primary B lymphopoiesis and enhances lymphocyte recovery after bone marrow transplantation. *J. Immunol.* **152,** 4320–4327.
139. Montecino-Rodriguez, E., Clark, R., Johnson, A., Collins, L., and Dorshkind, K. (1996) Defective B cell development in snell dwarf (*dw/dw*) mice can be corrected by thyroxine treatment. *J. Immunol.* **157,** 3334–3340.
140. Kincade, P. W., Medina, K. L., Smithson, G., and Scott, D. C. (1994) Pregnancy: a clue to normal regulation of B lymphopoiesis. *Immunol. Today* **15,** 539–544.
141. Han, S. H., Zheng, B., Schatz, D. G., Spanopoulou, E., and Kelsoe, G. (1996) Neoteny in lymphocytes: Rag1 and Rag2 expression in germinal center B cells. *Science* **274,** 2094–2097.

Chapter 11

Regulation of Lymphocyte Development by Microenvironmental and Systemic Factors

Encarnacion Montecino-Rodriguez and Kenneth Dorshkind

1. Introduction

Lymphocyte development is a dynamic process in which committed lymphoid precursors progress through a series of defined maturational stages before generating B- and T-cells that express immunoglobulin and the T-cell receptor (TCR), respectively *(1–4)*. This process is regulated by a variety of increasingly well-defined extracellular signals that influence the growth and differentiation of developing lymphoid progenitors.

One source of these stimuli is the hematopoietic microenvironment that supports B- and T-cell development in the bone marrow and thymus, respectively *(5–10)*. The nonhematopoietic stromal cells that constitute these microenvironments mediate their effects by secretion of various cytokines and/or through direct cell-cell interactions with lymphoid progenitors. In addition, there is emerging evidence that lymphopoiesis can be regulated by extramedullary and extrathymic signals, and particular attention has focused on the endocrine system in this regard *(11–13)*.

The aim of this chapter is to provide an overview of these microenvironmental and systemic stimuli, with particular emphasis on those shown to play a critical role in lymphopoiesis.

2. Microenvironmental Regulation of Lymphopoiesis

Much of what is known about the microenvironmental regulation of lymphopoiesis has been learned from the use of various in vitro systems. The development of the Whitlock-Witte culture system was of particular value in dissecting stromal cell regulation of B-cell development. These cultures duplicate aspects of the hematopoietic microenvironment found in the bone marrow in vivo and maintain B lineage cells, ranging from immature precursors to surface IgM-expressing cells, for periods up to several months *(14)*. Comparable culture systems able to support the full range of

From: *Molecular Biology of B-Cell and T-Cell Development*
Edited by: J. G. Monroe and E. V. Rothenberg © Humana Press Inc., Totowa, NJ

intrathymic T-cell development have not been described, although it has been possible to reproduce specific stages of thymopoiesis in vitro by plating thymocyte subpopulations onto heterogeneous thymic stromal cell layers or clonal populations of thymic stroma (reviewed in refs. *15,16*). In the absence of a long-term thymocyte culture system, many laboratories have relied on the fetal thymic organ culture (FTOC) assay. The basic FTOC protocol involves culturing intact murine fetal thymic lobes or lobes depleted of endogenous precursors and reseeded with a source of T-cell precursors. After various periods of time, lobes are dissociated, and the extent of T-cell development is determined *(17)*. The FTOC is the only in vitro system that preserves the three-dimensional organization of the thymus, which is apparently necessary for the full process of T-cell differentiation to take place. These in vitro systems have been of particular value in the identification of cell–cell interactions and soluble signals that regulate lymphocyte development.

2.1. Cell-Cell Interactions

Morphologic observations of the intact bone marrow and thymus clearly demonstrate that developing lymphoid cells are intimately associated with stromal cells *(8,18)*, and these direct cell contacts have been shown to be critical during early lymphoid development. For example, separation of $CD45R^{+/-}$ B-cell progenitors or $CD4^-CD8^-$ thymocyte progenitors from the stroma by culture in diffusion chambers results in marked inhibition of cell growth *(16,19)*.

Multiple cell adhesion molecules are expressed by lymphoid progenitors and stromal cells, and some of these mediate interactions between lymphoid cells and extracellular matrix components *(20)* (Table 1) (Fig. 1), whereas others are involved in lymphocyte-stromal cell binding (Table 1) *(8,9,21–23)*. For example, CD44, the cell surface hyaluronate receptor, is widely distributed on hematopoietic cells, including B- and T-cell progenitors. The addition of anti–CD44 antibodies, or excess amounts of the CD44 ligand hyaluronate, to long-term bone marrow cultures inhibited the binding of developing B lineage cells to the stroma and suppressed their further maturation *(24)*. CD44 is also expressed on immature $CD4^-CD8^-$ thymocytes and has been proposed to be a homing receptor that facilitates entry of bone marrow derived prothymocytes into the thymus *(5)*. BST-1, a glycosyl phosphatidylinositol-anchored protein, is expressed by stromal cells able to support pre–B-cell growth *(25)* and has been implicated in potentiating the growth and maturation of $CD4^-CD8^-$ thymocytes *(26)*. Finally, another cell surface determinant implicated in B and T lymphopoiesis is the VLA-4 integrin. Addition of antibodies to VLA-4 or its ligand VCAM-1 inhibited B lymphopoiesis in long-term bone marrow cultures *(27–29)* and interfered with the binding of $CD4^-CD8^-$ thymocytes to thymic stromal cells and fibronectin *(30,31)*, suggesting an important role for these integrins during lymphopoiesis.

Additional cell surface molecules have been implicated in the regulation of either thymopoiesis or B lymphopoiesis. For example, the KMI-6 determinant is expressed by bone marrow stromal cells at the site of their interaction with pre-B-cells *(32)*. Within the thymus, contacts between developing thymocytes and major histocompatibility complex antigens expressed by thymic epithelial cells are recognized to be critical in the development of the T-cell repertoire *(5)*, and additional cell adhesion molecules that regulate thymocyte growth and maturation are being identified. Addition of antibodies to CD81, a protein expressed by stromal cells in the thymic cortex that has been postulated to be the pre–T-cell receptor ligand, to FTOC blocked the development of TCR $\alpha\beta^+$ thymocytes *(33)*. Similarly, galectin-1, a lectin-like molecule expressed by thymic epithelial cells, has been shown to mediate thymocyte binding to the stroma *(34)*. Finally,

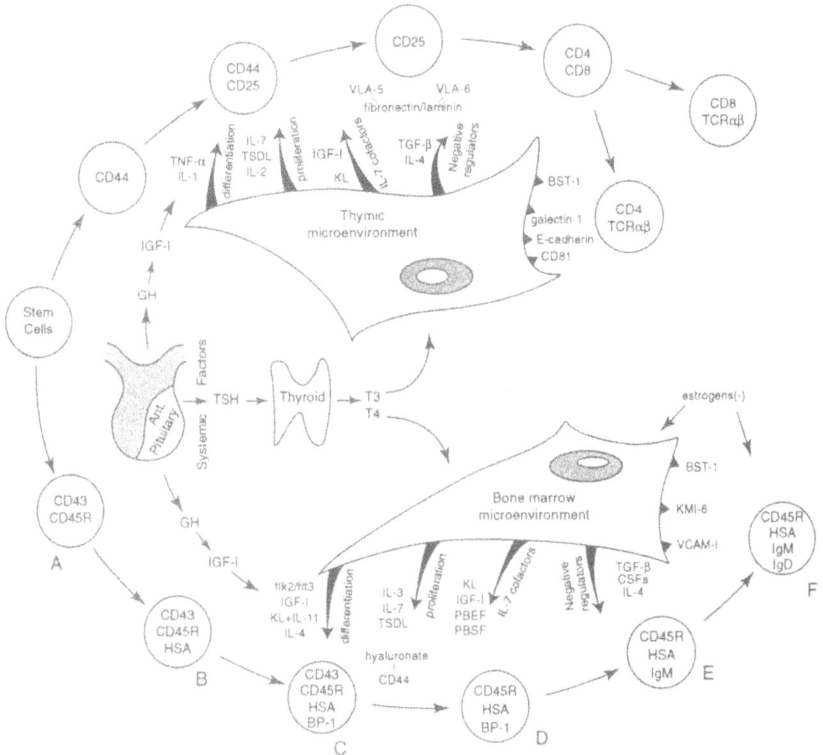

Fig. 1. Regulation of T- and B-cell development by microenvironmental and systemic factors. Cell surface determinants expressed on developing thymocytes and bone marrow B lineage cells at various stages of development are indicated. The definition of B lineage fractions A–F is based on the scheme developed by Hardy et al. *(42)*. Selected cytokines produced by the lymphoid microenvironment and endocrine system implicated in regulation of lymphocyte development are indicated. "Microenvironment" in the figure is used generically to refer to any thymic or marrow population with the potential to secrete factors that regulate B- or T-cell development.

Muller et al. have suggested that homotypic interactions mediated by E-cadherin, a counterpart for the integrin $\alpha_E\beta_7$, which is expressed on both immature thymocytes and thymic epithelial cells, play an important role in early thymocyte development *(35)*. The identification of additional molecules involved in adhesion of lymphoid progenitors to stromal cells can be expected as proteins recognized by antibodies generated against marrow and thymic stromal cells are characterized in more detail.

The aforementioned studies provide circumstantial evidence for the involvement of specific cell adhesion molecules in lymphopoiesis, but whether or not their role is critical for that process is best assessed by analyzing lymphocyte development in knockout mice in which their expression is impaired. Such an analysis demonstrated that α4 integrins are essential for both B- and T-cell development. Arroyo et al. *(36)* disrupted the gene encoding the α4 integrin chain. Although this mutation resulted in embryonic lethality of α4 knockout mice, they were able to assess the role of α4 protein in lymphopoiesis by using the in vivo RAG complementation assay. Analysis of adult $\alpha4^{-/-}$/$RAG^{-/-}$ chimeric mice demonstrated that production of bone marrow B lineage cells was blocked at the pro–B-cell stage, and that their thymus was atrophied and consisted primarily of

Table 1
Selected Cell Adhesion Molecules Involved in Lymphoid Development

Adhesion molecules[a]	Site of expression	Ligand	Function
CD44 *(24)*	B and T lineage cells	Hyaluronate	Adhesion to stroma during early stages of of B and T (?) lymphopoiesis
KMI-6 *(32)*	Stromal cells	*Unknown*	Mediates pre-B-cell adhesion to stroma (?)
CD81 (TAPA-1) *(33)*	Thymic cortical stroma	Pre-T-cell receptor (?)	Necessary for $\alpha\beta$ T-cell development in FTOC
BST-1 *(25)*	Stromal and hematopoietic cells	*Unknown*	Stimulates pre-B-cell and thymocyte growth and development
Galectin-1 *(34)*	Thymic epithelium	Oligosaccharides on thymocytes	Adhesion to stroma
VLA-4 *(27)*	B lineage cells and thymocytes	VCAM-1 and Fibronectin	Adhesion to stroma and extracellular matrix
VLA-5 *(23)*	Thymocytes	Fibronectin	Adhesion to extracellular matrix
VLA-6 *(23)*	Thymocytes	Laminin	Adhesion to extracellular matrix
E-cadherin *(35)*	Thymocytes and thymic epithelium	$\alpha_E\beta_7$–integrin	Homotypic interactions between thymocytes and thymic epithelium

[a] Relevant references regarding these adhesion molecules are given in parenthesis.

double negative thymocytes with few $CD4^+$ $CD8^+$ cells. Although fetal T-cell development progressed normally in the chimeric mice, they showed a reduced number of B-1 (CD5) B-cells in their peritoneal cavity, suggesting that α4 integrins also play a role in the development, migration, and/or survival of these fetal B lineage cells.

2.2. Cytokines

Extensive work performed over the last decade has resulted in the identification of a variety of bone marrow and thymic stromal cell-derived cytokines that can arbitrarily be separated into functional categories based on their ability to stimulate the proliferation of lymphoid progenitors, promote their differentiation, or inhibit those processes *(8,9,37–39)*.

2.2.1. Proliferation Factors

The characterization of stromal cells present in the adherent layer of Whitlock-Witte long-term B-cell cultures revealed that they were the source of an activity, named IL-7, that stimulated the proliferation of B-cell progenitors. The gene encoding IL-7 was subsequently cloned from a transformed stromal cell line *(40)*, and studies with the recombinant cytokine demonstrated that it was able to stimulate thymocyte growth as well *(41)*.

Within the B-cell lineage, progenitors that have undergone D-J rearrangements at the immunoglobulin-heavy chain gene are highly IL-7 responsive *(42)*. Pro-B-cells that have not yet rearranged their immunoglobulin genes may express the IL-7 receptor, but they do not proliferate in response to the factor *(43)*, and pre-B-cells in which the cytoplasmic immunoglobulin μ heavy chain protein is present no longer express the IL-7 receptor *(44)*. Interestingly, in addition to stimulating proliferation of murine B-cell progenitors, IL-7 also plays a distinct role in their differentiation through its apparent ability to potentiate Ig heavy chain gene rearrangements. A single cytoplasmic tyrosine residue in the IL-7 receptor (IL-7R) α chain is essential for cell cycle entry and PI-3 dependent proliferation, whereas a separate and distinct cytoplasmic motif is involved in transmission of signals necessary for differentiation *(44a)*.

In the thymus, IL-7 stimulates the growth of triple negative thymocyte progenitors that do not express CD4, CD8, or the T-cell receptor *(3)*, and acts as a maintenance factor for these thymocytes, which are the most immature intrathymic precursors *(45,46)*. There is recent evidence suggesting that both of these IL-7 functions are a result of the ability of IL-7 to induce bcl-2 gene expression, resulting in an antiapoptotic effect that leads to enhanced cell survival *(46a–d)*. It has also been proposed that IL-7 can promote thymocyte differentiation by potentiating rearrangement of genes that encode the T-cell receptor *(47,47a)*. There is evidence that IL-7 may have a direct effect on TCR-γ rearrangements *(48)*. However, although IL-7 expression by MHC class II^+ epithelial cells is important in creating conditions necessary for TCR-β gene rearrangements *(49)*, the ability of IL-7 to directly potentiate the latter process is controversial *(16,45)*.

The analysis of mice treated with anti-IL-7 *(50)* or anti-IL-7R *(51)* neutralizing antibodies or transgenic animals in which the genes encoding IL-7 *(52)* or its receptor *(53)* have been disrupted demonstrated that IL-7 is an obligate lymphopoietic factor in mice. Although the point at which B-cell development is arrested differs slightly in IL-7 and IL-7R knockout mice, the frequency of $CD45R^+$ IgM^+ cells is severely depressed in their bone marrow. The thymus is also lymphopenic in these mice. Despite this severe effect on primary lymphopoiesis, some mature lymphocytes do accumulate in the absence of IL-7 stimulation and accumulate in peripheral lymphoid organs. However, they are functionally abnormal *(53a)*. Interestingly, human B-cell development does not appear to be dependent upon IL-7 *(53b)*, suggesting that it is controlled by different stimuli *(47a)*.

Additional cytokine(s) with the potential to stimulate the growth of B- and T-cell progenitors have also been reported. Some of these, like thymic stromal cell-derived lymphopoietin *(54)*, can stimulate the growth of both thymocytes and pro-B-cells *(55)*, whereas other factor(s) appear to have differential effects on B- or T-lineage cells. For example, IL-3 has been reported to stimulate the growth of B-cell progenitors. Initial reports of its effects on pre-B-cells *(56)* were controversial, but a key to demonstrating its B lymphopoietic activity appears to be the use of purified B lineage targets *(57,58)*. If heterogeneous populations that contain myeloid precursors are used, IL-3, which is a known growth factor for myeloid progenitors, preferentially stimulates myelopoiesis. There are also numerous reports indicating the potential of various cytokines, such as IL-1, IL-2, IL-3, IL-6, IL-12, and/or c-kit ligand (KL), to stimulate the growth of the most immature $CD4^{lo}$ and $CD44^{+}CD25^{+}$ triple negative thymocytes alone or in combination with IL-7 *(37,45)*. However, the response of B- and T-cell progenitors to one or more of these factors in vitro does not necessarily indicate that they have a critical role in vivo. In fact, the observation that T- and B-cell development in IL-7 and IL-7R knockout mice is severely compromised indicates that none of these cytokines can compensate for the absence of IL-7 during B or T lymphopoiesis.

2.2.2. Proliferation Cofactors

Several additional factors are able to potentiate the proliferative response of lymphoid progenitors to IL-7 in vitro (Fig. 1). In general, these molecules are not able to stimulate significant cell growth when used alone. It is not clear why so many factors that can synergize with IL-7 exist and whether this in vitro activity in fact reflects their role in vivo. Thus, although additional work is required to elucidate their physiologic function, it is clear that at least some of these mediators, such as pre-B-cell growth stimulatory factor (PBSF)/stromal cell-derived factor-1 (SDF-1), play a critical role during early B lymphopoiesis.

The gene encoding PBSF/SDF-1, a member of the CXC group of chemokines, was cloned from a bone marrow stromal cell line that secreted a factor able to stimulate proliferation of a pre-B-cell line *(59)*. Despite this activity on cell lines, PBSF/SDF-1 has little effect on the growth of freshly isolated marrow cells but can potentiate their proliferative response to IL-7. Mice lacking PBSF/SDF-1 as a result of targeted gene inactivation die perinatally and exhibit a number of abnormalities that include a significant reduction of $CD43^{+}CD45R^{+}$ pro-B-cells and pre-B-cells in fetal liver *(60)*. The production of B lineage and myeloid cells in the bone marrow is also impaired. These abnormalities could result from defects in the ability of hematopoietic stem cells to seed to the marrow microenvironment *(61)*. However, since T lymphopoiesis appears to be normal in the PBSF/$SDF^{-/-}$ mice, PBSF/SDF-1 does not seem to be involved in homing of progenitors to the thymus *(60)*.

Several additional factors that can potentiate the response of B- and T-cell progenitors to IL7 have been described and include KL *(62–67)*, pre-B-cell colony enhancing factor *(68)*, Insulin-like growth factor-I (IGF-I) *(69–71)*, and Flk-2/Flt-3 ligand *(72)*.

2.2.3. Differentiation Factors

The extrinsic signals that regulate commitment of hematopoietic precursors to the B- and T-cell lineages are not as well-defined as those that stimulate their proliferation, although the marrow and thymic microenvironments are thought to be the source of such molecules.

It has been relatively easy to demonstrate that thymic stromal cells produce multiple cytokines that include IL-1, IL-3, IL-6, IL-7, IL-12, KL, TNF-α, and various colony stimulating factors *(37,45)* and that some of these factors are critical for normal thymopoiesis in FTOC *(64,73)*. However, the nature of the FTOC system makes it difficult to define the cellular target or stages of development sensitive to these factors. In addition, thymic stromal cells are also the source of various thymic hormones that are thought to affect thymopoiesis *(74,75)*. However, despite an extensive literature describing their effects on developing T-cell progenitors, the function of these thymic peptides during thymopoiesis and whether or not they are necessary for that process has not been demonstrated *(76)*.

Although further studies are needed to identify T-cell differentiation factors, several cytokines have been implicated in early B-cell differentiation. Binding of KL to its receptor, c-kit, has been reported to induce the differentiation of $CD45R^-$ cells to a $CD45R^+$ stage *(65)*. However, this is controversial, and there is much stronger evidence supporting its role as an early B-cell differentiation factor in combination with other cytokines such as IL-7 and IL-11 *(77,78)*. IGF-I, a bone marrow stromal cell-derived factor *(79)*, has been shown to potentiate maturation of lymphohematopoietic precursors into B lineage cells in vitro *(71)*. Finally, Flk-2/Flt-3 ligand was shown to support the differentiation of purified $CD45R^-$ hematopoietic precursors into $CD45R^+$ pro-B-cells *(72)*, and in combination with IL-7 it is also a cofactor for the growth of primitive $CD43^+CD45R^{lo}HSA^-$ B-cell progenitors *(80)*.

Attempts have been made to determine whether one or more of these factors is required for normal B and T lymphopoiesis. Analysis of Flk-2/Flt-3 receptor knockout mice has established that signaling through this receptor is critical for early B lymphopoiesis, since the frequency of cells in the pro-B-cell (Fractions A–C; Fig. 1) compartment was significantly reduced, and pre-B-cells in Fraction D were somewhat reduced. The fact that early B lymphopoiesis in the Flk-2/Flt-3 receptor knockout mice is only partially depressed could be explained by the presence of compensatory cytokines such as IGF-I or KL. In support of this premise was the finding that B lymphopoiesis was more severely impaired in mice with defects in both the Flk-2/Flt-3 and KL pathways *(81)*. However, whereas the c-kit/KL pathway may compensate for deficiencies in the Flk-2/Flt-3 ligand/receptor signaling, it does not appear to be an obligate factor for B lymphopoiesis, since injection of anti-c-kit antibodies into mice does not compromise marrow B-cell production *(66,82)*.

Transient reductions in numbers of immature thymocytes were also observed in Flk-2/Flt-3 receptor knockout mice, and this effect was much more pronounced in animals produced by breeding Flk-2/Flt-3 $receptor^{-/-}$ and c-kit receptor defective W/W^V mice *(81)*. Thus, the expression of both receptors appears to be necessary for the generation of normal thymocyte numbers and frequencies *(81)*. This finding is consistent with studies showing that inclusion of anti–c-kit antibodies in FTOC inhibits thymopoiesis *(64)*. Additional evidence that the c-kit/KL pathway is involved in thymocyte development was obtained by analysis of mice deficient in expression of both c-kit and the common cytokine receptor γ chain. The latter molecule forms complexes with receptors for IL-2, IL-4, IL-7, IL-9, and IL-15. Although B-cells could still be detected in mice deficient in c-kit and γ chain expression, thymocyte development was completely abrogated in mice with mutations in both receptors. The latter result indicates that signaling through both c-kit and γ-chain associated cytokine pathways is required during the earliest stages of normal T-cell development *(83)*.

2.2.4. Inhibitors of Lymphopoiesis

It is becoming increasingly clear that cell production in the hematopoietic system is also regulated by various inhibitory molecules. These factors, which can be of microenvironmental or systemic origin, can act directly on lymphoid precursors or mediate their effects indirectly through actions on cells of the hematopoietic microenvironment *(84)*. For example, transforming growth factor-β *(85,86)*, gamma interferon *(87,88)*, and IL-1 *(84,89)* may act through both mechanisms. The study of negative regulators is further complicated by the fact that even within a single hematopoietic lineage the same factor may stimulate some stages of development and at the same time inhibit others. In this regard, IL-4 has been proposed to potentiate the pre-B to B-cell transition as well as inhibit pro-B-cell growth *(90,91)*. A detailed discussion of this emerging topic is beyond the scope of the present discussion and has recently been reviewed *(39)*.

3. Regulation of Lymphopoiesis by Systemic Factors

In addition to regulatory signals of microenvironmental origin, there is an extensive, and often confusing, literature describing the potential for hormones to affect the development and function of B and T lymphocytes *(11–13)*. However, many of these reports do not distinguish hormonal effects on primary lymphopoiesis from those on secondary differentiation and were performed prior to the development of modern flow cytometric techniques that permit detailed analysis of lymphocyte subpopulations. Renewed interest in defining immune-endocrine interactions has triggered a number of recent studies that have provided new insights into the hormonal regulation of primary lymphocyte development.

3.1. Hormones as Positive Regulators of Lymphopoiesis

There is considerable circumstantial evidence that hormones derived from the anterior pituitary gland are involved in the regulation of primary lymphopoiesis, and much of the data supporting this hypothesis were generated by analysis of the Snell dwarf mouse. These mice are deficient in the production of anterior pituitary-derived growth hormone (GH), thyroid stimulating hormone (TSH), and prolactin *(92,93)*, because of a mutation in the gene encoding the *pit-1* transcription factor, which is required for normal function of hormone-secreting cells in the anterior pituitary gland *(94)*. Since the production of IGF-I and thyroid hormones are regulated by GH and TSH, respectively, dwarf mice are deficient in these hormones as well. The frequency of B lineage cells at stages B-F as defined by Hardy et al. *(42)* (Fig. 1) is significantly depressed in the bone marrow of dwarf mice *(95,96)*, and recent work from the authors' laboratory demonstrating that thyroid hormones can restore B-lymphopoiesis to normal in the mice, has established a key role for the pituitary/thyroid axis in B-cell development *(95)*. This conclusion was confirmed by data showing that B-lymphopoiesis is deficient in the hypothyroid strain of mice, which is selectively deficient in thyroid hormone production as a result of the incapacity of thyroid epithelial cells to respond to TSH, and can be restored to normal by thyroxine treatment *(95)*. Prolactin, GH, or IGF-I failed to restore B lymphopoiesis to normal in dwarf mice (*95* and unpublished observations). The inability of GH, IGF-I, and prolactin to do so was consistent with observations made on Little mice, which are deficient in GH and IGF-I *(97)*, IGF-I knockout mice *(98)*, which have a selective IGF-I deficiency, and prolactin knockout mice *(98a)*, which are deficient in prolactin production. The cellularity of hematopoietic tissue in these mice was normal relative to their size, and the frequencies of the different subpopulations of marrow B lineage cells were not significantly different from values in their +/? littermates *(95,98a)*.

Although these observations suggest that the GH/IGF-I axis does not specifically regulate B-cell development, they do not necessarily exclude a potential effect of GH and/or IGF-I on B lymphopoiesis. Indeed, in vivo studies have demonstrated that the absolute number, but not the frequency, of B lineage cells increases in IGF-I treated mice *(99,100)*. However, these increases in cell numbers occur in parallel with increases in the absolute number of myeloid cells and overall weight gains of the hormone treated mice. In view of these findings, GH and IGF-I would appear to act as general anabolic/somatogenic hormones that have growth promoting effects on cells in multiple tissues, including the hematopoietic system.

There is also an extensive literature suggesting that thyroxine, GH, and IGF-I are thymopoietic factors *(12,13,101–103)*. Indeed, treatment of mice with these hormones can increase thymus cellularity *(99,104)*. Similar to what was observed in the B-cell lineage, this effect parallels the overall growth of the treated mice, and the relative proportions of CD4 and/or CD8 expressing thymocytes were unaffected *(95,103)*. These results thus suggest that the effects of these hormones on T-cell production also result from their general growth promoting properties and that they are not specific regulators of thymopoiesis. Additional studies are needed to determine what role prolactin might play in thymocyte development. Prolactin receptors are expressed intrathymically *(74)*, and there are reports that prolactin-treated dwarf mice have a reduced number of thymocytes *(105)*. However, this effect was not observed in our studies *(98a)*.

The analysis of thymopoiesis in various mice deficient in the production of one or more anterior pituitary hormones further suggests that they are not obligate thymopoietic factors. The frequency of CD4 and/or CD8 expressing thymocyte subpopulations is normal in mice with deficiencies in prolactin GH, IGF-I, and/or thyroid hormone production and, when normalized to the size of the mouse, their thymic cellularity is also normal *(95,98a)*. A report that the frequency of $CD4^+CD8^+$ thymocytes declines at an accelerated rate in dwarf mice *(106)* is not in agreement with these observations. However, the latter effects were not observed in the authors' studies *(100)* or even in additional reports from the same laboratory *(105)*.

3.2. Hormones as Negative Regulators of Lymphopoiesis

The aforementioned information has focused on positive regulation of lymphopoiesis by hormones. However, it has long been recognized that steroid hormones have negative effects on thymopoiesis, and Kincade and colleagues have described the potent negative effects of estrogens on bone marrow B lymphopoiesis *(107–110)*. These negative effects could be mediated directly on B-cell progenitors or indirectly through actions on stromal cells *(107,111)*. Interestingly, the DNA domains to which the thyroid hormone receptor and the estrogen receptor bind are overlapping *(112)*, but whether or not this explains why the estrogens and thyroid hormones seem to have opposite effects on B lymphopoiesis requires further analysis.

3.3. Mechanisms of Hormone Action

The mechanism(s) of action of hormones identified as critical regulators of lymphopoiesis remain to be defined. They could directly affect the growth and/or differentiation of developing lymphoid cells. In support of this premise are results showing that lymphoid progenitors express receptors for GH, prolactin, IGF-I, and thyroid hormones *(13,74,113)*. Alternatively, hormonal effects could be mediated indirectly via induction of other systemic mediators, or through actions on cells of the lymphopoietic microenvironment, since bone marrow and thymic stromal cells express receptors for multiple hormones *(74)*. Binding of a particular hormone to these could then determine whether the stromal cell(s) deliver positive or negative regulatory signals to developing lymphoid cells. In view of this possibility, defining the mechanisms of how hormones regulate lymphoid development will be extremely challenging.

4. Comparative Analysis of B and T Lymphopoiesis

It is evident from the aforementioned information that many of the regulatory signals that control primary B- and T-cell development in the bone marrow and thymus are the same. Thus, both processes are dependent upon direct cell contacts with cells of the lymphoid microenvironment, particularly at the earliest stages of differentiation, and the $\alpha 4$ integrin expressed on developing B- and T-cell progenitors may mediate these interactions. It is clear that murine B- and T-cell development are also strictly dependent upon IL-7, and that other cytokine(s) cannot compensate for the absence of IL-7. However, as noted *(53b)*, IL-7 may not be an essential human lymphopoietic cytokine.

However, despite these many similarities, analysis of the various mutant mice deficient in the production of particular cytokines and hormones indicates that the parameters that regulate B- and T-cell development are not identical. For example, IL-7 actions on developing B- and T-cell progenitors may not be the same. Thus, although IL-7 may induce antiapoptotic signals through bcl-2 gene expression in immature thymocytes, there is no evidence for similar effects in developing B lineage cells *(46b,c)*. Initial analysis of the PBSF/SDF-$1^{-/-}$ and Flk-2/Flt-3 receptor$^{-/-}$ mice indicates that PBSF/SDF-1 and Flk-2/Flt-3 ligand seem to be more critical for B lymphopoiesis than T-cell development, and c-kit/KL signaling pathways appear to more crucial for normal thymopoiesis. Similarly, the study of the various hormone deficient mice indicated that B lymphopoiesis, and not T-cell development, was strictly dependent on thyroid hormones.

These observations may be of relevance when considering strategies to boost the normal production of B- and T lineage cells, as might be necessary during periods of immunodeficiency, or in the design of protocols to inhibit the growth of malignancies that develop in the B- and T-cell developmental pathways.

References

1. Dorshkind, K. (1997) B cell development, in *Comprehensive Toxicology* (Gleen Sipes, I., Jay Gandolfi, A., and McQueen, C. A., eds.), Elsevier, New York, NY, Vol. 5, 57–76.
2. Godfrey, D. I., Kennedy, J., Suda, T., and Zlotnik, A. (1993) A developmental pathway involving four phenotypically distinct subsets of CD3⁻ CD4⁻ CD8⁻ triple-negative adult mouse thymocytes defined by CD44 and CD25 expression. *J. Immunol.* **150,** 4244–4252.
3. Godfrey, D. I. and Zlotnik, A. (1993) Control points in early T cell development. *Immunol. Today* **14,** 547–553.
4. Rothenberg, E. V. (1992) The development of functionally responsive T cells. *Adv. Immunol.* **51,** 85–214.
5. Anderson, G., Moore, N. C., Owen, J. J. T., and Jenkinson, E. J. (1996) Cellular interactions in thymocyte development. *Annu. Rev. Immunol.* **14,** 73–100.
6. Boyd, R. L., Tucek, C. L., Godfrey, D. I., Izon, D. J., Wilson, T. J., Davidson, N. J., Bean, A. G. D., Ladyman, H. M., Ritter, M. A., and Hugo, P. (1993) The thymic microenvironment. *Immunol. Today* **14,** 445–459.
7. Deryugina, E. I. and Muller-Sieburg, C. E. (1993) Stromal cells in long-term cultures: Keys to the elucidation of hematopoietic development? *Crit. Rev. Immunol.* **13,** 115–150.
8. Dorshkind K. (1990) Regulation of hemopoiesis by bone marrow stromal cells and their products. *Annu. Rev. Immunol.* **8,** 111–137.
9. Kincade, P. W., Lee, G., Pietrangeli, C. E., Hayashi, S. I., and Gimble, J. M. (1989) Cells and molecules that regulate B lymphopoiesis in bone marrow. *Annu. Rev. Immunol.* **7,** 111–143.

10. van Ewjik, W. (1991) T-cell differentiation is influenced by thymic microenvironments. *Annu. Rev. Immunol.* **9,** 591–615.
11. Clark, R. (1997) The somatogenic hormones and insulin-like growth factor-I: Stimulators of lymphopoiesis and immune function. *Endocrine Rev.* **18,** 1–23.
12. Hooghe-Peters, E. L. and Hooghe, R. (1995) Growth hormone, prolactin, and IGF-I as lymphohemopoietic cytokines, R. G. Lancles, Austin, Tx.
13. Kooijman, R., Hooghe-Peters, E. L., and Hooghe, R. (1996) Prolactin, growth hormone, and insulin-like growth factor-I in the immune system. *Adv. Immunol.* **63,** 377–454.
14. Whitlock, C. and Witte, O. N. (1982) Long-term culture of B lymphocytes and their precursors from murine bone marrow. *Proc. Natl. Acad. Sci. USA* **79,** 3608–3512.
15. Montecino-Rodriguez, E. and Dorshkind, K. (1997) Thymocyte development in vitro: implications for studies of ageing and thymic involution. *Mech. Ageing Dev.* **93,** 47–57.
16. Montecino-Rodriguez, E. and Dorshkind, K. (1996) Long-term culture of triple negative thymocytes. *J. Immunol.* **156,** 957–962.
17. Jenkinson, E. and Owen, J. J. T. (1990) T cell differentiation in thymus organ cultures. *Semin. Immunol.* **16,** 12–19.
18. Dorshkind, K., Schouest, L., Fletcher, W. H. (1985) Morphologic analysis of long-term bone marrow cultures that support B-lymphopoiesis or myelopoiesis. *Cell Tissue Res.* **239,** 375–382.
19. Kierney, P. C. and Dorshkind, K. (1987) B lymphocyte precursors and myeloid progenitors survive in diffusion chamber cultures but B cell differentiation requires close association with stromal cells. *Blood* **70,** 1418–1424.
20. Lannes-Vicira, J., Dardenne, M., and Savino, W. (1991) Extracellular matrix components of the mouse thymus microenvironment: Ontogenetic studies and modulation by glucocorticoid hormones. *J. Histochem. Cytochem.* **39,** 1539–1546.
21. Le, P. T. and Singer, K. H. (1993) Human thymic epithelial cells: Adhesion molecules and cytokine production. *Int. J. Clin. Lab. Res.* **23,** 56–60.
22. Oritani, K. and Kincade, P. W. (1996) Identification of stromal cell products that interact with pre-B cells. *J. Cell Biol.* **134,** 771–782.
23. Patel, D. D. and Haynes, B. F. (1993) Cell adhesion molecules involved in intrathymic T cell development. *Sem. Immunol.* **5,** 283–292.
24. Miyake, K., Underhill, C. B., Lesley, J., and Kincade, P. W. (1990) Hyaluronate can function as a cell adhesion molecule and CD44 participates in hyaluronate recognition. *J. Exp. Med.* **172,** 69–75.
25. Kaisho T., Ishikawa, J., Oritami, K., Inazawa, J., Tomizawa, H., Muraoka, O., Ochi, T., and Hirano, T. (1994) BST-1, a surface molecule of bone marrow stromal cell lines that facilitates pre-B-cell growth. *Proc. Natl. Acad. Sci. USA* **91,** 5325–5329.
26. Vicari, A. P., Bean, A. G., and Zlotniik, A. (1996) A role for BP-3/BST-1 antigen in early T cell development. *Int. Immunol.* **8,** 183–191.
27. Kina T., Majumdar, A. S., Heimfeld, S., Kaneshima, H., Holzmann, B., Katsura, Y., and Weissman, I. L. (1991) Identification of a 107 kD glycoprotein that mediates adhesion between stromal cells and hematolymphoid cells. *J. Exp. Med.* **173,** 373–381.
28. Miyake, K., Medina, K., Ishihara, K., Kimoto, M., Auerbach, R., and Kincade, P. W. (1994) A VCAM like adhesion molecule on murine bone marrow stromal cells mediates binding of lymphocyte precursors in culture. *J. Cell. Biol.* **114,** 557–565.
29. Miyake K., Weissman, I. L., Greenberger, J. S., and Kincade, P. W. (1991) Evidence for a role of the integrin VLA-4 in lympho-hemopoiesis. *J. Exp. Med.* **173,** 599–607.
30. Sawada, M., Nagamine, J., Takeda, K., Utsumi, K., Koshugi, A., Tatsumi, Y., Hamaoka, T., Miyake, K., Nakajima, K., Watanabe, T., Sakakibara, S., and Fujiwara, H. (1992) Expression of VLA-4 on thymocytes: maturation state-associated transition and its correlation with their capacity to adhere to thymic stromal cells. *J. Immunol.* **149,** 3517–3524.
31. Utsumi, K., Sawada, M., Narumiya, S., Namamine, J., Sakata, T., Iwagami, S., Kita, Y., Teraoka, H., Hirano, H., Ogata, M., Hamaoka, T., and Fujiwara, H. (1991) Adhesion of immature thymocytes to thymic stromal cells through fibronectin molecules and its significance for the induction of thymocyte differentiation. *Proc. Natl. Acad. Sci. USA* **88,** 5685–5689.
32. Jacobsen K., Miyake, K., Kincade, P. W., and Osmond, D. G. (1992) Highly restricted expression of a stromal cell determinant in mouse bone marrow in vivo. *J. Exp. Med.* **176,** 927–935.
33. Boismenu, R., Rhein, M., Fischer, W. H., and Havran, W. L. (1996) A role for CD81 in early T cell development. *Science* **271,** 198–200.

34. Baum, L. G., Pang, M., Perillo, N. L., Wu, T., Delegeane, A., Uittenbogaart, C. H., Fukuda, M., and Seilhamer, J. J. (1995) Human thymic epithelial cells express an endogenous lectin, galectin-1, which binds to core 2 O-glycans on thymocytes and T lymphoblastoid cells. *J. Exp. Med.* **181,** 877–887.
35. Muller, K. M., Luedecker, C. J., Udoy, M. C., and Farr, A. G. (1997) Involvement of E-cadherin in thymus organogenesis and thymocyte maturation. *Immunity* **6,** 257–264.
36. Arroyo, A. G., Yang, J. T., Rayburn, H., and Hynes, R. O. (1996) Differential requirements for α4 integrins during fetal and adult hematopoiesis. *Cell* **85,** 997–1008.
37. Carding, S. R., Hayday, A. C., and Bottomly, K. (1991) Cytokines in T-cell development. *Immunol. Today* **12,** 239–245.
38. Dorshkind, K. (1997) Growth and differentiation factors that regulate B lymphocyte development. *Weir's Handbook of Experimental Immunology.* 5th ed., 81.1–81.12.
39. Marshall, E. and Lord, B. I. (1996) Feedback inhibitors in normal and tumor tissues. *Int. Rev. Cytol.* **167,** 185–261.
40. Namen, A. E., Lupton, S., Hjerrild, K., Wagnall, J., Mochizuki, D. Y., Schmierer, A., Mosley, B., March, C., Urdal, D., Gillis, S., Cosman, D., and Goodwin, R. G. (1988) Stimulation of B cell progenitors by cloned murine interleukin-7. *Nature* **333,** 571–573.
41. Morrissey, P. J., Goodwin, R. G., Norda, R. P., Anderson, D., Grabstein, K. H., Cosman, D., Sims, J., Lupaton, S., Acres, B., Reed, S. G., Mochizuki, D., Eisenman, J., Conlon, P. J., and Namen, A. E. (1989) Recombinant interleukin-7, pre-B cell growth factor, has costimulatory activity on purified mature T cells. *J. Exp. Med.* **169,** 707–716.
42. Hardy, R. R., Carmack, C. E., Shinton, S. A., Kemp, J. D., and Hayakawa, K. (1991) Resolution and characterization of pro-B and pre-pro-B cell stages in normal mouse bone marrow. *J. Exp. Med.* **173,** 1213–1225.
43. Faust, E. A., Saffran, D. C., Toksoz, D., Williams, D. A., and Witte, O. N. (1993) Distinctive growth requirements and gene expression patterns distinguish progenitor B cells from pre-B cells. *J. Exp. Med.* **177,** 915–923.
44. Henderson, A. J., Narayanan, R., Collins, L., and Dorshkind, K. (1992) Status of kL chain gene rearrangements and c-kit and IL-7 receptor expression in stromal cell-dependent pre-B cells. *J. Immunol.* **149,** 1973–1979.
44a. Corcoran, A. E., Smart, F. M., Cowling, R. J., Crompton, T., Owen, M. J., and Venkitaraman, A. R. (1996) The interleukin-7 receptor α chain transmits distinct signals for proliferation and differentiation during B lymphopoiesis. *EMBO J.* **15,** 1924–1932.
45. Moore, T. A. and Zlotnik, A. (1995) T-cell lineage commitment and cytokine responses of thymic progenitors. *Blood* **86,** 1850–1860.
46. Suda, T. and Zlotnik, A. (1991) IL-7 maintains the T cell precursor potential of $CD3^-$ $CD4^-$ $CD8^-$ thymocytes. *J. Immunol.* **146,** 3068–3073.
46a. von Freeden-Jeffry, U., Solvasson, N., Howard, M., and Murray, R., (1997) The earliest T lineage-committed cells depend on IL-7 for bcl-2 expression and normal cell cycle progression. *Immunity* **7,** 147–154.
46b. Kondo, M., Akashi, K., Domen, J., Sugamura, K., and Weissman, I. L. (1997) Bcl-2 rescues T lymphopoiesis, but not B or NK cell development, in common γ chain-deficient mice. *Immunity* **7,** 155–162.
46c. Akashi, K., Kondo, M., von Freeden-Jeffry, U., Murray, R., and Wiessman, I. L. (1997) Bcl-2 rescues T lymphopoiesis in interleukin-7 receptor-deficient mice. *Cell* **89,** 1033–1041.
46d. Maraskovski, E., O'Reilly, L. A., Teepe, M., Corcoran, L. M., Peschon, J. J., and Strasser, A. (1997) Bcl-2 can rescue T lymphocyte development in interleukin-7 receptor-deficient mice but not in mutant rag-$1^{-/-}$ mice. *Cell* **89,** 1011–1019.
47. Muegge, K., Vila, M., and Durum, S. (1993) Interleukin 7: a cofactor for V(D)J rearrangement of the T cell receptor gene. *Science* **261,** 923–96.
47a. Candeias, S., Muegge, K., and Durum, S. K. (1997) IL-7 receptor and VDJ recombination: trophic versus mechanistic actions. *Immunity* **6,** 501–508.
48. Appasamy, P. M., Kenniston, T. W., Weng, Y., Holt, E. C., Kost, J., and Chambers, W. H. (1993) Interleukin-7 induced expression of specific T cell receptor γ variable region genes in murine fetal liver cultures. *J. Exp. Med.* **178,** 2201–2206.
49. Oosterwegel, M. A., Haks, M. C., Jeffry, U., Murray, R., and Kruisbeek, A. M. (1997) Induction of TCR gene rearrangements in uncommitted stem cells by a subset of IL-7 producing, MHC class II-expressing thymic stromal cells. *Immunity* **6,** 351–360.

50. Grabstein K. H., Waldschmidt, T. J., Finkelman, F. D., Hess, B. W., Alpert, A. R., Bolani, N. E., Namen, A. E., and Morrissey, P. J. (1993) Inhibition of murine B and T lymphopoiesis in vivo by an anti-interleukin 7 monoclonal antibody. *J. Exp. Med.* **178,** 257–264.
51. Sudo, T., Nishikawa, S., Ohno, N., Aklyama, N., Tamakoshi, M., Yoshida, H., and Nishikawa, S. (1993) Expression and function of the interleukin 7 receptor in murine lymphocytes. *Proc. Natl. Acad. Sci. USA* **90,** 9125–9129.
52. von Freeden-Jeffry, U., Vieira, P., Lucian, L. A., McNeil, T., Burdach, S. E. G., and Murray, R. (1995) Lymphopenia in interleukin (IL)-7, gene-deleted mice identifies IL-7 as a nonredundant cytokine. *J. Exp. Med.* **181,** 1519–1526.
53. Peschon, J. J., Morrissey, P. J., Grabstein, K. H., Ramsdell, F. J., Maraskovsky, E., Gliniak, B. C., Park, L. S., Ziegler, S. F., Williams, D. E., Ware, C. B., Meyer, D., and Davison, B. L. (1994) Early lymphocyte expansion is severely impaired in interleukin 7 receptor-deficient mice. *J. Exp. Med.* **180,** 1955–1960.
53a. Maraskovsky, E., Teepe, M., Morrissey, P. J., Braddy, S., Miller, R. E., Lynch, D. H., and Peschon, J. J. (1996) Impaired survival and proliferation in IL-7 receptor-deficient peripheral T cells. *J. Immunol.* **157,** 5315–5323.
53b. Pribyl, J. A. R. and LeBien, T. W. (1996) Interleukin 7 independent development of human B cells. *Proc. Natl. Acad. Sci. USA* **93,** 10,348–10,353.
54. Friend, S. L., Hosier, S., Nelson, A., Foxworthe, D., Williams, D. E., and Farr, A. (1994) A thymic stromal cell line supports in vitro development of surface IgM$^+$ B cells and produces a novel growth factor affecting B and T lineage cells. *Exp. Hematol.* **22,** 321–328.
55. Ray, R. J., Furlonger, C., Williams, D. E., and Paige, C. J. (1996) Characterization of thymic stromal-derived lymphopoietin (TSLP) in murine B cell development in vitro. *Eur. J. Immunol.* **26,** 10–16.
56. Palacios, R. G., Henson, G., Steinmetz, M., and McKearn, J. P. (1984) Interleukin-3 supports growth of mouse pre-B cell clones in vitro. *Nature* **309,** 126–131.
57. Rennick, D., Jackson, J., Moulds, C., Lee, F., and Yang, G. (1989) IL-3 and stromal cell derived factor synergistically stimulate the growth of pre-B cell lines cloned from long-term lymphoid bone marrow cultures. *J. Immunol.* **142,** 161–166.
58. Winkler, T. H., Melchers, F., and Rolink, A. G. (1995) Interleukin-3 and Interleukin-7 are alternative growth factors for the same B-cell precursors in the mouse. *Blood* **85,** 2045–2051.
59. Nagasawa, T., Kikutani, H., and Kishimoto, T. (1994) Molecular cloning and structure of a pre-B cell growth stimulating factor. *Proc. Natl. Acad. Sci. USA* **91,** 2305–2309.
60. Nagasawa, T., Hirota, S., Tachibana, K., Takakura, N., Nishikawa, S., Kitamura, Y., Yoshida, N., Kikutani, H., and Kishimoto, T. (1996) Defects of B-cell lymphopoiesis and bone-marrow myelopoiesis in mice lacking the CXC chemokine PBSF/SDF-1. *Nature* **382,** 635–638.
61. Aiuti, A., Webb, I. J., Bleul, C., Springer, T., and Gutierrez-Ramos, J. C. (1997) The chemokine SDF-1 is a chemoattractant for human CD34$^+$ hematopoietic progenitor cells and provides a new mechanisms to explain the mobilization of CD34$^+$ progenitors to peripheral blood. *J. Exp. Med.* **185,** 111–120.
62. Billips, L. G., Petitte, D., Dorshkind, K., Narayanan, R., Chiu, C. P., and Landreth, K. S. (1992) Differential roles of stromal cells, interleukin-7, and kit-ligand in the regulation of B lymphopoiesis. *Blood* **79,** 1185- 1192.
63. Funk, P. E., Varas, A., Witte, P. L. (1993) Activity of stem cell factor and IL-7 in combination on normal bone marrow B lineage cells. *J. Immunol.* **150,** 748–752.
64. Godfrey, D. I., Zlotnik, A., and Suda, T. (1992) Phenotypic and functional characterization of c- kit expression during intrathymic T cell development. *J. Immunol.* **149,** 2281–2285.
65. McNeice, I. K., Langley, K. E., and Zsebo, K. M. (1991) The role of recombinant stem cell factor in early B cell development. *J. Immunol.* **146,** 3785–3790.
66. Ogawa, M., Matsuzaki, Y., Nishikawa, S., Hayashi, S. I., Kunisada, T., Sudo, T., Kina, T., Nakauchi, H., and Nishikawa, S. I. (1991) Expression and function of c-kit in hemopoietic progenitor cells. *J. Exp. Med.* **174,** 63–71.
67. Rolink, A., Streb, M., Nishikawa, S. I., and Melchers, F. (1991) The c-kit encoded tryrosine kinase regulates the proliferation of early pre-B cells. *Eur. J. Immunol.* **21,** 2609–2612.
68. Samal, B., Sun, Y., Stearns, G., Xie, C., Suggs, S., and McNiece, I. (1994) Cloning and characterization of the cDNA encoding a novel human pre-B cell-colony enhancing factor. *Mol. Cell. Biol.* **14,** 1431–1437.

69. Funk, P., Kincade, P. W., Witte, P. L. (1994) Native associations of early hematopoietic stem cells and stromal cells involved in cell aggregates. *Blood* **83,** 361–369.
70. Gibson, L. F., Piktel, D., and Landreth, K. S. (1993) Insulin like growth factor-I potentiates expansion of interleukin-7 dependent pro-B cells. *Blood* **82,** 3005–3011.
71. Landreth, K. S., Narayanan, R., and Dorshkind, K. (1992) Insulin-like growth factor-I regulates pro-B cell differentiation. *Blood* **80,** 1207–1212.
72. Hirayama, F., Lyman, S. D., Clark, S. C., and Ogawa, M. (1995) The flt3 ligand supports proliferation of lymphohematopoietic progenitors and early B-lymphoid progenitors. *Blood* **85,** 1762–1768.
73. Zuniga-Pflucker, J. C., Jiang, D., and Lenardo, M. (1995) Requirement for TNF-α and IL-1α in fetal thymocyte commitment and differentiation. *Science* **268,** 1906–1909.
74. Dardenne, M. and Savino, W. (1994) Control of thymus physiology by peptidic hormones and neuropeptides. *Immunol. Today* **15,** 518–523.
75. Millington, G. and Buckingham, J. C. (1995) Thymic peptides and neuroendocrine-immune communication. *J. Endocrinol.* **133,** 163–168.
76. Cordero, O. J., Maurer, H. R., and Nogueira, M. (1997) Novel approaches to immunotherapy using thymic peptides. *Immunol. Today* **18,** 10–13.
77. Cumano, A., Kee, B. L., Ramsden, D. A., Marshall, A., Paige, C. J., and Wu, G. E. (1994) Development of B lymphocytes from lymphoid committed and uncommitted progenitors. *Immunol. Rev.* **137,** 5–33.
78. Kee, B. L., Cumano, A., Iscove, N. N., and Paige, C. J. (1994) Stromal cell independent growth of bipotent B cell-macrophage precursors from murine fetal liver. *Int. Immunol.* **6,** 401–407.
79. Abboud S. L., Bethel C. R., and Aron D. C. (1991) Secretion of insulin-like growth factor I and insulin-like growth factor-binding proteins by murine bone marrow stromal cells. *J. Clin. Invest.* **88,** 470–475.
80. Hunte, B. E., Hudak, S., Campbell, D., Su, Y., and Rennick, D. (1995) flk2/flt3 ligand is a potent cofactor for the growth of primitive B cell progenitors. *J. Immunol.* **156,** 489–496.
81. Mackarehtschian, K., Hardin, J. D., Moore, K. A., Boest, S., Goff, S. P., and Lemischka, I. R. (1995) Targeted disruption of the flk2/flt/3 gene leads to deficiencies in primitive hematopoietic progenitors. *Immunity* **3,** 147–161.
82. Rico-Vargas, S. A., Weiskopf, B., Nishikawa, S., and Osmond, D. G. (1994) c-kit expression by B cell precursors in mouse bone marrow: stimulation of B cell genesis by in vivo treatment with anti-c-kit antibody. *J. Immunol.* **152,** 2845–2852.
83. Rodewald, H.-R., Ogawa, M., Haller, C., Waskow, C., and DiSanto, J. P. (1997) Prothymocyte expansion by c-kit and the common cytokine receptor γ chain is essential for repertoire formation. *Immunity* **6,** 265–272.
84. Dorshkind K. (1988) IL-1 inhibits B cell differentiation in long term bone marrow cultures. *J. Immunol.* **141,** 531–538.
85. Hayashi, S. I., Gimble, J. M., Henley, A., Ellingsworth, L. R., and Kincade, P. W. (1989) Differential effects of TGF-β on lymphohemopoiesis in long-term bone marrow cultures. *Blood* **74,** 1711–1717.
86. Lee G., Namen, A. E., Gillis, S., Ellingsworth, L. R., and Kincade, P. W. (1989) Normal B cell precursors responsive to recombinant IL-7 and inhibition of IL-7 activity by transforming growth factor-β. *J. Immunol.* **142,** 3875–3883.
87. Gimble, J. M., Medina, K., Hudson, J., Robinson, M., and Kincade, P. W. (1993) Modulation of lymphohematopoiesis in long-term cultures by gamma interferon: direct and indirect action on lymphoid and stromal cells. *Exp. Hematol.* **21,** 224–230.
88. Grawunder U., Melchers, F., and Rolink, A. (1993) Interferon-gamma arrests proliferation and causes apoptosis in stromal cell/interleukin-7-dependent normal murine pre-B cells lines and clones in vitro, but does not induce differentiation to surface immunoglobulin-positive B cells. *Eur. J. Immunol.* **23,** 544–551.
89. Suda T., Okada, S., Suda, J., et al. (1989) A stimulatory effect of recombinant murine interleukin-7 (IL-7) on B cell colony formation and an inhibitory effect of IL-1α. *Blood* **74,** 1936–1941.
90. Billips, L. G., Petitte, D., and Landreth, K. S. (1990) Bone marrow stromal cell regulation of B lymphopoiesis: Interleukin-1 (IL-1) and IL-4 regulate stromal cell support of pre-B cell production in vitro. *Blood* **75,** 611–619.
91. King, A., Wierda, D., and Landreth, K. S. (1988) Bone marrow stromal cell regulation of B lymphopoiesis: I. The role of macrophages, interleukin-1, and interleukin-4 in pre-B cell maturation. *J. Immunol.* **141,** 2016–2026.

92. Cross, R. J., Bryson, J. S., and Roszman, T. L. (1992) Immunologic disparity in the hypopituitary dwarf mouse. *J. Immunol.* **148,** 1347–1352.
93. Fabris, N., Pierpaoli, W., and Sorkin, W. (1971) Hormones and the immunological capacity. III. The immunodeficiency disease of the hypopituitary Snell-bagg dwarf mouse. *Clin. Exp. Immunol.* **9,** 209–225.
94. Li, S., Crenshaw 3d, E. B., Rawson, E. J., Simmons, D. M., Swanson, L. W., and Rosenfeld, M. G. (1990) Dwarf locus mutants lacking three pituitary cell types result from mutations in the pou-domain gene pit-1. *Nature* **347,** 528–533.
95. Montecino-Rodriguez, E., Clark, R., Powell-Braxton, L., and Dorshkind, K. Primary B cell development is impaired in mice with defects of the pituitary/thyroid axis. *J. Immunol.* **159,** 2712–2719.
96. Murphy, W. J., Durum, S. K., Anver, M. R., and Longo, D. L. (1992) Immunologic and hematologic effects of neuroendocrine hormones: studies on Dw/J Dwarf Mice. *J. Immunol.* **148,** 3799–3805.
97. Lin, S. C., Lin, C. R., Gukovsky, I., Lusis, A. J., Sawchenko, P. E., and Rosenfeld, M. G. (1993) Molecular basis of the little mouse phenotype and implications for cell type-specific growth. *Nature* **364,** 208–213.
98. Powell-Braxton, L., Hollingshead, P., Warburton, C., Dowd, M., Pittes-Meek, S., Dalton, D., Gillett, N., and Stewart, T. A. (1993) IGF-I is required for normal embryonic growth in mice. *Genes Dev.* **7,** 2609–2617.
98a. Horseman, N. D., Zhao, W., Montecino-Rodriguez, E., Tanaka, M., Nakashima, K., Engle, S. J., Smith, F., Markoff, E., and Dorshkind, K. (1997) Defective mammopoiesis, but normal hematopoiesis, in mice with a targeted in disruption of the prolactin gene. *EMBO J.* **16,** 6926–6935.
99. Jardieu, P., Clark, R., Mortensen, D., and Dorshkind, K. (1994) In vivo administration of insulin-like growth factor-1 stimulates primary B lymphopoiesis and enhances lymphocyte recovery after bone marrow transplantation. *J. Immunol.* **152,** 4320–4327.
100. Montecino-Rodriguez, E., Clark, R., Johnson, A., Collins, L., and Dorshkind, K. (1996) Defective B cell development in Snell dwarf (dw/dw) mice can be corrected by thyroxine treatment. *J. Immunol.* **157,** 3334–3340.
101. Savino, W., Mello-Cohelo, V., and Dardenne, M. (1995) Control of the thymic microenvironment by growth hormone/insulin-like growth factor-I-mediated circuits. *Neuroimmunomodulation* **2,** 313–318.
102. Taub, D. D., Tsarfaty, G., Lloyd, A. R., Durum, S. K., Longo, D. L., and Murphy, W. J. (1994) Growth hormone promotes human T cell adhesion and migration to both human and murine matrix proteins and directly promotes xenogeneic engraftment. *J. Clin. Invest.* **94,** 293–300.
103. Villa-Verde, D. M. S., De Mello-Cohelo, V., Farias-De-Olivera, D. A., Dardenne, M., and Savino, W. (1993) Pleitropic influence of triiodothyronine on thymus physiology. *Endocrinology* **133,** 867–875.
104. Clark, R., Strasser, J., McCabe, S., Robbins, K., and Jardieu, P. (1993) Insulin-like growth factor-I stimulation of lymphopoiesis. *J. Clin. Invest.* **92,** 540–548.
105. Murphy, W. J., Durum, S. K., and Longo, D. L. (1993) Differential effects of growth hormone and prolactin on murine T cell development and function. *J. Exp. Med.* **178,** 231–236.
106. Murphy, W. J., Durum, S. K., and Longo, D. L. (1992) Role of neuroendocrine hormones in murine T cell development. *J. Immunol.* **149,** 3851–3857.
107. Kincade, P. W., Medina, K., and Smithson, G. (1994) Sex hormones as negative regulators of lymphopoiesis. *Immunol. Rev.* **137,** 119–134.
108. Masuzawa, T, Miyaura, C, Onoe, Y, Kusano, K, Ohta, H., Nozawa, S. C., and Suda, T. (1994) Estrogen deficiency stimulates B lymphopoiesis in mouse bone marrow. *J. Clin. Invest.* **94,** 1090–1097.
109. Medina, K. L., Kincade, P. W. (1994) Pregnancy-related steroids are potential negative regulators of B lymphopoiesis. *Proc. Natl. Acad. Sci. USA* **91,** 5382–5386.
110. Medina, K. L, Smithson, G., Kincade, P. W. (1993) Suppression of B lymphopoiesis during normal pregnancy. *J. Exp. Med.* **178,** 1507–1515.
111. Smithson, G., Medina, K., Ponting, I., and Kincade, P. W. (1995) Estrogen suppresses stromal cell dependent lymphopoiesis in culture. *J. Immunol.* **155,** 3409–3417.
112. Jameson, L. J. and DeGroot, L. J. (1995) Mechanisms of thyroid hormone action, in *Endocrinology* (DeGroot, L. J., ed.), W. B. Saunders Co., Philadelphia, pp. 583–616.
113. Gagnerault, M. C., Postel-Vinay, M. C., and Dardenne, M. (1996) Expression of growth hormone receptors in murine lymphoid cells analyzed by flow cytofluorometry. *Endocrinology* **137,** 1719–1726.

Chapter 12

Cytokines and Chemokines in T-Cell Development

Albert Zlotnik, Myriam Capone, and Alain P. Vicari

1. Introduction

1.1. T-Cell Development in the Last 15 Years

The history of T-cell development is highly connected to the physiology of the thymus. Following the pioneering observations of J. F. A. P. Miller on the role of the thymus in T lymphocyte production, many laboratories have studied the events that take place in this gland. As shall be reviewed in this chapter and elsewhere in this book, the events known to take place in the thymus have remained fundamentally unchanged and include: colonization of the thymus by bone-marrow derived precursors; commitment to the T-cell lineage; rearrangement of the TCR genes; selection of T-cells according to their MHC and antigenic specificity, and finally, export from the thymus to the periphery. However, new molecular insights obtained more recently have reaffirmed these events. During the 1980s, the main interest of most T-cell development labs focused on the selection mechanisms that resulted in the T-cell repertoire. This was prompted by the molecular characterization of the T-cell receptor, as well as the availability of reagents (monoclonal antibodies, and so forth), which allowed the demonstration of positive and negative selection. Only a few labs focused instead on the earlier events of T-cell development, before positive and negative selection take place. More recently, this situation has changed with more labs studying the early events of T-cell development in the thymus. We have really only begun to understand the basic events that take place before the $CD4^+CD8^+$ (double positive [DP]) stage. This situation means that many basic and important developments await to be discovered and understood in early T-cell development.

From: *Molecular Biology of B-Cell and T-Cell Development*
Edited by: J. G. Monroe and E. V. Rothenberg © Humana Press Inc., Totowa, NJ

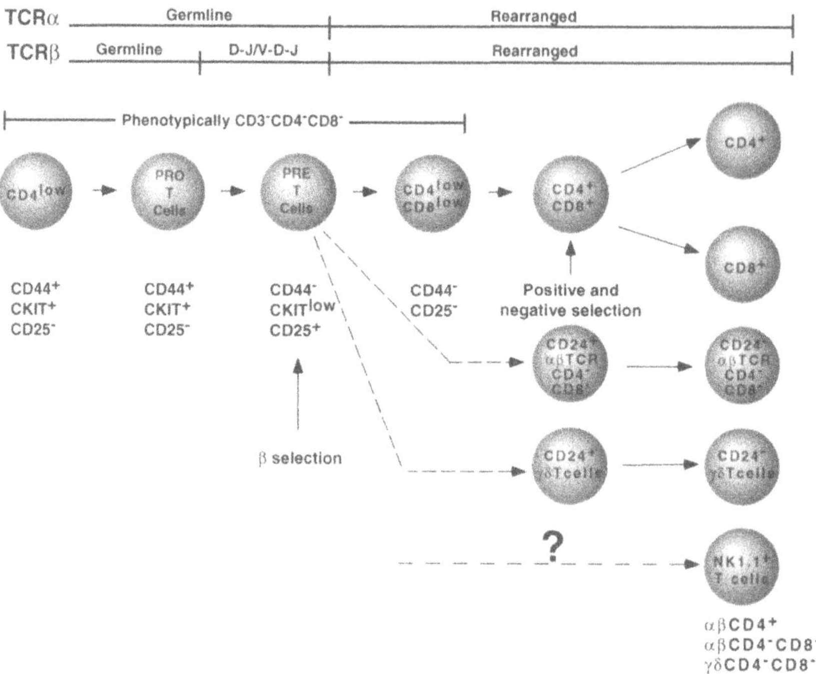

Fig. 1. Intrathymic T-cell development.

1.2. Developing Thymocytes Spend Most of their Time in the Thymus at the CD3⁻CD4⁻CD8⁻ (Triple Negative) Stage

Several developments have renewed interest in early T-cell development. These include the production of knockout mice using homologous recombination, the increased understanding of the events that take place during this period, and finally, the fact that, following 10 years of intense research, the current thinking on positive and negative selection involves the affinity/avidity model, which envisions that the resulting T-cell repertoire is selected from a population of T-cells with moderate (but not high) affinity for self major histocompatability (MHC), whereas negative selection aims at the elimination of cells recognizing self antigens (or at least those present in the thymus at the time) with high affinity (reviewed elsewhere in this book). The relative acceptance of this model has redirected several T-cell development labs to other areas where the understanding of the events that take place is still poor. Such is the case of early T-cell development where increased understanding of the events that take place here points to very interesting unanswered questions for which no real clues exist. Another important clue to the importance of the triple negative (TN) stage of T-cell development comes from the fact that T-cells are likely to spend most of their time in the thymus at this stage. If a fetal thymus depleted of thymocytes (using 2-deoxyguanosine, in an in vitro model of T-cell development called fetal thymus organ culture (FTOC) *(1)* is repopulated with a very early stage of T-cell precursor from the TN stage, it is necessary to wait several weeks (depending on which specific stage is used) before single positive (SP; $CD3^+CD4^+$ or $CD3^+CD8^+$) mature T-cells are detected. The latter cells include the cells that will eventually be exported from the thymus. A schematic representation of the known main events in intrathymic T-cell development are depicted in Fig. 1. In contrast, if $CD3^{lo}$ DP thymocytes are used to repopulate the same FTOC, SP thymocytes can be detected within one week. This observation strongly suggests that developing T-cells spend most of their time at the TN stage, a conclusion that gets further support from the complexity of events that occur at this stage.

1.3. Three Distinct T-Cell Sublineages Develop in the Thymus

Three T-cell sublineages have been identified in the thymus and elsewhere in the body. The first one is the classic CD4 and CD8 SP T-cells, the second is the $\gamma\delta$ T-cells, and the third one is the NK1.1$^+$ T-cells, which include the $\alpha\beta$TCR$^+$ DN and the CD4+NK1.1$^+$ T-cells *(2)*, as well as a subset of $\gamma\delta$TCR$^+$ DN NK1.1+ T-cells that the authors recently identified in the thymus *(3)*. As will be detailed in this chapter, each one of these sublineages exhibits specific cytokine production patterns, as well as distinct proliferation patterns in response to specific cytokines or combinations thereof. Indeed, these three sublineages of T-cells probably exit the thymus at a stage where they will be functionally very close to their peripheral counterparts and exert their specific physiological function. Pro-T-cells (described in Subheading 2.1.2.) are the precursors of all these sublineages. Thus, several questions arise: when and how are these characteristics acquired during T-cell development? As in other fields, various investigators have specific biases, depending on their particular expertise. Given that the authors' initial interest in T-cell development came from the study of cytokines there, we will show how the analysis of cytokine production and responsiveness may help to understand the dynamics of the events that drive the differentiation of early progenitors to the T-cell lineage and then to particular T-cell sublineages.

2. Cytokines and Commitment to the T-Cell Lineage

2.1. When Does T-Cell Lineage Commitment Take Place?

One of the most important events in the life of a T-cell is when it becomes committed to the T-cell lineage. It is widely believed that this event occurs to a lymphoid-committed cell, which probably arises in the bone marrow. There is ample evidence for a lymphoid-committed cell that can no longer give rise to myeloid cells in the bone marrow, and, as will be discussed in Subheading 2.1.1., also in the thymus.

2.1.1. T-Cell Commitment Takes Place in the Thymus: The CD4^{lo} Precursors that First Arrive in the Thymus Are Not Yet Committed to the T-Cell Lineage

Why would developing T-cells spend most of their time at the TN stage? The answer to this question lies in the complexity of events that occur here. To understand these events the different stages that have been identified within the TN stage must be reviewed, which are outlined in Fig. 1. Shortman and coworkers *(4)* have identified what is currently considered to be the first cells that arrive in the thymus from the bone marrow. This is a very small subset of CD4^{lo}CD3$^-$CD8$^-$CD44$^+$CD25$^-$c-kit$^+$TSA-1/Sca-2$^+$ cells. These cells shall be referred to as CD4^{lo} precursors in this chapter. Several lines of evidence support the premise that these are the first cells to arrive in the thymus. Their TCR genes are in germline configuration *(4)*. Furthermore, these cells are not yet committed to become T-cells. They can yield B-cell progeny in vitro and in vivo *(5)*, NK cells *(5)*, and they can also give rise to thymic dendritic cells in vivo *(6,7)*. The latter subset is very important, as it is likely to represent a specific lineage of dendritic cells called the lymphoid-derived (as opposed to myeloid-derived) dendritic cells *(8–10)*. These two dendritic cell subsets have different characteristics and probably will be shown to have different functions. For example, lymphoid-derived dendritic cells are likely to play a role during negative selection in the thymus *(11)*. Importantly, however, $CD4^{lo}$ cells do not give rise to macrophages, neutrophils, or other myeloid cells *(5)*. Thus, they are likely to represent a "real" lymphoid-committed precursor. There is no evidence that such a precursor becomes committed to the lymphoid lineage in the adult thymus; it most likely arrives there already committed to the lymphoid lineage. As such, it must express surface molecules specific to lymphoid cells, that, in turn, should facilitate its specific entry into the thymus. This precursor will be discussed in detail elsewhere in this book. However, we want to emphasize that we still know very little about this stage of T-cell development.

2.1.2. Progenitor (Pro)-T-Cells: A Pivotal Stage in the Life of a Developing T-Cell

As shown in Fig. 1, the next step of T-cell development is the pro-T-cell stage, composed of thymocytes that express concomitantly the CD44 and CD25 antigens in combination with the c-kit marker, and are thus defined as $CD44^{+}ckit^{+}CD25^{+}TN$ cells. Although it had been previously described as an early T-cell precursor *(12)*, we identified the pro–T-cell stage as a key step in the life of a developing thymocyte *(13)*. One of the important characteristics of this subset is that its T-cell receptor (TCR) β chain genes were found in germline configuration by Southern Blot analysis *(14)*, underlying the immature phenotype of this precursor (the $CD4^{lo}$ cells are germline as well). Indeed, expression of TCR rearranged genes is a pivotal event in the life of a T-cell, since it indicates irreversible commitment to the T-cell lineage. Interestingly, the appearance of TCR β rearrangements was concomitant to the downregulation of the CD44 and c-kit antigens, as pro-T-cells were in the process to become pre-T-cells ($CD44^{lo}\,ckit^{lo}CD25^{+}$ TN) *(15)*. Moreover, this latest subset delineates the first stage in which complete TCR V-DJ β rearrangements could be detected, leading to the expression of a rearranged TCR β chain *(14)*. These observations prompted the question as to whether pro-T-cells (as the early $CD4^{lo}$ progenitors) could yield lineages other than T-cells. To test this hypothesis, repopulation assays were set up with both $CD4^{lo}$ and pro–T-cells, isolated from adult thymuses, and transferred into severe combined immunodeficiency (SCID) mice *(5)*. Interestingly, the progeny from pro-T-cells was composed of a majority of T-cells as well as a few NK cells, but did not include cells from the B lineage. These findings were confirmed by Wu and Shortman, who showed in similar experiments that pro-T thymocytes could give rise to T-cells, as well as some dendritic thymic cells *(7)*. Taken together, these results indicate that at the beginning of their thymic life, T-cell progenitors are subjected to selective pressures leading to the acquisition of a T-cell phenotype; most of these changes occur between the $CD4^{lo}$ and the pro T-cell stages, with the striking observation that pro-T-cells have lost the potential to give rise to B-cells.

Are pro-T-cells committed to the T-cell lineage? According to these comments, as well as elsewhere in this book, it will probably be concluded that the "exact" stage marking T-cell commitment within the TN populations is controversial. Foremost, it is unclear whether a single pro-T-cell can still give rise to T and NK cells, for example, T and dendritic cells, or other combinations, for that matter. The identification of such "missing links" in the T-cell development pathway is likely to be very difficult as these are very small populations to begin with. The analyses will have to be done at a single cell level, probably using new strategies in cellular biology. However, there are some molecular aspects that are worth keeping in mind. Indeed, our studies by Southern Blot suggested that pro-T-cells still had their TCR β locus in germline configuration. Further analyses showed that the accessibility to the VDJ recombinase occurs at the same time for the TCRβ, TCRγ, and

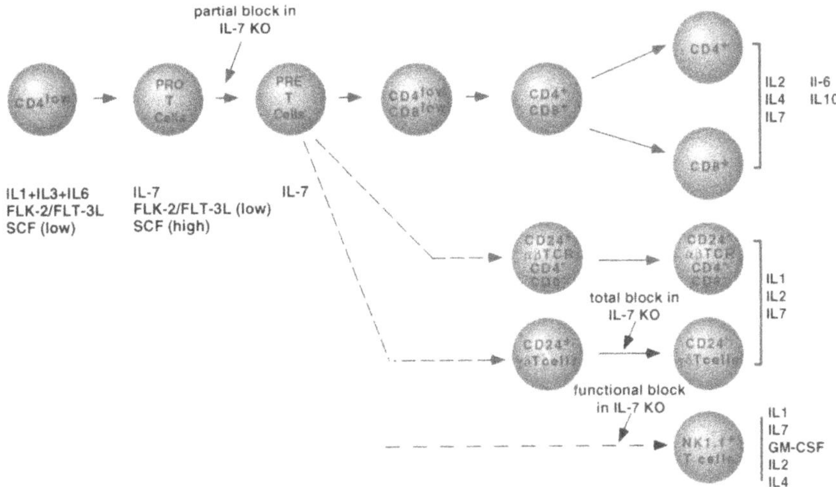

Fig. 2. Cytokine responsiveness of thymocyte subsets.

TCRδ loci, at a stage close to the pro-T-cells. If these cells are already (at least partially) committed to the T lineage, then the signal(s) that induce commitment to the T-cell lineage are not the same as the one(s) that induce TCR rearrangements. We will see now how the analysis of the cytokine responsiveness and of the cytokine production by these early subsets support this hypothesis.

2.2. Cytokine Production/Responsiveness as Markers of T-Lineage Commitment

2.2.1. In Vitro Studies

2.2.1.1. CD4^{lo} and Pro-T-cells show independent patterns of cytokine responsiveness. Despite the preceding observation that both CD4^{lo} and pro-T-cells have (at least for their vast majority) their TCR genes in germline configuration, the authors will give in the following paragraphs, two examples to illustrate that each population presents a particular pattern of cytokine responsiveness. The first example concerns their different ability to respond to SCF and Flt-2/Fk3 ligand. When Flt-2/Fk3 ligand was identified and cloned, it was observed that it was capable of costimulating proliferation of CD25$^+$ TN T-cells. This was an activity very much like another cytokine, SCF, which was identified as a signal for the proliferation of early thymic precursors *(16)*, an observation which was confirmed later *(17)*. It has not been clear whether the signals delivered by SCF and Flt-2/Flk-3 ligand are interchangeable. It has been observed *(5)* that CD4^{lo} or pro-T-cells can be cultured with a variety of cytokine combinations and will still repopulate FTOC following culture in vitro. However, more careful analysis of these conditions, comparing specifically SCF and Flt-2/Flk-3 ligand on CD4^{lo} or pro-T-cells, indicated that Flt-2/Flk-3 ligand results in more physiological effects on CD4^{lo} cells than SCF (Fig. 2) *(18)*. CD4^{lo} cells cultured with Flt-2/Flk-3 ligand repopulate FTOC with developmental kinetics resembling those of freshly isolated CD4^{lo}, whereas similar cells cultured with SCF show altered (faster) kinetics of repopulation when compared with freshly isolated cells. These results suggest that Flt-2/Flk-3 ligand is a physiological signal at the CD4^{lo} stage of thymocyte development, whereas SCF may be more of a developmental signal for pro-T-cells (Fig. 2). The relationship of these results to T-cell commitment remains an area for future research.

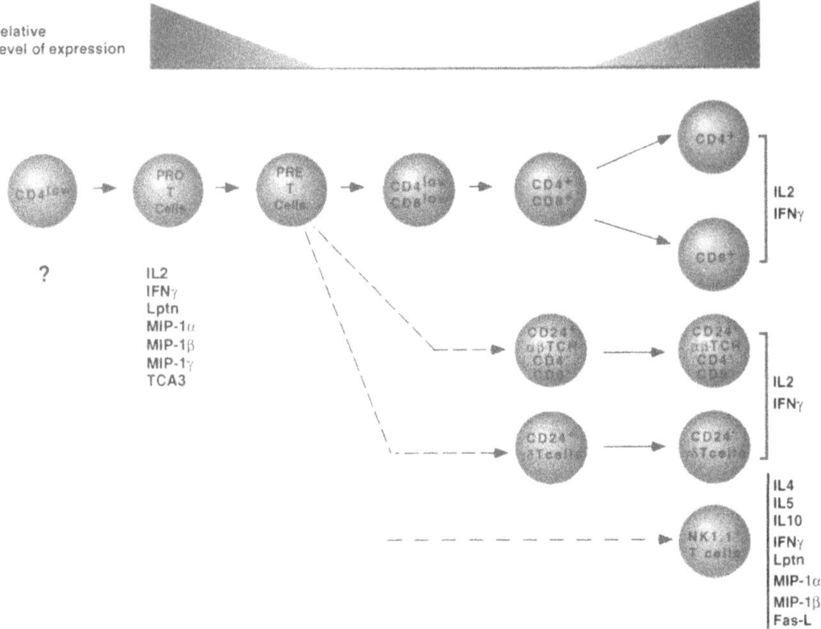

Fig. 3. Cytokine production potential of thymocyte subsets.

The second example concerns the different effect that IL-7 exerts on CD4^{lo} and pro-T-cells. In contrast to the CD4^{lo} population, pro-T-cells display a marked preference for IL-7 in their cytokine responses *(19)* (Fig. 2). In fact, pro-T-cells can be cultured in IL-7 for several days in vitro, and then reintroduced into a fetal thymus in FTOC, and they will go on to differentiate and form a normal thymus like freshly isolated pro-T-cells *(5)*.

2.2.1.2. Pro-T-cells are potent cytokine and chemokine producers. Figure 3 shows some characteristics of CD4^{lo}, Pro, Pre, and "Post-Pre" thymocytes in terms of cytokine production. The latter subset is the CD44^{-}CD25^{-}c-kit^{-}"TN", which are direct precursors of DP. In fact, they are called them "TN" because they are already transcribing CD4 and CD8, in other words, they are already CD4^{low} and CD8^{low}, but appear phenotypically (by flow cytometry) as "TN." As shown in Figure 3, it is not known at this time what are the cytokines and chemokines produced by CD4^{lo} cells. However, we found that pro-T-cells are able to produce large titers of some cytokines and chemokines, including IL-2, IFNγ, and lymphotactin (Lptn). In fact, we cloned Lptn from an activated pro–T-cell cDNA library *(20)*. They have also shown that freshly isolated pro-T-cells transcribe these genes *(21)*, indicating that (at least some) pro-T-cells are activated in vivo. In vitro, we activated pro-T-cells with a combination of calcium ionophore, phorbol ester, and IL-1. The response of pro-T-cells to IL-1 is a particular feature of these cells *(21)*. Now, only T and NK cells are known to produce IFNγ, whereas IL-2 and Lptn are mainly T-cell products. In addition, pro-T-cells produce granzymes and a variety of other chemokines (MIP-1α, MIP-1β, Rantes, TCA-3) known to be produced by mature T-cells *(21)*.

In conclusion, the cytokine and chemokine production/responsiveness of CD4^{lo} and pro-T-cells reflect the roles that have been postulated for these progenitors: CD4^{lo} cells represent the earliest precursors to arrive in the thymus and, as such, still exhibit the cytokine responses of their bone marrow progenitors; in contrast, pro-T-cells (as cells that have already differentiated along the T-cell commitment pathway) show a marked preference for IL-7 in their cytokine responsiveness and produce cytokines and chemokines produced by $CD8^+CD3^+$ thymocytes and splenocytes. In other words, pro-T-cells already have some characteristics of mature T-cells, despite their immature phenotype (illustrated by the lack of TCR gene rearrangement). It is possible that these responses represent the expression of a "T-cell genetic program" already triggered in pro-T-cells. Importantly, however, this T-cell genetic program is not random. For example, pro-T-cells do not produce Th2 cytokines (IL-4, IL-5, IL-10, IL-13). Therefore, it is possible that this repertoire represents an "original" T-cell effector program that could have arisen early during evolution.

2.2.2. In Vivo Studies

The production of gene-targeted mice with mutations affecting cytokines and their receptors has provided fresh insight about the importance of these molecules for host defenses *(22)*. In contrast, few knockouts have, to date, provided information about lymphoid development *(22)*. Although mice lacking IL-2 die prematurely because of a dysregulated immune system, the T-cell subset composition is apparently unaffected. In addition, the development of cells from the B lineage is normal, as observed in the IL-4 knockout mice. Interestingly, we will see that mice lacking IL-7 and its receptor were more informative, since they exhibit impaired development of B, T, as well as NK cells, depending on the targeted gene. Indeed, three knockout mouse models were produced to analyze the role(s) of IL-7 during lymphoid development. These include, the IL-7 *(23)*, IL-7 receptor α chain (IL-7Rα) *(24)*, and IL-7 receptor γ (IL-7Rγ) *(25)* chain knockouts. These mice show very interesting phenotypes. The IL-7 knockout has no mature B-cells, containing instead only precursor B-cells until the pre-B-cell stage, where development of this lineage stops. Initial examination of the T-cell lineage indicated that the thymus is reduced in size, but all main subsets are present *(23)*. In contrast, the IL-7Rα knockout has no mature B-cells, or T-cells, but has NK cells. The last knockout, the IL-7Rγ chain (a common chain between the IL-4, IL-7 and IL-15 receptors) lacks NK cells as well *(25)*. Taken at face value, this would indicate that although IL-7 is not absolutely necessary for T-cell development, there are other factors required for T and NK development whose receptors use these chains as well. One such candidate is thymic stroma derived lymphopoietin (TSLP) *(26)*, which has been shown to be able to replace IL-7 in B-cell development, and which has been described to use the IL-7Rα chain. A factor that is probably very important in NK cell development is IL-15, which shares the γ chain of its receptor with the IL-7R. In fact, in the human system, IL-15 has been shown to influence NK cell development *(27)*. We would predict that IL-15 would have similar effects on either $CD4^{lo}$ or Pro T-cells as well.

3. Cytokines and Commitment to the T-Cell Sublineages

In this part, the different steps necessary to the acquisition of a T-cell phenotype characterized by the expression of a TCR and the specific features particular to each T-cell sublineage will briefly be described. Then the cytokine production and responsiveness of the three distinct sublineages of T-cells: αβ SP T-cells, γδ T-cells and NK1.1 + T-cells will be reviewed. Finally, several reports will be analyzed that strongly suggest that the commitment to one of these sublineages is independent of TCR usage.

3.1. Development of T-Cell Sublineages

As mentioned previously, three different lineages of T-cells have been identified in the thymus. Each of these sub populations exhibits specific functions depending on their

TCR ($\alpha\beta$ or $\gamma\delta$). Interestingly, NK1.1$^+$ T-cells can express one or the other receptor and thus exhibit features in common with both $\alpha\beta$ and $\gamma\delta$ T-cells. As we will later describe, the acquisition of a specific repertoire is a tightly regulated process; it implies both molecular and cellular selective events, which occur at different stages of the differentiation pathway.

3.1.1. Development of $\alpha\beta$ and $\gamma\delta$ T-Cells

Past studies done in different laboratories, including ours, have arrived to the present concept that $\alpha\beta$ and $\gamma\delta$ T-cells arise from a common precursor. Nevertheless, despite the significant amount of attention this question has received recently, the exact stage at which $\gamma\delta$ T-cells branch away from the main $\alpha\beta$ differentiation pathway remains controversial; for this reason, and although it is being covered elsewhere in this book, we will review the current knowledge necessary for understanding of their analysis.

3.1.1.1. The Pre T-cells are a critical stage in the $\gamma\delta$/$\alpha\beta$ T-cell pathways. We reported initially that CD25$^+$ TN T-cells (a subset that we now know includes Pro and Pre T-cells) when cultured in vitro in IL-7–containing media give rise, within 24–48 hours, to $\gamma\delta$ TCR$^+$ DN T-cells and to $\alpha\beta$TCR+ DN *(28)*. Importantly, the cells that appear in these cultures are CD24$^+$, indicating that they are still immature versions of these lineages. Nevertheless, these observations indicate that these cells respond to IL-7, and that precursors of these cells are already present among the pre-T-cells. Thus, we believe that most $\gamma\delta$ T-cells split from the main $\alpha\beta$ T-cell pathway prior to or at the pre-T-cell stage (Fig. 1). Interestingly,we found that it was even possible to delineate pre-T-cells giving rise to an almost exclusive $\alpha\beta$ T-cell progeny in FTOC by sorting those expressing BP-3, a surface molecule related to CD38 and expressed exclusively in pre-T-cells during T-cell differentiation *(29)*.

The importance of the pre-T-cell stage in the life of a developing thymocyte was further demonstrated by the discovery of β selection *(30,31)*. This subject will be reviewed in detail elsewhere (*see* Chapters 22 and 23), but its nature and implications for T-cell development will briefly be described. As mentioned previously, Pre-T-cells represent the first stage of the differentiation pathway where complete TCR V-DJ β rearrangements are detected. Nevertheless, pre-T-cells have not yet rearranged the α TCR locus and is the stage where the β chain is first associated with a surrogate α chain *(32)*. The reason for expressing this pre-T receptor is probably to have a "quality control" step for cells destined to become $\alpha\beta$ TCR+. Indeed, this process ensures that only T-cells capable of expressing a correctly (in-frame) rearranged TCR β chain will advance to the DP stage. This was shown by the large increase of in-frame TCR β rearrangements found at the post-pre-T-cell stage, represented by CD44^{lo}ckit^{lo}CD25$^-$TN thymocytes (Fig. 1) *(30,33)*. These positively selected cells will then rearrange the TCR α variable gene segments, whereas those cells that have failed to rearrange β chain in frame will be deleted. As a consequence, T-cell differentiation is blocked at the pre T-cell stage in both β-TCR *(34)* and pTα KO mice *(35)*. Interestingly, the development of $\gamma\delta$ T-cells is normal in these mice, indicating that there is no need for β-TCR gene rearrangement or β-selection to become a $\gamma\delta$ T-cell.

3.1.1.2. TCR Gene Rearrangements. During their thymic life, T-cell precursors submit to both cellular and molecular selective pressures, which lead to the acquisition of a functional repertoire. The variability of this repertoire is guaranteed by the rearrangements/expression of TCR genes, which occur at the early stages of the differentiation pathway. For each α, β, γ, and δ locus, the concurrent activity of trans and *cis*-regulatory elements ensure the specific expression of these genes in a particular subset. Thus, analysis of the TCRα and β loci in thymocytes revealed that rearrangements at the TCRβ locus occur before rearrangements at the TCRα locus. In contrast, the exact order of TCRγ and δ (in relationship to TCRβ rearrangements) has never been clearly demonstrated. We will summarize in the following paragraph, new findings deduced from both quantitative and qualitative PCR analyses done recently in their laboratory.

Previous analysis by Southern blot showed that pro-T-cells had still their TCRβ loci in germline configuration *(14)*. Interestingly, amplification of Dβ-Jβ joints by PCR revealed that some of these cells had initiated the first step in the rearranging process, whereas no V-DJ TCRβ rearrangements had occurred at this early stage (M. Capone and A. Zlotnik, unpublished observations). Similar experiments at the TCRγ and δ loci showed that V-J γ, as well as complete V-DJ δ rearrangements could also be detected in pro-T-cells, at least for the Vγ2-Jγ1 and Vδ5-Jδ1 chains (M. Capone and A. Zlotnik, unpublished observations). In contrast, rearrangements of the Vγ5-Jγ1 and Vδ4-Jδ1 chains were not detected before the pre-T-cell stage. However, it is possible that the amount of Dβ-Jβ, Vγ2-Jγ1 and Vδ5-Jδ1 joints present in the pro-T-cell subset represented only a few alleles. In contrast, TCR γ and δ rearrangements are abundant in pre-T-cells, for all the different chains analyzed. The implications of these findings are the following:

1. γδ T-cells can split from the main αβ cells at the earliest (pro-T-cell) stage of the T-cell differentiation pathway in the adult thymus (Fig. 1).
2. Complete TCRβ rearrangements occur after Vγ2-Jγ1 and Vδ5-Jδ1 rearrangements, suggesting that there is a window of time where no competition exists between the generation of αβ and γδ T-cells.
3. For both TCRγ and δ loci, rearrangements of the different chains are sequential. Thus, as demonstrated previously in the embryo, the appearance of the different subpopulations of γδ cells follow some "waves" during T-cell differentiation in the adult thymus.
4. Finally, the opening of the chromatin for the three TCRβ, γ, and δ loci occurs concomitantly and, thus, probably depends on the activation of factors expressed at this time (unkown). Since $CD25^+c\text{-}kit^+CD44^+$ (pro-T-) cells are no longer able to give rise to B-cells, commitment to the T-cell lineage (or at least the loss of the ability to commit to the B-cell lineage) implies the expression of a genetic program involving molecules that remain to be discovered.

3.1.2. Development of $NK1.1^+$ T-Cells

$NK1.1^+$ T-cells belong to a more hetereogeneous sublineage of T-cells: they can express or not CD4 and use either αβ or γδ TCR and are, therefore, better defined by other markers including NK1.1, Ly49-A, IL-2R-β, as well as by specific biological properties *(2)*. Similarly, to the classical αβ and γδ sublineages, they can differentiate from pro-T-cells when these cells are reintroduced in FTOC (A. Vicari, T.A. Moore, unpublished observations). A very specific feature of αβ $NK1.1^+$ T-cells is that they seem to be dependent of the expression of β2 microglobulin-associated nonclassical MHC molecules for their development, since they are present only at very low numbers in β2 microglobulin-deficient mice *(36)*, as well as in CD1-deficient mice *(37)*. This may explain why they use a restricted set of Vβ and Vα TCR gene segments *(2)*. However, this dependence on β2 microglobulin-associated molecules is not valid for γδ $NK1.1^+$ T-cells *(3)*. It can be seen in more detail how this observation along with others suggests that T-cell sublineage commitment is, to some extent, independent of TCR usage.

3.2. Cytokine Production/Responsiveness and Commitment to the T-Cell Sublineages

3.2.1. In Vitro *Studies*

3.2.1.1. Cytokine production and characteristics of the responses to cytokines of CD4 and CD8 SP αβ TCR^+ thymocytes. The precursors of the CD4 and CD8 SP cells fail to proliferate in response to cytokines or produce cytokines during the DP stage, and only regain responses after they have undergone positive and negative selection to become SP *(38)*. This phenomenon probably represents a "fail-safe" mechanism designed to prevent an immature, nonselected T-cell from escaping with immune function. Such a cell would have the potential of being autoreactive, for example, leading to autoimmunity. By waiting until the cells have undergone positive and negative selection (which represent, by this model, quality control steps) to become SP before regaining immune function, this mechanism ensures that these cells will not cause havoc were they to be released prematurely from the thymus. It is also worth noting that the CD4 SP thymocytes are not the same as those found in the periphery *(39)*. Many of them are still $CD24^+$ and cannot yet make cytokines. This indicates that there are further differentiation steps that these cells undergo in the thymus before being released to the periphery. Interestingly, CD4 SP thymocytes exhibit cytokine responses different from peripheral CD4 SP. They respond very well to IL-6 in combination with IL-2 *(40)*, and can be inhibited completely in their proliferation by IFNγ *(41)*. Interestingly, the latter characteristic is present in Th2, but not Th1 T-cell clones *(42)*. $CD4^+CD24^-$SP thymocytes, therefore, represent cells ready for export from the thymus, and are the precursors of cells that will eventually differentiate into Th1 and Th2 T-cells. However, at this stage, they only produce some IL-2 and IFNγ, but no significant IL-4 *(38)*. This is also the phenotype of the Thp (for Th precursors) found in the periphery. In contrast, $CD8^+CD3^+$ SP thymocytes produce larger amounts of IL-2 and IFNγ upon activation, and already show a closer phenotype to mature $CD8^+$ cytotoxic lymphocytes *(38,43)*.

3.2.1.2. Cytokine production and proliferation in response to cytokines of γδ TCR^+ thymocytes. The γδ TCR^+DN T-cells exhibit specific responses *(44)*, and are specifically dependent on IL-7 for their development *(45)*. Only the $CD24^-$ subset of γδ TCR^+ thymocytes produce cytokines, as these are the mature cells. Some of their other responses are interesting. Activation of γδ TCR^+ thymocytes on solid phase anti-CD3 leads to massive apoptosis. However, the presence of IL-7 eliminates this effect and leads instead to proliferation (T. Suda and A. Zlotnik, unpublished observation). Interestingly, we initially reported that αβ TCR^+DN thymocytes produce large amounts of IL-4 and IFNγ upon activation *(46)*. We have now observed that only the $NK1.1^+$ fraction within the $\alpha\beta TCR^+$ DN produce IL-4 (A. Vicari and A. Zlotnik, unpublished observations). We made similar observations for the γδ TCR^+ thymocytes, showing that only the $NK1.1^+$ fraction of this subset produces IL-4. Thus, the γδ $NK1.1^-$ T-cells found in the thymus are functional, rather similar to the αβ TCR^+DN $NK1.1^-$ thymocytes and produce mainly limited amounts of IL-2 and IFNγ upon activation.

3.2.1.3. Cytokine production and proliferation in response to cytokines of $NK1.1^+$ thymocytes. $NK1.1^+$ T-cells are likely to be the most active in the thymus as far as cytokine responsiveness and production. Indeed, if unseparated thymocytes are cultured with IL-7 for several days, these cells will eventually make up virtually all the responding cells *(47)*. The cytokine production pattern of αβ TCR^+ $NK1.1^+$T-cells is very unusual, considering also that it can be observed in the absence of antigen-specific priming: they produce IL-4, IL-5, IL-10 (all Th2 cytokines) *(48)*, but also IFNγ, Lymphotactin (Lptn) and granzymes, which are part of the CD8 cytokine production pattern (J. Kennedy, A. Zlotnik, unpublished observations). Thus, they appear to be a combination of Th2 × CD8 in their cytokine production pattern. The possible implications of these unusual biological properties in immune responses and regulation have been reviewed elsewhere *(2)*. Interestingly, the $NK1.1^+$ thymocytes that express a γδ

TCR seem to have similar biological properties than those expressing an αβ TCR, for example, the potential to produce high levels of IL-4 upon stimulation *(3)*.

3.2.2. In Vivo Studies

In this part, the case of the IL-7 KO mice will be re-examined, which brought more interesting insight to the role of this cytokine in T-cell development.

3.2.2.1. IL-7 KO mice show impaired development of αβ, γδ, and NK1.1$^+$T-cells. Initial examination of the T-cell lineages in these mice indicated that all main subsets are present in the thymus, but the cellularity was very low. More detailed analysis uncovered a partial block in development between the pro- and the pre-T-cell development stages *(45)*. However, this block is not complete, and a significant number of cells move on to the pre–T-cell stage and beyond, arguably much less dependent on IL-7 than the pro-T-cell step. Indeed, our in vitro observations indicated that IL-7 could maintain the viability of pro-T-cells, whereas their dependence on IL-7 diminishes as these cells progress towards the pre–T-cell stage *(49)*. Interestingly, the IL-7–deficient mouse does not have mature γδ T-cells *(45)*. The only γδ T-cells detectable are CD24$^+$, a stage that is known to be immature and to probably represent a preselection stage in this lineage *(28)*. No mature intraepithelial (IEL) γδ T-cells are detectable in the gut. This may indicate that either all IEL are IL-7–dependent, or that the CD24$^+$ population in the gut is very small and, therefore, very difficult to identify using conventional flow cytometry. Finally, it was found that NK1.1$^+$ T-cells from IL-7 KO mice were functionally impaired, suggesting a very important role for IL-7 in the functional differentiation of NK1.1$^+$ T-cells *(50)*.

The authors conclude from these analyses that IL-7 is a physiological signal for the survival of pro-T-cells, and thus plays an important role at the beginning of the differentiation pathway, between the pro and the pre-T-cell stages. Interestingly, we showed previously that it is at this stage where TCRβ, γ, and δ rearrangements are initiated.

3.2.2.2. TCRγ rearrangements are reduced in IL-7 knockout mice. Since the early block of T-cell development in IL-7 KO mice, we sought to determine if TCR rearrangements were affected in these mice. Detection of γδ TCR$^+$ thymocytes in the IL-7 knockout would indicate that IL-7 is not strictly necessary for TCR γ or δ rearrangements, however, such an observation does not rule out that IL-7 may modulate TCR rearrangements. Indeed, despite the efforts made by different teams in the last few years, a direct role of IL-7 in inducing TCR rearrangements has not been proven to date. In addition, most of the experiments were performed in vitro using cultured cells, making it difficult to analyze the role of IL-7 because of its ability to maintain the survival of pro-T-cells. Interestingly, our semiquantitative analysis by PCR showed that TCRγ rearrangements were drastically reduced in early T-cell progenitors from IL-7 knockout adult thymuses, whereas the amount of D-J β as well as TCRδ rearrangements were comparable to the amounts observed in normal mice (M. Capone and A. Zlotnik, unpublished observations). Taken at face value, this observation strongly suggests that in addition to its maintenance/viability role, IL-7 may regulate the rate of rearrangements at the TCRγ locus. Nevertheless, the presence of some γδ T-cells (the CD24+ subset) in IL-7 knockout mice, as well as the failure to induce in vitro TCRγ rearrangements in IL-7–cultivated pro T from normal mice, indicates that rearrangements at the TCRγ locus involves other factors that remain to be defined.

3.3. Is the Functional T-Cell Sublineage Commitment Dependent on TCR Usage?

Two examples of the flexibility T-cells display during T-cell development in the thymus will be described. The first involves the development of γδ TCR$^+$ NK1.1$^+$ in a mouse that cannot express the αβTCR. The second example is the development of T-cells bearing αβTCR, but with characteristics of γδ T-cells in αβTCR transgenic mice.

3.3.1. Development of γδNK1.1⁺ T-Cells in Absence of αβNK1.1⁺ T-Cells

A small population of thymic NK1.1⁺ T-cells that express a γδ TCR have been described *(3)*. These cells are so far functionally identical to αβNK1.1 + T-cells since they produce IL-4 and IFN-γ. However, unlike αβNK1.1 + T-cells *(2)*, they do not depend on the expression of β2-microglobulin associated Class I or Class I-like MHC molecules for their selection since they are present in β2-microglobulin KO mice. We observed that these cells were present in higher proportion and cell number in α-TCR KO mice, but in normal proportion in β-TCR KO mice. It was then found that the proportion of in-frame β-TCR rearrangements was higher in γδNK1.1⁺ T-cells from α-TCR KO mice than from normal mice *(3)*. This strongly suggested that these additional γδNK1.1⁺ T-cells became committed to the γδ lineage after β selection, probably because they were not able to express αβ TCR. Since NK1.1⁺ T-cells expressing a αβ or a γδ TCR do not have the same selection requirements, these observations also mean that the functional commitment to express the very particular biological properties of NK1.1⁺ T-cells is independent of the choice of TCR usage.

3.3.2. αβ TCR⁺ DN Cells in α and β TCR Transgenic Mice That Should Have Been γδ TCR+ T-Cells Instead

It has been known for some time that many (but not all) transgenic mouse models where the α and β TCR have been introduced express the predicted transgene positive SP T-cells, but also contain a relatively large population of DN T-cells expressing the α and β transgene. The nature of these cells remains obscure as does the reason why they exist in these mice. However, seen again from the point of view of cytokines, they exhibit characteristics of γδ T-cells. This conclusion is supported by recent observations by Bruno et al. *(51)*. That is, they express upon activation some IL-2, some IFNγ, and proliferate with cytokine combinations that are reminiscent of γδ T-cell responses. Normal αβTCR⁺DN from normal mice produce large amounts of IL-4 instead, and no IL-2 since they most are part of the NK1.1⁺T-cells. Thus, it appears that the αβTCR⁺ DN cells found in these transgenics are actually γδTCR⁺ DN T-cells in their characteristics, although they express the αβ TCR. Thus, these cells represent γδ "wannabes" as well, constituting the second example of "mixed phenotype" T-cells induced by a mutation. The reason these cells arise is linked to the model accounting for the "split" of the γδ lineage from the main αβ lineage and the NK1.1 T-cell lineage. It is believed that γδ T-cells split from the main αβ TCR pathway somewhere between the pro and the pre-T-cell stages. In fact, some may split even at the pro-T-cell stage. As mentioned previously, we have recently obtained evidence using PCR that some Pro T-cells have already rearranged some γ and/or δ TCR genes (M. Capone and A. Zlotnik, unpublished observations). Thus, the presence of the "γδ wannabe" cells in the αβ TCR transgenic mice probably depends on the promoter used to express the transgene, and the time at which the transgene is expressed during T-cell development. If the transgene is already expressed at the pro-T-cell stage, more "γδ wannabes" will be produced. However, if the transgene is expressed later towards the pre-T-cell stage in a more physiological way, then fewer "γδ wannabes" will arise.

3.3.3. Implications of This Model: The Finger of God

The number of "γδ wannabe" cells will depend on the timing of the expression of the transgene promoter, and the time when the developing T-cell received a signal to become a $\gamma\delta$ T-cell. The latter conclusion is a very important new concept: there must exist signal(s) not only to commit precursors to the T-cell lineage, but also to commit such a developing T-cell to either the $\gamma\delta$ T-cell sublineage, and in the adult thymus, the NK1.1$^+$ T-cell lineage. These signals probably target cells between the Pro and the Pre T-cell stages. The model that arises is as follows: A developing T-cell will receive a signal(s) to become committed to the $\gamma\delta$ lineage, and this cell will go on to express a certain genetic program that will give it certain cytokine production/response characteristics and to try to rearrange a $\gamma\delta$ TCR. In those cases where rearrangement of a $\gamma\delta$ TCR has been prevented, as in the case of the $\alpha\beta$TCR transgenics, then the cell can end up using an $\alpha\beta$ TCR. The reason behind this change is that it is likely that the expression of a rearranged $\alpha\beta$TCR will result in down regulation of RAG-1 and RAG-2, thus rendering the T-cell unable to rearrange any more genes. Since the authors have no clue at present as to the nature of the signal that programs the T-cell to the $\gamma\delta$ T-cell lineage, we refer to it in our lab as the "finger of God." We envisage a signal, most likely from the thymic stroma, that will induce (randomly selected?) developing T-cells to acquire this genetic program.

Similar signals must exist for the other main T-cell lineages, the NK1.1$^+$ T-cells, as well as the main TCR $\alpha\beta^+$ subsets of SP. It is possible that under conditions where a particular TCR cannot be expressed (as in the various KOs studied), the developing T-cells are actually able to "default" and express instead a different TCR. This model envisages a developing T-cell where the commitment to a given T-cell lineage is independent of the TCR rearrangement signals.

4. Emergence of Novel Thymic Factors: The Chemokine Paradigm

4.1. Many Chemokines are Expressed in the Thymus

As mentioned above, we originally cloned Lymphotactin from a pro-T-cell library. In the same study, they observed that a large number of other chemokines are produced by pro-T-cells. These include MIP-1α, MIP-1β, Rantes, TCA-3, MIP-1γ/CCF18/MMRP2, and Lptn. Therefore, the question arises: what are the function of these chemokines in T-cell development? Indeed, as far as we know, these observations suggest, for the first time, a link between chemokines and T-cell development. Recent advances in genomics and bioinformatics have resulted in the discovery of a large number of new chemokines *(52)* and we are likely to see many new chemokines reported as this book appears in print. However, virtually nothing is known about the role that these mediators may have in T-cell development.

4.2. SDF-1 is Required for Normal B-Cell Development

An important example of the potential importance of chemokines in lymphopoiesis comes from the recent report of Nagasawa et al. *(53)*; who produced and analyzed a SDF-1 knockout mouse. SDF-1 is a CXC chemokine and a ligand for CXCR4 (otherwise known as fusin) and was initially described as a growth factor for pre-B-cells *(54)*. The important and surprising phenotype of this mutant mouse is that it exhibits profound defects in B-cell development, with no mature B-cells exiting the bone marrow. SDF-1 is known to be produced by bone marrow stromal cells *(55)*, and is chemotactic for lymphocytes, including CD34$^+$ precursor cells *(55)*. Again, at this point it is unclear why SDF-1 is required for normal B-cell development, but some clues arise from the examination of the knockout mouse. The architecture of the stromal compartment appears abnormal. This is an area where chemokines are very likely to have effects. In addition, the effects of the absence of SDF-1 may include bone marrow stromal cells, as well as lymphoid precursors. The development of the bone marrow stroma is likely to depend as well on the presence of developing lymphocytes, which may, in turn, influence the differentiation and/or influx of stromal elements.

4.3. Which Chemokines Play a Role in T-Cell Development in the Thymus?

The bone marrow developmental process outlined above mirrors what happens in the thymus, where the whole organ develops from the initial interaction of lymphoid precursors with thymic stroma. As pointed out before, pro-T-cells transcribe MIP-1α, MIP-β, RANTES, MIP-1γ/CCF18/MMRP2, TCA-3, and Lptn (Fig. 3). However, none of these represent a thymus-specific chemokine since they are largely present elsewhere in the body. However, they are other recently identified chemokines that are more likely to have a role in T-cell development.

4.3.1. TARC

Yoshie et al. described the chemokine called thymus and activation regulated chemokine (TARC) *(56)*, which is expressed preferentially in the thymus, most likely by stromal cells. This chemokine appears to be produced only by dendritic cells (T. MacClanahan et al. unpublished observations). Such an observation makes TARC an important candidate to have a role in T-cell development.

4.3.2. TECK

We have recently isolated a novel chemokine that is the most thymic-specific chemokine reported so far. For this reason it is called thymus expressed chemokine (TECK). TECK is expressed only in the thymus, and to a lesser extent, in the small intestine. Its main source within the thymus is the thymic dendritic cells. Importantly, we did not detect TECK production by myeloid-derived human dendritic cells. As mentioned in Subheading 2.1.1., two kinds of dendritic cells have been identified: those that are lymphoid-derived (from bone marrow lymphoid precursors in human) *(10)* and from $CD4^{lo}$ or pro-T-cells in the mouse *(7)*, or the myeloid-derived dendritic cells that are derived from $CD34^{+}$ progenitors or peripheral blood monocytes *(9)*. The former subset represents probably the majority of dendritic cells in the thymus, whereas the latter is more widespread. Hence, TECK may represent a lymphoid-dendritic cell specific chemokine. If this is the case, it suggests that it may play a role in negative selection, as thymic dendritic cells are likely to play a role in this process. Interestingly, TECK is also expressed in the small intestine, a site that is generally considered capable of extrathymic differentiation. Thus, the expression pattern of TECK most closely parallels the sites of T-cell development, further suggesting a role for this chemokine in T-cell development. TECK is chemotactic for thymocytes and dendritic cells, indicating that it can have a role in the differentiation and traffic of cells within the thymus. These observations make TECK a very interesting candidate to explore further in the context of T-cell development.

4.4. Chemokines: A Developing Area of Research

Until now, virtually no attention has focused on a potential role for chemokines in T-cell development. However, recent findings make this a field that deserves more work. Chemokines, in general, are molecules that have received scant attention, not only from immunologists working in the field of T-cell development, but from immunologists in general. One common finding from groups applying bioinformatics and genomics to cells of importance in immunology has been the discovery of many new chemokines. In contrast to most chemokines that are already known and have been cloned from peripheral leukocytes, the new chemokines may exhibit a more selective production pattern (like TECK). We should expect reports on a number of new, selectively produced chemokines in the future. The molecules will likely have important roles to play not only in T-cell development, but also in other areas of immunology such as the control of Th1 and Th2 responses, delayed type hypersensitivity, and autoimmunity, as well as related phenomena including angiogenesis, metastasis and apoptosis.

5. Conclusion

We have reviewed T-cell development from various angles. The image that arises is that the thymus is indeed a critical organ for the production, not only of the main pathway of T-cells, but for other sublineages as well, including the $\gamma\delta$ and the NK1.1$^+$ T-cells. We still know very little about the function of these cells. We are still in the early stages of their understanding of the events that go on in the thymus. The model proposed shows a non-TCR dominant scheme of T-cell development. The value of this T revised model is that it predicts other signals, present in the thymus, which we know nothing about. The picture presented by this model is that the thymus is the place where T-cells are made, first by commitment to the T-cell lineage, then by commitment to a particular sublineage, and then by the expression of a TCR. This sequence of events, as well as the examples of alterations presented, gives a picture of a developing T-cell, that once committed to a particular sublineage, tries very hard to express a TCR, and in the cases of the mutations discussed, can in some cases end up with a different TCR than it normally would. These examples underscore the resolve that T-cells have for the expression of a TCR, and make us wonder if some pathological conditions may indeed involve T-cell sublineage/TCR alterations. The importance of this emerging information is that, as more and more new molecules expressed in the thymus are discovered, they will need to have models like this in mind in order to understand their biology. We hope that this review will contribute to this process.

References

1. Jenkinson, E. J. and Anderson, G. (1994) Fetal thymic organ cultures. *Curr. Opin. Immunol.* **6,** 293–297.
2. Vicari, A. and Zlotnik, A. (1995) NK1.1$^+$ T cells: a new family of T cells. *Immunol. Today* **17,** 71–76.
3. Vicari, A. P., Mocci, S., Openshaw, P., O'Garra, A., and Zlotnik, A. (1996) Mouse $\gamma\delta$ TCR$^+$NK1.1$^+$ thymocytes specifically produce interleukin-4, are major histocompatibility complex class I independent, and are developmentally related to $\alpha\beta$ TCR$^+$NK1.1$^+$ thymocytes. *Eur. J. Immunol.* **26,** 1424–1429.
4. Shortman, K. and Wu, L. (1996) Early T lymphocyte precursors. *Ann. Rev. Immunol.* **14,** 29–47.
5. Moore, T. and Zlotnik, A. (1995) T cell lineage commitment and cytokine responses of thymic progenitors. *Blood* **86,** 1850–1860.
6. Ardavin, C., Wu, L., Li, C. L., and Shortman, K. (1993) Thymic dendritic cells and T cells develop simultaneously in the thymus from a common precursor population. *Nature* **362,** 761–763.
7. Wu, L. and Shortman, K. (1996) Thymic dendritic cell precursors: relationship to the T lymphocyte lineage and phenotype of the dendritic cell progeny. *J. Exp. Med.* **184,** 903–911.
8. Caux, C., Vanbervliet, B., Massacrier, C., Dezutter-Dambuyant, C., de Saint-Vis, B., Jacquet, C., Yoneda, K., Imamura, S., Schmitt, D., and Banchereau, J. (1996) CD34$^+$ hematopoietic progenitors from human cord blood differentiate along two independent dendritic cell pathways in response to GM-CSF$^+$TNF alpha. *J. Exp. Med.* **184,** 695–706.
9. Cella, M., Sallusto, F., and Lanzavecchia, A. (1997) Origin, maturation and antigen presenting function of dendritic cells. *Curr. Opin. Immunol.* **9,** 10–16.
10. Galy, A., Travis, M., Cen, D., and Chen, B. (1995) Human T, B, natural killer and dendritic cells arise from a common bone marrow progenitor cell subset. *Immunity* **3,** 459–473.

11. Suss, G. and Shortman, K. (1996) A subclass of dendritic cells kills CD4 T cells via Fas/Fas-ligand-induced apoptosis. *J. Exp. Med.* **183,** 1789–1796.
12. Lesley, J., Schulte, R., Trotter, J., and Hyman, R. (1988) Kinetics of thymic repopulation by intrathymic progenitors after intravenous injection: evidence for successive repopulation by an IL-2R+, Pgp1+ progenitor. *Cell Immunol.* **117,** 378–385.
13. Godfrey, D., Kennedy, J., Suda, T., and Zlotnik, A. (1992) Evidence for a developmental pathway involving four subsets of phenotypically and functionally distinct subsets of $CD4^-CD8^-CD3^-$ triple negative adult mouse thymocytes defined by CD44 and CD25 expression. *J. Immunol.* **150,** 4244–4252.
14. Godfrey, D., Kennedy, J., Mombaerts, P., Tonegawa, S., and Zlotnik, A. (1994) Onset of T cell receptor (TCR) β gene rearrangement and role of TCR-β expression during $CD3^-CD4^-CD8^-$ thymocyte differentiation. *J. Immunol.* **152,** 4783–4792.
15. Godfrey, D. and Zlotnik, A. (1993) Control points in early T cell development. *Immunol. Today* **14,** 5457–5453.
16. Godfrey, D., Zlotnik, A., and Suda, T. (1992) Phenotypic and functional characterization of c-kit expression during intrathymic T cell development. *J. Immunol.* **149,** 2281–2285.
17. Rodewald, H., Kretzschmar, K., Swat, W., and Takeda, S. (1995) Intrathymically expressed c-kit ligand (stem cell factor) is a major driving factor for expansion of very immature thymocytes in vivo. *Immunity* **3,** 313–319.
18. Moore, T. A. and Zlotnik, A. (1997) Differential effects of Flk-2/Flt-3 ligand and stem cell factor on murine thymic progenitor cells. *J. Immunol.* **158,** 4187–4192.
19. Suda, T. and Zlotnik, A. (1991) IL-7 maintains the T cell precursor potential of $CD3^-CD4^-CD8^-$ thymocytes. *J. Immunol.* **146,** 3068–3073.
20. Kelner, G., Kennedy, J., Bacon, K., Kleyensteuber, S., Largaespada, D., Jenkins, N., Copeland, N., Bazan, J. F., Moore, K., Schall, T. J., and Zlotnik, A. (1994) Lymphotactin: a novel cytokine which represents a new class of chemokine. *Science* **266,** 1395–1399.
21. Kelner, G. and Zlotnik, A. (1995) Cytokine profile of early thymocytes and the characterization of a new class of chemokine. *J. Leuk. Biol.* **57,** 778–781.
22. Brandon, E. P., Idzerda, R. L., and McKnight, G. S. (1995) Targeting the mouse genome: a compendium of knockouts (partII). *Current Biol.* **7,** 758–765.
23. von Freeden-Jeffry, U., Vieira, P., Lucian, L. A., McNeil, T., Burdach, S. E. G., and Murray, R. (1995) Lymphopenia in interleukin (IL)-7 gene-deleted mice identifies IL-7 as a non-redundant cytokine. *J. Exp. Med.* **181,** 1519–1526.
24. Peschon, J., Morrissey, P., Grabstein, K., Ramsdell, F., Maraskovsky, E., Gliniak, B., Park, L., Ziegler, S., Williams, D., and Ware, C. (1994) Early lymphocyte expansion is severely impaired in interleukin 7 receptor-deficient mice. *J. Exp. Med.* **180,** 1955–1960.
25. Cao, X., Shores, E. W., Hu-Li, J., Anver, M. R., Kelsall, B. L., Russell, S. M., Drago, J., Noguchi, M., Grinberg, A., and Bloom, E. T. (1995) Defective lymphoid development in mice lacking expression of the common cytokine receptor chain. *Immunity* **2,** 223–238.
26. Ray, R., Furlonge, R. C., Williams, D., and Paige, C. (1996) Characterization of thymic stromal-derived lymphopoietin (TSLP) in murine B cell development in vitro. *Eur. J. Immunol.* **26,** 10–16.
27. Leclercq, G., Debacker, V., de Smedt, M., and Plum, J. (1996) Differential effects of interleukin-15 and interleukin-2 on differentiation of bipotential T/natural killer progenitor cells. *J. Exp. Med.* **184,** 325–336.
28. Suda, T. and Zlotnik, A. (1993) Origin, differentiation and repertoire selection of CD3+CD4–CD8- thymocytes bearing either αβ or γδ T cell receptors. *J. Immunol.* **150,** 447–455.
29. Vicari, A., Bean, A., and Zlotnik, A. (1996) A role for BP-3/BST-1 antigen in early T cell development. *Int. Immunol.* **8,** 183–191.
30. Dudley, E. C., Petrie, H. T., Shah, L. M., Owen, M. J., and Hayday, A. C. (1994) T cell receptor β chain rearrangement and selection during thymocyte development in adult mice. *Immunity* **1,** 83–93.
31. Groettrup, M. and Boehmer, H. V. (1993) A role for a pre-T-cell receptor in T-cell development. *Immunol. Today* **14,** 610–614.
32. Saint-Ruf, C., Ungewiss, K., Groettrup, M., Bruno, L., Fehling, H. J., and von Boehmer, H. (1994) Analysis and expression of a cloned pre-T receptor gene. *Science* **266,** 1208–1212.
33. Mallick, C. A., Dudley, E. C., Viney, J. L., Owen, M. J., and Hayday, A. C. (1993) Rearrangement and diversity of T cell receptor β chain genes in thymocytes: a critical role for the β chain in development. *Cell* **73,** 513–519.

34. Mombaerts, P., Clarke, A. R., Rudnicki, M. A., Iacomini, J., Itohara, S., Lafaille, J. J., Wang, L., Ichikawa, Y., Jaenisch, R., Hooper, M. L., and Tonegawa, S. (1992b) Mutations in T-cell antigen receptor genes α and β block thymocyte development at different stages. *Nature* **360,** 225–231.
35. Fehling, H., Krotkova, A., Saint-Ruf, C., and von Boehmer, H. (1995) Crucial role of the pre-T-cell receptor alpha gene in development of αβ but not γδ T cells. *Nature* **375,** 795–798.
36. Bix, M., Coles, M., and Raulet, D. (1993) Positive selection of Vβ8+CD4-CD8- thymocytes by class I molecules expressed by hematopoietic cells. *J. Exp. Med.* **178,** 901–908.
37. Chen, Y., Chiu, N., Mandal, M., Wang, N., and Wang, C. (1997) Impaired NK1+ T cell development and early IL-4 production in CD1-deficient mice. *Immunity* **6,** 459–67.
38. Fischer, M., MacNeil, I., Suda, T., Cupp, J. E., Shortman, K., and Zlotnik, A. (1991) Cytokine production by mature and immature thymocytes. *J. Immunol.* **146,** 3452–3456.
39. Ramsdell, F., Jenkins, M., Dinh, Q., and Fowlkes, B. J. (1991) The majority of CD4+CD8– thymocytes are functionally immature. *J. Immunol.* **147,** 1779–1785.
40. Hodgkin, P. D., Bond, M. W., O'Garra, A., Frank, G., Lee, F., Coffman, R. L., Zlotnik, A., and Howard, M. (1988) Identification of IL-6 as a T-cell derived factor that enhances the proliferative response of thymocytes to IL-4 and phorbol myristate acetate. *J. Immunol.* **141,** 151–157.
41. Hodgkin, P., Cupp, J., Zlotnik, A., and Howard, M. (1990) IL-2, IL-6, and IFNg have distinct effects on the IL-4plus PMA-induced proliferation of thymocyte subpopulations. *Cell. Immunol.* **126,** 57–68.
42. Fitch, F., Mckisic, M. D., Lancki, D. W., and Gajewski, T. F. (1993) Differential regulation of murine T lymphocyte subsets. *Ann. Rev. Immunol.* **11,** 29–48.
43. Chen, W.-F., Fischer, M., Frank, G., and Zlotnik, A. (1989) Distinct patterns of lymphokine requirement for the proliferation of various subpopulations of activated thymocytes in a single cell assay. *J. Immunol.* **143,** 1598–1605.
44. Roberts, K. and Shevach, E. (1991) Immunoregulatory role of γδ T cells. *Ann. N. Y. Acad. Sci.* **636,** 1–8.
45. Moore, T., Murray, R., and Zlotnik, A. (1996) Inhibition of γδ T cell development and early thymocyte maturation in IL-7$^{-/-}$ mice. *J. Immunol.* **157,** 2366–2373.
46. Zlotnik, A., Godfrey, D., Fischer, M., and Suda, T. (1992) Cytokine production by $CD4^-CD8^-$ thymocytes: $CD4^-CD8^-$ $abTCR^+$ thymocytes produce IL-4. *J. Immunol.* **149,** 1211–1215.
47. Vicari, A., Moraes, M. C. L. D., Gombert, J. M., Dy, M., Penit, C., Papiernik, M., and Herbelin, A. (1994) Interleukin-7 induces a preferential expansion of $V\beta 8.2^+CD4^-CD8^-$ and $V\beta 8.2^+CD4^+CD8^-$ thymocytes positively selected by class I molecules. *J. Exp. Med.* **180,** 653–661.
48. Arase, H., Arase, N., Nagakawa, K., Good, R. A., and Onoe, K. (1993) $NK1.1^+$ $CD4^+$ $CD8^-$ thymocytes with specific lymphokine secretion. *Eur. J. Immunol.* **23,** 307–310.
49. Suda, T. and Zlotnik, A. (1992) Interleukin 7: its pleiotropic biological activities. *Adv. Neuroimmunol.* **2,** 99–108.
50. Vicari, A., Herbelin, A., Leite-de-Moraes, M., Freeden-Jeffry, U. V., Murray, R., and Zlotnik, A. (1996) $NK1.1^+$ T cells from IL-7-deficient mice have a normal distribution and selection but exhibit impaired cytokine production. *Int. Immunol.* **8,** 1759–1766.
51. Bruno, L., Fehling, H. J., and von Boehmer, H. (1996) The αβ T cell receptor can replace the γδ receptor in the development of γδ lineage cells. *Immunity* **5,** 343–352.
52. Rossi, D., Vicari, A. P., Franz-Bacon, K., McClanahan, T., and Zlotnik, A. (1997) Identification through bioinformatics of 2 new human chemokines: MIP3alpha and MIP-3 beta. *J. Immunol.* **158,** 1033–1036.
53. Nagasawa, T., Hirota, S., Tabubana, K., Takakura, K., Nishikawa, S., Kitamura, Y., Yoshida, N., Kikutani, H., and Kishimoto, T. (1996) Defects of B cell hemopoiesis and bone marrow myelopoiesis in mice lacking the CXC chemokine PBSF/SDF-1. *Nature* **382,** 635–638.
54. Nagasawa, T., Kikutani, H., and Kishimoto, T. (1994) Molecular cloning and struture of a pre-B-cell growth-stimulating factor. *Proc. Natl. Acad. Sci. USA* **91,** 2305–2309.
55. Aiuti, A., Webb, I. J., Bleul, C., Springer, T., and Gutierrez-Ramos, J. C. (1997) The chemokine SDF-1 is a chemoattractant for human $CD34^+$ hematopoietic progenitor cells and provides a new mechanism to explain the mobilization of $CD34^+$ progenitors to peripheral blood. *J. Exp. Med.* **185,** 111–120.
56. Imai, T., Yoshida, T., Baba, M., Nishimura, M., Kakizaki, M., and Yoshie, O. (1996) Molecular cloning of a novel T cell-directed CC chemokine expressed in thymus by signal sequence trap using Epstein-Barr virus vector. *J. Biol. Chem.* **271,** 21,514–21,521.

Chapter 13

Cytokine and Stromal Influences on Early B-Cell Development

Lisa J. Jarvis and Tucker W. LeBien

1. Introduction

Mammalian bone marrow (BM) is a complex milieu of rare pluripotent stem cells, developmentally restricted stem cells, a range of immature to mature cells in distinct lymphohematopoietic lineages, and nonlymphohematopoietic cells *(1)*. The latter category consists of several cell types, including adventitial reticular cells, barrier cells, endothelial cells, adipocytes, osteoblasts, and osteoclasts. The adventitial reticular cells line the abluminal surface of the marrow vascular sinus, and the cytoplasmic processes that extend from these cells are in direct contact with lymphohematopoietic cells *(2)*. Whether adventitial reticular cells constitute a single cell type with origin in a common mesenchymal precursor is not known, but they manifest many attributes of fibroblast-like cells *(3)*. The term BM stromal cells is also used to describe the adherent cell population established from the in vitro culture of BM, and the predominant cell present in such an adherent cell population is generally the adventitial reticular/fibroblast-like cell. In this chapter, the authors will employ the term BM stromal cell to describe the adventitial reticular/fibroblast-like cell that predominates cultures established from mouse or human BM plated in tissue culture medium supplemented with fetal bovine serum.

The authors' laboratory *(4–10)*, and others *(11–18)*, have employed nontransformed human BM stromal cells as an in vitro microenvironment to evaluate the adhesion, survival, growth, differentiation, and death of human B-cell precursors. The B-cell compartment in human BM encompasses several developmental stages characterized by sequential changes in gene expression, and the term B-cell precursor shall be used to define all $CD19^+$ cells not expressing cell surface light chains. Although there were differences in the source (e.g., age of the donor) of the BM specimens and culture conditions used to establish the stromal cell cultures in the individual studies, it seems likely that the predominant cell present in all studies was the adventitial reticular/fibro-

From: *Molecular Biology of B-Cell and T-Cell Development*
Edited by: J. G. Monroe and E. V. Rothenberg © Humana Press Inc., Totowa, NJ

blast-like cell. One of the major logistical problems in using nontransformed human BM stromal cells is that they do not survive beyond three to four passages following successful establishment of a confluent adherent population in vitro *(19)*. Hence, repetitive long-term use of the same stromal cell population is not possible, although in the authors' experience they can be preserved in a resting (G0) state for months in serum-free medium *(19)*. Interestingly, long-term murine BM stromal cell clones can be established with relative ease *(1)*, and the widely used murine S17 BM stromal cell line has been shown to support the growth of very early $CD19^+$ human B-cell precursors *(19a)*. With these issues in mind, the discussion will be focused on recent studies that used human stromal cells, but comment on circumstances in which these data are supported by, or contrast with, data generated in murine systems.

BM stromal cells can influence B-cell development by at least three different mechanisms. First, BM stromal cells produce cytokines, which positively and negatively affect B-cell growth and development *(1,20)*, and the local concentration and physical disposition (i.e., stromal cell membrane bound or bound to the extracellular matrix) of these cytokines at the BM stromal cell/B-cell precursor interface may be a critical factor. Second, murine *(21)* and human *(4,16)* B-cell precursors and stromal cells adhere primarily through the interaction of VLA-4 (very late antigen-4 or CD49d/CD29) and VCAM-1 (vascular cell adhesion molecule-1 or CD106) on their respective surfaces. This VLA-4/VCAM-1 interaction could potentially activate signaling pathways in both cell types. Third, noncytokine, VLA-4/VCAM-1-independent interactions between B-cell precursors and stromal cells may influence BM stromal cell function and/or the response of B-cell precursors to stromal cell contact. It is likely that components of all three mechanisms play a role in B-cell development.

2. Role of Cytokines

Analysis of cytokines that positively and negatively regulate murine and human B lymphopoiesis has been studied in detail, and it is not the authors' intent to provide an exhaustive review of this subject. However, a brief summary of the physiologic significance of some studies will be presented, with a specific emphasis on the role of IL-7.

There is no substitute for studying B lymphopoiesis in vivo *(22)*, but this is obviously not feasible in humans, except for the lessons learned from congenital immunodefiency diseases, which affect the B-lineage. A major challenge in the development of any in vitro system for studying B lymphopoiesis is to effect an accurate recapitulation of the specialized three-dimensional in vivo BM microenvironment encompassing lymphohematopoietic cells, stromal cells, and the extracellular matrix. The physical association of secreted cytokines with the extracellular matrix is well known *(23)*, particularly the association of molecules such as GM-CSF, IL-3, IL-7, and basic fibroblast growth factor with heaparan sulfate proteoglycans. Cytokine/heparan sulfate proteoglycan interactions serve to concentrate cytokines in stromal cell niches, potentially preventing diffusion and enhancing the optimal physical presentation of the cytokine to cognate receptors on B-cell precursors (and other lymphohematopoietic cells). Extensively studied molecules such as kit ligand (KL) and Flt-3/Flk-2 ligand (FL) are expressed in the membrane of human BM stromal cells, but are probably more active as extracellular cleavage products *(24–27)*. Interestingly, a family of metalloproteinases (designated disintegrins or adamalysins) that enzymatically cleave tumor necrosis factor-α (TNF-α) from the cell surface have recently been described *(28,29)*. One member of this family is the TNF-α-converting enzyme (TACE), which is expressed in a variety of tissues, including the marrow, and mediates release of soluble TNF-α from cells expressing the transmembrane form of TNF-α *(28,29)*. It seems possible that other disintegrins or cell surface proteases could be identified that cleave the extracellular domain of KL or FL, resulting in a potential extracellular source for stimulation of lymphohematopoiesis. KL and FL are members of the same structural protein family. FL (potentially acting with IL-7 and IL-11) can support the commitment of stem cells into early B-lineage cells in the mouse *(26,30–33)*, and can promote limited growth of human pro-B-cells in concert with IL-7 *(34)*. The importance of FL in murine B-cell development has also been realized in mice with a targeted disruption of the gene encoding the FL receptor; these mice have a subtle decrease in the BM pro-B-cell compartment (Hardy fractions A, B, and C) and impaired development of B-cells following transplantation *(35)*. All these results are compatible with a role for FL in promoting survival of stem cells with the immediate developmental potential of becoming B-lineage cells.

2.1. Role of IL-7

An understanding of human B lymphopoiesis is attained largely through in vitro culture systems, or through insight gleaned from analysis of B-cell development in congenital immunodeficiency diseases. Human and murine B lymphopoiesis exhibit marked similarities in patterns of gene expression, regulation of immunoglobulin gene rearrangement, fates of developing B-cells, and so forth. However, one striking difference appears to be the role of IL-7.

IL-7 was discovered by Namen and his colleagues at Immunex almost 10 years ago *(36)*. An IL-7 cDNA was cloned from a murine BM stromal cell line *(36)*, and was reported to act as a growth factor for murine B-cell precursors *(37)*. Nishikawa's laboratory developed highly defined in vitro culture conditions that support the growth of c-kit$^+$/IL-7 receptor$^+$ murine B-cell precursors in the absence of BM stromal cells *(38)*. Essential components include KL, IL-7, transferrin, and insulin. Importantly, IL-7 starvation led to G1 arrest, strongly suggesting that IL-7 plays a major role in regulating the G1/S phase transition in murine B-cell precursors *(38)*. Additional studies using IL-7 receptor α chain deficient mice *(39)*, IL-7 deficient mice *(40)*, mice treated with anti–IL-7 *(41)*, or mice treated with anti–IL-7 receptor α chain *(42)* all yielded comparable results (i.e., B-cell development in the BM was severely impaired). The discovery that the so-called gamma chain (γc) component of the IL-2 receptor was a common subunit for the receptors for IL-2, IL-4, IL-7, IL-9, and IL-15 was a landmark in our understanding of interleukin function (reviewed in ref. *43*). Not surprisingly, mice deficient in γc, and, therefore, unable to signal through the IL-7 receptor, exhibited a disruption in B-cell development *(44,45)*, very similar to IL-7 receptor α chain or IL-7-deficient mice. Additional evidence that IL-7 signaling is critical for murine B lymphopoiesis was confirmed by the discovery that Jak3-deficient mice failed to develop B-cells *(46,47)*. These results are consonant with the known physical association between Jak3 and γc *(48,49)*. Thus, an impressive convergence of observations from many laboratories has demonstrated that IL-7 signaling through the IL-7 receptor/γc complex, and subsequent activation of Jak3, is an essential nonredundant growth stimulus for murine B-cell development.

The role of IL-7 in human B-cell development is different from the role in murine B-cell development. The first report on the effect of IL-7 on normal human B-cell precursors was published by Saeland and his colleagues *(50)*. Short-term analysis (< 7 days) of adult or fetal BM-derived B-cell precursors by ^{3}H-TdR incorporation or cell cycle status revealed that IL-7 exerted an effect on B-cell precursors, but it was difficult to distinguish whether IL-7 induced cell proliferation or merely potentiated cell survival *(50)*. Moreover, these studies were conducted in the absence of an in vitro BM stromal cell microenvironment. At the same time, the authors' laboratory *(10)* was in the process of evaluating the effect of IL-7 on human B-cell precursors using an in vitro BM stromal cell microenvironment. The authors initially reported that CD19$^+$ surface IgM- B-cell precursors would undergo an approximately 10-fold expansion when cultured on BM stromal cells in the presence of IL-7. Expansion ceased after three weeks of culture, and the IL-7/stromal cell-responsive B-cell precursor population could not be transferred to fresh BM stromal cells and be successfully re-expanded. These results were subsequently confirmed by others *(14)*. Interestingly, during the authors' initial studies *(10)*, they could only demonstrate a marginal effect of IL-7 on B-cell precursors in the absence of BM stromal cells (manifesting as a two to threefold increase in ^{3}H-TdR incorporation), and IL-7 did not exert a bona fide mitogenic effect, (i.e., there was no evidence that B-cell precursors in G0/G1 could be induced to divide). Billips and colleagues reached a similar conclusion *(51)*, and in the authors' opinion there is no evidence that IL-7 functions as a true growth factor in human B-cell development. Supplementation of BM stromal cells with IL-7 convincingly enhances growth of B-cell precursors *(6,10,14)*, but IL-7 most likely cooperates with an unknown BM stromal cell molecule(s). The BM stromal cell stimulus could include the FL *(34)*, but the authors believe there are additional unknown molecules as well.

What, then, are other potential roles of IL-7 in human B-cell development, and what is the evidence that cells in the human BM microenvironment produce IL-7 *in situ*? Regarding the issue of IL-7 production, the best evidence is an interesting report that detected IL-7 expression by reverse transcriptase–polymerase chain reaction (RT-PCR) in human BM biopsies from normal donors *(20)*. This study only utilized RT-PCR; consequently production of IL-7 protein in the normal human BM microenvironment is likely, but unproven. However, more direct evidence exists in the mouse on this issue. Funk and colleagues *(52)* purified VCAM-1$^+$ murine BM reticular cells (presumably BM stromal cells) by an immunomagnetic separation procedure, and detected cytoplasmic IL-7 protein in VCAM-1$^+$ cells by immunohistochemical staining. Assuming IL-7 protein is expressed in the human BM microenvironment, it follows from the murine studies that the fibroblast-like advential reticular cells, which dominate in vitro BM cultures *(10,13,15,16)*, may be the source of IL-7 in the BM microenvironment. The authors have used enzyme-linked immunosorbent assay (ELISA) to quantify IL-7 protein in BM stromal culture supernatants. This assay is sensitive to approx 1 pg IL-7/mL, and the authors have detected 1–2 pg/mL concentrations in the authors' BM stromal cell cultures *(6)*. However, this level of endogenous IL-7 production appears to have little (if any) direct effect on growth of human B-cell precursors on BM stromal cells. Indeed, cultures must be supplemented with exogenous IL-7 to a concentration of 10 ng/mL to obtain optimal growth of B-cell precursors *(6)*. It is possible that IL-7 produced by human BM stromal cells *in situ* is synthesized or expressed in a molecular form that cannot be achieved (or detected) in the authors' BM stromal cell cultures; possibly in association with an extracellular matrix component such as heparan sulfate proteoglycans, or cooperatively with other BM stromal cell-derived growth factors.

The authors' laboratory plated FACS-purified CD19$^+$/CD34$^+$/cytoplasmic μ^- pro-B-cells and CD19$^+$/CD34$^-$/cytoplasmic μ^+ pre-B-cells onto BM stromal cells to examine IL-7 receptor function *(6)*. Flow cytometric quantitation indicated that pre-B-cells expressed comparable levels of IL-7 receptors compared to pro-B-cells, but only the latter were responsive to IL-7 stimulation *(6)*. Furthermore, IL-7/BM stromal cell enhanced expansion of pro-B-cells was accompanied by the loss of CD34 and TdT, and acquisition of cytoplasmic μ heavy chains. Consistent with these observations, Billips et al. *(51)* reported that IL-7 downregulated RAG-1, RAG-2, and TdT mRNA expression in human pro-B-cells. Interestingly, the effect of IL-7 on RAG-1/RAG-2 was blocked by crosslinking CD19. Since IL-7 enhances CD19 expression on pro-B-cells *(51,53)*, Billips et al. proposed that IL-7, via upregulation of CD19 and subsequent binding of CD19 to a putative BM stromal cell ligand, would maintain RAG enzymatic activity and Ig heavy chain rearrangements *(51)*.

The authors' laboratory has used the serum-free BM stromal cell culture that supports the growth of human B-cell precursors *(6,10,14)*, to analyze B-cell development from pluripotent stem cells *(8)*. FACS-purified $CD34^+$/lineage$^-$ stem cells were isolated from fetal BM and cultured on fetal BM stromal cells in serum-free conditions, without the addition of exogenous cytokines. Evaluation of these cultures over a three-week period indicated that the $CD34^+$/lineage$^-$ cells underwent commitment, differentiation, and expansion into the B-lineage *(8)*; culminating in cells expressing μ/κ or μ/λ Ig receptors. Importantly, B-cell development in this culture system was not influenced by the addition of exogenous IL-7, or by the addition of neutralizing goat anti–IL-7 antibody (to neutralize the 1–2 pg/mL levels of IL-7 produced by stromal cells in this culture).

The results described above *(8)* are in accord with the apparent IL-7-independent development of human B-cells in patients with X-linked severe combined immunodeficiency disease (XSCID) *(54,55)*. The mutation in the γc subunit potentially influences signaling via IL-2, IL-4, IL-7, IL-9, and IL-15; although γc is more essential for signaling by IL-2 and IL-7 *(56)*, than IL-4 *(57,58)*. T and NK cell development are severely impaired in XSCID, but B-cell numbers are normal or even elevated *(54,55)*. Since γc is a critical subunit for IL-7 signaling *(56,59,60)*, it is reasonable to conclude that B-cell precursors in XSCID are incapable of responding to IL-7. The authors would emphasize, however, that the IL-7 responsiveness of B-cell precursors isolated from the BM of patients with XSCID has not been reported (undoubtedly because of the difficulty, indeed the ethical limitations, in obtaining enough BM from infants with this disease). Additional evidence for a negligible role of the IL-7 receptor/γc in human B-cell development are severe combined immunodeficiency (SCID) patients with mutations in Jak3. These patients also exhibit normal or elevated numbers of circulating B-cells *(61,62)*. Collectively, the authors' in vitro results *(8)* and the congenital immunodeficiences with mutations in Jak3 or γc indicate little or no role for IL-7 in at least the numerical development of human B-cells.

3. Role of B-Cell Precursor VLA-4 Adhesion to Stromal Cell VCAM-1

The interaction of B-cell VLA-4 with stromal cell VCAM-1 represents the primary mechanism of adhesion between these two cell types *(4,16,21)*. Standard adhesion assays have demonstrated almost complete inhibition of human B-cell precursor adhesion to BM stromal cells by addition of antibodies that block either the α4 or the β1 subunit of VLA-4, and at least partial inhibition by VCAM-1 antibodies *(4,16)*. In contrast, antibodies specific for fibronectin, or the fibronectin (CS-1)-binding domain of the α4 subunit, do not block adhesion. The authors have reported that cytokines that increase (IL-1β, IL-4) or decrease (TGF-β) stromal cell VCAM-1 expression enhance or inhibit B-cell precursor adhesion, respectively *(4)*. The authors have also noted a correlation between VCAM-1 expression on stromal cells from BM transplant recipients and the capacity of the stromal cells to support the in vitro growth of B-cell precursors, suggesting that the level of stromal cell VCAM-1 expression may influence B-cell development *(5)*. In contrast, variations in BM stromal cell ICAM-1 expression did not correlate with either adhesion or growth support of B-cell precursors *(5)*, and antibodies to ICAM-1 did not block B-cell precursor adhesion to BM stromal cells *(4)*, most likely because human B-cell precursors express very low levels of LFA-1 *(4)*. VLA-4/VCAM-1 interactions could potentially influence several aspects of B-cell development, including embryonic migration of pluripotent stem cells and commitment to the B-lineage, modulation of B-cell precursor/stromal cell interactions, and cell signaling in B-cell precursors.

Several studies in mice have demonstrated the requirement for VLA-4 in the trafficking of stem cells from fetal liver to the marrow, as well as and growth and differentiation of lymphocytes within the BM microenvironment. Chimeric mice derived from injection of ES cells containing a targeted deletion of the VLA $\alpha4$ subunit (CD49d) gene into wild type, RAG-$1^{-/-}$, or RAG-$2^{-/-}$ blastocysts showed a dramatic deficiency of $\alpha4^{-/-}$ B-cells in the adult BM, blood, and lymphoid organs *(63)*, but a milder deficiency was observed in $\alpha4^{-/-}$ chimeras younger than three months. Although circulating T-cell numbers and phenotype were normal at birth, postnatal production of $\alpha4^{-/-}$ T-cells was severely compromised. The authors proposed that embryonic lymphopoiesis did not require $\alpha4$ expression, but a profound dependency on $\alpha4$ occurred once lymphopoiesis shifted to the marrow in adult mice. In a study on the influence of VLA-4 in a murine BM transplant model *(64)*, BM lodgement of transplanted hematopoietic progenitors in irradiated recipients was decreased by precoating transplanted progenitors with anti–VLA-4, or administering anti–VCAM-1 to the recipients. Three possible explanations for these results were proposed *(64)*: decreased adhesion of precursors to BM endothelium, decreased transmigration into the BM, or decreased retention in the stromal cell microenvironment. In experiments analyzing mice chimeric for deletion of the $\beta1$ integrin subunit (CD29) *(65)*, $\beta1^{-/-}$ lymphoid cells were entirely absent postnatally, and $\beta1^{-/-}$ hematopoietic stem cells could be detected in the yolk sac and fetal blood, but not in the fetal liver and marrow. Since the lack of $\beta1$ did not alter the differentiation ES cells into IgM-producing B-cells in vitro, the authors concluded that deficient trafficking of progenitors from the yolk sac to the fetal liver and BM might represent the major defect in $\beta1^{-/-}$ lymphoid cell expression *(65)*. Results from these three studies illustrate the general importance of VLA-4 in lymphoid development, although distinguishing a role for VLA-4 in trafficking versus a role for VLA-4 in signaling B lymphoid cells in the niche of a BM stromal cell, was not accomplished.

In vitro culture systems have been instructive for evaluating the functional significance of VLA-4/VCAM-1 interactions in mice and men. Miyake and colleagues first reported that a rat MAb to the $\alpha4$ subunit completely ablated murine B lymphopoiesis in the Whitlock-Witte *(66)* culture system *(67)*. Whitlock-Witte cultures are initiated using total nucleated BM cell populations. It is, therefore, unclear at what stage of B-cell development (i.e., stem cell commitment to B220$^+$ B lineage cells or proliferation and expansion of B220$^+$ B lineage cells) the anti-$\alpha4$ reagent was exerting an effect. Ryan and his colleagues developed a lymphoid progenitor colony assay to examine the role of VLA-4 in the early stages of human lymphopoiesis *(17)*. In this assay, FACS-purified CD34$^+$/CD10$^-$ or affinity isolated CD34$^+$ cells from adult BM were cultured on adult BM stromal cells, and TdT$^+$ lymphoid colonies were detected at day 14. Interestingly, phenotypic analysis of the TdT$^+$ colonies indicated that only about one-third of the cells expressed CD19 *(17)*. TdT$^+$ colony formation required direct contact with BM stromal cells, and was blocked by a mouse MAb to the human $\alpha4$ subunit *(17)*. These results suggest that the clonogenic cell in this assay is a very early lymphoid progenitor, potentially similar to the $CD10^+$ common lymphoid progenitor described by Galy and colleagues *(68)*. Thus, the reports by Ryan *(17)* and Miyake *(67)* are consistent with a role for VLA-4 in stem cell → lymphoid progenitor or lymphoid progenitor → B-lineage cell commitment and differentiation. In a study that examined the survival capacity of normal and leukemic B-cell precursors on human BM stromal cells, murine MAb to human $\alpha4$ and $\beta1$ subunits inhibited the survival of $CD34^+$/$CD19^+$ pro-B-cells by > 50%, but had only a minor effect on the survival of $CD19^+$/$CD34^-$ pre-B and $CD19^+$/surface μ^+ immature B-cells *(11)*.

In analyzing B-cell precursor adhesion to BM stromal cells, the predominance of VLA-4–mediated adhesion may mask detection of weaker or quantitatively more minor adhesive interactions. The majority of in vitro adhesion assays typically employ a rather forceful washing procedure to remove nonadherent B-cells from stromal cells. These assays may select for integrin-mediated adhesion, which is relatively strong and takes place in static conditions (as opposed to selectins, which bind under conditions of flow). Significantly, Patrick and coworkers have reported biphasic adhesion of B-cell precursor leukemic cell lines to BM stromal cells, with the first 15 min of the adhesion assay completely inhibitable by VLA-4 MAb, but the subsequent phase being independent of the presence of antibodies to VLA-4, VCAM-1, LFA-1, CD44, E-selectin, or L-selectin *(67)*. These results were obtained using a parallel-flow detachment assay in which the shear force used to remove B-cells can be controlled. Therefore, additional molecular interactions may mediate the retention of lymphoid cells in the BM microenvironment, an event that would be crucial as B-cell precursors are undergoing heavy and light chain immunoglobulin gene rearrangement.

4. Role of VLA-4 Engagement During B-Cell Development

Cell signaling associated with VLA-4 engagement has been reported for many cell types, including B-cells. Signals transduced following B-cell VLA-4 activation via stromal cell VCAM-1 or the CS-1 domain of fibronectin may be important in B-cell precursor growth and development. Characterization of the signaling pathways downstream of integrin engagement are being intensely studied (reviewed in refs. *70,71*). Protein tyrosine kinases are activated in B-cells following crosslinking VLA-4 using MAb, recombinant/soluble VCAM-1, or the FN-40 cleavage fragment of fibronectin *(72)*. Tyrosine phosphorylated proteins include focal adhesion kinase (also known as FAK or p125FAK) *(72a)*, the related adhesion focal tyrosine kinase (also known as RAFTK or PYK2) *(73)*, and the human enhancer of differentiation (also known as HEF1 or p105HEF1) *(74)*. Tyrosine phosphorylation of all these proteins are potentially coupled to changes in cytoskeletal organization, cell shape, and cell motility in fibroblasts *(70,71)*, but the mechanistic outcome of these tyrosine phosphorylation events in B-cells is unknown. Microvilli, membrane ruffles, and filopodia have been identified on the surface of B-cells at points of contact with BM stromal cells or extracellular matrix, where VLA-4 and VLA-5 are also concentrated *(75)*. Activation of FAK may play a role in the developmental migration of B-cell progenitors (from the para-aortic splanchnopleura to the yolk sac, fetal liver, and BM), migration of transplanted progenitors into the BM, or even transit of developing B-cell precursors along BM stromal cell pathways.

A link between anchorage-dependent cell cycle progression (or inhibition of apoptosis) and integrin engagement has been reported. Although these studies were conducted in fibroblasts or other adherent cell lines, the results may be relevant to human B-cell precursors, which are dependent on contact with BM stromal cells for survival and growth. Wary and coworkers have proposed a mechanism that links engagement of some integrins (including VLA-5) to cell cycle progression *(76)*. Crosslinking of selected integrins was followed by calveolin-mediated association of the integrin with the adapter protein Shc, leading to activation of the Ras pathway *(76)*. Integrin-Shc association was then correlated with activation of ERK-2, replication of DNA (as measured by incorporation of BrdU), and protection of cells from apoptosis. Activation of ERK2 following integrin engagement was also demonstrated by others *(77)*. Anchorage-dependent transcription of cyclins D, E, and A, and phosphorylation of the retinoblastoma protein (pRb) have been reported by several groups *(78–82)*, so that results from different laboratories now link adhesion with cell cycle progression and transcriptional regulation.

The fate of developing B-cell precursors is influenced by a hierarchy of endogenous and external factors. In particular, the presence of a functional heavy chain gene rearrangement is absolutely required for the transition of a pro-B-cell to a pre-B-cell *(22,83)*. There has been considerable interest, but no success in identifying putative ligands for the pre-BCR (μ heavy chain expressed with ψ-light chain) and CD19 (which modulates signaling through surface μ) on the surface of stromal cells. Activation of these two receptors is crucial for early B-cell development to proceed normally, although disruption of the λ5 component of the ψ light chain *(84)* has a much more severe effect than disruption of CD19 *(85,86)*. Assuming that contact with stromal cells activates signaling through μ/ψ light chain and/or CD19, changes in pre-BCR and BCR/CD19 signal transduction *(83,87–89)* could then reflect differential responses to stromal cell engagement at different stages of development. Recent reports linking BCR or CD19 signaling to integrin-mediated adhesion may represent a mechanism of BCR-related cell signaling by stromal cell contact, without a CD19 ligand on the stromal cell surface. Crosslinking of VLA-4 and VLA-5 reportedly enhances tyrosine phosphorylation of CD19 in B-cell lines *(90)*. In addition, crosslinking of either integrins or the BCR induced tyrosine phosphorylation of the FAK-like signaling molecule RAFTK *(73)*. Hence, adhesion of B-lineage cells to BM stromal cells can potentially activate signaling pathways that intersect with those activated by BCR-related signaling. Consistent with this view, TAPA-1 (CD81), which is involved in CD19 receptor signaling *(91)*, colocalized and could be coimmunoprecipitated with VLA-4 in human B- and T-cell lines *(92,93)*. It remains to be demonstrated, however, that integrin activation subsequent to adhesion of B-cells to BM stromal cells can activate similar signaling pathways in normal B-cell precursors, or that integrin-mediated adhesion can influence cell fate decisions that are based on expression of a functional μ heavy chain.

5. B-Cell/Stromal Cell Interactions That Do Not Involve VLA-4 and VCAM-1

As discussed in Subheadings 3 and 4, a considerable volume of data supports a role for VLA-4/VCAM-1 in the growth and development of B-lineage cells. Surprisingly, however, stromal cells from VCAM-1 null mice, or stromal cells isolated from wild-type mice that do not express VCAM-1, can support B-cell growth and differentiation in vitro and in vivo *(94)*. This suggests that whereas VLA-4 is essential *(63)*, VCAM-1 is necessary, but not essential for normal murine B-lymphopoiesis. The authors recently conducted a series of experiments testing the hypothesis that human BM stromal cells receive signals from B lymphoid cells via a VLA-4/VCAM-1 signaling pathway. This hypothesis is outlined in Fig. 1. As discussed in Subheading 4, there is considerable evidence that VLA-4 engagement of either of its ligands (VCAM-1 or the CS-1 domain

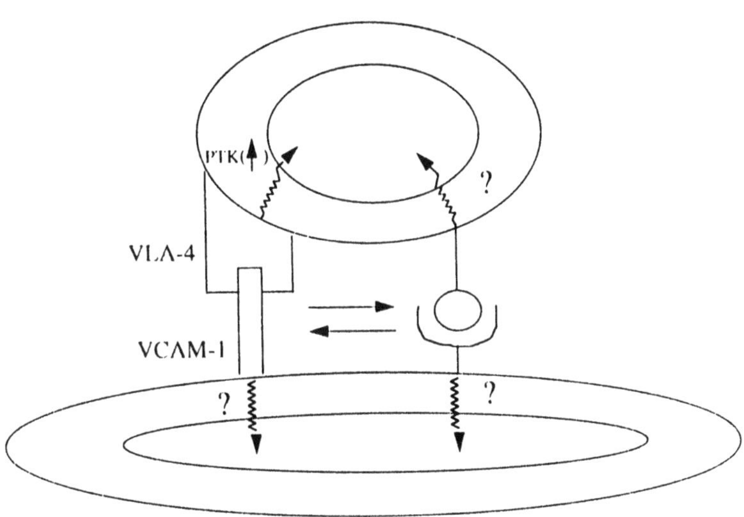

Fig. 1. Model demonstrating potential signaling events occurring subsequent to VLA-4/VCAM-1 adhesive interaction between B-cell precursors and BM stromal cells. VCAM-1 binding to VLA-4 leads to protein tyrosine kinase activation and phosphorylation of several substrates in B-cell precursors; putative downstream events (i.e., induction or suppression of gene expression) have not been characterized. The ultimate effect on B-cell precursors could be at the level of proliferation, survival, differentiation, or apoptosis. Conversely, VLA-4 crosslinking of VCAM-1 could transduce signals to the BM stromal cell. The other ligand/receptor pair is meant to encompass the sum of all other potential interactions that occur at the B-cell precursor/BM stromal cell interface. The horizontal arrows indicate that modification of signaling could occur via cross-talk between VLA-4/VCAM-1 and other unknown receptor/ligand pairs.

of fibronectin) leads to protein tyrosine kinase activation in B-lineage cells, but there is no evidence that VCAM-1 engagement transduces a signal to the stromal cell (or to the authors' knowledge, any other cell that expresses VCAM-1, e.g., inflammatory cytokine-activated endothelial cells). In fact, the VCAM-1 cytoplasmic tail contains no conserved amino acid sequences (e.g., tyrosines, poly proline sequences) that could serve as potential docking sites for signaling molecules containing SH2 or SH3 domains. Nonetheless, it was conceivable that VCAM-1 crosslinking could transduce a signal to the stromal cell by an unknown mechanism, possibly by altering the signaling function of an unknown receptor/ligand interaction (Fig. 1).

The authors approached this problem by developing an assay to detect stromal cell protein tyrosine kinase activation, and used the RAMOS B-cell line as a lymphoid cell stimulus *(7)*. RAMOS was chosen because it does not express the α5 integrin subunit, and hence signaling through VLA-5/fibronectin could not contribute to the results. The authors generated an α4-deficient RAMOS subclone by low dose (300 rads) gamma irradiation and subsequent selection by FACS. The α4 subclone was completely negative for VLA-4 by flow cytometry, and no α4 mRNA was detected by Northern blotting. Tyrosine phosphorylation of several stromal cell proteins occurred within 5–10 min of contact by either $\alpha 4^{+}$ or $\alpha 4^{-}$ RAMOS cells *(7)*. Tyrosine phosphorylation was not detected following MAb crosslinking of stromal cell VCAM-1. it was further demonstrated that brief contact (5–10 minutes) was sufficient to increase tyrosine phosphorylation of the stromal cell proteins FAK and paxillin by two- to threefold, and enhance the kinase activity and phosphorylation of ERK2 *(95)*. This was detectable, despite the presence of substantial constitutive tyrosine phosphorylation of stromal cell FAK and paxillin, which was presumed to be caused by their adhesion to extracellular matrix in the tissue culture flask *(95)*. These collective results persuasively argue that the interaction of VLA-4 with VCAM-1 (or fibronectin) is not needed to activate stromal cell protein tyrosine kinases.

Intriguingly, studies by Jacobsen and coworkers identified an antibody (KMI6), which localized to murine BM stromal cell membranes at points of contact with lymphoid precursors in vivo *(96)*. This antibody was later shown to be specific for an unusual epitope of the β1 integrin subunit, which is dependent on disulfide bonding and is not expressed on most primary cells *(97)*. The capacity of this antibody to bind stromal cells at points of lymphoid contact may indicate a role for stromal cell β1 integrins during lymphoid development. Human BM stromal cells express VLA-3 and VLA-5, and very low levels of VLA-1 and VLA-2 *(19)*. The lack of adhesion of the α4-deficient RAMOS *(7)*, and the almost complete abrogation of normal human B-cell precursor adhesion to stromal cells by antibodies to VLA-4 (which is expressed on B-cell precursors, but not on stromal cells) *(4,16)*, makes it unlikely that stromal cell β1 plays a role in the adhesion of B-cells to stromal cells in our culture system. It follows that although the contact-mediated activation of stromal cell FAK, paxillin, and ERK2 is reminiscent of integrin-mediated signaling (reviewed in refs. *70,71*), it is unlikely that engagement of stromal cell β1 integrins plays a role in B-cell-stimulated stromal cell signaling. The authors' data argue for the existence of a receptor/ligand interaction with no adhesive function, which may be a factor in stromal cell signaling following B-cell contact.

The stromal cell signaling pathway identified can be activated by contact with several human B-lineage cell lines and normal pre- and pro-B-cells (Table 1). Although a detailed analysis of non–B-lineage cells has not been conducted, preliminary studies indicate that some myeloid and T-cell lines activate stromal cell tyrosine kinases as well. Thus, this is not a unique property of B-lineage cells. Moreover, not all cells tested activated stromal cell tyrosine kinases, most notably the myeloid leukemic cell line HL-60. Since several reagents have been shown to activate FAK in fibroblast cell lines, the authors tested whether direct stimulation of stromal cells would induce tyrosine phosphorylation profiles comparable to those observed following lymphoid cell contact (Table 1). Neither bombesin, lysophosphatidic acid, or sphingomyelinase induced additional tyrosine phosphorylation of stromal cell FAK above the constitutive level. In contrast, treatment of stromal cells with phorbol esters produced a protein tyrosine phosphorylation profile very similar to that detected following RAMOS cell contact, indicating that tyrosine phosphorylation of FAK, paxillin, and ERK2 was enhanced by this treatment and that protein kinase C was potentially involved.

The authors have evaluated several biochemical and chemical treatments that alter extracellular matrix, membrane proteins, or carbohydrates on the surface of the B-cell, or stromal cell, for their effect on contact-mediated stromal cell signaling (Table 2). The possibility was considered that a cytokine presented by B-cell surface proteoglycans could initiate signaling. Therefore, both stromal cells and B-cells were treated with chlorate, which inhibits formation of sulfated proteoglycans. Removal of the majority of stromal cell and B-cell proteoglycans did not block the ability of RAMOS cells to

Table 1
Cells and Agents Evaluated for their Ability
to Stimulate Stromal Cell Tyrosine Phosphorylation

Cells	Description	Stimulation
RAMOS	B lymphoma cell line	+
RAMOS-4c	CD49d/VLA-4 negative RAMOS	+
NALM-6	Pre-B ALL	+
BLIN-1	Pre-B ALL	+
BLIN-2	Pre-B ALL	+
Normal human pre-B-cells	$CD10^+/sIgM^-/CD34^-$	+
Normal human pro-B-cells	$CD10^+/sIgM^-/CD34^+$	+
HL-60	Myeloid leukemia cell line	–
Agents[a]	**Desired Effect**	
Bombesin	Neuropeptide stimulus	–
Lysophosphatidic acid	Stimulates tyrosine phosphorylation of FAK	–
Sphingomyelinase	Hydrolyzes sphingomyelin	–
Phorbol esters	Activates PKC	+

[a]Bombesin - 10 n*M*, 5 min-5 h; lysophosphatidic acid - 20 μ*M*, 5–10 min; sphingomyelinase - 10 mU/mL, 1–10 min; PMA - 100 n*M*, 5–10 min

Table 2
Agents Evaluated for their Ability to Inhibit
RAMOS Cell Stimulation of Stromal Cell Protein Tyrosine Kinase Activation

Treatment (cell type treated)[a]	Desired effect	Inhibition of stimulation
Chlorate (stromal cells + RAMOS)	Inhibits proteoglycan sulfation	–
Suramin (stromal cells)	Inhibits HSPG-dependent signaling	–
Pronase (RAMOS)	Surface protein cleavage	–
Trypsin (RAMOS)	Surface protein cleavage	–
Paraformaldehyde (RAMOS)	Cell fixation	+
N-glycosidase F (RAMOS)	Cleaves N-linked sugars	–
Neuraminidase (RAMOS)	Cleaves sialic acid	–
Tunicamycin (RAMOS)	Blocks N-linked glycosylation	–

[a]Chlorate - 30 m*M*, 4 days; suramin - 1 mg/mL, 16 h; pronase - 2.5 U/mL, 2 h; trypsin - 0.05%, 15 min; paraformaldehyde - 0.15%; N-glycosidase F - 1 U/mL, 4–16 h; neuraminidase - 38 mU/mL, 1 h; tunicamycin - 0.1 - 1.0 μg/mL, 16 h

stimulate stromal cell signaling. Treatment of stromal cells with suramin, which blocks signaling induced by some cytokines (e.g., bFGF) that are dependent on proteoglycans for presentation, also had no effect. RAMOS was protease-treated to screen for involvement of B-cell surface proteins in stromal cell stimulation. Treatment with pronase or trypsin cleaved specific B-cell proteins, but had no effect on the ability of the RAMOS cells to stimulate the stromal cell signaling pathway. Fixation of B-cells with paraformaldehyde completely ablated stromal cell stimulation, indicating that a protein-protein interaction may be involved, but one that does not involve protein epitopes on the B-cell surface that can be cleaved by pronase or trypsin. Glycosylation of B-cell surface proteins may be essential for stabilizing binding to stromal cell receptors. Therefore, whether treatment of B-cells with N-glycosidase F or neuraminidase, which cleave specific cell surface carbohydrate structures, or tunicamycin, which inhibits N-linked glycosylation of newly formed proteins, altered their ability to stimulate stromal cell signaling was tested. Treatment of B-cells with these reagents had no effect on stromal cell signaling, although alteration of the electrophoretic mobility of specific B-cell proteins was observed, indicating that glycosylation was indeed affected. These preliminary results provide preliminary insight into the identity of the cell surface molecules on RAMOS and BM stromal cells that mediate signaling, and suggest that oligosaccharides or proteoglycans may not be crucial.

In testing the effect of B-cell contact on stromal cell function, it was found that contact with RAMOS cells ($\alpha4^+$ or $\alpha4^-$), BLIN-1 cells, or normal human B-cell precursors, enhanced stromal cell production of IL-6 (*7* and unpublished data). Culturing RAMOS cells in transwell inserts that prevented direct contact with stromal cells, or fixation of RAMOS cells with 0.15% paraformaldehyde, completely eliminated contact enhanced IL-6 production by stromal cells. Furthermore, fixation of stromal cells ablated all IL-6 production, even in the presence of unfixed RAMOS cells. Thus, cell-to-cell contact and conformationally intact RAMOS membrane molecules are crucial for enhancing synthesis of stromal cell IL-6. Contact with RAMOS cells, FACS-purified normal human pro-B-cells, or CD34$^+$/lineage- hematopoietic stem cells did not enhance the very small amount of IL-7 secreted by stromal cells *(7,8)*. The authors' results with human B-cell stimulation of primary human BM stromal cells are in general contrast to results of Sudo and coworkers, who reported that contact with a murine IL-7–dependent B-cell line enhanced IL-7 production by the ST2 murine stromal cell line *(98)*. However, several laboratories have reported that myeloma cell contact enhances human stromal cell IL-6 production *(99–101)*. Similarly, CD34$^+$ hematopoietic stem cells or myeloma cells can enhance osteoblast IL-6 production *(102–103)*. Thus, IL-6 production is particularly sensitive to contact-dependent enhancement. Chauhan and coworkers have identified a role for the transcription factor NFκB in myeloma cell-stimulated enhancement of stromal cell IL-6 production *(104)*. Therefore, it seems likely that a diverse array of signaling pathways initiated at points of contact between stromal cells and several distinct lymphohematopoietic cells could converge at NFκB, leading (amongst several possible changes in gene expression) to enhanced IL-6 production. A model that portrays the results of the authors' stromal cell studies is shown in Fig. 2. In this model, B-cell precursor/BM stromal cell interactions proceed through three phases. The first phase is the adhesion process mediated by VLA-4 and VCAM-1, and the signal transduced through VLA-4. The second phase is an unknown receptor/ligand interaction that leads to stromal cell signaling. The third phase is the outcome of stromal cell signaling, (i.e., cytoskeletal reorganization or AP-1 activation of gene expression [cytokine genes?]).

In addition to the B-cell-signaling events that follow VLA-4 crosslinking, other signaling pathways potentially activated in B-cells by stromal cell contact have been reported. Tagoh and coworkers described a potential role for stromal cells in human B-cell precursor differentiation *(105,106)*. In their studies, RAG-1 and RAG-2 gene expression were induced in the EBV-transformed human lymphoid progenitor cell line FL8.2 following contact with the PA6 murine BM stromal cell line *(106)*. IL-3, IL-6, and IL-7 could augment, but not substitute for, stromal cell contact. The stromal cell surface molecule potentially responsible for RAG-1 induction in FL8.2 cells has been cloned, and contains four putative transmembrane-spanning domains, but no significant homology to the tetraspans membrane protein family *(105)*. Although instructive, these studies are potentially limited by the use of an EBV transformant, since the EBV latent gene products could induce or repress genes normally silent or activated, respectively, in normal B-cell precursors.

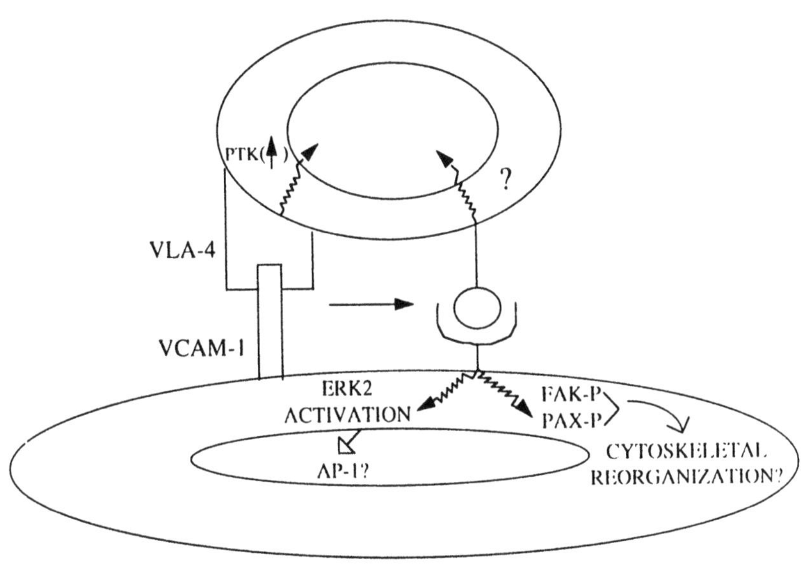

Fig. 2. Outcome of B-cell precursor/stromal cell adhesion in the BM microenvironment. In this model, VLA-4/VCAM-1 interaction is the initial event that results in protein tyrosine kinase activation following VLA-4 crosslinking (which is induced by VCAM-1 or CS-1 domain of fibronectin). The authors' data *(7)* does not provide evidence that a signal is transduced through VCAM-1. The second event that occurs simultaneous with, or subsequent to, VLA-4/VCAM-1 interaction is the binding of an unknown receptor/ligand (one or more) pair. The unknown stromal cell receptor(s) transduce a signal that leads to protein tyrosine phosphorylation of FAK, paxillin, and ERK2; and activation of ERK2. The potential downstream events could include activation of AP-1 and/or cytoskeletal reorganization.

Various B-cell precursor or stromal cell surface membrane molecules have been postulated to play a role in stromal cell-mediated B-cell development, but the precise role of these molecules and their specific function have not been elucidated. Campana and coworkers proposed a role for CD38 in human B-cell development, based on the observation that anti-CD38 inhibited the growth of freshly isolated human B-cell precursor ALL cells and cell lines on unpassaged primary BM adherent cells *(107)*. Crosslinking CD38 on B-cell precursors induced phosphorylation of proteins including syk, phospholipase C-γ, and PI-3kinase *(108)*, and PI-3kinase activation and its association with c-cbl was involved in CD38-mediated growth suppression *(109)*. A ligand for B-cell CD38 on BM adherent cells has not been identified, but CD38 binds hyaluronate *(110)* and appears to mediate weak adhesion of T- and B-cells to endothelium *(111)*. Significantly, it was necessary to minimize integrin-mediated adhesion before CD38-mediated adhesion could be detected *(110)*. Two other cell surface molecules, BST-1 *(112)* and BST-2 *(113)*, are expressed on the surface of human BM stromal cells, and reportedly enhance the growth of the stromal cell-dependent murine pre–B-cell line, DW34. BST-1 and BST-2 have been cloned. Whereas the transmembrane protein BST-2 exhibits no significant homology with known proteins, the glycosyl phosphatidylinositol-anchored BST-1 has homology to CD38. To the authors' knowledge, no ligand has yet been identified for either protein, and there is no published evidence that human BM stromal cell BST-1 or BST-2 can stimulate human B-cell precursors. The CXC chemokine pre-B-cell growth-stimulating factor/stromal cell-derived factor 1 (PBSF/SDF-1), whose receptor LESTR/fusin is expressed on lymphoid cells and is essential for HIV infection *(114)*, was originally identified as a pre-B-cell growth factor *(115)*. PBSF/SDF-1 is produced by BM stromal cells and is a potent chemoattractant, as demonstrated in experiments using human CD34+ hematopoietic progenitors *(116)* and peripheral blood lymphocytes *(117)*. PBSF/SDF-1 also transiently increases actin polymerization in peripheral blood lymphocytes (as measured by FITC-phalloidin staining), which may be a prerequisite for motility during extravasation or recirculation to the BM *(117)*. Variability in PBSF/SDF-1 and chemotactic responses produced by different stromal cell clones has suggested a role for PBSF/SDF-1 in migration of developing B-cells from one "developmental niche" in the marrow to the next *(116)*. Furthermore, PSF-1/SDF-1 deficient mice exhibit severe impairment of B-lymphopoiesis in fetal liver and BM *(117)*. Further analysis of the role of this protein in the migration and growth of human lymphohematopoietic cells is needed, but data already reported suggests interesting possibilities for the role of PBSF/SDF-1 in B-cell development, mobilization, and recirculation.

6. Conclusions

How will the mechanisms and outcomes of these B-cell precursor/stromal cell interactions be elucidated, and how will new molecular interactions be identified? Regarding the latter challenge, several cloning and protein expression strategies have been applied to stromal cells. Honjo and coworkers devised a method designated signal sequence trap to identify novel secreted and/or type I transmembrane proteins produced by stromal cells *(119)*. Indeed, PBSF/SDF-1 was originally isolated by this strategy *(119)*. Several additional molecules of largely unknown function in the context of their effect on lymphopoiesis have been identified *(120)*. Zannettino and colleagues have used retroviral expression cloning of a stromal cell cDNA library, and screening with antibody-coated magnetic beads, to identify cDNAs encoding cell surface molecules *(121)*. Monoclonal antibodies recognizing cell surface antigens are used in this expression cloning technique *(121)*, and, hence, one disadvantage is that cell surface molecules for which no MAb has been produced cannot be identified. Oritani and Kincade have devised a screening technique that identified murine BM stromal cell surface molecules that specifically interact with pre-B-cells *(122)*. The stromal cell cDNA was first screened with a signal sequence trap, then selected cDNAs were expressed as soluble Ig fusion proteins and used to stain the surface of murine pre-B-cells. This technique is particularly attractive, since it "selects" for cDNAs encoding secreted or transmembrane stromal cell molecules that bind to pre-B-cells, but MAb are not a requirement in the screening strategy. One of the molecules identified by this technique is designated SC1/ECM2 *(123)*. SC1/ECM2 contains 650 amino acids, lacks a hydrophobic membrane spanning domain, and is probably secreted by BM stromal cells into an extracellular matrix-bound form. Importantly, SC1/ECM2 fusion protein binds to pre-B-cells, augments the IL-7-dependent cloning of pre-B-cells, but has no effect on myeloid progenitors *(123)*. A human homolog designated hevin has been identified *(124)*, and hevin exerts an antiadhesive effect on endothelial cells *(125)*. It will be extremely interesting to determine the role of hevin in human B lymphopoiesis.

In conclusion, considerable progress has been made in elucidating the role of cytokines and adhesion in B-cell development. The essential role of VLA-4 during embryonic development and adhesion of B-cell precursors to BM stromal cells have been well-characterized. Some initial insight into the cell signaling pathways activated following VLA-4 crosslinking have emerged, but the more distal outcome of these signaling events on survival, growth, differentiation, and death ofB-cell precursors are unknown. The converse side of the relationship is even less developed, but the authors' laboratory has provided strong evidence that human B-cells can activate signaling pathways in adventitial reticular BM stromal cells. Studies of the thymus have indicated that the integrity of thymic epithelial cells is dependent on the presence of early prothymocytes and T-cell receptor-positive cells, underscoring the notion that the thymic microenvironment can be shaped by developing thymocytes *(126–128)*. Therefore, it is conceivable that some comparable symbiosis exists between BM stromal cells and B-cell precursors (or more broadly, lymphohemtopoietic cells in the marrow). A major goal of future studies will be to complete the characterization of receptor/ligand interactions that occur at the B-cell precursor/BM stromal cell interface, the signaling pathways activated in both cell types, and the outcome of these signaling pathways in altering gene expression. These studies will be coupled to an already impressive body of knowledge regarding the role and regulation of Ig gene rearrangement during B-cell development and will collectively deepen our understanding of the developmental biology of the immune system.

References

1. Dorshkind, K. (1990) Regulation of hemopoiesis by bone marrow stromal cells and their products. *Ann. Rev. Immunol*. **8,** 111–137.
2. Abboud, C. N. and Lichtman, M. A. (1995) Structure of the marrow, in *Williams Hematology* (Beutler, E., Lichtman, M. A., Coller, B. S., and Kipps, T. J., eds.), McGraw-Hill, Inc., New York, NY, pp. 25–38.
3. Liesveld, J. L., Abboud, C. N., Duerst, R. E., Ryan, D. H., Brennan, J. K., and Lichtman, M. A. (1989) Characterization of human marrow stromal cells: role in progenitor cell binding and granulopoiesis. *Blood* **73,** 1794–1800.
4. Dittel, B. N., McCarthy, J. B., Wayner, E. A., and LeBien, T. W. (1993) Regulation of human B-cell precursor adhesion to bone marrow stromal cells by cytokines that exert opposing effects on the expression of vascular cell adhesion molecule-1 (VCAM-1). *Blood* **81,** 2272–2282.
5. Dittel, B. N. and LeBien, T. W. (1995) Reduced expression of vascular cell adhesion molecule-1 on bone marrow stromal cells isolated from marrow transplant recipients correlates with a reduced capacity to support human B lymphopoiesis in vitro. *Blood* **86,** 2833–2841.
6. Dittel, B. N. and LeBien, T. W. (1995) The growth response to Il-7 during human B cell ontogeny is restricted to B-lineage cells expressing CD34. *J. Immunol.* **155,** 2359–2368.
7. Jarvis, L. J. and LeBien, T. W. (1995) Stimulation of human bone marrow stromal cell tyrosine kinases and IL-6 production by contact with B lymphocytes. *J. Immunol.* **155,** 2359–2368.
8. Pribyl, J. A. R., and LeBien, T. W. (1996) Interleukin 7 independent development of human B cells. *Proc. Natl. Acad. Sci. USA* **93,** 10348–10353.
9. Villablanca, J. G., Anderson, J. M., Moseley, M., Law, C.-L., Elstrom, R. L., and LeBien, T. W. (1990) Differentiation of normal human pre-B cells in vitro. *J. Exp. Med.* **172,** 325–334.
10. Wolf, M. L., Buckley, J., Goldfarb, A., Law, C.-L., and LeBien, T. W. (1991) Development of a bone marrow culture for maintenance and growth of normal human B cell precursors. *J. Immunol.* **147,** 3324–3330.
11. Manabe, A., Murti, K. G., Coustan-Smith, E., Kumagai, M., Behm, F. G., Raimondi, S. C., and Campana, D. (1994) Adhesion-dependent survival of normal and leukemic human B lymphoblasts on bone marrow stromal cells. *Blood* **83,** 758–766.
12. McGinnes, K., Quesniaux, V., Hitzler, J., and Paige, C. (1991) Human B lymphopoiesis is supported by bone marrow-derived stromal cells. *Exp. Hematol.* **19,** 294–303.
13. Moreau, I., Duvert, V., Caux, C., Galmiche, M.-C., Charbord, P., Banchereau, J., and Saeland, S. (1993) Myofibroblastic stromal cells isolated from human bone marrow induce the proliferation of both early myeloid and B-lymphoid cells. *Blood* **82,** 2396–2405.

14. Moreau, I., Duvert, V., Banchereau, J., and Saeland, S. (1993) Culture of human fetal B-cell precursors on bone marrow stroma maintains highly proliferative CD20dim cells. *Blood* **81,** 1170–1178.
15. Ryan, D. H., Nuccie, B. L., Abboud, C. N., and Liesveld, J. L. (1990) Maturation-dependent adhesion of human B cell precursors to the bone marrow microenvironment. *J. Immunol.* **145,** 477–484.
16. Ryan, D. H., Nuccie, B. L., Abboud, C. N., and Winslow, J. M. (1991) Vascular cell adhesion molecule-1 and the integrin VLA-4 mediate adhesion of human B cell precursors to cultured bone marrow adherent cells. *J. Clin. Invest.* **88,** 995–1004.
17. Ryan, D. H., Nuccie, B. L., and Abboud, C. N. (1992) Inhibition of human bone marrow lymphoid progenitors by antibodies to VLA integrins. *J. Immunol.* **149,** 3759–3764.
18. Ryan, D. H., Nuccie, B. L., Ritterman, I., Liesveld, J. L., and Abboud, C. N. (1994) Cytokine regulation of early human lymphopoiesis. *J. Immunol.* **152,** 5250–5258.
19. Pribyl, J. A. R., Shah, N., Dittel, B. N., and LeBien, T. W. (1997) Methods for purification and growth of human B cell precursors in bone marrow stromal cell-dependent cultures, in *Immunology Methods Manual* (Lefkovits, I., ed.), Academic Press Ltd, pp. 902–923.
19a. Rawlings, D. J., Quan, S. G., Kato, R. M., and Witte, O. N. (1995) Long-term culture system for selective growth of human B-cell progenitors. *Proc. Natl. Acad. Sci. USA* **92,** 1570–1574.
20. Cluitmans, F. H. M., Esendam, B. H. J., Landegent, J. E., Willemze, R., and Falkenburg, J. H. F. (1995) Constitutive in vivo cytokine and hematopoietic growth factor gene expression in the bone marrow and peripheral blood of healthy individuals. *Blood* **85,** 2038–2044.
21. Miyake, K., Medina, K., Ishihara, K., Kimoto, M., Aeurbach, R., and Kincade, P. W. (1991) A VCAM-like adhesion molecule on murine bone marrow stromal cells mediates binding of lymphocyte precursors in culture. *J. Cell Biol.* **114,** 557–565.
22. Rajewsky, K. (1996) Clonal selection and learning in the antibody system. *Nature* **381,** 751–758.
23. Verfaillie, C., Hurley, R., Bhatia, R., and McCarthy, J. B. (1994) Role of bone marrow matrix in normal and abnormal hematopoiesis. *Crit. Rev. Onc. Hem.* **16,** 201–224.
24. Heinrich, M. C., Dooley, D. C., Freed, A. C., Band, L., Hoatlin, M. E., Keeble, W. W., Peters, S. T., Silvey, K. S., Ey, F. S., Kabat, D., Maziarz, R. T., and Bagby, G. C., Jr. (1993) Constitutive expression of Steel factor gene by human stromal cells. *Blood* **82,** 771–783.
25. Lisovsky, M., Braun, S. E., Ge, Y., Takahira, H., Lu, L., Savchenko, V. G., Lyman, S. D., and Broxmeyer, H. E. (1996) Flt3-ligand production by human bone marrow stromal cells. *Leukemia* **10,** 1012–1018.
26. Rosnet, O., Buhring, H. J., DeLapeyriere, O., Beslu, N., Lavagna, C., Marchetto, S., Rappold, I., Drexler, H. G., Birg, F., Rottapel, R., Hannum, C., Dubreuil, P., and Birnbaum, D. (1996) Expression and signal transduction of the FLT3 tyrosine kinase receptor. *Acta Haematol.* **95,** 218–223.
27. Toksoz, D., Zsebo, K. M., Smith, K. A., Hu, S., Brankow, D., Suggs, S. V., Martin, F. H., and Williams, D. A. (1992) Support of human hematopoiesis in long-term bone marrow cultures by murine stromal cells selectively expressing the membrane-bound and secreted forms of the human homolog of the steel gene product, stem cell factor. *Proc. Natl. Acad. Sci. USA* **89,** 7350–7354.
28. Black, R. A., Rauch, C. T., Kozlosky, C. J., Peschon, J. J., Slack, J. L., Wolfson, M. F., Castner, B. J., Stocking, K. L., Reddy, P., Srinivasan, S., Nelson, N., Boiani, N., Schooley, K. A., Gerhart, M., Davis, R., Fitzner, J. N., Johnson, R. S., Paxton, R. J., March, C. J. and Cerretti, D. P. (1997) A metalloproteinase disintegrin that releases tumor necrosis factor-α from cells. *Nature* **385,** 729–733.
29. Moss, M. L., Jin, S. L. C., Milla, M. E., Burkhart, W., Carter, H. L., Chen, W. J., Clay, W. C., Didsbury, J. R., Hassler, D., Hoffman, C. R., Kost, T. A., Lambert, M. H., Leesnitzer, M. A., McCauley, P., McGeehan, G., Mitchell, J., Moyer, M., Pahel, G., Rocque, W., Overton, L. K., Schoenen, F., Seaton, T., Su, J. L., Warner, J., Willard, D. and Becherer, J. D. (1997) Cloning of a disintegrin metalloproteinase that processes precursor tumor necrosis factor-α. *Nature* **385,** 733–736.
30. Hirayama, F., Lyman, S. D., Clark, S. C., and Ogawa, M. (1995) The flt3 ligand supports proliferation of lymphohematopoietic progenitors and early B-lymphoid progenitors. *Blood* **85,** 1762–1768.
31. Ray, R. J., Paige, C. J., Furlonger, C., Lyman, S. D., and Rottapel, R. (1996) Flt3 ligand supports the differentiation of early B cell progenitors in the presence of interleukin-11 and interleukin-7. *Eur. J. Immunol.* **26,** 1504–1510.

32. Veiby, O. P., Jacobsen, F. W., Cui, L., Lyman, S. D., and Jacobsen, S. E. W. (1996a) The flt3 ligand promotes the survival of primative hemopoietic progenitor cells with myeloid as well as B lymphoid potential. *J. Immunol.* **157,** 2953–2960.
33. Veiby, O. P., Lyman, S. D., and Jacobsen, S. E. W. (1996b) Combined signaling through interleukin-7 receptors and flt3 but not c-kit potently and selectively promotes B-cell commitment and differentiation from uncommitted murine bone marrow progenitor cells. *Blood* **88,** 1256–1265.
34. Namikawa R., Muench, M. O., deVries, J. E., and Roncarolo, M. G. (1996) The Flk2/Flt3 ligand synergizes with interleukin-7 in promoting stromal-cell-independent expansion and differentiation of human fetal pro-B cells in vitro. *Blood* **87,** 1881–1890.
35. Mackarehtschian, K., Hardin, J. D., Moore, K. A., Boast, S., Goff, S. P., and Lemischka, I. R. (1995) Targeted disruption of the flk2/flt3 gene leads to deficiencies in primitive hematopoietic progenitors. *Immunity* **3,** 147–161.
36. Namen, A. E., Lupton, S., Hjerrild, K., Wignall, K., Mochizuki, D. Y., Schmierer, A., Mosley, B., March, C. J., Urdal, D., Gillis, S., Cosman, D., and Goodwin, R. G. (1988) Stimulation of B cell progenitors by cloned murine interleukin-7. *Nature* **333,** 571–573.
37. Lee, G., Namen, A. E., Gillis, S., Ellingsworth, L. R., and Kincade, P. W. (1989) Normal B cell precursors responsive to recombinant murine IL-7 and inhibition of IL-7 activity by transforming growth factor-β. *J. Immunol.* **142,** 3875–3883.
38. Yasunaga, M., Wang, F. H., Kunisada, T., Nishikawa, S., and Nishikawa, S.-I. (1995) Cell cycle control of c-kit$^+$IL-7R$^+$ B precursor cells by two distinct signals derived from IL-7 receptor and c-kit in a fully defined medium. *J. Exp. Med.* **182,** 315–323.
39. Peschon, J. J., Morrissey, P. J., Grabstein, K. H., Ramsdell, F. J., Maraskovsky, E., Gliniak, B. C., Park, L. S., Ziegler, S. F., Williams, D. E., Ware, C. B., Meyer, J. D., and Davison, B. L. (1994) Early lymphocyte expansion is severely impaired in interleukin-7 receptor-deficient mice. *J. Exp. Med.* **180,** 1955–1960.
40. von Freeden-Jeffrey, U., Vieira, P., Lucian, L. A., McNeil, T., Burdach, S. E., and Murray, R. (1995) Lymphopenia in interleukin (IL-7)-7 gene-deleted mice identifies IL-7 as a non-redundant cytokine. *J. Exp. Med.* **181,** 1519–1526.
41. Grabstein, K. H., Waldschmidt, T. J., Finkelman, F. D., Hess, B. W., Alpert, A. R., Boiani, N. E., Namen, A. E., and Morrissey, P. J. (1993) Inhibition of murine B and T lymphopoiesis in vivo by an anti-interleukin 7 monoclonal antibody. *J. Exp. Med.* **178,** 257–264.
42. Sudo, T., Nishikawa, S., Ohno, N., Akiyama, N., Tamakoshi, M., Yoshida, H., and Nishikawa, S.-I. (1993) Expression and function of the interleukin 7 receptor in murine lymphocytes. *Proc. Natl. Acad. Sci. USA* **90,** 9125–9129.
43. Sugamura, K., Asao, H., Kondo, M., Tanaka, N., Ishii, N., Ohbo, K., Nakamura, M., and Takeshita, T. (1996) The interleukin-2 receptor γ chain: its role in the multiple cytokine receptor complexes and T cell development in XSCID. *Ann. Rev. Immunol.* **14,** 179–205.
44. Cao, X., Shores, E. W., Hu-Li, J., Anver, M. R., Kelsall, B. L., Russell, S. M., Drago, J., Noguchi, M., Grinberg, A., Bloom, E. T., Paul, W. E., Katz, S. I., Love, P. E., and Leonard, W. J. (1995) Defective lymphoid development in mice lacking expression of the common cytokine receptor γ chain. *Immunity* **2,** 223–238.
45. DiSanto, J. P., Muller, W., Guy-Grand, D., Fischer, A., and Rajewsky, K. (1995) Lymphoid development in mice with a targeted deletion of the interleukin-2 receptor γ chain. *Proc. Natl. Acad. Sci. USA* **92,** 377–381.
46. Nosaka, T., van Deursen, J. M. A., Tripp, R. A., Thierfelder, W. E., Witthuhn, B. A., McMickle, A. P., Doherty, P. C., Grosveld, G. C., and Ihle, J. N. (1995) Defective lymphoid development in mice lacking Jak3. *Science* **270,** 800–802.
47. Thomis, D. C., Gurniak, C. B., Tivol, E., Sharpe, A. H., and Berg, L. J. Defects in B lymphocyte maturation and T lymphocyte activation in mice lacking Jak3. *Science* **270,** 794–797.
48. Miyazaki, T., Kawahara, A., Fujii, H., Nakagawa, Y., Minami, Y., Z.-Liu, J., Oishi, I., Silvennoinen, O., Goldman, A. S., Schmalstieg, F. C., Ihle, J. N., O'Shea, J. J., and Leonard, W. J. (1994) Functional activation of Jak1 and Jak3 by selective association with IL-2 receptor subunits. *Science* **266,** 1045–1047.
49. Russell, S. M., Johnston, J. A., Noguchi, M., Kawamura, M., Bacon, C. M., Friedmann, M., Berg, M., McVicar, D. W., Witthuhn, B. A., Silvennoinen, O., Goldman, A. S., Schmalstieg, F. C., Ihle, J. N., O'Shea, J. J., and Leonard, W. J. (1994) Interaction of IL-2Rβ and γc chains with Jak1 and Jak3: Implications for XSCID and XCID. *Science* **266,** 1042–1045.

50. Saeland, S., Duvert, V., Pandrau, D., Caux, C., Durand, I., Wrighton, N., Wideman, J., Lee, F., and Banchereau, J. (1991) Interleukin-7 induces the proliferation of normal human B-cell precursors. *Blood* **78,** 2229–2238.
51. Billips, L. G., Nunez, C. A., Bertrand, F. E., Stankovic, A. K., Gartland, G. L., Burrows, P. D., and Copper, M. D. (1995) Immunoglobulin recombinase gene activity is modulated reciprocally by interleukin 7 and CD19 in B cell progenitors. *J. Exp. Med.* **182,** 973–982.
52. Funk, P. E., Stephan, R. P., and Witte, P. L. (1995) Vascular cell adhesion molecule 1-positive reticular cells express interleukin-7 and stem cell factor in the bone marrow. *Blood* **86,** 2661–2671.
53. Wolf, M. L., Weng, W.-K., Stieglbauer, K. T., Shah, N., and LeBien, T. W. (1993) Functional effect of IL-7-enhanced CD19 expression on human B cell precursors. *J. Immunol.* **151,** 138–148.
54. Noguchi, M., Yi, H., Rosenblatt, H. M., Filipovich, A. H., Adelstein, S., Modi, W. S., McBride, O. W., and Leonard, W. J. (1993a) Interleukin-2 receptor β chain mutation results in X-linked severe combined immunodeficiency in humans. *Cell* **73,** 147–157.
55. Schmalstieg, F. C., Leonard, W. J., Noguchi, M., Berg, M., Rudloff, H. E., Denny, R. M., Dave, S. K., Brooks, E. G., and Goldman, A. S. (1995) Missense mutation in exon 7 of the common γ chain gene causes a moderate form of x-linked combined immunodeficiency. *J. Clin. Invest.* **95,** 1169–1173.
56. Lai, S. Y., Molden, J., and Goldsmith, M. A. (1997) Shared γc subunit within the human interleukin-7 receptor complex. A molecular basis for the pathogenesis of X-linked severe combined immunodeficiency. *J. Clin. Invest.* **99,** 169–177.
57. Lai, S. Y., Molden, J., Liu, K. D., Puck, J. M., White, M. D., and Goldsmith, M. A. (1996) Interleukin 4-specific signal transduction events are driven by homotypic interactions on the interleukin-receptor (subunit. *EMBO J.* **15,** 4506–4514.
58. Taylor, N., Candotti, F., Smith, S., Oakes, S. A., Jahn, T., Isakov, J., Puck, J. M., O'Shea, J. J., Weinberg, K., and Johnston, J. A. (1997) Interleukin-4 signaling in B lymphocytes from patients with X-linked severe combined immunodeficiency. *J. Biol. Chem.* **272,** 7314–7319.
59. Kondo, M., Takeshita, T., Higuchi, M., Nakamura, M., Sudo, T., Nishikawa, S., and Sugamura, K. (1994) Functional participation of the IL-2 receptor β chain in IL-7 receptor complexes. *Science* **262,** 1453–1455.
60. Noguchi, M., Nakamura, Y., Russell, S. M., Ziegler, S. F., Tsang, M., Cao, X., and Leonard, W. J. (1993b) Interleukin-2 receptor β chain: a functional component of the interleukin-7 receptor. *Science* **262,** 1877–1880.
61. Macchi, P., Villa, A., Giliani, S., Sacco, M. G., Frattini, A., Porta, F., Ugazio, A. G., Johnston, J. A., Candotti, F., O'Shea, J. J., Vezzoni, P., and Notarangelo, L. D. (1995) Mutations of Jak-3 gene in patients with autosomal severe combined immune deficiency (SCID). *Nature* **377,** 65–68.
62. Russell, S. M., Tayebi, N., Nakajima, H., Riedy, M. C., Roberts, J. L., Aman, M. J., Migone, T.-S., Noguchi, M., Markert, M. L., Buckley, R. H., O'Shea, J. J., and Leonard, W. J. (1995) Mutation of Jak3 in a patient with SCID: essential role of Jak3 in lymphoid development. *Science* **270,** 797–800.
63. Arroyo, A. G., Yang, J. T., Rayburn, H., and Hynes, R. O. (1996) Differential requirements for α4 integrins during fetal and adult hematopoiesis. *Cell* **85,** 997–1008.
64. Papayannopoulou, T., Craddock, C., Nakamoto, B., Priestley, G. V., and Wolf, N. S. (1995) The VLA4/VCAM-1 adhesion pathway defines contrasting mechanisms of lodgement of transplanted murine hemopoietic progenitors between bone marrow and spleen. *Proc. Natl. Acad. Sci. USA* **92,** 9647–9651.
65. Hirsch, E., Iglesias, A., Potocnik, A. J., Hartman, U., and Fassler, R. (1996) Impaired migration but not differentiation of haematopoietic stem cells in the absence of β1 integrins. *Nature* **380,** 171–175.
66. Whitlock, C. A. and Witte, O. N. (1982) Long-term culture of B lymphocytes and their precursors from murine bone marrow. *Proc. Natl. Acad. Sci. USA* **79,** 3608–3612.
67. Miyake, K., Weissman, I. L., Greenberger, J. S., and Kincade, P. W. (1991) Evidence for a role of the integrin VLA-4 in lympho-hemopoiesis. *J. Exp. Med.* **173,** 599–607.
68. Galy, A., Travis, M., Cen, Z., and Chen, B. (1995) Human T, B, natural killer, and dendritic cells arise from a common bone marrow progenitor cell subset. *Immunity* **3,** 459–473.
69. Patrick, C. W., Juneja, H. S., Lee, S., Schmalstieg, F. C., and McIntire, L. V. (1995) Heterotypic adherence between human B-lymphoblastic and pre-B lymphoblastic cells and marrow stromal cells is a biphasic event: integrin very late antigen-4α mediates only the early phase of the heterotypic adhesion. *Blood* **85,** 168–178.

70. Clark, E. A. and Brugge, J. S. (1995) Integrins and signal transduction pathways: the road taken. *Science* **268,** 233–239.
71. Richardson, A. and Parsons, J. T. (1995) Signal transduction through integrins: a central role for focal adhesion kinase? *Bioessays* **17,** 229–236.
72. Freedman, A. S., Rhynhart, K., Nojima, Y., Svahn, J., Eliseo, L., Benjamin, C. D., Morimoto, C., and Vivier, E. (1993) Stimulation of protein tyrosine phosphorylation in human B cells after ligation of the β1 integrin VLA-4. *J. Immunol.* **150,** 1645–1652.
72a. Manie, S. N., Astier, A., Wang, D., Phifer, J. S., Chen, J., Lazarovits, A. I., Morimoto, C., and Freedman, A. S. (1996) Stimulation of tyrosine phosphorylation after ligation of β7 and β1 integrins on human B cells. *Blood* **87,** 1855–1861.
73. Astier, A., Avraham, H., Manie, S. N., Groopman, J., Canty, T., Avraham, S., and Freedman, A. S. (1997) The related adhesion focal tyrosine kinase is tyrosine-phosphorylated after β1-integrin stimulation in B cells and binds to p130cas. *J. Biol. Chem.* **272,** 228–232.
74. Manie, S. N., Beck, A. R. P., Astier, A., Law, S. F., Canty, T., Hirai, H., Drucker, B. J., Avraham, H., Haghayeghi, N., Sattler, M., Salgia, R., Griffin, J. D., Golemis, E. A., and Freedman, A. S. (1997) Involvement of p130Cas and p105HEF1, a novel cas-like docking protein, in a cytoskeleton-dependent signaling pathway initiated by ligation of integrin or antigen receptor on human B cells. *J. Biol. Chem.* **272,** 4230–4236.
75. Murti, K. G., Brown, P. S., Kumagai, M. A., and Campana, D. (1996) Molecular interactions between human B cell progenitors and the bone marrow microenvironment. *Exp. Cell Res.* **226,** 47–58.
76. Wary, K. K., Mainiero, F., Isakoff, S. J., Marcantonio, E. E., and Giancotti, F. G. (1996) The adaptor protein Shc couples a class of integrins to the control of cell cycle progression. *Cell* **87,** 733–743.
77. Schlaepfer, D. D., Hanks, S. K., Hunter, T., and van der Geer, P. (1994) Integrin-mediated signal transduction linked to Ras pathway by GRB2 binding to focal adhesion kinase. *Nature* **372,** 786–791.
78. Bohmer, R. M., Scharf, E., and Assoian, R. K. (1996) Cytoskeletal integrity is required throughout the mitogen stimulation phase of the cell cycle and mediates the anchorage-dependent expression of cyclin D1. *Mol. Biol. Cell* **7,** 101–111.
79. Fang, F., Orend, G., Watanabe, N., Hunter, T., and Ruoslahti, E. (1996) Dependence of cyclin E-CDK2 kinase activity on cell anchorage. *Science* **271,** 449–502.
80. Guadano, T. M., Ohtsubo, M., Roberts, J. M., and Assoian, R. K. (1993) A link between cyclin A expression and adhesion-dependent cell cycle progression. *Science* **262,** 1572–1575.
81. Shulze, A., Zerfass-Thome, K., Berges, J., Middendorp, S., Jansen-Durr, P., and Henglein, B. (1996) Anchorage-dependent transcription of the cyclin A gene. *Mol. Cell. Biol.* **16,** 4632–4638.
82. Zhu, X., Ohtsubo, M., Bohmer, R. M., Roberts, J. M., and Assoian, R. K. (1996) Adhesion-dependent cell cycle progression linked to the expression of cyclin D1, activation of cyclin E-cdk2, and phosphorylation of the retinoblastoma protein. *J. Cell Biol.* **133,** 391–403.
83. Burrows, P. D. and M.D Cooper. (1997) B cell development and differentiation. *Current Opin. Immunol.* **9,** 239–244.
84. Kitamura, D., Kudo, A., Schaal, S., Muller, W., Melchers, F., and Rajewsky, K. (1992) A critical role of lambda 5 protein in B cell development. *Cell* **69,** 823–831.
85. Engel, P., Zhou, L.-J., Ord, D. C., Sato, S., Koller, B., and Tedder, T. F. (1995) Abnormal B cell development, activation, and differentiation in mice that lack or overexpress the CD19 signal transduction molecule. *Immunity* **3,** 39–50.
86. Rickert, R. C., Rajewsky, K., and Roes, J. (1995) Impairment of T-cell-dependent B-cell responses and B-1 cell development in CD19-deficient mice. *Nature* **376,** 352–355.
87. Krop, I., Schaffer, A. L., Fearon, D. T., and Schissel, M. S. (1996) The signaling activity of murine CD19 is regulated during B cell development. *J. Immunol.* **157,** 48–56.
88. Wasserman, R., Li, Y. S., and Hardy, R. R. (1995) Differential expression of the Blk and Ret tyrosine kinases during B lineage development is dependent on Ig rearrangement. *J. Immunol.* **155,** 644–651.
89. Weng, W. K., Jarvis, L., and LeBien, T. W. (1994) Signaling through CD19 activates vav/mitogen-activated protein kinase pathway and induces formation of a CD19/vav/phosphatidylinositol 3-kinase complex in human B cell precursors. *J. Biol. Chem.* **269,** 32,514–32,521.
90. Xiao, J., Messinger, Y., Jin, J., Myers, D. E., Bolen, J. B., and Uckun, F. M. (1996) Signal transduction through the β1 integrin family surface adhesion molecules VLA-4 and VLA-5 of human B-cell precursors activates CD19 receptor-associated protein tyrosine kinases. *J. Biol. Chem.* **271,** 7659–7664.

91. Matsumoto, A. K., Martin, D. R., Carter, R. H., Klickstein, L. B., Ahern, J. M., and Fearon, D. T. (1993) Functional dissection of the CD21/CD19/TAPA-1/Leu-13 complex of B lymphocytes. *J. Exp. Med.* **178,** 1407–1417.
92. Mannion, B. A., Berditchevski, F., Kraeft, S. K., Chen, L. B., and Hemler, M. E. (1996) Transmembrane-4 superfamily proteins CD81 (TAPA-1), CD82, CD63, and CD53 specifically associate with integrin α4β1 (CD49d/CD29). *J. Immunol.* **157,** 2039–2047.
93. Rubinstein, E., LeNaour, F., Lagaudriere-Gesbert, C., Billard, M., Conjeaud, H., and Boucheix, C. (1996) CD9, CD63, CD81, and CD82 are components of a surface tetraspan network connected to HLA-DR and VLA integrins. *Eur. J. Immunol.* **26,** 2657–2665.
94. Friedrich, C., Cybulski, M. I., and Gutierrez-Ramos, J. C. (1996) Vascular cell adhesion molecule-1 expression by hematopoiesis-supporting stromal cells is not essential for lymphoid or myeloid development. *Eur. J. Immunol.* **26,** 2773–2780.
95. Jarvis, L. J., Maguire, J. E., and LeBien, T. W. (1997) Contact between human bone marrow stromal cells and B lymphocytes enhances VLA-4/VCAM-1-independent tyrosine phosphorylation of focal adhesion kinase, paxillin and ERK2 in stromal cells. *Blood* **90,** 1626–1635.
96. Jacobsen, K., Miyake, K., Kincade, P. W., and Osmond, D. G. (1992) Highly restricted expression of a stromal cell determinant in mouse bone marrow in vivo. *J. Exp. Med.* **176,** 927–935.
97. Wu, X., Miyake, K., Medina, K. L., Kincade, P. W., and Gimble, J. M. (1994) Recognition of murine integrin β1 by a rat anti-stromal cell monoclonal antibody. *Hybridoma* **13,** 409–416.
98. Sudo, T., Ito, M., Ogawa, Y., Iizuka, M., Kodama, H., Kunisada, T., Hayashi, S. I., Ogawa, M., Sakai, K., Nishikawa, S., and Nishikawa, S. I. (1989) Interleukin 7 production and function in stromal cell-dependent B cell development. *J. Exp. Med.* **170,** 333–338.
99. Caligaris-Cappio, F., Bergui, L., Gregoretti, M. G., Gaidoano, G., Gaboli, M., Schena, M., Zallone, A. Z., and Marchisio, P. C. (1991) Role of bone marrow stromal cells in the growth of human multiple myeloma. *Blood* **77,** 2688–2693.
100. Lokhorst, H. M., Lamme, T., deSmet, M., Klein, S., deWeger, R. A., van Oers, R., and Bloem, A. C. (1994) Primary tumor cells of myeloma patients induce interleukin-6 secretion in long-term bone marrow cultures. *Blood* **84,** 2269–2277.
101. Uchiyama, H., Barut, B. A., Mohrbacher, A. F., Chauhan, D., and Anderson, K. C. (1993) Adhesion of human myeloma-derived cell lines to bone marrow stromal cells stimulates interleukin-6 secretion. *Blood* **82,** 3712–3720.
102. Barille, S., Collette, M., Bataille, R., and Amiot, M. (1995) Myeloma cells upregulate interleukin-6 secretion in osteoblastic cells through cell-to-cell contact but downregulate osteocalcin. *Blood* **86,** 3151–3159.
103. Taichman, R. S., Reilly, M. J., Verma, R. S., and Emerson, S. G. (1997) Augmented production of interleukin-6 by normal human osteoblasts in response to CD34+ hematopoietic bone marrow cells in vitro. *Blood* **89,** 1165–1172.
104. Chauhan, D., Uchiyama, H., Akbarali, Y., Urashima, M., Yamamoto, K. I., Liebermann, T. A., and Anderson, K. C. (1996) Multiple myelome cell adhesion-induced interleukin-6 expression in bone marrow stromal cells involves activation of NF-κB. *Blood* **87,** 1104–1112.
105. Tagoh, H., Kishi, H., and Muraguchi, A. (1996) Molecular cloning and characterization of a novel stromal cell-derived cDNA encoding a protein that facilitates gene activation of recombinase activating gene (RAG)-1 in human lymphoid progenitors. *Biochem. Biophys. Res. Comm.* **221,** 744–749.
106. Tagoh, H., Kishi, H., Okumura, A., Kitagawa, T., Nagata, T., Mori, K., and Muraguchi, A. (1996) Induction of recombinase activating gene expression in a human lymphoid progenitor cell line: requirement of two separate signals from stromal cells and cytokines. *Blood* **88,** 4463–4473.
107. Kumagai, M., Coustan-Smith, E., Murray, D. J., Silvennoinen, O., Murti, K. G., Evans, W. E., Malavasi, F., and Campana, D. (1995) Ligation of CD38 suppresses human B lymphopoiesis. *J. Exp. Med.* **181,** 1101–1110.
108. Silvennoinen, O., Nishigaki, H., Kitanaka, A., Kumagai, M., Ito, C., Malavasi, F., Lin, Q., Conley, M. E., and Campana, D. (1996) CD38 signal transduction in human B cell precursors: Rapid induction of tyrosine phosphorylation, activation of syk tyrosine kinase and phosphorylation of phospholipase C-γ and phosphatidylinositol 3-kinase. *J. Immunol.* **156,** 100–107.
109. Kitanaka, A., Ito, C., Nishigaki, H., and Campana, D. (1996) CD38-mediated growth suppression of B-cell progenitors requires activation of phosphatidylinositol 3-kinase and involves its association with the protein product of the c-cbl proto-oncogene. *Blood* **88,** 590–598.

110. Nishina, H., Inageda, K., Takahashi, K., Hoshino, S., Ikeda, K., and Katada, T. (1994) Cell surface antigen CD38 identified as ecto-enzyme of NAD glycohydrolase has hyaluronate-binding activity. *Biochem. Biophys. Res. Comm.* **203,** 1318–1323.
111. Dianzani, U., Funaro, A., DiFranco, D., Garbarino, G., Bragardo, M., Redoglia, V., Buonfiglio, D., DeMonte, L. B., Pileri, A., and Malavasi, F. (1994) Interaction between endothelium and CD4+CD45RA+ lymphocytes. *J. Immunol.* **153,** 952–959.
112. Kaisho, T., Ishikawa, J., Oritani, K., Inazawa, J., Tomizawa, H., Muraoka, O., Ochi, T., and Hirano, T. (1994) BST-1, a surface molecule of bone marrow stromal cell lines that facilitates pre-B cell growth. *Proc. Natl. Acad. Sci. USA* **91,** 5325–5329.
113. Ishikawa, J., Kaisho, T., Tomizawa, H., Lee, B. O., Kobune, Y., Inazawa, J., Oritani, K., Itoh, M., Ochi, T., Ishihara, K., and Hirano, T. (1995) Molecular cloning and chromosomal mappiong of a bone marrow stromal cell surface gene, BST-2, that may be involved in pre-B-cell growth. *Genomics* **26,** 527–534.
114. Oberlin, E., Amara, A., Bachelerie, F., Bessia, C., Virelizier, J. L., Arenzana-Seisdedos, F., Schwartz, O., Heard, J. M., Clark-Lewis, I., Legler, D. F., Loetscher, M., Baggiolini, M., and Moser, B. (1996) The CXC chemokine SDF-1 is the ligand for LESTR/fusin and prevents infection by T-cell-line-adapted HIV-1. *Nature* **382,** 833–835.
115. Nagasawa, T., Kikutani, H., and Kishimoto, T. (1994) Molecular cloning and structure of a pre-B-cell growth-stimulating factor. *Proc. Natl. Acad. Sci. USA* **91,** 2305–2309.
116. Aiuti, A., Webb, I. J., Bleul, C., Springer, T., and Gutierrez-Ramos, J. C. (1997) The chemokine SDF-1 is a chemoattractant for human $CD34^+$ hematopoietic progenitor cells and provides a new mechanism to explain mobilization of $CD34^+$ progenitors to peripheral blood. *J. Exp. Med.* **185,** 111–120.
117. Bleul, C. C., Fuhlbrigge, R. C., Casasnovas, J. M., Aiuti, A., and Springer, T. A. (1996) A highly efficacious lymphocyte chemoattractant, stromal cell-derived factor 1 (SDF-1). *J. Exp. Med.* **184,** 1101–1109.
118. Nagasawa, T., Hirota, S., Tachibana, K., Takakura, N., Nishikawa, S.-I., Kitamura, Y., Yoshida, N., Kikutani, H., and Kishimoto, T. (1996) Defects in B-cell lymphopoiesis and bone marrow myelopoiesis in mice lacking the CXC chemokine PBSF/SDF-1. *Nature* **382,** 635–638.
119. Tashiro, K., Tada, H., Heilker, R., Shirozu, M., Nakano, T., and Honjo, T. (1993) Signal sequence trap: a cloning strategy for secreted proteins and type I membrane proteins. *Science* **261,** 600–603.
120. Shirozu, M., Tada, H., Tashiro, K., Nakamura, T., Lopez, N. D., Nazarea, M., Hamada, T., Sato, T., Nakano, T., and Honjo, T. (1996) Characterization of novel secreted and membrane proteins isolated by the signal sequence trap method. *Genomics* **37,** 273–280.
121. Zannettino, A. C. W., Rayner, J. R., Ashman, L. K., Gonda, T. J., and Simmons, P. J. (1996) A powerful new technique for isolating genes encoding cell surface antigens using retroviral expression cloning. *J. Immunol.* **156,** 611–620.
122. Oritani, K. and Kincade, P. W. (1996) Identification of stromal cell products that interact with pre-B cells. *J. Cell Biol.* **134,** 771–782.
123. Oritani, K., Kanakura, Y., Aoyama, K., Yokota, T., Copeland, N. G., Gilbert, D. J., Jenkins, N. A., Tomiyama, Y., Matsuzawa, Y., and Kincade, P. W. (1997) Matrix glycoprotein SC1/ECM2 augments B lymphopoiesis. *Blood* **90,** 3404–3413.
124. Girard, J. P. and Springer, T. A. (1995) Cloning from purified high endothelial venule cells of hevin, a close relative of the antiadhesive extracellular matrix protein SPARC. *Immunity* **2,** 113–123.
125. Girard, J. P. and Springer, T. A. (1996) Modulation of endothelial cell adhesion by hevin, an acidic protein associated with high endothelial venules. *J. Biol. Chem.* **278,** 4511–4517.
126. Shores, E. W., VanEwijk, W., and Singer, A. (1991) Disorganization and restoration of thymic medullary epithelial cells in T cell receptor-negative scid mice: evidence that receptor-bearing lymphocytes influence maturation of the thymic microenvironment. *Eur. J. Immunol.* **21,** 1657–1661.
127. Ritter, M. A. and Boyd, R. L. (1993) Development in the thymus: it takes two to tango. *Immunol. Today* **14,** 462–469.
128. Hollander, G. A., Wang, B., Nichogiannopoulou, A., Platenburg, P. O., van Ewijk, W., Burakoff, S. J., Gutierrez-Ramos, J. C., and Terhorst, C. (1995) Developmental control point in induction of thymic cortex regulated by a subpopulation of prothymocytes. *Nature* **373,** 350–353.

Part IV

Commitment and Ordered Progression in Development of Lymphoid Lineages

Chapter 14

Staging B-Cell Development and the Role of Ig Gene Rearrangement in B Lineage Progression

Richard R. Hardy, Susan Shinton, Robert Wasserman, and Yue-Sheng Li

1. Introduction

As B lymphocytes are generated from hematopoietic stem cells, they pass through several intermediate stages that are characterized by distinctive molecular and functional features. The earliest stage is distinguished by accessibility of the immunoglobulin (Ig) heavy chain locus, indicating chromatin changes preparatory to heavy chain rearrangement. Upon activation of the recombinase complex, first a diversity (D) region segment rearranges to one of four joining (J) segments (usually on both chromosomes), and then one of 50–100 variable (V) region genes rearranges to the D-J segment. If this first attempt fails to generate a productive (inframe) heavy chain protein coding sequence, a second V to DJ rearrangement can occur on the other chromosome. Expression of heavy chain protein in the cytoplasm marks the classical pre-B-cell and signals the cell to progress to the next stage of B-cell differentiation—clonal expansion followed by light chain rearrangement. V to J rearrangement at the light chain locus results in expression of a complete IgM molecule, which is rapidly transported to the surface of the immature B-cell. Further differentiation (and possibly selection) finally generates the $IgM^{+}IgD^{+}$ mature B-cell.

This emerging picture of the ordered stage-by-stage progression of increasingly specialized cell function requires a careful separation of the intermediate populations. Here the authors present a framework for identifying these cell fractions based on surface phenotype, a subsetting scheme that has proved useful in characterizing B-cell development in both normal and mutant mice. Some of the distinctive functional changes that occur as cells begin to express Ig heavy chain protein are also described.

From: *Molecular Biology of B-Cell and T-Cell Development*
Edited by: J. G. Monroe and E. V. Rothenberg © Humana Press Inc., Totowa, NJ

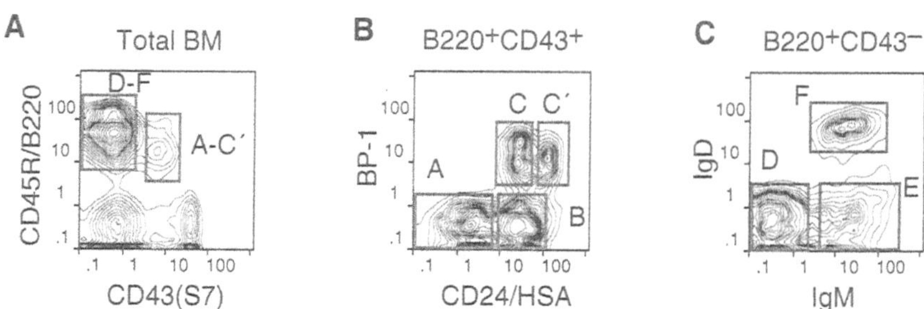

Fig. 1. Multicolor flow cytometry analysis of B lineage stages in mouse bone marrow. Contour plots show that the correlated expression of CD43(S7) and CD45R(B220) divides B220$^+$ cells into earlier (CD43$^+$) and later (CD43$^-$) stage cells **(A)**. The earlier cells can be further subdivided on the basis of correlated expression of CD24(HSA) and BP-1/6C3 **(B)**. The more mature cells can be resolved into small pre-B, immature B and mature B-cells based on the correlated expression of IgM and IgD **(C)**.

2. Phenotypic Subdivision

B lineage cells in mouse can be identified by expression of the high molecular mass isoform of the CD45 common leukocyte antigen, a specificity termed "B220" *(1)*. Staining of mouse bone marrow with antibodies to B220 and IgM clearly delineates two populations of B220$^+$ cells: one IgM$^+$ (a mixture of immature and mature B-cells), the other IgM$^-$ (early B lineage cells, including pre-B-cells). Several years ago, the authors showed that expression of CD43 (variously referred to as leukosialin or sialophorin) divides IgM$^-$ pre-B-cells into two fractions (*see* Fig. 1A) *(2)*. Since most IgM$^+$ cells in bone marrow (and spleen) express low to undetectable levels of CD43, and since all B220$^+$ cells in severe combined immunodeficiency (SCID) mice (immunodeficient animals incapable of efficiently completing Ig rearrangements) *(3)* were CD43$^+$, it appeared likely that CD43$^-$ pre-B-cells represented the more mature stage and CD43$^+$ the earlier stage.

Analysis of two additional markers revealed further complexity in the B220$^+$CD43$^+$ population. One, the heat stable antigen (CD24), increases generally during early stages of hematopoiesis *(4,5)*, and analysis of CD24 expression revealed low, intermediate, and high levels on B220$^+$CD43$^+$ cells *(6)*. Interestingly, all B220$^+$CD43$^-$ pre-B-cells show the high level, suggesting a progression from the lowest through the intermediate to the highest levels during early stages of B-cell development. The second molecule, BP-1/6C3, is a cell surface aminopeptidase *(7–10)*, typically found at high levels on transformed pre–B-cell lines, and at lower levels on normal B220$^+$CD43$^-$ pre-B-cells. BP-1 expression on the B220$^+$CD43$^+$ population is heterogeneous, with some cells lacking it, and others expressing amounts equal to or greater than that found on pre-B-cells. Simultaneous analysis of B220, CD43, HSA, and BP-1 delineated four fractions of B220$^+$CD43$^+$ cells: HSA$^-$BP-1$^-$ cells, HSA$^+$BP-1$^-$ cells, HSA$^+$BP-1$^+$ cells, and HSA^{++}BP-1$^+$ cells. The increased level of HSA on the latter fraction is comparable to that on CD43$^-$ pre-B-cells and this, together with a somewhat reduced amount of CD43, suggests that these cells are intermediate between the CD43$^+$ and CD43$^-$ B220$^+$ cell populations (*see* Fig. 1B).

B220$^+$CD43$^+$ cells will persist and even proliferate in stromal cell-dependent B lineage cultures *(11,12)*. If cells from each fraction are deposited onto pre-established stromal cell layers, recovered after short-term culture (4 days), phenotypic progression is evident. That is, cultures seeded with HSA$^-$BP-1$^-$ cells yield HSA$^+$BP-1$^-$ and HSA$^+$BP-1$^+$

Table 1
Ordering and Extent of Rearrangement in B Lineage Fractions

Cell fraction	Fr. A	Fr. B	Fr. C	Fr. C'	Fr. D	Fr. E
Description	pre-pro-B	early pro-B	late pro-B	large pre-B	small pre-B	immature B
Ig heavy chain status	D → J initiating	DJ predominant (low level)	V → DJ initiating (low level)	VDJ complete (low level)		
Ig light chain status					$V_\kappa \rightarrow J_\kappa$ ongoing	$V_\kappa J_\kappa$ complete

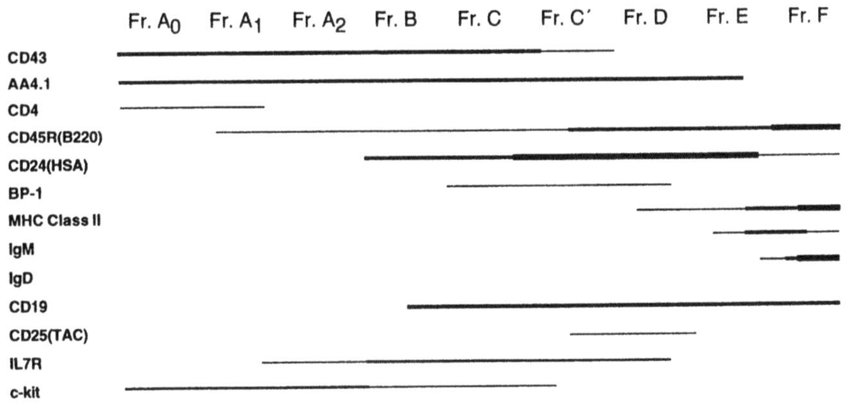

Fr. A0 Fr. A1 Fr. A2 Fr. B Fr. C Fr. C′ Fr. D Fr. E Fr. F
CD43
AA4.1
CD4
CD45R(B220)
CD24(HSA)
BP-1
MHC Class II
IgM
IgD
CD19
CD25(TAC)
IL7R
c-kit

Fig. 2. Diagram showing expression of cell surface proteins on stages of B lineage cells described in this review. Relative expression level is indicated by line thickness. Data taken from refs. *(6,18,20,51,66–69)*.

cells. Cultures seeded with $HSA^+BP\text{-}1^-$ cells yield predominantly $HSA^+BP\text{-}1^+$ cells. Cultures seeded with $HSA^+BP\text{-}1^+$ cells yield predominantly $B220^+CD43^-$ cells, some even expressing IgM. This supports an ordering of the early stage fractions summarized in Table 1.

As shown in Fig. 1, $B220^+CD43^-$ cells include both pre-B-cells and B-cells. Further analysis of the two immunoglobulin isotypes expressed on naive B-cells, IgM, and IgD, divides the B-cells into two subsets, newly formed or immature IgM^+IgD^- cells and mature IgM^+IgD^+ B-cells (*see* Fig. 1C). These latter cells resemble recirculating naive B-cells found in spleen and lymph nodes, based on expression of many other surface molecules, and may in fact represent recirculating B-cells transiting back through bone marrow. These $B220^+CD43^-$ fractions are also summarized in Table 1. Together with the $B220^+CD43^+$ fractions, the authors have labeled these subsets alphabetically, Fr. A through Fr. E. Figure 2 summarizes cell surface protein expression of a number of differentiation stage-specific markers, with relative level indicated by line thickness.

3. Ordered Rearrangement/Role of MU Heavy Chain

Work with transformed B lineage cell lines has defined major milestones in the development of B-cells: completion of heavy chain D-J rearrangement, productive V-DJ rearrangement, and productive light chain rearrangement *(13–16)*. Therefore, determination of the extent of DJ, VDJ, and VκJκ rearrangement serves to clarify the nature of the phenotypic stages described in Figs. 1 and 2 and also tests the extent to which rearrangement is an ordered process. A severe limitation of working with these normal populations is the small numbers of cells obtainable, typically on the order of 10^5. Nevertheless, PCR-based analysis of the loss of germline DNA between the D-J and V-D segments of heavy chain and between Vκ and Jκ segments demonstrates a largely ordered rearrangement program *(6)*. There is relatively little rearrangement in Fr. A and extensive D-J rearrangement in Fr. B, but little V-DJ rearrangement. V-DJ rearrangement becomes apparent in Fr. C (5–20%) and plateaus in Fr. D. Thus, the B220$^+$CD43$^+$HSA$^+$ fractions (B and C) consist of D-J rearranged cells in the process of V-DJ rearrangement. The authors have termed this stage "pro-B" to distinguish it from the pre-B stage where heavy chain rearrangement is complete and heavy chain protein is expressed in the cytoplasm. Comparable analyses using PCR assays that amplify the DNA segments generated by rearrangement have confirmed this analysis *(17,18)*.

Similar analysis shows that kappa light chain rearrangement occurs predominantly in the CD43$^-$ Fr. D stage, although low level light chain rearrangement (a few percent) is detected as early as Fr. B *(17,18)*. Thus, although not absolute, rearrangement is largely ordered with D-J preceding V-DJ and heavy chain preceding light chain (*see* Table 1), as previously deduced from studies with transformed cells *(19)*. Mice in which the heavy chain locus has been inactivated by gene targeting contain some light chain rearrangement *(20)*, demonstrating that this ordering is not absolute. The level of rearrangement at each locus is summarized in Table 1.

4. Stage-Dependent Functional Alterations

Interesting functional differences become apparent by comparing the growth of these fractions in stromal cell culture (*see* Fig. 3). The CD43$^-$ fractions do not survive even four days in stromal cell culture, whereas the CD43$^+$ fractions either survive (Fr. A) or proliferate (Fr. B, C). Early stages of B lymphopoiesis depend on cell contact signals, whereas later stages only require soluble mediators, notably IL-7. Comparison of the extent of cell recovery from cultures of these fractions maintained on a stromal line versus in diffusion chambers (that block stromal contact, but allow diffusion of soluble mediators) shows absolute contact dependence of Fr. A, but very substantial proliferation in the absence of contact with Fr. B and C. Results similar to diffusion chamber culture are also obtained by growth in simple medium supplemented with IL-7. A comparison of the growth of cells isolated from bone marrow of animals incapable of making Ig heavy chain (SCID, Rag-1/2 knockout) with cells from such mice bearing Ig heavy chain transgenes (thus all cells expressing heavy chain protein) reveals a critical role for heavy chain in this transition: cells from Ig$^-$ mice proliferate in contact, but then die in its absence, whereas cells from Ig$^+$ mice grow well in contact-independent cultures, including simple medium supplemented with IL-7 *(21,22)*.

In fact, comparison of bone marrow cells from recombination-deficient mice with those from Ig transgenic recombination-deficient mice *(21–24)* also reveals a sharp transition in phenotypic stages (Fig. 4). Cells lacking heavy chain are blocked at the B220$^+$CD43$^+$ stage. Moreover,B220$^+$CD43$^+$ cells reach the HSA$^+$BP-1$^+$ stage (Fr. C), but do not upregulate HSA. In contrast, B220$^+$CD43$^+$ cells from Ig transgenic mice show upregulated levels of HSA and also significant numbers of B220$^+$CD43$^-$ cells (Fr. D). Thus, for normal B lineage cells, progression of B220$^+$CD43$^+$ cells from the HSA$^+$ to HSA^{++} stage (and beyond) requires the presence of Ig heavy chain, likely interacting with surrogate light chain *(25–27)* (*see below*).

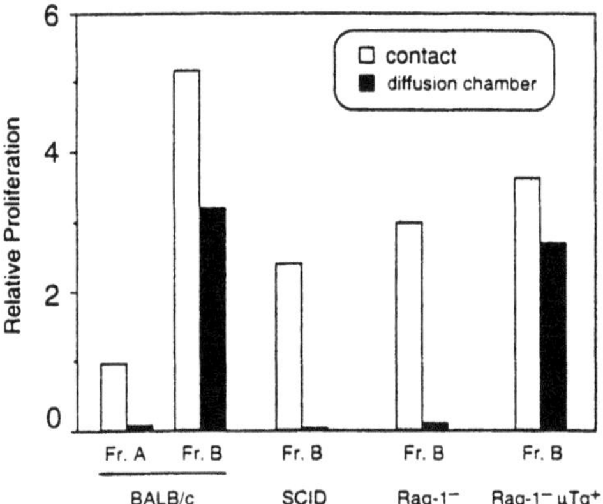

Fig. 3. Relative increase in cell number after four day culture, either in stromal cell contact or in a diffusion chamber separating cells from the stromal layer. Comparison of Fr. A and Fr. B from normal (BALB/c) with Fr. B cells from recombination-deficient (SCID and Rag-1⁻) and recombination deficient (Rag-1⁻) μ Ig transgenic mice. Contact independent growth in Fr. B is restored in recombination deficient cells by expression of the heavy chain transgene.

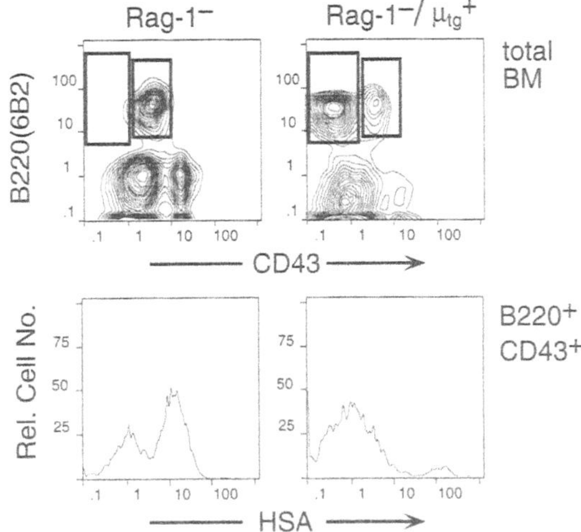

Fig. 4. Populations of B lineage cells in Rag-1⁻ and Rag-1⁻ Ig μ transgene⁺ bone marrow as revealed by correlated expression of CD45R(B220), CD43(S7) and CD24(HSA). Note the appearance of B220⁺CD43⁺HSA⁺⁺⁺ and B220⁺CD43⁻ cells in heavy chain transgene⁺ bone marrow.

Stromal culture can yield significant numbers of pre-B and immature B-cells, but few mature B-cells. Injection of cells into SCID immunodeficient mice, animals that lack all B220⁺CD43⁻ fractions *(2)*, allows generation of mature B-cells. Comparison of mice injected iv either with a hematopoietic stem cell (HSC) enriched fraction, (Thy-1^low^Lineage⁻) *(28,29)* or with pro-B-cells, shows that the HSC-injected mice develop T- and B-cells, whereas the pro–B-injected mice contain B-cells without significant numbers of T-cells (Fig. 5). Analysis of bone marrow shows that B lymphopoiesis is established within three to four weeks after HSC injection, but occurs only transiently after pro-B-cell injection. Thus, cells at the B220⁺CD43⁺HSA⁺ pro-

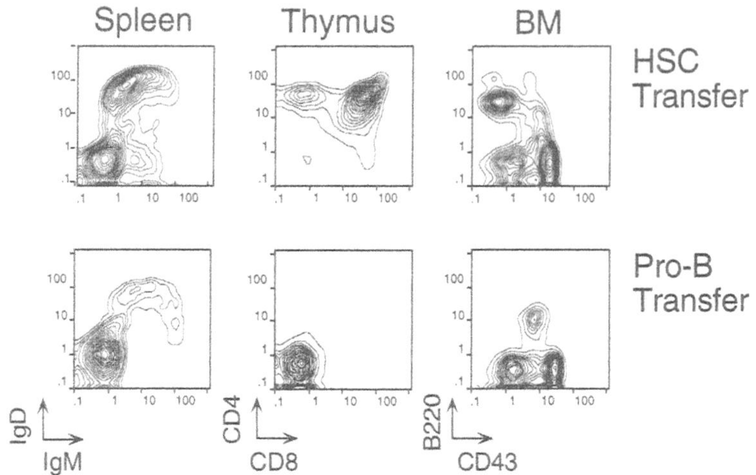

Fig. 5. Extent of reconstitution of lymphoid cells in SCID mice after transfer of either stem cell (HSC) or pro-B-cell fractions. Whereas both B- and T-cells are apparent in HSC-transferred recipients, only B-cells are seen in animals given pro-B-cell. Note that in bone marrow, whereas small pre-B-cells (Fr. D) are present in mice given HSC, these cells are absent from pro-B injected animals.

B stage are largely B-lineage committed and do not extensively self-renew; instead, they differentiate into resting mature B-cells.

5. Stage-Dependent Changes in Gene Expression

Analysis of B lineage associated genes serves to further substantiate the order of B lineage stages described above and also provides new information (Table 2). Mb-1, the gene encoding Ig-α (one of the CD3–like Ig accessory molecules) *(30–32)*, is found at high levels from Fr. B and serves to confirm the B lineage nature of most of the fractions. The distinctive timing of the recombinase activating genes (Rag-1 and Rag-2) and terminal deoxynucleotidyl transferase (TdT) explains a difference between the joints of heavy and light chain genes: TdT an enzyme that is responsible for adding nongermline nucleotides (N-sequence) at the heavy chain D-J and V-D junctions *(33–35)*, and the relative rarity of such N-sequence in light chain junctions is explained by the absence of TdT expression after Fr. C, since most light chain rearrangement occurs in Fr. D.

The sharp downregulation of TdT expression is dependent on expression of Ig heavy chain, as demonstrated by transfection of a pro-B-cell line with heavy chain genes *(36)*. After transfection, TdT levels decreased 5–10-fold. This effect likely results from assembly of heavy chain with the surrogate light chain components, λ5 and VpreB, molecules previously shown to associate with heavy chain prior to expression of conventional light chain *(37)*. Interestingly, these molecules are present at high levels during the pro-B stage, then decrease at the late pre-B (Fr. D) stage. Thus, it is possible that the surrogate light may function very early in B lymphopoiesis, prior to productive heavy chain rearrangement. One possibility is that it serves as a signaling mechanism to detect productive rearrangement, perhaps by competition with the recently described surrogate heavy chain *(38)*. One consequence of this signal appears to be the transition from contact dependence to independence described in Subheading 4 and entry into rapid cell

Table 2
Gene Expression in Bone Marrow B Lineage Fractions

	Fr. A	Fr. B	Fr. C	Fr. C'	Fr. D	Fr. E	Fr. F
Rag-1/2	+/-	+++	+++	–	+++	+/-	–
TdT	+/-	+++	+++	–	–	–	–
λ5/VpreB	+/-	+++	+++	+	–	–	–
Ig-β	+	++	+++	+++	+++	+++	+++
Ig-α	+/-	+	++	+++	+++	+++	+++
μ	–	–	–	+++	++	++	++
Bcl-2	+++	++	+	+/-	–	–	++
Bcl-x_L	–	++	++	++	+++	+	–

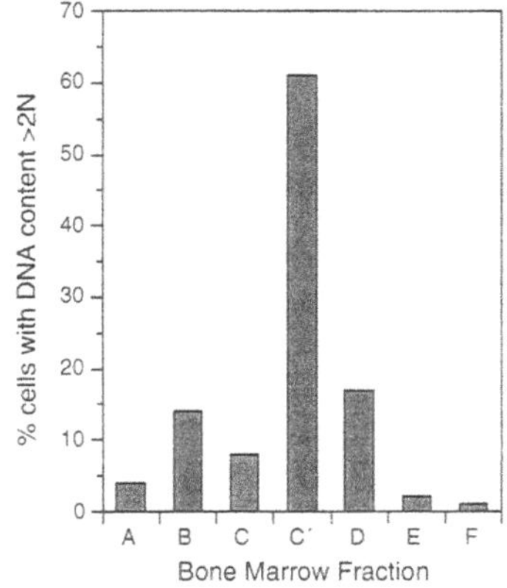

Fig. 6. Percent of cells with DNA content greater than G_0/G_1 in bone marrow B lineage fractions as determined by staining permeabilized sorted cells with propidium iodide.

cycle. The cell cycle status of these fractions (Fig. 6) shows some proliferation in Fr. A–C, a majority of cells in Fr. C' in cycle, and most having exited cycle at Fr. D.

Analysis of the expression of molecules potentially important in signaling changes in growth properties of B lineage cells, such as tyrosine kinases, has also revealed distinctive patterns of expression, particularly for blk and ret *(39)*. Using the degenerate PCR primer approach, the authors screened for protein tyrosine kinases (PTKs) that might play a role in progression beyond the pro-B stage, and identified five differentially regulated PTKs and compared their gene expression in defined stages of early B lineage cells from normal, recombination-deficient, and Ig transgenic recombination-deficient mice. Three PTKs (fgr, Flk-2/Flt-3, and tsk) showed comparable decreases at an early stage. In contrast, the decreasing expression of ret and the increasing expression of blk seen in differentiating B-cells from normal mice were not observed in recombination-deficient mice, unless they carried Ig transgenes. Thus, the expression of these PTKs appears dependent on productive Ig rearrangement and suggests important roles for both ret and blk at distinct stages in the Ig-dependent progression of B-cell differentiation.

The generation of B-cells involves several stages of cell selection, first for productive Ig rearrangement, then likely testing the newly formed antibody for self-reactivity. Thus, autoreactive B-cells have been shown to be either deleted or rendered unresponsive ("anergized") at the immature stage (Fr. E) in bone marrow by using several transgenic mouse model systems *(22,40–44)*. Elimination of developing B-cells by programmed

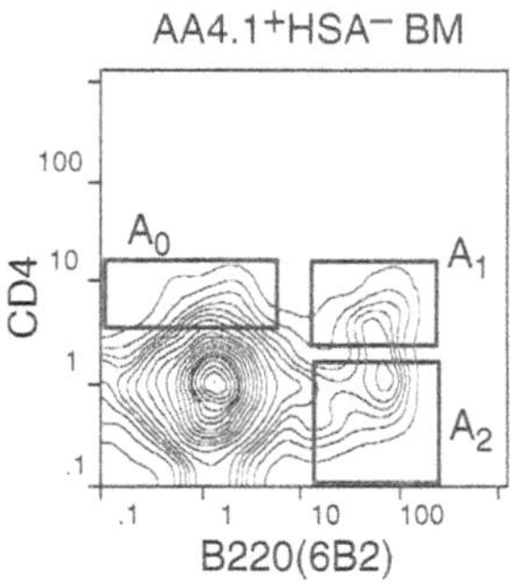

Fig. 7. Earliest stages of B lineage cells as revealed by staining with AA4.1, CD24(HSA), CD45R(B220), and CD4. Panel shows the correlated expression of CD45R(B220), and CD4 on AA4.1$^+$HSA$^-$ cells in bone marrow.

cell death (apoptosis) likely depends on levels of antiapoptotic molecules such as Bcl-2 and Bcl-x *(45–48)*. In fact, Bcl-2 decreases from the earliest stage, reaching a nadir at the pre-B/immature B-cell stage and rises sharply at the mature B-cell stage. This high-low-high pattern is highly reminiscent of that seen with Bcl-2 during T-cell development in thymus, in which minimal levels are found at the CD4/CD8 double positive stage. Analysis with monoclonal antibody to Bcl-2 has confirmed that protein expression is also very low at the Pre-B/immature B stage compared to that in mature B-cells *(49)*.

In contrast with the pattern of Bcl-2 expression, Bcl-x expression is low at the earliest stages and rises at the pre-B/immature B stage, decreasing in mature B-cells. Bcl-x transgenic mice that constitutively overexpress this protein accumulate large numbers of B220$^+$CD43$^+$ cells in bone marrow, many of which harbor aberrant heavy chain rearrangements *(50)*. It is possible that productive rearrangement and heavy chain expression serves to maintain Bcl-x expression during the stages when Bcl-2 is very low, sparing such cells from apoptotic death. In this scheme, expression from the Bcl-x transgene would allow the persistence of cells lacking productive rearrangements, presumably the expanded population detected in such mice.

6. Earliest Stages of B Lineage Development

The earliest fraction described above, Fr. A, shows little evidence of rearrangement and low expression of B lineage-associated genes. In order to determine the extent of B lineage cells within this population, the authors have analyzed bone marrow cells for the expression of B220 and HSA along with two additional surface markers, AA4.1 and CD4 *(51)*. AA4.1 is expressed on HSC *(52)*, B-cell /myeloid bipotential progenitors *(52,55)*, and early B lineage cells *(38,39)*. CD4, usually considered as restricted to T lineage cells, is expressed at low levels on lymphoid progenitors *(56–59)*. About half of the B220$^+$CD43$^+$HSA$^-$ cells (previously termed Fr. A) *(6)* express AA4.1, and only the AA4.1$^+$ subfraction proliferates in stromal cell culture, providing evidence that only this subfraction includes B lineage precursors. Quantitating expression of CD4 refines this analysis, since only primitive multilineage hematopoietic precursors bear low levels of this molecule, and its expression is extinguished during the earliest stages of B lineage development. Among the CD43$^+$HSA$^-$AA4.1$^+$ cells, three cell fractions can be determined, termed A_0, A_1, and A_2, identified by the expression patterns B220$^-$CD4$^+$, B220$^+$CD4$^+$, and B220$^+$CD4$^-$ respectively (Fig. 7). The A_0 fraction resembles the

Table 3
Gene Expression in Earliest B Lineage Fractions

	Fr. A_0	Fr. A_1	Fr. A_2	Fr. B
μ_0	–	+++	+++	–
Rag-1/2	–	+/-	+	+++
λ5/VpreB	–	–	+	+++
Ig-β	–	+	++	+++
Ig-α	–	–	+	+++

common lymphoid progenitor population reported by others *(56,57,58)*, whereas A_1 and A_2 represent the earliest identifiable populations of B lineage cells.

Analysis of transcription from the unrearranged IgH locus, μ_0 *(60,61)*, provides evidence for B lineage commitment. Simultaneous measurement of levels of Rag-1 and Rag-2 *(62,63)* mRNA further refines this analysis, since transcription of these recombinase genes should initiate before or coincident with IgH rearrangement *(18,64,65)*. Using semi-quantitative reverse transcriptase–polymerase chain reaction (RT-PCR), it is found A_1, and A_2 have high levels of μ_0 transcripts, but very low levels of Rag-1 and Rag-2 expression when compared to more differentiated $B220^+CD43^+HSA^+$ Pro-B-cells (Table 3). These data are consistent with the idea that locus accessibility precedes functional recombinase activity. Additional analysis of the pattern of expression of a set of B lineage-restricted genes further establishes the B lineage character of these fractions and provide evidence to support the ordering of A_0, A_1, and A_2.

7. Summary and Conclusions

Differentiating B lineage cells in mouse bone marrow can be staged based on the expression of distinctive combinations of cell surface molecules. The authors have characterized eight fractions of $B220^+$ cells, the earliest expressing high levels of heavy chain germline transcript, intermediate stages showing D-J and then V-DJ rearrangement, later stages possessing cytoplasmic heavy chain protein and kappa light chain rearrangements and terminal stages resembling peripheral B-cells. The expression of heavy chain μ protein allows the developing cells to pass a critical checkpoint, presumably through assembly with surrogate light chains and the Ig accessory molecules to form the pre-B-cell receptor complex. Further analysis of the assembly and function of this complex in the intermediate stages delineated here should facilitate our understanding of the specific interactions and events required for normal B-cell development. A more thorough understanding of this process will also help design rational treatment strategies for B leukemias and lymphomas that represent transformed counterparts of distinctive stages in B-cell development. In this regard, it is also interesting to note the sharp changes in expression of genes that block programmed cell death, Bcl-2 and Bcl-x, through this pathway. Their potential regulation by signals through the pre–B-cell receptor provide a possible mechanism for selection of pre-B-cells with "appropriate" heavy chain structures and their disregulation a possible contributing factor to B lymphoma.

References

1. Coffman, R. L. and Weissman, I. L. (1981) B220: a B cell-specific member of the T200 glycoprotein family. *Nature* **289,** 681–683.

2. Hardy, R. R., Kemp, J. D., and Hayakawa, K. (1989) Analysis of lymphoid populations in scid mice: detection of a potential B lymphocyte progenitor population present at normal levels in scid mice by three color flow cytometry with B220 and S7. *Curr. Top. Microbiol. Immunol.* **152,** 19–25.
3. Bosma, M. J. and Carroll, A. M. (1991) The SCID mouse mutant: definition, characterization and potential uses. *Annu. Rev. Immunol.* **9,** 323–350.
4. Kay, R., Takei, F., and Humphries, R. K. (1990) Expression cloning of a cDNA encoding M1/69–J11d heat-stable antigens. *J. Immunol.* **145,** 1952–1959.
5. Symington, F. W. and Hakomori, S.-I. (1984) Hematopoietic subpopulations express cross-reactive, lineage-specific molecules detected by monoclonal antibody. *Mol. Immunol.* **21,** 507.
6. Hardy, R. R., Carmack, C. E., Shinton, S. A., Kemp, J. D., and Hayakawa, K. (1991) Resolution and characterization of pro-B and pre-pro-B cell stages in normal mouse bone marrow. *J. Exp. Med.* **173,** 1213–1225.
7. Cooper, M. D., Mulvaney, D., Coutinho, A., and Cazenave, P. A. (1986) A novel cell surface molecule on early B-lineage cells. *Nature* **321,** 616–618.
8. Ramakrishnan, L., Wu, Q., Yue, A., Cooper, M. D., and Rosenberg, N. (1990) BP-1/6C3 expression defines a differentiation stage of transformed pre-B cells and is not related to malignant potential. *J. Immunol.* **145,** 1603–1608.
9. Wu, Q., Lahti, J. M., Air, G. M., Burrows, P. D., and Cooper, M. D. (1990) Molecular cloning of the murine BP-1/6C3 antigen: a member of the zinc-dependent metallopeptidase family. *Proc. Natl. Acad. Sci. USA* **87,** 993–997.
10. Wu, Q., Tidmarsh, G. F., Welch, P. A., Pierce, J. H., Weissman, I. L., and Cooper, M. D. (1989) The early B lineage antigen BP-1 and the transformation-associated antigen 6C3 are on the same molecule. *J. Immunol.* **143,** 3303–3308.
11. Whitlock, C. A., Tidmarsh, G. F., Muller-Sieburg, C., and Weissman, I. L. (1987) Bone marrow stromal cell lines with lymphopoietic activity express high levels of a pre-B neoplasia-associated molecule. *Cell* **48,** 1009–1021.
12. Whitlock, C. A. and Witte, O. N. (1982) Long-term culture of B lymphocytes and their precursors from murine bone marrow. *Proc. Natl. Acad. Sci. USA* **79,** 3608–3612.
13. Alt, F., Rosenberg, N., Lewis, S., Thomas, E., and Baltimore, D. (1981) Organization and reorganization of immunoglobulin genes in A-MULV-transformed cells: rearrangement of heavy but not light chain genes. *Cell* **27,** 381–390.
14. Alt, F. W., Blackwell, T. K., DePinho, R. A., Reth, M. G., and Yancopoulos, G. D. (1986) Regulation of genome rearrangement events during lymphocyte differentiation. *Immunol. Rev.* **89,** 5–30.
15. Alt, F. W., Oltz, E. M., Young, F., Gorman, J., Taccioli, G., and Chen, J. (1992) VDJ recombination. *Immunol. Today* **13,** 306–314.
16. Alt, F. W., Yancopoulos, G. D., Blackwell, T. K., Wood, C., Thomas, E., Boss, M., Coffman, R., Rosenberg, N., Tonegawa, S., and Baltimore, D. (1984) Ordered rearrangement of immunoglobulin heavy chain variable region segments. *EMBO J* **3,** 1209–1219.
17. Ehlich, A., Schaal, S., Gu, H., Kitamaru, D., Muller, W., and Rajewsky, K. (1993) Immunoglobulin heavy and light chain genes rearrange independently at early stages of B cell development. *Cell* **72,** 695–704.
18. Li, Y.-S., Hayakawa, K., and Hardy, R. R. (1993) The regulated expression of B lineage associated genes during B cell differentiation in bone marrow and fetal liver. *J. Exp. Med.* **178,** 951–960.
19. Reth, M. G., Ammirati, P., Jackson, S., and Alt, F. W. (1985) Regulated progression of a cultured pre-B-cell line to the B-cell stage. *Nature* **317,** 353–355.
20. Loffert, D., Schaal, S., Ehlich, A., Hardy, R. R., Zou, Y.-R., Muller, W., and Rajewsky, K. (1994) Early B-cell development in the mouse: insights from mutations introduced by gene targeting. *Immunol. Rev.* **137,** 135–153.
21. Reichman-Fried, M., Bosma, M. J., and Hardy, R. R. (1993) B-lineage cells in mu-transgenic scid mice proliferate in response to IL-7 but fail to show evidence of immunoglobulin light chain gene rearrangement. *Int. Immunol.* **5,** 303–310.
22. Spanopoulou, E., Roman, C. A., Corcoran, L. M., Schlissel, M. S., Silver, D. P., Nemazee, D., Nussenzweig, M. C., Shinton, S. A., Hardy, R. R., and Baltimore, D. (1994) Functional immunoglobulin transgenes guide ordered B-cell differentiation in Rag-1–deficient mice. *Genes Dev.* **8,** 1030–1042.

23. Reichman-Fried, M., Hardy, R. R., and Bosma, M. J. (1990) Development of B-lineage cells in the bone marrow of scid mice following the introduction of functionally rearranged immunoglobulin transgenes. *Proc. Natl. Acad. Sci. USA* **87,** 2730–2739.
24. Young, F., Ardman, B., Shinkai, Y., Lansford, R., Blackwell, T. K., Mendelsohn, M., Rolink, A., Melchers, F., and Alt, F. W. (1994) Influence of immunoglobulin heavy-and light-chain expression on B-cell differentiation. *Genes Dev.* **8,** 1043–1057.
25. Karasuyama, H., Kudo, A., and Melchers, F. (1990) The proteins encoded by the VpreB and lambda 5 pre-B cell-specific genes can associate with each other and with mu heavy chain. *J. Exp. Med.* **172,** 969–972.
26. Karasuyama, H., Rolink, A., and Melchers, F. (1993) A complex of glycoproteins is associated with VpreB/lambda 5 surrogate light chain on the surface of mu heavy chain-negative early precursor B cell lines. *J. Exp. Med.* **178,** 469–478.
27. Sakaguchi, N. and Melchers, F. (1986) $\lambda 5$, a new light-chain-related locus selectively expressed in pre-B lymphocytes. *Nature* **324,** 579–582.
28. Muller-Sieburg, C. E., Whitlock, C. A., and Weissman, I. L. (1986) Isolation of two early B lymphocyte progenitors from mouse marrow: a committed pre-pre-B cell and a clonogenic Thy-1-lo hematopoietic stem cell. *Cell* **44,** 653–662.
29. Spangrude, G. J., Heimfeld, S., and Weissman, I. L. (1988) Purification and characterization of mouse hematopoietic stem cells. *Science* **241,** 58–62.
30. Hombach, J., Leclercq, L., Radbruch, A., Rajewsky, K., and Reth, M. (1988) A novel 34-kd protein co-isolated with the IgM molecule in surface IgM-expressing cells. *EMBO J.* **7,** 3451–3456.
31. Hombach, J., Lottspeich, F., and Reth, M. (1990) Identification of the genes encoding the IgM-alpha and Ig-beta components of the IgM antigen receptor complex by amino-terminal sequencing. *Eur. J. Immunol.* **20,** 2795–2799.
32. Reth, M. (1993) Antigen receptors on B lymphocytes. *Ann. Rev. Immunol.* **10,** 98–121.
33. Gilfillan, S., Dierich, A., Lemeur, M., Benoist, C., and Mathis, D. (1993) Mice lacking TdT: Mature animals with an immature lymphocyte repertoire. *Science* **261,** 1175–1178.
34. Komori, T., Okada, A., Stewart, V., and Alt, F. W. (1993) Lack of N regions in antigen receptor variable region genes of TdT-deficient lymphocytes. *Science* **261,** 1171–1175.
35. Landau, N. R., Schatz, D. G., Rosa, M., and Baltimore, D. (1987) Increased frequency of N-region insertion in a murine pre-B-cell line infected with a terminal deoxynucleotidyl transferase retroviral expression vector. *Mol. Cell. Biol.* **7,** 3237–3243.
36. Wasserman, R., Li, Y.-S., and Hardy, R. R. (1997) Down-regulation of terminal deoxynucleotidyl transferase by Ig heavy chain in B lineage cells. *J. Immunol.* **158,** 1133–1138.
37. Melchers, F., Karasuyama, H., Haasner, D., Bauer, S., Kudo, A., Sakaguchi, N., Jameson, B., and Rolink, A. (1993) The surrogate light chain in B-cell development. *Immunol Today* **14,** 60–68.
38. Karasuyama, H., Rolink, A., Shinkai, Y., Young, F., Alt, F. W., and Melchers, F. (1994) The expression of Vpre-B/lambda 5 surrogate light chain in early bone marrow precursor B cells of normal and B cell-deficient mutant mice. *Cell* **77,** 133–143.
39. Wasserman, R., Li, Y.-S., and Hardy, R. R. (1995) Differential expression of the blk and ret tyrosine kinases during B lineage development is dependent on Ig rearrangement. *J. Immunol.* **155,** 644–651.
40. Chen, C., Nagy, Z., Radic, M. Z., Hardy, R. R., Huszar, D., Camper, S. A., and Weigert, M. (1995) The site and stage of anti-DNA B-cell deletion. *Nature* **373,** 252–255.
41. Goodnow, C. C. (1992) Transgenic mice and analysis of B-cell tolerance. *Annu. Rev. Immunol.* **10,** 489–518.
42. Hartley, S. B., Cooke, M. P., Fulcher, D. A., Harris, A. W., Cory, S., Basten, A., and Goodnow, C. C. (1993) Elimination of self-reactive B lymphocytes proceeds in two stages: arrested development and cell death. *Cell* **72,** 325–335.
43. Nemazee, D. and Burki, K. (1989) Clonal deletion of autoreactive B lymphocytes in bone marrow chimeras. *Proc. Natl. Acad. Sci. USA* **86,** 8039–8043.
44. Nemazee, D., Russell, D., Arnold, B., Haemmerling, G., Allison, J., Miller, J. F., Morahan, G., and Buerki, K. (1991) Clonal deletion of autospecific B lymphocytes. *Immunol. Rev.* **122,** 117–132.
45. Boise, L. H., Gonzalez-Garcia, M., Postema, C. E., Ding, L., Lindsten, T., Turka, L. A., Mao, X., Nunez, G., and Thompson, C. B. (1993) *bcl-x*, a bcl-2–related gene that functions as a dominant regulator of apoptotic cell death. *Cell* **74,** 597–608.

46. Hockenbery, D., Nunez, G., Milliman, C., Schreiber, R. D., and Korsmeyer, S. J. (1990) Bcl-2 is an inner mitochondrial membrane protein that blocks programmed cell death. *Nature* **348,** 334–336.
47. Strasser, A., Harris, A. W., Vaux, D. L., Webb, E., Bath, M. L., Adams, J. M., and Cory, S. (1990) Abnormalities of the immune system induced by dysregulated bcl-2 expression in transgenic mice. *Curr. Top. Microbiol. Immunol.* **166,** 175–181.
48. Vaux, D. L., Cory, S., and Adams, J. M. (1988) Bcl-2 gene promotes haemopoietic cell survival and cooperates with c-myc to immortalize pre-B cells. *Nature* **335,** 440–442.
49. Merino, R., Ding, L., Veis, D. J., Korsmeyer, S. J., and Nunez, G. (1994) Developmental regulation of the Bcl-2 protein and susceptibility to cell death in B lymphocytes. *EMBO J.* **13,** 683–691.
50. Fang, W., Mueller, D. L., Pennell, C. A., Rivard, J. J., Li, Y.-S., Hardy, R. R., Schlissel, M. S., and Behrens, T. W. (1996) Frequent aberrant immunoglobulin gene rearrangements in pro-B cells revealed by a Bcl-xL transgene. *Immunity* **4,** 291–299.
51. Li, Y.-S., Wasserman, R., Hayakawa, K., and Hardy, R. R. (1996) Identification of the earliest B lineage stage in mouse bone marrow. *Immunity* **5,** 527–535.
52. McKearn, J. P., McCubrey, J., and Fagg, B. (1985) Enrichment of hematopoietic precursor cells and cloning of multipotential B-lymphocyte precursors. *Proc. Natl. Acad. Sci. USA* **82,** 7414–7418.
53. Cumano, A. and Paige, C. (1992) Enrichment and characterization of uncommitted B-cell precursors from fetal liver at day 12 of gestation. *EMBO J.* **11,** 593–601.
54. Cumano, A., Paige, C. J., Iscove, N. N., and Brady, G. (1992) Bipotential precursors of B cells and macrophages in murine fetal liver. *Nature* **356,** 612–615.
55. Loken, M. R., Shah, V. O., Hollander, Z., and Civin, C. I. (1988) Flow cytometric analysis of normal B lymphoid development. *Pathol. Immunopathol. Res.* **7,** 357–370.
56. Chervenak, R., Dempsey, D., Soloff, R., Wolcott, R. M., and Jennings, S. R. (1993) The expression of CD4 by T cell precursors resident in both the thymus and the bone marrow. *J. Immunol.* **151,** 4486–4493.
57. Fredrickson, G. G. and Basch, R. S. (1989) L3T4 antigen expression by hemopoietic precursor cells. *J. Exp. Med.* **169,** 1473–1478.
58. Wu, L., Antica, M., Johnson, G. R., Scolly, R., and Shortman, K. (1991) Developmental potential of the earliest precursor cells from the adult mouse thymus. *J. Exp. Med.* **174,** 1617–1627.
59. Wu, L., Scolly, R., Egerton, M., Pearse, M., Spangrude, G. J., and Shortman, K. (1991) CD4 expressed on earliest T-lineage precursor cells in the adult murine thymus. *Nature* **349,** 71–74.
60. Alessandrini, A. and Desiderio, S. (1991) Coordination of immunoglobulin DJ_H transcription and D-to-J_H rearrangement by promoter-enhancer approximation. *Mol. Cell. Biol.* **11,** 2096–2107.
61. Schlissel, M. S., Corcoran, L. M., and Baltimore, D. (1991) Virus-transformed Pre-B cells show ordered activation but not inactivation of immunoglobulin gene rearrangement and transcription. *J. Exp. Med.* **173,** 711–720.
62. Oettinger, M. A., Schatz, D. G., Gorka, C., and Baltimore, D. (1990) RAG-1 and RAG-2, adjacent genes that synergistically activate V(D)J recombination. *Science* **248,** 1517–1523.
63. Schatz, D. G., Oettinger, M. A., and Baltimore, D. (1989) The V(D)J recombination activating gene, RAG-1. *Cell* **59,** 1035–1048.
64. Alt, F., Blackwell, T., and Yancopoulos, G. (1987) Development of the primary antibody repertoire. *Science* **238,** 1079–1087.
65. Schatz, D. G., Oettinger, M. A., and Schlissel, M. S. (1992) V(D)J recombination: molecular biology and regulation. *Ann. Rev. Immunol.* **10,** 359–383.
66. Chen, J., Ma, A., Young, F., and Alt, F. W. (1994) IL-2 receptor alpha chain expression during early B lymphocyte differentiation. *Int. Immunol.* **6,** 1265–1268.
67. Hayakawa, K., Tarlinton, D., and Hardy, R. R. (1994) Absence of MHC class II expression distinguishes fetal from adult B lymphopoiesis in mice. *J. Immunol.* **152,** 4801–4807.
68. Krop, I., de Fougerolles, A. R., Hardy, R. R., Allison, M., Schlissel, M. S., and Fearon, D. T. (1996) Self-renewal of B-1 lymphocytes is dependent on CD19. *Eur. J. Immunol.* **26,** 238–242.
69. Rolink, A., Grawunder, U., Winkler, T. H., Karasuyama, H., and Melchers, F. (1994) IL-2 receptor alpha chain (CD25, TAC) expression defines a crucial stage in pre-B cell development. *Int. Immunol.* **6,** 1257–1264.

Chapter 15

Lineage Relationships Between B Lymphocytes and Macrophages

Barbara L. Kee and Christopher J. Paige

1. Introduction

B lymphocytes, like all members of the hematopoietic system, develop from a common hematopoietic stem cell (HSC) in the bone marrow and fetal liver *(1)*. Restricted stem cells, apparently able to give rise to myeloid lineage cells but not to B and T lymphocytes, have also been identified *(2,3)*. However, lymphoid restricted stem cells have proven more difficult to identify conclusively, despite widespread belief that they exist (*see* refs. *4* and *5*). The development of hematopoietic cells committed to a single lineage is thought to occur through the progressive restriction of the differentiation options of multipotent progenitors. For example, multipotent myeloid stem cells develop into nonself-renewing progenitors that give rise to granulocytes, erythrocytes, macrophages, and megakaryocytes (GEMM progenitors) and subsequently into granulocytes and macrophages (GM progenitors) under conditions that support the development of all myeloid cell types *(6)*. Recently, bipotent progenitors, which develop into both B lymphocytes and macrophages, have been identified in the fetal liver of mice by the twelfth day of gestation (Fig. 1) *(7)*.

The existence of a B-cell/macrophage progenitor, although not suggested by the classical studies used to identify HSC, was implied by leukemias that exhibit phenotypic characteristics of both B lymphocytes and macrophages. The properties of these leukemic cells attest to the possibility of a close developmental relationship between the B lymphocyte and macrophage differentiation pathway. However, it was also suggested that the transformation process itself may have resulted in aberrant expression of lineage traits that would not be associated with those cells under normal developmental conditions *(8)*. The identification of a bipotent B-cell/macrophage progenitor lent credence to the hypothesis that these leukemic cells might represent transformed versions of an existing cell type. Furthermore, the coexpression of B-lineage and myeloid traits within a single

From: *Molecular Biology of B-Cell and T-Cell Development*
Edited by: J. G. Monroe and E. V. Rothenberg © Humana Press Inc., Totowa, NJ

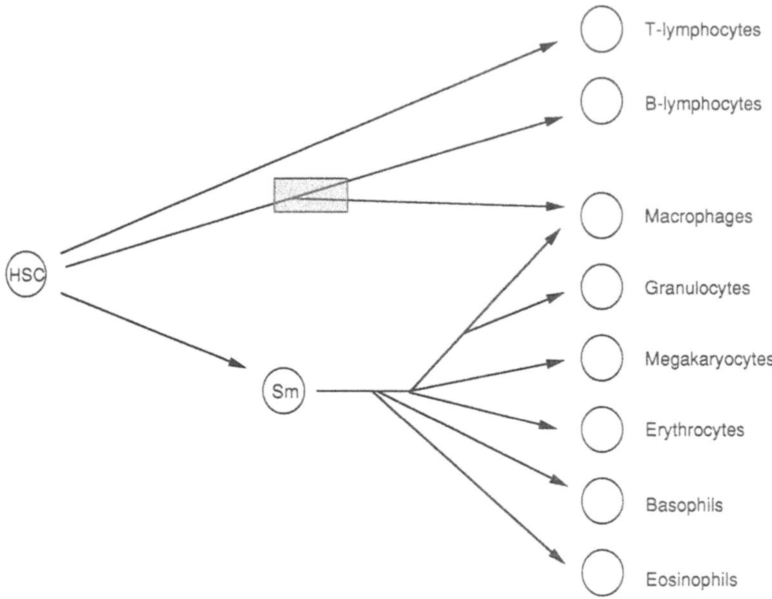

Fig. 1. Schematic outline of the development of mature hematopoietic cells from multipotent progenitors and stem cells. Self-renewing, mulitpotent stem cell have been identified, which gives rise to either all myeloid lineages or all of the mature cell types of the hematopoietic system (designated Sm, myeloid stem cell, or HSC). Additional multipotent myeloid progenitors, which lack self-renewal capacity, have been identified as the precursors to macrophage and granulocytes or macrophages, granulocytes, megakaryocytes and erythroid cells. More recently a bipotent precursor of B-lymphocytes and macrophages has been identified (shaded area).

cell may reflect the plasticity of normal cells prior to lineage determination. This possibility has recently been demonstrated in primary multilineage progenitors, which prime expression of genes associated with multiple developmental pathways prior to definitive lineage determination *(9)*.

A further indication that B lymphocytes and macrophages share a close developmental relationship is the finding that many transformed B-lineage cell lines are able to differentiate into macrophages (reviewed in ref. *10*). These B-lineage–derived macrophage cell lines demonstrate many functional characteristics of macrophages including expression of myeloid specific genes, proliferation in response to macrophage colony stimulating factor (M-CSF), and phagocytosis. Differentiation to the macrophage phenotype is accompanied by the a characteristic loss of specific B-lineage traits, whereas expression of other B-lineage traits does not appear to be incompatible with macrophage development. These findings suggest that expression of lineage associated traits does not necessarily result in the irrevocable commitment of a cell to differentiation through a particular developmental pathway. These lineage plastic cell lines have provided an excellent model system in which to study the requirements for lineage determination. In addition, advances in cell isolation and in vitro culture techniques and the ability to disrupt individual genes in the mouse genome have greatly facilitated the analysis of the role of specific proteins in the development of the hematopoietic system. In this review current understanding of the factors that regulated commitment of hematopoietic progenitors to the B-lymphocyte differentiation pathway will be discussed.

2. Development of B-Lymphocytes from Bipotent Progenitors

2.1. Identification of B-Lineage Cells

2.1.1. B-Lineage-Associated Genes

A number of gene products have been identified that are expressed in committed B-lineage cells and can be used to determine the relative stage of differentiation of a progenitor. The hallmark of a mature B lymphocyte is the ability to express immunoglobulin (Ig) on the cell surface, and to secrete Ig in response to antigenic or mitogenic stimulation. Cells committed to differentiation through the B lineage can further be identified by the presence of rearrangements of the DNA segments coding for the heavy- and light-chains of Ig. B-cell progenitors, although containing rearrangements at the Ig loci, can be distinguished from mature B-cells by the absence of detectable levels of IgM on the cell surface. In general, rearrangements at the Ig loci occur in a temporal order during the development of a B-cell and are, therefore, useful in determining the relative stage of differentiation of the cell. Rearrangement of a D (diversity) to J_H (joining) segment precedes rearrangement of a V (variable) segment to the existing DJ_H. Furthermore, rearrangement of the Ig heavy chain loci generally precedes rearrangement of Ig light chains (for review *see* ref. *11*). Although Ig rearrangements can be used to define the stage of development of a B-lineage cell, occasional DJ_H rearrangements have been found in T lymphocytes as well.

A number of genes whose products function in the rearrangement and/or expression of Ig are also useful for the identification of cells committed to differentiation through the B lineage (*see* Fig. 2). However, as with D-J_H rearrangements, some of these genes are expressed in other cell types; therefore, they are not conclusive markers of a B-lineage cell on their own. The recombinase activating genes Rag-1 and Rag-2 are expressed in B- and T-cell progenitors very early in the differentiation pathway and are required for the development of mature cells of both lineages *(12)*. Rag-1 and Rag-2 function in the site-specific cleavage of V, D, and J gene segments during the recombination of the Ig heavy and light chain loci (reviewed in ref. *13*). λ5 and VpreB, which, together, form a surrogate light chain found in association with Ig, are found in the most immature B-cell progenitors prior to expression of conventional light chains. This surrogate pre–B-cell receptor appears to play a critical role in B-lineage progression; however, the mechanism by which it functions is not well understood (reviewed in ref. *14*). Two additional proteins, mb-1 and B29, are found in B-cell progenitors at all stages of development with the exception of terminally differentiated plasma cells, and function in signal transduction through the Ig receptors. Recent studies indicate that B29 mRNA may be a very early marker of B-lymphocyte potential and is likely expressed prior to definitive lineage commitment *(15)*. For a review of the functions and distributions of each of these B-lineage–associated markers *see* Kee and Paige *(16)* or Loffert et al. *(12)*.

2.1.2. Cell Surface Markers of B-Lineage Cells

The identification of cell surface proteins expressed on progenitors at distinct stages of differentiation has increased biologists' ability to identify and purify these cells (Fig. 2). Markers associated with committed B-lymphocytes include two "pan" B-lineage markers CD19 and B220, an isoform of CD45. Both CD19 and B220 are transmembrane proteins that modulate signal transduction in B-lineage cells. These proteins are first detected on B-cell progenitors shortly after lineage commitment and are expressed through the mature B-cell stage. Expression of CD19 is restricted to B-lineage cells,

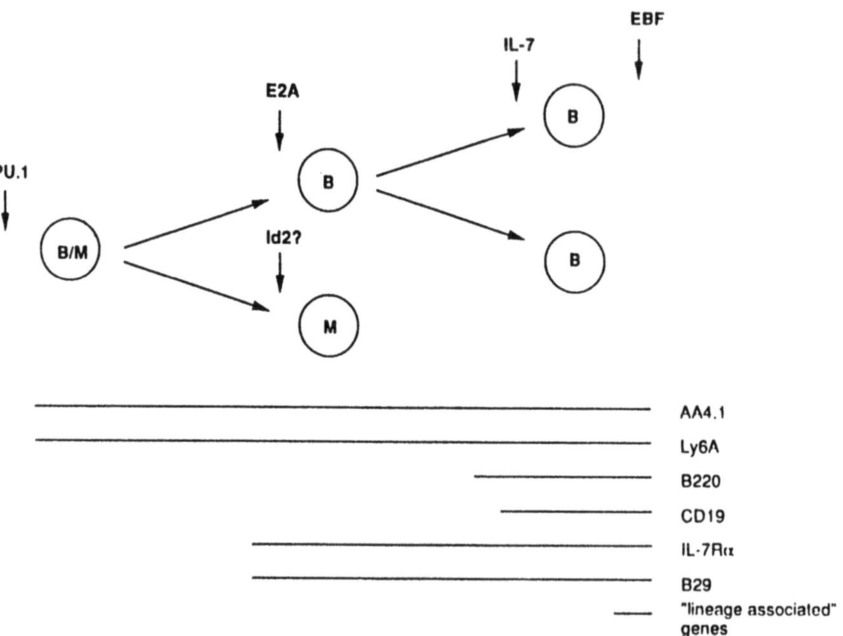

Fig. 2. Development of B-lymphocytes from bipotent B/macrophage progenitors. The pattern of cell surface protein expression on B/macrophage progenitors as they undergo restriction to the B lineage is shown on the bottom portion of the figure. In addition, the approximate timing of the requirement for the transcription factors PU.1, E2A, and EBF and for the cytokine IL-7 during the developmental process is depicted. The placement of Id2 prior to emergence of definitive macrophages is hypothetical and its correct placement requires further investigation.

whereas B220 is expressed on a small number of $CD43^+$ cells in bone marrow, which are not B-cell progenitors *(17)*. A number of additional proteins have been used to estimate the stage of development of committed B-cell progenitors *(18)*. In the bone marrow, pro-B-cells have been characterized as expressing both B220 and CD43. However CD43, also called leukosialin, is expressed on multipotent progenitors and committed progenitors of many cell lineages *(19)*. During B-lineage progression CD43 is downregulated at the transition of large cycling pro–B-cells to small pre–B-cells, and in vivo, the majority of $B220^+CD43^+$ cells do not contain Ig light chain gene rearrangements. The $CD43^+$ pro-B-cell stage has been subdivided further by the sequential acquisition of heat stable antigen (HSA) and aminopeptidase N (BP-1/6C3) *(18)*.

2.1.3. Cell Surface Markers for the Identification of Bipotent B-Cell/Macrophage Progenitors

Two additional markers, AA4.1 and Ly6A, have been very useful for the identification and purification of lineage unrestricted progenitors from early stages of gestation *(7,20)*. The antigen recognized by monoclonal antibody AA4.1 has not yet been identified; however, its expression is detected on multipotent hematopoietic cells, including stem cells as early as day 7.5 of gestation *(21,22)*. AA4.1 continues to be expressed on immature cells of many lineages, including B-lymphocytes and macrophages *(23–26)*. Expression of AA4.1 on B220 negative cells from bone marrow that can differentiate into B-lineage cells in vitro, has been demonstrated *(27)*; however it is not a marker of

HSC in bone marrow *(28,29)*. In combination with AA4.1, Ly6A, also known as stem cell antigen (Sca-1), is a useful marker for enrichment of bipotent progenitors from fetal liver. Ly6 is not expressed on multipotent cells prior to day 11 of gestation, although its expression can be detected on HSC in adult bone marrow in some strains of mice *(23,30)*.

2.2. Extrinsic Factors Regulating B-Cell Development from Bipotent Progenitors

2.2.1. Stromal Cells

Numerous laboratories have developed in vitro culture conditions in which B-lineage cells can be cloned and observed to differentiate *(31–35)*. All of these assays are dependent on the presence of adherent stromal cells or their products. In vivo, these cells are present in the hematopoietic microenvironment and are thought to provide the signals necessary for growth and differentiation of progenitors at multiple stages of development. The number and nature of these signals has not been resolved, but the production of cytokines is clearly one mechanism by which stromal cells support hematopoiesis (for review, *see* ref. *36* and Chapters 9–11, and 13). One of the crucial cytokines produced by stromal cells that support B lymphopoiesis is interleukin 7 (IL-7) *(37)*, the properties of which are discussed in Subheading 2.2.3. However, stromal cells provide factors in addition to IL-7 that are required at two distinct stromal cell-dependent phases of B-cell development. First, multipotent and bipotent cells are dependent on stromal cell-derived signals to reach a stage at which they can respond to IL-7 alone; second, IL-7 responsive progenitors are dependent on stromal cell-derived signals for maturation into surface Ig^+ and mitogen responsive B-cells *(38)*.

Three stromal cell-derived factorshave been identified, interleukin 11 (IL-11), mast cell growth factor (MGF), and IL-7, which are sufficient to replace the requirements for stromal cells in supporting the development of IL-7 responsive pre-B-cells from bipotent progenitors *(39)*. All of these factors can be made by stromal cells in vitro; however, it is not certain that these are the factors that they use to support B lymphopoiesis in vivo. Furthermore, the combination of IL-11 + MGF + IL-7 is not sufficient to support the development of bipotent progenitors, or pre-B lymphocytes, from multilineage progenitors isolated at earlier stages of gestation. In addition IL-11 + MGF + IL-7 are not sufficient to support the transition of pre-B lymphocytes into mitogen-responsive B-cells *(38)*.

2.2.2. IL-11+MGF and Flt-3/Flk-2 (FL) Act on Bipotent Progenitors and Their Direct Progeny

Both IL-11 and MGF are pleiotropic factors produced by stromal cells in bone marrow and fetal liver that synergize to promote the survival and proliferation of multilineage progenitors and stem cells. IL-11 is a 20-kDa soluble protein that elicits its biological responses by binding to a receptor composed of gp130 and a 151-kDa protein, both of which belong to the hematopoietic growth factor receptor family *(40,41)*. MGF, also known as stem cell factor (SCF), Steel factor or c-kit ligand, is 25-kDa protein that can exist in a transmembrane or a soluble form *(42)*. The receptor for MGF is a member of the protein tyrosine kinase receptor family *(43,44)*. As mentioned previously, IL-11 + MGF are sufficient to replace the requirement for stromal cells in the supporting the development of pre-B lymphocytes from bipotent B-cell/macrophage progenitors. Interestingly, substitution of IL-11 + MGF for stromal cells does not alter the kinetics of development of B lymphocytes or macrophages from bipotent progenitors. For example, the length of time required for the development of the first mitogen responsive cells, or for commitment to expression of one of the two Ig heavy chain alleles, is not altered by this change in culture conditions (*39* and unpublished data). These observations indicate that exogenous addition of IL-11 + MGF does not affect the self-renewal or differentiation potential of bipotent progenitors.

The requirement for IL-11 and MGF in the development of B lymphocytes from bipotent progenitors were assessed by delaying the addition of each of these cytokines at the initiation of culture *(15)*. Remarkably, it was found that both cytokines are required at the initiation of culture for the development of optimal numbers of either B-cells or macrophages. Furthermore, the combination IL-11 + MGF is sufficient to support the survival of bipotent cells the first three days of culture. During this time, a considerable expansion of cell numbers occurs, almost all of which are caused by cells that develop into macrophages. B-cell numbers do not begin to increase significantly until day three of culture, by which time commitment to the B lineage has already occurred (*see* section IL-7). This would appear to indicate that bipotent cells commit rapidly to the B or macrophage lineages, and that the B-cell progenitors remain quiescent until they are competent to respond to IL-7. In contrast, the macrophages continue to proliferate under the influence of IL-11 + MGF. However, preliminary data suggest that the precursors of B-cells are cycling rapidly at these early stages of culture (unpublished data). Therefore, an alternate model, in which bipotent progenitors proliferate in response to IL-11 + MGF, seems to be required. In such a model, the constant number of B-lineage progenitors could be explained only if, at each successive division, the probability of giving rise to a B-cell is decreasing. Regardless of which interpretation is correct, IL-11 + MGF support the proliferation of immature cells, but these cells do not maintain their multilineage potential.

Recent studies have indicated that, in many cases, the function of MGF can be replaced by Flt-3/Flk-2 ligand (FL) *(45–47)*. FL is a 25-kDa protein that, like MGF, can exist in a transmembrane or soluble form and also binds to a transmembrane receptor containing an intracellular domain possessing protein tyrosine kinase activity *(48)*. Both FL and its receptor have a cellular distribution remarkably similar to that of MGF and its receptor. The addition of IL-11 + FL + IL-7 to cultures of bipotent cells results in the development of B-cells and macrophages with similar kinetics to IL-11 + MGF + IL-7 containing cultures *(45)*. Interestingly, although the frequency of responding bipotent cells is the same under either set of conditions, the total number of cells present in a clone after expansion is greater in the presence of FL. This observation indicates that FL is a more potent proliferative stimulus than MGF for B-cell progenitors. In addition, whereas IL-11 + MGF + IL-7 is insufficient to support the development of B-lineage cells from multipotent progenitors isolated prior to day 12 of gestation, some of these cells are able to develop into B lymphocytes in the presence of IL-11 + FL + IL-7 *(45)*. A recent report by Veibry et al. *(47)* demonstrated a similar increase in B-lineage colony size when Lin-Sca + bone marrow cells were cultured in the presence of FL + IL-7 compared to MGF + IL-7. Interestingly, the development of B lymphocytes from these progenitors is dependent on the presence of both MGF (or FL) +IL-7 from the initiation of culture, suggesting that the colony initiating cells in this population are more mature than bipotent progenitors isolated on day 12 of gestation (*see* next section).

2.2.3. IL-7

IL-7 is a 25-kDa stromal cell-derived cytokine, which functions as a growth factor for pre-B lymphocytes *(37)*. The IL-7 receptor is composed of two proteins, both of which are members of the hematopoietic growth factor receptor family. IL-7Rα is a 68-kDa protein specific to the IL-7R, which associates with the common γ chain found in the receptors for IL-2, IL-4, IL-9, and IL-15 *(49–52)*. When added to cultures of murine bone marrow or fetal liver cells, IL-7 promotes the outgrowth of B220$^+$CD43$^+$, Ig heavy chain rearranged, pre-B lymphocytes *(53,54)*. IL-7 can synergize with MGF to promote the development of IL-7 responsive pre-B-cells from AA4.1$^+$B220$^-$ progenitors; however, all of these cells appear to be restricted to the B lineage (*39,55* and unpublished data). Over the past few years, the range of responses attributable to IL-7 has been extended to include several distinct aspects of B lymphopoiesis such as survival, proliferation, and differentiation.

In vitro, bipotent B-cell/macrophage progenitors are not dependent on the presence of IL-7 at the initiation of culture *(15)*. However, by day three of culture, the first cells are detected that have progressed to a stage where IL-7 becomes required for survival. Remarkably, some of the cells survive for as long as six days in the presence of IL-11 + MGF only. Under bulk-culture conditions, the timing of the requirement for IL-7 corresponds to the onset of expansion of clonable B-cell progenitors. This expansion of clonable B-cell progenitors is dependent on the presence of IL-7 in the culture medium *(15)*. Taken together, these results indicate that IL-7 is required for both the survival and proliferation of the progeny of bipotent B-cell/macrophage progenitors.

The authors questioned whether IL-7 might function in promoting commitment of bipotent progenitors to the B lineage. Single-cell cloning experiments indicated that these progenitors undergo lineage restriction by the third day of culture, concomitant with the requirement for IL-7 *(15)*. However, the frequency of progenitors that developed into B lymphocytes was identical in the presence or absence of IL-7, arguing that IL-7 is not required for B-lineage determination. Remarkably, these experiments still revealed an effect of IL-7 on progenitors prior to lineage restriction. In cultures containing IL-7, the number of Ly6A$^+$ cells was increased twofold compared with cultures that lacked IL-7. All of the B-lineage progenitors were found within the Ly6A$^+$ population *(15)*. If IL-7 promotes the expansion of cells after commitment to the B-lineage exclusively, the authors would predict an increase in the frequency of B-lineage cells within the Ly6A$^+$ population. However, the frequency of B-lineage cells in this population was similar in every experiment performed *(15)*. This result implies that the expansion of Ly6A$^+$ cells precedes the commitment event. Consistent with this model, an increase in the frequency of B-lineage cells in the Ly6A$^+$ population at later stages of culture was detected. The conclusion that IL-7 promotes the expansion of progenitors prior to definitive B-lineage commitment is further strengthened by the finding that AA4.1$^+$B220$^-$ cells are overrepresented in the bone marrow of IL-7 transgenic mice *(56)*.

The aforementioned studies are consistent with observations made from IL-7- and IL-7Rα-deficient mice *(57,58)*. These animals demonstrate a dramatic reduction in the development of B lineage, and T lineage cells. The arrest in B-cell development in these mice occurs at the B220$^+$CD43$^+$ pro–B-cell stage, prior to expression of BP-1/6C3. However, some mature B-cells do develop. Currently, it is not known whether this leakiness is the result of a redundancy in the IL-7 receptor-mediated signaling system. For example, a related cytokine, perhaps sharing the common γ chain of the IL-7 receptor, may compensate for the absence of IL-7 by activating a similar signaling pathway. Alternatively, if the only role of IL-7 were in promoting survival and proliferation, a small number of cells may survive long enough in the absence of IL-7 to complete the differentiation program. Either situation is consistent with the inability to detect leakiness under defined culture conditions, since alternative growth factors are not provided, and the number of clonable cells is limited.

Recent evidence suggests that the role of IL-7 may extend beyond survival and proliferation. In the authors' studies, they noted that IL-7 was required for the development of B-cell progenitors expressing a number of B lineage-associated genes including mb-1, λ5, VpreB, Rag-1, and BP-1/6C3 *(15)*. This finding is consistent with the hypothesis that IL-7 regulates the expression of these B lineage-associated genes. However, it is equally plausible that in the absence of IL-7 B-lineage progenitors die prior to attaining the stage of differentiation at which these genes are expressed. Evidence is accumulating that suggests that the signaling pathways elicited by IL-7 may regulate the expression of some B lineage-associated genes. For example, lymphocytes in the bone marrow of IL-7Rα-deficient mice do not express BP-1/6C3, despite the fact that B-cell progenitors transit though this stage to become mature B-cells *(56)*. However, a more convincing role for IL-7 in differentiation was provided by Corcoran et al., when they tested the ability of chimeric, or mutated, IL-7 receptors to rescue growth and differentiation of B-cell progenitors isolated from IL-7Rα-deficient mice *(59)*. In this study, a single tyrosine residue was identified in the cytoplasmic domain of the IL-7Rα (Y449), which is critical for the proliferative response to IL-7 but is not required for IL-7 mediated cell survival. Remarkably, the entire cytoplasmic domain of IL-7Rα was not required for cell survival, and this property may then be attributed to the common γ chain of the receptor. However, those B-lineage cells expressing the Y449 mutant receptor express cμ, whereas few B-lineage cells expressing the IL-7R lacking the cytoplasmic domain express this protein. This result suggests that the cytoplasmic domain of IL-7Rα provides a signal resulting in expression of cμ which is not dependent on Y449.

2.2.4. SDF-1

An essential role for SDF-1, a chemokine of the CXC family, in B-cell development has been demonstrated, since mice lacking this cytokine fail to develop any B-lineage cells *(59)*. However, this factor does not seem to play an essential role in B-cell development from bipotent progenitors under the authors' in vitro conditions. Nagasawa et al. speculate that the SDF-1 mutation may affect colonization of the bone marrow by HSC *(60)*. Since SDF-1 is a chemokine, it may also affect recruitment of progenitors into the appropriate microenvironment during fetal development. It has previously been demonstrated that B-cell development, unlike myelopoiesis, occurs in lymphoblastic islands in the fetal liver, suggesting that a specialized lymphopoietic microenvironment may exist in this organ *(61)*. Therefore, this chemokine may play a role in directing progenitors to the appropriate location for further development. If this is the case, this factor would not be required when culturing bipotent cells under optimal conditions in vitro.

2.3. Intrinsic Factors Regulating the Development of B-Lineage Cells

The development of B-lineage cells is dependent on the collective action of a manifold of transcriptional regulatory proteins (reviewed in ref. *62*). Several of these factors are required for the emergence of more than a single lineage; therefore, they may function in the development of multilineage progenitors. Alternatively, these transcription factors may perform a function that is required in the committed progenitors of many different lineages. Among the transcription factors that influence the development of multiple cell lineages, is the helix-loop-helix protein SCL/tal-1, which is required for the development of the entire hematopoietic system *(63,64)*. SCL/tal-1 has been proposed to regulate the decision of mesodermal cells to initiate formation of hematopoietic stem cells. Myb-1 appears to function downstream of SCL/tal-1, since targeted disruption of this gene results in the loss of all hematopoietic lineages with the exception of megakaryocytes *(65)*. The *ets*-related transcription factor PU.1 has been proposed to function even further downstream than myb-1, since the absence of this protein affects the development of lymphoid and some myeloid cells with the exception of megakaryocytes and erythrocytes *(66,67)*.

To date, no transcription factor has been identified, which exclusively affects the development of bipotent B-cell/macrophage progenitors. However, at least three transcription factors have been shown to be required for proper development through the early stages of the B lineage. One of these factors, the pair-rule protein Pax-5, is not required for B-lineage determination or the development of pro-B-cells, which can respond to IL-7 in the presence of stromal cell derived signals *(68)*. In the absence of Pax-5, B lymphopoiesis is arrested prior to the expression of BP-1/6C3, and prior to the accumulation of detectable V-DJ_H rearrangements *(69)*. The absence of early B-cell factor (EBF) results in an even earlier developmental arrest during B-lineage progression *(70)*. The bone marrow of EBF-deficient mice contains normal numbers of $B220^+CD43^+HSA^-BP\text{-}1^-$ pro-B-cells, suggesting that B-lineage commitment may have occurred; however, no B-lineage associated genes or Ig gene rearrangements can be detected in these cells. As discussed in Subheading 2.3.1., the transcription factors encoded by the E2A gene appear to be the most likely candidates for proteins that function in B-lineage commitment, because few, if any, B-cell progenitors can be identified in the bone marrow of E2A-deficient mice *(71,72)*.

2.3.1. Regulation of B-Cell Development by the Basic Helix-Loop-Helix Proteins E12 and E47

The E2A gene codes for two proteins, E12 and E47 that belong to the basic helix-loop-helix (bHLH) family of transcription factors. E12 and E47 differ from each other by the use of an alternatively spliced exon coding for the bHLH domain. These alternate bHLH domains share 83% sequence identity, and both proteins bind as dimers to the canonical E-box motif, CANNTG, found in the enhancers of many B lineage-associated genes *(73)*. The HLH domain is required for protein dimerization, whereas the basic region is required for binding to DNA.

E12 and E47 are class I HLH proteins, which are thought to have a wide tissue distribution, and to form heterodimers with cell-type specific, class II HLH proteins (reviewed in ref. *74*). In vertebrates, the E2A proteins, in conjunction with their cell-type restricted dimerizing partners, are known to function in cell fate decisions. For example, heterodimers of E2A with myoD, myf-5, or myogenin function directly in the specification of myocytes from mesodermal cells and E2A:NeuroD heterodimers are involved in the induction of neurons from ectoderm *(75–77)*. However, no tissue-restricted HLH partners for E2A have been identified in B-lymphocytes. Furthermore, E47 has been shown to function as a homodimer in these cells *(78)*. Homo- vs hetero-dimerization of E2A proteins may be regulated by phosphorylation of a serine residue in the conserved C terminal region of the protein which inhibits the formation of homodimers in non–B-lineage cells *(79)*.

The E2A proteins are required for B lymphopoiesis. Targeted disruption of E2A results in an arrest in B-lineage progression prior to the expression of CD19 and only a small number of $B220^+CD43^+HSA^-BP\text{-}1^-$ cells are present in the bone marrow of these mice *(80)*. In addition, few B lineage-associated genes can be detected by PCR in the bone marrow of these animals, and those that can are either not B lineage-restricted, such as IL-7Rα and EBF (which is also expressed in bone marrow stromal cells) or are known to be expressed prior to definitive lineage commitment, such as B29. The phenotype of

E2A deficient mice suggests that E12 or E47 is required for—or close to the time of—commitment to the B-lineage.

The high degree of sequence similarity between E12 and E47 has raised the question as to whether they are functionally distinct. Both proteins share the same cellular distribution, dimerize with the same proteins, and can bind to the same DNA sequence motif. The individual roles of E12 and E47 in promoting B lymphopoiesis was investigated recently by expressing transgenes for either E12 or E47 in E2A-deficient mice *(80)*. These experiments demonstrated that either protein alone is able to promote the development of cells that express B-lineage-associated genes such as Rag-1 and Rag-2, λ5, VpreB, mb-1, and undergo rearrangements of the Ig heavy chain loci. Surprisingly, however, mature B-cells were detected only in E47 transgenic mice. Therefore, it appears that E12, in the absence of E47, is not able to support the pre-B to B-cell transition. Importantly, optimal numbers of mature splenic B-cells are produced only when both transgenes are expressed, arguing that both E12 and E47 contribute significantly to the development of B-lineage cells.

2.3.2 A Role for E2A in the B-Cell/Macrophage Decision

Having clearly established a role for E2A in the development of committed B-lineage cells, it seems reasonable to consider that these proteins might play a role in the decision between the B-lymphocyte and macrophage cell fates from bipotent precursors. A number of papers have documented the differential expression of E2A proteins in B-lymphocytes and myeloid cells. For example, long-term cultures of myeloid progenitors initiated from rat bone marrow express very low levels of E2A; however, E2A levels increase when these cultures are switched to lymphoid supporting conditions *(81,82)*. The expression of E2A occurs just prior to the emergence of B220$^+$, cytoplasmic μ^+ pre-B-cells in these lymphoid long-term cultures. In contrast, a number of class V HLH proteins, known as Id proteins (inhibitors of differentiation), have been documented in immature myeloid cells, whereas their expression decreases early during B lymphopoiesis *(83,84)*. The Id proteins are HLH proteins that lack a basic region and are, therefore, capable of dimerizing with class I HLH proteins, but cannot bind to DNA. Consequently, Id proteins function as negative regulators of transcription by class I HLH proteins. Four Id proteins have been identified in the mouse, which have distinct but overlapping distributions and all of which heterodimerize with E2A proteins.

The opposing actions of E2A and Id appear to play a central role in lineage decisions in the well-characterized transition of 70Z/3 pre-B-cells to macrophages *(85,86)*. In the 70Z/3 pre–B-cell line, both E12 and E47 are expressed. However, upon differentiation to the macrophage, phenotype expression of both proteins is extinguished and the protein levels of Id2 increase *(87)*. Conditions have not yet been identified that allow this macrophage line, or any other B-cell derived macrophage, to revert to the B-lineage phenotype. However, remarkably, forced expression of E12 in 70Z/3 macrophages results in the activation of the B-lineage program *(87)*. This lineage conversion was evidenced by a decrease in adherence to plastic, an increase in expression of mRNA encoding IL-7Rα, λ5, μ, and Rag-1, as well as the ability to induce kappa light chain expression in response to mitogenic stimulation. The macrophage lines expressing E12 cease to express the myeloid antigen Mac-1, but they do retain a few macrophage traits such as expression of c-*fms*, Ly6 and Id2, as well as the ability to upregulate Ly6 in response to LPS.

3. B-Lineage Commitment

During the past five years, our knowledge of the diverse array of proteins that influence the development of committed B-lymphocytes from multipotent progenitors has increased dramatically. These proteins include the cytokines that promote the growth, survival, and differentiation of progenitors during the commitment process and transcription factors, which may function in choosing a particular cell fate. However, our understanding of the mechanism by which lineage commitment is achieved is still in its infancy. Previously, the authors proposed two models of lineage determination to use as a basis for interpreting the functions of potential lineage specifying genes *(16)*. The concatenation, or directed model, suggests that expression of a single gene is sufficient to initiate lineage determination. This lineage-specifying protein could function in a number of different ways; for example, through its ability to regulate the expression of all of the genes required for lineage determination or alternatively by initiating a cascade of events which leads to the committed state. The conjunction model suggests that commitment to a lineage is the result of the expression of a number of lineage-specifying genes at the right time in the correct cellular context. Cellular differentiation events may well encompass both of these models during the course of lineage determination and evidence in favor of both of these models has been published.

A recent paper by Hu et al. demonstrated that genes associated with distinct hematopoietic lineages can be expressed in multipotent cells prior to definitive lineage commitment *(9)*. These authors found expression of β-globin, a marker of erythroid cells, and myeloperoxidase, a marker of myeloid cells, as well as expression of a number of lineage-associated cytokine receptors in single cells from both a multipotent cell line (FDCP-mix) and multipotent populations of cells from murine bone marrow. Although this study provides some support for the conjunction model, the requirement for early multilineage gene expression in the commitment process remains to be demonstrated.

The ability of E12 to induce the conversion of 70Z/3 macrophages into pre-B-cells suggests that E12 may indeed be a protein that functions directly in the commitment process (Fig. 3). The simplest interpretation of these results is that increasing the expression of E12 allows the activation of E2A responsive genes that culminate in the progression of a cell through the B-lineage developmental pathway. Conversely, increasing the amount of Id2 would decrease the activity of E2A responsive genes and drive differentiation toward the macrophage developmental pathway. At the present time, the authors have no information regarding the genes that are regulated directly by E2A during this conversion and, which might, therefore, function in the lineage decision.

This E2A "dosage" model is similar to the mechanism by which the proneural genes (encoding HLH proteins) regulate the development of the sensory organ precursor (SOP) from ectoderm in Drosophila melanogaster *(88)*. This cell fate decision is regulated by the dose of HLH genes encoded by the achaete-scute complex (ASC) and daughterless, the Drosophila homolog of E2A. Furthermore, the development of the SOP is under the negative regulation of the HLH proteins, *hairy* and *extra-macrochaetae* (emc). Interestingly, the HLH domain of emc is related to the mammalian Id proteins. Given these striking similarities, it seems likely that the development of B-lymphocytes from multipotent progenitors may share other features with the development of the SOP in Drosophila. The development of the SOP is known to be regulated by cell–cell interactions mediated through the cell surface receptors Notch and Delta *(89)*. A number of mammalian homologs of these proteins have been identified, however, the potential role of any of these proteins in the development of the hematopoietic system is just beginning to be examined. Recent studies by Robey et al. have demonstrated that an activated form of Notch can influence the decision of T-cell progenitors to become $CD4^+$ vs $CD8^+$ T-cells, and that targeted disruption of one of the two Notch 1 alleles results in the preferential development of γδ T-cells as compared to αβ T-cells *(90,91)*. However, the

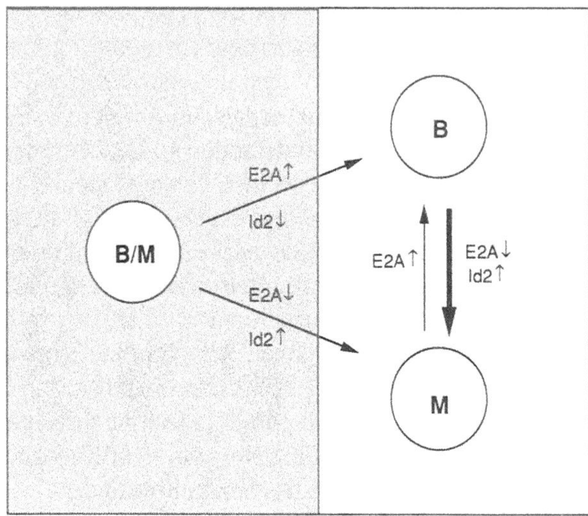

Fig. 3. The activity of E2A is a critical determinant of the B-lymphocyte fate. The open portion of the figure represent the potential relationship of E2A and Id2 to the development of B-lymphocytes or macrophages as suggested by experiments in the 70Z/3 cell line. In this case, increasing the functional activity of E2A favors the development of B-lineage cells whereas a decrease in activity, either through decreased levels of E2A or increased levels of Id2, is associated with the development of macrophages. The shaded area of the figure represents a hypothetical model of the requirements for E2A for the development of B-lymphocytes or macrophage from bipotent progenitors.

mechanisms that regulate the intracellular protein levels of E2A or Id in multipotent cells remain to be elucidated. The role of the E2A proteins in B-lymphopoiesis is further complicated by the finding that loss of expression of either of two other class I HLH proteins, HEB and E2-2, can also affect the development of B-lineage cells, although their effect is much less severe than absence of E2A *(92)*. Therefore, a complicated network of different positive and negative regulatory HLH proteins is likely to function in a combinatorial manner to influence differentiation through the B lineage.

Although the E2A proteins clearly play a central role in B-lineage determination, the mechanism by which they function remains to be fully elucidated. Identification of the genes activated by E2A during the commitment process will be essential to understanding the mechanism that effects the committed state. Furthermore, it remains to be determined how the activity of these transcription factors becomes restricted to the immediate progenitors of B-lineage cells. The pursuit of the answers to these questions is likely to reveal some unexpected findings regarding the interplay of extrinsic and intrinsic factors in the development of lineage restricted cells from multipotent hematopoietic progenitors.

Acknowledgments

The authors are grateful to Drs. Gretchen Bain and Cornelius Murre for many helpful discussions and comments on this manuscript. B.L.K. was supported by a fellowship from the Medical Research Council of Canada. This work was supported by work from the Medical Research Council of Canada and the National Cancer Institute of Canada.

References

1. Wu, A. M., Till, J. E., Siminovitch, L., and McCulloch, E. A. (1967) Cytological evidence for a relationship between normal hemopoietic colony-forming cells and cells of the lymphoid system. *J. Exp. Med.* **127,** 455–463.
2. Abramson, S., Miller, R. G., and Phillips, R. A. (1977) The identification in adult bone marrow of pluripotent and restricted stem cells of the myeloid and lymphoid systems. *J. Exp. Med.* **145,** 1567–1579.
3. Paige, C. J., Kincade, P. W., Moore, M. A. S., and Lee, G. (1979) The fate of fetal and adult B-cell progenitors grafted into immunodeficient CBA/N mice. *J. Exp. Med.* **150,** 548–563.
4. Lemischka, I. R., Raulet, D. H., and Mulligan, R. C. (1986) Developmental potential and dynamic behavior of hemopoietic stem cells. *Cell* **45,** 917–927.
5. Phillips, R. A. (1991) Hematopoietic stem cells: concepts, assays, and controversies. *Sem. Immunol.* **3,** 337–347.
6. Metcalfe, D. (1989) The molecular control of cell division, differentiation, commitment and maturation in haematopoietic cells. *Nature* **339,** 27–30.
7. Cumano, A., Paige, C. J., Iscove, N. N., and Brady, G. (1992) Bipotential precursors of B cells and macrophages in murine fetal liver. *Nature* **356,** 612–615.
8. Greaves, M. F., Chan, L. C., Furley, A. J., Watt, S. M., and Molgaard, H. V. (1986) Lineage promiscuity in hemopoietic differentiation and leukemia. *Blood* **67,** 1–11.
9. Hu, M., Krause, D., Greaves, M., Sharkis, S., Dexter, M., Heyworth, C., and Enver, T. (1997) Multilineage gene expression precedes commitment in the hemopoietic system. *Genes Dev.* **11,** 774–785.
10. Kee, B. L. and Paige, C. J. (1995) In vitro models of B lineage commitment. *Semin. Immunol.* **7,** 143–154.
11. Alt, F. W., Blackwell, T. K., DePinho, R. A., Reth, M. G., and Yancopoulos, G. D. (1986) Regulation of genome rearrangement events during lymphocyte differentiation. *Immunol. Rev.* **89,** 5–30.
12. Loffert, D., Schaal, S., Ehlich, A., Hardy, R. R., Zou, Y.-R., Muller, W., and Rajewsky, K. (1994) Early B-cell development in the mouse: insights from mutations introduced by gene targeting. *Immunol. Rev.* **137,** 135–153.
13. Ramsden, D. A., van Gent, D. C., and Gellert, M. (1997) Specificity in V(D)J recombination: new lessons from biochemistry and genetics. *Curr. Opin. Immunol.* **9,** 114–120.
14. Rolink, A., Haasner, D., Melchers, F., and Andersson, J. (1996) The surrogate light chain in mouse B-cell development. *Int. Rev. Immunol.* **13,** 341–356.
15. Kee, B. L. and Paige, C. J. (1996) In vitro tracking of IL-7 responsiveness and gene expression during commitment of bipotent B-cell/macrophage progenitors. *Curr. Biol.* **6,** 1159–1169.
16. Kee, B. L. and Paige, C. J. (1995) Murine B cell development: commitment and progression from multipotential progenitors to mature B lymphocytes. *Int. Rev. Cytol.* **157,** 129–179.
17. Rolink, A., ten Boekel, E., Melchers, F., Fearon, D. T., Krop, I., and Andersson, J. (1996) A subpopulation of B220+ cells in murine bone marrow does not express CD19 and contains natural killer cell progenitors. *J. Exp. Med.* **183,** 187–194.
18. Hardy, R. R., Carmack, C. E., Shinton, S. A., Kemp, J. D., and Hayakawa, K. (1991) Resolution and characterization of pro-B and pre-pro-B cell stages in normal mouse bone marrow. *J. Exp. Med.* **173,** 1213–1225.
19. Pallant, A., Eskenazi, A., Mattei, M. G., Fournier, R. E. K., Carlsson, R., Fukuda, M., and Frelinger, J. G. (1992) Characterization of cDNAs encoding human leukosialin and localization of the leukosialin gene to chromosome 16. *Proc. Natl. Acad. Sci. USA* **86,** 1328–1331.
20. Cumano, A. and Paige, C. J. (1992) Enrichment and characterization of uncommitted B-cell precursors from fetal liver a day 12 of gestation. *EMBO J.* **11,** 593–601.
21. Cumano, A., Dieterlen, F., and Godin, I. (1996) Lymphoid potential, probed before circulation in mouse, is restricted to caudal intraembryonic splanchnopleura. *Cell* **86,** 907–916.
22. Godin, I., Dieterlen-Lievre, F., and Cumano, A. (1995) Emergence of multipotent hematopoietic cells in the yolk sac and para-aortic splanchnopleura of 8. 5 dpc mouse embryos. *Proc. Natl. Acad. Sci. USA* **92,** 773–777.

23. Cumano, A., Furlonger, C., and Paige, C. J. (1993) Differentiation and characterization of B-cell precursors detected in the yolk sac and embryo body of embryos beginning at the 10- to 12- somite stage. *Proc. Natl. Acad. Sci. USA* **90,** 6429–6433.
24. Huang, H. and Auerbach, R. (1993) Identification and characterization of hematopoietic stem cells from the yolk sac and early mouse embryo. *Proc. Natl. Acad. Sci. USA* **90,** 10,110–10,114.
25. Jordan, C. T., McKearn, J. T., and Lemischka, I. R. (1990) Cellular and developmental properties of fetal hematopoietic stem cells. *Cell* **61,** 953–963.
26. McKearn, J. P., McCubrey, J., and Fagg, B. (1985) Enrichment of hematopoietic precursor cells and cloning of multipotential B-lymphocyte precursors. *Proc. Natl. Acad. Sci. USA* **82,** 7414–7418.
27. Li, Y.-S., Wasserman, R., Hayakawa, K., and Hardy, R. R. (1997) Identification of the earliest B lineage stage in mouse bone marrow. *Immunity* **5,** 527–535.
28. Szilvassy, S. J. and Cory, S. (1993) Phenotypic and functional characterization of competitive long-term repopulating hematopoietic stem cells enriched from 5-fluorouracil-treated murine marrow. *Blood* **81,** 2310–2320.
29. Trevisan, M. and Iscove, N. N. (1995) Phenotypic analysis of murine long term hemopoietic reconstituting cells quantitated competitively in vivo and comparison with more advanced colony-forming progeny. *J. Exp. Med.* **181,** 93–103.
30. Spangrude, G. J. and Brooks, D. M. (1993) Mouse strain variability in the expression of the hematopoietic stem cell antigen Ly-6A/E by bone marrow cells. *Blood* **82,** 3327–3332.
31. Hayashi, S.-I., Kunisada, T., Ogawa, M., Sudo, T., Kodama, H., Suda, T., Nishikawa, S., and Nishikawa, S.-I. (1990) Stepwise progression of B lineage differentiation supported by interleukin 7 and other stromal cell molecules. *J. Exp. Med.* **171,** 1683–1695.
32. Henderson, A. J., Johnson, A., and Dorshkind, K. (1990) Functional characterization of two stromal cell lines that support B lymphopoiesis. *J. Immunol.* **145,** 423–428.
33. Paige, C. J. (1983. Surface immunoglobulin-negative B-cell precursors detected by formation of antibody-secreting colonies in agar. *Nature* **302,** 711–713.
34. Rolink, A., Kudo, A., Karasuyama, H., Kikuchi, Y., and Melchers, F. (1991) Long-term proliferating early pre-B cell lines and clones with the potential to develop to surface Ig-positive, mitogen reactive B cells *in vitro* and *in vivo*. *EMBO J.* **10,** 327–336.
35. Whitlock, C. A. and Witte, O. N. (1982) Long-term culture B lymphocytes and their precursors from murine bone marrow. *Proc. Natl. Acad. Sci. USA* **79,** 3608–3612.
36. Kincade, P. W. (1991) Molecular interactions between stromal cells and B lymphocyte precursors. *Sem. Immunol.* **3,** 379–390.
37. Namen, A. E., Lupton, S., Hjerrild, K., Wignall, J., Mochizuki, D. Y., Schmierer, A., Mosley, B., March, C. J., Urdal, K., Gillis, S., Cosman, D., and Goodwin, R. G. (1988) Stimulation of B cell progenitors by cloned murine interleukin 7. *Nature* **333,** 571–573.
38. Cumano, A., Kee, B. L., Ramsden, D. A., Marshall, A., Paige, C. J., and Wu, G. E. (1994) Development of B lymphocytes from lymphoid committed and uncommitted progenitors. *Immunol. Rev.* **137,** 5–33.
39. Kee, B. L., Cumano, A., Iscove, N. N., and Paige, C. J. (1994) Stromal cell independent growth of bipotent B cell-macrophage precursors from murine fetal liver. *Int. Immunol.* **6,** 401–407.
40. Hilton, D. J., Hilton, A. A., Raicevic, A., Rakar, S., Harrison-Smith, M., Gough, N. M., Begley, C. G., Metcalf, D., Nicola, N. A., and Willson, T. A. (1994) Cloning of a murine IL-11 receptor alpha-chain; requirement for gp130 for high affinity binding and signal transduction. *EMBO J.* **13,** 4765–4775.
41. Yin, T., Yaga, T., Tsang, M. L.-S., Yasukawa, D., Kishimoto, T., and Yang, Y.-C. (1993) Involvement of IL-6 signal transducer gp130 in IL-11 mediated signal transduction. *J. Immunol.* **151,** 2555–2561.
42. Zsebo, K. M., Williams, D. A., Geissler, E. N., Broudy, V. C., Martin, F. H., Atkins, H. L., Hsu, R.-Y., Birkett, N. C., Okino, K. H., Murdock, D. C., Jacobsen, F. W., Langley, K. E., Smith, K. A., Takeishi, T., Cattanach, B. M., Galli, S. J., and Sugges, S. V. (1990) Stem cell factor is encoded at the Sl locus of the mouse and is the ligand for the c-*kit* tyrosine kinase receptor. *Cell* **63,** 213–224.

43. Chabot, B., Stephenson, D. A., Chapman, V. M., Besmer, P., and Bernstein, A. (1988) The protooncogene c-*kit* encoding a transmembrane tyrosine kinase receptor maps to the mouse W locus. *Nature* **335,** 88,89.
44. Geissler, E. N., Ryan, M. A., and Houseman, D. E. (1988) The dominant white spotting locus of the mouse encodes the c-kit protooncogene. *Cell* **55,** 185–192.
45. Ray, R. J., Paige, C. J., Furlonger, C., Lyman, S. D., and Rottapel, R. (1996) Flt 3 ligand supports the differentiation of early B cell progenitors in the presence of interleukin-11 and interleukin-7. *Eur. J. Immunol.* **26,** 1504–1510.
46. Veibry, O. P., Jacobsen, F. W., Cui, L., Lyman, S. D., and Jacobsen, S. E. W. (1996) The flt3 ligand promotes the survival of primitive hemopoietic progenitor cells with myeloid as well as B lymphoid potential. *J. Immunol.* **157,** 2953–2960.
47. Veiby, O. P., Lyman, S. D., and Jacobsen, S. E. W. (1996) Combined signaling through interleukin-7 receptors and flt3 but not c-kit potently and selectively promotes B-cell commitment and differentiation from uncommitted murine bone marrow progenitor cells. *Blood* **88,** 1256–1265.
48. Matthews, W., Jordan, C. T., Gavin, M., Jenkins, N. A., Copeland, N. G., and Lemischka, I. R. (1991) A receptor tyrosine kinase cDNA isolated from a population of enriched primitive hematopoietic cells and exhibiting close genetic linkage to c-*kit*. *Proc. Natl. Acad. Sci. USA* **88,** 9026–9030.
49. Goodwin, R. G., Friend, D., Ziegler, S. F., Jerzy, R., Falk, B. A., Gimpel, S., Cosman, D., Dower, S. L., March, C. J., Namen, A. E., and Park, L. S. (1990) Cloning of the human and murine interleukin-7 receptors: demonstration of a soluble form and homology to a new receptor superfamily. *Cell* **60,** 941–951.
50. Kondo, M., Takeshita, T., Ishii, N., Nakamura, M., Watanabe, S., Arai, K.-I., and Sugamura, K. (1993) Sharing of the interleukin-2 (IL-2) receptor γ chain between receptors for IL-2 and IL-4. *Science* **262,** 1874–1876.
51. Noguchi, M., Nakamura, Y., Russell, S. M., Ziegler, S. F., Tsang, M., Cao, X., and Leonard, W. J. (1993) Interleukin-2 receptor γ chain: a functional component of the interleukin-7 receptor. *Science* **262,** 1877–1880.
52. Russell, S. M., Keegan, A. D., Harada, N., Nakamura, Y., Noguchi, M., Leland, P., Friedmann, M. C., Miyajima, A., Puri, R. K., Paul, W. E., and Leonard, W. J. (1993) Interleukin-2 receptor γ chain: a functional component of the interleukin-4 receptor. *Science* **262,** 1880–1883.
53. Cumano, A., Dorshkind, K., Gillis, S., and Paige, C. J. (1990) The influence of S17 stromal cells and interleukin 7 on B cell development. *Eur. J. Immunol.* **20,** 2183–2189.
54. Lee, G., Namen, A. E., Gillis, S., Ellingsworth, L. R., and Kincade, P. W. (1989) Normal B cell precursors responsive to recombinant murine IL-7 and inhibition of IL-7 activity by transforming growth factor-β. *J. Immunol.* **142,** 3875–3883.
55. McNiece, I. K., Langley, K. E., and Zsebo, K. M. (1991) The role of recombinant stem cell factor in early B cell development–synergistic interaction with IL-7. *J. Immunol.* **146,** 3785.
56. Fisher, A. G., Burdet, C., LeMeur, M., Haasner, D., Gerber, P., and Ceredig, R. (1992) Lymphoproliferative disorders in an IL-7 transgenic mouse line. *Leukemia* **2,** 566–568.
57. Peschon, J. J., Morrissey, P. J., Grabstein, K. H., Ramsdell, F. J., Maraskovsky, E., Gliniak, B. C., Park, L. S., Ziegler, S. F., Williams, D. E., Ware, C. B., Mayer, J. D., and Davison, B. L. (1994) Early lymphocyte expansion is severely impaired in interleukin 7 receptor-deficient mice. *J. Exp. Med.* **180,** 1955–1959.
58. von Freeden-Jeffrey, U., Vieira, P., Lucian, L. A., McNeil, T., Burdach, S. E. G., and Murray, R. (1995) Lymphopenia in IL-7 gene deleted mice identifies IL-7 as a nonredundant cytokine. *J. Exp. Med.* **181,** 1519–1526.
59. Corcoran, A. E., Smart, F. M., Cowling, R. J., Crompton, T., Owen, M. J., and Venkitaraman, A. R. (1996) The interleukin-7 receptor α chain transmits distinct signals for proliferation and differentiation during B lymphopoiesis. *EMBO J.* **15,** 1924–1932.
60. Nagasawa, T., Hirota, S., Tachibana, K., Takakura, M., Nishikawa, S.-I., Kitamura, Y., Yoshida, N., Kikutani, H., and Kishimoto, T. (1996) Defects of B-cell lymphopoiesis and bone-marrow myelopoiesis in mice lacking the CXC chemokine PBSF/SDF-1. *Nature* **382,** 635–638.

61. Rossant, J., Vijh, K. M., Grossi, C. E., and Cooper, M. D. (1986) Clonal origin of haematopoietic colonies in the postnatal mouse liver. *Nature* **319,** 507–511.
62. Singh, H. (1996) Gene targeting reveals a hierarchy of transcription factors regulating specification of lymphoid cell fates. *Curr. Opin. Immunol.* **8,** 160–165.
63. Porcher, C., Swat, W., Rockwell, K., Fujiwara, Y., Alt, F. W., and Orkin, S. H. (1996) The T cell leukemia oncoprotein SCL/tal-1 is essential for development of all hematopoietic lineages. *Cell* **86,** 47–57.
64. Robb, L., Elwood, N. J., Elefanty, A. G., Kontgen, F., Li, R., Farnett, L. D., and Begley, C. G. (1996) The SCL gene product is required for the generation of all hematopoietic lineages in the adult mouse. *EMBO J.* **15,** 4123–4129.
65. Mucenski, M. L., McLain, K., Kier, A. B., Swerdlow, S. H., Schreiner, C. M., Miller, T. A., Pietryga, D. W., Scott, W. J., Jr., and Potter, S. S. (1991) A functional c-myb gene is required for normal murine fetal hepatic hematopoiesis. *Cell* **65,** 677–689.
66. McKercher, S. R., Torbett, B. E., Anderson, K. L., Henkel, G. W., Vestal, D. J., Baribault, H., Klemsz, M., Feeney, A. J., Wu, G. E., Paige, C. J., and Maki, R. A. (1996) Targeted disruption of the PU. 1 gene results in multiple hematopoietic abnormalities. *EMBO J.* **15,** 5647–5658.
67. Scott, E., Simon, M., Anastasi, J., and Singh, H. (1994) Requirement of transcription factor PU. 1 in the development of multiple hematopoietic lineages. *Science* **265,** 1573–1577.
68. Nutt, S. L., Urbanek, P., Rolink, A., and Busslinger, M. (1997) Essential functions of Pax5 (BSAP) in pro-B cell development: difference between fetal and adult B lymphopoiesis and reduced V-to-DJ recombination at the IgH locus. *Genes Dev.* **11,** 476–491.
69. Urbanek, P., Wang, Z. Q., Fetka, I., Wagner, E. F., and Buslinger, M. (1994) Complete block of early B cell differentiation and altered patterning of the posterior midbrain in mice lacking Pax-5/BSAP. *Cell* **79,** 901–913.
70. Lin, H. and Grosschedl, R. (1995) Failure of B-cell differentiation in mice lacking the transcription factor EBF. *Nature* **376,** 263–267.
71. Bain, G., Robanus Maandag, E. C., Izon, D. J., Amsen, D., Kruisbeek, A. M., Weintraub, B. C., Krop, I., Schlissel, M. S., Feeney, A. J., van Roon, M., van der Valk, M., te Riele, H. P. J., Berns, A., and Murre, C. (1994) E2A proteins are required for proper B cell development and initiation of immunoglobulin gene rearrangements. *Cell* **79,** 885–892.
72. Zhuang, Y., Soriano, P., and Weintraub, H. (1994) The helix-loop-helix gene E2A is required for B cell formation. *Cell* **79,** 875–884.
73. Murre, C. and Baltimore, D. (1992) The helix-loop-helix motif: Structure and Function, in *Transcriptional Regulation* (McKnight, S. L. and Yamamoto, K. R., eds.), Cold Spring Harbor Laboratory, NY, pp. 861–879.
74. Murre, C., Bain, G., van Kijk, M. A., Engel, I., Furnari, B. A., Massari, M. E., Matthews, J. R., Quong, M. W., Rivera, R. R., and Stuiver, M. H. (1994) Structure and function of helix-loop-helix proteins. *BBA* **1218,** 129–135.
75. Lassar, A. B. and Weintraub, H. (1992) The myogenic helix-loop-helix family: regulators of skeletal muscle determination and differentiation, in *Transcriptional Regulation* (McKnight, S. L. and Yamamoto, K. R., eds.), Cold Spring Harbor Laboratory Press, Cold Spring Harbor, NY, pp. 1037–1061.
76. Lee, J. E., Hollenberg, S. M., Snider, L., Turner, D. L., Lipnick, N., and Weintraub, H. (1995) Conversion of Xenopus ectoderm into neurons by NeuroD, a basic helix-loop-helix protein. *Science* **268,** 836–844.
77. Tapscott, S. J., Davis, R. L., Thayer, M. J., Cheng, P.-F., Weintraub, H., and Lassar, A. B. (1988) MyoD1: a nuclear phosphoprotein requiring a myc homology region to convert fibroblasts to myoblasts. *Science* **242,** 405–411.
78. Shen, C.-P. and Kadesch, T. (1995) B-cell-specific DNA binding by an E47 homodimer. *Mol. Cell. Biol.* **15,** 4518–4524.
79. Sloan, S. R., Shen, C.-P., McCarrick-Walmsley, R., and Kadesch, T. (1996) Phosphorylation of E47 as a potential determinant of B-cell-specific activity. *Mol. Cell. Biol.* **16,** 6900–6908.

80. Bain, G., Robanus Maandag, E. C., te Riele, H. P. J., Feeney, A. J., Sheehy, A., Schlissel, M., Shinton, S. A., Hardy, R. R., and Murre, C. (1997) Both E12 and E47 allow commitment to the B cell lineage. *Immunity* **6,** 145–154.
81. Jacobs, Y., Xin, X.-Z., Dorshkind, K., and Nelson, C. (1994) Pan/E2A expression precedes immunoglobulin heavy-chain expression during B lymphopoiesis in nontransformed cells, and Pan/E2A proteins are not detected in myeloid cells. *Mol. Cell. Biol.* **14,** 4087–4096.
82. Xin, X. Q., Nelson, C., Collins, C., and Dorshkind, K. (1994) Kinetics of E2A HLH protein expression during myelopoiesis and primary B cell differentiation. *J. Immunol.* **152,** 16,351–16,356.
83. Kreider, B. L., Benezra, R., Rovera, G., and Kadesch, T. (1992) Inhibition of myeloid differentiation by the helix-loop-helix protein Id. *Science* **255,** 1700–1702.
84. Voronova, A. F. and Lee, F. (1994) The E2A and tal-1 helix-loop-helix proteins associate in vivo and are modulated by Id proteins during interleukin 6-induced myeloid differentiation. *Proc. Natl. Acad. Sci. USA* **91,** 5952–5956.
85. Hara, H., Sam, M., Maki, R. A., Wu, G. E., and Paige, C. J. (1990) Characterization of a 70Z/3 pre-B cell derived macrophage clone. Differential expression of hox family genes. *Int. Immunol.* **2,** 691–696.
86. Tanaka, T., Wu, G. E., and Paige, C. J. (1994) Characterization of the B cell-macrophage lineage transition in 70Z/3 cells. *Eur. J. Immunol.* **24,** 1544–1548.
87. Kee, B. L. and Murre, C. (1997) The basic helix-loop-helix protein E12 acts upstream of EBF and Pax-5 in a cascade of transcription factors that coordinately regulate B lineage development. Submitted.
88. Ghysen, A., Dambly-Chaudiere, C., Jan, L. Y., and Jan, Y.-N. (1993) Cell interaction and gene interactions in peripheral neurogenesis. *Genes Dev.* **7,** 723–733.
89. Nye, J. S. and Kopan, R. (1995) Vertebrate ligands for Notch. *Current Biol.* **5,** 966–969.
90. Robey, E., Chang, D., Itano, A., Cado, D., Alexander, H., Lans, D., Weinmaster, G., and Salmon, P. (1996) An activated form of Notch influences the choice between CD4 and CD8 T cell lineages. *Cell* **87,** 483–492.
91. Washburn, T., Schweighoffer, E., Gridley, T., Chang, D., Fowlkes, B. J., Cado, D., and Robey, E. (1997) Notch activity influences the αβ versus γδ T cell lineage decision. *Cell* **88,** 833–843.
92. Zhuang, Y., Cheng, P., and Weintraub, H. (1996) B-Lymphocyte development is regulated by the combined dosage of three basic helix-loop-helix genes, E2A, E2-2, and HEB. *Mol. Cell. Biol.* **16,** 2898–2905.

Chapter 16

TCR-Independent Development of Pluripotent T-Cell Precursors

Li Wu, Ferenc Livak, and Howard T. Petrie

1. Introduction

The various contributions to this book are intended to serve as a collection of opinions based on contemporary knowledge. The opinion the authors will seek to illustrate here, that T-cell differentiation is not driven by T-cell receptor (TCR) expression, is an unconventional view and in reality, will probably need to be tempered by nuance and circumstance. Nonetheless, most of the data that have lead to the conventional view (i.e., T-cell development that is directed by TCR expression) could be reinterpreted to support the proposal that TCR expression, although absolutely required for T-cell survival and function, does not drive differentiation, but rather, facilitates survival. It is noteworthy to point out that many of the early stages of intrathymic differentiation occur prior to any TCR gene recombination, illustrating the concept that differentiation can occur without a TCR. Further, what immunologists refer to as "selection" is, in fact, a common function among developing tissues: survival, mediated by the absolute requirement for a given gene product at some specific point during development. Given the absence of a required gene product, as can happen in the mutation of any gene, the affected cell dies. Nevertheless, other developmental events occur independently of such a defect, up to and including the point where its essential function is required. In the case of the TCR, the frequency of such "mutations" is abnormally high, because of the random nature of the recombination and recognition processes. As will be discussed, it is nevertheless conceivable and useful, to view T-cell development as occurring independently of TCR expression, with TCR^+ cells surviving the developmental process, whereas TCR^- cells die. Likewise, an attempt will be made to make the similar point that TCR-α/β versus γ/δ expression on a given cell does not induce T lineage divergence; rather, it facilitates the survival of those cells that express the appropriate TCR isotype. Finally, it is important to state that the concepts presented here are directed toward an understanding

From: *Molecular Biology of B-Cell and T-Cell Development*
Edited by: J. G. Monroe and E. V. Rothenberg © Humana Press Inc., Totowa, NJ

of T-cell development in the adult murine thymus. Fetal T-cell development, although similar to that of the adult, differs in many important ways *(1,2)*, and extrapolation between these models may not be accurate.

2. Phenotypic Identification of Immature T-Cells

2.1. Categories of Immature Thymocytes

In order to understand the evolution of current paradigms for T-cell development, it is useful to recapitulate the field from a rough chronological perspective. Traditionally, thymocyte subpopulations have been defined based on their expression of the two surface molecules that characterize most T-cells in the peripheral lymphoid system (i.e., CD4 [initially referred to as L3T4 in the mouse] and CD8 [initially called Ly 2]). In the adult mouse, approx 15% of all thymocytes phenotypically resemble peripheral T-cells (i.e., they are either $CD4^+$ or $CD8^+$ [CD4/8 single positive, SP], and are also $CD3/TCR^+$). Consistent with their phenotype, these cells represent the most mature major group of cells in the thymus, although it is worth noting that such cells are not functionally mature *(3)*. Of the remaining thymocytes, two main groups can be distinguished by CD4 and CD8 expression. Approximately 80% of all thymocytes are positive for both markers (i.e., CD4/8 double positive, DP), whereas 3–4% express neither (CD4/8 double negative, DN). Although it has been clear for some time that DN cells were the precursors to DP and SP cells *(4)*, it is remarkable to note that as recently as nine years ago, it was not clear whether DP cells were a terminal (i.e., aberrant) state of differentiation, or an intermediate between DN and SP, a relationship that now seems blasé. Definitive answers regarding these relationships, together with a wealth of information regarding the timing of TCR gene recombination, were eventually gained through the study of mutant and transgenic mouse models, as is discussed in Subheading 3.1.

2.2. Segregation of Early DN Subsets

The verification of DN cells as the precursors to DP (and SP) was temporarily obscured by the identification of diverse phenotypic heterogeneity among DN cells from normal mice *(5–7)*. Surface proteins expressed on DN cells included various permutations of CD2, CD5, CD24, CD25, CD44, CD90, MHC class I, PNA, and others. Fortunately, out of at least 11 discrete subsets that could be identified at the time *(8)*, many were eventually determined not to be in the mainstream of T-cell development. Several groups subsequently defined a lineage pathway for DN cells, which was based primarily on the expression of CD24, 25, and 44 *(6,7)*. Early cells in this lineage expressed high levels of CD44, followed by low-level expression at later stages; the intermediate stages also transiently expressed CD25. Thus, the first consensus DN lineage was defined as $CD25^-44^+ \rightarrow CD25^+44^{lo} \rightarrow CD25^-44^{lo}$ *(6)*. It was also shown by several groups that all lymphoid components of this pathway were $CD24^+$ *(9)*, an important distinction, since many thymic stromal cells were also $CD25^-44^+$. An addition to the DN lineage was provided approximately six years later by the definition of a $CD25^+44^+$ population *(10)*. Unlike previous studies, the precursor/progeny relationships of this subset to the others was not demonstrated. Instead, it was shown that these cells were similar to the least mature ($CD25^-44^+$) DN thymocytes, in that they expressed surface CD117 and had TCR genes in germline configuration (discussed in Subheading 3.2.). By reason of this and their expression of CD25, they are proposed to be intermediates between the earliest DN cells and the $CD25^+44^{lo}$ subset. Thus, the currently accepted DN lineage, still defined by early expression of CD44 and transient expression of CD25, is $CD25^-44^+ \rightarrow CD25^+44^+ \rightarrow$

$CD25^{+}44^{lo} \rightarrow CD25^{-}44^{lo}$. In the interest of brevity, these subsets will subsequently be referred to as DN1 through DN4, respectively.

The description of DN4 cells as being "DN" (i.e., $CD4^{-}$ and $CD8^{-}$) is technically a misnomer, as these cells must be considered to represent incipient DP cells for several reasons. First, they already exhibit trace but distinguishable surface levels of the TCR-β chain, as well as CD3, CD4, and CD8 *(11)*. Since these cells have only just begun TCR-α chain rearrangement *(12)*, it is assumed that CD3/TCR-β expression at this stage occurs in conjunction with the surrogate TCR-α chain (pTα or gp33) *(13–15)*. Second, these cells rapidly and spontaneously differentiate into DP thymocytes in vitro without any additional stimulation *(16,17)*, suggesting that they are already programmed to become DP. Finally, DN4 cells display a distinct bias toward selection for productive TCR-β gene rearrangements *(18)*, a process that is thought to mediate the DN–DP transition (discussed in Subheading 3.3.). Thus, DN4 cells actually represent very early DP cells that segregate together with DN during purification, because of minimal expression levels of the markers used for depletion (CD4 and CD8). However, this phenomenon is fortuitous as it permits the purification and analysis of cells that have just undergone the DP transition, as will be discussed at multiple points in this chapter.

2.3. Reconstitution of the Thymus by Bone Marrow Cells

The thymus is a nonself-renewing lymphopoietic tissue, in that self-renewing precursors do not reside within the thymus but are continuously replenished by precursors deriving from the bone marrow *(9,19)*. In the young adult mouse, it is estimated that 50–100 bone marrow cells enter the thymus per day *(9,19)*. A long-standing debate has persisted as to whether bone marrow cells first commit to differentiate (in our case, into T-cells) and then exit the marrow, or whether they randomly exit the marrow and then differentiate into T-cells by virtue of homing to the thymus. The most primitive bone marrow hematopoietic stem cell (HSC), which has multilineage (lymphoid, myeloid, erythroid) potential, is believed to present as $lineage^{-}$ (Lin; lymphoid, myeloid, and erythroid marker), $Sca\text{-}1^{+}$ $Sca\text{-}2^{-}$ $CD44^{+}$ $CD117^{+}$ (c-kit) and rhodamine (Rh)-123^{lo} *(20,21)*. The demonstration that multipotent bone marrow cells exhibiting accelerated thymic reconstitution activity also differ from more primitive HSC (being Rh-123^{hi} and/or $Sca\text{-}2^{+}$) suggests that HSC probably undergo at least some differentiation prior to leaving the marrow *(20,22)*. However, no cell that is absolutely restricted to the T (or T and B) lymphoid lineage has been identified in adult bone marrow. This does not mean that such a cell does not exist; as has been pointed out *(20,22,23)*, one or more of the lineage markers used to distinguish lineage-committed cells from HSC (described earlier in this section) might also define lymphoid-restricted cells otherwise resembling primitive HSC.

2.4. The Earliest Intrathymic Precursor

As described above, DN cells were historically defined as the least mature population of precursors found in the thymus. However, even the earliest of them is numerically too abundant to correlate with precursor input; DN1 cells represent about 0.1–0.2% of all thymocytes *(6)*, or $1\text{-}5 \times 10^{5}$ cells in normal mice, vs no more than a few hundred input cells from the bone marrow *(see* Subheading 2.3.*)*. One possible explanation for this is that precursors arriving from the bone marrow proliferate in an undifferentiated state. Consistent with this, it has been shown that at least some DN1 cells are proliferating *(24,25)* (*see* Subheading 3.3. for more detail). In any case, careful characterization has led to the identification of an even earlier thymic precursor to DN cells *(26)*. One of the most remarkable characteristics of this population is that it expresses CD4 at levels that are low but nonetheless sufficient to result in the elimination of this subset when selecting against CD4 to distinguish DN thymocytes. The very immature status of this population is demonstrated by its ability to give rise to the remainder of thymocytes (including DN cells), and its otherwise genetic and phenotypic similarity to HSC, with the exception of being Sca-2^+ and Rh-123^{hi}. In these latter respects, this population of cells (subsequently referred to as $CD4^{lo}$ precursors) resembles the more differentiated HSC exhibiting rapid thymic colonizing activity (described in Subheading 2.3.). Although $CD4^{lo}$ thymocytes are still too numerically prevalent to represent the direct input of cells from the bone marrow, their other characteristics are consistent with the proposition that they are the direct (and possibly undifferentiated) progeny of the earliest cells seeding the thymus.

2.5. Developmental Potential of Early T-Cell Precursors

The phenotypic identification of the aforementioned lineages, together with the data regarding their differentiative potential and other data discussed below, has led to the lineage diagram illustrated in Fig. 1. Some further details regarding the differentiative capacity of these various populations are worthy of emphasis. By definition, primitive HSC are capable of supporting the development of all blood lineages. Those bone marrow cells described as being Rh-123^{hi} and Sca-2^+ are likewise multipotent *(20,22)*, although their more rapid reconstitution of the various lineages ranks them as being slightly more differentiated. The fact that thymic precursors do not reside intrathymically but must emigrate from the bone marrow automatically implicates the blood as a potential source for T lineage-committed precursors. A population of $CD90^+CD117^{lo}$ (Thy-1^+, c-kit^{lo}) cells that are T lineage-restricted has been identified in day 15.5 fetal blood *(27)*. A bone marrow/thymus intermediate has not yet been identified in the adult bloodstream. Whatever the phenotype of such a cell is, the demonstration that $CD4^{lo}$ thymocyte precursors generate B as well as T-cells *(28)*, implies that blood-borne intermediates in the adult are unlikely to be committed to the T-cell lineage. In addition, this same $CD4^{lo}$ precursor population can also give rise to NK cells *(29)* and TCR-γ/δ cells *(28)* (discussed in more detail later in this chapter), but not myeloid or erythroid cells *(28)*, thus fulfilling the definition for a common lymphoid-restricted precursor. Remarkably, this $CD4^{lo}$ subset can also generate thymic dendritic cells (DC), and does so at the T-cell:DC ratio normally found in the thymus *(30,31)*. This finding has significant implications for T-cell development at later (DP) stages, since coupled T-cell and DC development may help to ensure the sensitivity and fidelity of self-tolerance through clonal deletion *(30)*. As with all studies in which limited proliferative potential precludes the analysis of single precursors, it is difficult to state unconditionally that an individual $CD4^{lo}$ precursor is capable of giving rise to T, B, NK, and DC lineages. However, given the phenotypic homogeneity of this population and the available data, it remains the best candidate for a lymphoid-restricted precursor closely related to the bone marrow cells that colonize the thymus.

The developmental potential of DN thymocyte subsets has likewise been assessed and provides fairly strong evidence that absolute commitment to the T-cell lineage does not occur until the onset of TCR gene rearrangement. Unlike the $CD4^{lo}$ thymic precursor, the lineage potential of DN1 cells from adult thymus has not been directly assessed. In day 15 fetal thymocytes, cells with the DN1 phenotype were capable of differentiating into T, B, and NK cells *(32)*, thus corroborating their juxtaposition to the $CD4^{lo}$ precursor. Again, the direct extension of findings from fetal thymocytes to adult T-cell development may be misleading, however, since this same study found that fetal cells with the DN2 phenotype were exclusively committed to the T-cell lineage, whereas DN2 cells

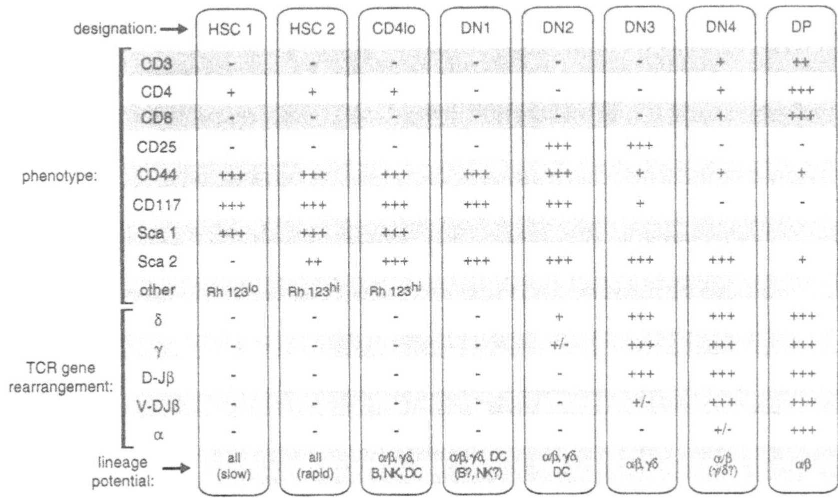

	designation: →	HSC 1	HSC 2	CD4lo	DN1	DN2	DN3	DN4	DP
phenotype:	CD3	-	-	-	-	-	-	+	++
	CD4	+	+	+	-	-	-	+	+++
	CD8	-	-	-	-	-	-	+	+++
	CD25	-	-	-	-	+++	+++	-	-
	CD44	+++	+++	+++	+++	+++	+	+	+
	CD117	+++	+++	+++	+++	+++	+	-	-
	Sca 1	+++	+++	+++					
	Sca 2	-	++	+++	+++	+++	+++	+++	+
	other	Rh 123^{lo}	Rh 123^{hi}	Rh 123^{hi}					
TCR gene rearrangement:	δ	-	-	-	-	+	+++	+++	+++
	γ	-	-	-	-	+/-	+++	+++	+++
	D-Jβ	-	-	-	-	-	+++	+++	+++
	V-DJβ	-	-	-	-	-	+/-	+++	+++
	α	-	-	-	-	-	-	+/-	+++
	lineage potential: →	all (slow)	all (rapid)	α/β, γδ, B, NK, DC	αβ, γδ, DC (B?, NK?)	αβ, γδ, DC	αβ, γδ	α/β (γ/δ?)	αβ

Fig. 1. Sequential development of murine T-cell precursors. Abbreviations: HSC, hematopoietic stem cell; DN, CD4/8-double negative. HSC1 and HSC2 cells are located in the bone marrow; remaining cells are found in the thymus. Descriptions refer to the corresponding population as a whole; individual cells or small proportions of the subset may vary from the description given.

from adult thymus can generate both DC and T-cells *(23)*. In contrast, DN3 cells are unable to generate any lineages other than T-cells in the adult *(23)*. Since DN3 are the first cells displaying detectable TCR gene rearrangements (*see* Subheading 3.2.), it appears that absolute commitment to the T-cell lineage in adult thymocytes is either obligated by TCR gene rearrangement or coincides with it.

3. TCR Gene Recombination During Development

3.1. Effects of Genetic Modification on Differentiation

Almost parallel with the studies described in Subheading 2., other studies assessing the relationship of TCR gene recombination to differentiation inspired new thinking about the inductive stimuli for this process, especially in the DN to DP transition. Specifically, the analysis of TCR-transgenic mice, or mice with defects in TCR gene recombination or expression, gave direct evidence that gene rearrangements at the various TCR loci were tightly correlated with developmental progression. One of the first clear demonstrations of this type was provided by introducing a TCR-β chain transgene into mice with severe combined immunodeficiency (SCID) *(33)*. SCID is a naturally occurring defect in gene recombination, which appears as a developmental arrest at DN3, a phenotype common to most recombination-deficient mutants. The expression of a TCR-β transgene in the thymus of SCID mice reconstituted development into the DP lineage *(34)*, revealing the dependence of this transition on the presence of a TCR-β chain. Comparable (and in many cases more dramatic) findings were subsequently published using other recombination-deficient mice and TCR transgenes. It is the TCR-β protein itself, and not the recombination process, which is required, since mice with mutations in TCR-β chain expression *(35)* present with essentially the same phenotype as recombination-deficient mice. Mice deficient in TCR-α gene expression, on the other hand, arrested later at the DP stage of development *(36,37)*, consistent with the analysis of TCR-α mRNA expression described earlier *(6)*. Since DN cells are the precursors of DP cells, a hierarchy of rearrangement is thus established, with TCR-β recombination occurring first (during the DN stage), followed by TCR-α recombination (in DP cells). This hierarchical pattern of rearrangement is not without biological relevance; if TCR-α and TCR-β loci rearranged independently, far fewer cells would successfully express both proteins *(38)*. By enforcing a requirement for TCR-β expression early in development, prior to the bulk of cell division in the thymus *(see* Subheading 3.3.*)*, the economy of TCR expression is maximized, as has been previously discussed *(12,38)*.

3.2. TCR Gene Recombination in Normal T-Cell Development

Molecular analyses of TCR genes during normal T-cell development supported the hierarchical model of TCR-β and TCR-α gene rearrangement (at the DN and DP stages of development, respectively) that had been deduced from recombination-deficient and/or transgenic mice. Using the DN lineage known at the time (including DN subsets 1, 3, and 4) (Fig. 1), it has been shown that rearrangements at the TCR-β locus were first detectable in DN3 cells *(6)*. This same study also demonstrated that DN3 cells mainly expressed mRNA transcripts associated with partial (i.e., D-J) rearrangements of the TCR-β locus, whereas full-length TCR-β mRNA (and TCR-α message) were primarily restricted to the DN4 stage of development *(6)*. These findings were later extended to show that the DN2 subset also exhibited germline TCR-β genes *(10,12)*. Given the knowledge that mice deficient in TCR-β expression abort T-cell development at the DN3 stage, it was assumed that D-Jβ and V-DJβ rearrangements occurred in rapid succession within the DN3 subset *(39)*. However, quantitative Southern blot analysis of D-J and V-DJβ rearrangements during normal T-cell development *(25)* suggest a different conclusion. First, these studies show that D-Jβ recombination cannot occur within cells at the DN3 stage, since cells of this phenotype display levels of D-J rearrangement equivalent to that found in mature T-cells, not the intermediate levels that must persist in cells actively undergoing D-J rearrangement. Thus, D-Jβ recombination in normal thymocytes must occur prior to the acquisition of the DN3 phenotype. This, in turn, suggests that thymocytes in recombination-deficient mice undergo developmental arrest after the point where recombination is initiated in normal mice. This apparent dissociation of developmental progression from the recombination process is contrary to the popular view that holds that the pre-TCR provides signals that are essential for the induction of the DN to DP transition. However, it is clear that all differentiative events preceding gene recombination (i.e., from bone marrow cells through the DN2 stage of development) (Fig. 1) must occur in the absence of a TCR signal. Thus, it is not impossible to envision that later stages of development might also be able to occur independently of TCR signalling. As will be discussed in the following paragraphs, TCR-independent differentiation during the DN to DP transition could explain the divergence of cell proliferation in TCR-β$^+$ cells versus programmed cell death (PCD) in TCR-β$^-$ cells that also occurs at this stage.

In contrast to the D-J locus, which is fully rearranged by the DN3 stage of development, V-DJ recombination is found in only about 10% of all TCR-β alleles in DN3 cells *(25)*. This finding is at odds with the popular view suggesting that D-J and V-DJβ rearrangements all occur in a burst during the DN3 stage *(39)*. However, these data are consistent with the direct analysis of temporal rearrangements in TCR-β genes during fetal thymus development *(24,40)*, as well as with the demonstration that DN3 express primarily the immature form of TCR-β mRNA *(6)*. If D-J and V-DJβ rearrangements are temporally separate, as the aforementioned results suggest, two additional conclusions can be made. The first is that cells that undergo V-DJβ rearrangement must exit relatively quickly from the DN3 stage, since complete rearrangements are infrequent but obligatory events within this population. The second is that the delay between D-Jβ and V-DJ β recombination must, therefore, be equivalent to the length of residence at the DN3 stage, since D-Jβ rearrangements occur prior to the acquisition of the DN3 phenotype. The estimated lifespan of DN3 cells is approximately two days *(9)*. The reason for a lag of this magnitude between D-J and V-DJβ rearrangement is not obvious. However, it is clear that developmental events other than gene rearrangement are required at this stage, since the inclusion of a fully rearranged TCR-β transgene does not significantly accelerate immature T-cell development *(24,41)*. Thus, the lag between D-J and V-DJβ recombination may represent the time required for other developmental events to occur, including and culminating with susceptibility of the V-DJβ locus to recombination, followed by rapid exodus from the DN compartment and differentiation into DP cells.

3.3. Consequences of TCR Recombination: Differentiation, Proliferation, and Programmed Cell Death (PCD)

During TCR gene recombination, discontinuous DNA segments encoding the variable (V, D, and J) portions of the TCR molecule are cut and relegated adjacent to each other to form a contiguous coding sequence (*42*; reviewed in ref. *43*). During this process, the broken ends can be modified in a variety of ways *(43)*. These modifications are believed to be essentially random, thus adding enormous diversity to the TCR repertoire without proportional genetic burden. However, random modifications to the DNA also mean that the number of DNA bases between initiation (V-region specific) and termination (J-region) codons may not be a multiple of three (i.e., they will be out-of-frame). Assuming random modifications to DNA ends, it can be predicted that for every three TCR-β genes being rearranged, two will terminate in out-of-frame configurations (reviewed in ref. *38*). This fact, together with the principle of allelic exclusion, means that an estimated 44% of all cells will fail to generate an inframe TCR-β gene rearrangement on either allele *(38)*. Since DN3 cells do not accumulate in the thymus with time, these aberrant cells must undergo PCD in order to maintain homeostasis. In contrast, those cells that make inframe TCR-β rearrangements express the pre-TCR at the cell surface, a process that (according to the popular view) induces proliferation and differentiation into DN4 and DP cells (reviewed in ref. *44*; *see* Chapters 22 and 23). This scenario obligates an active decision on the part of the cell, i.e., the induction of one genetic program (inducing differentiation and proliferation) in cells expressing the pre-TCR, versus the induction of an entirely different program (cell death) in those cells that fail to make a TCR. However, by assuming that development from DN3 to DN4 (i.e., DN to DP) occurs independently of TCR rearrangement or expression, as it does in the prior developmental stages (HSC through DN3), a very simple model can be proposed for the divergence of these two cell fates. The details for the revised and current models, as well as the experimental findings supporting them, are described immediately below.

Like most differentiating tissues, T-cells at different stages of development undergo cell division at profoundly different rates *(24,25)*. In particular, cells that are undergoing V-DJβ gene recombination (i.e., DN3 cells) are apparently more slowly dividing than either the preceding (DN2) or subsequent (DN4) developmental stages *(24,25)*, displaying a high proportion of cells with $2n$ DNA content (i.e., G_0 or G_1 phases). Based largely on this observation, together with data showing that one of the proteins required for recombination (RAG-2) is degraded upon entry into S phase *(45)*, a model coupling the cell cycle to TCR gene recombination has been proposed *(46)*. This model has its foundation in two well-documented phenomena: cell cycle arrest occurring in conjunction with DNA double strand breakage (double strand breakage is implicit in TCR gene recombination), and allelic exclusion, which precludes a single cell from assembling more than one inframe TCR-β gene. The model postulates that allelic exclusion could be enforced by restricting recombination to a population of cells that have undergone cell cycle arrest, ostensibly represented by the majority of DN3 cells, which exhibit $2n$ DNA content and are thus assumed to be arrested in G_0. Productive rearrangement at the TCR-β locus subsequently leads to pre-TCR expression, which transduces a mitogenic signal causing "arrested" cells to enter the cell cycle. Cell cycle progression, in turn, leads to the degradation of RAG-2, preventing further rearrangement of (potentially) germline genes. Concurrent transition to the DN4 stage, apparently through the same inductive signal, leads to silencing of the TCR-β locus, the accessibility of the TCR-α locus to recombination, and DP cell development.

Despite the appeal of this model, several lines of evidence argue against it. First, it is important to note that negative regulation of proliferation during the DN3 stage, as seen in normal mice *(24,25)*, is also seen in mice deficient in gene recombination *(25)*. This suggests that decreased mitotic activity during V-DJ recombination occurs independently of the recombination process per se, thus eliminating DNA strand breaks as a cause for decreased mitotic activity (i.e., arrest). Second, DNA strand breakage and coding joint relegation occur extremely rapidly during TCR gene recombination *(47)*, apparently reflecting a state of readiness to repair such genetically programmed DNA strand breakage. Consequently, an "arrest" (G_0) phase facilitating the induction of repair enzymes is not required during recombination, where relegation prior to subsequent mitosis is easily accommodated by the length of G_1. Third, a number of studies have shown that DN3 cells are not at all arrested in the cell division cycle, but in fact continue to divide as well as maintaining this phenotype *(24,48)*. Along these same lines, it can be seen that dividing cells are clearly present at the DN3 stage in recombination-deficient mice, albeit at lower numbers than in normal mice *(25)*. This suggests that not only are DN3 cells not arrested in cell cycle, but that proliferation in these cells is not dependent upon gene recombination or TCR-β/pre-TCR signaling. Finally, studies defining the extent of TCR-β recombination in cycling DN3 cells *(25)*, the effects of a targeted mutation of the pre-TCR *(49)*, and the effects of constitutive RAG-2 activity during cell cycle progression *(50)* all confirm that the induction of proliferation (through the pre-TCR or otherwise) is not responsible for the enforcement of allelic exclusion.

3.4. Cell Division/Cell Death Decisions and TCR-β Expression

Although the factors moderating allelic exclusion remain mysterious, the induction of proliferation at the DN3/DN4 transition may nonetheless play a critical role in T lymphopoiesis, through the coincidental regulation of either cell division or cell death. As mentioned in the previous section, the DN3/DN4 transition represents a dramatic increase in proliferative status *(24,25)*. DN4 cells in fact display a proportion of cycling cells that is rarely seen among primary tissues. This proliferative index is corroborated by the behavior of DN4 cells, which must undergo six to seven serial cell divisions over a period of approximately two days to generate the nondividing cortical DP cells, which constitute the bulk of the thymus *(9)*. It is well accepted that the induction of mitogenesis (as occurs during the DN3/DN4 transition) can lead to either cell division or cell death, the distinction between these fates being determined by the presence or absence (respectively) of a simultaneous survival signal. As described in Subheading 3., DN3 cells that make a productive TCR-β rearrangement must proliferate to generate the DP compartment; those which lack a TCR-β protein must be removed by PCD. If the DN3 to DN4 transition, together with the associated acceleration of cell cycle, occurred independently of TCR-rearrangement or expression, the difference between proliferation into DP cells or PCD could be determined by whether or not a signal is received through the pre-TCR. In this case, differentiation from DN to DP (and the coincident upregulation of cell cycle) would occur independently of TCR expression, as is the case for earlier stages of differentiation. Expression of the pre-TCR would still determine developmental fate, but in this case, the signal transmitted through the pre-TCR would lead to survival of mitogenically-stimulated cells, rather than differentiation per se.

The most appealing attribute of the model proposed above is that it eliminates the necessity for induction of two separate genetic programs leading to cell division or cell death, since in this case cell death would result from the induction of cell division in cells that do not receive a simultaneous (TCR-mediated) survival signal. In support of this hypothesis, recent studies from one of the authors' laboratories show that among thymocytes from recombination-deficient mice, those cells displaying membrane changes associated with death (i.e., Annexin V surface expression and/or permeability to DNA dyes) appear phenotypically as DN4 cells ($CD25^{-}CD44^{lo}CD90^{+}$; M. Tourigny and H. Petrie, in preparation). This suggests that such cells are attempting to become DP, but apparently die before completing the transition. The inference is that T-cell development proceeds, irrespective of TCR expression, through to the DN4 (i.e., DP) stage of development. The onset of new gene expression at this stage, including that of CD4 and CD8, leads to the activation of Src-family tyrosine kinases that in turn lead to proliferation and the divergence cell survival and cell death, based on the presence or absence of signaling through the pre-TCR. This concept has recently been documented by showing that CD4 can mediate the signals previously thought to be dependent on pre-TCR expression *(51)*, suggesting that differentiation to the DN4 stage, and concurrent activation of signaling pathways leading to proliferation, can occur independently of pre-TCR expression.

4. Non-TCR-Mediated Differentiation in T-Cell Development

The difference between TCR signaling as a stimulator of mitogenesis and differentiation versus survival is, in practice, academic; the end result is that cells without a TCR-β chain do not become DP. Since science is academic, such a distinction is nonetheless critical in identifying the authentic inductive stimuli for this transition. As described above, many transitions during early T-cell differentiation must occur independently of the TCR (Fig. 1), as TCR genes do not rearrange until the terminal stages of DN development. Thus, it is not impossible to propose that subsequent stages could occur independently of TCR as well. It is reassuring to note that if one eliminates the TCR from contention as an inductive stimulus in differentiation, it becomes possible to consider T-cell development as a more generic form of differentiation. As such, insights can be drawn from many other well-studied models of differentiation—from vertebrates to Drosophila. A number of gene products known to be influential in these other developmental systems have already been shown to have a role in T-cell development. Since most developmental signals are thought to originate from the extracellular environment, the authors will concentrate here on those interactions that involve cell surface molecules, and, which, likewise have been shown to have an effect on T-cell differentiation.

4.1. Paracrine Signaling

Molecules secreted systemically or locally are known to play an important role in many aspects of development, including proliferation, differentiation, and survival. Many paracrine signaling molecules are known to be important in the T-cell developmental pathway (reviewed in ref. *52*). Most noteworthy among these at present is signaling through the IL-7/IL-7R pathway. It has been known for some time that IL-7 enhances the survival of thymocytes in vitro *(53)*. The need for IL-7 in thymocyte survival has been underscored by recent studies using mice deficient in IL-7R expression *(54)*. T-cells from such mice arrest in development at the DN1 stage of development. However, constitutive *bcl-2* expression in IL-7R-deficient mice completely restores T-cell development throughout all phenotypes *(55,56)*. Thus, antagonism of PCD by *bcl-2* expression mimics signaling through the IL-7R, suggesting that engagement of this receptor in normal cells transmits a key survival signal. It is interesting to note that the transition from DN1 to DN2, which is blocked by mutation of the IL-7R, represents an apparent acceleration in proliferative status *(24,25)*, much like the one seen at the DN3/DN4 transition (discussed in Subheading 3.3.). Consequently, it is possible that (TCR-independent) induction of mitogenesis, together with antagonism of cell death (in this case, through the IL-7R) also plays a role at this stage of differentiation, as well as at the DN/DP transition.

The induction of cell survival may not be the only signal transmitted through the IL-7R, however. A number of studies have shown that IL-7/IL-7R interaction stimulates the induction of rearrangement at the TCR-β and -γ loci, at least in fetal T-cell precursors *(57,58)*, as well as the activation of RAG-1 and RAG-2 genes *(59)*. In support of this, it has been shown that IL-7-secreting thymic stromal cells are capable of inducing TCR-β and -δ recombination in fetal T-cell progenitors in vitro, whereas equivalent stromal cells from IL-7–deficient mice lack this capability *(60)*. Further, the introduction of a TCR-transgene into IL-7R–deficient mice reconstitutes development into DP and SP lineages *(61)*, again suggesting that induction of the gene recombination process may be a key function of signaling through the IL-7R. However, it remains possible that the cell survival aspects of IL-7R signalling described immediately above may be responsible for the recombination effects as well, by allowing differentiation into the DN2 stage, where recombination can subsequently occur. Further experimentation will be required to distinguish between these two possibilities. Nonetheless, such studies emphasize the importance of signaling through soluble factors during early T-cell development and commitment. The number of known cytokines, including those with known or proposed effects on T-cell development (reviewed in ref. *52*), makes this a fertile area for future research.

4.2. Juxtacrine Signaling

The importance of paracrine signals in lymphoid development has received considerable scrutiny. However, the role of juxtacrine interactions (i.e., those requiring intimate cell-cell contact), has received considerably less attention. This is surprising, given the broad importance of such signals in virtually all other developmental models—from whole invertebrates to mammalian tissues. As described in this section, it is clear from thymic morphology that communication between thymic parenchymal and/or stromal elements is critical for T-cell development *(62)*. A few potentially interesting mediators of juxtacrine signaling in T-cell development are described in the following section.

In addressing the question of which non–TCR-related molecules might influence the development of DN cells, it is informative to note the morphological localization of DN cells within the thymus, with respect to gross thymic architecture. Cells migrating into the thymus are thought to enter through blood vessels concentrated at the cortico–medullary junction *(2)*. From this point, DN cells migrate distally into the cortex in a distinct pattern, apparently maintaining intimate contact with stromal cells that compose the subcapsular layer of connective tissue surrounding the thymus *(2)*. These stromal components are of diverse origins, including bone marrow-derived cells, epithelial cells, and fibroblasts *(12)*. Cells of these types are known to be responsible for the generation of an extracellular matrix that is critically important for tissue differentiation in many developmental systems. Furthermore, these stromal cells also directly express receptors and the ligands for receptors with known roles in development. Some potentially critical interactions already known to be important in developing T-cells are further described below.

For juxtacrine (and, in many cases, paracrine) signaling to occur, cells must be maintained in proximity to one another. One of the best-known mediators of such interactions is represented by the cadherin family. Cadherins are transmembrane proteins known to be important in the formation of cell–cell junctions. Formation of junctions may serve two distinct purposes. The first and best understood function is to initiate and/or sustain the interactions of other receptor/ligand interactions, either paracrine (such as IL-7/IL-7R, discussed in the preceeding section) or other juxtacrine signals *(see immediately below)*. However, a large body of evidence is accumulating to suggest that cadherins and related molecules may also directly influence development through the control of gene transcription. For instance, β-catenin strongly associates with the intracellular domain of cadherins at focal points of cell adhesion. Catenins are key intermediates in cell fate determination after signaling through other surface receptors during development, ultimately interacting directly with transcription factors, including some with known roles in lymphoid development (reviewed in ref. *63*). It is not clear at this time whether cadherin signaling cooperates or competes with these other pathways for signaling through catenins or what transcriptional regulation might ensue. However, it is also known that catenins can be phosphorylated by Src-family tyrosine kinases, such as those activated during the DN/DP transition. Phosphorylation leads to the inability of catenins to interact with cadherins at cell–cell junctions, which may in turn lead to the breakdown of cellular adhesion, thus allowing DN cells to detach from the subcapsular epithelium. Consequently, any parallel signals dependent upon continued proximity with the stroma would also be disrupted, undoubtedly leading to differential gene transcription and further differentiative events, including proliferation and/or PCD (perhaps mediated through integrin signaling; *see immediately below*). It is known that at least one cadherin family member (E-cadherin) has a profound and obligatory role very early during T-cell development *(64)*. However, the precise role of cadherins in T-cell (and other) developmental processes remains to be elucidated.

Integrins are often thought to exhibit adhesive functions similar to those described above, a concept that is strengthened by the localization of many integrin ligands to the extracellular matrix (e.g., laminin, fibronectin, vitronectin). However, integrins differ from classical adhesion molecules (as discussed above) in a number of important ways. For one, integrins are not required for the formation of defined focal adhesions, although they are frequently concentrated at these foci. Another characteristic difference is that unlike dedicated adhesion molecules, integrins generate intracellular signals through the activation of tyrosine kinase activity. The paradigms for integrin signaling involve proliferation, differentiation, and survival. By virtue of these, signaling through integrins is an attractive candidate for non–TCR-mediated regulation of the DN to DP transition, since this transition is likewise characterized by proliferation and the divergence of survival and PCD fates. Not surprisingly, many integrins signal through the Ras/Raf/MAPK pathway, the induction of which is an important step in cell proliferation. Likewise, the activation of this pathway is an obligatory event in the DN to DP transition *(65)*. Activation of the Ras/Raf pathway can also act in a negative feedback loop to modulate integrin activation status *(66)*. Again, in support of the involvement of integrins, differential regulation of integrin activation has been shown to occur during the DN to DP transition *(67)*. Since the affinity of integrins for their ligands changes with activation status, this effect could potentially play a role in the release of DN cells from the subcapsular region and in further differentiation into DP cells. In addition, receptor tyrosine kinase activity (such as that mediated through integrins) can lead to the activation of phosphoinositide 3-kinase (PI3-K); such activation has recently been shown to be critical in the moderation of cell survival through Akt *(68)*. Thus, the known roles for integrin signaling in proliferation, differentiation, and cell survival correlate convincingly with the behavior of cells at the DN to DP transition. The diverse patterns of integrin expression seen during T-cell development (*see* refs. *67*, *69*, and *70* for examples) strongly implicate integrins as potential mediators of this change. However, given the complexity of integrin expression patterns and downstream signals, a clear assessment of the role of integrins in T-cell development is likely to require substantially more effort than is currently being given to this promising field of endeavor.

5. TCR-Independent Divergence of TCR-α/β and -γ/δ Lineages

Like the induction of differentiation in the mainstream of intrathymic development, the differential expression of TCR-α/β or -γ/δ isotypes has been suspected to be responsible for the divergence of these lineages in the thymus. The reasons for this assumption are discussed in detail below but relate primarily to the fact that expression of these receptors is mutually exclusive in T-cells of the respective lineages. Since TCR expression requires rearrangement of the corresponding loci, and since the genes encoding γ/δ and α/β-TCRs rearrange in hierarchical fashion, the majority of studies have focused on the competitive nature of TCR gene recombination, and lineage commitment by TCR expression. The authors will, therefore, begin their discussion of T-cell lineage divergence from this perspective.

Although many variants exist, two primary models have been used to explain the divergence of discrete lineages from a single progenitor. The "stochastic-selective" model presumes that lineage commitment occurs randomly among such precursors, and that subsequent selective pressures (mediated through the local environment) perpetuate only those cells that have properly committed. The "instructive-selective" model proposes that commitment is induced by selective influences, presumably those mediated by molecular interactions relevant to the given lineage. In the case of α/β vs γ/δ T lineage commitment, the most relevant molecular interaction is likely to be mediated by the TCR. By virtue of economy, the instructive-selective model has historically been the most appealing, particularly for T-cell development, where losses caused by rearrangement errors and receptor diversity are already high.

5.1. Sequential Rearrangement of the TCR-γ/δ and -α/β Genes

From ontogenic studies of fetal thymus, it has been shown that TCR-γ and TCR-δ gene rearrangements occur prior to TCR-β gene recombination *(40)*. As has been discussed both here and elsewhere *(1,62)*, these findings cannot necessarily be extended to adult

T-cell development; for instance, fetal TCR-γ and -δ gene rearrangements are highly conservative *(71)* and do not resemble the diverse pattern seen in the adult *(72)*. The hierarchy of TCR gene rearrangements in the adult thymus has not been extensively described to date, although some data suggest that TCR-γ and -β gene rearrangements occur simultaneously in DN3 cells *(10)*. Recent studies from the authors' laboratories indicate that DN2 cells have initiated TCR-δ, but not TCR-β locus recombination (*25*, and F. L. and H. T. P., in preparation). Moreover, it is found that most DN3 cells possess extensive and complete TCR-δ gene rearrangements, whereas only a fraction show V-DJβ rearrangements. Thus, recombination of the TCR-δ (and probably -γ) loci appear to precede those at TCR-β during adult, as well as fetal T-cell development.

In contrast to rearrangements of the TCR-δ, -γ and -β loci, which occur sequentially but are nonetheless restricted to DN cells, TCR-α gene recombination does not initiate until thymocytes become DP *(12)*. Since there are very few (if any) TCR-γ/δ$^+$ DP cells in the adult thymus *(73)*, and because there is no evidence for an obligatory DP intermediate in γ/δ cell development, the transition to the DP stage and the onset of TCR-α gene rearrangement appears to signal commitment to the TCR-α/β lineage for most cells. It has also been shown that the latest point at which TCR-α/β and -γ/δ thymocytes can diverge is after V-DJβ rearrangement, but prior to rearrangement of TCR-α (i.e., at the DN3/DN4 transition; *74*). All the above arguments suggest that α/β vs γ/δ lineage divergence must occur during the DN stages of thymocyte development in normal mice. In the following section, the authors will focus on the status of TCR gene rearrangements in DN cells, and their effects on lineage divergence.

5.2. Rearrangement and Expression of TCR Genes in α/β and γ/δ T-Cells

As discussed previously, TCR-δ, -γ, and -β loci all rearrange during the DN stage of development. Unfortunately, with respect to the role of gene rearrangement in lineage commitment, all three loci can be found to be rearranged in cells of either lineage. TCR-α/β$^+$ T-cells and thymocytes, in addition to the obvious rearrangements of TCR-α and -β genes, display extensive rearrangements at the TCR-γ *(75)* and -δ loci *(76,77)*, although these gene products are not expressed at the cell surface *(40)* . Lack of γ and δ gene expression in DP and mature cells may be mediated through the actions of lineage-specific silencer elements, as has been shown to occur for the γ locus *(78)*. Many DN thymocytes, however, do transcribe rearranged TCR-γ and -δ genes *(79,80)*, consistent with studies suggesting that the γ locus silencer maintains, rather than imposes, lineage-specific TCR-γ expression *(81)*. The reason that α/β lineage-committed thymocytes do not express these γ/δ TCRs at the cell surface has recently been determined to reflect the fact that many of these rearrangements are nonproductive (out-of-frame) at one or the other (TCR-γ or the -δ) locus, resulting in the inability to assemble a functional heterodimeric complex *(76,82)*.

Similar to the TCR-δ and -γ rearrangements found in thymic α/β T-cells, TCR-β rearrangements are common in thymic γ/δ T-cells. In fact, D-Jβ rearrangements are as frequent in thymic γ/δ cells as they are in mature TCR-α/β$^+$ T-cells *(18,83)*. Complete V-DJβ rearrangements are less common but still occur at least one-third as frequently as they do in TCR-α/β$^+$ cells, and a significant proportion of these rearrangements are found to be inframe *(83)*. It is not clear whether the fully rearranged TCR-β genes are transcribed, or what functions they may serve. However, selection for productive V-DJβ joints in γ/δ T-cells suggests that the TCR-β protein (with or without pTα) may have some effects on the maturation of γ/δ as well as α/β T-cells. As described in Subheading 3.3., TCR-α gene rearrangement is primarily limited to TCR-α/β-committed cells, since such rearrangements are undetectable in thymic γ/δ cells by quantitative Southern blotting. However, rearranged TCR-α genes can apparently be amplified from thymic γ/δ cells using PCR, and in these cases, TCR-α mRNA appears to be expressed at levels comparable to those found in α/β cells *(84)*. Together, the data described above thus suggest that TCR gene rearrangements are promiscuous, and are not exclusive to the lineages ultimately defined by TCR expression. The mutually exclusive expression of α/β or γ/δ TCRs is likely due to a combination of preferential rearrangements (particularly of the TCR-α locus in α/β T-cells), transcriptional silencing of inappropriate genes in cells of the alternate lineage, and selection for those rearrangements which are consistent with other (TCR-independent) programs of lineage commitment.

5.3. Genetic Studies of Lineage Commitment

As mentioned earlier, the literal implications of the instructive model are that α/β lineage development would be blocked by constitutive expression of a γ/δ TCR transgene. In similar fashion, genetic elimination of the TCR-β protein would be expected to preclude development of the α/β, but not the γ/δ lineage. The study of numerous genetically modified mouse models has led to the following findings. In TCR-β mutant mice, a small, but substantial number of DP cells develop *(36)*. Recent studies from the authors' laboratories show that these DP cells have productive TCR-γ and -δ gene rearrangements (F. L., submitted), consistent with the demonstration that these DP cells are eliminated if the TCR-δ locus is likewise mutated *(36)*. Furthermore, in most of the γ/δ-TCR transgenic models that have been described, DP thymocytes still develop in varying proportions *(81,85–87)*. In at least some instances, these DP cells appear to develop by virtue of selection through endogenous TCR-β proteins, and ultimately become genuine α/β lineage cells *(81,86)*. In other strains of γ/δ-TCR transgenic mice, there is no evidence for endogenous V-DJβ rearrangement, but expression of the transgenic γ/δ-TCR is repressed, and TCR-α gene rearrangement initiated *(86,87)*. These findings suggest that DP thymocytes from TCR-γ/δ transgenic mice are actually in the TCR-α/β lineage, despite the presence of the γ/δ transgene. Thus, neither transgenic nor endogenous TCR-γ/δ expression is sufficient to preclude the development of cells into the TCR-α/β lineage.

Recent studies regarding the effects of enforced TCR-β transgene expression have led to mixed conclusions for the development of the TCR-γ/δ lineage. The initial analysis of TCR-β transgenic mice showed partial isotypic exclusion of TCR-γ gene rearrangements *(88,89)*, with an apparent inhibition of intrathymic γ/δ T-cell development *(89)*. However, recent studies in the H-Y reactive α/β-TCR transgenic model suggests that the unusual $CD4^-8^-$ transgenic TCR-α/β^+ peripheral T-cells, which develop, may be γ/δ- rather than α/β-lineage cells *(90)*. These latter findings suggest that expression of an α/β-TCR transgene does not prevent the development of TCR-γ/δ lineage cells.

5.4. A Revised Model of α/β and γ/δ T-Cell Lineage Commitment

As described in the preceeding sections, genetic experiments do not support a purely instructive model of T lineage commitment. Based on the available data, the authors propose an integration of the stochastic and selective models described earlier (F. L., submitted elsewhere). Commitment to the various T-cell lineages would occur stochastically, independent of and prior to TCR gene rearrangement and expression. Through locus-specific control mechanisms that remain to be elucidated, TCR gene rearrangement then occurs in hierarchical fashion in cells of either lineage, beginning with the δ and then the γ loci. The first rearrangements of the β locus (D-J) probably coincide with the timing of γ gene rearrangements, whereas V-DJβ rearrangements occur substantially later, followed even later by α gene rearrangements. Those cells, which are both successful in TCR-γ and -δ gene rearrangements and are γ/δ-lineage committed (by other genetic criteria), eventually mature into TCR-γ/δ cells. Because of the coincidence of γ- and D-Jβ rearrangements, many of these γ/δ cells have D-Jβ rearrangements, and some cells make V-DJβ rearrangements as well. However, the assembly of a productive TCR-β chain gene does not induce TCR-α/β lineage development in cells otherwise committed to the γ/δ lineage. Likewise, the assembly of a functional TCR-γ/δ receptor does not preclude differentiation into the DP stage in TCR-α/β lineage cells. Although TCR-γ/δ expression may facilitate the transition into DP cells in some instances, TCR-γ/δ$^+$ thymocytes do not proliferate as TCR-β/pTα$^+$ cells do; therefore, they contribute only a small fraction of DP thymocytes. The majority of DP thymocytes thus derive from α/β lineage-committed precursors, which may express rearrangements of the γ-and/or δ-genes, but nonetheless do not become γ/δ T-cells. Thus, T-cell lineage commitment appears to bear characteristics of both stochastic and instructive models, since lineage commitment is essentially stochastic, although subsequent survival (i.e., selection) is instructive, ultimately being restricted to the expression of the proper isotype of the TCR.

Acknowledgments

The authors wish to thank Drs. Filippo Giancotti and Barry Gumbiner (MSKCC) for helpful discussions, Ms. Teodora Staeva (Cornell) and Dr. M. Wright (WEHI) for comments regarding the manuscript, and Ms. Laurie Ketzenberg (MSKCC) and Jill Van Es (WEHI) for assistance in preparation of the manuscript. Ference Livak also wishes to acknowledge the long-term support of Dr. David Schatz (Yale).

References

1. Shortman, K. and Wu, L. (1996) Early T lymphocyte progenitors. *Ann. Rev. Immunol.* **14,** 29–47.
2. Boyd, R. L., Tucek, C. L., Godfrey, D. I., Izon, D. J., Wilson, T. J., Davidson, N. J., Bean, A. G. D., Ladyman, H. M., Ritter, M. A., and Hugo, P. (1993) Inside the thymus. *Immunol. Today* **14,** 445–459.
3. Petrie, H. T., Strasser, A., Harris, A. W., Hugo, P., and Shortman, K. (1993) CD4$^+$8$^-$ and CD4$^-$8$^+$ mature thymocytes require different post-selection processing for final development. *J. Immunol.* **151,** 1273–1279.
4. Fowlkes, B. J., Edison, L., Mathieson, B. J., and Chused, T. M. (1985) Early T lymphocytes: differentiation in vivo of adult intrathymic precursor cells. *J. Exp. Med.* **162,** 802–822.
5. Lesley, J., Trotter, J., Schulte, R., and Hyman, R. (1990) Phenotypic analysis of the early events during repopulation of the thymus by the bone marrow prothymocyte. *Cell. Immunol.* **128,** 63–78.
6. Pearse, M., Wu, L., Egerton, M., Wilson, A., Shortman, K., and Scollay, R. (1989) An early thymocyte development sequence marked by transient expression of the IL-2 receptor. *Proc. Natl. Acad. Sci. USA* **86,** 1614–1618.
7. Shimonkevitz, R. P., Husmann, L. A., Bevan, M. J., and Crispe, I. N. (1987) Transient expression of IL-2 receptor precedes the differentiation of immature thymocytes. *Nature* **329,** 157–159.
8. Wilson, A., D'Amico, A., Ewing, T., Scollay, R., and Shortman, K. (1988) Subpopulations of early thymocytes: a cross-correlation flow cytometric analysis of adult mouse Ly-2$^-$L3T4$^-$ (CD8$^-$CD4$^-$) thymocytes using eight different surface markers. *J. Immunol.* **140,** 1461–1469.
9. Shortman, K., Egerton, M., Spangrude, G. J., and Scollay, R. (1990) The generation and fate of thymocytes. *Sem. Immunol.* **2,** 3–12.

10. Godfrey, D. I., Kennedy, J., Mombaerts, P., Tonegawa, S., and Zlotnik, A. (1994) Onset of TCR-β gene rearrangement and role of TCR-β expression during $CD3^-CD4^-CD8^-$ thymocyte differentiation. *J. Immunol.* **152,** 4783–4792.
11. Petrie, H. T., Pearse, M., Scollay, R., and Shortman, K. (1990) Development of immature thymocytes: initiation of CD3, CD4 and CD8 acquisition parallels down-regulation of the interleukin-2 receptor α-chain. *Eur. J. Immunol.* **20,** 2813–2816.
12. Petrie, H. T., Livak, F., Burtrum, D., and Mazel, S. (1995) T cell receptor gene recombination patterns and mechanisms: cell death, rescue, and T cell production. *J. Exp. Med.* **182,** 121–127.
13. Bruno, L., Rocha, B., Rolink, A., Von Boehmer, H., and Rodewald, H. R. (1995) Intra- and extra-thymic expression of the pre-T cell receptor alpha gene. *Eur. J. Immunol.* **25,** 1877–1982.
14. Groettrup, M., Ungewiss, K., Azogui, O., Palacios, R., Owen, M. J., Hayday, A. C., and von Boehmer, H. (1993) A novel disulfide-linked heterodimer on pre-T-cells consists of the T-cell receptor beta chain and a 33 kd glycoprotein. *Cell* **75,** 283–294.
15. Saint-Ruf, C., Ungewiss, K., Groettrup, M., Bruno, L., Fehling, H. J., and von Boehmer, H. (1994) Analysis and expression of a cloned pre-T cell receptor gene. *Science* **266,** 1208–1212.
16. Nikolic-Zugic, J., Moore, M. W., and Bevan, M. J. (1989) Characterization of the subset of immature thymocytes which can undergo rapid in vitro differentiation. *Eur. J. Immunol.* **19,** 649–653.
17. Petrie, H. T., Hugo, P., Scollay, R., and Shortman, K. (1990) Lineage relationships and developmental kinetics of immature thymocytes: CD3, CD4 and CD8 acquisition in vivo and in vitro. *J. Exp. Med.* **172,** 1583–1590.
18. Dudley, E. C., Petrie, H. T., Shah, L. M., Owen, M. J., and Hayday, A. C. (1994) T cell receptor beta chain gene rearrangement and selection during thymocyte development in adult mice. *Immunity* **1,** 83–93.
19. Spangrude, G. J. and Scollay, R. (1990) Differentiation of hematopoietic stem cells in irradiated mouse thymic lobes: kinetics and phenotype of progeny. *J. Immunol.* **145,** 3661–3668.
20. Li, C., Wu, L., Antica, M., Shortman, K., and Johnson, G. R. (1995) Purified murine long-term in vivo hemopoietic repopulating cells are not prothymocytes. *Exp. Hematol.* **23,** 21–25.
21. Spangrude, G. J., Heimfeld, S., and Weissman, I. L. (1988) Purification and characterization of mouse hematopoietic stem cells. *Science* **241,** 58–62.
22. Antica, M., Wu, L., Shortman, K., and Scollay, R. (1994) Thymic stem cells in the mouse bone marrow. *Blood* **84,** 111–117.
23. Wu, L., Li, C. L., and Shortman, K. (1996) Thymic dendritic cell precursors: relationship to the T-lymphocyte lineage and phenotype of the dendritic cell progeny. *J. Exp. Med.* **184,** 903–911.
24. Pénit, C., Lucas, B., and Vasseur, F. (1995) Cell expansion and growth arrest phases during the transition from precursor $CD4^-8^-$ to immature $CD4^+8^+$ thymocytes in normal and genetically modified mice. *J. Immunol.* **154,** 5103–5113.
25. Tourigny, M. R., Mazel, S., Burtrum, D. B., and Petrie, H. T. (1997) T Cell receptor (TCR)-β gene recombination: dissociation from cell cycle regulation and developmental progression during T cell ontogeny. *J. Exp. Med.* **185,** 1549–1556.
26. Wu, L., Scollay, R., Egerton, M., Pearse, M., Spangrude, G. J., and Shortman, K. (1991) CD4 expressed on earliest T-lineage precursor cells in the adult murine thymus. *Nature* **349,** 71–74.
27. Rodewald, H., Kretzschmar, K., Takeda, S., Hohl, C., and Dessing, M. (1994) Identification of pro-thymocytes in murine fetal blood: T lineage commitment can precede thymus colonization. *EMBO J.* **13,** 4229–4240.
28. Wu, L., Antica, M., Johnson, G. R., Scollay, R., and Shortman, K. (1991) Developmental potential of the earliest precursor cells from the adult mouse thymus. *J. Exp. Med.* **174,** 1617–1627.
29. Matsuzaki, Y., Gyotoku, J., Ogawa, M., Nishikawa, S., Katsura, Y., Gachelin, G., and Nakauchi, H. (1993) Characterization of c-kit positive intrathymic stem cells that are restricted to lymphoid differentiation. *J. Exp. Med.* **178,** 1283–1291.
30. Ardavin, C., Wu, L., Li, C., and Shortman, K. (1993) Thymic dendritic cells and T cells develop simultaneously within the thymus from a common precursor population. *Nature* **362,** 761–763.

31. Wu, L., Vremec, D., Ardavin, C., Winkel, K., Suss, G., Georgiou, H., Maraskovsky, E., Cook, W., and Shortman, K. (1995) Mouse thymus dendritic cells: kinetics of development and changes in surface markers during maturation. *Eur. J. Immunol.* **25,** 418–425.
32. Zúñiga-Pflücker, J. C., Jiang, D., and Lenardo, M. J. (1995) Requirement for TNF-alpha and IL-1 alpha in fetal thymocyte commitment and differentiation. *Science* **268,** 1906–1909.
33. Bosma, G. C., Custer, R. P., and Bosma, M. J. (1983) A severe combined immunodeficiency mutation in the mouse. *Nature* **10,** 527–530.
34. von Boehmer, H. (1990) Developmental biology of T cells in T cell-receptor transgenic mice. *Ann. Rev. Immunol.* **8,** 531–556.
35. Mombaerts, P., Clarke, A. R., Hooper, M. L., and Tonegawa, S. (1991) Creation of a large genomic deletion at the T-cell antigen receptor β-subunit locus in mouse embryonic stem cells by gene targeting. *Proc. Natl. Acad. Sci. USA* **88,** 3084–3087.
36. Mombaerts, P., Clarke, A. R., Rudnicki, M. A., Iacomini, J., Itohara, S., Lafaille, J. J., Wang, L., Ichikawa, Y., Jaenisch, R., Hooper, M. L., and Tonegawa, S. (1992) Mutations in T-cell antigen receptor genes α and β block thymocyte development at different stages. *Nature* **360,** 225–231.
37. Philpott, K. L., Viney, J. L., Kay, G., Rastan, S., Gardiner, E. M., Chae, S., Hayday, A. C., and Owen, M. J. (1992) Lymphoid development in mice congenitally lacking T-cell receptor-α/β expressing cells. *Science* **256,** 1448–1452.
38. Malissen, M., Trucy, J., Jouvin-Marche, E., Cazenave, P.-A., Scollay, R., and Malissen, B. (1992) Regulation of TCR α and β gene allelic exclusion during T-cell development. *Immunol. Today* **13,** 315–322.
39. Godfrey, D. I. and Zlotnik, A. (1993) Control points in early T-cell development. *Immunol. Today* **14,** 547–553.
40. Pardoll, D. M., Fowlkes, B. J., Bluestone, J. A., Kruisbeek, A., Maloy, W. L., Coligan, J. E., and Schwartz, R. H. (1987) Differential expression of two distinct T-cell receptors during thymocyte development. *Nature* **326,** 79–81.
41. Dillon, S. R. and Fink, P. J. (1995) Thymic selection events mediated by the pre-TCR do not depend upon a limiting ligand. *Int. Immunol.* **7,** 1363–1373.
42. Tonegawa, S. (1983) Somatic generation of antibody diversity. *Nature* **302,** 575–581.
43. Schatz, D. G., Oettinger, M. A., and Schlissel, M. S. (1992) VDJ recombination: molecular biology and regulation. *Annu. Rev. Immunol.* **10,** 359–383.
44. Anderson, S. J. and Perlmutter, R. M. (1996) A signalling pathway governing early thymocyte maturation. *Immunol. Today* **16,** 99–105.
45. Lin, W. C. and Desiderio, S. (1994) Cell cycle regulation of VDJ recombination-activating protein RAG-2. *Proc. Natl. Acad. Sci. USA* **91,** 2733–2737.
46. Hoffman, E. S., Passoni, L., Crompton, T., Leu, T. M. J., Schatz, D. G., Koff, A., Owen, M. J., and Hayday, A. C. (1996) Productive T-cell receptor β-chain gene rearrangement: coincident regulation of cell cycle and clonality during development in vivo. *Genes Dev.* **10,** 948–962.
47. Roth, D. B., Nakajima, P. B., Menetski, J. P., Bosma, M. J., and Gellert, M. (1992) VDJ recombination in mouse thymocytes: double-strand breaks near T cell receptor δ rearrangement signals. *Cell* **69,** 41–53.
48. Egerton, M., Shortman, K., and Scollay, R. (1990) The kinetics of immature murine thymocyte development in vivo. *Int. Immunol.* **24,** 1903–1907.
49. Xu, Y., Davidson, L., Alt, F. W., and Baltimore, D. (1996) Function of the pre-T-cell receptor α chain in T-cell development and allelic exclusion at the T-cell receptor β locus. *Proc. Natl. Acad. Sci. USA* **93,** 2169–2173.
50. Li, Z., Dordai, D. I., Lee, J., and Desiderio, S. (1996) A conserved degradation signal regulates RAG-2 accumulation during cell division and links V(D)J recombination to the cell cycle. *Immunity* **5,** 575–589.
51. Norment, A. M., Forbush, K. A., Nguyen, N., Malissen, M., and Perlmutter, R. M. (1997) Replacement of pre-T cell receptor signalling functions by CD4 coreceptor. *J. Exp. Med.* **185,** 121–130.

52. Zlotnik A. and Moore, T. A. (1995) Cytokine production and requirements during T-cell development. *Curr. Opin. Immunol.* **7,** 206–213.
53. Shortman K. and Petrie, H. T. (1990) Interleukins and T-cell development in the thymus. *Res. Immunol.* **141,** 280.
54. Peschon, J. J., Morrissey, P. J., Grabstein, K. H., Ramsdell, F. J., Maraskovsky, E., Gliniak, B. C., Park, L. S., Ziegler, S. F., Williams, D. E., Ware, C. B., Meyer, J. D., and Davison, B. L. (1994) Early lymphocyte expansion is severely impaired in interleukin 7 receptor-deficient mice. *J. Exp. Med.* **180,** 1955–1960.
55. Akashi, K. M., Von Freeden-Jeffrey, U., Murray, R., and Weissman, I. L. (1997) Bcl-2 rescues T lymphopoiesis in IL-7 receptor deficient mice. *Cell* **89,** 1033–1041.
56. Maraskovsky, E., O'Reilly, L. A., Teepe, M., Corcoran, L. M., Peschon, J. J., and Strasser, A. (1997) Bcl-2 can rescue T lymphocyte development in interleukin-7 receptor-deficient mice but not in mutant rag-$1^{-/-}$ mice. *Cell* **89,** 1011–1019.
57. Appasamy, P. M., Kenniston, T. W., Jr., Weng, Y., Holt, E. C., Kost, J., and Chambers, W. H. (1993) Interleukin 7-induced expression of specific T cell receptor-γ variable region genes in murine fetal liver cultures. *J. Exp. Med.* **178,** 2201–2206.
58. Muegge, K., Vila, M. P., and Durum, S. K. (1993) Interleukin-7: a cofactor for V(D)J rearrangement of the T cell receptor β-gene. *Science* **261,** 93–95.
59. Billips, L. G., Nuñez, C. A., Bertrand, F. E. I., Stankovic, A. K., Gartland, G. L., Burrows, P. D., and Cooper, M. D. (1995) Immunoglobulin recombinase gene activity is modulated reciprocally by interleukin 7 and CD19 in B cell progenitors. *J. Exp. Med.* **182,** 973–982.
60. Oosterwegel, M. A., Haks, M. C., Jeffry, U., Murray, R., and Kruisbeek, A. M. (1997) Induction of TCR gene rearrangements in uncommitted stem cells by a subset of IL-7 producing, MHC class II-expressing thymic stromal cells. *Immunity* **6,** 351–360.
61. Crompton, T., Outram, S. V., Buckland, J., and Owen, M. J. (1997) A transgenic T cell receptor restores thymocyte differentiation in interleukin-7 receptor α chain-deficient mice. *Eur. J. Immunol.* **27,** 100–104.
62. Li, Y., Pezzano, M., Philp, D., Reid, V., and Guyden, J. (1992) Thymic nurse cells exclusively bind and internalize $CD4^+CD8^+$ thymocytes. *Cell. Immunol.* **140,** 495–506.
63. Peifer, M. (1997) β-Catenin as oncogene: the smoking gun. *Science* **275,** 1752,1753.
64. Müller, K. M., Luedecker, C. J., Udey, M. C., and Farr, A. G. (1997) Involvement of E-cadherin in thymus organogenesis and thymocyte maturation. *Immunity* **6,** 257–264.
65. Crompton, T., Gilmour, K. C., and Owen, M. J. (1996) The MAP kinase pathway controls differentiation from double-negative to double-positive thymocyte. *Cell* **86,** 243–251.
66. Hughes, P. E., Renshaw, M. W., Pfaff, M., Forsyth, J., Keivens, V. M., Schwartz, M. A., and Ginsberg, M. H. (1997) Suppression of integrin activation: a novel function of a ras/raf-initiated MAP kinase pathway. *Cell* **88,** 521–530.
67. Wadsworth, S. A., Halvorson, M. J., and Coligan, J. E. (1992) Developmentally regulated expression of the β_4 integrin on immature mouse thymocytes. *J. Immunol.* **149,** 421–428.
68. Hemmings, B. A. (1997) Akt signaling: linking membrane events to life and death decisions. *Science* **275,** 628–630.
69. Salomon, D. R., Mojcik, C. F., Chang, A. C., Wadsworth, S., Adams, D. H., Coligan, J. E., and Shevach, E. M. (1994) Constitutive activation of integrin α_4/β_1 defines a unique stage of human thymocyte development. *J. Exp. Med.* **179,** 1573–1584.
70. Wadsworth, S. A., Chang, A. C., Hong, M.-J. P., Halvorson, M. J., Otto, S., and Coligan, J. E. (1995) Expression of a novel integrin β_1 chain epitope and anti-β_1 antibody-mediated enhancement of fibronectin binding are dependent on the stage of T cell differentiation. *J. Immunol.* **154,** 2125–2133.
71. Asarnow, D. M., Kuziel, W. A., Bonyhadi, M., Tigelaar, R. E., and Tucker, P. W. Allison, J. P. (1988) Limited diversity of γδ antigen receptor genes of $Thy\text{-}1^+$ dendritic epidermal cells. *Cell* **55,** 837–847.
72. Elliott, J. F., Rock, E. P., Patten, P. A., Davis, M. M., and Chien, Y. (1988) The adult T-cell receptor δ-chain is diverse and distinct from that of fetal thymocytes. *Nature* **331,** 627–631.
73. Itohara, S., Nakanishi, N., Kanagawa, O., Kubo, R., and Tonegawa, S. (1989) Monoclonal antibodies specific to native murine T-cell receptor gamma delta: analysis of gamma delta

T cells during thymic ontogeny and in peripheral lymphoid organs. *Proc. Natl. Acad. Sci. USA* **86,** 5094–5098.
74. Petrie H. T., Scollay, R., and Shortman, K. (1992) Commitment to the TCR-α/β or γ/δ lineages can occur just prior to the onset of CD4 and CD8 expression among immature thymocytes. *Eur. J. Immunol.* **22,** 2185.
75. Hayday, A. C., Saito, H., Gillies, S. D., Kranz, D. M., Tanagawa, G., Eisen, H. N., and Tonegawa, S. (1985) Structure, organization, and somatic rearrangement of the T cell gamma genes. *Cell* **40,** 259–269.
76. Livak, F., Petrie, H. T., Crispe, I. N., and Schatz, D. G. (1995) In-frame TCR d gene rearrangements play a critical role in the αβ/γδ T cell lineage decision. *Immunity* **2,** 617–627.
77. Nakajima, P. B., Menetski, J. P., Roth, D. B., Gellert, M., and Bosma, M. J. (1995) V-D-J rearrangements at the T cell receptor δ locus in mouse thymocytes of the αβ lineage. *Immunity* **3,** 609–621.
78. Ishida, I., Verbeek, S., Bonneville, M., Itohara, S., and Berns, A. (1990) T-cell receptor γδ and γ transgenic mice suggest a role of a γ gene silencer in the generation of αβ T cells. *Proc. Natl. Acad. Sci. USA* **87,** 3067–3071.
79. Wilson, A., Held, W., and Macdonald, H. R. (1994) Two waves of recombinase gene expression in developing thymocytes. *J. Exp. Med.* **179,** 1355–1360.
80. Wilson, A., de Villartay, J. P., and MacDonald, H. R. (1996) T cell receptor δ gene rearrangement and T early α (TEA) expression in immature αβ lineage thymocytes: implications for αβ/γδ lineage commitment. *Immunity* **4,** 37–45.
81. Sim, G., Olsson, C., and Augustin, A. (1995) Commitment and maintenance of the αβ and γδ T cell lineages. *J. Immunol.* **154,** 5821–5831.
82. Dudley, E. C., Girardi, M., Owen, M. J., and Hayday, A. C. (1995) Alpha-beta and gamma-delta T cells can share a late common precursor. *Curr. Biol.* **5,** 659–669.
83. Burtrum, D. B., Kim, S., Dudley, E. C., Hayday, A. C., and Petrie, H. T. (1996) TCR gene recombination and α/β-γ/δ lineage divergence: productive TCR-β rearrangement is neither exclusive nor preclusive of γ/δ cell development. *J. Immunol.* **157,** 4293–4296.
84. Mertsching, E., Wilson, A., MacDonald, H. R., and Ceredig, R. (1997) T cell receptor α gene rearrangement and transcription in adult thymic γδ cells. *Eur. J. Immunol.* **27,** 389–396.
85. Bonneville, M., Ishida, I., Mombaerts, P., Katsuki, M., Verbeek, S., Berns, A., and Tonegawa, S. (1989) Blockage of αβ T-cell development by TCR γδ transgenes. *Nature* **342,** 931–934.
86. Dent, A. L., Matis, L. A., Hooshmand, F., Widacki, S. M., Bluestone, J. A., and Hedrick, S. M. (1990) Self-reactive γδ cells are eliminated in the thymus. *Nature* **343,** 714–719.
87. Kersh, G. J., Hooshmand, F. F., and Hedrick, S. M. (1995) Efficient maturation of alpha-beta lineage thymocytes to the $CD4^+CD8^+$ stage in the absence of TCR-β rearrangement. *J. Immunol.* **154,** 5706–5714.
88. Fenton, R. G., Marrack, P., Kappler, J. W., Kanagawa, O., and Seidman, J. G. (1988) Isotypic exclusion of γδ T cell receptors in transgenic mice bearing a rearranged β-chain gene. *Science* **241,** 1089–1092.
89. von Boehmer, H., Bonneville, M., Ishida, I., Ryser, S., Lincoln, G., Smith, R. T., Kishi, H., Scott, B., Kisielow, P., and Tonegawa, S. (1988) Early expression of a T-cell receptor beta-chain transgene suppresses rearrangement of the V gamma 4 gene segment. *Proc. Natl. Acad. Sci. USA* **85,** 9729–9732.
90. Bruno, L., Fehling, H. J., and von Boehmer, H. (1996) The α/β T cell receptor can replace the γ/δ receptor in the development of γ/δ lineage cells. *Immunity* **5,** 343–352.

Chapter 17

T-Cell Development from Hematopoietic Stem Cells

Koichi Akashi, Motonari Kondo, Annette M. Schlageter, and Irving L. Weissman

1. Introduction

The central cells of the immune system include three major populations of lymphocytes with distinct antigen recognition receptors: T-cells, B-cells, and natural killer (NK) cells. All lymphocyte populations, as well as other blood cell types, are derived from hematopoietic stem cells (HSC). HSC have been successfully isolated and characterized from mice *(1–5)* and humans *(6–9)*.

The functional criteria for HSC were provided by Siminovitch et al. *(10)* who showed that HSC at a single cell level are capable of self-renewal, as well as giving rise to greatly expanded numbers of blood cells of all lineages. Self-renewal, a fundamental property of stem cells, occurs when a cell enters the cell cycle, divides, and gives rise to at least one daughter cell that has a developmental potential equal to that of the parent. The self-renewal activity is required for HSC to maintain hematopoiesis for the lifetime of the host. During hematolymphoid differentiation, cells undergo orderly changes that include the progressive loss of HSC self-renewal capacity, and the commitment to one or more lineages; some regenerative capacity at the stage of lineage-committed precursors may be preserved. Although the intracellular events that direct HSC commitment to particular lineages remains unclear, HSC are probably undergoing a sequential activation or silencing of genes that encode specific cytokine receptors, transcription factors, and signal transduction molecules.

Recombinant cytokines have been useful both in vitro and in vivo to study the development of progenitors, and these experimental models have been especially useful in defining the progenitors that are committed to the myeloid lineages—granulocytes, monocyte/macrophages, erythrocytes, and platelets. However, it has been difficult to identify progenitors that are committed to lymphoid lineages, because the assays that are

From: *Molecular Biology of B-Cell and T-Cell Development*
Edited by: J. G. Monroe and E. V. Rothenberg © Humana Press Inc., Totowa, NJ

used to evaluate differentiation potential do not allow detectable differentiation to particular lineages; this may be because cells fail to reach a suitable microenvironment in vivo such as the thymus, or because there is an insufficient expansion for detection in vivo, or because of the stochastic nature of lineage commitment, at least in vitro (for review, *see* ref. *11*). As a result, the existence of common lymphoid progenitors that can only give rise to T-, B-, and NK cells has been controversial, and constituted an important gap in the hematopoietic lineage maps. It is important to know whether T- and B-cells arise directly from a pluripotent stem cells, or from a common lymphoid progenitor, or from lymphoid stem cells that can give rise to all lymphoid lineages. In this chapter, adult T lymphopoiesis is reviewed, with emphasis on the regulation of self-renewal and differentiation in progenitors. Figure 1 represents a model of differentiation sequences from HSC to lymphoid cells based on currently available data, that should be used as a guide to this chapter.

2. Hematopoietic Stem Cells

Adult bone marrow contains multipotent progenitors and HSC that can give rise to all lineages of blood cells for life (reviewed in ref. *12*). Till and McCulloch *(13)* discovered that mouse bone marrow contains highly proliferative progenitor cells that are capable of giving rise to individual colonies of myeloid, erythroid, and megakaryocytic cells within the spleens of irradiated hosts (CFU-S). The same cell type could give rise to lymphoid cells *(14)*. Till et al. *(15)* found that in a CFU-S assay there was heterogeneity in the ability of HSC to form spleen colonies, and they proposed that the self-renewal or differentiation of HSC is stochastically determined. Metcalf and Moore *(16)* suggested that HSC may have intrinsic differences in self-renewal potential *(17,18)*, and that the microenvironment probably influences the decision of self-renewal and differentiation. Subsequently, it was proposed that the stem cell pool is heterogenous in terms of self-renewal potential. With the invention of the fluorescence-activated cell sorter, cells that express specific surface antigens could be purified, and HSC populations with high reconstitution activity were identified from mice *(1–5)* and humans . Further characterization of HSC has revealed that distinct HSC populations have different self-renewal activity in vivo.

2.1. Mouse HSC

The efforts to identify the mouse HSC have been reviewed previously *(19,20)*. Spangrude et al. *(3)* purified a population of cells from bone marrow of C57BL-Thy1.1 mice that was highly enriched for HSC activity and represents approx 0.05% of mouse bone marrow. The phenotype of this population is Thy-1^{lo}Sca-1^{+} Lineage(Lin)$^{-/lo}$. Although the Thy-1^{lo}Sca^{+}1+ Lin$^{-/lo}$ population contains all of the hematopoietic progenitors in the bone marrow, it is still heterogeneous by a variety of criteria including self-renewal activity, CFU-S activity, and cell-cycle status *(1)*. The most striking heterogeneity was demonstrated with limit-dilution transplantation assays; most of the cells from this population exhibit transient multilineage reconstitution in which the number of donor-derived myeloid cells declines after four weeks and becomes undetectable by eight weeks after reconstitution (short-term HSC). Only a minority of these cells could reconstitute more than 16 wk (long-term HSC) at a single cell level *(21)*.

We have subdivided three HSC subpopulations within the Thy-1^{lo}Sca-1^{hi} Lin$^{-/lo}$ population: Thy-1^{lo}Sca-1^{hi} Lin^{-}Mac-1^{-}CD4^{-} cells (referred to as Mac-1^{-}CD4^{-}), Thy-1^{lo}Sca-1^{hi} Lin^{-}Mac-1^{lo}CD4^{-}cells (Mac-1^{lo}CD4^{-}), and Thy-1^{lo}Sca-1^{hi} Lin^{-}Mac-1^{lo}CD4^{lo} cells

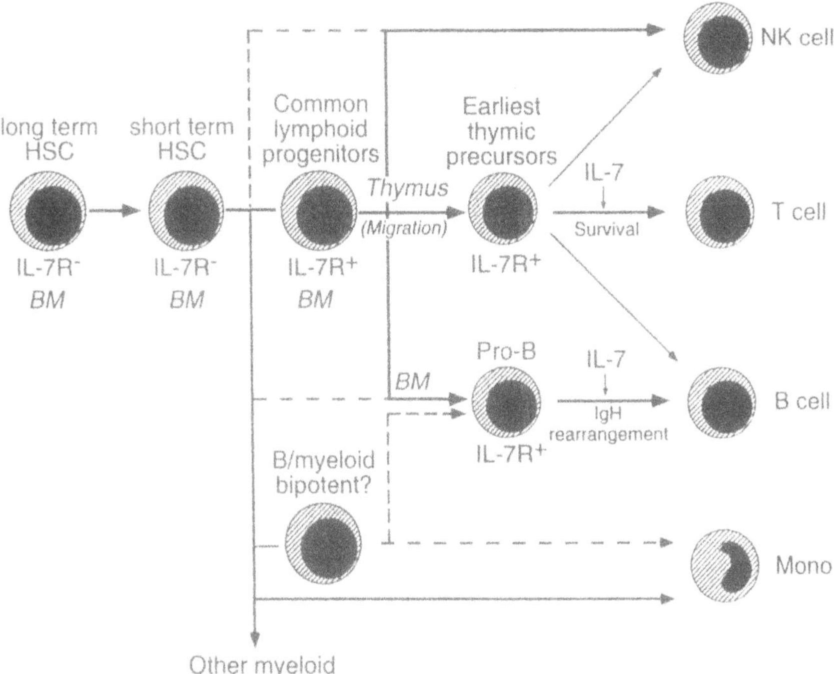

Fig. 1. The proposed differentiation sequences from HSC to lymphoid cells in adult mice. The HSC population including both long-term and short-term HSCs does not express IL-7R. Commitment to lymphoid lineages (possibly by internal gene programs) might be associated with immediate expression of IL-7R, and become common lymphoid progenitors that are able to generate all lymphoid classes (62a). The common lymphoid progenitors that successfully reach the thymic microenvironment can read out T-cell differentiation. The common lymphoid progenitors can differentiate into pro-B-cells in the bone marrow (BM). The earliest thymic precursor population might be heterogenous; a majority of them have already committed to T-cell lineages, but may contain rare common lymphoid progenitors that have just homed to the thymus, and still possess differentiation protential into B and NK cells. IL-7 plays different roles in T- and B-cell development; the principal role of IL-7 in T-cell development is to maintain cell survival (83,85) but that in B-cell development is other than maintenance of cell survival (85). The principal role of IL-7 in B lymphopoiesis is probably to promote rearrangement of IgH genes. Some of lymphoid cells may be developed directly from short-term HSC or multipotent progenitors. It is still unclear whether B-cells can also be derived from bipotent B-cell/myeloid progenitors.

(Mac-1^{lo}CD4^{lo}) *(1)*. The Mac-1^{-}CD4^{-} population exhibits a long-term reconstitution profile. The Mac-1^{lo}CD4^{-} population shows transient multipotent reconstitution, with some clones exhibiting only B and myeloid lineage reconstitution. Some cells in the Mac-1^{lo}CD4^{lo} population exhibit transient multilineage reconstitution, whereas others reconstitute B only or B plus myeloid lineage. The difference in the ability among these subsets to reconstitute a mouse for more than four months indicates that they are arranged in a lineage with a hierarchical relationships *(22)*. Consistent with this hypothesis, the Mac-1^{-}CD4^{-} population gives rise to the transiently reconstituting Mac-1^{lo}CD4^{-} population, whereas the Mac-1^{lo}CD4^{-} population gives rise to Mac-1^{lo}CD4^{lo} population, but not the long-term reconstituting Mac-1^{-}CD4^{-} population *(22)*. Accordingly, these three populations might be arranged in a lineage in terms of the progressive loss of self-renewal potential. HSC having long-term and the short-term reconstituting potential have also been successfully isolated using other markers such as incorporation of mitochondrial vital dye Rhodamine-123 (Rh123) *(23–25)* and CD34 *(2)*. Osawa et al. *(2)* reported that $CD34^-Sca\text{-}1^+c\text{-}Kit^+$ cells could reconstitute all lineages in a long-term, that $CD34^{lo}Sca\text{-}1^+c\text{-}Kit^+$ cells were a mixture of multipotent long-term and short-term cells, and $CD34^+Sca\text{-}1^+c\text{-}Kit^+$ cells exhibit multilineage reconstitution activity only in the short term.

The progressive loss of self-renewal potential in these discrete HSC compartments as evaluated by transplantation assays strongly suggests that the transition from long-term HSC to short-term HSC is intrinsically deterministic *(1)*. Among $Mac\text{-}1^{lo}$ HSC, the residual productive lifespans of these HSC clones (as measured by transplantation) are not widely disparate but, in fact, are mainly 8–12 wk. Retransfer of bone marrow of recipients of short-term HSC donors also centered around 8–12 wk, prompting the authors to propose that transplantation reveals or resets an intrinsic lifespan clock, with another 8–12 wk or long term (> 6 mo) as the two modal outcomes. The biochemical basis of such a clock remains a mystery. Telomerase expression widely correlates with self-renewal potential in many cell types *(26)*; thus the clock(s) might operate at least in part through telomerase action, and the authors would expect HSC to express telomerase. Recently, we have shown that approx 70% of fetal liver HSC, bone marrow HSC, and, only rarely non-self-renewing multipotent progenitors exhibit telomerase activity *(27)*. However, the different self-renewal fates may also be affected by extrinsic factors; for example, after transplantation, different HSC subsets may home to and be influenced by distinct hematopoietic niches.

Cytokines also influence HSC subsets. An important example is the c-kit ligand, steel factor (Slf; or stem cell factor), which is genetically defective in mice with a mutation in the Sl locus *(28)*. The homozygous Sl/Sl mouse has a defect in hematopoiesis, mast cells, primordial germ cells, and melanoblasts. The importance of c-Kit, which is expressed on HSC subsets, was demonstrated when mice were injected with neutralizing anti–c-Kit antibody, thereby eliminating most hematopoietic progenitors *(29)*. However, Slf is not necessary for the fetal generation, maintenance, or self-renewal of HSC *(30,31)*; rather, it synergizes with other early acting cytokines to promote the formation of all lineages. Similar to the c-Kit/Slf interaction is the interaction of the Flk-1 and Flk-2/Flt-3 receptors *(32,33)*, with their respective ligands, vascular endothelial growth factor, and Flt-3 ligand (FL) *(34,35)*. HSC respond little to FL alone, but FL synergizes with several other growth factors to promote proliferation. Flk-1 is required for hematopoiesis *(36)*. Flk-2 receptor-deficient mice exhibit only a relatively mild defect in B lymphopoiesis, but the double mutant of Flk-2 and c-Kit has a more extreme defect of hematopoiesis than that in the c-Kit mutant *(37)*. Although a number of growth factors can drive quiescent HSC into cycle, the factors that are capable of maintaining self-renewing division of these stem cells in vitro have not yet been identified. This is a problem that limits the use of HSC as a target of gene transfection, because current retroviral technologies require cell division for viral integration *(38)*.

Eighty percent of the cells in the $CD4^-Mac\text{-}1^-$ long-term HSC subset respond to the cytokine combination of Slf, IL-3 plus IL-6, and form colonies on methylcellulose *(39)*. The HSC subsets express various cytokine receptors, including IL-3, c-Kit, IL-6, and IL-1α. The common β chain, which is an indispensable subunit of IL-3, GM-CSF, and IL-5 receptors, are also expressed in this population *(40)*. The numbers of these cytokine receptors per cells are lowest in long-term ($Rh^{lo}Lin^-Sca\text{-}1^+c\text{-}Kit^+$) subset, and progressively increased to $Rh^{hi}Lin^-Sca\text{-}1^+c\text{-}Kit^+$ short-term HSC to $Lin^-Sca\text{-}1^-c\text{-}Kit^+$ progenitors *(41)*, corresponding to their hierarchical relationships.

The hierarchy of HSC subsets suggest that lineage commitment occurs within a short-term HSC population, such as the Mac-1^{lo}CD4^{lo} population. It is unclear whether the limited reconstitution patterns such as B lymphoid/myeloid, B/T lymphoid, or B lymphoid only, observed in this population represent clones that are rigorously committed to the observed lineages, or simply a failure to detect myeloid and T-lineage reconstitution. Homing to the thymus may be the critical step for HSC to differentiation into T-cells. The Mac-1^{lo}CD4^{lo} subset of cells, which have limited self-renewal capacity, may not be as successful at homing to the thymus as the long-term HSC, since the short-term HSC may not be able to expand enough for in vivo detection, maintaining their T-cell differentiation potential.

Cell survival is a prerequisite for self-renewal. Recently, several proteins that can sustain cell survival, such as Bcl-2 and Bcl-X_L, have been reported. HSC express both Bcl-2 and Bcl-x_L (unpublished data) and the expression of these antiapoptotic proteins is important for maintaining hematopoiesis as illustrated in the following examples. In Bcl-2-deficient mice, hematopoiesis develops normally, at least until the second post-natal week of life *(42,43)*; Bcl-2 deficient HSC are not able to engraft as well as normal HSC when transplanted into irradiated normal hosts *(44)*; and the disruption of *bcl-x* resulted in embryonic death with massive loss of hematopoietic cells and impairment of nervous system development *(45)*. However, the precise role of these survival proteins on HSC still needs to be clarified.

2.2. Human HSC

Primitive human hematopoietic progenitors are enriched in the CD34^+ population. Similar to mouse HSC, human HSC from fetal bone marrow, adult bone marrow, umbilical cord blood, and mobilized peripheral blood can be further defined by absence of expression of lineage markers and by Thy-1 expression as CD34^+Thy-1^+Lin$^-$cells *(7)*; several independent experiments have confirmed the expression of human Thy-1 *(46)*. The differentiation activity of the candidate human HSC along myeloerythroid and B lymphoid pathways have been extensively evaluated in vitro by long-term culture-initiating cell assay (LTC-IC), which initially includes the formation of cobblestone area-forming colonies (CAFC). Virtually all of the LTC-IC activity from adult bone marrow is contained in the CD34^+Thy-1^+Lin-Rh123^{lo} subset, which is both highly enriched for CAFC activity *(47)*, and is a subset of the CD34^+Lin$^-$Rh$123^{lo/med}$ *(48)*.

Xenogenic reconstitution systems using sheep, nonhuman primate, or mouse models have proven to be useful as in vivo models of human hematopoiesis. The SCID-hu mouse model is the most readily available, and modified thymus/liver SCID-hu models have been used for studying HIV infection *(49)*. In the original SCID-hu model, SCID mice are implanted with human fetal thymic grafts, injected with human fetal liver cells, and these mice can then support human hematopoiesis *(50)*. Successful differentiation of human HSC leads to the appearance of mature human CD4^+ and CD8^+ T-cells and human immunoglobulin in peripheral blood and all stages of human thymic maturation *(51)*. In another modification of the SCID-hu model, DiGuisto et al. showed that SCID mice that are implanted with human fetal thymus or bone fragments, can support the differentiation of CD34^+ fetal bone marrow cells to T-, B-, and myeloid cells *(8)*. Human hematopoiesis in SCID-recipient mice can be improved by the administration of human cytokines *(52)*; and by the use of NOD-SCID mice that have the relative NK deficiency of NOD mice. Although murine models of human hematopoiesis have provided the critical in vivo assay and allowed for the isolation of human HSC *(7)*, significant barriers need to be resolved before long-term multilineage reconstitution from single human HSC can be assayed, since engraftment requires high number of cells in this model, which involves HLA disparate transplants. Because of the limitation of these assay systems, there are no reported studies of clonogenic bursts in vivo; therefore, the delineation of subsets such as short-term and long-term HSC has not yet been achieved.

Recently, several studies have confirmed that HSC are contained in the CD34$^+$ or CD34$^+$Thy-1$^+$ fraction of bone marrow or mobilized blood stem cells by successful autologous stem cell transplantation for patients suffering from neuroblastoma, breast cancer *(53)*, lymphoma *(54)*, or multiple myeloma *(55)*. In these settings, the CD34$^+$ HSC might be useful for autologous transplantation, because this fraction is less contaminated with neoplastic cells *(55)*.

3. Commitment of HSC to Lymphoid Lineage

Mouse HSC with either long-term or short-term reconstitution potential can give rise to all blood cell types *(20)*. Commitment of HSC to specific lineages is probably regulated by elements in the bone marrow microenvironment, as well as by the intrinsic orchestration of developmentally specific gene programs. During a stepwise commitment process, bipotential or oligopotential progenitors might exist in sites of early hematopoiesis *(56)*. The identification of such clonal progenitors is essential for understanding particular hematological malignancies, as well as normal hematopoiesis.

An unresolved issue in the sequential commitment of HSC to lymphoid cells is whether lymphoid cells are derived directly from certain HSC subsets—from bipotential (T-cell/myeloid or B-cell/myeloid) progenitors, or from progenitors that exclusively give rise to all lymphoid cells, including T-, B-, NK, and lymphoid-derived antigen-presenting dendritic cells. Such oligopotent progenitors might have limited or no self-renewal capacity, since they should be downstream of short-term HSC in a developmental scheme. A common lymphoid progenitor has been characterized using expression markers for early thymic progenitors such as Sca-2, or for cytokine receptors such as IL-7 receptors (IL-7R). The existence of a common lymphoid progenitor has been supported by several lines of evidence: the disruption of genes that encode certain cytokines, cytokine receptors, and transcription factors exclusively eliminates lymphoid cells. However, the lesson that mutations of adenosine deaminase, a ubiquitous enzyme in all human tissues, can cause SCID in humans gives one pause when interpreting these experiments *(57)*. More promising, the earliest thymic progenitors can give rise to all lymphoid classes when a considerable number of these cells ($1–3 \times 10^4$) are injected *(58,59)*. However, because of the nature of the assays, the presence of a single clonogenic precursor giving rise to all lymphoid lineages was difficult to confirm.

3.1. Common Lymphoid Progenitors

Committed B-cell precursors that express B220 and CD43 and that have germline immunoglobulin genes are referred to as pro-B-cells. The pro-B-cells are mainly found in bone marrow, and are B lineage-restricted. The major sites for T- and B-cell development are thymus and bone marrow, respectively. Accordingly, it is reasonable to search for the "putative" common lymphoid progenitor within bone marrow cells.

The antigen Sca-2 *(60)*, which is present on T precursors within the thymus, but absent from long-term HSC subsets *(4)*, has been used by Antica et al. *(61)* to search for lymphoid-restricted cells in the bone marrow. They identified a Sca-1$^+$Sca-2$^+$Thy-1$^+$ population. However, although lymphoid reconstitution was enhanced in this population, the Sca-1$^+$Sca-2$^+$Thy-1$^+$ population also possessed multipotent reconstituting activity.

IL-7 is a nonredundant cytokine for both T- and B-cell development. The interaction between IL-7 and IL-7R induces survival signals for T lymphopoiesis (*see* Subheading 4.3.). The authors recently isolated a $Lin^{-/lo}$ IL-$7R^+$ Thy-1^-Sca-1^+c-Kit^+ population from bone marrow *(61a)*. This population possesses rapid T, B and NK cell-restricted reconstitution potential. The numbers of donor-derived T- and B-cells that were derived from these IL-$7R^+$Sca-1^+c-Kit+ cells begin to decline after four to six weeks, suggesting that this population has no or limited self-renewal activity. The authors could not detect myeloid lineage differentiation from this population by in vivo reconstitution assays or in vitro methylcellulose assays. This population can give rise to T- and B-cells after injection of 20 cells intrathymically and intravenously, respectively. Furthermore, cells from a three-day colony that was seeded on methylcellulose containing Slf, IL-7, and FL, with a single IL-$7R^+$Sca-1^+c-Kit^+ cell can give rise to both T- and B-cells after intrathymic and intravenous injection, respectively. These results indicate that the IL-$7R\alpha^+$Sca-1^+c-Kit^+ population contains common lymphoid progenitors that can differentiate at least into both T- and B-cells *(61a)*.

Hakoda et al. traced the potential lineage origin of peripheral blood lymphocytes from an atomic bomb survivor by using mutations in the hypoxanthine guanine phosphoribosyltransferase gene *(62)*. The results suggested that T-, B-, and NK cells were the differentiated progeny of a common progenitor. However, they were unable to check myeloid cells. These clones probably differentiated from HSC, since the clonal lymphopoiesis in this patient had persisted for more than 20 yr.

There is evidence of a T/NK bipotential precursor in human fetal thymus *(63)*, although clonal analysis was not reported. Gore et al. *(64)* identified a terminal deoxytransferase (TdT) positive population in the $CD34^+$ bone marrow fraction as a candidate lymphoid precursor population *(64)*, but functional analysis was not reported. A subpopulaton of these $CD34^+TdT^+$ cells express the neutral endopeptidase CD10 *(65)*. Recently, Galy et al. *(66)* found that the $Lin^-CD34^+CD10^+$ human bone marrow cells had a common lymphoid precursor activity. The developmental potential for lymphoid lineages was determined by in vitro and in vivo assays. The $Lin^-CD34^+CD10^-$Thy-1^+ multipotential HSC were $CD45RA^-$, whereas the $CD45RA^+Lin^-CD34^+CD10^+$Thy-$1^-$ population differentiated only into T-, B-, NK, and dendritic cells. The clonal origin of the progeny was shown in B-, NK, and dendritic cells, although the common origin of T- and B-cells was not completely demonstrated.

Thus, common lymphoid progenitors might exist in sites of early hematopoiesis in both mice and humans. It is important to clarify whether this stage is a required intermediate for lymphoid differentiation from HSC, since if HSC commit to lymphoid or myeloid lineages in a stochastic manner, immediate products of (short-term) HSC would include B-cell/myeloid and T-cell/myeloid bipotential progenitors as well as common lymphoid progenitors.

3.2. Bipotent (B-Cell/Myeloid and T-Cell/Myeloid) Progenitors

Several reports revealed a "close" relationship between the development of B and monocyte lineages. Klinken et al. demonstrated that the transfection of the oncogene v-raf into B-cell lines that were established from c-myc transgenic mice can result in production of macrophages that maintain the rearrangement of immunoglobulin heavy chain (IgH) genes *(67)*. Although this does not prove that the B-cells and monocytes are derived from bipotent progenitors, it indicates that B-cell commitment might be reversible, at least for macrophages, even after the completion of rearrangement of IgH genes. Cumano et al. reported that a population in fetal liver could give rise to both B-cells and macrophages from a single cells in vitro *(68)*. Hirayama et al. *(69)* also reported that B-cells can develop from myeloid colony-forming cells in mouse bone marrow. However, it is possible that these cells are pluripotent, since their in vivo differentiation activity including their T-cell developmental potential was not tested in these cases. Also, the bipotent B-cell/macrophage precursor could not give rise to the other myeloid cells, such as granulocytes, erythrocytes, and megakaryocytes in vitro *(68)*. The in vitro bipotency exhibited may not reflect a physiological differentiation process, but may simply reflect regenerative capacity of B-cell precursors for differentiation into macrophages, when provided with the S17 stromal cells and exogenous M-CSF. It remains unclear whether B-cells actually develop from the "bipotent" B-cell/macrophage precursor in vivo.

The close relationship between B- and myelomonocytic cell development is also found in human hematopoietic malignancies. The simultaneous expression of myeloid and B lymphoid antigens has been reported in B-cell acute lymphoblastic leukemia (ALL) and acute myelogenous leukemia (AML) *(70)*. Multiple myeloma is a mature B-cell malignancy, which sometimes expresses myelomonocytic antigens *(71)*. The authors reported a case with concomitant multiple myeloma and myelomonocytic leukemia *(72)*. In this case, the myeloma cells and monocytic leukemia cells had identical patterns of IgH gene rearrangement, and colonies obtained after a long-term methylcellulose culture of bone marrow cells contained both types of neoplastic cells, indicating that common B-cell/myelomonocytic leukemic progenitors gave rise to both neoplastic clones. The clonal origin of coexisting acute myelomonocytic leukemia and acute lymphoblastic leukemia has also been reported *(73)*. These cases collectively suggest that myeloid/B-cell bipotent progenitors might be involved in leukemic transformation.

Several reports suggest that T-cell/myeloid bipotent precursors are involved in human leukemias *(74)*; progressive lineage conversion of T-cell ALL to AML has been demonstrated in patients receiving 2'-deoxycoformycin *(75,76)*, and $CD34^+CD7^+$ ALL cells can differentiate into myeloerythroid cells under certain in vitro conditions *(77,78)*. However, there have been no data supporting the existence of T-cell/myeloid bipotent precursors in mice.

Leukemias that express antigens from multiple lineages may offer a snapshot of early hematopoietic progenitors that are transformed just prior to lineage commitment (lineage promiscuity) *(79)*. However, the transforming event itself may perturb the differentiation potential of the transformed progenitors into certain lineages, or may induce aberrant expression of sets of irrelevant lineage-associated genes (lineage infidelity) *(80)*. Further clonal analysis of progenitor activity of normal cells is required to understand this issue.

3.3. Cytokines

One of the important extracellular elements that affect the differentiation of hematopoietic progenitors are the cytokines present in microenvironments. The interaction between cytokines and cytokine receptors can induce variety of intracellular signals including phosphorylation of various signal transduction molecules that lead to the expression of a set of lineage-associated genes *(81,82)*. However, although cytokines may instruct the differentiation of some progenitors, there is no convincing evidence that cytokines can instruct lineage commitment of HSC or immature progenitors. Ogawa *(11)* has suggested that cytokines may influence the survival and proliferation of progenitors after commitment, but they do not determine the commitment of HSC. Indeed, it is implied that the self-renewal or differentiation of the progenitors was regulated by intrinsic factors, and not by cytokines *(83–87)*.

Nonetheless, defects in specific cytokine/cytokine receptor interactions lead to loss of specific lineages of cells, indicating that some cytokines are nonredundant for cell maturation. For example, the common cytokine receptor γ chain (γc) is an indispensable subunit of cytokine receptors including IL-2, IL-4, IL-7, IL-9, and IL-15 *(88–94)* and a defect in γc results in X-linked severe combined immunodeficiency (X-SCID) in humans *(95,96)*. Jak3, one of the Janus kinase members is a signal transduction molecule associated with γc *(97–99)*. Genetic defects of Jak3 in patients cause a congenital form of immunodeficiency that is identical to that seen in X-SCID patients, although it transmits as an autosomal recessive trait *(100,101)*. Mice with a disruption of γc by gene targeting exhibit a loss of T-, B-, and NK cells *(102–104)*, whereas mice with a null IL-7Rα chain or IL-7 mutation exhibit a loss of T- and B-cells, but NK cell development remains intact *(105–108)*, indicating that the signals from IL-7R are nonredundant for T- and B-cell development. NK cell development was inhibited in mice deficient for IL-2Rβ *(109)*, which is an indispensable subunit of the functional IL-2R and IL-15R complexes *(88)*. Since the IL-2-deficient mice have normal NK cells, the impaired development of NK cells in γc-deficient mice might be caused by a lack of functional IL-15R *(110)*. Jak3-deficient mice also exhibit a similar defect in T- and B-cell development *(111–113)*.

The other striking example of a missing lineage caused by defective cytokines is in osteopetrotic *op/op* mice that fail to form osteoclasts and most classes of macrophages because of the lack of functional macrophage colony-stimulating factor (M-CSF) *(114)*. In both cases, it was unclear whether cytokines are critical for commitment of progenitors (i.e., IL-7 for common lymphoid progenitor, and M-CSF for monocyte as a macrophage precursor), or for promoting cell survival or proliferation after commitment.

Recently, it has been shown that missing lineages could be restored by enforced expression of a survival protein, Bcl-2. The murine promoters, *Eμ* and *H-2K*, are used to express Bcl-2 in T-cells and all hematopoietic cells, respectively, in IL-7Rα-deficient and/or γc-deficient mice *(83,85)*. The enforced expression of Bcl-2 in T-cell progenitors resulted in a significant recovery of mature T-cells in both SCID strains. The rescue of mature T-cells results from the recovery in numbers of immature thymic progenitors and from the restoration of thymic positive selection (*see* Subheading 4.2.).

However, Bcl-2 could not rescue B-cell and NK cell development in γc deficient mice *(85)*. In *H-2K-bcl-2* γc-deficient mice, there is an impairment of the transition from pro-B to pre-B stage in the bone marrow, suggesting an important role for IL-7 in μ heavy chain gene rearrangement or in the formation of the pre-B receptor complex in vivo. This nonredundancy could be ascribed to the critical role of IL-7 in two stages of B-cell development; it has been shown that IL-7 promotes rearrangement of the μ heavy chain gene of pro-B-cells at least in vitro *(115)*, and stimulates proliferation of pre-B-cells *(116–118)*. Bcl-2 apparently could not substitute for γc (mainly IL-15R)-mediated signals for NK cell development *(85)*.

The authors have also reported that M-CSF delivers a survival signal for monocytes in vivo, and that enforced expression of Bcl-2 using human MRP8 promoter *(119)* in monocytes in *op/op* mice can rescue the differentiation of macrophage subsets and significantly reverses their osteopetrosis *(86)*.

These data collectively indicate that the principal role of IL-7 for T lymphopoiesis and that of M-CSF for formation of macrophage compartments is to provide survival signals for differentiating cells. The apparent difference in the role of IL-7 between T and B lymphopoiesis illustrates that the disruption of a single gene can block differentiation of a variety of cells through different mechanisms, and the lack of different lineage cells in mice with a single-gene knockout does not necessarily mean the elimination or inhibition of bipotent or oligopotent progenitors. In this context, IL-7 is not a critical factor for commitment of a common lymphoid progenitor.

In human AML, chromosomal aberrations are seen that are related to cytokines and/or cytokine receptors. For example, the deletion of the long arm of chromosome 5 ($5q^-$) that contains the genes for IL-3, IL-5, IL-6, GM-CSF, M-CSF, and fms (M-CSF receptor) is frequently found in myeloproliferative disorder and AML *(120,121)*. However, it is intriguing, because a copy of each gene can probably still be found on the other intact chromosome 5. The growth of leukemic progenitors is positively and negatively regulated by various cytokines, including cytokines secreted by the leukemic cells themselves *(122–125)*. Whether this disease results from a disruption, loss or unmasking of a "normal" growth factor or their receptor, or from the loss of a closely linked leukemia suppressor gene is currently unclear. Interestingly, heterozygous mutation in one of the important lymphoid-related transcription factors, Ikaros, leads to T lymphoproliferation with rapid development of T-cell leukemia and lymphoma *(126)* (*see* Subheading 3.4. in this chapter). A heterozygous disruption might decrease the level of proteins that are needed for differentiation (i.e., cytokine/cytokine receptors, and transcription factors), resulting in the accumulation of progenitors that are presumably susceptible to transformation. However, a disruption of the lymphoid-restricted cytokine/cytokine receptors has not been reported for lymphoid malignancies.

3.4. Transcriptional Factors

Intracellular events of lineage commitment are associated with silencing or activating genes. DNA-binding proteins that regulate transcription of these lineage-associated genes might bind to distinct promoters and/or enhancers of genes, and function as important controls in the commitment of HSC and/or lymphoid progenitors. Most of the transcription factors have been identified by studies of the promoters and enhancers of structural genes that are specifically expressed in individual hematopoietic lineages. Other factors have been identified through studies on oncogenic retroviruses or on translocations in hematological malignancies. In certain hematological malignancies, specific chromosome translocations result in a constitutive expression of new hybrid transcription factors that lead to the transformation of specific lineages. Many transcription factors have been studied, and this will be discussed elsewhere in this volume.

Knockout mice with disruptions in transcription factors that drive lymphoid cell development genes have a variety of immunodeficiencies. For example, the GATA3 knockout mouse lacks T-cells *(127)*, whereas the BSAP *(128)*, EBF *(129)*, and E2A *(130,131)* knockout mice have no B-cells, but so far, only the Ikaros knockout mice lack all lymphoid lineages *(132)*. Ikaros is a zinc-finger protein, and was originally cloned because of the affinity of its product for the CD3δ enhancer *(133)*. It is expressed almost exclusively in early fetal liver and in the fetal thymus. However, the authors have recently demonstrated that HSCs express Ikaros, with Ikaros RNA isoform profiles that distinguish long-term HSC from short-term HSC from lymphoid-committed progenitors (C. Klug et al., submitted). Disruption of Ikaros results in mice that lack T-, B- and NK cells, but not myeloid cells, suggesting that Ikaros is involved in the control of maturation of common lymphoid progenitors *(132)*. However, as in the cases of γc knockout, this may be a result of the block of distinct differentiation steps in each of the three lymphoid classes. Because of its RNA-splicing complexity, Ikaros might be involved in the control of distinct cellular events in the proliferation of hematolymphoid cells such as T-cells, since mice carrying a particular mutant allele exhibit a general T lymphoproliferation *(126)*.

Chromosomal translocations involving genes that encode transcription factors result in lineage specific hematological malignancies; for example, TAL1 or SCL in T-cell ALL with t(1;14)(p32;q11) *(134–137)*, Rbtn2/Ttg-2 in T-cell ALL with t(11;14)(p13;q11) *(138)*, and AML1 in AML with t(8;21)(q22;q22) or t(3;21)(q26;q22) *(139–141)*. In most cases, these translocations result in the constitutive expression of new hybrid proteins, probably driven by their transcription activity. The reasons that these translocations result in lineage-specific malignancies are largely unknown. In t(8;21) AML, the products of this translocation, AML1/ETO, is expressed in multipotential myeloid progenitors *(142)*, and AML1 is expressed in human $CD34^+$ hematopoietic progenitors *(143)*. The disruption of either TAL1, Rbtn2, or AML1 *(139–141)* is lethal to murine embryos, and these embryos display multilineage defects including both lymphoid and myeloid development. These transcription factors are thought to be critical in primary hematopoiesis, but they are not related to lineage commitment. Mice heterozygous for an AML1/ETO allele generated by the "knock-in" strategy die during gestation from impaired hematopoiesis in fetal liver. Since this phenotype resembles that in homozygous disruption of AML1, AML1/ETO seems to block normal AML1 function *(144)*. This suggests that lineage specificity in certain chromosomal translocation may result from the inhibition of normal function of transcription factors involved in the translocation.

4. T Lymphopoiesis in the Thymus

Lymphoid progenitors from the bone marrow seed the thymus, the major site for T-cell maturation. The characteristics of the earliest thymic progenitors are discussed in Chapter 16. The earliest thymic precursor is contained in the $CD4^-$ or lo $CD8^-$ CD3 $(TCR\alpha\beta)^-$ (triple negative; TN) c-Kit^+ fraction that, as a population, still has the potential to differentiate into NK cells, B-cells, and dendritic cells but has almost lost the ability to differentiate into the myeloid lineage *(58,59,145)*. This supports the hypothesis that there are intermediate progenitors, such as common lymphoid progenitors, in the developmental process between HSC and the earliest thymic progenitor. The earliest thymic precursor has different surface phenotypes from the common lymphoid progenitors *(69)*. In addition, an intravenous injection of more than 1×10^4 thymic precursors to lethally-irradiated congenic mice was required to detect B-cell progeny *(58,59)*, whereas the injection of as few as ~20 cells of common lymphoid progenitors resulted in the appearance of B-cell progeny *(61a)*. Accordingly, the earliest thymic precursor population may be heterogenous. This population may contain rare common lymphoid progenitors that have just homed to the thymus or a small number of oligopotent or monopotent progenitors for B-, NK, or dendritic cells as well as T-cell-committed progenitors.

Both $\gamma\delta$ and $\alpha\beta$ T-cells develop in the thymus. For $\alpha\beta$ T-cells, a number of control points regulating development have been defined. The thymic precursor population acquires various cell surface molecules, including CD4, CD8, and the TCR associated with the invariant CD3 polypeptides, during their intrinsic developmental program. This process is extrinsically influenced by the thymic microenvironment (reviewed by refs. *146–148*), which consists of thymic epithelial cells, macrophages, B-cells, and dendritic cells of bone marrow origin, and dendritic cells presumably from thymic precursor *(149)*. The thymic epithelial cells secrete a number of cytokines, including IL-1, IL-4, IFN-γ, TGF-α, Slf, and IL-7 *(150–154)*. The framework of the thymic microenvironment provides the appropriate cell to cell interactions in distinct thymic regions such as the cortical and medullary regions *(155,156)*. These interactions control the commitment, differentiation, and survival of developing thymocytes.

The expression of the TCR along with CD4 or CD8 is necessary for the thymocytes to interact with self-major histocompatibility complex (MHC) proteins and the eventual maturation into CD4 or CD8 T-cells. The cells that express the proper TCR combination undergo "positive selection" and can advance to the next stage. To get a TCR expressed, the germline locus that contains the β chain of the TCR is rearranged. TCRβ is expressed on the cell surface as a pre-TCRα/TCRβ complex *(157)*. At this stage, the TN cells are extensively proliferating, contributing to the expansion of thymic precursors. After a certain number of cell divisions, cells rearrange the TCRα chain forming TCRα/β complexes, and express CD4 and CD8 coreceptors.

The first thymocytes to express the TCRα/β chain are the $CD4^+CD8^+$ (double positive; DP) TCRα/β^{lo} cortical thymocytes. The fate of the DP TCRα/β^{lo} thymocytes is determined by positive and/or negative selection; cells that corecognize self MHC class II molecules with CD4 and TCR develop into or are educated to become $CD4^+CD8^-$ single positive (SP) cells *(158–161)*, and cells that corecognize self MHC class I with CD8 and TCR can become $CD4^-CD8^+$ SP cells *(162,163)*. The TCR^{lo} DP thymocytes can continuously rearrange and express alternative TCRα chains and form other TCRα/β chains to maximize the efficiency of selection *(164)*. However, the majority of TCR^{lo} DP thymocytes fail to express selectable TCRα/β, and are destined to die of neglect within 3–3.5 d *(166,167)*. Autoreactive cells are eliminated during this process by negative selection, although the sequential relationship between positive and negative selection is still controversial. Only 1–4% of DP thymocytes survive the stringent selection process, and downregulate either coreceptor in a complex manner *(168)*. This process requires a continuous engagement of TCR *(169)*. The molecular mechanism of these selections will be discussed elsewhere in this volume (*see* Chapters 23 and 24). The major issue discussed here is survival signals and cytokines that regulate the cells' fate during positive selection driven by TCR-MHC interaction.

4.1. Transition from $CD3^-CD4^-CD8^-$ TN Cells to $CD3^{lo}CD4^+CD8^+$ DP Cells

The molecules that initiate the recombination of VDJ for TCRβ or of VJ for TCRγ genes remain unclear *(170)*. This rearrangement requires the two tightly-regulated lymphoid-specific proteins RAG-1 and RAG-2, which specifically cleave DNA, which codes for TCR and immunoglobulin *(171,172)*. Mice that lack RAG-1 or RAG-2 genes have a complete block of early T- (and early B-) cell development *(173,174)*. The expression of transfected RAG-1 and RAG-2 in non-lymphoid tissue does not result in rearrangement of the genes *(175)*, indicating that commitment (for T-cell TCR recombination capacity) has already occurred in the thymic progenitors. IL-7 and/or thymic stromal cell-derived lymphopoietin (TSLP) whose receptor complexes use IL-7Rα *(176,177)* plays a critical role in processes leading to rearranging the TCRγ locus, since IL-7Rα-deficient mice completely lack T-cells that show the rearrangement of the TCRγ gene *(106)*. On the other hand, the TCRβ rearrangement can be seen in the IL-7Rα-deficient mice, although the number of mature TCRαβ T-cells are reduced. Cytokines that critically control the TCRβ rearrangement have not been reported, though the rearrangement of TCRβ locus may be supported by IL-1α, TNFα *(178)*, and IL-7 *(179)*.

The next step in thymic development is the expression of gp33, the pre-TCRα chain that forms a surrogate pre-TCRα/TCRβ complex with TCRβ chain *(157)*. Although the ligand(s) for this receptor complex has not been identified, the pre-TCR complex plays an important role for expansion of TN cells, since pre-TCRα knockout mice have a severe decrease in numbers of thymocyte and mature T-cells *(180)*. The tyrosine kinase *lck* may also play a role in the expression of functional TCRβ chain to form the pre-TCRα/TCRβ complex, since thymic maturation in *lck*-deficient mice is inhibited at this stage *(181)*. The TN cells also express high levels of Bcl-2, a survival protein *(182–184)*. The majority of these proliferating TN cells express various kinds of cytokine receptors, including IL-2Rα (CD25), IL-2Rγ (γc), IL-4Rα, IL-7Rα, and c-Kit *(185–187)*. A few cells in this population express the indispensable subunit of IL-2Rβ chain which is required for functional IL-2R and IL-15R *(187)*. Mice lacking either IL-2 *(188)*, IL-4 *(189)*, or both *(190)* have normal thymic development, although IL-4 can stimulate thymocyte expansion in vitro. On the other hand, both IL-7 and Slf are used for the expansion of the TN population. Genetic ablation of either IL-7, IL-7Rα, or γc gene results in the profound loss of thymocytes (*see* above), and the introduction of a γc deletion onto Sl/Sl mice induces a profound loss of thymic precursors *(192)*. IL-7 maintains survival of these TN cells, which proliferate in the presence of the pre-TCRα/TCRβ complex *(83)* at least by upregulating Bcl-2 *(83)*, and the Slf/c-Kit signals might induce cell mitosis.

These proliferating $CD25^+$ $c\text{-}Kit^+$ thymocytes gradually express both CD4 and CD8 coreceptors, and become DP cells. The proliferation and coreceptor expression of DP cells does not appear to depend on signals from the pre-TCRα/TCRβ complex, since administration of anti-CD3 antibody, or of a dose of γ-irradiation to RAG-1 or RAG-2-deficient mice *(193–195)* induces a rapid expansion of thymocytes and results in the development of DP cells. TN cells can easily become DP cells in suspension cultures in the absence of MHC-presenting thymic stromal cells. Accordingly, expression of CD4 and CD8 are intrinsically controlled, and not directly controlled by signals from the TCR genes.

4.2. Positive Selection at the DP Stage

The DP cell population is made up of different cell types that express CD4 and CD8 coreceptors at different levels, including cells prior to selection, cells undergoing positive selection, and cells that have failed selection. The TCR^{lo} DP subset are poised to receive selection depending upon the affinity or reactivity of their TCR coreceptor complex to self-MHC peptide complex. The signal from the TCRα/β complex is necessary for the DP cells to become SP cells (positive selection). Bcl-2-deficient (*bcl-2*$^{-/-}$) mice showed a gradual disappearance of T- (and B-) cells after the second postnatal week of life *(196,197)*. This suggests that Bcl-2 protects thymocytes undergoing positive selection *(198–200)*, as well as peripheral T-cells, from apoptotic stimuli, such as levels of endogenous glucocorticoid reached in the diurnal cycle *(148)* or stress. Bcl-x_L is expressed at the DP stage (but not in TN and SP cells) *(201)*, but its physiological role for the survival of DP cells is unclear.

The first stage of positive selection includes the upregulation of TCRs to medium-high levels *(148,202–205)*. A fraction of DP cells are $CD69^+$ and $TCR^{med\text{-}hi}$ *(167)*. This population can differentiate into SP cells with high efficiency, and has shown an increase in cells bearing certain Vβs that seem to be enriched by positive selection *(167,206)*. The positively selected DP cells upregulate Bcl-2 in TCR transgenic mice *(207)*, though most DP cells are largely negative for Bcl-2 in normal mice *(184)*. If positive selection does not occur, all developing thymocytes become DP cells, and die by apoptosis *(208)*.

Cells receiving positive selection are viable and are supported by signals from cytokine/cytokine receptor interactions. The small number of DP cells poised for selection or undergoing selection may express IL-7R, c-Kit, and Bcl-2. The authors recently found that the DP cells undergoing positive selection express c-Kit and/or IL-7R *(208a)*.

Figure 2 shows the distribution of c-Kit$^+$ and IL-7R$^+$ cells in MHC-deficient and normal mice. The c-Kit$^+$ thymocytes are continuously developing from DN → DP^{lo} → DP^{int} → transitional intermediates → SP cells, but DP^{hi} cells do not express c-Kit. The level of TCR on the surface increases during this development; TCR$^+$c-Kit$^+$ cells are DN to DP^{lo}; TCR^{lo}c-Kit$^+$ cells are DP^{int}, TCR$^{med\text{-}hi}$c-Kit$^+$ cells are CD4$^+$CD8^{lo} or CD4^{lo}CD8$^+$ transitional intermediates; and TCR^{hi}c-Kit$^-$ cells are SP cells (Fig. 3). The DP^{int}TCR^{lo}c-Kit$^+$ cells are negative for CD69, a T-cell activation marker, but the TCR$^{med\text{-}hi}$ transitional intermediates are CD69$^+$, and the majority of these c-Kit$^+$ populations express Bcl-2. Most TCR$^{lo\text{-}med}$c-Kit$^+$ cells are cycling, indicating that the positively selected cells proliferate. These c-Kit$^+$ cells express IL-7R, and an injection of either neutralizing anti-c-Kit or anti–IL-7Rα antibody can eliminate the c-Kit$^+$ population, suggesting that cells on this pathway depend on both Slf and IL-7. This pathway is tentatively called the c-Kit$^+$ pathway *(208a)*.

None of the thymocytes in MHC cl. I$^{-/-}$ cl. II$^{-/-}$ (MHC-DKO) mice can receive positive selection, therefore, they are destined to die by neglect. In these mice, more than 96% of thymocytes are DP^{hi} cells, there are not any TCR$^{lo\text{-}hi}$ c-Kit$^+$ cells, and thymocytes downregulate c-Kit at the DN to DP^{lo} stage (Fig. 2). This suggests that the DP^{int} TCR^{lo} c-Kit$^+$ cells are poised for positive selection and the TCR$^{med\text{-}hi}$ c-Kit$^+$ cells are products of positive selection.

The distribution of IL-7R$^+$ cells is considerably different from that of c-Kit$^+$ cells. Although the IL-7R$^+$ cells include the cells on the c-Kit$^+$ pathway, the IL-7R$^+$ thymocytes also include a minor population at the DP^{hi} stage. This small fraction of IL-7R$^+$c-Kit$^-$ DP^{hi} cells express medium levels of TCR and CD69 suggesting that DP cells immediately upregulate IL-7R after receiving positive selection. The IL-7R$^+$ cells are seen continuously from the DP^{hi} stage (transitional intermediates) → SP cells (the c-Kit$^-$ pathway). The DP^{hi} cells in MHC-DKO mice are negative for IL-7R, indicating that the DP^{hi}IL-7R$^+$c-Kit$^-$ cells in normal mice are receiving positive selection (Fig. 2). This fraction corresponds to the small positively-selected DP population that was previously reported *(167)*.

Indeed, the DP^{int} TCR^{lo} c-Kit$^+$ cells can differentiate into SP cells both in vivo on intrathymic injection and in vitro in a heterogenous thymic stroma culture *(209)*, whereas a small percentage of the DP^{hi} c-Kit$^-$ cells can also differentiate into SP cells in vivo. Both pathways generate similar numbers of SP cells *(198)*, although the c-Kit$^-$ pathway seems to contribute more to the generation of CD4 SP cells than CD8 SP cells *(83)*.

The difference in TCR/c-Kit profiles of thymocytes of normal mice and MHC-DKO mice reveals a sequence of events during positive selection on these two pathways. The MHC-DKO thymus completely lacks the TCR$^+$c-Kit$^+$ fraction, but TCR$^{lo\text{-}med}$c-Kit$^-$ cells (that are DP^{hi} cells) accumulate. These cells include a subset that should be absent in DP^{hi}c-Kit$^-$ cells from normal thymus cells bearing TCRα/β receptors that could respond to that strain's MHC alleles, if they could be expressed. Positive selection can occur from the DP^{hi} c-Kit$^-$ cells on the c-Kit$^-$ pathway, and DP^{hi}c-Kit$^-$ blast cells are more efficient in this process. This suggests that thymocytes might be first selected at the DP^{int} TCR^{lo} c-Kit$^+$ stage, and the cells that fail to receive positive selection to transitional intermediates become DP^{hi}c-Kit$^-$ cells, but a subset of DP^{hi}c-Kit$^-$ cells become available to be salvaged for positive selection. This second chance for positive selection may be a result of an alternative expression of TCRαβ receptor by continuous TCRα rearrangement, since the DP^{hi} cells in MHC-DKO mice express multiple TCRα chains in high frequencies *(208a)*.

Accordingly, two different, but successive positive selection pathways for thymic development exist; one begins from TCR^{lo}DP^{int}c-Kit$^+$IL-7Rα$^+$ cells (c-Kit$^+$ pathway) and the other from TCR^{lo}DP^{hi}c-Kit$^-$IL-7Rα$^-$ cells (c-Kit$^-$ pathway). On the c-Kit$^+$ path-

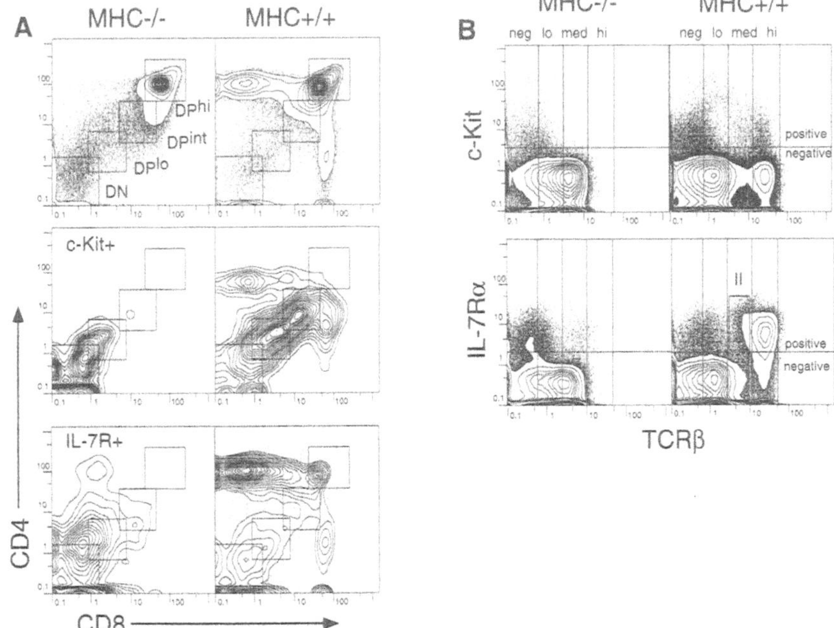

Fig. 2. Distribution of thymocytes that express c-Kit$^+$ or IL-7R$^+$ in normal and MHC-deficient mice. **(A)** The CD4/CD8 expression profiles of total thymocytes (upper panels), and c-Kit$^+$ thymocytes and IL-7R$^+$ thymocytes (middle panels). Squares indicate the DN, DP^{lo} DP^{int} and DP^{hi} stages as defined in this chapter. Note that the c-Kit$^+$ population does not include DP^{hi} cells, whereas the IL-7R$^+$ population includes a small DP^{hi} population. This population expresses medium levels of TCRβ and CD69 (data not shown). **(B)** The TCRβ/c-Kit, and TCRβ/IL-7R expression profiles of total thymocytes. Note that MHC-deficient mice completely lack the TCR^{hi} c-Kit population, part of the c-Kit$^+$ pathway.

way, the process of down regulation of CD4 and CD8 coreceptors is rather complex as discussed later (Fig. 4). The scheme showing relationships between these two pathways and their lineages is presented in Fig. 5.

4.3. The Role of Bcl-2 and IL-7 on Positive Selection

Bcl-2 does not by itself stimulate cell proliferation *(84,210,211)*. Bcl-2 does not substitute for signals generated during positive selection driven by TCR-MHC interactions, as illustrated by the fact that in *lck^{pr}-bcl-2* MHC$^{-/-}$ mice there are no SP cells *(199,207)*. T-cells are also not rescued by *bcl-2* transgenes in *lck^{pr}-bcl-2* RAG1$^{-/-}$ or *Eμ-bcl-2* SCID mice *(212)*.

Several studies have shown a potential link between IL-7 and Bcl-2 expression. The developing thymocytes in either IL-7R- or IL-7-deficient mice express only low levels of Bcl-2, and the ligation of IL-7R induces high levels of expression of Bcl-2 in splenic T-cells from IL-7-deficient mice *(83)*. Low level expression of Bcl-2 is also found in T-cells from γc-deficient mice *(213)*. This suggests that the signals from IL-7R maintain Bcl-2 levels in developing thymocytes.

Signals from the IL-7R play an important role in positive selection, since cells on either of the c-Kit pathways described above express IL-7R, and a neutralizing anti-IL–7Rα antibody inhibits the transition from DP to SP cells in vivo *(83,208a)*. This inhibition can be reversed by introducing transgenic Bcl-2 to the DP cells *(83)*. Introduction of an *Eμ-bcl-2*

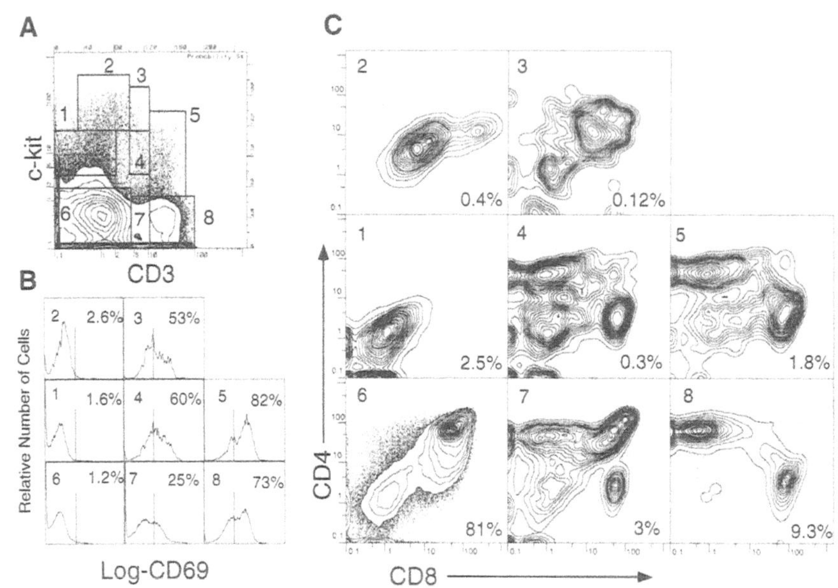

Fig. 3. CD4/CD8 and CD69 profiles of thymocytes defined by CD3 and c-Kit expression. **(A)** CD3/c-Kit profile of thymocytes. **(B)** CD69, and **(C)** CD4/CD8 profiles of each subset as gated in panel A. Note that thymic development from DN to SP cells is sequential and can be followed by tracking Areas 1 to 6, and CD69 expression that marks the engagement of TCR can be seen in Areas 3 to 6, indicating that positive selection begins at Area 2. If cells cannot receive positive selection at Area 2, cells progress to Area 7 down regulating c-Kit, and become DP cells. The sequence in this default pathway can be seen in the TCRβ/c-Kit profile in MHC-DKO mice in Fig. 2. Data from 300,000 cells were analyzed by flow cytometry and are presented as 5% probability plots. Each dot represents a single cell. Each box has a number which corresponds to the numbers in all panels.

transgene, which is selectively expressed in T-cells, into IL-7R$\alpha^{-/-}$ mice resulted in a significant restoration of T-cell numbers in the thymus and blood *(83)*. The introduction of a *H-2K-bcl-2* transgene into γc-deficient mice can induce a significant recovery of TN c-Kit$^+$ T-cell progenitors, as well as of thymocytes and mature T-cells *(85)*. This indicates that a principal role of IL-7 during thymic positive selection is to maintain cell survival.

Cell proliferation signals may depend on signals from c-Kit and the pre-TCRα complex. This trophic effect of IL-7 on T-cells is not only by induction of Bcl-2, but also involves other survival proteins. This is demonstrated by the fact that IL-7 can reinforce the survival of T-cells from Bcl-2-deficient mice *(196)*. However, the enforced expression of IL-7R on DP cells—this was accomplished by introducing both IL-7R and γc transgenes driven by the κ chain promoter and the IgH enhancer—does not affect the efficiency of positive selection, and the ligation of the transgenic IL-7R with IL-7 cannot induce Bcl-2 expression in the IL-7R-transgenic DP cells (C. Klug, K. Akashi, and I. L. Weissman, unpublished data). The positive selection signals induced by TCR engagement might be prerequisite for the activation of survival signals from IL-7R engagement.

4.4. Negative Selection

For the analysis of molecular events during negative selection, the purification of cells that are receiving negative selection is important, but difficult because the negatively

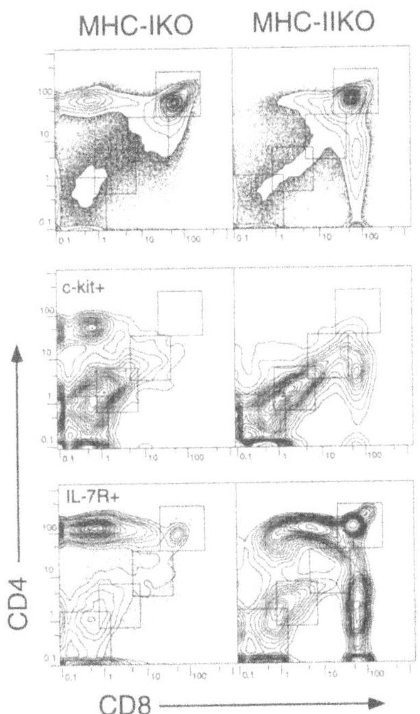

Fig. 4. Distribution of c-Kit$^+$ and IL-7R$^+$ cells in MHC-I- or II-deficient mice. Top panels show the CD4/CD8 profile of the whole thymocytes. The middle and bottom panels show the distribution of c-Kit$^+$ and IL-7R$^+$ cells in MHC-I deficient (MHC-IKO) or II-deficient (MHC-IIKO) mice. Note that c-Kit$^+$CD4^{lo}CD8$^+$ and CD4$^+$CD8^{lo} transition intermediates are not found in the MHC-IKO and MHC-IIKO thymus, respectively. On the other hand, the IL-7R$^+$CD4$^+$CD8^{lo} population can be seen in MHC-IIKO mice, indicating that a transient down regulation of CD8 is involved during positive selection for CD8 lineage from DP^{hi} c-Kit$^-$ cells on the c-Kit$^-$ pathway.

selected cells appear to be quickly removed from thymus *(165)*. The majority of apoptotic cells in the thymus are cells neglected by selection and are going to die by default. The sequence of events during positive and negative selection is controversial. Various models show that different signals evoked by affinity or avidity of TCR-MHC plus peptide interaction decide the cells' fate *(204,215)*.

The sequence of events that take place during negative selection has been studied using mouse strains that express superantigens *(216)* or antigen-specific TCR transgene. It appears that the negative selection of T-cells, which are reactive to superantigens, operates at the level of the TCR^{med} CD4$^+$8^{lo} or CD4^{lo}8$^+$ transitional intermediates, because a decrease in the number of T-cells bearing superantigens-specific Vβs begins at this stage *(203)*. In contrast, most TCR transgenic mice lack DP cells in the thymus when self-MHC plus peptide is present, implying that negative selection operates at or before the DP stage *(205,217)*. However, in most transgenic models, the TCR is expressed at medium to high levels during the CD4$^-$CD8$^-$ and DP stages, indicating that the "DP" stage in the TCR transgenic mice does not correspond to the TCR^{lo} DP stage in normal mice. The knock-in mice of the future might be useful to knock-in TCR genes and study this inconsistency.

In both the superantigen and TCR transgene models, enforced expression of Bcl-2 does not rescue the cells receiving negative selection *(218)*. This indicates that negative

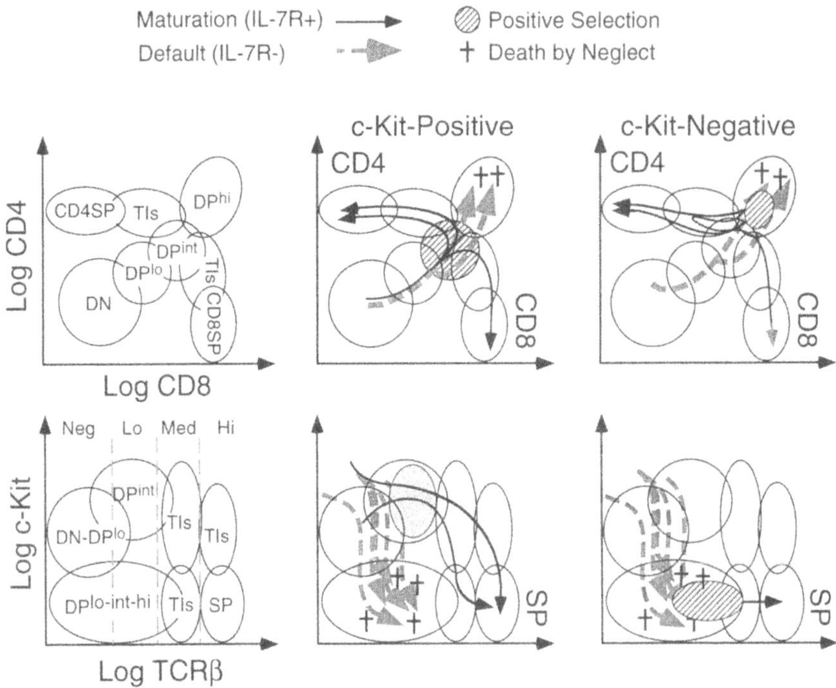

Fig. 5. Model of positive selection pathways for thymocytes. Positive selection first occurs at the $DP^{int}TCR^{lo}$ c-Kit^{+}IL-$7R^{+}$ stage on the c-Kit^{+} pathway. After positive selection, cells up regulate TCR, while maintaining IL-7R expression, and gradually losing c-Kit expression. The $DP^{int}TCR^{lo}$ c-Kit^{+}IL-$7R^{+}$ cells progress to TCR^{hi} c-Kit^{+}IL-$7R^{+}$ or TCR^{med} c-Kit^{-}IL-$7R^{+}$ transition intermediates (TIs), and become TCR^{hi} c-Kit^{-}IL-7R+ SP cells. During this transition, cells express selectable TCRs that are restricted to MHC class I and MHC class II and down regulate CD4 and CD8 coreceptor, respectively. Cells that have failed to receive positive selection at the $DP^{int}TCR^{lo}$ c-Kit^{+}IL-$7R^{+}$ stage immediately lose both c-Kit and IL-7R, and become the $DP^{int}TCR^{lo}$ c-Kit^{-}IL-$7R^{-}$ blasts. These cells continue to proliferate, up regulating both CD4 and CD8 coreceptors, and become the $DP^{hi}TCR^{lo}$ c-Kit^{-}IL-$7R^{-}$ blasts. The $DP^{hi}TCR^{lo}$ c-Kit^{-}IL-$7R^{-}$ blasts continue to express alternative TCRα/β complexes by alternative TCRα chain rearrangements and some of them can express selectable TCRα/β chain. By the second stage of positive selection, these "rescued" cells immediately up regulate IL-7R, but not c-Kit, and enter the TCR^{med} $CD4^{+}CD8^{lo}$-med c-Kit^{-} IL-$7R^{+}$ stage. At this stage, cells that express MHCII-restricted TCR continue to down regulate CD8, and become TCR^{hi} CD4 SP cells, whereas cells that express MHC I-restricted TCR begin to down regulate CD4, and become TCR^{hi} CD8 SP cells. The majority of $DP^{hi}TCR^{lo}$ c-Kit^{-}IL-$7R^{-}$ blasts that failed to receive positive selection cease cell division, become small $DP^{hi}TCR^{lo\text{-}med}$ c-Kit^{-}IL-$7R^{-}$ cells, and die by apoptosis.

selection need not result from a loss of viability during positive selection. It also indicates that the induction of apoptosis of DP cells by anti-CD3 antibody does not reflect the process of negative selection, because Bcl-2 could antagonize the anti-CD3 antibody-induced apoptosis. However, in the Mls-1^{a} positive bcl-2 transgenic AKR mice, there is an accumulation of TCR^{med} c-Kit^{+} cells that are DP^{int} to $CD4^{+}8^{lo}$ or $CD4^{lo}8^{+}$ transitional intermediates. In contrast, no TCR^{hi} SP cells express superantigen-specific Vβs. These cells lose IL-7R expression (unpublished data). The accumulation of superantigen-specific Vβ-positive cells might be because the *bcl-2* transgene prolongs the survival of these negatively selected cells at the TCR^{med} c-Kit^{+} stages, although cells cannot receive survival signals from IL-7R. The accumulation of negatively selected cells by the enforced expression of Bcl-2 suggests that the rapid downregulation of IL-7R by negative selection is critical: loss of IL-7R results in the decrease of endogenous Bcl-2 levels, and these events may lead the negatively selected cells to become sensitive to apoptosis in normal mice.

The molecular pathways that induce apoptosis in these negatively selected cells remain unclear. The transcription factor, Nur77 is an orphan member of the nuclear hormone receptor superfamily *(219)*, and is highly expressed during T-cell receptor–signaled apoptosis in vitro *(220,221)*. The transgenic introduction of a dominant-negative Nur77 mutant to mice perturbs T-cell development, and inhibits antigen-induced negative selection in TCR transgenic mice, suggesting the possible role of Nur77 in the downstream signaling events in antigen-induced negative selection *(222,223)*. Fas, a member of the TNF receptor family, has been shown to induce apoptosis in mature T-cells. The blockade of Fas-Fas ligand interactions inhibited apoptosis of Fas-expressing TCR^{med} DP cells in the cortex and the cortico-medullary junction, suggesting that Fas/Fas ligand interactions can modulate apoptosis of thymocytes during negative selection *(224)*. It is also possible that the *bcl-2*-protected negatively selected thymocytes are removed by a redundant programmed cell removal mechanism similar to the programmed removal of aging neutrophils by macrophages that occurs even if the neutrophils do not undergo apoptosis because of enforced Bcl-2 expression *(119)*. Further studies are required to elucidate the mechanisms of negative selection.

4.5. TCR Signaling

TCR-mediated signaling has been well-studied in mature T-cells. A number of important signal transduction molecules have been reported including tyrosine phosphorylation mediated by p56^{lck}, p59^{Fyn}T, Syk, and ZAP-70, dephosphorylation mediated by CD45, and activation of p21^{ras}. These molecules are discussed in Chapters 21 and 23.

Both Fyn, a member of the Src family, and ZAP70, a member of the Syk family, are associated with the TCR complex *(225,226)*. In either fyn-deficient mice *(227,228)* or fyn-dominant negative transgenic mice *(229)*, thymic T-cell development remains normal, although SP cells have impaired TCR-induced signaling. ZAP-70 plays a more important role in thymic development. Patients that fail to express ZAP-70 because of mutations in the structural gene *(230–232)* exhibit a loss of mature CD8 SP cells and a functional impairment of CD4 SP cells, although the number of CD4 SP cells are normal. These data indicate ZAP-70-mediated signals are necessary for CD8 maturation, but not for the generation of CD4 SP cells, suggesting that positive selection signals can be different between CD4 and CD8 SP cell maturation.

One possible approach for clarifying the difference between signals for CD4 and CD8 maturation is the identification of specified signal transduction molecules associated with either CD4 or CD8 coreceptors. The Src family tyrosine kinase lck has been shown to be associated with CD4 and CD8 coreceptors, but lck is associated with CD4 more than with CD8 *(233,234)*. However, although mice lacking *lck* showed a partial impairment in the development from DN to DP cells *(181,235)*, *lck* seems to be dispensable in positive selection for both CD4 SP and CD8 SP maturation *(235–237)*.

4.6. Coreceptor Downregulation

Positive selection of DP cells results in complete down regulation of a coreceptor to become SP cells. Recent studies showed that this process is not a simple shut-down of either coreceptor, but is rather complex *(168)*. The first evidence came from the analysis of MHC-I knockout and MHC-II knockout mice. In both mouse strains, both $TCR^{hi}CD4^{med}8^{+}$ and TCR^{hi} $CD4^{+}8^{med}$ transitional intermediate thymocytes are seen. These findings were interpreted to mean that the generation of these transitional intermediates was caused by stochastic downregulation of either coreceptor *(239–241)*, rather than "instructive" down regulation of one coreceptor (e.g., CD8) following recognition of the appropriate class of MHC (e.g., MHC class II) with both TCR and the other coreceptor (CD4). These cells express CD69, suggesting that these "coreceptor skewed" thymocytes could represent a transitional differentiation step from DP cells to mature SP cells *(239,240)*. A recent extensive analysis of these populations showed the presence of medium-sized TCR^{med} $CD4^{med}8^{med\text{-}hi}$ and TCR^{hi} $CD4^{med}8^{med\text{-}hi}$ thymocytes with MHC-I restricted TCR undergoing positive selection to the CD8 lineage *(242)*.

Lucas et al. *(168,243)* showed that $TCR^{int}CD4^{med}8^{+}$ thymocytes do not necessarily belong to the CD8 lineage pathway, but may include a MHC class II-restricted dead end subset. This contrasts with the authors' findings that TCR^{int} $CD4^{med}8^{+}$ $ckit^{+}$ cells are largely committed to CD8 SP maturation *(198)*. Lucas et al. suggests that commitment to the CD8 lineage may be instructive *(168)*. On the other hand, TCR^{med} $CD4^{+}8^{med}$ cells *(244)* or TCR^{med} $CD4^{med\text{-}hi}8^{med}$ cells *(245)* in normal and MHC II knockout mice have been reported to possess the capability of differentiation into CD8 SP cells as well as CD4 SP cells. These authors postulate that CD4 lineage commitment occurs regularly, whereas the CD8 lineage commitment requires an instructive signal by MHC class I-TCR interaction. Figure 4 shows the distribution of IL-$7R^{+}$ thymocytes in MHC-I knockout and MHC-II knockout mice. As described above, positively selected thymocytes immediately express IL-7R. The IL-$7R^{+}$ coreceptor skewed cells were only seen in $CD4^{+}CD8^{lo\text{-}med}$ transitional intermediates in MHC-II knockout mice, and IL-$7R^{+}$ $CD4^{lo}CD8^{+}$ transitional intermediates were not seen in MHC-I knockout mice. It is important to recognize that events that occur in gene-altered mice may reveal adaptive developmental potentials and lineage skewings that do not occur at significant levels in normal mice. Recently, Itano et al. proposed a new "instructive/selective" model in which the stronger signal favors CD4, but the weaker signal favors the CD8 lineage commitment, and a following "confirmatory" step ensures the survival of these committed T-cells with the appropriate TCR *(246)*. It is fair to say that we do not have the final answers for the stochastic versus instructive models of T-cell (and B-cell) selection. Unfortunately, we are still at the stage that we are forced to study T-cell maturation in model systems that are departures from physiological T-cell maturation in normal vertebrates. By attempting to throw light on the subject by using powerful but unphysiologic models, we are doomed to interpret the different kinds of shadows that are cast when light falls on our created objects[1].

5. Summary

Studying the development of hematopoietic stem cells and intermediate progenitors is essentially an attempt to understand the processes that lead to the development of clonogenic progenitors of increasingly narrower commitments; and to map the lineages (and stages within the lineages) when these clonogenic progenitors read out their developmental programs that are intrinsic and those that are affected by microenvironmental cells. That means we must isolate to homogeneity each progenitor and each stage of proposed lineal progression, and study the full developmental outcome when these cells are placed in physiological microenvironments. Here the authors have tried to report (from their view) the stem cells, progenitors, and lineages of cells as HSC eventually give rise to mature T-cells.

[1]Plato, from the *Allegory of the Caves*.

References

1. Morrison, S. J. and Weissman, I. L. (1994) The long-term repopulating subset of hematopoietic stem cells is deterministic and isolatable by phenotype. *Immunity* **1,** 661–673.
2. Osawa, M., Hanada, K., Hamada, H., and Nakauchi, H. (1996) Long-term lymphohematopoietic reconstitution by a single CD34- low/negative hematopoietic stem cell. *Science* **273,** 242–245.
3. Spangrude, G. J., Heimfeld, S., and Weissman, I. L. (1988) Purification and characterization of mouse hematopoietic stem cells. *Science* 241, 58–62.
4. Spangrude, G. J. and Scollay, R. (1990) Differentiation of hematopoietic cells in irradiated mouse thymic lobes. *J. Immunol.* **145,** 3661–3668.
5. Visser, J. W. M., Gauman, J. G. J., Mulder, A. H., Eliason, J. F., and de Leeuw, A. W. (1984) Isolation of murine pluripotent hemopoietic stem cells. *J. Exp. Med.* **59,** 1576–1590.
6. Andrews, R. G., Singer, J. W., and Bernstein, I. D. (1986) Monoclonal antibody 12-8 recognizes a 115-kd molecule present on both unipotent and multipotent hematopoietic colony-forming cells and their precursors. *Blood* **67,** 842–845.
7. Baum, C. M., Weissman, I. L., Tsukamoto, A. S., Buckle, A. M., and Peault, B. (1992) Isolation of a candidate human hematopoietic stem-cell population. *Proc. Natl. Acad. Sci USA* **89,** 2804–2808.
8. DiGiusto, D., Chen, S., Combs, J., Webb, S., Namikawa, R., Tsukamoto, A., Chen, B. P., and Galy, A. H. (1994) Human fetal bone marrow early progenitors for T, B, and myeloid cells are found exclusively in the population expressing high levels of CD34. *Blood* **84,** 421–432.
9. Strauss, L. C., Rowley, S. D., La Russa, V. F., Sharkis, S. J., Stuart, R. K., and Civin, C. I. (1986) Antigenic analysis of hematopoiesis. V. Characterization of My-10 antigen expression by normal lymphohematopoietic progenitor cells. *Exp. Hematol.* **14,** 878–886.
10. Siminovitch, L., McCulloch, E., and Till, J. 1963. The distribution of colony-forming cells among spleen colonies. *J. Cell Comp. Physiol.* **62,** 327–336.
11. Ogawa, M. (1993) Differentiation and proliferation of hematopietic stem cells. *Blood* **81,** 2844–2853.
12. Thomas, E. D. (1991) Frontiers in bone marrow transplantation. *Blood Cells* **17,** 259–267.
13. Till, J. and McCulloch, E. (1961) A direct measurement of the radiation sensitivity of normal mouse bone marrow cells. *Radiat. Res.* **14,** 1419–1430.
14. Wu, A., Till, J., Siminovitch, L., and McCulloch, E. (1968) Cytological evidence for a relationship between normal hematopoietic colony-forming cells and cells of the lymphoid system. *J. Exp. Med.* **127,** 455–467.
15. Till, J. and McCulloch, E. (1963) A stochastic model of stem cell proliferation, based on the growth of spleen colony-forming cells. *Proc. Natl. Acad. Sci. USA* **51,** 29–36.
16. Metcalf, D. and Moore, M. A. S. (1971) *Hematopoietic Cells.* New York, Elsevier.
17. Helman, S., Botnick, L. E., Hannon, E. C., and Vigneulle, R. M. (1978) Proliferative capacity of murine hematopoietic stem cells. *Proc. Natl. Acad. Sci. USA.* **75,** 490–494.
18. Micklem, H., and Ogden, D. (1976) Ageing of haematopoietic stem cell populations in the mouse, in *Stem Cells of Renewing Cell Populations* (Cairnie, A., Lala, P., and Osmond, D., eds.). Academic, New York, pp. 331–341.
19. Ikuta, K., Uchida, N., Friedman, J., and Weissman, I. L. (1992) Lymphocyte development from stem cells. *Annu. Rev. Immunol.* **10,** 759–783.
20. Morrison, S. J., Uchida, N., and Weissman, I. L. (1995) The biology of hematopoietic stem cells. *Ann. Rev. Cell Dev. Biol.* **11,** 35–71.
21. Smith, L. G., Weissman, I. L., and Heimfeld, S. (1991) Clonal analysis of hematopoietic stem-cell differentiation in vivo. *Proc. Natl. Acad. Sci USA* **88,** 2788–2792.
22. Morrison, S. J., Wandycz, A. M., Hemmati, H. D., Wright, D. E., and Weissman, I. L. (1997) Identification of a lineage of multipotent hematopoietic progenitors. *Development* **124,** 1929–1939.
23. Bertoncello, I., Hodgson, G. S., and Bradley, T. R. (1985) Multiparameter analysis of transplantable hemopoietic stem cells: I. The separation and enrichment of stem cells homing to marrow and spleen on the basis of rhodamine-123 fluorescence. *Exp. Hematol.* **13,** 999–1006.

24. Mulder, A. H. and Visser, J. W. M. (1987) Separation and functional analysis of bone marrow cells separated by Rhodamine-123 fluorescence. *Exp. Hematol.* **15,** 99–104.
25. Ploemacher, R. E. and Brons, R. H. C. (1989) Separation of CFU-S from primitive cells responsible for reconstitution of the bone marrow hemopoietic stem cell compartment following irradiation: Evidence for a pre-CFU-S cells. *Exp. Hematol.* **17,** 263–266.
26. Lundblad, V. and Wright, W. E. (1996) Telomeres and telomerase: a simple picture becomes complex. *Cell* **87,** 369–375.
27. Morrison, S. J., Prowse, K. R., Ho, P., and Weissman, I. L. (1996) Telomerase activity in hematopoietic cells is associated with self- renewal potential. *Immunity* **5,** 207–216.
28. Williams, D. E., de Vries, P., Namen, A. E., Widmer, M. B., and Lyman, S. D. (1992) The steel factor. *Dev. Biol.* **151,** 368–376.
29. Ogawa, M., Matsuzaki, Y., Nishikawa, S., Hayashi, S., Kunisada, T., Sudo, T., Kina, T., Nakauchi, H., and Nishikawa, S. (1991) Expression and function of c-kit in hemopoietic progenitor cells. *J. Exp. Med.* **174,** 63–71.
30. Ikuta, K. and Weissman, I. L. (1992) Evidence that hematopoietic stem cells express mouse c-kit but do not depend on steel factor for their generation. *Proc. Natl. Acad. Sci USA* **89,** 1502–1506.
31. Wineman, J. P., Nishikawa, S., and Muller-Sieburg, C. E. (1993) Maintenance of high levels of pluripotent hematopoietic stem cells in vitro: effect of stromal cells and c-kit. *Blood* **81,** 365–372.
32. Matthews, W., Jordan, C. T., Wiegand, G. W., Pardoll, D., and Lemischka, I. R. (1991) A receptor tyrosine kinase specific to hematopoietic stem and progenitor cell-enriched populations. *Cell* **65,** 1143–1152.
33. Rosnet, O., Marchetto, S., de Lapeyriere, O., and Birnbaum, D. (1991) Murine Flt3, a gene encoding a novel tyrosine kinase receptor of the PDGFR/CSF1R family. *Oncogene* **6,** 1641–1650.
34. Hannum, C., Culpepper, J., Campbell, D., McClanahan, T., Zurawski, S., Bazan, J. F., Kastelein, R., Hudak, S., Wagner, J., Mattson, J., et al. (1994) Ligand for FLT3/FLK2 receptor tyrosine kinase regulates growth of haematopoietic stem cells and is encoded by variant RNAs. *Nature* **368,** 643–648.
35. Lyman, S. D., James, L., Vanden Bos, T., de Vries, P., Brasel, K., Gliniak, B., Hollingsworth, L. T., Picha, K. S., McKenna, H. J., Splett, R. R., et al. (1993) Molecular cloning of a ligand for the flt3/flk-2 tyrosine kinase receptor: a proliferative factor for primitive hematopoietic cells. *Cell* **75,** 1157–1167.
36. Shalaby, F., Ho, J., Stanford, W. L., Fischer, K. D., Schuh, A. C., Schwartz, L., Bernstein, A., and Rossant, J. (1997) A requirement for Flk1 in primitive and definitive hematopoiesis and vasculogenesis. *Cell* **89,** 981–990.
37. Mackarehtschian, K., Hardin, J. D., Moore, K. A., Boast, S., Goff, S. P., and Lemischka, I. R. (1995) Targeted disruption of the flk2/flt3 gene leads to deficiencies in primitive hematopoietic progenitors. *Immunity* **3,** 147–161.
38. Varmus, H., Padgett, T., Heasley, S., Simon, G., and Bishop, J. 1977. Cellular functions are required for the synthesis and integrantion of avian sarcoma virus-specific DNA. *Cell* **11,** 307–319.
39. Morrison, S. J., Wandycz, A. M., Akashi, K., Globerson, A., and Weissman, I. L. (1996) The aging of hematopoietic stem cells. *Nat. Med.* **2,** 1011–1016.
40. Miyajima, A., Kitamura, T., Harada, N., Yokota, T., and Arai, K. (1992) Cytokine receptors and signal transduction. *Annu. Rev. Immunol.* **10,** 295–331.
41. McKinstry, W. J., Li, C. L., Rasko, J. E., Nicola, N. A., Johnson, G. R., and Metcalf, D. (1997) Cytokine receptor expression on hematopoietic stem and progenitor cells. *Blood* **89,** 65–71.
42. Nakayama, K., Nakayama, K., Negishi, I., Kuida, K., Sawa, H., and Loh, D. Y. (1994) Targeted disruption of Bcl-2 alpha beta in mice, occurrence of gray hair, polycystic kidney disease, and lymphocytopenia. *Proc. Natl. Acad. Sci USA* **91,** 3700–3704.
43. Veis, D. J., Sorenson, C. M., Shutter, J. R., and Korsmeyer, S. J. (1993) Bcl-2-deficient mice demonstrate fulminant lymphoid apoptosis, polycystic kidneys, and hypopigmented hair. *Cell* **75,** 229–240.
44. Matsuzaki, Y., Nakayama, K., Nakayama, K., Tomita, T., Isoda, M., Loh, D. Y., and Nakauchi, H. (1997) Role of bcl-2 in the development of lymphoid cells from the hematopoietic stem cell. *Blood* **89,** 853–862.
45. Motoyama, N., Wang, F., Roth, K. A., Sawa, H., Nakayama, K., Nakayama, K., Negishi, I., Senju, S., Zhang, Q., Fujii, S., et al. (1995) Massive cell death of immature hematopoietic cells and neurons in Bcl-x- deficient mice. *Science* **267,** 1506–1510.

46. Craig, W., Kay, R., Cutler, R. L., and Lansdorp, P. M. (1993) Expression of Thy-1 on human hematopoietic progenitor cells. *J. Exp. Med.* **177,** 1331–42.
47. Uchida, N., Combs, J., Chen, S., Zanjani, E., Hoffman, R., and Tsukamoto, A. (1996) Primitive human hematopoietic cells displaying differential efflux of the rhodamine 123 dye have distinct biological activities. *Blood* **88,** 1297–1305.
48. Udomsakdi, C., Eaves, C. J., Sutherland, H. J., and Lansdorp, P. M. (1991) Separation of functionally distinct subpopulations of primitive human hematopoietic cells using rhodamine-123. *Exp. Hematol.* **19,** 338–342.
49. Namikawa, R., Kaneshima, H., Lieberman, M., Weissman, I. L., and McCune, J. M. (1988) Infection of the SCID-hu mouse by HIV-1. *Science* **242,** 1684–1686.
50. McCune, J. M., Namikawa, R., Kaneshima, H., Shultz, L. D., Lieberman, M., and Weissman, I. L. (1988) The SCID-hu mouse: murine model for the analysis of human hematolymphoid differentiation and function. *Science* **241,** 1632–1639.
51. Kraft, D. L., Weissman, I. L., and Waller, E. K. (1993) Differentiation of CD3-4-8- human fetal thymocytes in vivo: characterization of a CD3-4+8- intermediate. *J. Exp. Med.* **178,** 265–277.
52. Lapidot, T., Pflumio, F., Doedens, M., Murdoch, B., Williams, D. E., and Dick, J. E. (1992) Cytokine stimulation of multilineage hematopoiesis from immature human cells engrafted in SCID mice. *Science* **255,** 1137–1141.
53. Berenson, R. J., Bensinger, W. I., Hill, R. S., Andrews, R. G., Garcia-Lopez, J., Kalamasz, D. F., Still, B. J., Spitzer, G., Buckner, C. D., Bernstein, I. D., et al. (1991) Engraftment after infusion of CD34+ marrow cells in patients with breast cancer or neuroblastoma. *Blood* **77,** 1717–1722.
54. Marin, G. H., Dal Cortivo, L., Cayuela, J. M., Marolleau, J. P., Pautier, P., Cojean-Zelek, I., Brice, P., Makke, J., Benbunan, M., and Gisselbrecht, C. (1997) Peripheral blood stem cell CD34+ autologous transplant in relapsed follicular lymphoma. *Hematol. Cell Ther.* **39,** 33–40.
55. Archimbaud, E., Philip, I., Coiffier, B., Michallet, M., Salles, G., Sebban, C., Roubi, N., Lopez, F., Bessueille, L., Mazars, P., Juttner, C., Atkinson, K., and Philip, T. (1996) $CD34^{+}Thy1^{+}Lin^{-}$ peripheral blood stem cells (PBSC) transplantation after high dose therapy for patients with multiple myeloma. *Blood* **88,** 595a.
56. Dexter, T. M. and Spooncer, E. (1987) Growth and differentiation in the hemopoietic system. *Annu. Rev. Cell. Biol.* **3,** 423–441.
57. Weissman, I. L. (1994) Stem cells, clonal progenitors, and commitment to the three lymphocyte lineages: T, B, and NK cells. *Immunity* **1,** 529–531.
58. Wu, L., Antica, M., Johnson, G. R., Scollay, R., and Shortman, K. (1991) Developmental potential of the earliest precursor cells from the adult mouse thymus. *J. Exp. Med.* **174,** 1617–1627.
59. Matsuzaki, Y., Gyotoku, J., Ogawa, M., Nishikawa, S., Katsura, Y., Gachelin, G., and Nakauchi, H. (1993) Characterization of c-kit positive intrathymic stem cells that are restricted to lymphoid differentiation. *J. Exp. Med.* **178,** 1283–1292.
60. Aihara, Y., Buhring, H. -J., Aihara, M., and Klein, J. (1986) An attempt to produce "pre–T" cell hybridomas and to identify their antigens. *Eur. J. Immunol.* **16,** 1391–1399.
61. Antica, M., Wu, L., Shortman, K., and Scollay, R. (1994) Thymic stem cells in mouse bone marrow. *Blood* **84,** 111–117.
61a. Kondo, M., Weissman, I. L., and Akashi, K. (1997) Identification of clonogenic common lymphoid progenitors in mouse bone marrow. *Cell* **91,** 661–672.
62. Hakoda, M., Hirai, Y., Shimba, H., Kusunoki, Y., Kyoizumi, S., Kodama, Y., and Akiyama, M. (1989) Cloning of phenotypically different human lymphocytes originating from a single stem cell. *J. Exp. Med.* **169,** 1265–1276.
63. Sanchez, M. J., Muench, M. O., Roncarolo, M. G., Lanier, L. L., and Phillips, J. H. (1994) Identification of a common T/natural killer cell progenitor in human fetal thymus. *J. Exp. Med.* **180,** 569–576.
64. Gore, S. D., Kastan, M. B., and Civin, C. I. (1991) Normal human bone marrow precursors that express terminal deoxynucleotidyl transferase include T-cell precursors and possible lymphoid stem cells. *Blood* **77,** 1681–1690.
65. LeBien, T. W. and McCormack, R. T. (1989) The common acute lymphoblastic leukemia antigen (CD10)—emancipation from a functional enigma. *Blood* **73,** 625–635.
66. Galy, A., Travis, M., Cen, D., and Chen, B. (1995) Human T, B, natural killer, and dendritic cells arise from a common bone marrow progenitor cell subset. *Immunity* **3,** 459–473.
67. Klinken, S. P., Alexander, W. S., and Adams, J. M. (1988) Hemopoietic lineage switch: v-raf oncogene converts Eμ-myc transgenic B cells into macrophages. *Cell* **53,** 857–867.

68. Cumano, A., Paige, C. J., Iscove, N. N., and Brady, G. (1992) Bipotential precursors of B cells and macrophages in murine fetal liver. *Nature* **356,** 612–615.
69. Hirayama, F., Shih, J. P., Awgulewitsch, A., Warr, G. W., Clark, S. C., and Ogawa, M. (1992) Clonal proliferation of murine lymphohemopoietic progenitors in culture. *Proc. Natl. Acad. Sci USA* **89,** 5907–5911.
70. Gale, R. P. and Ben Bassat, I. (1987) Hybrid acute leukaemia. Br J Haematol. **65,** 261–264.
71. Barlogie, B., Epstein, J., Selvanayagam, P., and Alexanian, R. (1989) Plasma cell myeloma: new biological insights and advances in therapy. *Blood* **73,** 865–879.
72. Akashi, K., Harada, M., Shibuya, T., Fukagawa, K., Kimura, N., Sagawa, K., Yoshikai, Y., Teshima, T., Kikuchi, M., and Niho, Y. (1991) Simultaneous occurrence of myelomonocytic leukemia and multiple myeloma: involvement of common leukemic progenitors and their developmental abnormality of "lineage infidelity." *J. Cell Physiol.* **148,** 446–456.
73. Akashi, K., Taniguchi, S., Nagafuji, K., Harada, M., Shibuya, T., Hayashi, S., Gondo, H., and Niho, Y. (1993) B-lymphoid/myeloid stem cell origin in Ph-positive acute leukemia with myeloid markers. *Leuk. Res.* **17,** 549–555.
74. Akashi, K., Shibuya, T., Harada, M., Morioka, E., Oshima, K., Kimura, N., Takeshita, M., Kurokawa, M., Kikuchi, M., and Niho, Y. (1990) Acute 'bilineal-biphenotypic' leukaemia. *Br. J. Haematol.* **74,** 402–407.
75. Hershfield, M. S., Kurtzberg, J., Harden, E., Moore, J. O., Whang-Peng, J., and Haynes, B. F. (1984) Conversion of a stem cell leukemia from a T-lymphoid to a myeloid phenotype induced by the adenosine deaminase inhibitor 2'- deoxycoformycin. *Proc. Natl. Acad. Sci USA.* **81,** 253–257.
76. Murphy, S. B., Stass, S., Kalwinsky, D., and Rivera, G. (1983) Phenotypic conversion of acute leukaemia from T-lymphoblastic to myeloblastic induced by therapy with 2'-deoxycoformycin. *Br. J. Haematol.* **55,** 285–293.
77. Griesinger, F., Arthur, D. C., Brunning, R., Parkin, J. L., Ochoa, A. C., Miller, W. J., Wilkowski, C. W., Greenberg, J. M., Hurvitz, C., and Kersey, J. H. (1989) Mature T-lineage leukemia with growth factor-induced multilineage differentiation. *J. Exp. Med.* **169,** 1101–1120.
78. Kurtzberg, J., Waldmann, T. A., Davey, M. P., Bigner, S. H., Moore, J. O., Hershfield, M. S., and Haynes, B. F. (1989) CD7+, CD4-, CD8- acute leukemia, a syndrome of malignant pluripotent lymphohematopoietic cells. *Blood* **73,** 381–390.
79. Greaves, M. F., Chan, L. C., Furley, A. J., Watt, S. M., and Molgaard, H. V. (1986) Lineage promiscuity in hemopoietic differentiation and leukemia. *Blood* **67,** 1–11.
80. McCulloch, E. A. (1987) Lineage infidelity or lineage promiscuity? *Leukemia* **1,** 235.
81. Ihle, J. N., Witthuhn, B. A., Quelle, F. W., Yamamoto, K., and Silvennoinen, O. (1995) Signaling through the hematopoietic cytokine receptors. *Annu. Rev. Immunol.* **13,** 369–398.
82. Watowich, S. S., Wu, H., Socolovsky, M., Klingmuller, U., Constantinescu, S. N., and Lodish, H. F. (1996) Cytokine receptor signal transduction and the control of hematopoietic cell development. *Ann. Rev. Cell Dev. Biol.* **12,** 91–128.
83. Akashi, K., Kondo, M., von Freeden-Jeffry, U., Murray, R., and Weissman, I. L. (1997) Bcl-2 rescues T lymphopoiesis in interleukin 7 receptor-deficient mice. *Cell* **89,** 1033–1041.
84. Fairbairn, L. J., Cowling, G. J., Reipert, B. M., and Dexter, T. M. (1993) Suppression of apoptosis allows differentiation and development of a multipotent hemopoietic cell line in the absence of added growth factors. *Cell* **74,** 823–832.
85. Kondo, M., Akashi, K., Domen, J., Sugamura, K., and Weissman, I. L. (1997) Bcl-2 rescues T lymphopoiesis, but not B or NK cell development in the common cytokine receptor g chain deficient mice. *Immunity* **17,** 2026–2030.
86. Lagasse, E. and Weissman, I. L. (1997) Enforced expression of Bcl-2 in monocytes rescues macrophages and partially reverses osteopetrosis in op/op mice. *Cell* **89,** 1–20.
87. Wu, H., Liu, X., Jaenisch, R., and Lodish, H. F. (1995) Generation of committed erythroid BFU-E and CFU-E progenitors does not require erythropoietin or the erythropoietin receptor. *Cell* **83,** 59–67.
88. Giri, J. G., Ahdieh, M., Eisenman, J., Shanebeck, K., Grabstein, K., Kumaki, S., Namen, A., Park, L. S., Cosman, D., and Anderson, D. (1994) Utilization of the beta and gamma chains of the IL-2 receptor by the novel cytokine IL-15. *EMBO J.* **13,** 2822–2830.
89. Kimura, Y., Takeshita, T., Kondo, M., Ishii, N., Nakamura, M., Van Snick, J., and Sugamura, K. (1995) Sharing of the IL-2 receptor gamma chain with the functional IL-9 receptor complex. *Int. Immunol.* **7,** 115–120.

90. Kondo, M., Takeshita, T., Higuchi, M., Nakamura, M., Sudo, T., Nishikawa, S., and Sugamura, K. (1994) Functional participation of the IL-2 receptor gamma chain in IL-7 receptor complexes. *Science* **263,** 1453–1454.
91. Kondo, M., Takeshita, T., Ishii, N., Nakamura, M., Watanabe, S., Arai, K., and Sugamura, K. (1993) Sharing of the interleukin-2 (IL-2) receptor gamma chain between receptors for IL-2 and IL-4. *Science* **262,** 1874–1877.
92. Noguchi, M., Nakamura, Y., Russell, S. M., Ziegler, S. F., Tsang, M., Cao, X., and Leonard, W. J. (1993) Interleukin-2 receptor gamma chain, a functional component of the interleukin-7 receptor. *Science* **262,** 1877–1880.
93. Russell, S. M., Keegan, A. D., Harada, N., Nakamura, Y., Noguchi, M., Leland, P., Friedmann, M. C., Miyajima, A., Puri, R. K., Paul, W. E., et al. (1993) Interleukin-2 receptor gamma chain: a functional component of the interleukin-4 receptor. *Science* **262,** 1880–1883.
94. Takeshita, T., Asao, H., Ohtani, K., Ishii, N., Kumaki, S., Tanaka, N., Munakata, H., Nakamura, M., and Sugamura, K. (1992) Cloning of the gamma chain of the human IL-2 receptor. *Science* **257,** 379–382.
95. Noguchi, M., Yi, H., Rosenblatt, H. M., Filipovich, A. H., Adelstein, S., Modi, W. S., McBride, O. W., and Leonard, W. J. (1993) Interleukin-2 receptor gamma chain mutation results in X-linked severe combined immunodeficiency in humans. *Cell* **73,** 147–157.
96. Puck, J. M., Deschenes, S. M., Porter, J. C., Dutra, A. S., Brown, C. J., Willard, H. F., and Henthorn, P. S. (1993) The interleukin-2 receptor gamma chain maps to Xq13.1 and is mutated in X-linked severe combined immunodeficiency, SCIDX1. *Hum. Mol. Genet.* **2,** 1099–1104.
97. Asao, H., Tanaka, N., Ishii, N., Higuchi, M., Takeshita, T., Nakamura, M., Shirasawa, T., and Sugamura, K. (1994) Interleukin 2-induced activation of JAK3, possible involvement in signal transduction for c-myc induction and cell proliferation. *FEBS Lett.* **351,** 201–206.
98. Miyazaki, T., Kawahara, A., Fujii, H., Nakagawa, Y., Minami, Y., Liu, Z. J., Oishi, I., Silvennoinen, O., Witthuhn, B. A., Ihle, J. N., et al. (1994) Functional activation of Jak1 and Jak3 by selective association with IL- 2 receptor subunits. *Science* **266,** 1045–1047.
99. Russell, S. M., Johnston, J. A., Noguchi, M., Kawamura, M., Bacon, C. M., Friedmann, M., Berg, M., McVicar, D. W., Witthuhn, B. A., Silvennoinen, O., et al. (1994) Interaction of IL-2R beta and gamma c chains with Jak1 and Jak3: implications for XSCID and XCID. *Science* **266,** 1042–1045.
100. Macchi, P., Villa, A., Gillani, S., Sacco, M. G., Frattini, A., Porta, F., Ugazio, A. G., Johnston, J. A., Candotti, F., O'Shea, J. J., et al. (1995) Mutations of Jak-3 gene in patients with autosomal severe combined immune deficiency (SCID). *Nature* **377,** 65–68.
101. Russell, S. M., Tayebi, N., Nakajima, H., Riedy, M. C., Roberts, J. L., Aman, M. J., Migone, T. S., Noguchi, M., Markert, M. L., Buckley, R. H., et al. (1995) Mutation of Jak3 in a patient with SCID: essential role of Jak3 in lymphoid development. *Science* **270,** 797–800.
102. Cao, X., Shores, E. W., Hu-Li, J., Anver, M. R., Kelsall, B. L., Russell, S. M., Drago, J., Noguchi, M., Grinberg, A., Bloom, E. T., et al. (1995) Defective lymphoid development in mice lacking expression of the common cytokine receptor gamma chain. *Immunity* **2,** 223-238.
103. DiSanto, J. P., Rieux-Laucat, F., Dautry-Varsat, A., Fischer, A., and de Saint Basile, G. (1994) Defective human interleukin 2 receptor gamma chain in an atypical X chromosome-linked severe combined immunodeficiency with peripheral T cells. *Proc. Natl. Acad. Sci USA* **91,** 9466–9470.
104. Ohbo, K., Suda, T., Hashiyama, M., Mantani, A., Ikebe, M., Miyakawa, K., Moriyama, M., Nakamura, M., Katsuki, M., Takahashi, K., Yamamura, K., and Sugamura, K. (1996) Modulation of hematopoiesis in mice with a truncated mutant of the interleukin-2 receptor gamma chain. *Blood* **87,** 956–967.
105. He, Y. W. and Malek, T. R. (1996) Interleukin-7 receptor alpha is essential for the development of gamma delta + T cells, but not natural killer cells. *J. Exp. Med.* **184,** 289–293.
106. Maki, K., Sunaga, S., and Ikuta, K. (1996) The V-J recombination of T cell receptor-gamma genes is blocked in interleukin-7 receptor-deficient mice. *J. Exp. Med.* **184,** 2423–2427.
107. Peschon, J. J., Morrissey, P. J., Grabstein, K. H., Ramsdell, F. J., Maraskovsky, E., Gliniak, B. C., Park, L. S., Ziegler, S. F., Williams, D. E., Ware, C. B., et al. (1994) Early lymphocyte expansion is severely impaired in interleukin 7 receptor-deficient mice. *J. Exp. Med.* **180,** 1955–1960.
108. von Freeden-Jeffry, U., Vieira, P., Lucian, L. A., McNeil, T., Burdach, S. E., and Murray, R. (1995) Lymphopenia in interleukin (IL)-7 gene-deleted mice identifies IL-7 as a nonredundant cytokine. *J. Exp. Med.* **181,** 1519–1526.

109. Suzuki, H., Duncan, G. S., Takimoto, H., and Mak, T. W. (1997) Abnormal development of intestinal intraepithelial lymphocytes and peripheral natural killer cells in mice lacking the IL-2 receptor beta chain. *J. Exp. Med.* **185,** 499–505.
110. Kundig, T. M., Schorle, H., Bachmann, M. F., Hengartner, H., Zinkernagel, R. M., and Horak, I. (1993) Immune responses in interleukin-2-deficient mice. *Science* **262,** 1059–1061.
111. Nosaka, T., van Deursen, J. M., Tripp, R. A., Thierfelder, W. E., Witthuhn, B. A., McMickle, A. P., Doherty, P. C., Grosveld, G. C., and Ihle, J. N. (1995) Defective lymphoid development in mice lacking Jak3. *Science* **270,** 800–802.
112. Park, S. Y., Saijo, K., Takahashi, T., Osawa, M., Arase, H., Hirayama, N., Miyake, K., Nakauchi, H., Shirasawa, T., and Saito, T. (1995) Developmental defects of lymphoid cells in Jak3 kinase-deficient mice. *Immunity* **3,** 771–782.
113. Thomis, D. C., Gurniak, C. B., Tivol, E., Sharpe, A. H., and Berg, L. J. (1995) Defects in B lymphocyte maturation and T lymphocyte activation in mice lacking Jak3. *Science* **270,** 794–797.
114. Yoshida, H., Hayashi, S., Kunisada, T., Ogawa, M., Nishikawa, S., Okamura, H., Sudo, T., Shultz, L. D., and Nishikawa, S. (1990) The murine mutation osteopetrosis is in the coding region of the macrophage colony stimulating factor gene. *Nature* **345,** 442–444.
115. Corcoran, A. E., Smart, F. M., Cowling, R. J., Crompton, T., Owen, M. J., and Venkitaraman, A. R. (1996) The interleukin-7 receptor alpha chain transmits distinct signals for proliferation and differentiation during B lymphopoiesis. *EMBO J.* **15,** 1924–1932.
116. Reichman-Fried, M., Bosma, M. J., and Hardy, R. R. (1993) B-lineage cells in mu-transgenic scid mice proliferate in response to IL-7 but fail to show evidence of immunoglobulin light chain gene rearrangement. *Int. Immunol.* **5,** 303–310.
117. Spanopoulou, E., Roman, C. A., Corcoran, L. M., Schlissel, M. S., Silver, D. P., Nemazee, D., Nussenzweig, M. C., Shinton, S. A., Hardy, R. R., and Baltimore, D. (1994) Functional immunoglobulin transgenes guide ordered B-cell differentiation in Rag-1-deficient mice. *Genes Dev.* **8,** 1030–1042.
118. Young, F., Ardman, B., Shinkai, Y., Lansford, R., Blackwell, T. K., Mendelsohn, M., Rolink, A., Melchers, F., and Alt, F. W. (1994) Influence of immunoglobulin heavy- and light-chain expression on B-cell differentiation. *Genes Dev.* **8,** 1043–1057.
119. Lagasse, E. and Weissman, I. L. (1994) bcl-2 inhibits apoptosis of neutrophils but not their engulfment by macrophages. *J. Exp. Med.* **179,** 1047–1052.
120. Lowenthal, R. M. and Marsden, K. A. (1997) Myelodysplastic syndromes. *Int. J. Hematol.* **65,** 319–338.
121. Van den Berghe, H. and Michaux, L. (1997) 5q-, twenty-five years later: a synopsis. *Cancer Genet. Cytogenet.* **94,** 1–7.
122. Akashi, K., Harada, M., Shibuya, T., Eto, T., Takamatsu, Y., Teshima, T., and Niho, Y. (1991) Effects of interleukin-4 and interleukin-6 on the proliferation of CD34+ and CD34- blasts from acute myelogenous leukemia. *Blood* **78,** 197–204.
123. Akashi, K., Shibuya, T., Harada, M., Takamatsu, Y., Uike, N., Eto, T., and Niho, Y. (1991) Interleukin 4 suppresses the spontaneous growth of chronic myelomonocytic leukemia cells. *J. Clin. Invest.* **88,** 223–230.
124. Geissler, K., Ohler, L., Fodinger, M., Virgolini, I., Leimer, M., Kabrna, E., Kollars, M., Skoupy, S., Bohle, B., Rogy, M., and Lechner, K. (1996) Interleukin 10 inhibits growth and granulocyte/macrophage colony- stimulating factor production in chronic myelomonocytic leukemia cells. *J. Exp. Med.* **184,** 1377–1384.
125. Oehler, L., Foedinger, M., Koeller, M., Kollars, M., Reiter, E., Bohle, B., Skoupy, S., Fritsch, G., Lechner, K., and Geissler, K. (1997) Interleukin-10 inhibits spontaneous colony-forming unit-granulocyte- macrophage growth from human peripheral blood mononuclear cells by suppression of endogenous granulocyte-macrophage colony-stimulating factor release. *Blood* **89,** 1147–1153.
126. Winandy, S., Wu, P., and Georgopoulos, K. (1995) A dominant mutation in the Ikaros gene leads to rapid development of leukemia and lymphoma. *Cell* **83,** 289–299.
127. Ting, C. N., Olson, M. C., Barton, K. P., and Leiden, J. M. (1996) Transcription factor GATA-3 is required for development of the T-cell lineage. *Nature* **384,** 474–478.
128. Urbanek, P., Wang, Z. Q., Fetka, I., Wagner, E. F., and Busslinger, M. (1994) Complete block of early B cell differentiation and altered patterning of the posterior midbrain in mice lacking Pax5/BSAP. *Cell* **79,** 901–912.
129. Lin, H. and Grosschedl, R. (1995) Failure of B-cell differentiation in mice lacking the transcription factor EBF. *Nature* **376,** 263–267.

130. Bain, G., Maandag, E. C., Izon, D. J., Amsen, D., Kruisbeek, A. M., Weintraub, B. C., Krop, I., Schlissel, M. S., Feeney, A. J., van Roon, M., et al. (1994) E2A proteins are required for proper B cell development and initiation of immunoglobulin gene rearrangements. *Cell* **79,** 885–892.
131. Zhuang, Y., Soriano, P., and Weintraub, H. (1994) The helix-loop-helix gene E2A is required for B cell formation. *Cell* **79,** 875–884.
132. Georgopoulos, K., Bigby, M., Wang, J. -H., Molnar, A., Wu, P., Winandy, S., and Sharpe, A. (1994) The Ikaros gene is required for the development of all lymphoid lineages. *Cell* **79,** 143–156.
133. Georgopoulos, K., Moore, D. D., and Derfler, B. (1992) Ikaros, an early lymphoid-specific transcription factor and a putative mediator for T cell commitment. *Science* **258,** 808–812.
134. Porcher, C., Swat, W., Rockwell, K., Fujiwara, Y., Alt, F. W., and Orkin, S. H. (1996) The T cell leukemia oncoprotein SCL/tal-1 is essential for development of all hematopoietic lineages. *Cell* **86,** 47–57.
135. Robb, L., Elwood, N. J., Elefanty, A. G., Kontgen, F., Li, R., Barnett, L. D., and Begley, C. G. (1996) The scl gene product is required for the generation of all hematopoietic lineages in the adult mouse. *EMBO J.* **15,** 4123–4129.
136. Robb, L., Lyons, I., Li, R., Hartley, L., Kontgen, F., Harvey, R. P., Metcalf, D., and Begley, C. G. (1995) Absence of yolk sac hematopoiesis from mice with a targeted disruption of the scl gene. *Proc. Natl. Acad. Sci USA.* **92,** 7075–7079.
137. Shivdasani, R. A., Mayer, E. L., and Orkin, S. H. (1995) Absence of blood formation in mice lacking the T-cell leukaemia oncoprotein tal-1/SCL. *Nature* **373,** 432–434.
138. Warren, A. J., Colledge, W. H., Carlton, M. B., Evans, M. J., Smith, A. J., and Rabbitts, T. H. (1994) The oncogenic cysteine-rich LIM domain protein rbtn2 is essential for erythroid development. *Cell* **78,** 45–57.
139. Okuda, T., van Deursen, J., Hiebert, S. W., Grosveld, G., and Downing, J. R. (1996) AML1, the target of multiple chromosomal translocations in human leukemia, is essential for normal fetal liver hematopoiesis. *Cell* **84,** 321–330.
140. Wang, Q., Stacy, T., Binder, M., Marin-Padilla, M., Sharpe, A. H., and Speck, N. A. (1996) Disruption of the Cbfa2 gene causes necrosis and hemorrhaging in the central nervous system and blocks definitive hematopoiesis. *Proc. Natl. Acad. Sci USA* **93,** 3444–3449.
141. Wang, Q., Stacy, T., Miller, J. D., Lewis, A. F., Gu, T. L., Huang, X., Bushweller, J. H., Bories, J. C., Alt, F. W., Ryan, G., Liu, P. P., Wynshaw-Boris, A., Binder, M., Marin-Padilla, M., Sharpe, A. H., and Speck, N. A. (1996) The CBFβ subunit is essential for CBFα2 (AML1) function in vivo. *Cell* **87,** 697–708.
142. Miyamoto, T., Nagafuji, K., Akashi, K., Harada, M., Kyo, T., Akashi, T., Takenaka, K., Mizuno, S., Gondo, H., Okamura, T., Dohy, H., and Niho, Y. (1996) Persistence of multipotent progenitors expressing AML1/ETO transcripts in long-term remission patients with t(8;21) acute myelogenous leukemia. *Blood* **87,** 4789–4796.
143. Erickson, P. F., Dessev, G., Lasher, R. S., Philips, G., Robinson, M., and Drabkin, H. A. (1996) ETO and AML1 phosphoproteins are expressed in CD34+ hematopoietic progenitors: implications for t(8;21) leukemogenesis and monitoring residual disease. *Blood* **88,** 1813–1823.
144. Yergeau, D. A., Hetherington, C. J., Wang, Q., Zhang, P., Sharpe, A. H., Binder, M., Marin-Padilla, M., Tenen, D. G., Speck, N. A., and Zhang, D. E. (1997) Embryonic lethality and impairment of haematopoiesis in mice heterozygous for an AML1-ETO fusion gene. *Nat. Genet.* **15,** 303–306.
145. Wu, L., Scollay, R., Egerton, M., Pearse, M., Spangrude, G. J., and Shortman, K. (1991) CD4 expressed on earliest T-lineage precursor cells in the adult murine thymus. *Nature* **349,** 71–74.
146. Adkins, B., Mueller, C., Okada, C. Y., Reichert, R. A., Weissman, I. L., and Spangrude, G. J. (1987) Early events in T-cell maturation. *Annu. Rev. Immunol.* **5,** 325–365.
147. Anderson, G., Moore, N. C., Owen, J. J., and Jenkinson, E. J. (1996) Cellular interactions in thymocyte development. *Annu. Rev. Immunol.* **14,** 73–99.
148. Weissman, I. L. (1994) Developmental switches in the immune system. *Cell* 76(2), 207–218.
149. Wu, L., Li, C. L., and Shortman, K. (1996) Thymic dendritic cell precursors: relationship to the T lymphocyte lineage and phenotype of the dendritic cell progeny. *J. Exp. Med.* **184,** 903–911.
150. Galy, A. H. and Spits, H. (1991) IL-1, IL-4, and IFN-γ differentially regulate cytokine production and cell surface molecule expression in cultured human thymic epithelial cells. *J. Immunol.* **147,** 3823–3830.
151. Le, P. T., Lazorick, S., Whichard, L. P., Haynes, B. F., and Singer, K. H. (1991) Regulation of cytokine production in the human thymus: epidermal growth factor and transforming growth

factor alpha regulate mRNA levels of interleukin 1 alpha (IL-1 alpha), IL-1 beta, and IL-6 in human thymic epithelial cells at a post-transcriptional level. *J. Exp. Med.* **174,** 1147–1157.
152. Le, P. T., Lazorick, S., Whichard, L. P., Yang, Y. C., Clark, S. C., Haynes, B. F., and Singer, K. H. (1990) Human thymic epithelial cells produce IL-6, granulocyte-monocyte-CSF, and leukemia inhibitory factor. *J. Immunol.* **145,** 3310–3315.
153. Namen, A. E., Lupton, S., Hjerrild, K., Wignall, J., Mochizuki, D. Y., Schmierer, A., Mosley, B., March, C. J., Urdal, D., and Gillis, S. (1988) Stimulation of B-cell progenitors by cloned murine interleukin-7. *Nature* **333,** 571–573.
154. Rodewald, H. R., Kretzschmar, K., Swat, W., and Takeda, S. (1995) Intrathymically expressed c-kit ligand (stem cell factor) is a major factor driving expansion of very immature thymocytes in vivo. *Immunity* **3,** 313–319.
155. Adkins, B., Gandour, D., Strober, S., and Weissman, I. (1988) Total lymphoid irradiation leads to transient depletion of the mouse thymic medulla and persistent abnormalities among medullary stromal cells. *J. Immunol.* **140,** 3373–3379.
156. Adkins, B., Tidmarsh, G. F., and Weissman, I. L. (1988) Normal thymic cortical epithelial cells developmentally regulate the expression of a B-lineage transformation-associated antigen. *Immunogenetics* **27,** 180–186.
157. Saint-Ruf, C., Ungewiss, K., Groettrup, M., Bruno, L., Fehling, H. J., and von Boehmer, H. (1994) Analysis and expression of a cloned pre-T cell receptor gene. *Science* **266,** 1208–1212.
158. Bikoff, E. K., Huang, L. Y., Episkopou, V., van Meerwijk, J., Germain, R. N., and Robertson, E. J. (1993) Defective major histocompatibility complex class II assembly, transport, peptide acquisition, and $CD4^+$ T cell selection in mice lacking invariant chain expression. *J. Exp. Med.* **177,** 1699–1712.
159. Gosgrove, D., Gray, D., Dierich, A., Kaufman, J., Lemeur, M., Benoist, C., and Mathis, D. (1991) Mice lacking MHC class II molecules. *Cell* **66,** 1051–1066.
160. Grusby, M. J., Johnson, R. S., Papaioannou, V. E., and Glimcher, L. H. (1991) Depletion of CD4+ T cells in major histocompatibility complex class II- deficient mice. *Science* **253,** 1417–1420.
161. Viville, S., Neefjes, J., Lotteau, V., Dierich, A., Lemeur, M., Ploegh, H., Benoist, C., and Mathis, D. (1993) Mice lacking the MHC class II-associated invariant chain. *Cell* **72,** 635–648.
162. Koller, B. H., Marrack, P., Kappler, J. W., and Smithies, O. (1990) Normal development of mice deficient in beta 2M, MHC class I proteins, and $CD8^+$ T cells. *Science* **248,** 1227–1230.
163. Zijlstra, M., Bix, M., Simister, N. E., Loring, J. M., Raulet, D. H., and Jaenisch, R. (1990) Beta 2-microglobulin deficient mice lack $CD4^-8^+$ cytolytic T cells. *Nature* **344,** 742–746.
164. McCormack, W. T., Liu, M., Postema, C., Thompson, C. B., and Turka, L. A. (1993) Excision products of TCR V alpha recombination contain in-frame rearrangements, evidence for continued V(D)J recombination in TCR^+ thymocytes. *Int. Immunol.* **5,** 801–804.
165. Surh, C. D. and Sprent, J. (1994) T-cell apoptosis detected in situ during positive and negative selection in the thymus. *Nature* **372,** 100–103.
166. Huesmann, M., Scott B., Kisielow, P., and von Boehmer, H. (1991) Kinetics and efficacy of positive selection in the thymus of normal and T cell receptor transgenic mice. *Cell* **66,** 533–540.
167. Shortman, K., Vremec, D., and Egerton, M. (1991) The kinetics of T cell antigen receptor expression by subgroups of $CD4^+8^+$ thymocytes: delineation of $CD4^+8^+3^{2+}$ thymocytes as post-selection intermediates leading to mature T cells. *J. Exp. Med.* **173,** 323–332.
168. Lucas, B. and Germain, R. N. (1996) Unexpectedly complex regulation of CD4/CD8 coreceptor expression supports a revised model for $CD4^+CD8^+$ thymocyte differentiation. *Immunity* **5,** 461–477.
169. Spain, L. M., Yelon, D., and Berg, L. J. (1994) Do the CD4 and CD8 lineages represent parallel pathways? *Sem. Immunol.* **6,** 213–2120.
170. Willerford, D. M., Swat, W., and Alt, F. W. (1996) Developmental regulation of V(D)J recombination and lymphocyte differentiation. *Curr. Opin. Genet. Dev.* **6,** 603–609.
171. McBlane, J. F., van Gent, D. C., Ramsden, D. A., Romeo, C., Cuomo, C. A., Gellert, M., and Oettinger, M. A. (1995) Cleavage at a V(D)J recombination signal requires only RAG1 and RAG2 proteins and occurs in two steps. *Cell* **83,** 387–395.
172. van Gent, D. C., Ramsden, D. A., and Gellert, M. (1996) The RAG1 and RAG2 proteins establish the 12/23 rule in V(D)J recombination. *Cell* **85,** 107–113.
173. Mombaerts, P., Iacomini, J., Johnson, R. S., Herrup, K., Tonegawa, S., and Papaioannou, V. E. (1992) RAG-1-deficient mice have no mature B and T lymphocytes. *Cell* **68,** 869–877.
174. Shinkai, Y., Rathbun, G., Lam, K. P., Oltz, E. M., Stewart, V., Mendelsohn, M., Charron, J., Datta, M., Young, F., Stall, A. M., et al. (1992) RAG-2-deficient mice lack mature lymphocytes owing to inability to initiate V(D)J rearrangement. *Cell* **68,** 855–867.

175. Schatz, D. G., Oettinger, M. A., and Schlissel, M. S. (1992) V(D)J recombination: molecular biology and regulation. *Annu. Rev. Immunol.* **10,** 359–383.
176. Friend, S. L., Hosier, S., Nelson, A., Foxworthe, D., Williams, D. E., and Farr, A. (1994) A thymic stromal cell line supports in vitro development of surface IgM+ B cells and produces a novel growth factor affecting B and T lineage cells. *Exp. Hematol.* **22,** 321–328.
177. Ray, R. J., Furlonger, C., Williams, D. E., and Paige, C. J. (1996) Characterization of thymic stromal-derived lymphopoietin (TSLP) in murine B cell development in vitro. *Eur. J. Immunol.* **26,** 10–16.
178. Zuniga-Pflucker, J. C., Di, J., and Lenardo, M. J. (1995) Requirement for TNF-alpha and IL-1 alpha in fetal thymocyte commitment and differentiation. *Science* **268,** 1906–1909.
179. Crompton, T., Outram, S. V., Buckland, J., and Owen, M. J. (1997) A transgenic T cell receptor restores thymocyte differentiation in interleukin-7 receptor alpha chain-deficient mice. *Eur. J. Immunol.* **27,** 100–104.
180. Fehling, H. J., Krotkova, A., Saint-Ruf, C., and von Boehmer, H. (1995) Crucial role of the pre-T-cell receptor alpha gene in development of $\alpha\beta$ but not $\gamma\delta$ T cells. *Nature* **375,** 795–798.
181. Molina, T. J., Kishihara, K., Siderovski, D. P., van Ewijk, W., Narendran, A., Timms, E., Wakeham, A., Paige, C. J., Hartmann, K. U., Veillette, A., et al. (1992) Profound block in thymocyte development in mice lacking $p56^{lck}$. *Nature* **357,** 161–164.
182. Gratiot-Deans, J., Ding, L., Turka, L. A., and Nunez, G. (1993) bcl-2 proto-oncogene expression during human T cell development: evidence for biphasic regulation. *J. Immunol.* **151,** 83–91.
183. Moore, N. C., Anderson, G., Williams, G. T., Owen, J. J., and Jenkinson, E. J. (1994) Developmental regulation of bcl-2 expression in the thymus. *Immunology* **81,** 115–119.
184. Veis, D. J., Sentman, C. L., Bach, E. A., and Korsmeyer, S. J. (1993) Expression of the Bcl-2 protein in murine and human thymocytes and in peripheral T lymphocytes. *J. Immunol.* **151,** 2546–2554.
185. Godfrey, D. I., Kennedy, J., Suda, T., and Zlotnik, A. (1993) A developmental pathway involving four phenotypically and functionally distinct subsets of CD3-CD4-CD8- triple-negative adult mouse thymocytes defined by CD44 and CD25 expression. *J. Immunol.* **150,** 4244–4252.
186. Kondo, M., Ohashi, Y., Tada, K., Nakamura, M., and Sugamura, K. (1994) Expression of the mouse interleukin-2 receptor gamma chain in various cell populations of the thymus and spleen. *Eur. J. Immunol.* **24,** 2026–2030.
187. Sugamura, K., Asao, H., Kondo, M., Tanaka, N., Ishii, N., Nakamura, M., and Takeshita, T. (1995) The common gamma-chain for multiple cytokine receptors. *Adv. Immunol.* **59,** 225–277.
188. Schorle, H., Holtschke, T., Hunig, T., Schimpl, A., and Horak, I. (1991) Development and function of T cells in mice rendered interleukin-2 deficient by gene targeting. *Nature* **352,** 621–614.
189. Kuhn, R., Rajewsky, K., and Muller, W. (1991) Generation and analysis of interleukin-4 deficient mice. *Science* **254,** 707–710.
190. Sadlack, B., Kuhn, R., Schorle, H., Rajewsky, K., Muller, W., and Horak, I. (1994) Development and proliferation of lymphocytes in mice deficient for both interleukins-2 and -4. *Eur. J. Immunol.* **24,** 281–284.
191. Guidos, C., Ransom, J., Fischer, M., Weissman, I., and Zlotnik, A. (1989) Role of interleukin-4 in T-cell ontogeny, changes in cell surface phenotype and lymphokine production of immature thymocytes after culture with interleukin-4 and phorbol ester. *J. Autoimmun.* **2 Suppl.,** 141–153.
192. Rodewald, H. R., Ogawa, M., Haller, C., Waskow, C., and DiSanto, J. P. (1997) Pro-thymocyte expansion by c-kit and the common cytokine receptor gamma chain is essential for repertoire formation. *Immunity* **6,** 265–272.
193. Guidos, C. J., Williams, C. J., Wu, G. E., Paige, C. J., and Danska, J. S. (1995) Development of $CD4^+CD8^+$ thymocytes in RAG-deficient mice through a T cell receptor beta chain-independent pathway. *J. Exp. Med.* **181,** 1187–1195.
194. Jacobs, H., Vandeputte, D., Tolkamp, L., de Vries, E., Borst, J., and Berns, A. (1994) CD3 components at the surface of pro-T cells can mediate pre-T cell development in vivo. *Eur. J. Immunol.* **24,** 934–939.
195. Zuniga-Pflucker, J. C., Jiang, D., Schwartzberg, P. L., and Lenardo, M. J. (1994) Sublethal gamma-radiation induces differentiation of $CD4^-/CD8^-$ into $CD4^+/CD8^+$ thymocytes without T cell receptor beta rearrangement in recombinase activation gene $2^{-/-}$ mice. *J. Exp. Med.* **180,** 1517–1521.
196. Nakayama, K. -I., Nakayama, K., Dustin, L. B., and Loh, D. Y. (1995) T-B cell interaction inhibits spontaneous apoptosis of mature lymphocytes in Bcl-2-deficient mice. *J. Exp. Med.* **182,** 1101–1110.

197. Veis, D. J., Sorenson, C. M., Shutter, J. R., and Korsmeyer, S. J. (1993) Bcl-2-deficient mice demonstrate fulminant lymphoid apoptosis, polycystic kidneys, and hypopigmented hair. *Cell* **75,** 229–240.
198. Akashi, K. and Weissman, I. L. (1996) The c-kit+ maturation pathway in mouse thymic T cell development: lineages and selection. *Immunity* **5,** 147–161.
199. Linette, G. P., Grusby, M. J., Hedrick, S. M., Hansen, T. H., Glimcher, L. H., and Korsmeyer, S. J. (1994) Bcl-2 is upregulated at the $CD4^+ CD8^+$ stage during positive selection and promotes thymocyte differentiation at several control points. *Immunity* **1,** 197–205.
200. Tao, B. and Fultz, P. N. (1995) Molecular and biological analyses of quasispecies during evolution of a virulent simian immunodeficiency virus, SIVsmmPBj14. *J. Virol.* **69,** 2031–2037.
201. Grillot, D. A., Merino, R., and Nunez, G. (1995) Bcl-XL displays restricted distribution during T cell development and inhibits multiple forms of apoptosis but not clonal deletion in transgenic mice. *J. Exp. Med.* **182,** 1973–1983.
202. Guidos, C. J. (1996) Positive selection of $CD4^+$ and $CD8^+$ T cells. *Curr. Opin. Immunol.* **8,** 225–232.
203. Guidos, C. J., Danska, J. S., Fathman, C. G., and Weissman, I. L. (1990) T cell receptor-mediated negative selection of autoreactive T lymphocyte precursors occurs after commitment to the CD4 or CD8 lineages. *J. Exp. Med.* **172,** 835–846.
204. Jameson, S. C., Hogquist, K. A., and Bevan, M. J. (1995) Positive selection of thymocytes. *Annu. Rev. Immunol.* **13,** 93–126.
205. von Boehmer, H. (1994) Positive selection of lymphocytes. *Cell* **76,** 219–28.
206. Lucas, B., Vasseur, F., and Penit, C. (1994) Production, selection, and maturation of thymocytes with high surface density of TCR. *J. Immunol.* **153,** 53–62.
207. Tao, W., Teh, S. J., Melhado, I., Jirik, F., Korsmeyer, S. J., and Teh, H. S. (1994) The T cell receptor repertoire of $CD4^-8^+$ thymocytes is altered by overexpression of the BCL-2 protooncogene in the thymus. *J. Exp. Med.* **179,** 145–153.
208. Grusby, M. J., Auchincloss, H., Jr., Lee, R., Johnson, R. S., Spencer, J. P., Zijlstra, M., Jaenisch, R., Papaioannou, V. E., and Glimcher, L. H. (1993) Mice lacking major histocompatibility complex class I and class II molecules. *Proc. Natl. Acad. Sci USA* **90,** 3913–3917.
208a. Akashi, K., Kondo, M., and Weissman, I. L. (1998) Two distinct pathways of positive selection for thymocytes. *Proc. Natl. Acad. Sci. USA*, in press.
209. Sen-Majumdar, A., Guidos, C., Kina, T., Lieberman, M., and Weissman, I. L. (1994) Characterization of preneoplastic thymocytes and of their neoplastic progression in irradiated C57BL/Ka mice. *J. Immunol.* **153,** 1581–1592.
210. Mazel, S., Burtrum, D., and Petrie, H. T. (1996) Regulation of cell division cycle progression by *bcl*-2 expression: a potential mechanism for inhibition of programmed cell death. *J. Exp. Med.* **183,** 2219–2226.
211. Vaux, D. L., Cory, S., and Adams, J. M. (1988) Bcl-2 gene promotes haemopoietic cell survival and cooperates with c- myc to immortalize pre-B cells. *Nature* **335,** 440–442.
212. Strasser, A., Harris, A. W., Corcoran, L. M., and Cory, S. (1994) Bcl-2 expression promotes B- but not T-lymphoid development in *scid* mice. *Nature* **368,** 457–460.
213. Nakajima, H., Shores, E. W., Noguchi, M., and Leonard, W. J. (1997) The common cytokine receptor gamma chain plays an essential role in regulating lymphoid homeostasis. *J. Exp. Med.* **185,** 189–195.
214. Sudo, T., Nishikawa, S., Ohno, N., Akiyama, N., Tamakoshi, M., Yoshida, H., and Nishikawa, S. (1993) Expression and function of the interleukin 7 receptor in murine lymphocytes. *Proc. Natl. Acad. Sci USA* **90,** 9125–9129.
215. Fowlkes, B. J. and Schweighoffer, E. (1995) Positive selection of T cells. *Curr. Opin. Immunol.* **7,** 188–195.
216. Winslow, G. M., Marrack, P., and Kappler, J. W. (1994) Processing and major histocompatibility complex binding of the MTV7 superantigen. *Immunity* **1,** 23–33.
217. Ohashi, P. S., Pircher, H., Burki, K., Zinkernagel, R. M., and Hengartner, H. (1990) Distinct sequence of negative or positive selection implied by thymocyte T-cell receptor densities. *Nature* **346,** 861–863.
218. Sentman, C. L., Shutter, J. R., Hockenberry, D., Kanagawa, O., and Korsmeyer, S. J. (1991) bcl-2 inhibits multiple forms of apoptosis but not negative selection in thymocytes. *Cell* **67,** 879–888.

219. Hazel, T. G., Nathans, D., and Lau, L. F. (1988) A gene inducible by serum growth factors encodes a member of the steroid and thyroid hormone receptor superfamily. *Proc. Natl. Acad. Sci. USA* **85,** 8444–8448.
220. Liu, Z. G., Smith, S. W., McLaughlin, K. A., Schwartz, L. M., and Osborne, B. A. (1994) Apoptotic signals delivered through the T-cell receptor of a T-cell hybrid require the immediate-early gene nur77. *Nature* **367,** 281–284.
221. Woronicz, J. D., Calnan, B., Ngo, V., and Winoto, A. (1994) Requirement for the orphan steroid receptor Nur77 in apoptosis of T- cell hybridomas. *Nature* **367,** 277–281.
222. Calnan, B. J., Szychowski, S., Chan, F. K., Cado, D., and Winoto, A. (1995) A role for the orphan steroid receptor Nur77 in apoptosis accompanying antigen-induced negative selection. *Immunity* **3,** 273–282.
223. Zhou, T., Cheng, J., Yang, P., Wang, Z., Liu, C., Su, X., Bluethmann, H., and Mountz, J. D. (1996) Inhibition of nur77/nurr1 leads to inefficient clonal deletion of self-reactive T cells. *J. Exp. Med.* **183,** 1879–1892.
224. Castro, J. E., Listman, J. A., Jacobson, B. A., Wang, Y., Lopez, P. A., Ju, S., Finn, P. W., and Perkins, D. L. (1996) Fas modulation of apoptosis during negative selection of thymocytes. *Immunity* **5,** 617–627.
225. Chan, A. C., Iwashima, M., Turck, C. W., and Weiss, A. (1992) ZAP-70: a 70 kd protein-tyrosine kinase that associates with the TCR ζ chain. *Cell* **71,** 649–662.
226. Samelson, L. E., Phillips, A. F., Luong, E. T., and Klausner, R. D. (1990) Association of the fyn protein-tyrosine kinase with the T-cell antigen receptor. *Proc. Natl. Acad. Sci USA* **87,** 4358–4362.
227. Appleby, M. W., Gross, J. A., Cooke, M. P., Levin, S. D., Qian, X., and Perlmutter, R. M. (1992) Defective T cell receptor signaling in mice lacking the thymic isoform of p59fyn. *Cell* **70,** 751–763.
228. Stein, P. L., Lee, H. M., Rich, S., and Soriano, P. (1992) pp59fyn mutant mice display differential signaling in thymocytes and peripheral T cells. *Cell* **70,** 741–750.
229. Cooke, M. P., Abraham, K. M., Forbush, K. A., and Perlmutter, R. M. (1991) Regulation of T cell receptor signaling by a src family protein- tyrosine kinase (p59fyn). *Cell* **65,** 281–291.
230. Arpaia, E., Shahar, M., Dadi, H., Cohen, A., and Roifman, C. M. (1994) Defective T cell receptor signaling and $CD8^+$ thymic selection in humans lacking zap-70 kinase. *Cell* **76,** 947–958.
231. Chan, A. C., Kadlecek, T. A., Elder, M. E., Filipovich, A. H., Kuo, W. L., Iwashima, M., Parslow, T. G., and Weiss, A. (1994) ZAP-70 deficiency in an autosomal recessive form of severe combined immunodeficiency. *Science* **264,** 1599–1601.
232. Elder, M. E., Lin, D., Clever, J., Chan, A. C., Hope, T. J., Weiss, A., and Parslow, T. G. (1994) Human severe combined immunodeficiency due to a defect in ZAP-70, a T cell tyrosine kinase. *Science* **264,** 1596–1599.
233. Veillette, A., Zuniga-Pflucker, J. C., Bolen, J. B., and Kruisbeek, A. M. (1989) Engagement of CD4 and CD8 expressed on immature thymocytes induces activation of intracellular tyrosine phosphorylation pathways. *J. Exp. Med.* **170,** 1671–1680.
234. Wiest, D. L., Yuan, L., Jefferson, J., Benveniste, P., Tsokos, M., Klausner, R. D., Glimcher, L. H., Samelson, L. E., and Singer, A. (1993) Regulation of T cell receptor expression in immature $CD4^+CD8^+$ thymocytes by $p56^{lck}$ tyrosine kinase: basis for differential signaling by CD4 and CD8 in immature thymocytes expressing both coreceptor molecules. *J. Exp. Med.* **178,** 1701–1712.
235. Anderson, S. J., Levin, S. D., and Perlmutter, R. M. (1993) Protein tyrosine kinase p56lck controls allelic exclusion of T-cell receptor beta-chain genes. *Nature* **365,** 552–554.
236. Chan, I. T., Limmer, A., Louie, M. C., Bullock, E. D., Fung-Leung, W. P., Mak, T. W., and Loh, D. Y. (1993) Thymic selection of cytotoxic T cells independent of CD8 alpha-Lck association. *Science* **261,** 1581–1584.
237. Fung-Leung, W. P., Louie, M. C., Limmer, A., Ohashi, P. S., Ngo, K., Chen, L., Kawai, K., Lacy, E., Loh, D. Y., and Mak, T. W. (1993) The lack of CD8 alpha cytoplasmic domain resulted in a dramatic decrease in efficiency in thymic maturation but only a moderate reduction in cytotoxic function of $CD8^+$ T lymphocytes. *Eur. J. Immunol.* **23,** 2834–2840.
238. Killeen, N. and Littman, D. R. (1993) Helper T-cell development in the absence of CD4-p56lck association. *Nature* **364,** 729–732.
239. Chan, S. H., Cosgrove, D., Waltzinger, C., Benoist, C., and Mathis, D. (1993) Another view of the selective model of thymocyte selection. *Cell* **73,** 225–236.

240. Crump, A. L., Grusby, M. J., Glimcher, L. H., and Cantor, H. (1993) Thymocyte development in major histocompatibility complex-deficient mice: evidence for stochastic commitment to the CD4 and CD8 lineages. *Proc. Natl. Acad. Sci USA* **90,** 10739–10743.
241. van Meerwijk, J. P. and Germain, R. N. (1993) Development of mature $CD8^+$ thymocytes: selection rather than instruction? *Science* **261,** 911–915.
242. van Meerwijk, J. P., O'Connell, E. M., and Germain, R. N. (1995) Evidence for lineage commitment and initiation of positive selection by thymocytes with intermediate surface phenotypes. *J. Immunol.* **154,** 6314–6323.
243. Lucas, B., Vasseur, F., and Penit, C. (1995) Stochastic coreceptor shut-off is restricted to the CD4 lineage maturation pathway. *J. Exp. Med.* **181,** 1623–1633.
244. Lundberg, K., Heath, W., Kontgen, F., Carbone, F. R., and Shortman, K. (1995) Intermediate steps in positive selection: differentiation of $CD4^+8^{int}$ TCR^{int} thymocytes into $CD4^-8^+TCR^{hi}$ thymocytes. *J. Exp. Med.* **181,** 1643–1651.
245. Suzuki, H., Punt, J. A., Granger, L. G., and Singer, A. (1995) Asymmetric signaling requirements for thymocyte commitment to the $CD4^+$ versus $CD8^+$ T cell lineages: a new perspective on thymic commitment and selection. *Immunity* **2,** 413–425.
246. Itano, A., Salmon, P., Kioussis, D., Tolaini, M., Corbella, P., and Robey, E. (1996) The cytoplasmic domain of CD4 promotes the development of CD4 lineage T cells. *J. Exp. Med.* **183,** 731–741.

Chapter 18

Gene Regulation in T-Cell Lineage Commitment

Ellen V. Rothenberg

1. Introduction

This chapter considers the molecular mechanisms that operate during the commitment of a pluripotent hematopoietic cell to differentiate within the T-cell lineage. This commitment event, or sequence of events, results in the establishment of a novel stable pattern of transcriptional regulation that can be inherited by the daughters of committed cells, which will define them as T-cells wherever they migrate in the body. Therefore, the essential changes in the cells during commitment are changes in gene regulation.

The progress of cells can be traced through T-lineage commitment by two complementary approaches. One approach is to consider the genes that need to be turned on in order to define the cell as a T-lineage cell. A cell that expresses a large number of genes that are not expressed by any mature cell type other than T-cells is very likely to have progressed down a developmental pathway unique to the T lineage. The regulators that induce expression of these genes, and those that block expression of lineage-inappropriate genes, are evidently key players in the conversion of a precursor into a T-cell. The other approach is to trace the history of the cells that become T-cells, and to determine what other fates, if any, they may adopt at various stages of their progress toward becoming T-cells. Irrespective of the number of T-cell properties that a cell may or may not be expressing at the time, a cell may be said to be committed to the T lineage when it can no longer give rise to anything else.

This chapter will attempt to draw together the two approaches, by defining the time course along which different T-lineage genes are turned on, by exploring the question of how genes of other lineages are turned off or kept off, and by relating these events to the cells' progress through T-lineage commitment. The expected and observed effects on this process caused by disrupting relevant transcriptional regulators will be compared with effects observed in other lineages. The results raise several issues about basic transcriptional strategies for lineage choice and the relationship of T-cells to their precursors.

From: *Molecular Biology of B-Cell and T-Cell Development*
Edited by: J. G. Monroe and E. V. Rothenberg © Humana Press Inc., Totowa, NJ

2. Molecular Landmarks for Progress in T-Lineage Differentiation

2.1. Discovery of Regulatory Mechanisms Starting from "Downstream Genes"

A starting point for understanding how T-cell precursors make their lineage choices is to ask how they meet the requirements for initiating the expression of genes that define a cell as a T-cell. Since expression of genes that are not expressed by other cell types marks a cell as having moved into a T-specific differentiation stage, the transcription factors that control expression of these genes are of great interest as potential players in the commitment process.

2.2. Genes That are Programmed for Expression in T-Cell Development

T-lineage genes that will be discussed throughout this chapter are grouped here into distinct "recognition" and "response" sets, based on their functions and their modes of regulation. A third set, constituting the growth control genes, is probably also important but is currently less well-characterized.

2.2.1. Genes Used in Antigen Recognition: The "Recognition Genes"

Mature T-cells recognize antigen through their expression of the heterodimeric $\alpha\beta$ or $\gamma\delta$ T-cell receptor (TCR), embedded in a transmembrane complex with the CD3 γ, δ, ε, and ζ (or η) signaling chains. All these chains are encoded by genes that are expressed constitutively in mature T-cells. In order to endow precursors with such receptors, however, several different sets of transcription units need to be activated during development. In detail, these genes are not coordinately regulated; as expected, their regulators include some nonoverlapping components.

2.2.1.1. CD3. Expression of CD3 components is initiated by the activation of the CD3 gene promoters and enhancers, very early in development *(1,2)*. This expression is largely T-lineage specific and, once initiated, appears to be completely stable. Transcription factors that are implicated in CD3 transcription are incompletely characterized, but appear to include CBF/Runt proteins, CREB family bZIP proteins, and Ikaros or related Zn finger proteins of the hunchback family *(3–6)*.

2.2.1.2. Recombinases. Because the TCR genes only encode biologically relevant products after undergoing rearrangement, the key developmental event that makes TCR expression possible is the induction of the recombinase genes RAG1 and RAG2. Terminal deoxynucleotidyl transferase (TdT), in postnatal lineages, also needs to be expressed in order to achieve a fully diverse TCR repertoire. These genes are expressed through much of thymocyte development, but they are turned off at positive selection *(7)*, and they are not T-lineage specific, since they are shared with B-cells. The transcription factors that drive expression of these genes are very slightly characterized, but they include Ikaros and related Zn finger proteins of the hunchback family, products of the E2A gene and other related bHLH factors, Ets family factors, and probably CBF/Runt domain factors in addition to more ubiquitous factors *(8,9)*.

2.2.1.3. TCR Enhancers. Activation of the enhancers of the TCR genes themselves, via T-cell specific suites of transcription factors, appears to be most important for focusing the activity of the recombinases on the appropriate loci *(10,11)*. TCR enhancer activities are largely T-lineage specific in mature cells, but they are not only developmentally activated in cells that are already T-lineage committed *(12–16)* (H. Wang and E. V. Rothenberg, unpublished data). The transcription factors that service the TCR gene enhancers arc partially characterized, and they share with the CD3 enhancers the use of

CBF/Runt and Ets family factors. Also used conspicuously are the sequence-specific HMG box factors TCF-1 or LEF-1, the Zn finger protein GATA-3, members of the CREB subfamily of bZIP transcription factors, and in some cases, C-Myb *(17–21)*. In the γ and δ chain enhancers, the CBF/Runt sites are associated with Myb sites, whereas in the α and β chain enhancers they are associated with Ets family sites *(17,19,22,23)*.

2.2.1.4. Pre-TCR Component. At least one temporary TCR component, the pTα surrogate light chain, is needed for appropriate selection and amplification of developing thymocytes that will use αβ-TCR (reviewed extensively in Chapters 22 and 23). It is expressed in a T-lineage specific way by purely transcriptional mechanisms, like CD3 components but is shut off at a late stage of αβ-TCR thymocyte development like the recombinase components *(24,25)*. Very little is known yet about the transcription factors responsible for its regulation.

2.2.1.5. Dedicated Signal Transduction Intermediates. Finally, there are several lineage-restricted cytoplasmic signaling components that are now known to be critical for T-cell development because of their unique roles in transducing antigen receptor and coreceptor signals. These components, including the Lck and Zap70 protein tyrosine kinases *(26,27)*, appear to be expressed in largely, if not completely, T-lineage specific ways *(28–30)*. Although Lck, at least, is expressed prior to full TCR gene rearrangement *(31,32)*, it is not clear exactly how early it is turned on, and most of the other candidate T-cell specific signaling genes are even less well studied. Therefore, it is unknown whether expression of any of these genes participates in the early events through which precursors are specified and then committed to develop as T-cells. There is evidence for involvement of TCF or LEF HMG box proteins, Myb, Ets family, and Ikaros family Zn finger proteins in the regulation of Lck expression *(33,33a)*, but the other key regulators of this gene remain unidentified.

2.2.2. Genes Used in T-Cell Effector Function: The "Response Genes"

The effector roles of mature T-cells in the immune system are triggered by TCR signaling but executed only by a separate set of "response" genes. T-cell development cannot be considered complete without establishing the competence to express at least some subset of response genes. These genes are normally expressed in mature T-cells only upon stimulation, but their expression is highly T-lineage restricted. Promoter/enhancer regions of several of these genes are becoming well-characterized. In most cases, however, these analyses have revealed a potent basis for the activation-dependence of the response gene expression without clearly defining what molecular features of T-cells give these cells the unique competence to express these genes upon activation, whereas other cells cannot. Three examples of response genes, which have been assayed for expression in early stages of T-cell development, are the following.

2.2.2.1. IL-2. The interleukin (IL)-2 gene is probably the best characterized of the T-cell response genes. It is expressed in $CD4^+$ T-cells, especially during early rounds of contact with antigen, and to a lesser extent in $CD8^+$ T-cells, but in few, if any, other cell types. In the mouse, it is not expressed by mature NK cells. Its regulatory mechanisms have recently been reviewed in detail *(34–36)*. IL-2 expression is completely stimulation-dependent in mature T-cells, demanding a complex signal from TCR and costimulatory activation pathways, and is subject to modulation through a variety of auxiliary signaling inputs. The transcription factors that are known to control its expression, NF-AT, NF-κB/c-Rel, AP-1, and possibly also the Ets family GABP factors *(37)*, are transducers of Ca^{2+}, protein kinase C, Ras, and stress-pathway signals. Other factors potentially implicated are Oct-1 or Oct-2, Sp1, and/or Egr-1. None is T-lineage restricted, and none is yet shown to play a role in lineage choice per se.

2.2.2.2. IL-4. IL-4 is regulated in mature T-cells by a combination of acute TCR signals, current cytokine responses, and the T-cell's previous activation history. Although expressed readily by mast cells as well as by CD4$^+$ T-cells, it is not expressed by most other cell types *(38)*. IL-4 is known to be regulated in large part by NF-AT, AP-1, and Oct-1 transcription factors *(39–41)*. What gives it a regulation pattern distinct from IL-2 is the lack of involvement of NF-κB/rel family factors in IL-4 expression, and instead, the use of additional factors. Among those recently suggested to play a role are the bZIP factor c-Maf, NF-Y, a member of the C/EBP family, an uncharacterized negative regulatory protein, and directly or indirectly, GATA-3 *(42–45)*. The exceptional role of GATA-3 is discussed below (*see* Subheading 5.2.), but the other factors are expressed in multiple cell types.

2.2.2.3. Perforin. Unlike the two cytokines described, perforin is expressed in CD8$^+$ killer T-cells and NK cells, instead of CD4$^+$ helper T-cells. Also in contrast to IL-2 and IL-4, perforin expression is not transient after stimulation. Induction of perforin expression elicits a sustained transcriptional response that extends for days, as the killer effectors arm themselves, and perforin expression is ongoing in active NK populations. Perforin transcriptional regulatory mechanisms are under investigation, but the critical transcription factors are still controversial *(46–50)*. There is no evidence that NF-AT plays a role, but Ets family factor(s) appear to be centrally involved, and negative regulatory elements appear to be critical to restrict expression to the appropriate cell types.

2.2.3. Genes Controlling T-Cell Growth and Survival Properties

Among the most distinctive features of T-cells are their abilities to proliferate extensively, or remain quiescent for long periods of time without loss of potential to proliferate, depending upon environmental circumstances. Multiple mechanisms are now known to be used by the cells to limit their expansion (the use of CTLA4, or Fas/FasL interactions; *[51,52]*). However, little is known about the unique molecular features of T-cells that endow them with this extensive growth capacity.

It is possible that the unlimited proliferative lifespan of T-cells is not a lineage-specific characteristic at all in the normal sense, but rather, an aspect of stem cell biology that is lost in most lineages, but preserved by cells undergoing T-lineage differentiation. For example, a potential component of this "legacy" might be the telomerase complex that repairs chromosome ends after each round of replication. Cells in most hematopoietic lineages lose telomerase activity as they differentiate *(53)*, but thymocytes and T-cells remain capable of reactivating telomerase indefinitely, whenever they are mitogenically stimulated *(54)*. T-cells also retain the ability to express HoxB cluster homeobox genes in a temporal wave immediately after stimulation *(55)*, including the HoxB4 gene, which has been linked to clonal expansion in pluripotent hematopoietic precursors *(56,57)*. One implication of this interpretation would be that T-lineage precursors must diverge from other developmental pathways at an early enough stage to precede any event that irreversibly shuts off expression of such "self-renewal" functions in other lineages.

The only two known growth factors or growth factor receptors, which appear to be required for the development of T-cells, are the stem cell factor receptor c-kit and the IL-7Rα, which may be involved in responses to both IL-7 and another factor designated TSLP *(58,59)*. This seems striking in light of the extraordinary expansion that can accompany thymocyte proliferation: up to 10^5-fold net growth per single input cell *(60)*. The expression of c-kit and responsiveness to its ligand can be viewed as another "legacy" from the pluripotent precursor, one that is shared by the earliest B-lineage precursors. IL-7Rα expression, although also shared with B-lineage cells, seems to be more acutely required for expansion of T-lineage cells from the earliest stages. Since T-cells continue to be responsive to IL-7 as a growth and survival factor into maturity, it is possible that the regulators of IL-7Rα expression will include critical lineage-determining transcription factors. These molecules remain to be discovered.

2.3. Developmental Regulation of Expression of T-Lineage Genes

The sequence in which the various T-lineage associated genes come to be expressed has been traced in fetal and postnatal murine thymocytes, using combinations of cell-surface markers to distinguish stages of thymocyte development. Some of the most useful markers to resolve different stage early in T-lineage differentiation are c-kit, CD44, and CD25, which are differentially expressed on subsets of thymocytes before expression of CD4, CD8, and the TCR. Cell transfer experiments, in which the phenotypes and yield of progeny of the donor cells were analyzed as a function of time, have established precursor/product relationships among cells in these stages, essentially as shown in Fig. 1 and reviewed elsewhere (*see* Chapter 16 and *61,62*). In Fig. 1, as in Chapter 16, successive stages are designated "CD4^{lo}," "DN1," "DN2," "DN3," and "DN4." The earliest subset can further be resolved into a precursor population and a set of apparently immature NK cells, by use of additional markers Sca-1, CD122, and NK1.1 in mice of the appropriate genetic background *(63,64)*. Recent studies from a number of laboratories have now used analysis of RNA expressed in these subsets to define the stages in which various T-lineage genes are first turned on. The results of these studies, summarized in Fig. 1A, B, establish a series of discrete landmarks in the progression through early T-lineage differentiation.

There are two major conclusions from this work. First, T-lineage genes are turned on independently in several stepwise events, not in a single coordinated induction event. Second, the developmental onset of expression of the "response" genes actually precedes expression of many of the "recognition" genes. As discussed in a later section, this response gene expression probably also precedes T-lineage commitment.

2.3.1. Expression of Different Recognition Genes Before and After the "Pro-T" Transition

TCR gene rearrangement does not begin until the "pro-T" or DN2 stage, which is a critical point in the progress of thymocytes towards a T-cell fate, as discussed extensively below *(62,65,66)*. Although the TCR genes in cells of this stage remain in germline configuration, this is when the RAG genes begin to be expressed *(64)*, and rearrangements of the TCRβ, γ, and δ loci follow shortly thereafter *(67–69)*. The transition from earlier stages to the pro-T, or DN2 stage, is accompanied by the onset of expression of RAG1 and of the pre–T-cell receptor component pTα (Fig. 1A, "DN2 to DN3" population).

Not all components of the TCR are coregulated with these molecules, however. Another component of the recombinase enzyme battery, TdT, is actually expressed before RAG1 *(64,68)*. Although the RAG genes and TdT are shared with B-cells, and thus are not strictly T-lineage specific, other, more conventionally T-lineage specific, components are also expressed earlier than the DN2 stage. The CD3 components, especially CD3ε, are clearly expressed before this transition *(2,64)*, in CD4^{lo} and DN1 cells. Transcriptional activation of the TCRβ enhancer region occurs even earlier, since germline transcripts from the TCRβ constant region appear to be expressed more broadly, not only in thymocyte subsets but also in bone marrow and fetal liver cell fractions with the phenotypes of pluripotent stem cells *(16,64)*. Germline expression of certain TCR Vβ promoters has also been observed in less well characterized prethymic cells *(70)*. This prethymic TCRβ expression is noteworthy because in adult mice it appears that most

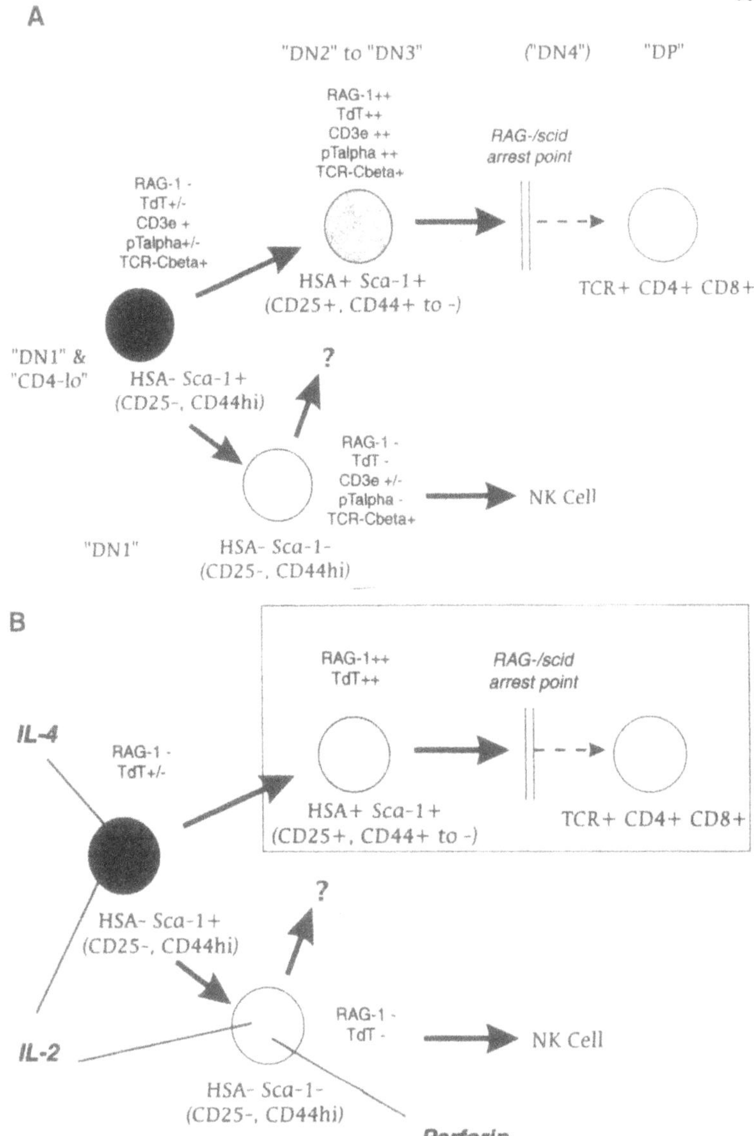

Fig. 1. Gene expression in primitive thymocyte subsets analyzed by reverse transcriptase-dependent polymerase chain reaction (RT-PCR). **(A)** Expression of T-cell "recognition" genes in phenotypically defined subsets of thymocytes. The acquisition of cell surface markers by primitive thymocytes prior to TCR surface expression is presented in a flow diagram, in which the combinations of cell surface markers expressed at different stages are indicated in a semi-italic font. Transcripts shown to be expressed in each of the stages, based on RT-PCR analysis, are listed in a sans-serif font. The data show that T-cell recognition genes are activated noncoordinately and that several are expressed in cells before the DN2 stage. The figure is based on work by Hua Wang, Rochelle Diamond, and the author (*63,64,71,* and unpublished data). The successive stages are thought to be first "$CD4^{lo}$", then DN1, DN2, DN3, DN4, the last of these converting rapidly to conventional $TCR^{low/+}$ $CD4^{+}$ $CD8^{+}$ thymocytes ("DP"), as indicated. The figure shows that in recombination-deficient animals, the cells do not progress beyond the DN3 stage. Also indicated is the division of the "DN1" population on the basis of Sca-1 expression, into Sca-1^{+} cells (referred to in the text as stem cell-like) and Sca-1- cells (referred to in the text as immature NK cell-like) *(63)*. Both "DN1" component populations express high levels of c-kit (not shown). Recent data

cells do not become committed to a T-lineage fate until after they arrive in the thymus, as discussed extensively below.

2.3.2. Precocious Expression of Response Genes

Very strikingly, the response genes are programmed for expression at the earliest stages. An example of this is shown in Fig. 2, where the ability to express IL-2 after pharmacological stimulation is tested in thymocyte subsets from recombination-deficient SCID mice. The most immature cells, the Sca-1^{high} HSA^{low} $CD44^{high}$ subset, are capable of expressing at least as much IL-2 after stimulation as are the more advanced, HSA^{+} cells *(71)*.

Since engagement of the TCR is normally required to trigger response gene activation in mature T-cells, the abilities of such early, TCR-negative precursors to express response genes might be expected to remain latent in vivo. Instead, recent work has shown that the response genes IL-2, IL-4, and perforin are all expressed at substantial levels by the most immature cells within the thymus of adult mice (H. Wang, R. A. Diamond, J. A. Yang-Snyder, and E.V.R., submitted). Results of these studies are summarized in Fig. 1B. However, different subsets within the $CD44^{high}$ $CD25^{-}$ "DN1" population show divergent response gene expression patterns, supporting the provisional separation of these cells into pluripotent precursors and immature NK cells. Whereas the "precursors" (Sca-1^{+} HSA^{-} $CD44^{high}$) express IL-2 and IL-4, but little perforin, the "immature NK" cells (Sca-$1^{-}$$HSA^{-}$ $CD44^{high}$) express perforin and IL-2, but no IL-4 (H. Wang, R. A. Diamond, J. A. Yang-Snyder, and E.V.R., submitted). It is a surprising but reproducible feature of the "immature NK" cells that they express substantial levels of IL-2 in vivo, although they apparently do not maintain this expression well when cultured in vitro (see Fig. 2B).

The most important feature of this expression is that the precursors become armed with T-lineage–associated response capacity prior to the activation of the recombinase machinery that will confer TCR upon them, and as discussed below, prior to T-lineage commitment. Furthermore, the expression of IL-2 by cells that resemble immature NK cells suggests that cells can express T-cell response genes, even if they are undergoing commitment to lineages in which the mature cells will not express these genes. These results open up the possibility that a number of "T-lineage restricted" response capabilities will be found to be present in multilineage hematopoietic precursors. In this case, T-lineage specificity of expression of these genes may be enforced generally by the negative regulation of these capabilities in cells that differentiate along other lineages.

2.4. Summary of Expression of T-Lineage Genes

Progression through early T-cell developmental stages is marked by developmentally regulated activation of T-lineage genes, and the sequence of these activation events

---

(137,138) suggest that at least in the fetus, some of the presumptive immature NK cells are bipotent and can give rise to T-cells, as indicated by an arrow with a question mark. **(B)** T-cell "response" genes are expressed in primitive thymocytes prior to lineage commitment. Populations are the same as in (A), but now the stages when the response genes IL-2, IL-4, and perforin are expressed are indicated (with RAG-1 and TdT expression repeated from (A) for comparison). In the same figure, the stages when T cells show evidence of lineage commitment are indicated (enclosed in a shaded box). The figure shows that the expression of IL-2, IL-4, and perforin in vivo precedes RAG-1 expression and is restricted to very primitive cell populations which appear not to be committed to the T-cell lineage (H. Wang, R. A. Diamond, J. A. Yang-Snyder, and E. V. R., submitted).

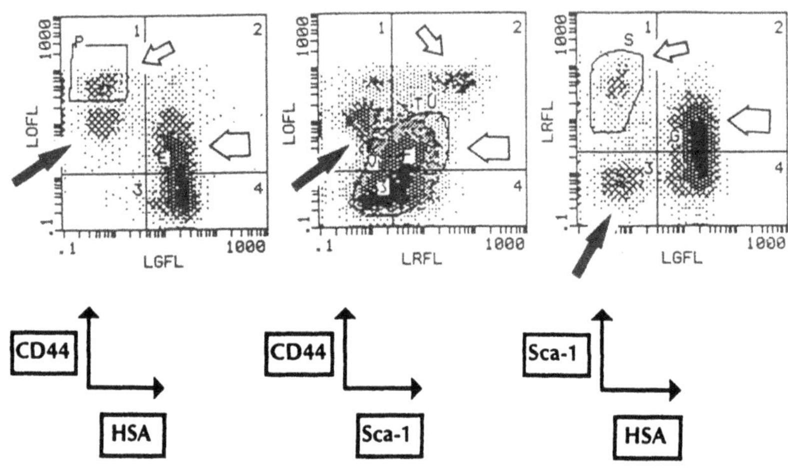

B

IL-2 EXPRESSION BY SCID THYMOCYTE SUBSETS

SUBSET	STIMULATION	IL-2/10^6 CELLS	
		Expt. 1	Expt. 2
Sca-1^{++} HSA^{low}	no IL-1	96	nd
	+ IL-1	93	120
HSA^+	no IL-1	5	<3
	+ IL-1	69	36
Sca-1^- HSA^{low}	+ IL-1	nd	8.3
Total SCID	no IL-1	5	10
	+ IL-1	57	64

Fig. 2. Functional responsiveness in vitro of immature *scid/scid* thymocytes. **(A)** Preparative sorting of three subsets of *scid/scid* thymocytes. Three-color immunofluorescent staining for Sca-1, HSA, and CD44 demarcates three populations, as indicated in the three two-color cytograms by different arrows. Wide white arrows in each panel indicate the HSA+ population, which is heterogeneous in CD44 and Sca-1 expression over a broad continuum (indicated by an amorphous region in middle cytogram). This subset, which represents all the $CD25^+$ cells *(71)*, includes DN2 ($CD44^{high}$) through DN3 ($CD44^{low}$) cells. Narrow black arrows in each panel indicate the Sca-1- HSA^{low} $CD44^{high}$ population, which corresponds to the immature NK-like component of the DN1 population, as shown in Fig. 1. Smaller shaded arrows in each panel indicate the Sca-1^+ HSA^{low} $CD44^{high}$ population, which includes the stem-cell like component of the DN1 population and most of the "$CD4^{lo}$" cells. The characteristics of this last subset are indicated by an amorphous region in both the leftmost and the rightmost panels. In the genetic background of the mice used here, though not in all strains, this population expresses distinctly higher levels of CD44 than even the immature NK-like cells within the DN1 population (*see* middle panel). **(B)** Ability of sorted *scid/scid* thymocyte subsets to express IL-2 after stimulation in vitro. The table shows the

establishes a series of landmarks for early differentiation. The effector or "response" genes in general are already expressed at the earliest discernible stages, then shut off and rendered dependent on acute induction signals for any re-expression, with the shutoff occurring at about the time that recombinase expression begins. Expression of certain TCR germline transcripts also turns on very early, indicating activation of enhancer-binding factors as early as in prethymic stages. Other "recognition" genes, not dependent on gene rearrangement for the function of their products, appear to be more stringently regulated, with expression limited to cells definitely within the thymus and progressing along a T-lineage path. Among the last of the "recognition" genes to be turned on is RAG1 itself.

This multistep gene activation program raises the possibility that T-cells acquire their identity by a cascade of choices, rather than by a single molecular event. The next section considers the relationship of this cascade to developmental commitment at the cellular level.

3. Commitment to the T Lineage

3.1. Specification and Commitment

The molecular landmarks for progress through T-lineage differentiation do not, in themselves, tell us anything about commitment. Strictly speaking, they tell us about "specification" *(72)*: the developmental program that is set in train so that, left to their own devices, primitive thymocytes will become T-cells.

A separate question is what the cells would do if they were not left to their own devices *(72)*. It is known that the thymic microenvironment is a highly potent inductive microenvironment for T-lineage differentiation. Spangrude and Scollay *(73)* showed that small numbers of presumptive hematopoietic stem cells, when forced to reside in the thymus, efficiently generated enormous numbers of T-cell progeny and failed to give rise to many cell types that they might otherwise have produced. However, as reviewed in Chapter 16 in this volume, small numbers of primitive thymocytes can give rise to non-T-lineage progeny, if they are removed from the thymic microenvironment *(65,74–79)*. Thus, the stepwise activation of T-lineage characteristics described in the next section remains open to interruption or diversion, until another kind of event "locks in" the differentiation program and makes it inescapable. The developmental stage at which the cells can no longer give rise to any viable progeny, but T-cells, no matter what the environment, is the stage at which they are committed to the T lineage.

None of the positive gene regulation events listed in Section 2.3. is necessarily connected with commitment to the T lineage in this sense, that is, the foreclosing of other options. (Successful TCR gene rearrangement, in a sense, is a "semantic" indicator of commitment, to the extent that we would classify any cell expressing TCRβ chains as a T-lineage cell of some kind no matter what its other properties were. However, this trivial case sidesteps the real mechanistic question of commitment.) The major issue is how a cell comes to regulate its gene expression so as to acquire a whole suite of T-cell properties and to block acquisition of other lineage properties. To explore the kinds of

---

biologically active IL-2 secreted by each of the three subsets indicated in the previous panel following stimulation overnight in culture with calcium ionophore plus phorbol ester, as described *(71)*. IL-1 was added because it is needed for induction of IL-2 from the great majority of immature thymocytes *(71,139)*. Data are from two experiments over two years apart (ref. *71* and unpublished results).

regulatory functions that may bring about commitment, one must consider further the pathway through which a cell becomes committed, and the options at each stage that the cell foregoes.

3.2. Commitment as an Extended Process

3.2.1. Timing of Commitment in the T Lineage

Thymocytes become committed to the T-lineage developmental program before TCR expression, even though some of the earliest thymocyte types are not committed to the T lineage. In the fetus, there is evidence that some T-lineage commitment may occur prethymically *(80,81)*. However, an advantage of the adult is that many T-lineage precursors appear to migrate to the thymus, where they can be easily studied, before their commitment is complete. Chapter 16 reviews evidence that commitment is thought to take place during the DN2 stage or in the DN2 → DN3 transition. The most primitive thymocytes (CD4^{lo} thymocytes) are able to give rise to dendritic cells, B-cells, NK cells, and T-cells upon adoptive transfer; cells past the DN2 stage can give rise only to T-cells. There must always be two caveats to the interpretation of the experiments from which these conclusions are drawn. One is that any heterogeneity in a precursor population could result in mixed types of progeny, so that the commitment could actually take place earlier than proposed. The other is that the cell-transfer protocol that is used to challenge the cells' state of specification may not allow all diverse progeny types to be recovered efficiently, so that a cell type that appeared committed might actually retain some alternative developmental potential (e.g., mast cell or eosinophil differentiation) that remained unmonitored. Further work will certainly address these caveats. However, even considering these caveats, the studies of commitment in postnatal thymocytes show a robust and highly interesting pattern of developmental choices, and this has serious implications for the molecular mechanisms through which specification and commitment occur.

3.2.2. Stepwise Loss of Developmental Alternatives

3.2.2.1. Alternative Developmental Potentials and the Regulation of Their Loss. Although the endpoint for commitment is relatively well-established, the thymus also appears to maintain small pools of intermediates, between the most primitive and the T-lineage–committed cell types, which are partially restricted in their developmental potential. The choices of developmental program that remain open to these cells contract as they progress along the T-lineage pathway, and the loss of potential appears to be hierarchical rather than stochastic. Thus, erythromyeloid potential is lost first, then B-lineage potential, then natural killer potential, and finally, or at the same time as the loss of NK potential, the cells lose the capacity to give rise to thymic dendritic cells, their last alternative *(65,78,79,82)*.

The sequential losses of developmental potential might be thought of as analogous to the frequent examples of binary choice through asymmetric division in other developmental systems *(83)*, but in fact, it is likely that they are quite different. One crucial difference is that, in contrast to examples like anchor cell determination in *C. elegans* or the morphogenesis of sensory bristles in *Drosophila* melanogaster, there is no evidence that one thymocyte's lineage choice constrains the fate of its sisters or neighbors in any way. A precursor cell that retains three developmental potentials is not required to generate all three cell types, but instead may give rise to a clone of progeny uniformly committed to any one of the three fates. In the human system, in vitro clonal analysis has shown that the same cell can give rise to T-cells and NK cells, or to NK cells and dendritic cells, in proportion depending mainly on environmental conditions *(84,85)*. Indeed, under normal circumstances, the overwhelming majority of pluripotent intrathymic precursors appear to adopt the same one, or perhaps two, lineage choices (i.e., T-cells and dendritic cells, with the T-lineage numbers greatly amplified by the proliferation that is incorporated into the αβ-TCR lineage differentiation program). Primitive thymocytes may thus be considered direct targets for any of at least four different specification processes. The question of commitment is exactly how progression down the T-lineage differentiation pathway shuts off access to these alternatives.

3.2.2.2. Hierarchies of Developmental Potential and Hierarchies of Molecular Sharing. The hierarchical way that options are closed off implies that the remaining options define clusters of molecularly related, or compatible, developmental fates. To the extent that this is true, the overlap in gene expression programs between the different progeny of hematolymphoid precursors may be traced to inheritance of those properties from a common, partially restricted progenitor.

The ability of the "$CD4^{lo}$" population to give rise to T and B (and NK) cells, but not conventional erythromyeloid cells, suggest that this might be a common lymphoid precursor distinct from other hematopoietic lineages. The unusually long lifetimes and common morphological and molecular features of lymphocytes that distinguish them from other hematopoietic cells make this a satisfying grouping, and the discovery that all three of these lineages are selectively eliminated in dominant negative mutants of the Ikaros transcription factor, which also exhibit virtual elimination of the thymus, reinforces this connection *(3)*. At a minimum, this precursor should have acquired (or, as suggested in Section 2.2.3., selectively preserved) the potential for long-term proliferation and a dependence on Ikaros function. Less obvious a priori, but still in accord with gene expression patterns, is the clear loss of B-cell developmental potential prior to the loss of NK developmental potential, suggesting that in spite of their sharing of the "exotic" recombinase functions, B-cells are more different from T-cells overall than NK cells are. Figure 3 shows, in detail, the discordance between recombinase gene expression and the fine structure of these developmental branchpoints. The expression of T-lineage genes like certain CD3 components, Lck, granzymes, and perforin in NK cells but not in B-cells can be viewed as consistent with this *(82)*.

3.2.2.3. The Problematic Case of the Thymic Dendritic Cell Connection. Much less easy to explain is the apparent retention by thymocytes of the ability to give rise to thymic dendritic cells—ostensibly a myeloid cell type—until the very last developmental choice point. The close relationship is further supported by the absence of dendritic cells in Ikaros null mice *(86)*, and yet there is presumably little overlap in gene expression patterns between T-cells and dendritic cells. By this stage, T-lineage genes like CD3ε, the TCRβ enhancer, and the response genes IL-2, IL-4, and perforin have already been activated in the developing thymocytes, and none of these are expected to be expressed in mature dendritic cells. A particularly striking feature of the developmental timing of these events is that RAG gene induction appears to overlap, and TdT gene induction appears to precede, the last stages in which thymocytes can still give rise to dendritic cells. Thus, if the induction of these genes should be uniform throughout the population, it would appear that recombinase-negative dendritic cells can be derived from a recombinase-positive precursor (*see* Fig. 3).

It is interesting to speculate that the late disappearance of the dendritic cell option is an indication that a myeloid-like cell fate may be preserved as a default along several hematopoietic pathways. Interesting in this connection is the fact that splenic dendritic

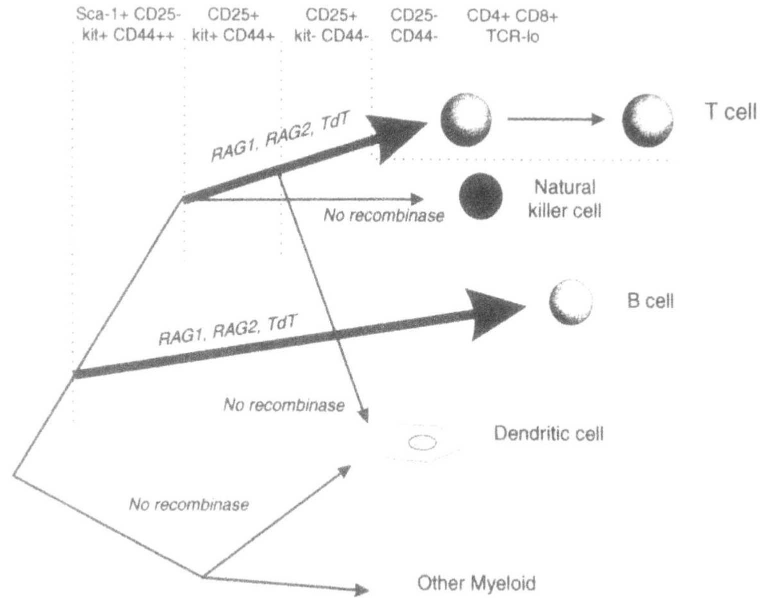

Fig. 3. Ordering of thymocyte lineage decisions relative to onset of recombinase expression and progression through phenotypic stages. The diagram summarizes the stages at which various alternative developmental potentials are lost *(65,77–79)*, in the context of the RNA-level expression of recombinase components (from Fig. 1). In this figure the cell-surface markers used to demarcate the stages include CD25, which correlates very highly with HSA expression in these populations, in place of HSA. The expression of c-kit, which is highly correlated with expression of CD44, is also indicated. The stages demarcated at the top of the figure apply only to cells retaining T-lineage developmental potential, and correspond to the following stages: CD4^{lo}/stem-cell like DN1; then DN2; then DN3; then DN4; and then DP.

cells appear to have two separate origins, in spite of sharing nearly homogeneous differentiated characteristics *(78)*. It may also be relevant that a specialized, bipotent macrophage/B-cell precursor is generated during hematopoiesis, which has lost the ability to give rise to T-cells or other types of erythromyeloid cells (*see* Chapter 15) *(87,88)*. Many leukemogenic processes, both spontaneous and induced, have immortalized fully interconverted B-derived macrophages, of which some even contain immunoglobulin gene rearrangements. Thus, even recombinase gene expression and activity do not necessarily prevent lymphoid cells from adopting certain types of "myeloid" fates.

The evidence for a close developmental link between T-cells and dendritic cells, in spite of minimal likely overlap in gene expression profiles, emphasizes that even though T-lineage genes may be expressed earlier, their expression is not stabilized until after the DN2 stage. Both this positive stabilization and the inhibition of alternative lineage characteristics, like those of dendritic cells, are essential features of the commitment process.

4. The Search for Mechanisms that Mediate Specification and Commitment of Pluripotent Precursors

4.1. Commitment Proper and Other Rate-Limiting Events in Hematolymphoid Development

To discuss mechanisms responsible for commitment, it is first necessary to dispel some confusion about what is meant by "commitment." Many kinds of perturbations of differentiation have been described as effects on "lineage commitment." Essentially, any mutation or intervention that blocks the production of a particular type of cell can be alleged to have prevented commitment to that lineage. In this discussion, however, several kinds of mechanism that could bring such an outcome about will be distinguished.

1. Cells can fail to differentiate a certain way because they indeed fail to execute the positive functions needed to specify them for a particular lineage.
2. Cells can undergo specification and commitment, but fail to survive because they are deprived of a survival or proliferation factor that is selectively needed in that lineage.
3. Cells can undergo specification and commitment to a particular lineage, but fail to mature to the stage at which their phenotype is scored.
4. Finally, cells could initiate a developmental pathway but fail to stabilize this choice, thus, they undergo aberrant differentiation or full transdifferentiation to another cell type.

Numerous gene disruption phenotypes in the hematopoietic system, when analyzed closely, have proven to be of types 2 or 3. The mechanism of type 1 comes close to addressing lineage choice but actually only measures specification—that is, a "forward" component of developmental progress along one lineage path. Only the last type of mechanism, 4, which is rarely scored, would be an effect on commitment proper. A return to interpretation of the effects of gene disruption phenotypes will be in the last section (Subheading 5). Here the kinds of mechanisms likely to drive cells from specification to commitment will be considered.

4.2. Specification and Commitment at the Level of Gene Regulation

4.2.1. A Model Illustrating Some Essential Features

It is likely that the process of lineage commitment involves some of the elements diagrammed in Fig. 4, as hypothetical components of a network that

1. Starts a cascade of lineage-specific gene expression,
2. Represses (or aborts, as in the figure) expression of lineage inappropriate genes, and
3. Stabilizes the resulting gene expression pattern so that it is no longer reversible.

There are several key elements in this hypothetical network. First, the initial lineage-specific genes (Fig. 4A,B) that are turned on during specification have to be inducible using transcription factors present prior to specification (1,2,3). Either an extracellular signal or an internal "stochastic" mechanism could be invoked to alter the factors in the unspecified, pluripotent precursor to give them this capability. Second, among the lineage-specific genes induced during initial specification must be genes that encode new lineage-specific transcription factors (or cofactors that modify transcription factor activity) (4^+, 5^-). Third, the new lineage-specific transcription factors should not only be able to turn on new downstream genes (Fig. 4C); they should also be able to stabilize the expression of lineage-specific "downstream" genes, so that they no longer depend on the state of signaling (i.e., the replacement of "2" by "4^+" at the promoter of gene B). Finally, the new lineage-specific transcription factors should include negative regulatory activities (5^-), to block induction or repress expression of any genes of an alternative lineage that might be derived from the same pluripotent precursor. The elements of the network that give it its ability to drive a lineage choice are the induction of both positive and negative transcription factors during the specification process.

4.2.2. Multistage Commitment in the Context of the Model

An unresolved aspect of the multistep loss of pluripotentiality observed in immature thymocytes is how individual losses of potential are connected with the overall drive

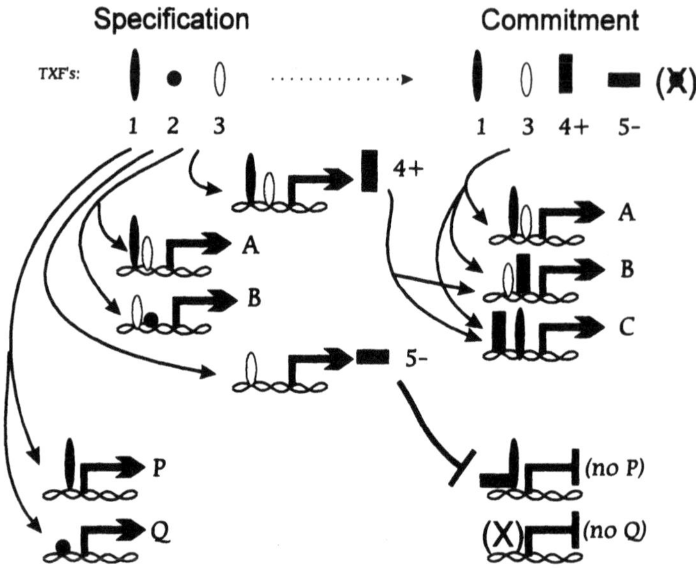

Fig. 4. Model of transcription factor interactions with target "downstream" genes during progression from developmental specification to commitment. The diagram portrays schematically two states of a precursor cell initiating a T-lineage gene expression program: specification and commitment. See text for discussion of the distinction between these two states (Section 3.1.). In the diagram, transcription factors active within a cell at a given time are listed at the top of the figure ("TXF's") and given designations by number (1–5). "Downstream genes," the genes that confer specific properties on T-cells, are designated by letter (A–C); these could represent genes encoding TCR or signaling components. Downstream genes used in mature cells of other lineages, such as B or dendritic cells, are exemplified by the genes labeled P and Q. In the initial state of specification, T-lineage genes A and B begin to be expressed through the activity of transcription factors 1, 2, and 3, but also non-T-lineage genes P and Q are activated because of the actions of factors 1 and 2. T-lineage transcription factors 4 and 5 are also induced de novo, and these give the system the ability to move to the state of commitment. Factor 4 (4+) is a positive regulatory factor with two activities: it allows additional T-lineage genes to be activated (here exemplified by C), and it also permits more stable (or stronger) activation of gene B, due to its ability to replace factor 2 on the promoter of B. Factor 2, which was originally present in the precursor state, is now dispensable and can be lost (see crossed out 2 on top list of factors in committed state). Factor 5 (5-), the other newly synthesized T-lineage factor, is a negative regulatory factor, which can now block ectopic expression of the non-T lineage gene P. The other non-T lineage gene Q can be shut off passively because of the loss of factor 2. Thus the conversion from the initial stages of specification to lineage commitment is accomplished here by the induced synthesis of two new factors, 4+ and 5–, and the loss (by dilution or a direct regulatory interaction) of one pre-existing factor, 2. The general features diagrammed here could very well be repeated for new downstream genes and new transcription factors at a succession of stages before commitment is complete.

toward T-lineage commitment. A priori, this does not seem to be much of a problem in explaining the T/NK lineage divergence, where the cells may be separated only—to our knowledge—by the expression of a set of functions that one possesses and the other lacks—namely, the recombination of the TCR genes. As the cell expresses genes like CD3, perforin, and presumably other shared T/NK characteristics, it becomes more and more like a T-cell or an NK cell and less and less like a B-cell, neutrophil, or megakaryocyte. As noted above, however, this simple view of the multistage process breaks down for explaining the persistence of dendritic cell developmental potential, since before the cells lose this potential, current data suggest that they have expressed a significant number of genes that are not expected to be typical dendritic cell products. A more robust mechanism is needed to affect not only the genes expressed at the time, but the cell's future potential for gene expression.

4.2.2.1. Repression and the Nature of Pluripotentiality. The model in Fig. 4 emphasizes that repression, or blockade of induction, is necessary to prevent expression of lineage-inappropriate characteristics, but repression is one function that has been starkly neglected in most studies of lymphoid cell differentiation. The underlying assumption has been that a pluripotent precursor, as long as it is uncommitted, is a cell with potential, but no actual downstream gene expression. In fact, strong evidence has been obtained for pluripotent precursors of other hematopoietic lineages, which shows that expression of "lineage-specific" downstream genes and "lineage-specific" transcription factors can substantially precede lineage choice *(89–91)*. A particularly powerful recent analysis has revealed that β-globin and myeloperoxidase, two downstream genes, which are considered mutually exclusive markers of the erythroid and myeloid lineages, can even be expressed, simultaneously, in individual pluripotent precursor cells *(90)*. Little is known about potential crosslineage gene expression in lymphoid cells, except some evidence that germline or partially rearranged Ig and TCR genes can be expressed ectopically *(10,15,92–94)*. Accordingly, the authors group has recently begun to look for evidence to indicate whether any other lineage-inappropriate genes are expressed ectopically in primitive thymocytes. Although these studies are in an early stage, it has been found that, indeed, one B-lineage specific downstream gene, B29 (Ig-β or CD79b), which is not expressed in mature T-cells, is expressed at low, but significant levels in thymocytes *(64)*. This initial example of clear ectopic expression, which is repressed later, is reminiscent of the evidence that IL-2 (H. Wang and E. V. R., unpublished data) and CD3 *(82)* may be expressed in immature, but not mature NK cells, and with the possibility that recombinase-negative dendritic cells may be derived from DN2 cells expressing RAG1, TdT, and CD3ε. These examples, although the latter two require confirmation at the single-cell level, suggest that multilineage gene expression may also occur in pluripotent $CD4^{lo}$ thymocytes. The implication is that progression to maturity in the T lineage will require active repression, either of the downstream genes themselves or of their regulators, to terminate the expression of such inappropriate genes.

An interesting point is that the activation of additional lineage-specific genes does not need to be tightly coordinated with the repression of lineage-inappropriate genes. Lineage commitment and the refinement of T-lineage specific gene expression are actually aspects of a sustained process. In the case of B29, which is extreme, the eventual repression that is detected is imposed long after all question of lineage commitment has been settled, at least in principle: B29 is shut off only when the cells are already TCR^+ thymocytes undergoing the last stages of positive selection *(64)*. This case may serve as an illustration of how separate mechanisms could be deployed noncoordinately to shut off the genes that control access to B-lineage, NK-lineage, and dendritic cell lineage specification mechanisms, in a cascade of separate regulatory events.

4.2.2.2. Stabilization of T-Lineage Gene Expression. The ability of thymocytes, apparently already expressing many T-lineage genes, to dismantle this gene expression program and revert to an existence as dendritic cells emphasizes the difference between gene activation per se and the stabilization of gene expression that accompanies commitment. Since most available information on T-lineage specific gene expression comes from examination of cells that have passed through this event, it gives little insight into any differences between the regulatory factors that may activate lineage-specific gene expression initially and those that make it a constitutive feature of a long-lived cell. However, an attractive and testable hypothesis is that the initial specification events induce expression of novel transcription factors that replace or supplement those present in the pluripotent precursors, converting low-affinity, highly conditional binding interactions into high-affinity binding interactions with enhancer sequences of T-lineage–specific genes. In this case, the mediators of the stabilization-aspect of commitment would be molecules that interact with or replace the mediators of specification.

Rendering this scenario more likely are two features of the mammalian hematopoietic system. One is the system "penchant" for assigning key roles in lineage-specific gene expression to transcription factors that are members of multigene families. In such families, similar or interchangeable DNA-binding specificities are coupled with subtle distinctions in transcriptional activation and protein-protein interaction. Since many of these family members are expressed in divergent developmental patterns, there are numerous candidates for carrying out such a substitution under precise developmental regulation. Good examples are the Ets family, with a minimum of 17 members *(95)*; the bHLH family; and the GATA family, all of which are important in aspects of TCR gene expression and rearrangement. The second feature is the fact that regulation of gene expression is profoundly combinatorial, requiring simultaneous inputs from a diverse array of positive regulatory factors. The ability of transcription factors to interact productively with others can dictate their biological role almost as much as their ability to interact with the target sequences in the DNA itself. Thus there are many possible gradations in the ability of factors with similar DNA-binding specificities to work on given promoters, in the context of given neighboring factors.

Factors of a given family can be associated in complex regulatory networks, with dramatically different developmental roles for different family members. The example par excellence is that of the relationship between GATA-1 and GATA-2 in the erythroid lineage *(96,97)*, reviewed in Chapter 3. Here, GATA-2, expressed in a precursor, helps to induce expression of GATA-1, the key regulator of multiple erythroid lineage genes, which is further upregulated by erythroid lineage-specific signals (e.g., from the erythropoietin receptor). GATA-1 then inhibits GATA-2 expression and differentiation proceeds. Although GATA-2, when expressed at high levels, can in principle service many erythroid promoters, it appears not to be able to sustain erythroid cell viability; in this sense at least it cannot "stabilize." Disruption of the GATA-1 gene thus leads to an irremediable loss of erythroid cells. On the other hand, all the other GATA genes together cannot compensate for a disruption of GATA-2, which leads to stem cell loss and arrest of all hematopoiesis.

The fundamental requirement for a system that drives cells to express a new set of genes stably is that the presence of the critical lineage-specific transcription factors must be sustained. One of the salient features of GATA-1, which contributes to its ability to stabilize erythroid commitment, is that it is positively autoregulated by its own binding *(96)*. Although the presence of potential autoregulatory sites is likely to be common in transcription factor genes, it is possible that the factors that play a key role in developmental stabilization are distinguished by the ability to bind better than other members of the same family to their own autoregulatory sites.

5. Effects of Transcription Factor Mutations on T-Lineage Differentiation

At the heart of the thymocyte lineage commitment should be the identification of the key transcription factors that control both the positive and negative aspects of T-lineage commitment. The central question is which factors, if any, might play the role of a GATA-1 homologue for the T lineage. As discussed in Section 2, the implementation of the T-lineage developmental program is relatively complex. Even so, the T-cell recognition genes, although not completely coordinate in their regulation, should represent a good case of a "gene battery," i.e., genes that should be coexpressed in a cell type-specific way because of their sharing of a common set of transcription factors. Those factors implicated in this regulatory coordination would seem likely to include CBF/Runt factors, GATA-3, Ets family factors, Ikaros family Zn finger factors, and the sequence-specific HMG box proteins TCF-1 or LEF-1 and Sox-4. Many of these transcription factor genes have now been experimentally disrupted or converted into dominant negative transgenes, and so it has become possible to begin to assess their roles in T-cell development *(98–101)*. A summary of these factors, their expression patterns, and the phenotypes of their mutations is presented in Table 1.

5.1. Complex Phenotypes of T-Lineage Factor Mutations

5.1.1. Contrasting Effects of Disrupting Genes Encoding T-Lineage vs B-Lineage Transcription Factors

At first analysis, results of T-lineage factor mutations seem disappointingly complex. Relatively few directed mutations thus far selectively block T-cell development, except for those that interfere with intrathymic selection checkpoints long past the point when T-lineage identity is established. The majority of cases thus far fall into one of two patterns. Either homozygous mutants exhibit severe effects extending to multiple lineages beyond T-cells, or they appear to have relatively little effect even on T-cell development. In some cases, the most conspicuous effects of the knockouts of these genes have been confined to other lineages, and the T-lineage effects have been minimal. CBFα2 (AML1) and Ikaros mutations do arrest development of T-cells but of other hematopoietic lineages as well *(3,86,102,103)*. GATA-3, Sox4, and LEF-1 mutations severely affect nonhematopoietic lineages, with GATA-3 causing fetal lethality associated with broad defects in definitive hematopoiesis and Sox4 having its most pronounced hematopoietic effects on early B-cell development *(104,105)*. Ets-1 mutations have a severe effect on mature T-cell responses to stimulation and on cortical thymocyte viability, but allow thymocyte differentiation to proceed to apparent completion. Mutations of a different Ets family factor, PU.1, do block or delay thymocyte development, but much more complete ablation is seen in the B-cell and macrophage lineages (for a comprehensive review of the role of Ets proteins, see ref. *95*, and for detailed discussion of PU.1, *see* Chapter 7). Only mutations of TCF-1 appear to give a clearly defined lineage-specific arrest, and that is seen at a fairly late stage, between the TCRβ-selection checkpoint and differentiation into CD4$^+$ CD8$^+$ cortical thymocytes *(106)*. These results do not immediately reveal ways that these regulators of T-lineage specific downstream genes might be needed to drive T-lineage commitment per se.

The perplexing results of these mutations contrast with the much clearer results obtained in a number of cases in which B-lineage transcription factors have been disrupted *(101,107,108)*. E2A, EBF, and Pax5/BSAP were all identified as factors that directly drive expression of B-lineage "downstream genes," and mutation of the gene encoding any one of these three factors arrests B-cell development at an early stage, prior to VDJ rearrangement of the Ig heavy chain genes (*see* Chapters 6 and 15 and *109–113*). In the case of EBF, the defect is lineage-specific as expected from the expression pattern of the targeted factor, and in the case of E2A, the defect appears B-lineage specific even

Table 1

Transcription Factors Active in T-Cell Development[a]

Transcription factor	Class	Targets	Expression	Phenotype of knockout mutant
CBFα2 (=AML1, PEBP2αB)	Runt	TCRα, β, γ, δ; RAG1; CD3δ; CD3ε	Thymocytes, T-cell lines, B-cell lines, myeloid cell lines, pluripotent precursors	Lack of definitive hematopoiesis: all lineages
TCF-1	HMG	TCRα, β, δ; CD3ε; CD4, CD8α, IL-4, IL-13, Lck proximal?	Thymocytes more than mature T-cells; also many non-hematopoietic embryonic cell types	T-cell development blocked during DN $\rightarrow$ DP transition
LEF-1	HMG	same as TCF-1	Pre-B-cells, thymocytes, many non-hematopoietic embryonic cell types	Lack of B-1 B-cell lineage; lack of whiskers, hair, teeth; neurological defects; most thymic populations appear OK
Sox-4	HMG	CD2, CD3ε	Thymocytes, gonads, and multiple embryonic tissues	Cardiac malformation, early B developmental defect. Also T-lineage slowdown
Ets family	Winged helix	TCRα, β, γ, δ, CD2, RAG1; TdT; CD3ε, CD4, CD8α, perforin, many B-lineage genes	Many expression patterns for different family members. Ets-1 in mature B- and T-cells, PU.1 in B-cells and macrophages	Ets-1 knockout: T-, B-cells develop but show accelerated cell death, plasma cell differentiation in response to activation. PU-1 knockout: elimination of B-cells and macrophages, early loss, late recovery of T-cell development
Ikaros	Zn finger (hunchback)	CD3δ, CD2, CD8α, TdT, RAG1, Lck proximal?	T-cells, thymocytes, early B-cells, hematopoietic stem cells	Dominant negative: complete block of lymphoid development (T, B, NK), and some myeloid abnormalities. Null mutation: block of B, NK, fetal T development but postnatal T development apparently unaffected

GATA-3	Zn finger (GATA)	TCRα, β, δ, CD2, CD8α	Hematopoietic precursors, T-cells, other embryonic tissues including midbrain and eye	Severe neurological abnormalities, gross defects in fetal liver hematopoiesis. T-lineage developmental block in $RAG^{-/-}$ chimera reconst.
C-Myb	bHLH (class C)	TCRγ, δ, CD4, Bcl-2?	Hematopoietic cells, some other embryonic tissues	Multilineage fetal hematopoiesis defect
E2A, HEB (or other bHLH)	bHLH (class A)	RAG1, CD4, CD8α, TCRγ, many B-lineage genes	Ubiquitous	E2A knockout severe B-lineage developmental arrest, slowdown of T-lineage devel due to early defect. E2A/HEB double heterozygotes show T-devel slowdown
CREB	bZIP (CREB /ATF family)	TCRα, β; CD2, CD8α	Ubiquitous, also many ubiquitous family members. Possible T-cell specific splice variants	Knockout: no detecteable effect on any hematopoietic cells due to redundancy. Dom. negative from T-cell specific promoter: normal T-cell development, inhibited response to activation

[a]Table adapted from data summarized in refs. *(21,95,98–100)*, supplemented with data from refs. *(3–6,8,9,19,20,22,33,86,102–106,113,114,116,117,119,124–136)*.

though the factor itself is expressed more broadly. E2A could fit nicely into the model presented in Fig. 4 as an example of a pluripotent precursor factor that initiates specification. The failure of Pax5 to be induced in B-lineage precursors in E2A and EBF mutant mice nicely positions it as a lineage-specific factor induced through the E2A-dependent specification process.

5.1.2. Distortions of Knockout Phenotypes in T Lineage Differentiation

Several mechanisms are likely to obscure effects of transcription factor mutations on the T lineages. Two examples for which there is evidence are the use of redundant transcription factors, and the masking of initial developmental defects by extensive proliferation later in thymocyte development.

Evidence for redundancy comes from analysis of E2A mutations, which block B-lineage development and RAG1 expression in the B lineage. If the ubiquitous transcription factor, E2A, is directly required to turn on RAG1 in B-cells, then it is noteworthy that T-cells in the same E2A-mutant mice do manage to express recombinase, and even to generate mature cells with normal TCR rearrangements. T-lineage cells could manage to express appropriate E2A target genes like RAG1 in the absence of E2A by expressing factors that are functionally redundant with E2A on such promoters. A candidate for the redundant factor is the related bHLH protein HEB, in that double heterozygotes of mutants in E2A and HEB do show a more severe developmental perturbation in the thymus than heterozygotes of either single mutation *(114)*. Thus T lineage cells are not independent of E2A, so much as buffered against the effects of E2A loss by redundancy. A similar mechanism presumably explains the weak T-lineage phenotypes of LEF-1 knockouts and Sox4 knockouts *(98)*, and the T-lineage leakiness of the Ikaros-null C-terminal mutant phenotype *(96,115)*. It is not clear yet whether the T lineage makes more extensive use of transcription factor intrafamily redundancy than other lineages.

T-lineage transcription factor knockout phenotypes are also likely to be obscured by the extreme use of developmental quality-control checkpoints and compensatory proliferation by the thymus, long after T-lineage commitment. Fairly detailed study can be required to focus on functions that specifically affect early lineage choice if they do not also play a role in later thymocyte clonal expansion. However, with this kind of care, some mutations that showed surprisingly small "quantitative" effects on thymocyte populations at first have recently been shown to exert very severe effects on T-lineage cell generation at the earliest stages. Thus, both Sox4 and E2A homozygous mutations in fact turn out to impose a significant kinetic barrier to thymocyte development after all *(116,117)*. The effects of these mutations could only be revealed in their full strength when they were examined in conditions where the kinetics of thymocyte development, as well as steady-state population sizes, were examined.

A final, more speculative factor, which may cause T-lineage factor mutations to appear to lack lineage-specific effects, could be a tendency of T-lineage cells to preserve characteristics otherwise found only in pluripotent or oligopotent precursors, as suggested in Subheading 2.2.3. Since gene disruptions tend to show their whole-animal phenotype in the earliest cell types that use the gene, such mutations would appear as effects on pluripotent precursors (cf. CBF/Runt, Myb, GATA-3 mutant phenotypes). It is interesting to speculate that both an unusually redundant use of multiple transcription factors of the same family and a high capacity for regulative proliferation could similarly be connected with such a precursor legacy.

5.2. The Case of a Potential Lineage Regulator: Recursive Use of GATA-3 from Pluripotent Precursors to Mature Effector Cells

Perhaps the best current candidate for a factor that helps dictate T-lineage commitment is GATA-3. GATA-3 is turned on in the earliest stages of fetal thymocyte development *(118)* and contributes importantly to the activity of all the known TCR enhancers and possibly other T-cell genes as well. Disruption of the GATA-3 gene leads to a severe effects on nonlymphoid cells and kills embryos by severe hemorrhage prior to the arrival of lymphocytes in the thymus *(104)*, but recent technical advances have made it possible to test whether GATA-3 disruption has any specific effect on T-lineage differentiation. Given the broad perturbations of fetal liver hematopoiesis observed in knockout animals, it was possible that no lymphoid precursors of any kind could be generated from GATA-3 deficient cells. However, when homozygous GATA-3 mutant embryonic stem cells were forced to contribute the lymphoid lineages in chimeras after injection into RAG-knockout blastocysts, donor-derived lymphocytes, as well as other hematopoietic cell types, were produced. Although the GATA-3 mutant ES cells gave rise to erythromyeloid cells and even B-cells very efficiently under these conditions, they could not generate any detectable T-lineage cells *(119)*. Thus, the GATA-3 function is absolutely required in a cell-autonomous way to give rise to T-cells, but is dispensable in cells destined to become B-cells and presumably in any common T/B precursor.

Making this result especially provocative is the suggestion that the T-lineage block in the GATA-3 mutant cells may be quite early. Incomplete characterization leaves some uncertainty as to the stage at which the donor GATA-3-mutant cells are blocked, but the cellularity of the thymus overall suggests that they do not undergo any significant proliferation. They contribute at most a negligible fraction to the size of the RAG-deficient thymus (~2-3% of normal thymic cellularity), and they remain $CD4^-CD8^-$ *(119)*. Thus, the lack of GATA-3 seems to have prevented the cells from taking any steps in thymocyte development that are detectable over the background of early stages seen in the RAG-host *(63,120)*. This is striking since the known target genes of GATA-3, the TCR genes, are not needed for progression to this checkpoint *(121)*. GATA-3 may, therefore, act as a regulator of a classic gene battery that includes survival and lineage-specific proliferation genes yet to be discovered, as well as the TCR genes themselves. It is interesting in this regard that GATA-1, the erythroid regulator in the GATA family, has been reported to influence cell proliferation rates and survival *(122,123)*.

At least some functions of GATA-3 are exercised in nonlymphoid hematopoietic lineages, as shown by the phenotypes of the GATA-3 knockout mice *(104)*. The earliest $CD3\varepsilon^+$ cells in the murine fetal thymus at E12 also express GATA-3 already *(118)*, raising the possibility that the expression of this gene is initially activated in a pluripotent precursor, and maintained rather than induced de novo in the early thymocytes. If so, it is likely to have a distinct spectrum of roles in the precursors from those it exercises in early T-lineage specification. Recently, GATA-3 has been shown to carry out yet a third kind of function, this time regulating, by its levels of expression, the choice of response genes turned on in response to activation in mature T-cells *(45)*. In other words, this transcription factor may be able to regulate qualitatively different kinds of gene expression, at up to three successive stages in the development of lymphohematopoietic cells. This example indicates that presumptive lineage-specification transcription factors need not be a special class: they can be serially deployed and redeployed to regulate different sets of downstream genes as the cells move from one type of lineage decision to another.

5.3. Concluding Remarks

This chapter has attempted to interpret cellular data on acquisition of a stable lineage commitment in the light of the molecular mechanisms needed to account for the establishment of a T-lineage gene expression pattern in early thymocyte differentiation. The focus has been on postnatal murine thymocytes, for which molecular and cellular analyses have been most frequent, and upon which the effects of targeted gene disruption have thus far been easiest to score. There are several conclusions that emerge from the overview.

First, T lineage gene expression is initiated in a series of steps, which may be dependent on some common components, but which do not represent a single, coordinated developmental transition.

Second, T-lineage gene expression begins substantially prior to the full establishment of T-lineage commitment. The initiation of expression of lineage-specific downstream genes, even in discordant combinations, while cells are at least oligopotent is likely to be a general feature of hematopoietic differentiation.

Third, actual commitment, as measured at the cellular level, is likely to be executed by distinct repressors and stabilizers of gene expression, which are needed to make the T-lineage gene expression program specific and sustainable over many months and many rounds of cell division. These are not necessarily factors that are conspicuous as activators of T-lineage downstream genes in established, mature cells, and thus need to become targets of direct study in the future.

Finally, a very interesting possibility is that many T-lineage properties are not specifically acquired through T-cell differentiation, so much as inherited from pluripotent precursors and specifically preserved from loss. T-lineage differentiation would then be distinct from differentiation along other hematopoietic lineages by using the stabilizing functions of commitment not only upon newly-induced, lineage-specific genes, but also upon genes active in the pluripotent precursor.

We do not know all that we need to know to focus on the most important regulatory factors at this point. T-lineage genes are activated in a way that is clearly noncoordinate at a fine scale, so many "layers" of transcription factor activation and repression are possible. To know at what point the T-lineage genes begin to be driven by maximally T-lineage specific transcription factors, one would have to know whether or not the factors present can still participate in activating lineage-inappropriate gene expression at that point. There is a great need for more work to determine which non–T-lineage genes are expressed in early T-cell precursors, what transcription factors are responsible for that expression, and to what extent the expression of those genes reflects retention of competence to activate a full, alternative differentiation program.

In essence, it is now possible to see that early T-cell development is not a simple forward progression but a succession of choices. The most exciting regulatory mechanisms for this process are to be found now by examining the progress of differentiation in light of the choices not taken.

Acknowledgments

This work was deeply influenced by critical scientific discussions with members of the Caltech Developmental Biology Colloquium and faculty of the Embryology Course of the Marine Biological Laboratory at Woods Hole, MA. Of many colleagues whose ideas helped to stimulate this article, the author especially wishes to thank Eric Davidson (Caltech), Michael Levine (University of California, Berkeley), and James Posakony (University of California, San Diego). Eric Davidson also provided illuminating advice and criticism, which have greatly improved the manuscript. The author also wishes to thank the members of her laboratory, whose valuable experiments, enthusiastic scholarship, and intelligent discussion contributed in many ways to this paper. Work in the author's laboratory reviewed here was supported by grants from the NIH (AI34041 and AG13108), from the State of California Tobacco-Related Disease Research Program, and funding from the Stowers Institute for Medical Research.

References

1. Malissen, M., Gillet, A., Ardouin, L., Bouvier, G., Trucy, J., Ferrier, P., Vivier, E., and Malissen, B. (1995) Altered T cell development in mice with a targeted mutation of the CD3-ε gene. *EMBO J.* **14,** 4641–4653.
2. Wilson, A. and MacDonald, H. R. (1995) Expression of genes encoding the pre-TCR and CD3 complex during thymus development. *Int. Immunol.* **7,** 1659–1664.
3. Georgopoulos, K., Bigby, M., Wang, J.-H., Molnar, A., Wu, P., Winandy, S., and Sharpe, A. (1994) The Ikaros gene is required for the development of all lymphoid lineages. *Cell* **79,** 143–156.
4. Georgopoulos, K., Morgan, B. A., and Moore, D. D. (1992) Functionally distinct isoforms of the CRE-BP DNA-binding protein mediate activity of a T-cell-specific enhancer. *Mol. Cell. Biol.* **12,** 747–757.
5. Hallberg, B., Thornell, A., Holm, M., and Grundstrom, T. (1992) SEF1 binding is important for T cell specific enhancers of genes for T cell receptor-CD3 subunits. *Nucleic Acids Res.* **20,** 6495–6499.
6. Ogawa, E., Maruyama, M., Kagoshima, H., Inuzuka, M., Lu, J., Satake, M., Shigesada, K., and Ito, Y. (1993) PEBP2/PEA2 represents a family of transcription factors homologous to the products of the *Drosophila* runt gene and the human *AML1* gene. *Proc. Natl. Acad. Sci. USA* **90,** 6859–6863.
7. Brandle, D., Muller, S., Muller, C., Hengartner, H., and Pircher, H. (1994) Regulation of RAG-1 and CD69 expression in the thymus during positive and negative selection. *Eur. J. Immunol.* **24,** 145–151.
8. Brown, S. T., Miranda, G. A., Galic, Z., Hartman, I. Z., Lyon, C. J., and Aguilera, R. J. (1997) Regulation of the RAG-1 promoter by the NF-Y transcription factor. *J. Immunol.* **158,** 5071–5074.
9. Ernst, P., Hahm, K., Trinh, L., Davis, J. N., Roussel, M. F., Turck, C. W., and Smale, S. T. (1996) A potential role for Elf-1 in terminal transferase gene regulation. *Mol. Cell. Biol.* **16,** 6121–6131.
10. Schatz, D. G., Oettinger, M. A., and Schlissel, M. S. (1992) V(D)J recombination, molecular biology and regulation. *Annu. Rev. Immunol.* **10,** 359–383.
11. Willerford, D. M., Swat, W., and Alt, F. W. (1996) Developmental regulation of V(D)J recombination and lymphocyte differentiation. *Curr. Opin. Gen. Devel.* **6,** 603–609.
12. Biassoni, R., Verdiani, S., Cambiaggi, A., Romeo, P.-H., Ferrini, S., and Moretta, L. (1993) Human $CD3^-CD16^+$ natural killer cells express the hGATA-3 T cell transcription factor and an unrearranged 2.3-kb TcR δ transcript. *Eur. J. Immunol.* **23,** 1083–1087.
13. Furley, A. J., Chan, L. C., Mizutani, S., Ford, A. M., Weilbaecher, K., Pegram, S. M., and Greaves, M. F. (1987) Lineage specificity of rearrangement and expression of genes encoding the T cell receptor-T3 complex and immunoglobulin heavy chain in leukemia. *Leukemia* **1,** 644–652.
14. Greenberg, J. M., Quertermous, T., Seidman, J. G., and Kersey, J. H. (1986) Human T cell γ-chain gene rearrangements in acute lymphoid and nonlymphoid leukemia: comparison with the T cell receptor β-chain gene. *J. Immunol.* **137,** 2043–2049.
15. Siden, E. J. (1993) Regulated expression of germline antigen receptor genes in mast cell lines from the murine embryo. *J. Immunol.* **150,** 4427–4437.
16. Soloff, R. S. K., Wang, T.-G., Lybarger, L., Dempsey, D., and Chervenak, R. (1995) Transcription of the TCR-β locus initiates in adult murine bone marrow. *J. Immunol.* **154,** 3888–3901.
17. Giese, K., Kingsley, C., Kirshner, J. R., and Grosschedl, R. (1995) Assembly and function of a TCRα enhancer complex is dependent on LEF-1-induced DNA bending and multiple protein-protein interactions. *Genes Dev.* **9,** 995–1008.
18. Henderson, A. J., McDougall, S., Leiden, J., and Calame, K. L. (1994) GATA elements are necessary for the activity and tissue specificity of the T-cell receptor β-chain transcriptional enhancer. *Mol. Cell. Biol.* **14,** 4286–4294.
19. Hernandez-Munain, C. and Krangel, M. S. (1994) Regulation of the T-cell receptor δ enhancer by functional cooperation between c-Myb and core-binding factors. *Mol. Cell. Biol.* **14,** 473–483.
20. Hsiang, Y. H., Spencer, D., Wang, S., Speck, N. A., and Raulet, D. H. (1993) The role of viral enhancer "core" motif-related sequences in regulating T cell receptor-γ and -δ gene expression. *J. Immunol.* **150,** 3905–3916.

21. Leiden, J. M. (1993) Transcriptional regulation of T cell receptor genes. *Ann. Rev. Immunol.* **11,** 539–570.
22. Hsiang, Y. H., Goldman, J. P., and Raulet, D. H. (1995) The role of c-Myb or a related factor in regulating the T cell receptor γ gene enhancer. *J. Immunol.* **154,** 5195–5204.
23. Wotton, D., Ghysdael, J., Wang, S., Speck, N. A., and Owen, M. J. (1994) Cooperative binding of Ets-1 and core binding factor to DNA. *Mol. Cell. Biol.* **14,** 840–850.
24. Bruno, L., Rocha, B., Rolink, A., von Boehmer, H., and Rodewald, H.-R. (1995) Intra- and extra-thymic expression of the pre-T cell receptor α gene. *Eur. J. Immunol.* **25,** 1877–1882.
25. Saint-Ruf, C., Ungewiss, K., Groettrup, L. B., Fehling, H. J., and von Boehmer, H. (1994) Analysis and expression of a cloned pre-T cell receptor gene. *Science* **266,** 1208–1212.
26. Nagishi, I., Motoyama, N., Nakayama, K.-I., Nakayama, K., Senju, S., Hatakeyama, S., Zhang, Q., Chan, A. C., and Loh, D. Y. (1995) Essential role for ZAP-70 in both positive and negative selection of thymocytes. *Nature* **376,** 435–438.
27. Wallace, V. A., Kawai, K., Levelt, C. N., Kishihara, K., Molina, T., Timms, E., Pircher, H., Penninger, J., Ohashi, P. S., Eichmann, K., and Mak, T. W. (1995) T lymphocyte development in p56lck deficient mice: allelic exclusion of the TcR β locus is incomplete but thymocyte development is not restored by TcR β or TcR αβ transgenes. *Eur. J. Immunol.* **25,** 1312–1318.
28. Biondi, A., Paganin, C., Rossi, V., Benvestito, S., Perlmutter, R. M., Mantovani, A., and Allavena, P. (1991) Expression of lineage-restricted protein tyrosine kinase genes in human natural killer cells. *Eur. J. Immunol.* **21,** 843–846.
29. Chan, A. C., Iwashima, M., Turck, C. W., and Weiss, A. (1992) ZAP-70, a 70 kd protein-tyrosine kinase that associates with the TCR ζ chain. *Cell* **71,** 649–662.
30. Perlmutter, R. M., Marth, J. D., Lewis, D. B., Peet, R., Ziegler, S. F., and Wilson, C. B. (1988) Structure and expression of lck transcripts in human lymphoid cells. *J. Cell. Biochem.* **38,** 117–126.
31. Anderson, S. J., Levin, S. D., and Perlmutter, R. M. (1993) Protein tyrosine kinase $p56^{lck}$ controls allelic exclusion of T-cell receptor β-chain genes. *Nature* **365,** 552–554.
32. Hattori, N., Kawamoto, H., and Katsura, Y. (1996) Isolation of the most immature population of murine fetal thymocytes that includes progenitors capable of generating T, B, and myeloid cells. *J. Exp. Med.* **184,** 1901–1908.
33. Allen, J. M., Forbush, K. A., and Perlmutter, R. M. (1992) Functional dissection of the *lck* proximal promoter. *Mol. Cell. Biol.* **12,** 2758–2768.
33a. McCracken, S., Leung, S., Bosselut, R., Ghysdael, J., and Miyamoto, N. G. (1994) Myb and Ets transcription factors are required for activity of the human lck type I promoter. *Oncogene* **9,** 3609–3615.
34. Jain, J., Loh, C., and Rao, A. (1995) Transcriptional regulation of the IL2 gene. *Curr. Opin. Immunol.* **7,** 333–342.
35. Rothenberg, E. V. and Ward, S. B. (1996) A dynamic assembly of diverse transcription factors integrates activation and cell-type information for interleukin-2 gene regulation. *Proc. Natl. Acad. Sci. USA* **93,** 9358–9365.
36. Serfling, E., Avots, A., and Neumann, M. (1995) The architecture of the interleukin-2 promoter: a reflection of T lymphocyte activation. *Biochem. Biophys. Acta* **1263,** 181–200.
37. Avots, A., Hoffmeyer, A., Flory, E., Cimanis, A., Rapp, U. R., and Serfling, E. (1997) GABP factors bind to a distal interleukin 2 (IL-2) enhancer and contribute to c-Raf-mediated increase in IL-2 induction. *Mol. Cell. Biol.* **17,** 4381–4389.
38. Brown, M. A. and Hural, J. (1997) Functions of IL-4 and control of its expression. *Crit. Rev. Immunol.* **17,** 1–32.
39. Chuvpilo, S., Schomberg, C., Gerwig, R., Heinfling, A., Reeves, R., Grummt, F., and Serfling, E. (1993) Multiple closely-linked NFAT/octamer and HMG I(Y) binding sites are part of the interleukin-4 promoter. *Nucl. Acids Res.* **21,** 5694–5704.
40. Rooney, J. W., Hoey, T., and Glimcher, L. H. (1995) Coordinate and cooperative roles for NF-AT and AP-1 in the regulation of the murine IL-4 gene. *Immunity* **2,** 473–483.
41. Szabo, S. J., Gold, J. S., Murphy, T. L., and Murphy, K. M. (1993) Identification of cis-acting regulatory elements controlling interleukin-4 gene expression in T cells: roles for NF-Y and NF-ATc. *Mol. Cell. Biol.* **13,** 4793–4805.
42. Ho, I.-C., Hodge, M. R., Rooney, J. W., and Glimcher, L. H. (1996) The proto-oncogene c-maf is responsible for tissue-specific expression of interleukin-4. *Cell* **85,** 973–983.

43. Li-Weber, M., Krafft, H., and Krammer, P. H. (1993) A novel enhancer element in the human IL-4 promoter is suppressed by a position-independent silencer. *J. Immunol.* **151,** 1371–1382.
44. Li-Weber, M., Salgame, P., Hu, C., Davydov, I. V., and Krammer, P. H. (1997) Differential interaction of nuclear factors with the PRE-I enhancer element of the human IL-4 promoter in different T cell subsets. *J. Immunol.* **158,** 1194–1200.
45. Zheng, W.-P. and Flavell, R. A. (1997) The transcription factor GATA-3 is necessary and sufficient for Th2 cytokine gene expression in CD4 cells. *Cell* **89,** 587–596.
46. Horta, M. D., Fu, K. C., Koizumi, H., Young, J. D., and Liu, C. C. (1996) Cell-free conversion of a ubiquitous nuclear protein into a killer-cell-specific form that binds to the NF-P enhancer element in the mouse perforin gene. *Eur. J. Biochem.* **238,** 639–646.
47. Lichtenheld, M. G. and Podack, E. R. (1992) Structure and function of the murine perforin promoter and upstream region. Reciprocal gene activation or silencing in perforin positive and negative cells. *J. Immunol.* **149,** 2619–2626.
48. Lichtenheld, M. G., Podack, E. R., and Levy, R. B. (1995) Transgenic control of perforin gene expression. *J. Immunol.* **154,** 2153–2163.
49. Youn, B. S., Kim, K. K., and Kwon, B. S. (1996) A critical role of Sp1- and Ets-related transcription factors in maintaining CTL-specific expression of the mouse perforin gene. *J. Immunol.* **157,** 3499–3509.
50. Zhang, Y. and Lichtenheld, M. G. (1997) Non-killer cell-specific transcription factors silence the perforin promoter. *J. Immunol.* **158,** 1734–1741.
51. Lynch, D. H., Ramsdell, F., and Alderson, M. R. (1995) Fas and FasL in the homeostatic regulation of immune responses. *Immunol. Today* **16,** 569–574.
52. Waterhouse, P., Penninger, J. M., Timms, E., Wakeham, A., Shahinian, A., Lee, K. P., Thompson, C. B., Griesser, H., and Mak, T. W. (1995) Lymphoproliferative disorders with early lethality in mice deficient in *Ctla-4*. *Science* **270,** 985–988.
53. Morrison, S. J., Prowse, K. R., Ho, P., and Weissman, I. L. (1996) Telomerase activity in hematopoietic cells is associated with self-renewal potential. *Immunity* **5,** 207–216.
54. Weng, N. P., Levine, B. L., June, C. H., and Hodes, R. J. (1996) Regulated expression of telomerase activity in human T lymphocyte development and activation. *J. Exp. Med.* **183,** 2471–2479.
55. Carè, A., Testa, U., Bassani, A., Tritarelli, E., Montesoro, E., Samoggia, P., Cianetti, L., and Peschle, C. (1994) Coordinate expression and proliferative role of HOXB genes in activated adult T lymphocytes. *Mol. Cell. Biol.* **14,** 4872–4877.
56. Helgason, C. D., Sauvageau, G., Lawrence, H. J., Largman, C., and Humphries, R. K. (1996) Overexpression of HOXB4 enhances the hematopoietic potential of embryonic stem cells differentiated in vitro. *Blood* **87,** 2740–2749.
57. Sauvageau, G., Thorsteinsdottir, U., Eaves, C. J., Lawrence, H. J., Largman, C., Lansdorp, P. M., and Humphries, R. K. (1995) Overexpression of HOXB4 in hematopoietic cells causes the selective expansion of more primitive populations in vitro and in vivo. *Genes Dev.* **9,** 1753–1765.
58. Candéias, S., Muegge, K., and Durum, S. K. (1997) IL-7 receptor and VDJ recombination: trophic versus mechanistic actions. *Immunity* **6,** 501–508.
59. Rodewald, H.-R., Ogawa, M., Haller, C., Waskow, C., and DiSanto, J. P. (1997) Pro-thymocyte expansion by c-kit and the common cytokine receptor γ chain is essential for repertoire formation. *Immunity* **6,** 265–272.
60. Kingston, R., Jenkinson, E. J., and Owen, J. J. T. (1985) A single stem cell can recolonize an embryonic thymus, producing phenotypically distinct T-cell populations. *Nature* **317,** 811–813.
61. Godfrey, D. I. and Zlotnik, A. (1993) Control points in early T-cell development. *Immunol. Today* **14,** 547–553.
62. Shortman, K. and Wu, L. (1996) Early T lymphocyte progenitors. *Annu. Rev. Immunol.* **14,** 29–47.
63. Diamond, R. A., Ward, S. B., Owada-Makabe, K., Wang, H., and Rothenberg, E. V. (1997) Different developmental arrest points in $RAG2^{-/-}$ and scid thymocytes on two genetic backgrounds: developmental choices and cell death mechanisms before TCR gene rearrangement. *J. Immunol.* **158,** 4052–4064.
64. Wang, H., Diamond, R. A., and Rothenberg, E. V. (1997) Cross-lineage expression of Ig-β (B29) in thymocytes: positive and negative gene regulation to establish T-cell identity, submitted.

65. Moore, T. A. and Zlotnik, A. (1995) T-lineage commitment and cytokine responses of thymic progenitors. *Blood* **86,** 1850–1860.
66. Zúñiga-Pflücker, J. C. and Lenardo, M. J. (1996) Regulation of thymocyte development from immature progenitors. *Curr. Opin. Immunol.* **8,** 215–224.
67. Godfrey, D. I., Kennedy, J., Mombaerts, P., Tonegawa, S., and Zlotnik, A. (1994) Onset of TCR-β gene rearrangement and role of TCR-β expression during CD3-CD4-CD8- thymocyte differentiation. *J. Immunol.* **152,** 4783–4792.
68. Ismaili, J., Antica, M., and Wu, L. (1996) CD4 and CD8 expression and T cell antigen receptor gene rearrangement in early thymic precursor cells. *Eur. J. Immunol.* **26,** 731–737.
69. Petrie, H. T., Livak, F., Burtrum, D., and Mazel, S. (1995) T cell receptor gene recombination patterns and mechanisms: cell death, rescue, and T cell production. *J. Exp. Med.* **182,** 121–127.
70. Candéias, S., Hardy, R. R., Li, Y. S., and Staerz, U. D. (1994) T cell receptor Vβ8.2 gene germline transcription: an early event of lymphocyte differentiation. *Eur. J. Immunol.* **24,** 3073–3081.
71. Rothenberg, E. V., Chen, D., and Diamond, R. A. (1993) Functional and phenotypic analysis of thymocytes in SCID mice: evidence for functional response transitions before and after the SCID arrest point. *J. Immunol.* **151,** 3530–3546.
72. Davidson, E. H. (1990). How embryos work: a comparative view of diverse modes of cell fate specification. *Development* **108,** 365–389.
73. Spangrude, G. J. and Scollay, R. (1990) Differentiation of hematopoietic stem cells in irradiated mouse thymic lobes: kinetics and phenotype of progeny. *J. Immunol.* **145,** 3661–3668.
74. Ardavin, C., Wu, L., Li, C. L., and Shortman, K. (1993) Thymic dendritic cells and T cells develop simultaneously in the thymus from a common precursor population. *Nature* **362,** 761–763.
75. Matsuzaki, Y., Gyotoku, J.-I., Ogawa, M., Nishikawa, S.-I., Katsura, Y., Gachelin, G., and Nakauchi, H. (1993) Characterization of c-kit positive intrathymic stem cells that are restricted to lymphoid differentiation. *J. Exp. Med.* **178,** 1283–1292.
76. Rodewald, H.-R., Moingeon, P., Lucich, J. L., Dosiou, C., Lopez, P., and Reinherz, E. L. (1992) A population of early fetal thymocytes expressing FcgammaRII/III contains precursors of T lymphocytes and natural killer cells. *Cell* **69,** 139–150.
77. Wu, L., Antica, M., Johnson, G. R., Scollay, R., and Shortman, K. (1991) Developmental potential of the earliest precursor cells from the adult mouse thymus. *J. Exp. Med.* **174,** 1617–1627.
78. Wu, L., Li, C.-L., and Shortman, K. (1996) Thymic dendritic cell precursors: relationship to the T lymphocyte lineage and phenotype of the dendritic cell progeny. *J. Exp. Med.* **184,** 903–911.
79. Zúñiga-Pflücker, J. C., Jiang, D., and Lenardo, M. J. (1995) Requirement for TNF-α and IL-1α in fetal thymocyte commitment and differentiation. *Science* **268,** 1906–1909.
80. Kawamoto, H., Ohmura, K., and Katsura, Y. (1997) Direct evidence for the commitment of hematopoietic stem cells to T, B, and myeloid lineages in murine fetal liver. *Int. Immunol.* **9,** 1011–1019.
81. Rodewald, H. R., Kretzschmar, K., Takeda, S., Hohl, C., and Dessing, M. (1994) Identification of pro-thymocytes in murine fetal blood: T lineage commitment can precede thymus colonization. *EMBO J.* **13,** 4229–4240.
82. Spits, H., Lanier, L. L., and Phillips, J. H. (1995) Development of human T and natural killer cells. *Blood* **85,** 2654–2670.
83. Morrison, S. J., Shah, N. M., and Anderson, D. J. (1997) Regulatory mechanisms in stem cell biology. *Cell* **88,** 287–298.
84. Res, P., Martinez-Caceres, E., Jaleco, A. C., Staal, F., Noteboom, E., Weijer, K., and Spits, H. (1996) $CD34^+$ $CD38^{dim}$ cells in the human thymus can differentiate into T, natural killer, and dendritic cells but are distinct from pluripotent stem cells. *Blood* **87,** 5196–5206.
85. Sanchez, M. J., Muench, M. O., Roncarolo, M. G., Lanier, L. L., and Phillips, J. H. (1994) Identification of a common T/natural killer cell progenitor in human fetal thymus. *J. Exp. Med.* **180,** 569–576.
86. Wang, J.-H., Nichogiannopoulou, A., Wu, L., Sun, L., Sharpe, A. H., Bigby, M., and Georgopoulos, K. (1996) Selective defects in the development of the fetal and adult lymphoid system in mice with an Ikaros null mutation. *Immunity* 5, 537–549.

87. Borrello, M. A. and Phipps, R. P. (1996) The B/macrophage cell: an elusive link between CD5+ B lymphocytes and macrophages. *Immunol. Today* **17,** 471–475.
88. Cumano, A., Paige, C. J., Iscove, N. N., and Brady, G. (1992) Bipotential precursors of B cells and macrophages in murine fetal liver. *Nature* **356,** 612–615.
89. Cross, M. A., Heyworth, C. M., Murrell, A. M., Bockamp, E. O., Dexter, T. M., and Green, A. R. (1994) Expression of lineage restricted transcription factors precedes lineage specific differentiation in a multipotent haemopoietic progenitor cell line. *Oncogene* **9,** 3013–3016.
90. Hu, M., Krause, D., Greaves, M., Sharkis, S., Dexter, M., Heyworth, C., and Enver, T. (1997) Multilineage gene expression precedes commitment in the hemopoietic system. *Genes Dev.* **11,** 774–785.
91. Sposi, N. M., Zon, L. I., Carè, A., Valtieri, M., Testa, U., Gabbianelli, M., Mariani, G., Bottero, L., Mather, C., Orkin, S. H., and Peschle, C. (1992) Cell cycle-dependent initiation and lineage-dependent abrogation of GATA-1 expression in pure differentiating hematopoietic progenitors. *Proc. Natl. Acad. Sci. USA* **89,** 6353–6357.
92. Blom, B., Res, P., Noteboom, E., Weijer, K., and Spits, H. (1997) Prethymic CD34$^+$ progenitors capable of developing into T cells are not committed to the T cell lineage. *J. Immunol.* **158,** 3571–3577.
93. McCubrey, J. A., Steelman, L. S., Risser, R. G., and McKearn, J. P. (1989) Structure and expression of the T cell receptor gamma locus in pre-B and early hemopoietic cells. *Eur. J. Immunol.* **19,** 2303–2308.
94. Okada, A., Mendelsohn, M., and Alt, F. (1994) Differential activation of transcription versus recombination of transgenic T cell receptor β variable region gene segments in B and T lineage cells. *J. Exp. Med.* **180,** 261–272.
95. Bassuk, A. G. and Leiden, J. M. (1997) The role of Ets transcription factors in the development and function of the mammalian immune system. *Adv. Immunol.* **64,** 65–104.
96. Bockamp, E.-O., McLaughlin, F., Murrell, A., and Green, A. R. (1994) Transcription factors and the regulation of haemopoiesis: lessons from GATA and SCL proteins. *BioEssays* **16,** 481–488.
97. Shivdasani, R. A. and Orkin, S. H. (1996) The transcriptional control of hematopoiesis. *Blood* **87,** 4025–4039.
98. Clevers, H. C. and Grosschedl, R. (1996) Transcriptional control of lymphoid development, lessons from gene targeting. *Immunol. Today* **17,** 336–343.
99. Clevers, H. C., Oosterwegel, M. A., and Georgopoulos, K. (1993) Transcription factors in early T-cell development. *Immunol. Today* **14,** 591–596.
100. Fitzsimmons, D. and Hagman, J. (1996) Regulation of gene expression at early stages of B-cell and T-cell differentiation. *Curr. Opin. Immunol.* **8,** 166–174.
101. Singh, H. (1996) Gene targeting reveals a hierarchy of transcription factors regulating specification of lymphoid cell fates. *Curr. Opin. Immunol.* **8,** 160–165.
102. Okuda, T., van Deursen, J., Hiebert, S. W., Grosveld, G., and Downing, J. R. (1996) AML1, the target of multiple chromosomal translocations in human leukemia, is essential for normal fetal liver hematopoiesis. *Cell* **84,** 321–330.
103. Wang, Q., Stacy, T., Binder, M., Marin-Padilla, M., Sharpe, A. H., and Speck, N. A. (1996) Disruption of the *Cbfa2* gene causes necrosis and hemorrhaging in the central nervous system and blocks definitive hematopoiesis. *Proc. Natl. Acad. Sci. USA* **93,** 3444–3449.
104. Pandolfi, P. P., Roth, M. E., Karis, A., Leonard, M. W., Dzierzak, E., Grosveld, F. G., Engel, J. D., and Lindenbaum, M. H. (1995) Targeted disruption of the *GATA3* gene causes severe abnormalities in the nervous system and in fetal liver haematopoiesis. *Nature Genetics* **11,** 40–44.
105. Schilham, M. W., Oosterwegel, M. A., Moerer, P., Ya, J., de Boer, P. A. J., Van de Wetering, M., Verbeek, S., Lamers, W. H., Kruisbeek, A. M., Cumano, A., and Clevers, H. (1996) Defects in cardiac outflow tract formation and pro-B-lymphocyte expansion in mice lacking Sox-4. *Nature* **380,** 711–714.
106. Verbeek, S., Izon, D., Hofhuis, F., Robanus-Maandag, E., te Riele, H., Van de Wetering, M., Oosterwegel, M., Wilson, A., MacDonald, H. R., and Clevers, H. (1995) An HMG-box-containing T-cell factor required for thymocyte differentiation. *Nature* **374,** 70–74.
107. Baker, S. J. and Reddy, E. P. (1995) B cell differentiation: role of E2A and Pax5/BSAP transcription factors. *Oncogene* **11,** 413–426.

108. Opstelten, D. (1996) B lymphocyte development and transcription regulation in vivo. *Adv. Immunol.* **63,** 197–268.
109. Bain, G., Robanus Maandag, E. C., Izon, D. J., Amsen, D., Kruisbeek, A. M., Weintraub, B. C., Krop, I., Schissel, M. S., Feeney, A. J., van Roon, M., van der Valk, M., te Riele, H. P. J., Berns, A., and Murre, C. (1994) E2A proteins are required for proper B cell development and initiation of immunoglobulin gene rearrangements. *Cell* **79,** 885–892.
110. Lin, H. and Grosschedl, R. (1995) Failure of B-cell differentiation in mice lacking the transcription factor EBF. *Nature* **376,** 263–267.
111. Nutt, S. L., Urbanek, P., Rolink, A., and Busslinger, M. (1997) Essential functions of Pax5 (BSAP) in pro-B cell development: difference between fetal and adult B lymphopoiesis and reduced V-to-DJ recombination at the IgH locus. *Genes Dev.* **11,** 476–491.
112. Urbanek, P., Wang, Z. Q., Fetka, I., Wagner, E. F., and Busslinger, M. (1994) Complete block of early B cell differentiation and altered patterning of the posterior midbrain in mice lacking Pax5/BSAP. *Cell* **79,** 901–912.
113. Zhuang, Y., Soriano, P., and Weintraub, H. (1994) The helix-loop-helix gene E2A is required for B cell formation. *Cell* **79,** 875–884.
114. Zhuang, Y., Cheng, P., and Weintraub, H. (1996) B-lymphocyte development is regulated by the combined dosage of three basic helix-loop-helix genes, *E2A*, *E2-2*, and *HEB*. *Mol. Cell. Biol.* **16,** 2898–2905.
115. Morgan, B., Sun, L., Avitahl, N., Andrikopoulos, K., Ikeda, T., Gonzales, E., Wu, P., Neben, S., and Georgopoulos, K. (1997) Aiolos, a lymphoid restricted transcription factor that interacts with Ikaros to regulate lymphocyte differentiation. *EMBO J.* **16,** 2004–2013.
116. Bain, B., Engel, I., Robanus Maandag, E. C., te Riele, H. P., Voland, J. R., Sharp, L. L., Chun, J., Huey, B., Pinkel, D., and Murre, C. (1997) E2A deficiency leads to abnormalities in T-cell development and to rapid development of T-cell lymphomas. *Mol. Cell. Biol.* **17,** 4782–4791.
117. Schilham, M. W., Moerer, P., Cumano, A., and Clevers, H. C. (1997) Sox-4 facilitates thymocyte differentiation. *Eur. J. Immunol.* **27,** 1292–1295.
118. Hattori, N., Kawamoto, H., Fujimoto, S., Kuno, K., and Katsura, Y. (1996) Involvement of transcription factors TCF-1 and GATA-3 in the initiation of the earliest step of T cell development in the thymus. *J. Exp. Med.* **184,** 1137–1147.
119. Ting, C.-N., Olson, M. C., Barton, K. P., and Leiden, J. M. (1996) Transcription factor GATA-3 is required for development of the T-cell lineage. *Nature* **384,** 474–478.
120. Zúñiga-Pflücker, J. C., Schwartz, H. L., and Lenardo, M. J. (1993) Gene transcription in differentiating immature T cell receptor^{neg} thymocytes resembles antigen-activated mature T cells. *J. Exp. Med.* **178,** 1139–1149.
121. Mombaerts, P., Clarke, A. R., Rudnicki, M. A., Iacomini, J., Itohara, S., Lafaille, J. J., Wang, L., Ichikawa, Y., Jaenisch, R., Hooper, M. L., and Tonegawa, S. (1992) Mutations in T-cell antigen receptor genes α and β block thymocyte development at different stages. *Nature* **360,** 225–231.
122. Dubart, A., Romeo, P. H., Vainchenker, W., and Dumenil, D. (1996) Constitutive expression of GATA-1 interferes with the cell-cycle regulation. *Blood* **87,** 3711–3721.
123. Weiss, M. J. and Orkin, S. H. (1995) Transcription factor GATA-1 permits survival and maturation of erythroid precursors by preventing apoptosis. *Proc. Natl. Acad. Sci. USA* **92,** 9623–9627.
124. Barton, K., Muthusamy, N., Chanyangam, M., Fischer, C., Clendenin, C., and Leiden, J. M. (1996) Defective thymocyte proliferation and IL-2 production in transgenic mice expressing a dominant-negative form of CREB. *Nature* **379,** 81–85.
125. Clausell, A. and Tucker, P. W. (1994) Functional analysis of the Vγ3 promoter of the murine $\gamma\delta$ T-cell receptor. *Mol. Cell. Biol.* **14,** 803–814.
126. Clevers, H. C., Dunlap, S., Wileman, T. E., and Terhorst, C. (1988) Human CD3-ε gene contains three miniexons and is transcribed from a non-TATA promoter. *Proc. Natl. Acad. Sci. USA* **85,** 8156–8160.
127. Hambor, J. E., Mennone, J., Coon, M. E., Hanke, J. H., and Kavathas, P. (1993) Identification and characterization of an Alu-containing, T-cell-specific enhancer located in the last intron of the human CD8α gene. *Mol. Cell. Biol.* **13,** 7056–7070.

128. Hernandez-Munain, C., Lauzurica, P., and Krangel, M. S. (1996) Regulation of T cell receptor δ gene rearrangement by c-Myb. *J. Exp. Med.* **183,** 289–293.
129. Hummler, C., Cole, T. J., Blendy, J. A., Ganss, R., Aguzzi, A., Schmid, W., Beermann, F., and Schutz, G. (1994) Targeted mutation of the CREB gene: compensation within the CREB/ATF family of transcription factors. *Proc. Natl. Acad. Sci. USA* **91,** 5647–5651.
130. Lauzurica, P., Zhong, X.-P., Krangel, M. S., and Roberts, J. L. (1997) Regulation of T cell receptor δ gene rearrangement by CBF/PEBP2. *J. Exp. Med.* **185,** 1193–1201.
131. Oosterwegel, M., Van de Wetering, M., and Clevers, H. (1993) HMG box proteins in early T-cell differentiation. *Thymus* **22,** 67–81.
132. Punturieri, A., Shirakata, Y., Bovolenta, C., Kikuchi, G., and Coligan, J. E. (1993) Multiple cis-acting elements are required for proper transcription of the mouse Vδ1 T cell receptor promoter. *J. Immunol.* **150,** 139–150.
133. Salomoni, P., Perrotti, D., Martinez, R., Franceschi, C., and Calabretta, B. (1997) Resistance to apoptosis in CTLL-2 cells constitutively expressing c-Myb is associated with induction of BCL-2 expression and Myb-dependent regulation of *bcl-2* promoter activity. *Proc. Natl. Acad. Sci. USA* **94,** 3296–3301.
134. Wotton, D., Lake, R. A., Farr, C. J., and Owen, M. J. (1995) The high mobility group transcription factor, SOX4, transactivates the human CD2 enhancer. *J. Biol. Chem.* **270,** 7515–7522.
135. Yamada, T., Hitomi, Y., Satake, M., and Oikawa, T. (1995) Differential expression of the T cell receptor/CD3 genes and their lymphoid-specific transcription factor genes in murine T cell x fibroblast and T cell x B cell hybrids. *Eur. J. Immunol.* **25,** 2710–2713.
136. Yang, L., Lanier, E. R., and Kraig, E. (1997) Identification of a novel, spliced variant of CREB that is preferentially expressed in the thymus. *J. Immunol.* **158,** 2522–2525.
137. Carlyle, J. R., Michie, A. M., Furlonger, C., Nakano, T., Lenardo, M. J., Paige, C. J., and Zúñiga-Pflücker, J. C. (1997) Identification of a novel developmental stage marking lineage commitment of progenitor thymocytes. *J. Exp. Med.* **186,** 173–182.
138. Leclercq, G., Debacker, V., De Smedt, M., and Plum, J. (1996) Differential effects of interleukin-15 and interleukin-2 on differentiation of bipotential T/natural killer progenitor cells. *J. Exp. Med.* **184,** 325–336.
139. Rothenberg, E. V., Diamond, R. A., Pepper, K. A., and Yang, J. A. (1990) Interleukin-2 gene inducibility in T cells prior to T-cell receptor expression: changes in signaling pathways and gene expression requirements during intrathymic maturation. *J. Immunol.* **144,** 1614–1624.

Chapter 19

The $\alpha\beta/\gamma\delta$ Lineage Decision

An Evaluation of the "T-Cell Receptor Determinant," "Progenitor Precommitment," or "Codeterminant" Models

Eric S. Hoffman, Lorena Passoni, Erastus C. Dudley, Michael Girardi, and Adrian Hayday

1. Introduction

An accident of molecular biology in 1984 *(1,2)* prefaced a roundly unanticipated fact, that vertebrates make two sets of qualitatively distinct T-cells: $\alpha\beta$ T-cells and $\gamma\delta$ T-cells *(3)*. There are many differences between these cell types, most notably in the antigen receptors that define them. Whereas $\alpha\beta$ T-cell receptors (TCRs) mostly recognize complexes of antigenic peptide and major histocompatibility complex (MHC) molecules, $\gamma\delta$TCRs recognize a spectrum of cell-associated antigens which seems as diverse as the antigen specificity of immunoglobulins *(4)*. Moreover, in mice lacking Syk kinase, sets of $\gamma\delta$ cells fail to develop, like B-cells, whereas $\alpha\beta$ T-cell development progresses apparently normally *(5,6)*. These observations suggest that $\gamma\delta$ cells and $\alpha\beta$ T-cells are extremely different, and likely to arise from progenitor cells that diverge early during lymphopoiesis. Conversely, there is an obligatory association of TCR$\gamma\delta$ and TCR$\alpha\beta$ with the polypeptide complex, CD3, that has been used as the defining feature of T-cells. Additionally, many (possibly most) $\gamma\delta$ cells arise from the thymus *(7,8)*. By these criteria, $\gamma\delta$ cells and $\alpha\beta$ T-cells may be sisters, arising from a late lineage decision of a common intrathymic precursor.

By now, several experiments and a volume of speculation have been directed at distinguishing between these two possibilities for the divergence of the $\alpha\beta$ and $\gamma\delta$ lineages. This review will summarize that speculation and review the findings of the relevant experiments. Although complete resolution of the issue is not yet at hand, the experimental data place clear constraints on models of lineage commitment. For example, in both humans and in mice, it now seems clear, that the fate of a T-cell progenitor is

From: *Molecular Biology of B-Cell and T-Cell Development*
Edited by: J. G. Monroe and E. V. Rothenberg © Humana Press Inc., Totowa, NJ

rapidly influenced by the nature of the T-cell receptor rearrangements successfully completed. Interestingly, this competition over a cell's fate may be between "complete TCRs," namely αβ or γδ, and "incomplete TCRs," namely the preTCR.

Nonetheless, the authors also conclude that none of the available data answer the fundamental question; do peripheral lymphoid γδ cells and peripheral lymphoid αβ T-cells derive from distinct or from common thymic progenitors? Hence, some attention is paid at the end of this chapter to future experiments that might clarify this issue.

2. Thymic Origins of γδ Cells and αβ T-Cells

Although γδ cells are distributed throughout the body's tissues, there is evidence to indicate that most originate in the thymus *(7,8)*. For example, athymic nude mice show complete depletion of epidermal γδ cells, significant depletion of spleen and lymph node γδ cells, and partial depletion of intestinal γδ cells *(9)*. Additionally, cells with inframe γδ TCR gene rearrangements can be found in the thymus throughout development, and adoptive transfer of a fetal thymus from an euthymic mouse will reconstitute epidermal γδ cells in nude mice *(10,11)*. Indeed, γδ cells that will seek the skin are apparently the first thymocytes to complete maturation in the mouse, closely followed by γδ cells that will seek the genital epithelium and tongue *(11,12)*. As would be expected, fluorescence-labeled γδ cells can be detected in the peripheral lymphoid organs of mice in which fluorescein isothiocyanate (FITC) has been injected intrathymically *(13)*. Given that many, possibly most, murine γδ cells derive from progenitors in the thymus, the issue arises as to how thymocytes give rise to two cell types: γδ T-cells and αβ T-cells.

3. Precedents for Lineage Commitment Decisions

The resolution of the γδ/αβ lineage commitment issue might be aided by the scrutiny of other developmental systems in which two distinct cell types arise from seemingly a single pool of precursors. For example, the development of oligodendrocytes and type 2 astrocytes from a single (O-2A) precursor in the rat optic nerve *(14)*. This system has illustrated the important interplay of a progenitor cell's intrinsic biological clock with its responsiveness to external growth and differentiation factors. Thus, if the O-2A is cultured in vitro, it will prematurely differentiate as an oligodendrocyte. By contrast, provision of platelet derived growth factor from Type I astrocytes maintains O-2A proliferation, and the cell differentiates as an oligodendrocyte according to an intrinsic clock that mimics the differentiation schedule seen in vivo. However, provision to the culture of ciliary neurotrophic factor, also from Type I astrocytes, provokes differentiation as a Type 2 astrocyte. In short, the fate of a bipotential precursor is both determined and scheduled by a dynamic balance of external factors and an intrinsic biological clock. This would seem a plausible scenario for the commitment of a common thymocyte progenitor toward an αβ(+) or a γδ(+) fate.

Equally interesting concepts have followed from the study of the development of neuronal and epidermal cells in the *Drosophila* nervous system *(15)*. This developmental system revealed the *Notch* pathway, and the critical role of interactions among equivalent progenitor cells. Thus, if cell A adopts fate X, this precludes cell B from adopting fate X, leaving it instead to adopt an alternative or default fate. In the development of the fly photoreceptor (reviewed in ref. *16*), the communication is slightly different: the first progenitor cell to adopt a specific fate, then actively instructs the fate of its neighboring progenitor. By extrapolation, the commitment of one thymocyte to a γδ(+) fate might significantly influence whether or not a neighboring progenitor cell can commit to the same fate.

Additional lessons may be available within the immune system itself: for example, the development of CD4$^+$ CD8$^-$ αβ T-cells and CD8$^+$ CD4$^-$ αβ T-cells from a CD4$^+$ CD8$^+$ ("DP") precursor population. The authors have come to appreciate this as an example of fate determined by avidity of ligand-cell receptor interactions *(17–19)*. Classic precedent for this concept lies in the different fates adopted by cells at different points on a gradient of morphogen, such as *bicoid (20)*.

Not withstanding the value of these parallels, the mechanism determining the two primary axes of polarity of the fly embryo (anterior-posterior and dorsal-ventral) are significantly different from each other *(20,21)*; moreover, although both mechanisms are utilized in vertebrates, neither determine polarity. Thus, it becomes difficult to predict what known mechanism will apply to a particular developmental pathway. Likewise, little help is available from old "rules;" for example, progenitors in vertebrates remain plastic whereas those in invertebrates show early precommitment. It has become clear that both paradigms are utilized across the phyla.

Furthermore, although there are components that seem common to many developmental transitions, among them *Notch* and *ras*, it is unclear, by the very fact of their ubiquitous expression that these molecules confer specificity. More likely, perhaps, they act as "permissive factors" required for cells to be able to respond to specific "instructive signals," the nature of which is in most cases not elucidated. The identity of such instructive signals is the critical issue in understanding the αβ/γδ lineage decision, and in particular, whether or not part of the instructive signaling is provided by products of successful T-cell receptor gene rearrangement.

In considering the development of αβ(+) versus γδ(+) T-cells, one should recognize from the outset that there is likely to be more than one pathway. For example, in B-cell development, most, but not all progenitors rearrange their heavy chain genes before their light chain genes *(22)*. Likewise, the maturation of most, but not all, B-cells is contingent on the pre–B-cell receptor composed of V-preB, lambda 5, and the immunoglobulin heavy chain *(23,24)*. T-cell development is no exception. For example, it has become clear that normal thymocytes developing in the thymus of a severe combined immunodeficient (SCID) mouse can induce in *trans* the partial maturation of SCID precursors that would otherwise show no developmental potential *(25)*.

Sometimes, such observations are taken to imply a second regulated pathway of development. But they may equally well represent "noise" in the system; "unlikely" developmental decisions might be provoked by low affinity receptor-ligand interactions that happen stochastically when two cells over-expressing the receptor and ligand respectively, are able to interact. Such unlikely events may be important in the development of disease. But their impact on our description of developmental biology has to be carefully considered. Highly manipulated experimental systems, for example, creating T-cell repertoires of a single specificity, seem likely to increase such biological "noise" both greatly and variably. In short, it may not be reasonable to expect a useful working model of development to explain every experimental result. With this in mind, we shall test hypotheses for how γδ cells and αβ T-cells develop, and the potential role(s) played in those events by the products of successful TCR gene rearrangement.

4. Temporal Separation of γδ T-Cell Development and αβ T-Cell Development

There is a potentially simple explanation for γδ/αβ lineage determination, namely that γδ cells develop from distinct progenitors in the thymus prior to the production of αβ

T-cells. The temporal separation of γδ T-cell development and αβ T-cell development is best indicated by the development of murine intraepithelial γδ cell subsets. At least a fraction of the γδ cells that seed the skin (and probably a sizable fraction notwithstanding data for some extrathymic development *[9,26]*) develop from thymocytes that mature at around E16- E17 *(10,11)*. These TCRγδ(+), skin T-cell progenitors are swiftly followed by γδ cells that seed the reproductive epithelium and tongue, all prior to the development of significant numbers of αβ T-cells *(10,12)*. The development of such intraepithelial T-cell repertoires requires fetal hematopoietic stem cells (HSC), a fetal thymic stroma (44, 45), and p72 Syk kinase *(5)*, whereas none of these are required for the development of lymphoid γδ T-cells or αβ T-cells.

These data seem to support the distinct, "precommitted progenitor model," at least for intraepithelial γδ cells, but they do not establish it. For example, the gene rearrangement mechanisms in the fetal thymus may first target particular V(D)J γ and δ segments, probably via activation of germline transcription. If the cells fail to produce in frame Vγ5 and Vδ1 rearrangements (commonly found in skin γδ cells *[4]*), they attempt other γ/δ rearrangements. Indeed, γδ cells that fail to make productive Vγ5 gene rearrangements can successfully rearrange the Vγ6 gene and exit to the reproductive epithelium *(29)*. Because TCR gene rearrangements in the fetus seem to be biased by short regions of V and J DNA sequence homology, and because such homologies in Vγ5, Vγ6, and Jγ1 are so positioned as to favor productive gene rearrangements, the generation of Vγ5-expressing cells and Vγ6-expressing cells may be quite efficient *(30)*. Thus, the fetal progenitors would appear to give rise almost exclusively to γδ cells. Nonetheless, by analogy to the O-2A progenitor, continued failure at Vγ6 and other γ/δ rearrangements might be followed by attempts to rearrange the α and β loci, if the cells' developmental clock is still ticking. In short, it is not clear that the early fetal HSC represent committed γδ cell progenitors.

The components in an early progenitor cell that bias gene rearrangement to particular Vγ and Vδ genes are likely to include chromatin-associated proteins *(31–35)*. The expression of these in early HSC rather then late HSC could be viewed as progenitor precommitment to the γδ phenotype. However, it might also reflect the age of a stem cell; i.e., as the clock ticks, there is an erosion of the balance of factors that bias the developmental outcome toward γδ cells *(14)*. By analogy, factors in αβ T-cell progenitors appear to regulate germline transcription so that rearrangement of 5' Jα elements to 3' Vα elements precedes that of 3' Jα elements to 5' Vα elements *(36)*; nonetheless, the cell is accepted to be a precursor for potentially all αβ T-cells. To clarify whether potent transcription factors confer on progenitors permanent precommitment or merely transient bias, HSC should be examined at the single cell level for the activity of factors such as E-box binding proteins *(31)*. Such studies demand an improved phenotypic description of different progenitor cell stages.

Additionally, the stromal environment can impose apparent limitations on the differentiation potential of early HSC. For example, when fetal liver stem cells were used to reconstitute adult SCID mice, the resultant TCR gene rearrangements showed evidence of high terminal deoxynucleotidyl transferase (TdT) activity, compared with the simple TdT-independent TCR gene rearrangements characteristic of fetal HSC developing in fetal thymi *(37)*. This is an important illustration of apparent progenitor precommitment being attributable to the cell's environment. Indeed, the postnatal thymic stroma has been shown to be nonpermissive for the development of epidermal γδ cells from fetal HSC *(27)*.

Mice rendered transgenic for the skin-associated, Vγ5, Vδ1 genes showed the almost exclusive development of TCR Vγ5Vδ1$^+$ cells, up until approximately two weeks postpartum, when it became apparent that γδ, αβ-double TCR$^+$ cells were developing *(38)*.

These cells are most likely progeny of late HSC. Although they express TCR γδ, they cannot adopt a γδ cell fate. This seemingly supports the idea of temporally distinct HSC, of different developmental potential. However, it is also possible that the complete maturation of TCR Vγ5Vδ1$^+$ cells requires "positive selection" based on engagement of nascent TCRs with some ligand(s) on the stroma. If the expression of this (putative) ligand(s) is downregulated at about two weeks postpartum, the postnatal progenitors will receive no signal that they have γδ potential and may attempt TCRα/β gene rearrangements *(39)*. In reviewing the potential influence of TCR gene expression on the γδ/αβ lineage decision, we remain ignorant of the ligands, if any, that are engaged by nascent TCRs to signal their successful production. Some possibilities are considered in a later section of this article.

In short, it can be difficult to assign progenitor precommitment as the main reason for bias in developmental outcomes, because the development of a cell type depends on an intricate balance of the stem cell potential, selecting elements expressed by the stroma, and the capacity of ligands in the periphery to support the cells' subsequent survival.

5. Spatial Distinction of γδ Cell Development and αβ T-Cell Development

Irrespective of the development of intraepithelial γδ cells, lymphoid γδ cells can be produced postnatally, coincident with the production of αβ T-cells. One straightforward explanation for the separate derivation of lymphoid γδ cells and αβ T-cells would be that γδ cells develop in the thymus in a different subanatomical location than αβ T-cells (i.e., the committed progenitors are physically separated). There are no direct data pertaining to this hypothesis. The γδ cell development can proceed normally in mice in which the thymic structure is highly disorganized, (e.g., in TCRα$^{-/-}$ mice, in which the conventional alignment of the thymic cortex and medulla is severely disrupted) *(40,41)*. However, this may reflect the fact that γδ cell development is completed at an earlier (premedullary) stage of development than is αβ T-cell development. Peripheral γδ cells commonly adopt different microanatomical locations than do αβ T-cells, for example, in the splenic sinusoids *(42)*. However, this is not necessarily of any developmental significance.

6. Coincident Development of γδ Cells and αβ T-Cells from Postnatal Thymocytes

Although lymphoid γδ cells and lymphoid αβ T-cells develop from the thymus at the same time, speculation about the lineage relationship between them was initially colored by the following:

1. The early ontogenetic appearance of intraepithelial γδ cells.
2. The evidence that in postnatal thymocytes, the order of gene rearrangement is δ,γ,β (occurring approximately at the same time), followed by α.
3. The fact that the TCRδ locus lies within the TCRα locus, and is, therefore, deleted by VJα rearrangements.
4. The observation that most γδ cells mature as CD4$^-$, CD8$^-$ "double negative" (DN) cells, akin to an early, intermediate stage in αβ T-cell development.

Together, these considerations led to the "TCR determinant model" *(27,43,44)* (Fig. 1A), in which a common progenitor for γδ cells and αβ T-cells first attempts to become a γδ cell, but, failing productive rearrangement of TCRγ and δ genes, deletes the TCRδ locus in subsequent attempts to become an αβ T-cell (Fig. 2A). Implicit in this progressive rearrangement hypothesis is that the successful recombination of γ and δ genes precludes the αβ T-cell fate, and, under most circumstances, directs a cell toward the γδ fate. (Note

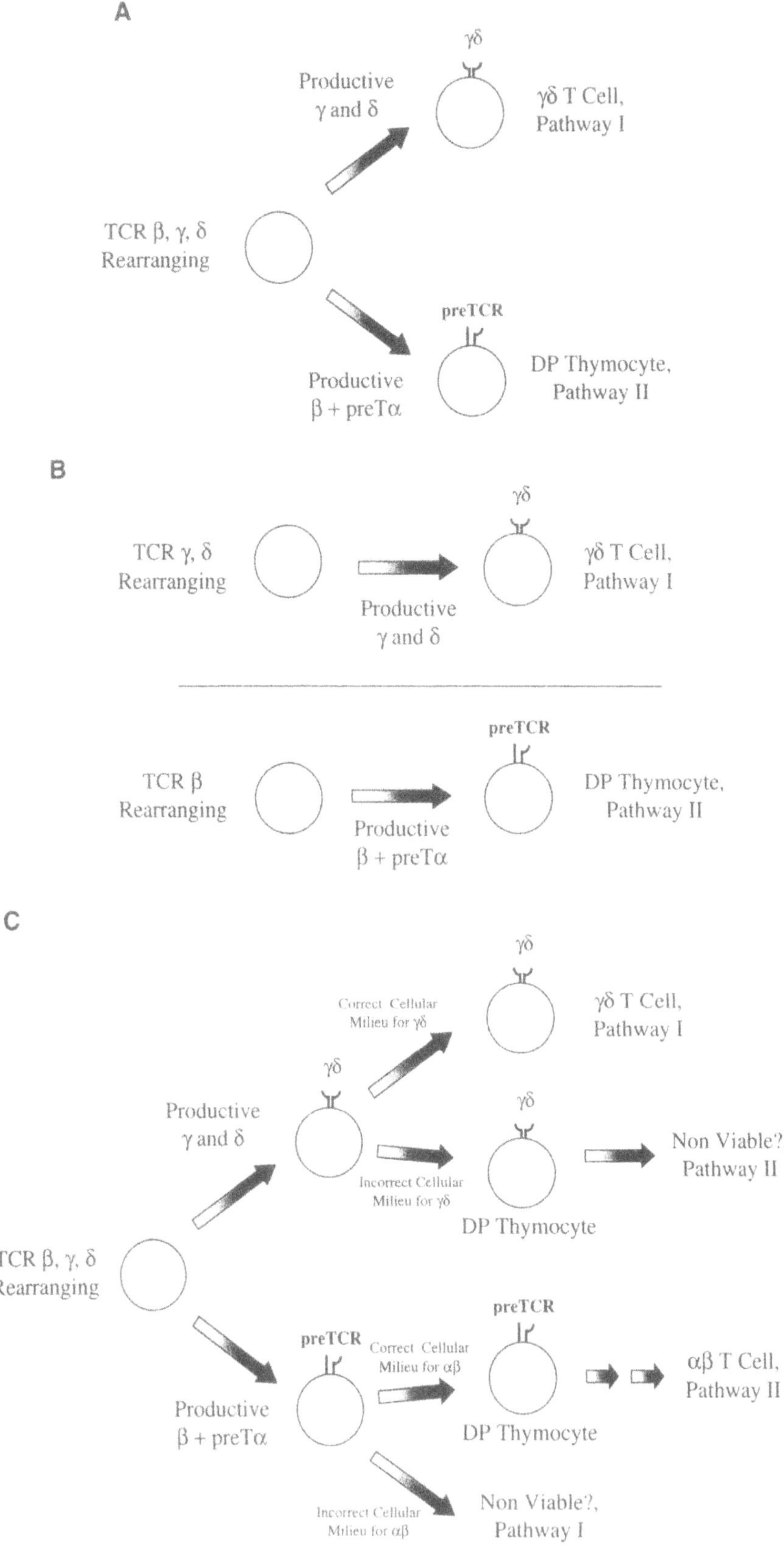
A
γδ
Productive
γ and δ
γδ T Cell,
Pathway I
TCR β, γ, δ
Rearranging
preTCR
Productive
β + preTα
DP Thymocyte,
Pathway II
B
γδ
TCR γ, δ
Rearranging
γδ T Cell,
Pathway I
Productive
γ and δ
preTCR
TCR β
Rearranging
DP Thymocyte,
Pathway II
Productive
β + preTα
C
γδ
Correct Cellular
Milieu for γδ
γδ T Cell,
Pathway I
γδ
γδ
Productive
γ and δ
Non Viable?,
Pathway II
Incorrect Cellular
Milieu for γδ
DP Thymocyte
TCR β, γ, δ
Rearranging
preTCR
preTCR
Correct Cellular
Milieu for αβ
αβ T Cell,
Pathway II
Productive
β + preTα
DP Thymocyte
Incorrect Cellular
Milieu for αβ
Non Viable?,
Pathway I

that in Fig. 1A, γδ cell differentiation is denoted as Pathway I, as proposed by Passoni et al. *[45]*, in recognition of the fact that it is completed earlier and in fewer steps than αβ T-cell differentiation). Likewise, early productive rearrangement of TCRβ chain genes, the products of which can combine with pTα to form a preTCR *(46–48)*, might draw some progenitors away from the γδ(+) fate, directing them instead into Pathway II. The essence of this model is competition: successful γ/δ rearrangements compete with successful β rearrangements to dictate cell fate. As depicted in Fig. 1A, this model is the epitome of the "single lineage" or "common precursor hypothesis."

Alternatively, the "progenitor pre-commitment model" *(45,49)* (Fig. 1B) proposes that precursors are already directed to either an αβ T-cell or γδ cell fate, prior to any signaling from the products of TCR gene rearrangements. Thus, one set of progenitors is precommitted to attempt VDJδ rearrangements, whereas the other set is precommitted to VJα rearrangements, which necessarily delete the TCRδ locus in its germline configuration *(49)*, either directly, or through the prior recombination of δ-rec and ψJα elements that flank DJCδ *(50,51)* (Fig. 2B). Thus, the only preclusion to a precommitted αβ T-cell differentiation pathway (Pathway II) is failure to complete TCRα/β gene rearrangements. The essence of this model is noncompetitive. Any form of dys-regulation at the TCR γ/δ loci should not affect the development of αβ T-cells along Pathway II, because the γ/δ products are benign or phenotypically neutral in a precommitted αβ progenitor. As depicted in Fig. 1B, this is the epitome of the "two lineage"/"distinct precursor" hypothesis.

Intermediate between the two preceding models is the "codeterminant model" *(45)* (Fig. 1C). This model resembles the TCR determinant model in that successful rearrangement at TCRγ/δ loci precludes αβ T-cell development, but it resembles the progenitor precommitment model in that successful TCRγ/δ rearrangements alone do not ensure differentiation as a γδ cell *(45)*. Rather, lineage is determined by a necessary combination of the TCR and other factors (Fig 1C). The predictions of these three major hypotheses and their resilience vis-a-vis experimental findings will be considered below.

A consideration of Fig. 2 makes it clear that the status of the excised TCRδ genes in αβ T-cell progenitors is a litmus test to distinguish between the "TCR determinant model" and the "progenitor precommitment model." An approach to characterizing the status of TCRδ genes in αβ T-cell progenitors was suggested by Yamagichi's finding that TCR locus elements lying between rearranging V [D] and J gene segments can be recovered on circles *(52)*.

7. DNA Libraries of Extrachromosomal TCRδ Gene Excision Products Demand Modification of the Progenitor Precommitment Model

TCR δ^+ clones recovered from libraries of high molecular weight extrachromosomal circles of thymus nuclei, appeared predominantly to retain the unrearranged, germline

---

Fig. 1. *(previous page)* Three models of αβ vs γδ T-cell lineage decision. Several models exist for αβ vs γδ T-cell lineage decisions. **(A)** TCR determinant model. The productive rearrangement of TCR loci determines the αβ vs. γδ T-cell lineage decision. **(B)** Progenitor precommitment model. The αβ vs γδ T-cell lineage decision is made independent of TCR loci rearrangement. Rearranging thymocytes are already precommited to the αβ or γδ T-cell lineage. **(C)** Codeterminant model. The αβ vs γδ T-cell lineage decision is made through a combination of TCR loci rearrangement, followed by correct support for that lineage decision, both internal and external of the cell.

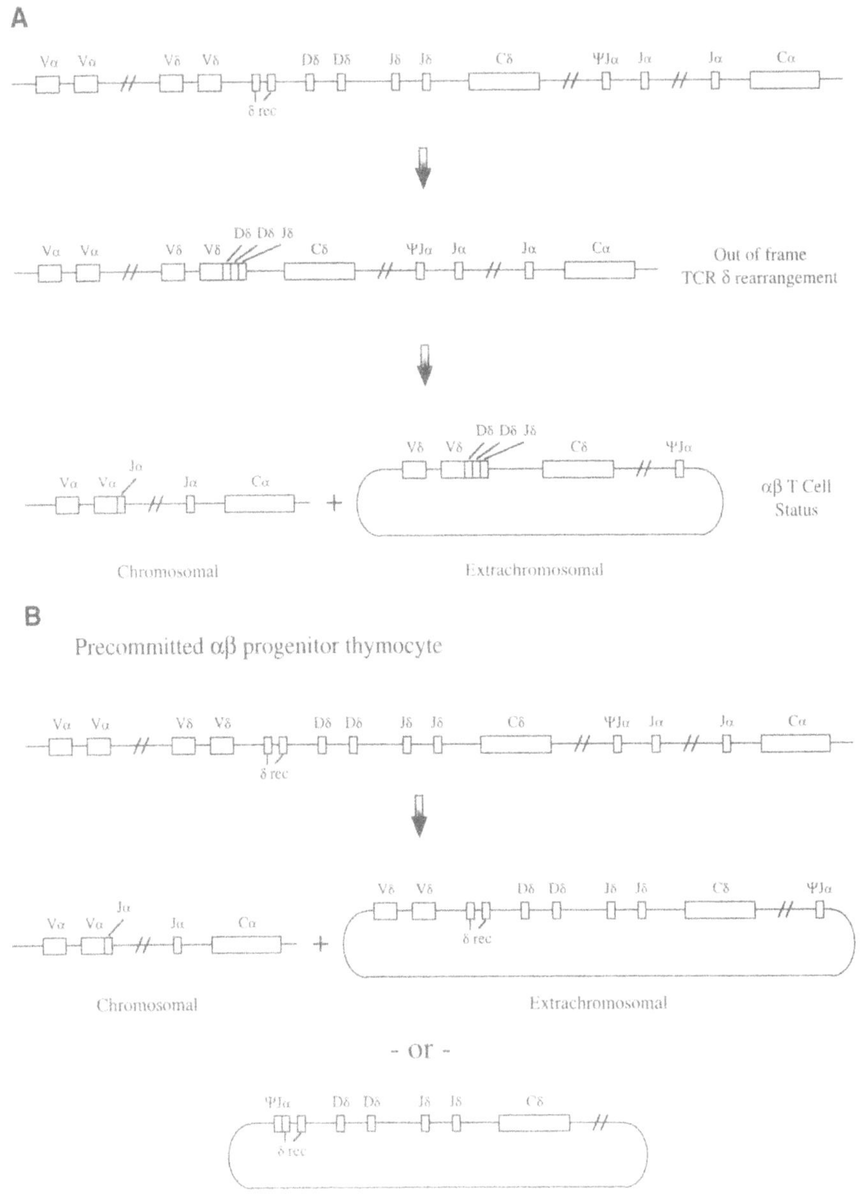

Fig. 2. TCR α/δ locus rearrangement in lineage decision. The TCR δ locus is excised from TCR α/δ locus rearrangement after TCR α rearrangement and can be detected as extrachromosomal circles. The rearrangement status of the TCR δ locus on these extrachromosomal circles can be predicted by several of the models. **(A)** TCR determinant model. One predicted outcome of TCR α/δ locus rearrangement in the TCR determinant model is predominantly out-of-frame TCR δ rearrangement on extrachromosomal circles in αβ T-cells. **(B)** Precommitment model. Two predicted outcomes of TCR α/δ locus rearrangement in the progenitor precommitment model are an unrearranged TCR δ loci or a δ rec to ΨJα rearrangement

configuration *(49)* (Fig. 2B). Since it can be reasonably argued that the bulk of thymocytes are αβ progenitors, this result was taken to mean that prior rearrangement of TCRδ is neither an obligatory nor common step in αβ progenitors. Thus, it was concluded that αβ

T-cells and γδ T-cells derive from different cell lineages, the former of which is precommitted to express and rearrange TCRα genes, rather than TCR δ genes *(49)*.

However, a similar analysis of DNA circles harvested from thymocytes and splenocytes, yielded V-D-D-Jδ rearrangements *(53)*, therefore favoring the progressive V-[D]-J rearrangement of TCRδ and TCRα (Fig. 2A), qualified by the occasional detection of germline δ sequences excised by the "δ-rec" mechanism *(50)* (Fig. 2B).

Since these two reports, other independent analyses have indicated that V-D-D-Jδ rearrangements are more common in αβ T-cell progenitors than δ deletion via δrec and ψJα *(54–59)*. Furthermore, Krangel and colleagues showed that TCRδ-locus transcriptional enhancer-dependent rearrangement of transgenic TCR gene segments occurred in all thymocyte subsets, irrespective of their being αβ T-cell or γδ-cell progenitors, whereas rearrangements dependent on the TCRα enhancer were limited to αβ cells *(32,33,35)*. Taken together, the population data, and the single cell data (provided by analysis of gene rearrangements in thymic hybridomas *[58]*) indicate that precommitted αβ progenitor cells, if they exist, are unlikely to preclude V-D-D-Jδ recombination at the TCRγ/δ loci.

To reconcile the obvious contradictions of such data with the earlier results of Winoto and Baltimore, Yamagishi suggested that the analysis of only nuclear circles (as performed by Winoto and Baltimore *[49]*) biased the recovered sample toward large genomic δ fragments that are retained in the nucleus, and excluded smaller V-D-D-Jδ "rearrangement-circles" that leak into the cytoplasm. An alternative explanation is that V-D-D-Jδ rearrangements are commonly detected in αβ T-cells and their progenitors, because excised germline TCRδ genes undergo subsequent, extrachromosomal V-D-D-J rearrangements when freed from the constraints of their chromosomal configuration. If this is the case, such rearrangements should show the random occurrence of inframe junctions, since the TCRδ product should be neutral in precommited αβ T-cell progenitors (Fig. 1B). Conversely, disproportionately out-of-frame δ rearrangements would suggest that cells expressing TCRδ products were selected away from the αβ T-cell fate (Figs. 1A, 1C). The authors, therefore, tested this hypothesis.

8. The Status of Rearranged TCRγ/δ Genes in αβ T-Cells Demonstrates that TCR Gene Rearrangements in Part Determine Cell Fate

The authors' experimental approach was to employ the polymerase chain reaction-restriction fragment length polymorphism (PCR RFLP) approach *(22,39,60)*. This technique displays on a sequencing gel the diversity of polyclonal gene rearrangements between particular V, [D], and J gene segments, sampling in a single lane probably ≥ 80 chromosomes. The results showed that TCRδ rearrangements in αβ T-cells and their progenitors were predominantly (78–81%) out of frame *(39)*, seemingly at odds with the progenitor precommitment model (*see* below). Similar results were obtained by others using either direct DNA sequencing of murine αβ T-cell and thymocyte genomic DNA *(54)*, or "spectratyping" (a technique similar to PCR.RFLP) of human thymocytes *(56)*.

By contrast, other reports noted randomly rearranged TCRδ genes in αβ T-cell progenitors, consistent with δ rearrangements being neutral events in αβ-committed progenitors *(59)*. The explanation for this discrepancy is unclear, but two points might be noted: first, the latter studies deduced random rearrangement by averaging of different V-D-J rearrangements, whereas several individual V-D-J rearrangement combinations were strikingly enriched in out-of-frame joins; second, the analysis was of RNA, and as such may have overestimated the frequency of inframe joins, because steady-state levels of transcripts of productively rearranged genes are usually greater than those of abortively rearranged genes. In short, the bulk of the data available indicates that TCRδ genes are disproportionately non-productively rearranged in αβ T-cell progenitors in humans and in mice.

It might be hypothesized that the TCRδ V-D-D-J rearrangement mechanism is simply not random, but for some reason yields disproportionately out-of-frame junctions. If this is the case, the same out-of-frame rearrangements should be seen in mice with null mutations in the δ coding region *(61)*. This was not the result: TCRδ rearrangements in αβ T-cells and their progenitors in TCRδ$^{-/-}$ mice were randomly rearranged *(39)*. These data strongly indicate that αβ progenitors pass through a cell type in which the products of successful TCRδ rearrangement are not neutral but can inhibit or preclude αβ T-cell differentiation. This would demand a significant qualification of the precommitment model (*see* below).

Nonetheless, not all TCRδ rearrangements in αβ T-cell progenitors were out-of-frame *(39)*. It is hypothesized that this was because successful TCRγ gene rearrangements are also required in order for TCRδ to interfere with αβ T-cell development. A quantitative modeling of the requirement for successful TCRγ and TCRδ rearrangements to preclude αβ T-cell development *(39)* predicts that in αβ progenitors, only 20% of rearranged δ chromosomes should be inframe, and ≤20% for γ. The authors' results for δ rearrangements (*see* above) ranged 19–22%, and interestingly, a review of the literature indicated that of 35 TCRγ gene rearrangements documented in αβ T-cells, ~14.5% were inframe (reviewed in ref. *39*). Consistent with this, 18–19% of TCRγ rearrangements were found by PCR.RFLP to be inframe in populations of αβ T-cells and their precursors *(39)*.

This capacity to preclude αβ T-cell development demonstrates that the products of successful TCRγ/δ gene rearrangements in part determine cell fate. Moreover, given the myriad approaches that have documented extensive γ/δ rearrangement in αβ T-cells and their precursors, it is believed that this is an active, physiologically relevant pathway. It clearly conflicts with the progenitor precommitment model as depicted in Fig. 1B. However, it fails to distinguish between the TCR determinant model (Fig. 1A) and the codeterminant model (Fig. 1C), because it does not test whether successful TCRγ/δ gene rearrangements guarantee γδ T-cell development, i.e., commitment to Pathway I. Moreover, it is also compatible with a modified precommitment model (Fig. 3), that both accommodates the fact that αβ-T-cell–committed progenitors seem able to rearrange TCR γ and δ genes, and recognizes that successful rearrangements at the TCRγ/δ loci can seemingly preclude successful development as αβ cells.

9. How Does TCRγ/δ Transduce a Signal in αβ-T-Cell Progenitors?

The inhibition of αβ T-cell development by TCRγδ might be caused by a shut-off of RAG-dependent TCRα/β gene rearrangement. Alternatively, or additionally, γ/δ chains might have other effects on the progenitors, for example, directing them toward another fate. This issue is returned to later in this chapter. Either way, the products of successfully rearranged TCR genes have somehow to transduce to their cell a signal. The nature of this signal transduction is a mystery. Invoking precedent, the products of TCR gene rearrangement would be expected to form a cell surface receptor that can engage a ligand on a second cell, most likely a stromal cell.

There is some, albeit limited, biochemical evidence that the product of successful TCRβ chain gene rearrangement forms a surface pre-TCR together with CD3 molecules and pre-Tα *(47)*, but there is no evidence as yet that this is the active biochemical form

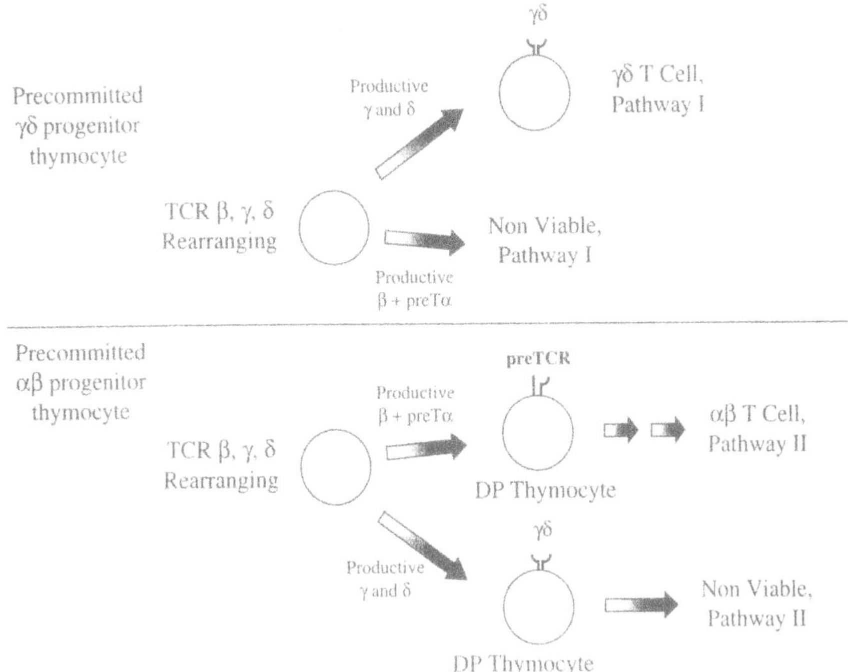

Fig. 3. Modified precommitment model. A modified version of the progenitor precommitment model allows for rearrangement of the TCR β, γ, and δ loci in a cell precommited to either lineage, but still requires any productive rearrangements to match the precommitment made by the precursor.

of the pre-TCR. A multi-protein cluster as complex as β.pTα.CD3 will presumably mature in the endoplasmic reticulum and then pass to the Golgi. Conceivably, its interaction with a particular molecule at that point within the cell could be sufficient to transduce a signal for the cells further development.

Conversely, surface engagement of a ligand may be necessary. The ligand cannot be conventional Class II or Class I MHC, because mutations in these do not block T-cell development at an early stage. Given that seemingly all cells that express a pre-TCR can be 'β-selected' toward the αβ(+) fate *(5,22)*, it seems unlikely that the pre-TCR ligand is specific for any Vβ region. Indeed, β selection can be mediated by a truncated chain lacking Vβ *(62)*. Possibly the ligand recognizes pTα, that is stabilized by pairing to a β chain. Likewise, there may be a generic ligand, not necessarily proteinaceous, for the products of successful TCR γ/δ rearrangements.

These considerations are not to rule out specific ligands for the positive or negative selection of specific γδ(+) thymocytes. The evidence is controversial for stringent positive and negative selection of γδ thymocytes bearing specific TCRs *(30,63)*. Notwithstanding, it may be that different ligands successively engage the nascent TCRs, with each engagement leading to different consequences (that will be reviewed later).

The question of whether successful TCRβ chain gene rearrangements likewise preclude Pathway I and γδ cell development, has also been approached in mice and humans using PCR.RFLP, DNA sequencing and spectratyping *(22,39,56,64)*. These studies have found that there are far fewer V-D-Jβ rearrangements in γδ cells and γδ(+) thymocytes than there are V(D)J γ/δ rearrangements in αβ cells; nonetheless, those present showed no consistent selection against inframe joinings. Thus, inframe β rearrangements alone are insufficient to commit cells away from a γδ(+) fate. This result is important because it requires further modification of the remaining viable models, depicted in Figs. 1A, 1C, and 3 (*see* below).

10. Limitations on Fate Determination by the Products of Successful TCR Gene Rearrangement Illustrated by TCR-Mutant Mice

The products of successful TCRγ/δ rearrangements can seemingly oppose the αβ(+) fate. To find out whether such products also actively determine the γδ(+) fate, T-cell development has been examined in TCRβ$^{-/-}$ mice (in which TCRγδ is the only TCR that can be successfully expressed), and in TCRγδ transgenic mice (in which TCRγ and δ genes are pre-rearranged inframe in all cells).

Progenitor development along Pathways I and II in these mice can be assessed by thymocyte phenotypes (Fig. 4). In brief, the signatory characteristic of Pathway II (and commitment toward an αβ(+) fate) is the acquisition by a thymocyte of both CD4 and CD8. Such double positives develop from final-stage (CD44^{lo}, CD25^{lo}, HSA^{hi}) DN cells that are rapidly cycling *(22,65–67)*. During the course of these events, widespread V-Jα rearrangement is induced. These coordinated proliferation and differentiation events *(67)* appear to be dependent on signaling from the preTCR *(46,48)*. The importance of this pathway is indicated by several results: most DPs in normal mice have productively rearranged TCRβ chain genes (63); and the transition of cells into final-stage DNs, and from there into DPs, is very poor in TCRβ$^{-/-}$ mice, and pTα$^{-/-}$ mice *(46,68)*.

The involvement of the pre-TCR in the DN to DP transition makes it the first demonstrated point at which the products of TCR genes have a critical effect on αβ T-cell development. Importance is also attached to the DN-to-DP transition because it is seen as the conspicuous divergence point for αβ T-cell development and γδ cell development. As stated above, most γδ progenitors developing along Pathway I enter a largely nonproliferating, final stage, DN subset, and complete maturation as DN cells (Fig. 4). Because inframe β rearrangements are not selected against in γδ cells (*see* above), Fig. 4 includes a putative γδ maturation pathway that post dates β-selection. This could reflect the development of cells that were selected for inframe β, while additionally harboring inframe rearrangements at either TCRγ or TCRδ. Following pre-TCR signaling, it is possible that the cognate γ or δ locus was successfully rearranged, prior to successful rearrangements at the α locus. However, the pathway is speculative: γδ(+) cells with inframe TCRβ chain genes might alternatively derive from precommitted γδ progenitors that do not express pTα and hence cannot assemble the pre-TCR (*see* below).

Because exit of αβ progenitors out of the DP subset is dependent on TCR engagement of either conventional MHC Class I or Class II, exit out of the final DN subset (along either Pathway I or Pathway II) effectively marks the last point at which T-cell development occurs in an MHC-independent fashion. Hence, the maturation of γδ cells at this point, prior to the DP transition, is consistent with their general lack of reactivity toward conventional Class I and/or Class II MHC. The question is whether productive rearrangement at the TCRγ/δ loci guarantees development by Pathway I, with maturation completed prior to the DP transition.

10.1. Results in TCRβ$^{-/-}$ Mice

The detailed analysis of genetically homogeneous TCRβ$^{-/-}$ littermates revealed only small and very variable numbers of DP cells, and most of the preceding final-stage DNs were not actively proliferating *(45)*. Hence, it seemed that most cells were committing

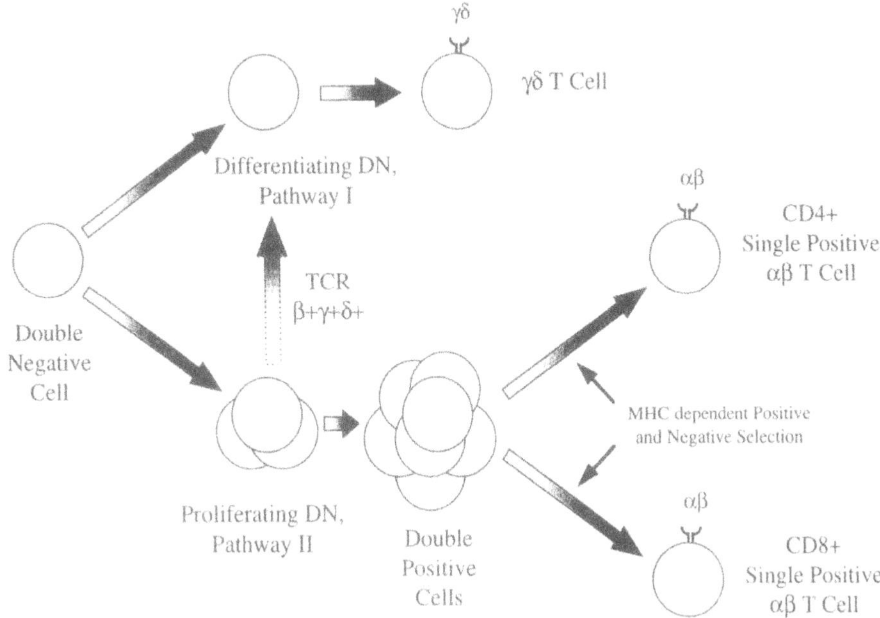

Fig. 4. Thymocyte development. Thymocytes go through a series of well defined surface marker changes and selective events during development. Here, the branch points and relationships between γδ, $CD4^+$ αβ, and $CD8^+$ αβ T-cell development are illustrated.

to Pathway I, consistent with the TCR determinant model as depicted in Fig. 1A. Nonetheless, the presence of some DPs together with small numbers of proliferating final-stage DN cells indicated that not all $TCR\beta^{-/-}$ thymocytes differentiate along Pathway I, and away from Pathway II. This, together with data derived from the initial analysis of genetically heterogenous $TCR\beta^{-/-}$ mice *(68)*, demonstrated that the $TCR\beta^{(+)}$.pre-TCR is not essential for the formation of DPs.

The DPs in $TCR\beta^{-/-}$ mice do not display significant developmental potential *(45)*. Hence, they may be small numbers of thymocytes that became DPs because of the 'background noise' of thymic dysregulation (the thymi in $TCR\beta^{-/-}$ mice are very small and irregular). Arguing against this, DPs do not form in $TCR(\beta x\delta)^{-/-}$ double mutant mice, or in $RAG^{-/-}$ mice. Alternatively, Buer et al. have speculated that DPs might form in $TCR\beta^{-/-}$ mice because of the influence in trans of γδ cells *(69)*: TCR^- SCID thymocytes can be provoked to mature as DPs by the presence of maturing TCR^+ cells *(25)*. However, this trans-acting pathway seems to support differentiation of only very few cells. To test whether there was, instead, an active effect of TCRγ/δ rearrangement on the maturation of $TCR\beta^-$ thymocytes as DPs, PCR.RFLP was applied to $TCR\beta^{-/-}$ mice *(45)*. It was found that the DPs were primarily selected for inframe TCRδ rearrangements. Some selection was evident for inframe γ rearrangements, although this was less convincing than the selection for γ in γδ(+) populations *(45)*. This issue is returned to below.

Notwithstanding the uncertainty over γ rearrangements, the data show that successful rearrangements at the TCRδ locus in $TCR\beta^{-/-}$ mice are associated with some, albeit few, cells adopting Pathway II. If the numbers of DPs in $TCR\beta^{-/-}$ mice are to be regarded as significant, the compatibility of productively rearranged TCRγ/δ genes with development along both Pathway I and Pathway II contradicts the TCR determinant model, as shown in Fig. 1A. Rather, it is consistent either with the codeterminant model (Fig. 1C), or the modified progenitor precommitment model (Fig. 3). Nevertheless, both of those models would have to accommodate the under-representation and poor developmental progression of TCRγ/δ-selected thymocytes along Pathway II *(45,68)* (*see* below).

10.2. Results in TCRγδ Transgenic Mice

Several different TCRγδ transgenic strains *(38,70–74)* are consistent with the analysis of TCRβ$^{-/-}$ mice. Although they commonly show significant over-representation of γδ cells, the representation of DPs can also be overt, indicating that Pathway II is active, not obviously precluded by the transgenic, inframe TCRγ/δ rearrangements. Moreover, many of the DPs express the rearranged TCRγ/δ transgenes, and have not obviously rearranged and activated the endogenous TCRβ locus *(72,73)*. Therefore, it has again been concluded that TCRγδ expression, in violation of the TCR-determinant model, can promote both a γδ(+) fate (Pathway I), and αβ(+) commitment (Pathway II). Furthermore, it was proposed that specific, locus-associated transcriptional silencer elements (*see* below) could extinguish γδ TCR transgene expression in the precommited αβ progenitors *(71)*.

Given these data, should one discard the TCR determinant model (Fig. 1A)? Only if one can still account for the fact that TCRγδ transgenes do have a major effect on T-cell development. Commonly, the ratio of γδ T-cells to αβ T-cells in TCRγδ transgenic mice increases from 1:50 to ~1:10–1:5, and in some TCRγδ transgenic mice, virtually no αβ T-cells are detected *(38,70)*. Additionally, thymus cellularity is usually very low, consistent with a major decrease in progenitor proliferation because of a reduced commitment to Pathway II (Fig. 4). Both these results are in keeping with the hypothesis that the developmental fate of a progenitor is significantly influenced by the nature of the successfully rearranged genes.

These data seem paradoxical, given the failure of some TCRγδ transgenes to preclude Pathway II. Moreover, the TCR transgenic results are astonishingly variable *(70,74)*, even for mice derived from the same founder *(70)*. To reconcile these seemingly different activities of TCRγδ transgenes in different mice, one should consider likely modifiers of TCRγδ action.

11. Potential Modifiers of TCR-Dependent Fate Determination

11.1. Avidity

Different results in different TCR transgenic mice may be a result of differences in expression of even the same transgenic TCR genes. Nonetheless, comparable transgene copy numbers in mice with very different phenotypes were taken as a challenge to this explanation *(74)*. Instead, the important variability in expression may be among the thymocytes within a single animal. To hypothesize, perhaps "high expressor" thymocytes readily commit to the γδ(+) fate (Pathway I), whereas "low expressor" thymocytes may not signal properly, hence failing to preclude TCRβ rearrangement, that then facilitates commitment to Pathway II. However, this explanation is challenged by the failure to find extensive TCRβ rearrangements in many of the γδTCR transgenic DPs *(72,73)*.

An alternative view of the effect of "TCR dosage" is based on the precedent for different avidities dictating the choice between fates for thymocytes undergoing MHC-αβTCR-mediated selection into CD4$^+$ and CD8$^+$ SPs. In that case, moderate avidity interactions determine differentiation, whereas high affinity interactions determine apoptosis *(17–19)*. Interestingly, a cell's capacity to interpret signals from a single signal transduction molecule can clearly vary with the stage of differentiation of the cell *(31)*.

Hence, it is plausible that progenitor DN thymocytes respond to moderate avidity interactions by differentiation, as do DPs, yet they respond to high avidity interactions by cell-cycling rather than by apoptosis (Fig. 5). In both DPs and DNs, the failure to receive any signal from the TCR/pre-TCR would also lead to death. In short, the TCR may be a prime determinant of fate, but the fate will vary as the TCR dose varies (Fig. 6). Under physiologic conditions, there may be much less variability in the level of expression of nascent γδTCR molecules, but nonetheless, some variability could explain the consistent presence of a small number of TCRδ$^{(+)}$ DPs *(45)*. In short, accommodating a strong effect of avidity resurrects the viability of the TCR determinant model (Fig. 1A).

11.2. Intracellular Signaling from the TCR

The assumption that the nascent TCR must engage a stromal ligand is not necessary for variable TCR expression to have a phenotypic consequence of the kind described. Compared to a low density of TCR, a high density of TCR may relay to the maturing thymocyte a stronger, more sustained or different signal. One aspect of this is the potential for overexpressed transgenic TCRγ/δ chains to compete for integration into different signal transduction webs. For example, the affinity of δ for pTα might ordinarily be very low, but with a sufficiently high concentration of δ, stable δ.pTα complexes may form. These might then relay a proliferative signal characteristic of the pre-TCR (Pathway II), rather than the differentiative signal, characteristic of TCR γδ signaling (Pathway I). Interestingly, this hypothesis could explain why δ-selection is more obvious than γ selection in DPs *(45)*. It would also predict that there would be higher numbers of γδ cells in pTα$^{-/-}$ mice, since there would, in this case, be no competition between pTα and γ for pairing with δ. This prediction is borne out experimentally *(46,69,75)*. Consistent with the hypothesis that γ/δ chains might be influenced by pTα independent of TCRβ, γδ levels are not noticeably increased in TCRβ$^{-/-}$ mice. Third, a putative δ.pTα complex might also explain why there seem to be remarkably few DPs in pTα–, TCRα–mice *(69)*, in which neither pTα.β complexes nor putative pTα.δ complexes could form.

11.3. Onset of Expression

A third component of TCR dosage, is variable onset of TCR expression, both between and within transgenic mice. Some thymocytes may experience the activity of a complete TCRγδ prior to the rearrangement and expression of any other TCR genes, e.g., TCRβ, whereas in others, β rearrangement and pairing with pTα may have occurred first. Although successful β rearrangement does not generally preclude the γδ fate (*see* above), it may be sufficient in some γδTCR transgenic mice to favor commitment to Pathway II. Nonetheless, this could not account for Pathway II in TCRβ$^{-/-}$ mice *(45)*.

11.4. Niches and a Putative Succession of Signals from TCRγδ

The most obvious deregulation introduced by TCR transgenes is the dose of thymocytes with successful TCR rearrangements relative to the number of potential interaction molecules ("niches") on the stromal cells. Niche limitation is a real and stringent phenomenon. It limits the capacity of B-cells to enter into follicles in the periphery *(76)*, and it sharply regulates the number of stem cells that can successfully enter the thymus each day *(77)*. It may also regulate the number of αβ(+) DP thymocytes that can positively select. Hence, it is possible that in TCRγδ transgenic mice, the potential sites for committing to Pathway I are saturated. What then happens to the remaining cells?

As was discussed earlier in this chapter, the potential intracellular and/or extracellular ligands for nascent TCRγδ and the pre-TCR are unelucidated. However, there may be

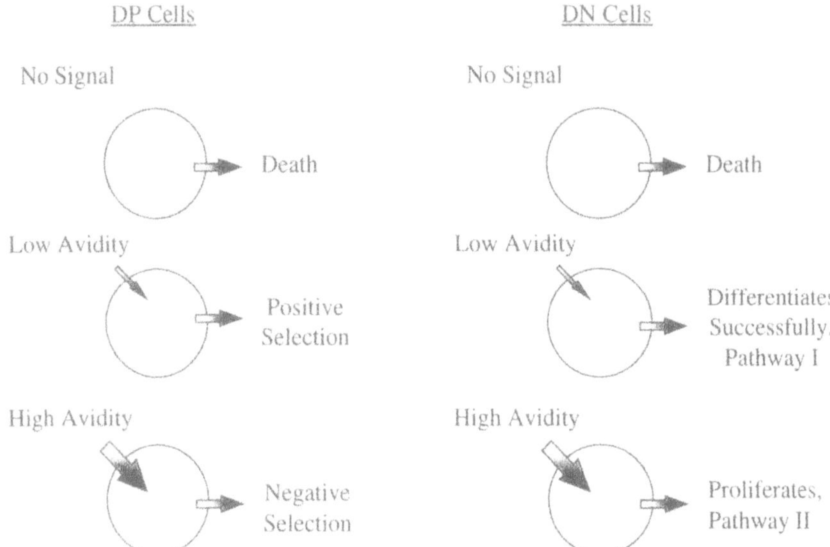

Fig. 5. Double negative and double positive cell parallels. Parallels may exist in selective signaling events between double negative and double positive cells. The avidity of the signal a double positive thymocyte receives can determine its fate. A similar avidity difference could determine the αβ vs γδ T-cell lineage decision.

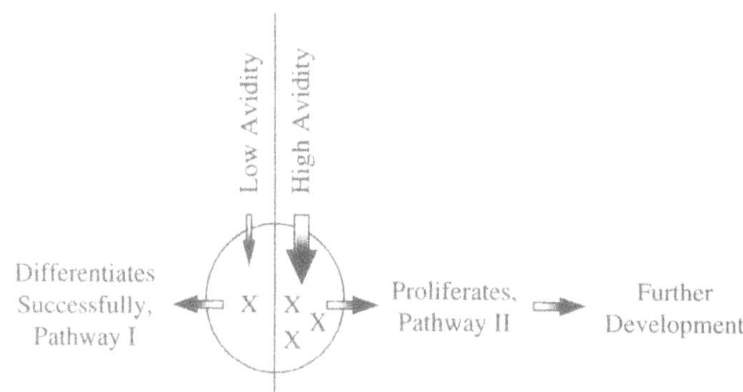

Fig. 6. Avidity determinant model. The relative avidity of a single kind of receptor/ligand interaction, rather than differing receptors or ligands, could determine the αβ vs γδ T-cell lineage decisions.

successive TCR/pre-TCR engagements with different outcomes. An experimental indication of this is provided by pTα-mutant mice, in which some, but not all, effects of productively rearranged TCRβ chain genes are lost *(78)*. Moreover, two recent hypotheses on the role of TCRαβ in the commitment of DPs to $CD4^+$ and $D8^+$ SPs both invoked two successive engagements of the TCR, each with distinct consequences (*79,80*; although *see* also ref. *81*).

Therefore, the remaining progenitor thymocytes, unable to engage a niche to complete γδ(+) maturation, may nonetheless have received some form of signal that renders them distinct from counterpart progenitors in $RAG^{-/-}$ or $TCR(\beta x\delta)^{-/-}$ mice. Possibly, this signal resets the developmental clock (e.g., by activation of Bcl2 or a related gene).

With extended lifetimes, some of the DN progenitors that cannot engage a niche may for stochastic reasons eventually commit to an alternative pathway of development, especially in the case that they have highly unusual levels (high or low) of TCR expression (*see* Aviditiy above). Such commitment of TCRγδ transgenic cells to Pathway II would give the misleading impression that the form of the TCR expressed does not play a major role in lineage commitment. The "niche hypothesis," rooted in precedent, could readily explain the development of significant numbers of DPs in TCRγδ transgenic mice, and the relatively small and variable numbers of DPs that form in TCRβ$^{-/-}$ mice and in normal mice *(45)*.

Interestingly, a 'generic' engagement of TCRγ/δ (entirely distinct from a stringent, TCR-specific "positive selection" signal) that precludes further rearrangement (e.g., of TCRβ genes), and initiates differentiation events, could explain why cells with productive rearrangements of TCRγ/δ loci seem to preclude αβ T-cell differentiation very efficiently in normal mice. If, by contrast, the preclusion of the αβ(+) fate (Pathway II) relied on a stringent positive selection process alone, one would predict that there would be many more inframe TCRγ/δ rearrangements in αβ T-cell progenitors, derived from cells that productively rearranged TCRγ/δ genes, but that had subsequently failed selection.

In conclusion, the finding in TCR transgenic mice and in TCR mutant mice that different fates can be adopted by cells with qualitatively the same or similar TCRs, does not rule out the viability of the TCR-determinant model, because there are too many putative modifiers of the actions of TCRγ/δ chains. These are not implausible modifiers, since examples of each can be found in other systems of fate determination. To gain further insight into the respective viabilities of the TCR determinant model (Fig. 1A), the codeterminant model (Fig. 1C), and the modified progenitor precommitment model (Fig. 3), data from TCRαβ transgenic mice shall be briefly reviewed.

12. TCRαβ Transgenic Mice: More Constraints on the Precommitment Model

The representation of γδ cells in TCRαβ(+) and TCRβ(+)transgenic mice is highly variable *(41,82–84)*. The most common observation is the retention of the TCRγδ (+) epidermal T-cell subset. This in itself does not imply progenitor precommittment, because these γδ cells may have derived from progenitor cells before the TCRαβ transgenes were active: hence, their fate would have been determined by TCRγδ. In short, the γδ cell phenotype in most TCRαβ transgenic mice can be explained by any of the three still-viable models, Figs. 1A, 1C, and 3.

However, there is an additional interesting aspect of TCRαβ transgenic mice that is germane to issues of fate determination—namely the unusual occurrence of significant numbers of DN TCRαβ(+) cells *(82,83)*. These cells apparently develop in the thymus on either positively selecting or negatively selecting backgrounds and can expand in the periphery in the presence of nominal antigen. Thus, they are not preapoptotic artifacts of negative selection. Moreover, the cells are not those that have undergone endogenous TCRα gene rearrangement, thereby altering the TCR specificity *(82)*, and indeed show little capacity to rearrange an ectopically integrated transgenic V-D-J recombination substrate *(83)*. By contrast, more conventional TCRαβ(+) SPs display a plethora of products of the recombination substrates *(83)*. These data suggest that the TCRαβ(+), DN cells complete maturation more quickly than their SP siblings, and phenotypically are γδ cells in every respect, but for their expression of TCRαβ *(82)*. Consistent with this, the cells show retention and V-D-J rearrangement of the endogenous TCRδ locus rather than its deletion by α rearrangement *(82)*.

Possibly, the product of the prerearranged TCRα chain competes with pTα for the product of the prerearranged β locus, thereby precluding Pathway II, and directing fate toward Pathway I. In this sense, the transgenic TCR is clearly determining fate, according to the competitive model depicted in Fig. 1A. Moreover, the failure of all αβTCR transgene-positive cells to become DN, "γδ-look-a-like" cells could again be explained by varying avidity of the TCR on high and low expressors; and/or a limited number of niches available. In fact, the differentiation of αβTCR transgene-positive cells along Pathway II operates at only about 5% of normal efficiency *(82,85)*. Again, the nature of the TCR chains expressed is a significant influence on cell fate.

Nonetheless, the demonstration that TCRαβ can substitute for TCRγδ demands further modification of the models presented in Figs. 1A, C, and 3. The modification of the TCR-determinant model is presented as the "Receptor Determinant" model in Fig. 7A. The distinct influences on cell fate are now seen not to be TCRγδ and TCRαβ, respectively, but a "Complete TCR" (either TCRγδ or TCRαβ) and an "Incomplete TCR" (the pre-TCR), respectively. It is plausible to invoke that complete TCRs transduce signals in immature thymocytes that are different from those transduced by incomplete TCRs, because pTα, the signatory chain of the preTCR, differs most noticeably from TCR chains α, β, γ, and δ, by virtue of a large cytoplasmic tail that could potentially be involved in unique signaling. Although it was recently reported that a version of pTα lacking the tail can rescue αβ T-cell development in $pT\alpha^{-/-}$ mice *(75)*, it was not clear that the rescued mice were indeed fully rescued. For example, there were still lower than normal numbers of DPs and higher than normal numbers of γδ cells.

According to Fig. 7, early expression of a complete TCR, be it αβ or γδ, connects with a signaling web X to promote differentiation as a DN cell. Conversely, the pre-TCR signals through signaling web Y to promote cell proliferation and commitment to Pathway II. Hence, this model retains the competitive essence of the TCR-determinant model. Additionally, the authors propose that the complete TCR can connect to signaling web Y, although not as effectively as the pre-TCR.

The basis for this is the very poor efficiency of Pathway II in many TCRαβ transgenic mice. Unlike the inhibition of Pathway II by productive rearrangement of TCRγ/δ chains, this cannot be attributed to allelic exclusion of the TCRα/β loci, since the prerearranged, α/β transgenes are naturally compatible with Pathway II. Rather, we propose that the complete TCR (be it TCRαβ [in this case] or TCRγδ [in other cases]) can signal weakly through web Y to induce Pathway II but without much coincident cell proliferation. The linkage of the complete TCR to Y rather than X could be governed by several variables including the relative amounts of X and Y over time. Again, this is reminiscent of the O-2A differentiation *(14)*.

The receptor determinant model depicted in Fig. 7A is reasonably powerful, because it can accommodate possibly all observations cited in this review, notably: the development of mature DN T-cells in TCRαβ transgenic mice (signaling from complete TCR through X); the reduced efficiency of DP development in TCRαβ transgenic mice (signaling from complete TCR through Y); the presence of low but variable numbers of DPs in $TCR\beta^{-/-}$ and TCRγδ transgenic mice (signaling from complete TCR through Y); and the increased number of γδ cells in $pT\alpha^{-/-}$ mice (these cells would derive from both an increased efficiency of Pathway I and from γδ-driven Pathway II, consistent with which, a significant fraction of the increased γδ cells are CD4[+]).

Nonetheless, most of the data could also be accounted for by a "further-modified precommitment model", depicted in Fig. 7B. In this case, signaling webs X and Y are presegregated into distinct progenitors (*see* Fig. 7B). Competition for Y between complete receptors and the pre-TCR could lead to variable outcomes for the Pathway II

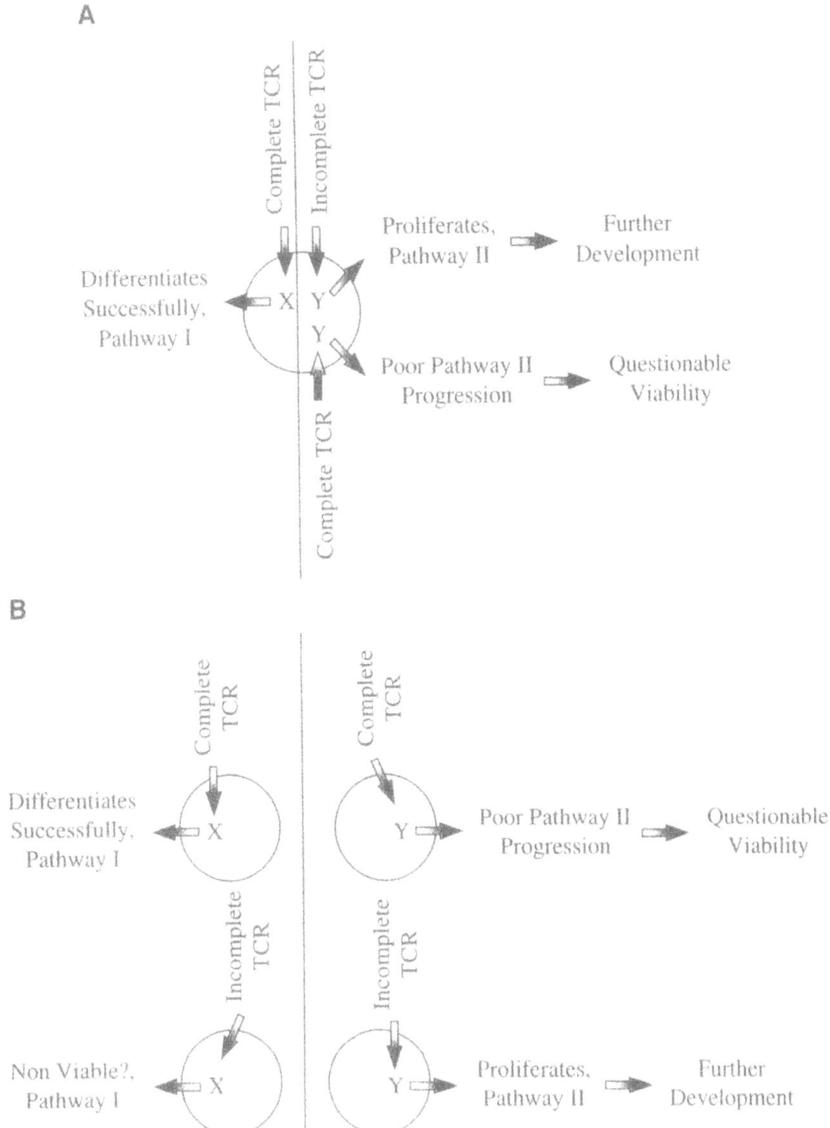

Fig. 7. Signal transduction in the receptor determinant and precommitment models. The signaling cascade downstream of a receptor/ligand interaction could determine the αβ vs γδ T-cell lineage decisions. Differential usage of signaling molecules in the TCR determinant model or differential expression of signaling molecules in the progenitor precommitment model could determine the αβ vs γδ T-cell lineage decisions. (A) Receptor determinant model. In the TCR determinant model, the αβ vs γδ T-cell lineage decision may depend on which of several signaling molecules expressed in an uncommitted precursor is activated. (B) Precommited signaling model. In the progenitor precommitment model, the αβ vs γδ T-cell lineage decision may depend on which signaling molecule is expressed in a precommited precursor. The correct signaling molecule for a receptor would have to be expressed to maintain viability.

progenitor, consistent with those observed in the different mice described. In addition, the data could likewise be accounted for by a modified codetermination model, that for reasons of parsimony is not shown.

An issue revisited by the models shown in Fig. 7 is that of the form of TCR/pre-TCR engagement. How could TCRαβ be seen equivalently to TCRγδ? In Fig. 8, two options for ligands are compared. In the top line, the ligand is specific for the conformation of the variable region of the nascent TCR. It will engage and facilitate "stringent positive selection" of cells bearing a limited number of TCRs, such as those on the left, but not those on the right. Conversely, the ligand in the second line recognizes a more basic epitope on the TCR (e.g., in the C-region). This ligand could effect "relaxed positive selection" of all complete γδ TCRs. Thus, only two such ligands would be required to effect "relaxed positive selection" of all complete TCRs. In an extreme case, a single ligand that recognizes CD3 could effect "relaxed positive selection" of all complete TCRs: the TCR chains might simply stabilize the CD3.

In conclusion, the available data do not distinguish between receptor determination, precommitment, or even codetermination for lymphoid αβ(+) and γδ(+) cells emerging from the postnatal thymus. Currently the authors know of no data that do. However, the survey that the authors have presented leads them to believe that competition is a significant factor in determining the development of thymocytes. Since most manipulations of the TCR change T-cell development patterns, one can state that fate is significantly influenced by the type of TCR genes successfully rearranged and expressed. Even in precommited progenitors, different TCRs would seem to be able to influence fate significantly and competitively, for example as depicted in Fig. 7B.

Nonetheless, the fundamental question remains: whether there is only one type of progenitor cell from which mature DN γδ cells emerge, and another type from which mature $CD4^+$ or $CD8^+$αβ T-cells emerge, or whether both cell types can emerge from one common, late-stage progenitor. In the following sections of this chapter, the authors consider factors that may either precommit progenitor cells, or that may, together with the TCR, codetermine the fate of a single common progenitor.

13. *Notch*–A Candidate Codeterminant of T-Cell Development

The widespread involvement of *Notch* in many developmental decision points was introduced at the beginning of this chapter. Notwithstanding, some attention should be paid to it here, because it is a candidate codeterminant of T-cell development. This statement stems from the capacity of *Notch* to modify T-cell development in a TCR-dependent fashion.

Robey and her colleagues found, in a series of imaginative experiments, that the expression of an activated *Notch* allele as a transgene could alter the fate of thymocytes in several ways *(86,87)*. Among these, transgenic TCRγδ cells on a *Notch* transgenic background more often differentiated as DP cells (toward an αβ(+) fate), than did so in unmanipulated TCRγδ transgenic mice. In terms of Fig. 7A, *Notch* could be increasing the level of Y. Likewise, there is an increased representation of DPs in $TCR\beta^{-/-}$ mice that express an activated *Notch* transgene. Again, an increase in the concentration of Y could accomplish this. The effects of *Notch* do not represent an alternative, TCR-independent pathway of lineage commitment, since the authors used PCR.RFLP to show that $TCR\beta^-$ thymocytes that developed as DPs were selected for inframe δ genes *(87)*.

A corollary experiment showed that proportionately more γδ cells developed from bone marrow heterozygous for *Notch*, than developed from $Notch^{+/+}$ bone marrow. In the context of Fig. 7A, heterozygosity at *Notch* may reduce the level of Y, giving a competitive advantage to the X signaling web. Consistent with this, the effects of *Notch* dosage are partial: even from $Notch^{+/-}$ bone marrow, more αβ T-cells than γδ cells developed.

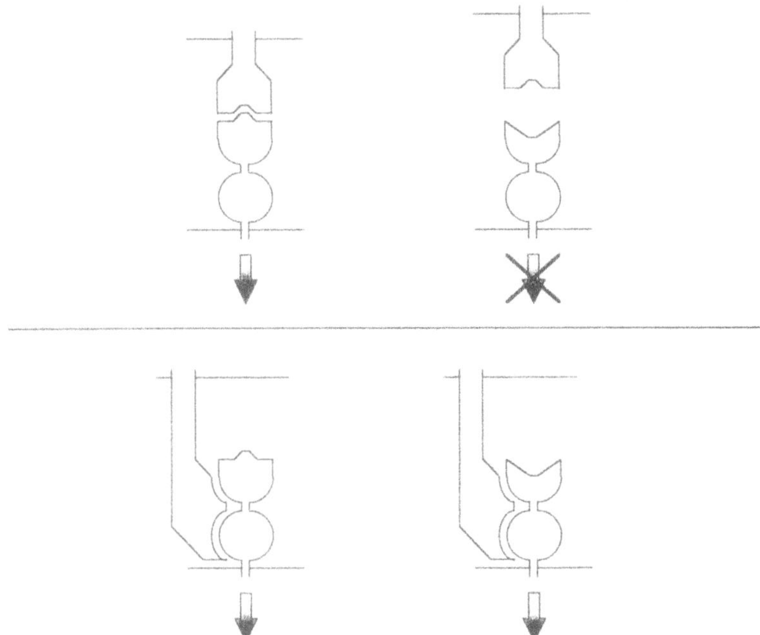

Fig. 8. Stringent vs relaxed positive selection. The traditional definition of positive selection of double positive, αβ T-cell lineage thymocytes is a stringent one, assuming ligand recognition of a minimum avidity at the antigen combining site. A relaxed definition may exist for double negative thymocytes and/or γδ T-cells, allowing selection based solely on surface expression of a receptor independent of specificity.

Alternatively, the correspondence of *Notch* and Y marks *Notch* as a precommitment factor, according to Fig. 7B.

Resolving the precise involvement of *Notch* in T-cell development may be difficult. First, the available antibody reagents against mouse *Notch* do not give clear and distinct patterns of *Notch* expression on thymocyte subsets. Second, and more importantly, the critical issue may not be heterogeneity in *Notch* expression but in *Notch* activity. This is likely regulated at multiple levels including the proteolytic processing of the primary *Notch* translation product (S. Artavanis-Tsakonis, personal communication) and the availability of any of several ligands such as jagged and serrate. Hence, determining differential activity of *Notch* in different cells within defined DN subsets is currently not easy. Another note of caution is that the genetic system so far used to analyze *Notch* is suboptimal. It is difficult to ensure that *Notch*$^{+/-}$ cells indeed have reduced *Notch* activity, and the activated *Notch* allele used is so powerful that it potentially introduces collateral dysregulation.

14. Heterogeneous Gene Expression Might Provide Support for a Precommitment Model

A testable prediction of the pre-commitment model (e.g., Fig. 7B) that distinguishes it from the receptor determinant model (Fig. 7A) is that progenitors of γδ cells and of αβ cells should display heterogeneity in gene expression from a relatively early time point, prior to (rather than a result of) signaling from complete or incomplete TCRs. There are some obvious candidates for molecules that may be markers of early lineage divergence within otherwise homogeneous thymocyte progenitors. First among these is preTα.

14.1. pTa—A Candidate Determinant of Proliferation Along Pathway II

One could propose that pTα+ cells in normal mice reflect progenitors commited to Pathway II. Although pTα signaling may not be required for Pathway II differentiation (i.e., appearance of DPs), it may induce cell proliferation. Thus, in $pT\alpha^{-/-}$ mice, there are small numbers of DPs *(69)*. Conversely, the $pT\alpha^-$ cells in normal mice, have the γδ(+) fate as their only developmental potential, irrespective of the status of TCRβ chain gene rearrangement. This could accommodate the inframe β-rearrangements reported in different analyses of γδ cells *(22,39,56,64)*. In TCRαβ transgenic mice, the ectopically early expression of TCRα could artifactually provide a chain to pair with β to confer an αβ(+) fate on what would otherwise be TCRγδ(+) cells *(69)*.

Encouraging the hypothesis that pTα determines T-cell development, is an heterogeneity in pTα expression *(46,88)*. Provocatively, pTα is absent from γδ(+) thymocytes. However, the absence of pTα may be a consequence of rather than a component of the cause of γδ differentiation. Examination of HSA^+ $\gamma\delta^+$ cells does not provide a window on immature γδ T-cells, since there is evidence from different experiments that HSA may downregulate only after emigration from the thymus and subsequent completion of γδ thymocyte development *(13,45,89)*. Hence, a better resolution of this will require the development of an antibody that can facilitate sorting of $pT\alpha^+$ and $pT\alpha^-$ immature thymocytes, so that their differentiation potential can be compared. If pTα is a lineage determinant, it might be predicted that constitutive expression of pTα in all early thymocytes (e.g., from the proximal *lck* promoter) might preclude development of thymocytes as γδ cells. The results of such a study have yet to be reported, although transgenic mice expressing mutant forms of pTα have been described *(75)*.

14.2. Differential Expression of Signal Transduction Molecules

It has been shown that the TCR-associated protein complex can be different in some γδ cells compared to most αβ T-cells. Thus, epithelial γδ cells in particular can utilize FcεRIγ in place of CD3ζ, and commonly connect the TCR signaling complex to p72.Syk rather than to ZAP70 (*see* refs. *5,90*). In similar vein, some γδ cells are observed in mice deficient for lck and fyn tyrosine kinases, whereas essentially all αβ T-cell development is compromised at the DN-DP transition *(91,92)*. Such results encourage the view that γδ-committed progenitors may be identified among HSC on the basis of the unique expression of particular signaling molecules. However, as for *Notch*, differential expression of signaling molecules may be manifest more at the level of activity rather than the presence of either the protein or RNA. The experimental demonstration that single cells within an apparently homogeneous population differ reproducibly in the active state of signal transduction enzymes cannot be readily undertaken at this time.

14.3 Differential Expression of Factors That Regulate Gene Rearrangement and/or Expression

There is evidence for the differential expression of nuclear factors that regulate gene activity and rearrangement. A case in point is the regulation of rearrangement between two elements, "δrec" and ψJα (mouse Jα61) that flank and thereby delete, Cδ *(50)* (Fig. 2). Factors binding to DNA adjacent to δrec have been identified in thymocytes *(51)*. Moreover, γδ cells show little rearrangement of a transgenic construct containing the germline configuration of δrec-Cδ-Jα61, whereas evidence of considerably more rearrangement is evident in αβ cells. When the binding site for the factors is deleted, the rearrangement occurs more promiscuously, ruling out the possibility that γδ (+) cells differentiated along Pathway I too rapidly to undertake appreciable DNA rearrangement *(51)*. Hence, it could be hypothesized that γδ progenitors exclusively express a factor that suppresses δrec-Jα61 rearrangement, whereas this is absent from αβ progenitors. Thus, differentiation in the latter cells is precommited toward an αβ(+) fate, because Cδ will commonly be deleted.

There are at least three facts that preclude the ready acceptance of this model as a mechanism of γδ/αβ lineage precommitment. First, most available evidence suggests that the δ locus in αβ T-cells is not often deleted via δrec-Jα61 recombination *(49,55)*. Second, mice deficient in TEA, a promoter/enhancer element that activates δrec-Jα61 recombination, show only reduced usage of some Vα-Jα rearrangements (as if the locus is not opening properly), but no fundamental changes in numbers of γδ(+) and αβ(+) cells *(93)*. Thus, successful commitment to the αβ(+) fate does not require progenitor-specific selective activation of TEA and δrec-Jα61 rearrangement. The third point is a more general one: namely, differences in δrec-, TEA-, or Jα61- activating factors may be a product not a determinant of progenitor commitment. Hence, a detailed analysis is required of the temporal onset of heterogeneity in gene expression, vis-a-vis the stage at which thymocytes receive signals through either complete or incomplete TCRs, as the case may be.

This same argument applies to the expression of locus "silencers." It has been argued, primarily through the study of transgenes that αβ T-cells silence TCRγ gene expression *(71)*, while γδ cells can silence TCRα expression *(94)*. Data for the latter case are the more substantially developed. However, the differential expression of such factors may enforce and/or maintain lineage commitment, once that commitment has been determined by other factors.

15. Different Requirements for γδ Cell and αβ T-Cell Development

One result commonly taken to support the hypothesis that αβ and γδ cells arise, respectively, from precommitted progenitors, is the distinct sensitivities of αβ T-cell development and γδ cell development, respectively, to particular mutations. An example of this is the complete sensitivity of γδ cell development to deficiency in either IL-7 or the IL-7R α chain, whereas αβ T-cell development occurs, although in significantly reduced numbers *(95,96)*. The important effect of IL-7 on αβ T-cell development proves to be rescue from apoptosis, since αβ T-cell development is restored by activated *bcl2* transgenes. By contrast, γδ cell development is not rescued by Bcl2, suggesting that IL-7 has additional and/or other effects. Whereas this would seem to support the precommitment hypothesis, the results can equally well be explained by the actions of IL-7 on a single precursor. First, IL-7 is required for TCRγ gene rearrangement. Thus, IL-7 deficiency precludes γδ cell development from either a common or a distinct progenitor. Second, a defining feature of the final stages of Pathway I, again irrespective of whether the cells arise from a common or precommitted precursor, may be a continuing requirement for IL-7. Support for this additional activity of IL-7 comes from the finding that TCR αβ(+) DN cells present in TCRαβ transgenic mice (*see* above) are also sensitive to IL-7 deficiency, even though they develop from cells with pre-rearranged genes.

16. Survival vs Commitment

Most often, the potential role of the TCR in lineage commitment is viewed as a positive developmental step, signaled by engagement of either the complete or incomplete TCR. Alternatively, these respective 'TCRs' might promote survival of the thymocyte while other factors instruct the pathway of development. In this sense, the TCR chains would be permissive rather than instructive for development. This distinction can be illustrated by consideration of TCR$\beta^{-/-}$ mice. The poor representation of proliferating final-stage DNs and the following DP subsets have been argued (above) to be compatible with either the TCR determinant model (in which most $\gamma\delta$ [+] cells commit to Pathway I) or the progenitor precommitment model (since cells commited to Pathway II will become DPs irrespective of the nature of the TCR).

A revised view of the TCR$\beta^{(-)}$ phenotype is that developing DN cells might enter pathways I and II with approximately equal efficiency, but that the subsequent survival of the cells requires signaling from the appropriate TCR. Thus, expression of TCR$\gamma\delta$ may be incompatible with the maintenance of the "$\alpha\beta$ differentiation pathway" hence, cells die in the absence of TCRβ. These two concepts are presented for the TCR determinant model in Fig. 9A, and for the modified progenitor precommitment model in Fig. 9B. To test these ideas requires assessment not simply of pool sizes ("snapshots," as has been presented in this chapter), but of the kinetics of entry into particular subsets ("moving pictures"). Although more difficult to undertake, these tests could be extremely informative, because the different models make different predictions regarding the outcomes. According to the TCR determinant model, the commitment of δ-selected cells to Pathway II should be inefficient compared to the commitment to Pathway I; this is why there are few DP cells in TCR$\beta^{-/-}$ mice. Conversely, the progenitor precommitment model predicts that the commitment of δ-selected cells to Pathway II should be as efficient as the commitment to Pathway I, since the nature of the TCR is irrelevant. The small numbers of Pathway II cells would be a result of the failure of the $\gamma\delta$TCR to sustain the cells during subsequent Pathway II development.

So far, there is no evidence that the function of either complete or incomplete TCRs during DN thymocyte development is to prevent apoptosis, and deregulated expression of Bcl-2 has failed to rescue development in RAG$^{-/-}$ mice. However, based on the specificities of pathways, it is possible that another gene that can inhibit apoptosis would rescue TCR deficiencies, and reveal the "normal numbers" of progenitors that committed to particular pathways. Such studies should be pursued.

17. A Challenging Future

The resolution of lineage commitment should be made by the assessment of differentiation potential of defined cells, for example, in fetal thymic organ culture, or after intrathymic injection in vivo. The differentiation of those progenitors into either $\alpha\beta$ cells or $\gamma\delta$ cells, or both, could potentially be assayed. To measure the developmental potential of a pure defined cell type, it is ideal to be able to follow the fate of a single progenitor cell. But such an analysis may be confounded by the potential of one cell to affect the development of another (*see* above).

For these reasons, there is a pressing need to apply biochemistry and other reductionist approaches. We will be able to speculate better on the respective signaling capacities of complete TCRs and incomplete TCRs when we have elucidated their ligands. And the pathways of development will be much easier to dissect, mechanistically, when we can

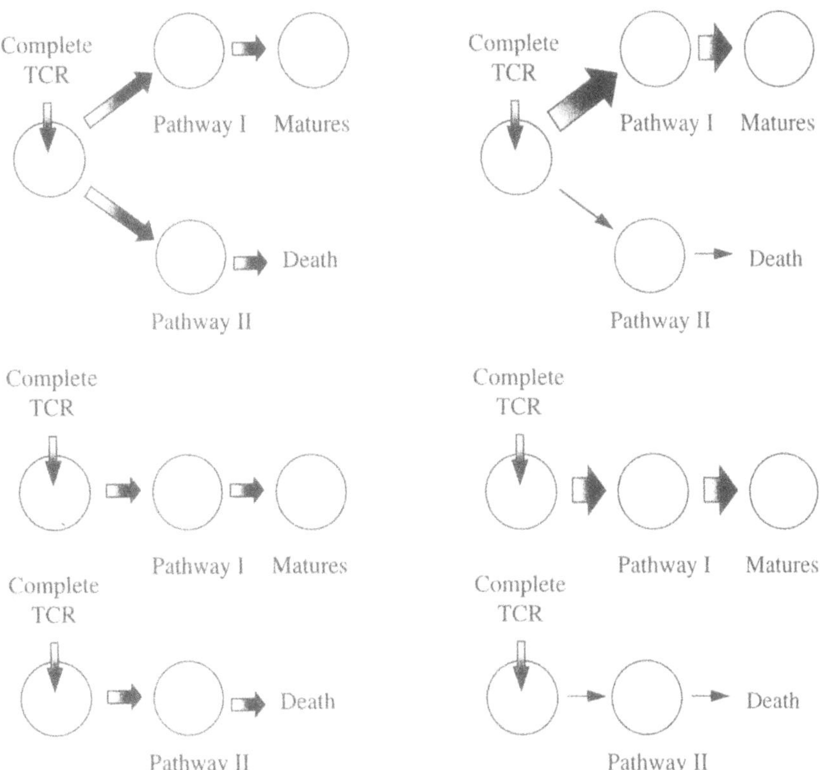

Fig. 9. Efficiency paradigms in the receptor determinant and precommitment models. Both the TCR determinant model and the progenitor precommitment model predict the existence of nonviable, dead-end thymocytes. However, the relative frequency of these nonviable thymocytes has not been determined. **(A)** Efficiency paradigm for the receptor determinant model. The relative frequency of nonviable thymocytes arising could be either frequent (left) or rare (right) in the TCR determinant model. **(B)** Efficiency paradigm for the progenitor precommitment model. Similarly, the relative frequency of nonviable thymocytes arising could be either frequent (left) or rare (right) in the progenitor precommitment model.

induce thymocytes to undergo even single transitions in culture, in defined conditions, without any other cells present. In such a system, the fate of progenitor cells could be related to their rate of cell division, to the levels of potential regulators such as $p27^{kip1}$, to their responsiveness to growth and differentiation factors, and to the engagement (through antibodies) of different molecules on the cell surface. Indeed, the kinetics of development—growth vs death—could be assessed. By the combination of pharmacological reagents and progenitors from different mutant mouse strains, one could dissect a thymocyte's active metabolism as it commits toward either an αβ(+) or a γδ(+) fate, and finally resolve the role(s) played by the products of successful TCR gene rearrangements.

Acknowledgments

This work was supported by NIH grant GM37759 to AH. The authors thank many individuals, particularly Bob Wyman, for discussions of various aspects of T-cell development, and of development in general.

References

1. Hayday, A. C., Saito, H., Gillies, S. D., Kranz, D. M., Tanigawa, G., Eisen, H. N., and Tonegawa, S. (1985) Structure, organization, and somatic rearrangement of T cell gamma genes. *Cell* **40,** 259–269.
2. Saito, H., Kranz, D. M., Takagaki, Y., Hayday, A. C., Eisen, H. N., and Tonegawa, S. (1984) The complete primary structure of an heterodimeric T cell receptor protein as deduced from cDNA sequences *Nature* **309,** 757–762.
3. Brenner, M. B., McLean, J., Dialynas, D. P., Strominger, J. L., Smith, J. A., Owen, F. L., Seidman, J. G., Ip, S., Rosen, F., and Krangel, M. S. (1986. Identification of a putative second T-cell receptor. *Nature* **322,** 145–149.
4. Hayday, A. and Pao, W. (1997) T cell receptor, γδ, in *Encyclopedia of Immunology*, 2nd ed. (Roitt, I. M. and Delves, P. J., eds.), Academic, London, UK, in press.
5. Mallick-Wood, C. A., Pao, W., Cheng, A. M., Lewis, J. M., Kulkarni, S., Bolen, J. B., Rowley, B., Tigelaar, R. E., Pawson, T., and Hayday, A. C. (1996) Disruption of epithelial γδ T cell repertoires in mice deficient in Syk tyrosine kinase. *Proc. Natl. Acad. Sci. USA* **93,** 9704–9709.
6. Turner, M., Mee, P. J., Costello, P. S., William, O., Price, A. A., Duddy, L. P., Furlong, M. T., Geahlen, R. L., and Tybulewicz, V. L. J. (1995) Perinatal lethality and blocked B-cell development in mice lacking the tyrosine kinase Syk. *Nature* **378,** 298–302.
7. Dunon, D., Cooper, M. D., and Imhof, B. A. (1993) Thymic origin of embryonic intestinal gamma/delta T cells. *J. Exp. Med.* **177,** 257–263.
8. Pardoll, D. M., Fowlkes, B. J., Lew, A. M., Maloy, W. L., Weston, M. A., Bluestone, J. A., Schwartz, R. H., Coligan, J. E., and Kruisbeek, A. M. (1988) Thymus-dependent and thymus-independent developmental pathways for peripheral T cell receptor-gamma delta-bearing lymphocytes. *J. Immunol.* **140,** 4091–4096.
9. Rocha, B., Vassalli, P., Guy-Grand, D. (1994) Thymic and extrathymic origins of gut intraepithelial lymphocyte populations in mice. *J. Exp. Med.* **180,** 681–686.
10. Havran, W. L. and Allison, J. P. (1988) Developmentally ordered appearance of thymocytes expressing different T-cell antigen receptors. *Nature* 335, 443–445.
11. Havran, W. L. and Allison, J. P. (1990) Origin of thy1$^{(+)}$ dendritic epidermal cells of adult mice from fetal precursors. *Nature* 344, 68–70.
12 Itohara, S., Farr, A. G., Lafaille, J. J., Bonneville, M., Takagaki, Y., Haas, W., and Tonegawa, S. (1990) Homing of a gamma delta thymocyte subset with homogeneous T-cell receptors to mucosal epithelia. *Nature* 343, 754–757.
13. Kelly, K., Pearse, M., Lefrancois, L., and Scollay, R. (1993) Emigration of selected subsets of $\gamma\delta^+$ T cells from the adult murine thymus. *Int. Immunol.* **5,** 331–335.
14. Raff, M. C. (1989) Glial cell diversification in the rat optic nerve. *Science* **243,** 1450–1455.
15. Heitzler, P. and Simpson, P. (1991) The choice of cell fate in the epidermis of *Drosophila. Cell* **64,** 1083–1092.
16. Wyman, R. J. (1986) Sequential induction and a homeotic switch of cell fate. *Trends Neuro Sci* **9,** 339–340.
17. Alam, S. M., Travers, P. J., Wung, J. L., Nasholds, W., Redpath, S., Jameson, S. C., and Gascoigne, N. R. J. (1996) T-cell-receptor affinity and thymocyte positive selection *Nasture* **381,** 616–620.
18. Ashton-Rickardt, P. G. and Tonegawa, S. (1994) A differential-avidity model for T-cell selection. *Immunol. Today* **15,** 362–366.
19. Jameson, S. C., Hogquist, K. A., and Bevan, M. J. (1995) Positive selection of thymocytes. *Ann. Rev. Immunol.* **13,** 93–126.
20. Struhl, G. (1989) Differing strategies for organizing anterior and posterior body pattern in *Drosophila* embryos. *Nature* **338,** 741–744.
21. Belvin, M. P., and Anderson K. V. (1996) A conserved signaling pathway: the Drosophila toll-dorsal pathway. *Ann. Rev. Cell Dev. Biol.* **12,** 393–416.
22. Dudley, E., Petrie, H. T., Shah, L. M., Owen, M. J., and Hayday, A. C. (1994) T cell receptor β chain gene rearrangement and selection during thymocyte development in adult mice. *Immunity* **1,** 83–93.

23. Karasuyama, H., Rolink, A., Shinkai, Y., Young, F., Alt, F. W., and Melchers, F. (1994) The expression of Vpre-B/lambda 5 surrogate light chain in early bone marrow precursor B cells of normal and B cell-deficient mutant mice. *Cell* **77,** 133–143.
24. Kitamura, D., Kudo, A., Schaal, S., Muller, W., Melchers, F., and Rajewsky, K. (1992) A critical role of l5 protein in B cell development. *Cell* **69,** 823–831.
25. Shores, E. W., Sharrow, S. O., Uppenkamp, I., and Singer, A. (1990) T cell receptor-negative thymocytes from SCID mice can be induced to enter the CD4/CD8 differentiation pathway. *Eur. J. Immunol. 20,* 69–77.
26. Elbe, A., Kilgus, O., Strohal, R., Payer, E., Schreiber, S., and Stingl, G. (1992) Fetal skin: a site of dendritic epidermal T cell development. *J. Immunol.* **149,** 1694–1701.
27. Ikuta, K., Kina, T., MacNeil, I., Uchida, N., Peault, B., Chien, Y.-H., and Weissman, I. L. (1990) A developmental switch in thymic lymphocyte maturation potential occurs at the level of hematopoietic stem cells. *Cell* **62,** 863–874.
28. Ikuta, K. and Weissman, I. L. (1991) The Junctional modifications of a T cell receptor g chain are determined at the level of thymic precursors. *J. Exp. Med.* **174,** 1279–1282.
29. Heyborne, K., Fu, Y. X., Kalataradi, H., Reardon, C., Roark, C., Eyster, C., Vollmer, M., Born, W., and O'Brien, R. (1993) Evidence that murine V gamma 5 and V gamma 6 gamma delta-TCR^+ lymphocytes are derived from a common distinct lineage. *J. Immunol.* **151,** 4523–4527.
30. Asarnow, D., Cado, D., and Raulet, D. (1993) Selection is not required to produce invariant T-cell receptor γ-gene junctional sequences *Nature* **362,** 158–160.
31. Galandrini, R., Henning, S. W., and Cantrell, D. A. (1997) Different functions of the GTPase Rho in prothymocytes and late pre-T cells. *Immunity* **7,** 163–174.
32. Lauzurica, P. and Krangel, M. S. (1994a) Enhancer-dependent and -independent steps in the rearrangement of a human T cell receptor delta transgene. *J. Exp. Med.* **179,** 43–55.
33. Lauzurica, P. and Krangel, M. S. (1994b) Temporal and lineage-specific control of T cell receptor alpha/delta gene rearrangement by T cell receptor alpha and delta enhancers. *J. Exp. Med.* **179,** 1913–1921.
34. Ohteki, T., Wilson, A., Verbeek, S., MacDonald, H. R., and Clevers, H. (1996) Selectively impaired development of intestinal T cell receptor γδ cells and liver $CD4^+$ $NK1^+$ T cell receptor αβ+ cells in T cell factor-1-deficent mice. *Eur. J. Immunol.* **26,** 351–355.
35. Roberts, J. L., Lauzurica, P., and Krangel, M. S. (1997) Developmental regulation of VDJ recombination by the core fragment of the T cell receptor alpha enhancer. *J. Exp. Med.* **185,** 131–140.
36. Thompson, S. D., Manzo, A. R., Pelkonen, J., Larche, M., and Hurwitz, J. L. (1991) Developental T cell receptor gene rearrangements: relatedness of the αβ and γδ T cell precursor. *Eur. J. Immunol.* **21,** 1939–1950.
37. Bogue, M., Mossmann, H., Stauffer, U., Benoist, C., and Mathis, D. (1993) The level of N-region diversity in T cell receptors is not pre-ordained in the stem cell. *Eur. J. Immunol.* **23,** 1185–1188.
38. Bonneville, M., Ishida, I., Mombaerts, P., Katsuki, M., Verbeek, S., Berns, A., and Tonegawa, S. (1989) Blockage of alpha beta T-cell development by TCR gamma delta transgenes. *Nature* **342,** 931–934.
39. Dudley, E. C., Girardi, M., Owen, M. J., and Hayday, A. C. (1995) αβ and γδ T cells can share a late common precursor. *Curr. Biol.* **5,** 659–669.
40. Palmer, D., Viney, J. L., Ritter, M. A., Hayday, A. C., and Owen, M. J. (1993) Expression of the αβ T cell receptor is necessary for the development of the thymic medulla. *Dev Immunol.* **3,** 175–179.
41. Philpott, K. L., Viney, J. L., Kay, G., Rastan, S., Gardiner, E. M., Chae, S., Hayday, A. C., and Owen, M. J. (1992) Lymphoid development in mice congenitally lacking T cell receptor alpha beta-expressing cells. *Science* **256,**1448–1452.
42. Bucy, R. P., Chen, C. L., Cihak, J., Losch, U., and Cooper, M. D. (1988) Avian T cells expressing gamma delta receptors localize in the splenic sinusoids and the intestinal epithelium. *J. Immunol.* **141(7),** 2200–2205.

43. Allison, J. P. and Lanier, L. L (1987) The T-cell antigen receptor γ gene:rearrangement and cell lineages. *Immunol. Today* 8, 293–296.
44. Pardoll, D. M., Fowlkes, B. J., Bluestone, J. A., Kruisbeek, A. M., Maloy, W. L., Coligan, J. E., and Schwartz, R. H. (1987) Differential expression of two disitnct T-cell receptors during thymocyte development. *Nature* **326,** 79–81.
45. Passoni, L., Hoffman, E., Kim, S., Crompton, T., Pao, W., Dong, M.-Q., Owen, M. J., and Hayday, A. C. (1997) Intrathymic δ selection events in γδ cell development. *Immunity* **7,** 83–95.
46. Fehling, H. J., Krotkova, A., Saint-Ruf, C., and von Boehmer, H. (1995) Crucial role of the pre-T-cell receptor a gene in development of αβ but not γδ T cells. *Nature* **375,** 795–798.
47. Groettrup, M., Ungewiss, K., Azogui, O., Palacios, R., Owen, M. J., Hayday, A., and von Boehmer, H. (1993. A novel disulfide-linked heterodimer on pre-T cells consists of the T cell receptor β chain and a 33kD glycoprotein. *Cell* 75, 283–294.
48. Saint-Ruf, C., Ungewiss, K., Groettrup, M., Bruno, L., Fehling, H. J., and von Boehmer, H. (1994) Analysis and expression of a cloned pre-T cell receptor gene. *Science* **266,** 1208–1212.
49. Winoto, A. and Baltimore, D. (1989) Separate lineages of T cells expressing the αβ and γδ receptors. *Nature* **338,** 430–432.
50. deVillartay, J.-P., Hockett, R. D., Coran, D., Korsmeyer, S. J., and Cohen, D. I. (1988) Deletion of the human T-cell receptor δ-gene by site-specific recombination. *Nature* **335,** 170–174.
51. Janowski, K. M., Ledbetter, S., Mayo, M. S., and Hockett, R. D. (1997) Identification of a DNA segment exhibiting rearrangement modifying effects upon transgenic δ-deleting elements. *J. Exp. Med.* **186,** 91–100.
52. Fujimoto, S. and Yamagishi, H. (1987) Isolation of an excision product of T-cell receptor α-chain gene rearrangements. *Nature* **327,** 242–243.
53. Takeshita, S., Toda, M., and Yamagishi, H. (1989) Excision products of the T cell receptor gene support a progressive rearrangement model of the α/δ locus. *EMBO J.* **8,** 3261–3270.
54. Livak, F., Petrie, H. T., Crispe, I. N., and Schatz, D. G. (1995) In-frame TCR δ gene rearrangements play a critical role in the αβ/γδ T cell lineage decision. *Immunity* **2,** 617–627.
55. Livak, F. and Schatz, D. G. (1996) T-cell receptor alpha locus V(D)J recombination by-products are abundant in thymocytes and mature T cells. *Mol. Cell. Biol.* **16,** 609–618.
56. Margolis, D., Yassai, M., Hlettko, A., McOlash, L., and Gorski, J. (1997) Concurrent or sequential δ and β TCR gene rearangement during thymocyte development. *J. Immunol.* **159,** 529–533.
57. Nakajima, P. B., Menetski, J. P., Roth, D. B., Gellert, M., and Bosma, M. J. (1995) V-D-J rearrangements at the T cell receptor delta locus in mouse thymocytes of the alpha beta lineage. *Immunity* **3,** 609–621.
58. Thompson, S. D., Pelkonen, J., and Hurwitz, J. L. (1990) Concomitant T-cell receptor α and δ gene rearrangements in individual T-cell precursors. *Proc. Natl. Acad. Sci USA* **87,** 5583–5586.
59. Wilson, A., de Villartay, J. P., and MacDonald, H. R. (1996) T cell receptor delta gene rearrangement and T early alpha (TEA) expression in immature alpha beta lineage thymocytes: implications for αβ/γδ lineage commitment. *Immunity* **4,** 37–45.
60. Mallick, C., Dudley, E. C., Viney, J. L., Owen, M. J., and Hayday, A. C. (1993) Rearrangement and diversity of T cell receptor β chain genes in thymocytes: a critical role for the β chain in development. *Cell* **73,** 513–519.
61. Itohara, S., Mombaerts, P., Lafaille, J., Iacomini, J., Nelson, A., Clarke, A. R., Hooper, M. L., Farr, A., and Tonegawa, S. (1993) T cell receptor delta gene mutant mice: independent generation of αβ T cells and programmed rearrangements of γδ TCR genes. *Cell* **72,** 337–348.
62. Ossendorp, F., Jacobs, H., van der Horst, G., de Vries, E., Berns, A., and Borst, J. (1992) T cell receptor αβ lacking the β chain V domain can be expressed at the cell surface but prohibits T cell maturation. *J. Immunol.* **148,** 3714–3722.
63. Itohara, S. and Tonegawa, S. (1990) Selection of γδ T cells with canonical T-cell antigen receptors in fetal thymus. *Proc. Natl. Acad. Sci. USA* **87,** 7935–7938.
64. Burtrum, D. B., Kim, S., Dudley, E. C., Hayday, A. C., and Petrie, H. T. (1996) TCR gene recombination and αβ-γδ lineage divergence: productive TCR-β rearrangement is neither exclusive nor preclusive of γδ cell development. *J. Immunol.* **157,** 4293–4296.

65. Fowlkes, B. J., Edison, L., Mathieson, B. J., and Chused, T. M. (1985) Early T lymphocytes: differentiation in vivo of adult intrathymic precursor cells. *J. Exp. Med* **162,** 802.
66. Godfrey, D., Kennedy, J., Suda, T., and Zlotnik, A. (1993) A developmental pathway involving four phenotypically and functionally distinct subsets of CD3-CD4-CD8- triple negative adult mouse thymocytes defined by CD44 and CD25 expression. *J. Immunol.* **150,** 4244–4252.
67. Hoffman, E. S., Passoni, L., Crompton, T., Leu, T. M. J., Schatz, D. G., Koff, A., Owen, M. J., and Hayday, A. C. (1996) Productive T cell receptor β chain gene rearrangement: coincident regulation of cell proliferation and clonality during T cell development in vivo. *Genes Dev.* **10,** 948–962.
68. Mombaerts, P., Clarke, A. R., Rudnicki, M. A., Iacomini, J., Itohara, S., Lafille, J., Wang, L., Ichikawa, Y., Jaenisch, R., Hooper, M. L., and Tonegawa, S. (1992) Mutations in T-cell receptor genes α and β block thymocyte development at different stages. *Nature* **360,** 225–231.
69. Buer J., Aifantis, I., DiSanto, J. P., Fehling, H. J., and von Boehmer, H. (1997) Role of different T cell receptors in the development of pre-T cells. *J. Exp. Med.* **185,** 1541–1547.
70. Dent, A. L., Matis, L. A., Hooshmand, F., Widacki, S. M., Bluestone, J. A., and Hedrick, S. M. (1990) Self reactive γδ T cells are eliminated in the thymus. *Nature* **343,** 714–719.
71. Ishida, I., Verbeek, S., Bonneville, M., Itohara, S., Berns, A., Tonegawa, S. (1990) T-cell receptor gamma delta and gamma transgenic mice suggest a role of a gamma gene silencer in the generation of alpha beta T cells. *Proc. Natl. Acad. Sci. USA* **87,** 3067–3071.
72. Kersh, G. J., Hooshmand, F. F., and Hedrick, S. M. (1995) Efficient maturation of αβ lineage thymoctes to the $CD4^+CD8^+$ stage in the absence of TCR-β rearrangement. J. *Immunol.* **154,** 5706–5714.
73. Livak, F., Wilson, A., MacDonald, H. R., and Schatz, D. G. (1997) αβ lineage commited thymocytes can be rescued by the γδ TCR in the absence of TCRβ. *Eur. J. Immunol.* in press.
74. Sim, G. K., Olsson, C, and Augustin, A. (1995) Commitment and maintenance of the alpha beta and gamma delta T cell lineages. *J. Immunol.* **154,** 5821–5831.
75. Fehling, H. J., Ititani, B. M., Krotkova, A., Forbusch, K., Laplace, C., Perlmutter, R. M., and von Boehmer, H. (1997) Restoration of thympoiesis in $pT\alpha^{-/-}$ mice by anti CD3ε antibody treatment or with transgenes encoding activated lck or tailless pTα. *Immunity* **6,** 703–714.
76. Cyster, J., Hartley, S. B., and Goodnow, C. C. (1994) Competition for follicular niches excludes self-reactive cells from the recirculating B-cell repertoire, *Nature* **371,** 389–395.
77. Donskoy, E. and Goldschneider, I. (1992) Thymocytopoiesis is maintained by blood-borne precursors throughout postnatal life. A study in parabiotic mice. *J. Immunol.* **148,** 1604–1612.
78. Xu, Y., Davidson, L., Alt, F. W., and Baltimore, D. (1996) Function of the pre T-cell receptor a chain in T-cell development and allelic exclusion at the T-cell receptor β locus. *Proc. Natl. Acad. Sci USA* **93,** 2169–2173.
79. Chan, S. H., Cosgrove, D., Waltzinger, C., Benoist, C., and Mathis, D. (1993) Another view of the selective model of thymocyte selection. *Cell* **73,** 225–236.
80. Davis, C. B., Killeen, N., Crooks, M. E., Raulet, D., Littman, D. R. (1993) Evidence for a stochastic mechanism in the differentiation of mature subsets of T lymphocytes. *Cell* **73,** 237–247.
81. Suzuki, H., Punt, J. A., Granger, L. G., and Singer, A. (1995) Asymmetric signaling requirements for thymocyte commitment to the $CD4^+$ versus $CD8^+$ T cell lineages: a new perspective on thymic commitment and selection. *Immunity* **2,** 413–425.
82. Bruno, L., Fehling, H. J., and von Boehmer, H. (1996) The αβ T cell receptor can replace the γδ receptor in the development of γδ lineage cells. *Immunity* **5,** 343–352.
83. Capone, M., Curnow, J., Bouvier, G., Ferrier, P., and Horvat, B. (1995) T cell development in TCR-alpha beta transgenic mice. Analysis using V(D)J recombination substrates. *J. Immunol.* 154, 5165–5172.
84. Pircher, H., Ohashi, P., Miescher, G., Lang, R., Zikopoulos, A., Burki, K., Mak, T. W., MacDonald, H. R., and Hengartner, H. (1990) T cell receptor (TcR) beta chain transgenic mice: studies on allelic exclusion and on the TcR+ gamma/delta population. *Eur. J. Immunol.* **20,** 417–424.
85. Kisielow, P., Bluthmann, H., Staerz, U., Steinmetz, M., and von Boehmer, H. (1988) Tolerance in T-cell-receptor transgenic mice involves deletion of nonmature $CD4^+8^+$ thymocytes. *Nature* **333,** 742–746.

86. Robey, E., Chang, D., Itano, A., Cado, D., Alexander, H., Lans, D., Weinmaster, G., Salmon, P. (1996) An activated form of Notch influences the choice between CD4 and CD8 T cell lineages. *Cell* **87,** 483–492.
87. Washburn, T., Schweighoffer, E., Gridley, T., Chang, D., Fowlkes, B. J., Cado, D., and Robey, E. (1997) Notch activity influences the αβ versus γδ T cell lineage decision. *Cell* **88,** 833–843.
88. Bruno, L., Rocha, B., Rolink, A., von Boehmer, H., and Rodewald, H.-R. (1995) Intra- and extra-thymic expression of the pre T cell receptor a gene *Eur. J Immunol* **25,** 1877–1882.
89. Zorbas, M. and Scollay, R. (1993) Development of γδ T cells in the adult murine thymus. *Eur J. Immunol.* **23,** 1655–1660.
90. Heiken, H., Schulz, R. J., Ravetch, J. V., Reinherz, E. L., and Koyasu, S. (1996) T lymphocyte development in the absence of Fc epsilon receptor I gamma subunit: analysis of thymic-dependent and independent αβ and γδ pathways. *Eur. J. Immunol.* **26,** 1935–1943.
91. Groves, T., Smiley, P., Cooke, M. P., Forbush, K., R. M., Guidos, C. J. (1996) Fyn can partially substitute for Lck in T lymphocyte development. *Immunity* **5,** 417–428.
92. van Oers, N. S. C., Lowin-Kropf, B., Finlay, D., Connolly, K., and Weiss, A. (1996) αβ T cell development is abolished in mice lacking both lck and fyn protein tyrosine kinases. *Immunity* **5,** 429–436.
93. Villey, I., Caillol, D., Selz, F., Ferrier, P., and de Villartay, J.-P. (1996) Defect in rearrangement of the most 5' TCR-J α following targeted deletion of T early α (TEA): implications for TCR a locus accessibility. *Immunity* **5,** 331–342.
94. Winoto, A. and Baltimore, D. (1989) αβ lineage-specific expression of the a T cell receptor gene by nearby silencers. *Cell* **59,** 649–655.
95. He, Y.-W. and Malek, T. R. (1996) Interleukin-7 receptor alpha is essential for the development of gamma delta + T cells, but not natural killer cells. *J. Exp. Med.* **184,** 289–293.
96. Maki, K., Sunaga, S., Komagata, Y., Kodaira, Y., Mabuchi, A., Karasuyama, H., Yokomuro, K., Miyazaki, J. I., and Ikuta, K. (1996) Interleukin 7 receptor-deficient mice lack γδ T cells. *Proc. Natl. Acad. Sci. USA* **93,** 7172–7177.

Part V

Selection Process Operating During B-Lymphocyte Development

Chapter 20

Structure and Function of the Pro- and Pre-B-Cell Receptors on B-Lymphoid Lineage Precursor Cells

Thomas H. Winkler and Fritz Melchers

1. Introduction

B lymphocytes develop from hematopoietic stem cells. In mouse and in man, B lymphocyte development takes place first during embryogenesis—mainly in the fetal liver and then during postnatal life in the bone marrow *(1–5)*. The development from progenitor (pro) and precursor (pre) B-cells to immature and mature B lymphocytes is characterized by proliferation, differentiation, and ordered rearrangements of immunoglobulin (Ig) heavy (H) and light (L) chain genes. As for the other hematopoietic lineages few lineage-committed progenitor cells give rise to large numbers of mature effector cells.

Progressive differentiation along the pathway of B-lymphocyte development can be characterized by intracellular and surface-bound molecular markers. A general marker for cells of the B lineage is the CD19 molecule that has long been recognized in man *(6)*, and recently, also in mice *(7)*. In addition, expression of a CD45 RO isoform, called B220, has been used to characterize B-lymphoid cells in the mouse *(8)*. The different stages of the B-cell development have been defined by work of Osmond et al. *(3,9)*, Hardy et al. *(1)*, Nishikawa et al. *(10)*, and Rolink et al. *(5,11)* for the mouse and by several groups in man *(12–14)*. A comparison of the different schemes has recently been published *(11,15)*.

The authors have suggested a nomenclature for the developmental stages of B-cell development based on the rearrangement status of the Ig heavy (H) and light (L) chain gene loci at the different progenitor and precursor cell stages *(5)*. In pro-B-cells, the immunoglobulin heavy and light chain loci are all in germline configuration (Fig. 1). Pre–B-I cells carry DJ_H rearrangements at the H chain loci, whereas pre–B-II cells have at least one allele in V_HDJ_H configuration. Both pre–B-I cells and pre–B-II cells have

From: *Molecular Biology of B-Cell and T-Cell Development*
Edited by: J. G. Monroe and E. V. Rothenberg © Humana Press Inc., Totowa, NJ

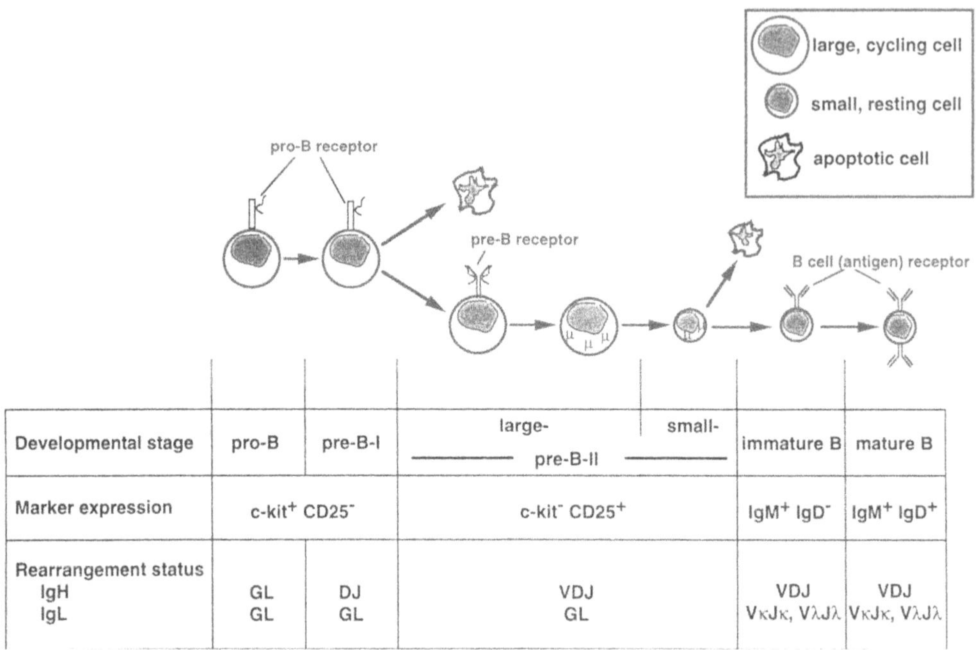

Developmental stage	pro-B	pre-B-I	large- pre-B-II	small- pre-B-II	immature B	mature B
Marker expression	c-kit⁺ CD25⁻		c-kit⁻ CD25⁺		IgM⁺ IgD⁻	IgM⁺ IgD⁺
Rearrangement status IgH IgL	 GL GL	 DJ GL	 VDJ GL		 VDJ VκJκ, VλJλ	 VDJ VκJκ, VλJλ

Fig. 1. A model of B-cell development in normal mouse bone marrow.

their light chain genes in germline configuration (Fig. 1). Immature and mature B-cells express IgM on the cell surface, whereas IgD is expressed only on mature B lymphocytes. The authors have characterized and experimentally separated the different stages of the development, mainly by use of the differential expression of the tyrosine kinase c-kit and the IL-2 receptor α chain (CD25) *(11)*. C-kit is expressed on pro–B- and pre–B-I cells, but not on pre–B-II cells. CD25 is expressed on pre–B-II cells, but not on pro–B and pre–B-I cells (Fig. 1). Apparently, CD25 expression correlates with the expression of μH chain in the cytoplasm *(11)*. The pre–B-II cells could be further divided according to their cell cycle status (i.e., their size). One can distinguish large cycling CD25⁺ pre–B-II cells from small resting CD25⁺ pre–B-II cells (Fig. 1).

Two proteins encoded by the pre-B-cell-specific genes V_{preB} *(16)* and λ5 *(17)* can associate with each other to form a light chain-like structure, the so-called surrogate light chain (Fig.2). The surrogate light chain can be found in association with a molecular complex of glycoproteins on the surface of μH chain negative pro–B-cells *(18,19)*. This complex is referred to as the pro-B-cell receptor. In the pre-B-cell receptor, the surrogate light chain is associated with μH chains *(20–23)* (Fig. 2). The pre-B-cell receptor has a structure similar to the B-cell receptor (BCR), which is composed of μH chain and L chains, since the accessory molecules Ig-α and Ig-β that function as signal transducer are found associated with both receptors *(23,24)* (Fig. 2).

In this chapter the structure of the pro-B and pre-B receptors is described and present evidence for the functions of these receptors in B-cell development is summarized.

2. Gene and Protein Structure of the Surrogate Light Chain

2.1. Structure and Evolution of the Surrogate Light Chain Genes

The V_{preB} and the λ5 genes are found on the same chromosomes as the λ light chain genes in both mouse (chromosome 16) and man (chromosome 22) *(25,26)*. In the mouse,

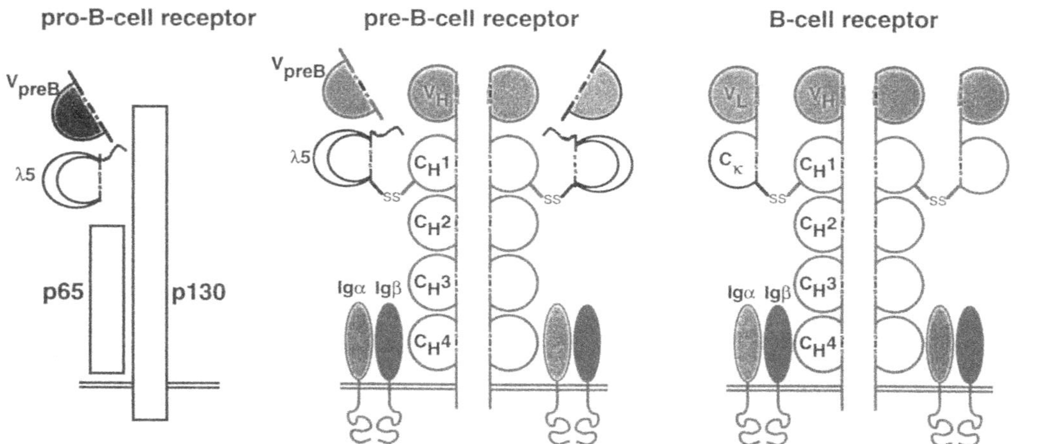

Fig. 2. Model structures of the pro–B-cell receptor, the pre-B-cell receptor, and the B-cell antigen receptor.

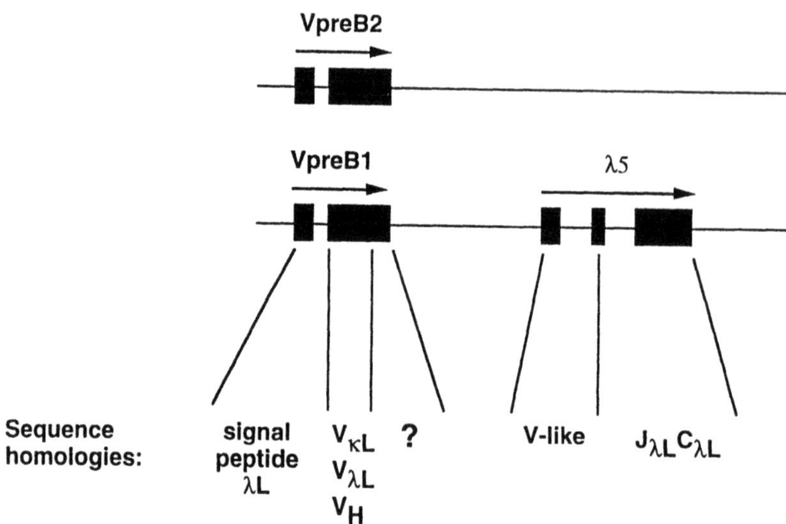

Fig. 3. Organization and sequence homologies of the mouse surrogate light chain genes on chromosome 16.

there are two functional V_{preB} genes with very high sequence homology *(16)*. The V_{preB1} and λ5 genes are located within 10 kb of each other with an unknown distance from V_{preB2} and from the λ L chain locus *(16)*.

Both the V_{preB} genes, as well as the λ5 gene, show regions of sequence homology to the λ light chain genes, as well as regions with no homology to known genes or proteins. The exon I and the 5' part of exon II of V_{preB} show sequence homology to V-regions of the heavy or the κ or λ light chain gene loci (Fig. 3). The sequence homology breaks off at the approximate position equivalent to the CDR3 region of the immunoglobulin V gene segments. The remaining 3' segment of the exon II shows no similarity to any known sequence. In the λ5 gene, the exon I and the 5' region of the exon II show no strong sequence homologies, although weak homology can be detected with Ig domains. The 3' region of exon II as well as exon III are highly homologous to the Jλ as well as the Cλ genes.

In contrast to the V and J genes of the light chain loci, the V_{preB} and the λ5 genes do not undergo rearrangement with each other during B-cell development. The typical rearrangement signal sequences present immediately 3' of the V_L chain genes, as well as immediately 5' of the J_L chain genes are missing in the V_{preB} and λ5 genes.

Another VpreB-like molecule has been found to be expressed in pre-B-cells (earlier called 8HS20) *(27)*, called V_{preB3} *(28)*. In contrast to V_{preB1} and V_{preB2} genes, the V_{preB3} gene contains an intron separating the V-like domain into two exons. The location of this gene within the genome of the mouse has not yet been determined.

In man, there is only one V_{preB} gene within a cluster of Vλ genes *(29)*, with 80% overall sequence identity to the mouse $V_{preB1/2}$ genes *(30)*. Multiple λ5-like genes have been found in man *(31–34)*. A cluster of three genes, 14.1, 16.1, and Fλ1 do not rearrange during B-cell development. Another gene, the Igλ1 gene that can rearrange during B-cell development, is also organized in a typical three-exon structure very similar to the λ5 and the 14.1 gene *(32)*. The 14.1 gene is transcribed and translated into a λ5-like protein. None of the other λ5-like genes have been found to be translated into protein. It is intriguing to speculate that the Igλ1 gene represents a descendent from a primordial λ5-like gene where the rearrangement signal sequences have been integrated. However, it remains

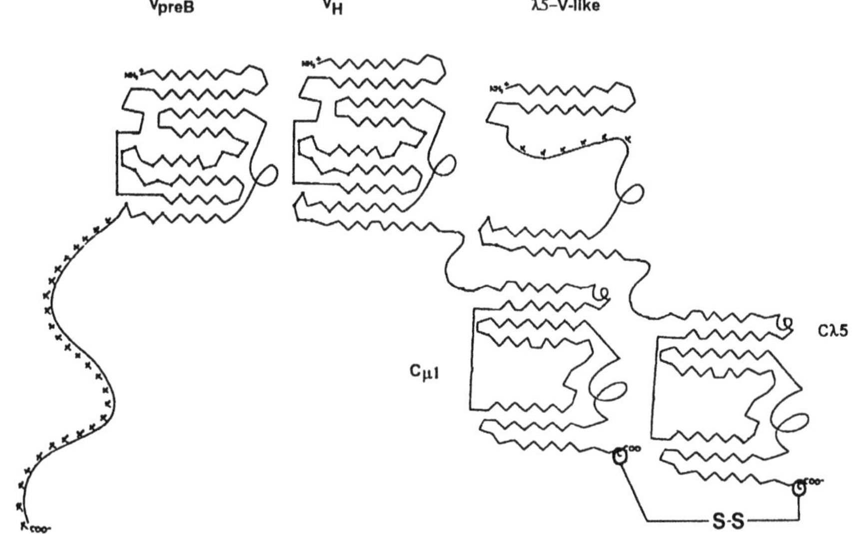

Fig. 4. Speculative structure of the pre-B receptor complex. V_{preB} is drawn as if it would be an Ig variable region with an unknown carboxy terminus protruding from the region analogous to the CDR3 of a variable region. λ5 is drawn with a constant region analogous to the Jκ and Cκ region and with a variable region-like amino terminal end, in which four (A, B, F, and G) of the seven β-strands of an Ig domain are present. V_{preB} and the V-like-domain of λ5 are modelled after the V_H-domain. Cμ1 and "C"λ5 are modelled after the Cκ-domain. The V_H and Cκ- domain structures are taken from Padlan, 1977, *(109)*, as redrawn by Klein, 1990 *(110)*. The CH1 domain and the Cλ domain of the λ5 protein are disulphide linked. Note that most likely the V_{preB}-, the V_H- and the λ5-V-like domains all make contact with each other.

unclear how the surrogate light chain genes evolved relative to the λ light chain loci, as well as to the V region clusters used in rearrangements of the Ig H and κL chain genes.

2.2. Predicted Structure of V_{preB} and λ5 Proteins and of the Complex with μH Chains

The proteins encoded by the V_{preB} and λ5 genes associate noncovalently but quite tightly with each other to form the V_{preB}/λ5 surrogate light chain. Formal proof that they, together with μH chains, can form a triple, and all possible double complexes come from cell lines into which either all genes or all possible combinations of two of these genes were stably transfected *(18)* (T. Seidl and F. Melchers, in preparation). Expression was accomplished in fibroblasts, myeloma cells, and *Drosophila* (Schneider-) cells. Surrogate L chain molecules are, in fact, secreted from these cells, and the same is true for the triple complex when expressed in either fibroblasts or *Drosophila* cells.

The three-dimensional structures of surrogate L chain, either alone, or associated with either μH chains or gp130 protein, have not yet been analyzed. The sequence homologies detected in the gene sequences with λ light chains, with Jλ and with V-regions have led us to speculate that V_{preB} might form the three-dimensional structure of an Ig-variable region with an unknown carboxy-terminal end protruding from the region analogous to the third complementarity determining region (CDR3), where homology with V-regions seen in the amino-terminal region of V_{preB} terminates (Fig. 4). The λ5 part of surrogate light chain is drawn as a constant (Cλ) and J (Jλ) region of λ L chains, as well as with a truncated, variable region-like amino-terminal portion in which four (A, B, F, G) of the seven (A→G) β-strands of an Ig-V-region domain are expected to be present. Furthermore, the aminoterminal domain of the λ5 protein appears to contain a signal peptide sequence with two potential cleavage sites, of which one appears to be used in pre-B-cells (K. Ohnishi and F. Melchers, unpublished observation). Note that the structures shown in Fig. 4 have not been obtained by X-ray crystallography but are speculations.

3. Regulation of the Expression of the Surrogate Light Chain Genes

3.1. The Expression of the Surrogate Light Chain Genes is Lineage and Stage Specific

The expression of the RNA trancripts from V_{preB} and λ5 genes has been studied in a series of transformed cell lines that appear frozen at a different stages of B-cell development. In general, V_{preB} and λ5 are always coexpressed in the same cells. Furthermore, the two V_{preB} genes, V_{preB1} and V_{preB2}, are coexpressed during B-cell development *(35)*. Northern analysis showed that V_{preB} and λ5 are expressed in Abelson Virus transformed pro- and pre-B-cell lines *(5,16,36)*. In the HAFTL-1 cell line that has the capacity to develop into pre-B-cells or into myeloid cells *(37)* Northern analysis of poly A^+ mRNA revealed that λ5 and V_{preB} are already expressed at the progenitor stage, and increase in expression as the progenitors differentiate to pre-B-cells, or are turned off as the progenitors differentiate to myeloid cells *(36)*. In NFS-5, pre-B-cells that express a functional μH chain *(38)*, λ5 and V_{preB} are still expressed. The latest transformed cells in the B-lineage pathway that express the λ5, and V_{preB} genes are immature sIg^+ cell lines, such as the B-cell lymphoma 38C-13 or sIg^+ variants of NFS-5 cells *(36)*. In more mature B-cell lines and Ig-secreting plasmacytomas, the expression of the λ5 and V_{preB} genes is undetectable.

The human V_{preB} and lambda-like genes follow this pattern of pre-B-cell specific expression *(30,33,34)*. The analysis of several B-cell lymphomas and leukemias showed that the expression of V_{preB} can serve as a lineage- and stage-restricted marker for B-cell precursor leukemias *(39)*.

The λ5 and V_{preB} genes have never been found to be expressed in other cell lineages including T-cells, myeloid cells, epithelial cells, or fibroblasts. Thus, these genes seem to be expressed in a strictly lineage-specific manner.

3.2. Cis-Acting Elements Controlling the Pre-B Specific Expression of the Surrogate Light Chain Genes

The pre-B-cell specific expression of the λ5 gene is regulated at the level of transcription. The promotor of the λ5 gene lacks a TATA box and the transcription is started at multiple sites *(40,41)*. Several genes expressed in the early stages of both B- and T-lymphocyte development contain TATA less promotors *(40,41)*, like the terminal deoxynucleotidyltransferase (TdT) gene *(42)*, the lck gene *(43)*, and the pre-Tα gene *(44)*. Recently the 5' regulatory region of the λ5 gene (5'λ5) has been analysed in detail *(45,46)*. The 5'λ5 region contains two separable elements, a 3' region with general promotor activity and a 5' region containing an enhancer that confers the specificity of expression, and was also found to act on heterologous promotors *(40,45–47)*. Apparently, the enhancer acts as a suppressing region in later B-cell stages and in other cells *(45)*. The transcription factor EBF (early B-cell factor) binds to a DNA motif in the λ5 enhancer *(47)*. Hence, it might be important for activating the λ5 gene in the proper lineage. Other factors and *cis* acting elements yet to be identified are likely to be involved in the activation of transcription, and further elements must be responsible for suppression in the later B-cell stages.

A more stringent characterisation of the 5'λ5 region that consists only of about 720 bp had been performed recently. The authors introduced a transgene containing the human CD25 gene under the control of the regulatory region located immediately 5' of the λ5 gene into the germline of mice *(48)*. The analysis of several founder mice showed that the 5' regulatory region of λ5 confers lineage and stage-specific expression of the marker transgene. The short stretch of the 722-bp long 5' regulatory region, therefore, contains the essential cis acting regulatory elements for lineage and differentiation stage-specific expression. Interestingly, a small, but distinct population of early B-cell progenitors became detectable in the transgenic mice that expressed the transgene and the endogenous λ5 gene, but they were negative for the expression of the lineage marker CD19 *(48)*. These results show that λ5 is expressed in B-cell development even earlier than CD19.

4. Expression of the Surrogate Light Chain Proteins in Cell Lines

Monoclonal antibodies specific for the V_{preB} and λ5 proteins detected surrogate light (SL) chain, even in the absence of μH chain on the surface of early precursor B-cell lines *(18,19,49)*. In the mouse, a complex of glycoproteins was coprecipitated with the SL chain. A 130 kDa protein was most consistently detected in noncovalent association with the SL chain. The surface expression of SL chain suggested a receptor structure present on early precursor B-cells that was termed pro-B receptor (Fig. 2).

Abelson-virus- or chemically transformed pre-B-cell lines, or human tumor cell lines with productively rearranged μH chain loci, were found to express the μ-chain disulfide-bonded to SL chains on the cell surface *(20,21,23,50)*. A Dμ protein, encoded by a $DJ_H\mu$ rearranged H-chain allele in reading frame 2, was also found to be accociated with the SL chain on the surface of an Abelson-virus–transformed cell line *(18,51)*. In certain cell lines coexpression of SL chain, conventional L-chain, and μH chain as Ig-like hybrid molecules is detectable *(50,52)*.

In conclusion, surrogate light chain proteins are expressed in transformed cell lines of the B-lymphocyte lineage from stages corresponding to the earliest precursors to the stage of an immature B-cell.

5. Expression of the SL Chain Proteins During B-Cell Development in Normal Bone Marrow

From the data of the pattern of SL chain expression on transformed cell lines, one would have expected to find the SL chain expressed on the surface of subpopulations of progenitor and precursor B lymphocytes in the fetal liver and bone marrow. Because of a lack of specific antibodies, the detection of the surrogate light chain proteins in vivo has been controversial in the beginning. With a polyclonal reagent the SL chain, in association with the μH chain, has been detected on the surface of some precursor and immature B-cells in the bone marrow *(53)*. However, the rather small population of cells expressing the surrogate light chain was not further characterized.

Monoclonal antibodies raised against the λ5 and the V_{preB} proteins first revealed a confusing pattern of expression of the SL chain on the surface of bone marrow cells. As described in the previous paragraph, these reagents were able to recognize the SL chain on transformed cell lines in association with a complex of glycoproteins, as well as in association with the μH chain *(18)*. Even normal pre-B-I cells cultivated in vitro in IL-7 on stromal cells showed clearly detectable cell surface expression of λ5 and V_{preB} in the absence of μH chain *(54)*. The expression of SL chain on the surface of pre-B-cells cultivated in vitro in IL-7 has been confirmed by others *(19)*. Subsequently, pro–B-cells and pre–B-I cells in mouse bone marrow were found to express the SL chain in the absence of μH chain on the surface *(55)*. Particularly, the pro–B-cell fraction of B-cell deficient RAG-2 $^{-/-}$ mice clearly stained positive with anti-λ5, as well as anti-V_{preB} antibodies. A small fraction of early B lymphocyte precursors in bone marrow of normal mice showed comparable staining patterns. In normal mice, the surface expression of SL was confined to the early stages (pro-B and pre-B-I) of pre-B-cell development and became undetectable in μH chain positive pre-B-II cells. However, a fraction of about 30% of all large cells expressing cytoplasmic μH chain coexpressed the surrogate light chain in the cytoplasm *(11,55)*.

The authors then showed that incubation of freshly prepared bone marrow cells for one hour at 37°C upregulates the surface expression of surrogate light chain on pro-B/pre-B-I cells, and on large pre-B-II cells *(56)*. Two different complexes with the SL chain were resolved on the surface of bone marrow cells with two different monoclonal antibodies. One recognizes the λ5 protein in free form, in association with the gp130/gp35–65 complex, as well as in association with the μH chain. This antibody stained nearly all c-kit$^+$ pro-B- and pre-B-I cells, as well as a small fraction of all large CD25+ pre-B-II cells. The antigenic determinant recognized by the second antibody, called SL156, is formed by the SL chain only when associated with the μH chain. The SL156 antibody was found to stain a small population of exclusively large pre-B-cells that have low or undetectable levels of c-kit, and that are positive for CD25 expression. About one third of all large CD25$^+$ pre-B-II cells expressed the surrogate light chain in association with the μH chain.

It is concluded that pro-B- and pre-B-I cells express the SL on the cell surface as a so called pro-B receptor. Single-cell PCR analysis of the configurations of the heavy and light chain loci established that the SL156 positive fraction of cells expressing the pre-B-cell receptor on the cell surface is the next developmental stage in B-cell development *(57)*. Further in development, the surrogate light chain genes are downregulated, and the expression of the pre-B-cell receptor becomes undetectable. Hence, the remaining two-thirds of the large pre–B-II cells and all small pre–B-II cells are negative for the expression of the surrogate light chain proteins.

The authors currently have no experimental data to explain the observed upregulation of the surrogate light chain after short incubation in vitro at 37°C. However, it is tempting to speculate that the downmodulation of the SL chain in vivo might be a consequence of an interaction of the SL chain with a putative ligand in the bone marrow microenvironment and that incubation of the cells in vitro (i.e., in the absence of the ligand allows re-expression on the surface).

The cell surface expression patterns of the surrogate light chain on human bone marrow pre-B-cells has been a similarly contentious issue. The work of Cooper and collegues, based on a series of monoclonal antibodies, indicated that, although SL chain production in the human bone marrow spans several developmental stages, cell surface expression is confined only to a μH chain positive stage *(50)*. In contrast to the findings in the mouse, the developmental stage of cells that coexpress SL chain and μH chain has been positioned later than in mouse, directly before the sIgM$^+$ immature B-cells *(50)*. Results that disagree with Lassoued et al. and agree with data obtained in mouse bone marrow have been published by others with different monoclonal antibodies *(49,58,59)*. In the latter publications, a population of human bone marrow pre-B-cells have been found that express the SL chain in the absence of μH chain. In the μ-chain negative cells, the SL has been found to be associated with a complex of glycoproteins similar in size to the associated proteins in the mouse *(58,59)*. These experiments suggest that in both mouse and man a similar molecular complex forms the so-called pro-B receptor. The pro-B receptor is expressed on a fraction of early B-cell progenitors expressing CD19, CD10, CD34, and TdT *(49,58–60)*. This fraction of cells has been recently shown to carry the immunoglobulin heavy chain loci DJ_H rearranged or in germline configuration *(60)*.

A subpopulation of pre-B-II cells expressing the SL chain in μH chain positive cells on the cell surface has been described by all groups *(49,50,58–60)*. This population of cells was found to be $CD34^-$ and TdT^- and single cell PCR analyses have positioned these cells after the $CD34^+$ pro/pre–B-I cells, just as in the mouse *(60)*.

The most likely explanation for the apparent discrepancy between the findings of Lassoued et al. and the other groups, is the specificity of the monoclonal antibodies used *(50,59)*. It may well be that the antibodies used by Lassoued et al. only recognize free SL chain (as present intracytoplasmically in pro-B-cells *[50]*) and SL chain in association with μH chain, but not SL chains in association with the gp130 glycoprotein complex on the pro-B receptor *(59)*. Interestingly, the monoclonal antibodies from Lassoued et al. were raised against μH chain-SL positive pre-B-cell lines, whereas the other groups used V_{preB} protein as immunogen.

In summary, the expression patterns of the surrogate light chain in mouse and man show striking similarities. An early cell population of pro–B and pre–B-I cells express the surrogate light chain on the cell surface in a complex with different glycoproteins with a major constituent of around 130 kDa as pro-B receptor. The associated proteins have also been termed "surrogate heavy chain" although the structure of the complex and its function(s) is yet to be determined. The cells expressing this complex carry B-lineage markers, such as B220 and CD19, express TdT and c-kit in mouse, and CD34 in human bone marrow. A second cell population expresses the SL on the cell surface in association with the μH chain as the pre-B-cell receptor. This population of cycling cells has lost the expression of c-kit (mouse) or CD34 (human). Later in the development, the surface expression of SL chain proteins becomes undetectable although low amounts of mRNA might still be detectable *(48,60,61)*.

6. Functions of the Pro-B Receptor

The function of the molecular complex of the surrogate light chain in association with the p130 molecule is unclear. Early pre-B-cell development prior to expression of the μH chain appears to be normal in λ5 knockout mice, and pre-B-I cells from those mice show normal in vitro growth on stromal cells in the presence of IL-7 (45, 84). One has to keep in mind, however, that VpreB is normally expressed in the λ5 deficient mouse. It is possible that an early receptor complex consisting of VpreB in association with gp130 and possibly other proteins functions normally in the absence of the λ5 protein. This hypothesis will become testable when all three genes on chromosome 16 of the mouse, i.e., VpreB1, VpreB2, and λ5, have been deleted on the same chromosome. It will be interesting to see whether in such triple-defective mice B-cell development up to the pre-B-I cell stage is still normal. Likewise the identification of the gene encoding for gp130 protein and the targeted disruption of this gene should shed light on the role of the early receptor complex in B-cell development. These studies are currently underway in our laboratory.

The recent analysis of mice with a targeted disruption of the Igβ gene suggested an earlier block of differentiation of B-cell development than that observed in λ5 knockout mice. The authors hypothesized that Igβ might be involved in signals neccessary for completing V_H to DJ_H rearrangement *(29)*. The pro-B receptor complex would be a candidate for a receptor associated with this signalling pathway. However, the Igα and Igβ signaling molecules, although they are expressed in these pro-B / pre-B-I cells, apparently do not associate with the pro-B receptor molecules (H. Karasuyama, pers. communication) in pro-B-cell lines.

7. Functions of the Pre-B-Cell Receptor

7.1. The Critical Role of the Pre-B-Cell Receptor to Establish the Pre-B-II Cell Compartments

The expression of a μ heavy chain on the surface B-cell precursors appears to be crucial for the further development of the cells at the transition from the pre–B-I to the pre–B-II stage. Several mouse mutants have clearly documented the critical role of a membrane-bound μH chain in B-cell development. In rearrangement-deficient mice such as the SCID mutant *(64)* or the RAG-1 *(65)* and RAG-2 *(66)* knockout mice, the development of B-cell precursors is blocked at the pro–B-cell stage. A functional μ heavy chain is sufficient and essential for the development of pre–B-II cells as the block of development of SCID and RAG knockout mice can be overcome by introducing different μH chain transgenes, all selected from the peripheral B-cell repertoire *(64,67,68)*. Finally, the targeted deletion of the membrane exon of the μ-chain gene (in μMT mice) leads to a complete block of development at the transition of pre–B-I to pre–B-II cells *(69)*. In all these mutant mice, no peripheral B-cells are made.

Almost the same phenotype is seen in λ5 deficient mice *(54,62,70)*. In the bone marrow of these mice, the pre–B-II compartment is reduced at least 40-fold as compared to normal mice. Essentially, all surface IgM negative B-lineage cells in bone marrow of λ5 knockout mice are c-kit positive. Similarly, immature B-cells are reduced at least as much as pre–B-II cells. The B-cells in the peripheral lymphatic organs are not completely absent, but the numbers are severely reduced in young animals and are filled to about half the normal content at 6-months of age. These findings highlight the important function of the λ5 protein as one constituent of the pre–B receptor in the pre–B-I to pre–B-II transition.

7.2. The Pre-B Receptor Signals Proliferative Expansion of Cells with In-Frame Rearranged μ Heavy Chains

In normal mice, the $CD25^+$ pre–B-II compartment contains approx 8–10 times more cells than the pre–B-I compartment *(11)*. Approximately one quarter of all these pre–B-II cells is large in size, with 60–70% of cells in S or G2 phase of the cell cycle *(11,55)*. The bone marrow pre-B-cells that coexpress SL chain and μH chain in the cytoplasm, or that express the pre–B receptor on the cell surface, are entirely large in size and all are cycling *(55,56)*. The SCID, $RAG^{-/-}$, μMT, and λ5 mutant mice all have a severely reduced number of pre–B-II cells, and none of them apparently are in cycle. The expression of a pre–B receptor thus appears to trigger proliferation and expansion of cells with a functional rearrangement of a μH chain.

The effect of this proliferative expansion is that it positively selects pre-B-cells with a functional heavy chain so that practically all pre–B-II cells express a μH chain in the cytoplasm. The pairing of μH chains and SL chains might be considered as a proofreading mechanism that also selects μH chains, which later are able to pair with L-chains

(71). Furthermore, the proliferative expansion of pre–B-II cells predicts that a given μH chain will be found in the peripheral B-cell repertoire associated with different L chains.

The number of divisions that a pre–B-II cell undergoes after expression of the pre-B-cell receptor is difficult to measure. According to estimations of Osmond a B-lineage cell undergoes approx six cell divisions during development from the time when B220 is expressed to the immature B-cell stage *(9)*. Most of the divisions appeared to precede μH chain expression *(9)*. These calculations were recently reexamined (D. G. Osmond, T. H. Winkler and F. Melchers, manuscript in preparation) using a CD19 specific monoclonal antibody as a marker for B-lineage cells. These experiments lead to the finding that a major fraction of the "late pro–B-cell fraction" as determined by Osmond's earlier work (i.e., $B220^+$, TdT^-, and cytoplasmic μ-chain negative) does not belong to the B-cell lineage at all; rather it consists of NK cell precursors and a second cell fraction of yet unknown function *(7)*. As this late pro–B-cell fraction was accounting for a major compartment of cycling cells in the earlier calculations *(3)*, the proliferative expansion of B-cell precursors at the μH chain positive stage now appears to be an underestimate. Preliminary calculations using CD19 as marker for all B-lineage cells suggested an average of four cell divisions of large pre–B-II cells (D. G. Osmond, T. H. Winkler and F. Melchers). Another analysis came to the conclusion that pre-B-cells may undergo five to six cell divisions after μH chain expression *(72)*.

The proliferative stimulus delivered by the pre–B receptor can be demonstrated in short-term cultures of sorted pre–B-I cells in vitro. Ex vivo sorted c-kit^+ $CD19^+$ pre–B-I cells from bone marrow of normal mice are able to expand in the absence of any further stimulus in plain culture medium in vitro (Fig. 5). At the time of the sort, less than 5% of the cells express the μH chain intracytoplasmically. Already after three days in culture, essentially all viable cells are cytoplasmic μ-chain positive and many of them are large in size (i.e., in the cell cycle). Observations under the microscope using time-lapse video recording showed that these cells divide every 12 hours in vitro. It suggests that heavy chain rearrangements are ongoing in these cultures, and that cells with an inframe μH chain rearrangement receive a proliferative stimulus, presumably through the pre-B-cell receptor. By contrast, sorted pre–B-I cells from λ5 knockout mice rapidly die under the same culture conditions and do not divide (Fig. 5). Only approx 15% of the cells were found to express cytoplasmic μH chain after three days, as well as after the six-day culture period. Both pre-B-I cells from normal and $\lambda5^{-/-}$ mice can proliferate on stromal cells in the presence of IL-7 (Fig. 5, insert).

Cells that carry nonproductive V_HDJ_H rearrangements on both IgH alleles apparently accumulate in part at a developmental stage earlier than the pre–B-receptor positive stage. These cells can be found in the bone marrow *(73)*. They appear to be out of the cell cycle *(1)*. The majority of cells that have undergone two nonproductive V_HDJ_H rearrangements probably die *in situ* by apoptosis. Interestingly, in mice that overexpress the anti-apoptosis protein Bcl-xL, the population of cells with nonproductively rearranged H-chain genes were found greatly expanded. In this population of cells, a panoply of aberrant rearrangements and deletions in the H chain locus were observed *(74)*.

A conventional κ light chain expressed as a transgene early in development, i.e., under the control of the Eμ-enhancer active already in pro–B/pre–B-I cells, can overcome the defect in B-cell maturation in the λ5 knockout mouse *(75,76)* (A. G. Rolink, J. Andersson and F. Melchers, unpublished). The same transgenic light chain under its own control, expressed later in small pre-B-II cells and immature B-cells, however, cannot. Apparently, a conventional light chain in association with the μH chain can signal proliferative expansion when expressed at the pre–B-I to pre–B-II transition, in the same way

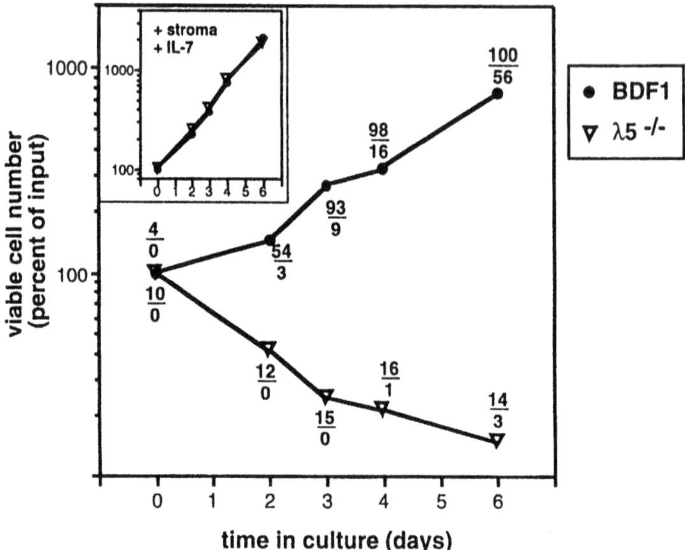

Fig. 5. Sorted pre-B-I cells from normal mice undergo proliferative expansion in vitro, whereas pre-B-I cells from $\lambda5^{-/-}$ mice do not. $CD19^{+}$ c-kit^{+} cells where sorted from bone marrow of normal mice (BDF1) as well as from $\lambda5^{-/-}$ mice and cultivated in cell culture medium without stromal cells. The same sorted cells were also put in cultures containing stromal cells and Interleukin-7 (figure insert). Cells were removed at the indicated time points and the number of viable cells were counted. At the same time the percentage of cells expressing cytoplasmic μH chain and IgM on the cell surface were determined by FACS analysis. The upper numbers close to the data points give the percentage of cytoplasmic μ-chain positive cells, the lower numbers give the percentage of surface IgM positive cells at the indicated time points.

as the pre-B-cell receptor consisting of μH chain and SL chain. The signal delivered from the conventional light chain in association with the μH chain in early cells therefore appears qualitatively different from the signal that such a receptor (i.e., the B-cell antigen receptor) normally delivers to the immature B-cell, where no proliferation, but arrest of differentiation and apoptosis, is induced. This finding might reflect different signaling pathways downstream of the B-cell receptor in pre–B-I/large pre–B-II cells and small pre–B-II cells. However, one has to consider that the V_{preB} molecule is still expressed in the early cell population of λ5 knockout mice. Therefore, one cannot formally rule out that μH chain, conventional light chain and V_{preB} form a molecular complex expressed in the light chain-transgenic λ5 knockout mice. Such a receptor might deliver a signal similar to the pre-B-cell receptor but different from the B-cell receptor, (for discussion of the pre–B receptor signal, *see* below).

7.3. The Role of the Pre–B Receptor in Allelic Exclusion

7.3.1. The Pre-B-Cell Receptor Signals Transient Shut Down of Recombination

Various analyses have suggested that a productive rearrangement at one H chain allele mediates H-chain allelic exclusion by preventing further V_H to DJ_H rearrangements at the other allele *(77,78)*. The expression of a membrane-bound μH chain appears neccessary for signalling allelic exclusion as mutants expressing only the secreted form of the μ-chain on one allele generate allelically "included" cells with two different μ-chains

(79). Allelic exclusion appears to be established at the earliest pre-B-cell stage where a productively rearranged H-chain locus becomes expressed *(73)*.

Part of the mechanisms to achieve allelic exclusion could be to turn off the expression of the *RAG* genes, as both RAG-1 and RAG-2 have been shown to be essential for the rearrangement process *(65,66)*. The authors have shown that, indeed, the expression of the pre-B-cell receptor correlates with a downregulation of RAG-1 and RAG-2 gene expression at RNA and protein levels *(61)*. The expression of the *RAG* genes during B-cell development follows a bimodal pattern. Expression is up in pro–B and pre–B-I cells, downregulated in pre–B receptor positive pre–B-II cells, and fully upregulated again in small pre–B-II cells. In immature B-cells, *RAG* gene expression begins to be downregulated again and is totally off in mature B-cells. The two waves of *RAG* gene expression correlate with the ordered rearrangement of the immunoglobulin genes at the heavy chain and the light chain loci. The two distinct stages of development are separated by a highly proliferative stage in which recombination is apparently completely shut down. Also, the direct measurement of recombinase activity using assays for broken-ended DNA intermediates of the V(D)J recombination in the developmental stages has reached the same conclusion *(80)*.

In addition to the transcriptional regulation of both the *RAG-1* and *RAG-2* genes, the RAG-2 protein accumulation is regulated across the cell cycle. In the G1 phase of the cell cycle RAG-2 protein accumulates and gets rapidly degraded in the S phase. This is presumably mediated by a cyclin dependent phosphorylation event *(81,82)*. In c-kit positive pre–B-I cells that are cycling in vivo, such a regulation can be demonstrated by assaying for RAG-2 protein content in fractions enriched for cells in the G1 phase versus cells in S, G2, and M phase of the cell cycle. RAG-2 protein is easily detectable in G1 cells, whereas it is apparently completely absent in cells enriched for the S, G2, and M phases *(61)*.

Both the transcriptional as well as the posttranslational regulation of the *RAG* genes may in part explain allelic exclusion of the heavy chain locus. However, *RAG* expression becomes upregulated again during light chain rearrangement when the cells are in a resting stage. L-chain gene rearrangements, but no further H-chain rearrangements are observed *(80)*. This suggests that a differential accessibility of heavy and light chain loci, possibly at the level of chromatin structure, might allow light chain rearrangements and might at the same time prevent further $V_H \rightarrow DJ_H$ rearrangement in the late stage pre–B-II cells *(83,84)*.

7.3.2. Allelic Exclusion in λ5 Deficient Mice

If the pre–B receptor controls *RAG* gene expression and opening and closing of IgH chain alleles at the chromatin structural level, then one might expect that the μMT and the λ5 mutant mouse could be deficient in these processes and, hence, allow the productive VDJ rearrangement at two alleles. This, in fact, was observed in μMT mice, which are incapable of depositing the pre–B receptor in membranes *(79)*.

A recent analysis of the rearrangement status at the single cell level, demonstrated that among early progenitor cells in λ5 knockout mice that were selected for μH chain expression in the cytoplasm 5 out of 16 cells contain two functional V_HDJ_H rearrangements *(85)*. In the same cell population of control mice, none of 21 sorted single cells showed two functional IgH chain rearrangements. This suggested that in the absence of λ5 protein IgH chain loci seemed to be allelically included in early progenitor cells. However, at the immature B-cell stage, those double-producing B-cells became undetectable by surface staining for IgM allotypes in the λ5 knockout mouse. Likewise, the spleen of λ5 knockout mice were found not to contain mature B-cells with two functional rearrangements of the heavy chain loci *(85)*.

From these data the question arose why allelically included B-cell progenitors do not contribute to the peripheral B-cell pool in λ5-deficient mice. A counterselection of double-producing progenitors at later developmental stages by mechanisms that are not yet understood might explain this discrepancy. A recent analysis of mice whose IgH alleles are engineered to encode two distinct antibody heavy (H) chains generate a normal sized B-cell compartment in which most cells stably express the two heavy chains *(86)*.

The results exclude the possibility that "heavy chain toxicity" *(87)* contributes significantly to the establishment of allelic exclusion. It has been suggested that in the λ5 knockout mouse, the contribution of allelically included progenitors to the peripheral B-cell pool is neglegible because of a failure of these cells to rearrange their light chain genes efficiently *(85)*. In such a scenario, the appropriate signal for light chain rearrangement is missing in the absence of the pre-B-cell receptor, and the generation of low numbers of B-cells would depend on a few cells that undergo light chain rearrangement before heavy chain rearrangement *(70)*. A limited life-span of early progenitors and a "slow" recombination process would favor the development of those B-cell progenitors, which have undergone V_H to DJ_H rearrangement only on one allele. This hypothesis would predict that most of the immature and mature B-cells in the periphery of λ5 knockout animals contain one allele of the IgH chain locus only DJ_H rearranged.

7.4. Can all Ig Heavy Chains Associate with the Surrogate Light Chain?

Pre–B-II cells, which have undergone a productive V_HDJ_H rearragement and express a μH chain, can only form a pre-B-cell receptor on the surface if this μH chain can associate with SL chain. All cells expressing a μH chain defective in association are expected not to participate in the proliferative expansion and allelic exclusion. Such defects might be the consequence of structural features of certain V_H-domains.

It is known that V_H-dependent selection processes can operate at the IgM^+ stage. The ratio of usage of V_H genes of the J558 family to V_H genes of the 7183 family is different between pre-B-cells in the bone marrow and peripheral B-cells *(88–90)*. The analysis of the ratio of productive (P) versus nonproductive (NP) rearrangements of certain VH genes revealed that VH-dependent selection processes may also occur at the pre-B-cell stage before normal light chain is expressed *(91,92)*. The best-studied example is the V_H81X gene, a member of the 7183 family, located most proximal to the D elements *(93)*. Whereas approx 10–40% of all V_H rearrangements of the bone marrow and the fetal liver utilize the V_H81X gene, it is rarely expressed in the peripheral repertoire of adult animals *(88,91,93–95)*. Only 20–30 % of the rearrangements involving the V_H81X gene are productive in bone marrow pre-B-cells, whereas up to 90% of the rearrangements of other V_H genes have been found to be productive in these cells *(91,92,94)*.

One way to explain the underrepresentation of productive V_H81X expressing pre-B-cells in the pre–B-II compartment would be that the majority of V_H81X/μH chains would not assemble with the SL chain as proposed initially by Decker et al. *(91)*. Indeed, it was shown that two V_H81X/μ chains with different V_H-D-J_H joining sequences are not assembled with SL chain in pre-B-cell lines, and consequently, cannot be expressed on the cell surface (44). The inability of V_H81X to pair with SL chain may depend on the CDR3 of the particular rearranged V_H81X gene *(96)*. It can be expected that μH chains with V_H domains that cannot form a pre-B-cell receptor cannot participate in proliferative expansion and allelic exclusion.

Another example is the case of certain V_H12-D-J_H joining sequences that are overrepresented in the periphery over other V_H12-D-J_H sequences. It has been shown that the former sequences are selected at the pre–B-I to pre–B-II cell transition *(97)*. However, the analysis has shown that the former as well as the latter μH chains containing the different V_H12-D-J_H joining sequences are able to assemble with the SL chain. In that case, the simple failure of certain V_H12-D-J_H joining sequences to pair with the SL chain does not explain the V_H dependent selection. Although the mechanism for that selection process remains entirely unclear, the authors have speculated that certain CDR3 regions do not allow binding of the pre-B receptor to a ligand in the bone marrow (*see* below).

7.5. The Role of the Pre-B Receptor in Cellular Maturation

During the transition from the pre–B-I cell stage to the pre–B-II cell stage, pre-B-cells undergo a program of differentiation that can be characterized by the loss or the gain of certain molecular markers. The early markers c-kit and CD43 are lost, and the expression of the genes for the surrogate light chain are downregulated *(5)*. *RAG* gene expression is downregulated and it is suspected that the non-VDJ-rearranged H chain alleles become inaccessible for futher rearrangement. In humans CD34 is downregulated at the transition from pre–B-I to pre–B-II *(60)*. At the pre–B-II cell stage the IL-2 receptor α chain (CD25) is upregulated in mice *(11,98)*. Most importantly, sterile transcription of the κL chain locus becomes detectable at the large pre–B-II cell stage and later at the small pre–B-II cell stage where light chain rearrangements take place *(61,80)*.

Does the pre–B receptor signal up-, respectively, downregulation of any of these events? In vitro pro–B-cell lines from RAG-$2^{-/-}$ mice can undergo significant differentiation including downregulation of expression of c-kit, CD43, and of the SL chain, upregulation of CD25 expression and upregulation of sterile κ-transcription in the absence of a signal from the pre–B receptor *(99)*. For these parts of the molecular program of early B-cell differentiation there is apparently no need for expression of the pre–B receptor. However, it still remains a possibility that the pre–B receptor directly downregulates RAG expression and the closure of the non-VDJ rearranged H-chain allele. Also, in vivo the expression of a μH chain in association with the SL chain is not absolutely necessary for the induction of light chain rearrangement as shown in JH, μMT, and λ5 knockout mice *(70)*.

The ordered rearrangement of the heavy and light chain loci observed in the major differentiation pathway of B-cell progenitors in normal mice in vivo suggests, however, that sequential accessibility first of H-chain and later of L-chain gene loci is an important element in the control of immunoglobulin gene rearrangements. Within this scenario, the pre–B receptor expression expands cells that are selected for expression of a functional μH chain, and thereby fills up the pre–B-II compartment where the light chain loci now become fully accessible. Hence, the pre-B-cell receptor enables the generation of cells in which these rearrangements can be induced by pre-B-cell receptor independent signalling pathways.

7.6. The Nature of the Signal Transmitted from the Pre-B Receptor

The signal transducing unit of the pre–B receptor is composed of the heterodimer of Igα and Igβ (Fig. 2). The crucial role of the Igα and Igβ molecules in pre-B-cell development has been recently demonstrated. A transgenic approach used a chimeric receptor consisting of a mutant μH chain, that on its own is unable to contact the Igα/Igβ complex, with the cytoplasmic domains of either Igα or Igβ. Both the μH chain/Igα and the μH chain/Igβ chimeric molecules were able to activate pre-B-cell development in vivo

(100,101). Targeted disruption of the Igβ gene in mice leads to a complete block in pre–B development *(63)*. Most likely, the formation of a pre-B-cell receptor complex is completely abolished in these mice. A mouse mutant that lacks only the Igα cytoplasmic tail forms a pre–B receptor complex on the cell surface, but also in these mice pre-B-cell development is impaired, albeit incompletely *(102)*.

The immunoreceptor tyrosine-based activation motifs (ITAMs) in the cytoplasmic domains of Igα and Igβ *(103)* couple the B-cell receptor, as well as the pre-B-cell receptor to cytoplasmic tyrosine kinases, in particular Src family kinases (Lyn, Fyn, Blk, and Lck) *(104)*. Also, the Syk kinase has been reported to be critically involved in the signaling cascade in the B-cell receptor (reviewed in ref. *104*). Whereas individual Src like kinases appear to be dispensable for pre-B-cell development, the Syk kinase has a bottleneck role in pre–B receptor signaling *(105,106)*. Irradiated mice reconstituted with *syk*$^{-/-}$ fetal liver cells developed almost no B-cells.

In summary, the signal triggered from the pre-B-cell receptor is initiated by the Igα/Igβ coreceptor molecules and leads, probably via several independent Src like kinases, to the activation of Syk. At the moment, it is not clear whether there is any difference in the signaling pathway downstream of the pre–B receptor vs the B-cell antigen receptor, and whether signaling to proliferative expansion and to allelic exclusion use different pathways.

7.7. Is There a Ligand for the Pre-B-Cell Receptor?

The signaling that the pre-B-cell receptor induces in pre–B-II cells is expected to be mediated by changes of the context and/or the conformations of the signal-transducing complex with μH chain, SL chain, and Igα and Igβ. One of the ways to induce such changes would be the binding, and possibly crosslinking, of the receptor to a ligand. So far, there is no genetic or biochemical evidence that such a ligand exists. If a ligand for the pre-B-cell receptor exists it is unlikely to bind to the V_H-region of the μH chains. This conclusion can be reached from experiments in which a series of transgenic μH chains containing different V_H regions have all been able to stimulate proliferative expansion to near normal numbers of pre–B-II cells in RAG-deficient animals. However, it cannot be rigorously ruled out that all these different μH chains share a common structural principle, which could be recognized by such a ligand. It is also unlikely that the λ5-protein is directly involved in binding to a putative ligand since normal L chains, expressed prematurely in pre-B-I cells as transgenes, can rescue the λ5$^{-/-}$ defect *(75,76)*. Again, it cannot be rigorously ruled out that these transgenic L chains share a common structure with the λ5 protein.

However, the V_{preB} protein is still a candidate for potential ligand binding. First, double transfectants producing μH chain and V_{preB} have revealed that the two proteins can associate with each other, i.e., even in the absence of the λ5 protein. Furthermore, purified V_{preB} protein was shown to be able to bind to V_H and V_L domains, to Fab fragments and to antibody molecules *(107)*. This suggests that transgenic L chains, which rescue the λ5-defect, could form triple complexes consisting of μH chain, transgenic L chains, and V_{preB} proteins. Therefore, the V_{preB} molecule could be the site where crosslinking by either a ligand or by self-association could occur.

8. Concluding Remarks

During B-cell development, pro–B and pre–B-I cells express a pro–B-cell receptor of a complex of glycoproteins associated with surrogate L chain. They are followed by cycling pre–B-II cells, which express a pre-B-cell receptor composed of μH chains, surrogate L chains, and the signal transducing Igα and Igβ molecules. Surrogate L chain is composed of two noncovalently associated proteins encoded by the V_{preB} and the λ5 genes, which form a light chain-like structure. The functions of the pro–B-cell receptor are unknown at present. The pre-B-cell receptor signals proliferative expansion of pre–B-II cells, thereby selecting μH chain-producing cells over nonproducing cells by factors of 10–50. It is likely that the pre-B-cell receptor is also involved in allelic exclusion, which in part is achieved by the downregulation of the V(D)J rearrangement machinery in pre-B-cell receptor-expressing cells. It appears not to be involved in the onset of L-chain gene transcription and rearrangement, and in the maturation of pre-B-cells to mature stages monitored by the expression of a series of marker molecules. It is striking how similar the expression pattern and functions of the pre-B-cell receptor in B-cell development are with those of the preTα/β-TCR chain containing pre-T-cell receptor in T-cell development *(108)*.

Acknowledgments

The authors would like to thank Drs. Antonius Rolink and Paschalis Sideras for critically reading our manuscript. The Basel Institute for Immunology was founded and is supported by F. Hoffmann - La Roche Ltd, Basel, Switzerland.

References

1. Hardy, R. R., Carmack, C. E., Shinton, S. A., Kemp, J. D., and Hayakawa, K. (1991) Resolution and characterization of pro–B and pre–pro–B cell stages in normal mouse bone marrow. *J. Exp. Med.* **173,** 1213–1225.
2. Ogawa, M., Nishikawa, S., Ikuta, K., Yamamura, F., Naito, M., Takahashi, K., and Nishikawa, S. I. (1988) B cell ontogeny in murine embryo studied by a culture system with the monolayer of a stromal cell clone, ST–2, B cell progenitor develops first in the embryonal body rather than in the yolk sac. *EMBO J.* **7,** 1337–1343.
3. Osmond, D. G. (1986) Population dynamics of bone marrow B lymphocytes. *Immunol. Rev.* **93,** 103–133.
4. Owen, J. J. T., Raff, M. C., and Cooper, M. D. (1975) Studies on the generation of B lymphocytes in the mouse embryo. *Eur. J. Immunol.* **5,** 468–473.
5. Rolink, A. and Melchers, F. (1991) Molecular and cellular origins of B lymphocyte diversity. *Cell* **66,** 1081–1094.
6. Nadler, L. M., Anderson, K. C., Marti, G., Batyes, M., Park, E., Daley, J. F., and Schlossman, S. F. (1983) B4, a human B lymphocyte–associated antigen expressed on normal, mitogen–activated, and malignant B lymphocytes. *J. Immunol.* **131,** 244–250.
7. Rolink, A., ten Boekel, E., Melchers, F., Fearon, D. T., Krop, I., and Andersson, J. (1996) A subpopulation of $B220^+$ cells in murine bone marrow does not express CD(19 and contains natural killer cell progenitors. *J. Exp. Med.* **183,** 187–194.
8. Coffman, R. L. and Weissman, I. L. (1981) A monoclonal antibody that recognizes B cells and B cell precursors in mice. *J. Exp. Med.* **153,** 269–279.
9. Osmond, D. G. (1991) Proliferation kinetics and the lifespan of B cells in central and peripheral lymphoid organs. *Curr. Opin. Immunol.* **3,** 179–185.
10. Tsubata, T. and Nishikawa, S.–I. (1991) Molecular and cellular aspects of early B–cell development. *Curr. Opin. Immunol.* **3,** 186–192.
11. Rolink, A., Grawunder, U., Winkler, T. H., Karasuyama, H., and Melchers, F. (1994) IL–2 receptor a chain (CD25, TAC) expression defines a crucial stage in pre–B cell development. *Int. Immunol.* **6,** 1257–1264.
12. Banchereau, J. B. and Rousset, F. (1992) Human B lymphocytes: phenotype, proliferation and differentiation. *Adv. Immunol.* **52,** 125–262.
13. Burrows, P. D. and Cooper, M. D. (1993) B–cell development in man. *Curr. Opin. Immunol.* **5,** 201–206.

14. LeBien, T. W., Wormann, B., Villablanca, J. G., Law, C. L., Steinberg, L. M., Shah, V. O., and Loken, M. R. (1990) Multiparameter flow cytometric analysis of human fetal bone marrow B cells. *Leukemia* **4,** 354–358.
15. Rolink, A., Karasuyama, H., Haasner, D., Grawunder, U., Martensson, I. L., Kudo, A., and Melchers, F. (1994. Two pathways of B–lymphocyte development in mouse bone marrow and the roles of surrogate L chain in this development. *Immunol. Rev.* **137,** 185–201.
16. Kudo, A. and Melchers, F. (1987) A second gene, VpreB in the lambda 5 locus of the mouse, which appears to be selectively expressed in pre–B lymphocytes. *EMBO J.* **6,** 2267–2272.
17. Sakaguchi, N. and Melchers, F. (1986) Lambda 5, a new light–chain–related locus selectively expressed in pre–B lymphocytes. *Nature* **324,** 579–582.
18. Karasuyama, H., Rolink, A., and Melchers, F. (1993) A complex of glycoproteins is associated with VpreB/lambda 5 surrogate light chain on the surface of μ heavy chain–negative early precursor B cell lines. *J. Exp. Med.* **178,** 469–478.
19. Shinjo, F., Hardy, R. R., and Jongstra, J. (1994) Monoclonal anti–λ5 antibody FS1 identifies a 130 kDa protein associated with λ5 and Vpre–B on the surface of early pre–B cell lines. *Intern. Immunol.* **6,** 393–399.
20. Karasuyama, H., Kudo, A., and Melchers, F. (1990) The proteins encoded by Vpre–B and λ5 pre–B cell–specific genes can associate with each other and with μ heavy chains. *J. Exp. Med.* **172,** 969–972.
21. Kerr, W. G., M. D. Cooper, L. Feng, P. D. Burrows, and L. M. Hendershot. (1989. Mu heavy chain can associate with a pseudo–light chain complex (ψL) in human pre–B cells "in vitro." *Proc. Natl. Acad. Sci. USA* **85,** 4473–4477.
22. Pillai, S. and Baltimore, D. (1987) Formation of disulphide–linked μ2ω2 tetramers in pre–B cells by the 18K ω–immunoglobulin light chain. *Nature* **329,** 172–174.
23. Tsubata, T. and Reth, M. (1990) The products of pre–B cell–specific genes (l5 and VpreB) and the immunoglobulin μ chain form a complex that is transported onto the cell surface. *J. Exp. Med.* **172,** 973–976.
24. Hombach, J., Tsubata, T., Leclercq, L., Stappert, H., and Reth, M. (1990) Molecular components of the B–cell antigen receptor complex of the IgM class. *Nature* **343,** 760–762.
25. Kudo, A., Pravtcheva, D., Sakaguchi, N., Ruddle, F. H., and Melchers, F. (1987) Localization of the murine λ5 gene on chromsome 16. *Genomics* **1,** 277–279.
26. Mattei, M. G., Fumoux, F., Roeckel, N., Fougereau, M., and Schiff, C. (1991) The human pre–B–specific lambda–like cluster is located in the 22q11.2–22q12.3 region, distal to the IgC lambda locus. *Genomics* **9,** 544–546.
27. Shirasawa, T., Ohnishi, K., Hagiwara, S., Shigemoto, K., Takebe, Y., Rajewsky, K., and Takemori, T. (1993) A novel gene product associated with mu chains in immature B cells. *EMBO J.* **12,** 1827–1834.
28. Ohnishi, K. and Takemori, T. (1994) Molecular components and assembly of μ–surrogate light chain complexes in pre–B cell lines. *J. Biol. Chem.* **269,** 28,347–28,353.
29. Bauer, S. R., Huebner, K., Budarf, M., Finan, J., Erikson, J., Emanuel, B. S., Nowell, P. C., Croce, C. M., and Melchers, F. (1988) The human VpreB gene is located on chromosome 22 near a cluster of Vλ1 gene segments. *Immunogenetics* **28,** 328–333.
30. Bauer, S. R., Kudo, A., and Melchers, F. (1988) Structure and pre–B lymphocyte restricted expression of the VpreB gene in humans and conservation of its structure in other mammalian species. *EMBO J.* **7,** 111–116.
31. Chang, H., Dmitrovsky, E., Hieter, P., Mitchell, Leder, P., Turoczi, L., Kirsch, I., and Hollis, G. (1986) Identification of three new Ig λ–like genes in man. *J. Exp. Med.* **163,** 425–435.
32. Evans, R. J. and Hollis, G. F. (1991) Genomic structure of the human Ig lambda 1 gene suggests that it may be expressed as an Ig lambda 14.1–like protein or as a canonical B cell Ig lambda light chain, implications for Ig lambda gene evolution. *J. Exp. Med.* **173,** 305–311.
33. Hollis, G. F., Evans, R. J., Stafford–Hollis, J. M., Korsmeyer, S. J., and McKearn, J. P. (1989) Immunoglobulin λ light chain–related genes 14.1 and 16.1 are expressed in pre–B cells and may encode the human immunoglobulin ω light chain protein. *Proc. Natl. Acad. Sci. USA* **86,** 5552–5556.
34. Schiff, C., Bensmana, M., Guglielmi, P., Milili, M., Lefranc, M. P., and Fougereau, M. (1990) The immunoglobulin lambda–like gene cluster (14.1, 16.1 and F lambda 1) contains gene(s) selectively expressed in pre–B cells and is the human counterpart of the mouse lambda 5 gene. *Int. Immunol.* **2,** 201–207.

35. Dul, J. L., Argon, Y., Winkler, T. H., ten Boekel, E., Melchers, F., and Martensson, I. L. (1996) The murine VpreB1 and VpreB2 genes both encode a VpreB protein of the surrogate light chain and are co–expressed during B cell development. *Eur. J. Immunol.* **26,** 906–913.
36. Kudo, A., Thalmann, P., Sakaguchi, N., Davidson, W. F., Pierce, J. H., Kearney, J. F., Reth, M., Rolink, A., and Melchers, F. (1992) The expression of the mouse VpreB/lambda 5 locus in transformed cell lines and tumors of the B lineage differentiation pathway. *Int. Immunol.* **4,** 831–840.
37. Holmes, K. L., Pierce, J. H., Davidson, W. F., and Morse, H. C. I. (1986) Murine hematopoietic cells with pre B/myeloid characteristics are generated by in vitro transformation with retroviruses containing res, ras, abl and src oncogenes. *J. Exp. Med.* **164,** 443.
38. Reth, M., Ammirati, P., Jackson, S., and Alt, F. (1985) Regulated progression of a cultured preB cell to the B–cell stage. *Nature* **317,** 353–355
39. Bauer, S. R., Kubagawa, H., MacLennan, I., and Melchers, F. (1991) VpreB gene expression in hematopoietic malignancies: a lineage– and stage–restricted marker for B cell precursor leukemias. *Blood 78,* 1581–1588.
40. Donohoe, M. E. and Blomberg, B. B. (1997) The 14.1 surrogate light chain promoter has lineage– and stage–restricted activity. *J. Immunol.* **158,** 1681–1691.
41. Kudo, A., Bauer, S. R., and Melchers, F. (1989) Structure, control of expression and putative function of the pre–B cell–specific genes VpreB and lambda 5. *Prog. Immunol.* **7,** 339–347.
42. Lo, K., Landau, N. R., and Smale, S. T. (1991) LyF–1, a transcriptional regulator that interacts with a novel class of promoters for lymphocyte–specific genes. *Mol. Cell. Biol.* **11,** 5229–5243.
43. Allen, J. M., Forbush, K. A., and Perlmutter, R. M. (1992) Functional dissection of the lck promotor. *Mol. Cell. Biol.* **12,** 2758–2768.
44. Fehling, H. J., Laplace, C., Mattei, M. G., Saint–Ruf, C., and von Boehmer, H. (1995) Genomic structure and chromosomal location of the mouse pre–T–cell receptor alpha gene. **42,** 275–281.
45. Mårtensson, I.–L. and Melchers, F. (1994) Pre–B cell specific λ5 gene expression due to suppression in non pre–B cells. *Int. Immunol.* **6,** 863–872.
46. Yang, J., Glozak, M. A., and Blomberg, B. B. (1995) Identification and localization of a developmentally stage–specific promoter activity from the murine lambda 5 gene. *J. Immunol.* **155,** 2498–2514.
47. Mårtensson, I.–L. and Mårtensson, A. (1997) Early B cell factor binds to a site critical for λ5 core enhancer activity. *Eur. J. Immunol.* **27,** 315–320.
48. Mårtensson, I.–L., Melchers, F., and Winkler, T. H. (1997) A transgenic marker for mouse B lymphoid precursors. *J. Exp. Med.* **185,** 653–662.
49. Guelpa–Fonlupt, V., Tonnelle, C., Blaise, D., Fougereau, M., and Fumoux, F. (1994) Discrete early pro–B and pre–B stages in normal human bone marrow as defined by surface pseudo–light chain expression. *Eur. J. Immunol.* **24,** 257–264.
50. Lassoued, K., Nunez, C., Billips, L., Kubagawa, H., Monteiro, R. C., Le Bien, T. W., and Cooper, M. D. (1993) Expression of surrogate light chain receptors is restricted to a late stage in pre B cell differentiation. *Cell* **73,** 73–86.
51. Tsubata, T., Tsubata, R., and Reth, M. (1991) Cell surface expression of the short immunoglobulin μ chain (Dμ–protein) in murine pre–B cells is differently regulated from that of the intact μ chain. *Eur. J. Immunol.* **21,** 1359–1363.
52. Bergman, Y., Haimovich, J., and Melchers, F. (1977) An IgM–producing tumor with biochemical characteristics of a small B lymphocyte. *Eur. J. Immunol.* **8,** 574–581.
53. Cherayil, B. J. and Pillai, S. (1991) The ω/λ5–surrogate immunoglobulin light chain is expressed on the surface of transitional B lymphocytes in murine bone marrow. *J. Exp. Med.* **173,** 111–116.
54. Rolink, A., Karasuyama, H., Grawunder, U., Haasner, D., Kudo, A., and Melchers, F. (1993) B cell development in mice with a defective lambda 5 gene. *Eur. J. Immunol.* **23,** 1284–1288.
55. Karasuyama, H., Rolink, A., Shinkai, Y., Young, F., Alt, F. W., and Melchers, F. (1994) The expression of Vpre–B/lambda 5 surrogate light chain in early bone marrow precursor B cells of normal and B cell–deficient mutant mice. *Cell* **77,** 133–143.
56. Winkler, T. H., Rolink, A., Melchers, F., and Karasuyama, H. (1995) Precursor B cells of mouse bone marrow express two different complexes with the surrogate light chain on the surface. *Eur. J. Immunol.* **25,** 446–450.
57. Ten Boekel, E., Melchers, F., and Rolink, A. (1995) The status of Ig loci rearrangements in single cells from different stages of B cell development. *Intern. Immunol.* **7,** 1013–1019.

58. Meffre, E., Fougereau, M., Argenson, J. N., Aubaniac, J. M., and Schiff, C. (1996) Cell surface expression of surrogate light chain (psi L) in the absence of mu on human pro–B cell lines and normal pro–B cells. *Eur. J. Immunol.* **26,** 2172–2180.
59. Sanz, E. and de la Hera, A. (1996) A novel anti–Vpre–B antibody identifies imunoglobulin–surrogate receptors on the surface of human pro–B cells. *J. Exp. Med.* 183, 2693–2698.
60. Ghia, P., ten Boekel, E., Sanz, E., de la Hera, A., Rolink, A., and Melchers, F. (1996) Ordering of human bone marrow B lymphocyte precursors by single–cell polymerase chain reaction analyses of the rearrangement status of the immunoglobulin H and L chain gene loci. *J. Exp. Med.* **184,** 2217–2229.
61. Grawunder, U., Leu, T. M. J., Schatz, D. G., Werner, A., Rolink, A. G., Melchers, F., and Winkler, T. H. (1995) Downregulation of RAG1 and RAG2 gene expression in preB cells after functional immunoglobulin heavy chain rearrangement. *Immunity* **3,** 601–608.
62. Kitamura, D., Kudo, A., Schaal, S., Muller, W., Melchers, F., and Rajewsky, K. (1992) A critical role of λ5 protein in B cell development. *Cell* **69,** 823–831.
63. Gong, S. and Nussenzweig, M. C. (1996) Regulation of an early developmental checkpoint in the B cell pathway by Ig beta. *Science* **272,** 411–414.
64. Reichmann–Fried, M., Hardy, R. R., and Bosma, M. J. (1990) Development of B lineage cells in the bone marrow of scid/scid mice following the introduction of functionally rearranged immunoglobulin transgenes. *Proc. Natl. Acad. Sci. USA* **87,** 2730–2734.
65. Mombaerts, P., Iacomini, J., Johnson, R. S., Herrup, K., Tonegawa, S., and Papaioannou, V. E. (1992) RAG–1 deficient mice have no mature B and T lymphocytes. *Cell* **68,** 869–877.
66. Shinkai, Y., Rathbun, G., Lam, K. P., Oltz, E. M., Stewart, V., Mendelsohn, M., Charron, J., Delta, M., Young, F., Stahl, A., and Alt, F. W. (1992) RAG–2 deficient mice lack mature lymphocytes owing to inability fo initiate V(D)J rearrangement. *Cell* **68,** 855–867.
67. Spanopoulou, E., Roman, C. A., Corcoran, L. M., Schlissel, M. S., Silver, D. P., Nemazee, D., Nussenzweig, M. C., Shinton, S. A., Hardy, R. R., and Baltimore, D. (1994) Functional immunoglobulin transgenes guide ordered B–cell differentiation in Rag–1–deficient mice. *Genes Dev.* **8,** 1030–1042.
68. Young, F., Ardman, B., Shinkai, Y., Lansford, R., Blackwell, T. K., Mendelsohn, M., Rolink, A., Melchers, F., and Alt, F. W. (1994) Influence of immunoglobulin heavy– and light–chain expression on B–cell differentiation. *Genes Dev.* **8,** 1043–1057.
69. Kitamura, D., Roes, J., Kuhn, R., and Rajewsky, K. (1991) A B cell–deficient mouse by targeted disruption of the membrane exon of the immunoglobulin mu chain gene. *Nature* **350,** 423–426.
70. Ehlich, A., Schaal, S., Gu, H., Kitamura, D., Muller, W., and Rajewsky, K. (1993) Immunoglobulin heavy and light chain genes rearrange independently at early stages of B cell development. *Cell* **72,** 695–704.
71. Keyna, U., Beck–Engeser, G. B., Jongstra, J., Applequist, S. E., and Jäck, H.–M. (1995) Surrogate light chain–dependent selection of Ig heavy chain V regions. *J. Immunol.* **155,** 5536–5542.
72. Decker, D. J., Boyle, N. E., Koziol, J. A., and Klinman, N. R. (1991) The expression of the Ig H chain repertoire in developing bone marrow B lineage cells. *J. Immunol.* B 350–361.
73. Ehlich, A., Martin, V., Müller, W., and Rajewsky, K. (1994) Analysis of the B–cell progenitor compartment at the level of single cells. *Curr. Biol.* **4,** 573–583.
74. Fang, W., Mueller, D. L., Pennel, C. A., Rivard, J. J., Li, Y. S., Hardy, R. R., Schlissel, M. S., and Behrens, T. W. (1996) Frequent aberrant immunoglobulin rearrangements in pro–B cells revealed by a bcl–xL transgene. *Immunity* **4,** 291–299.
75. Papavasiliou, F., Jankovic, M., and Nussenzweig, M. C. (1996) Surrogate or conventional light chains are required for membrane immunoglobulin mu to activate the precursor B cell transition. *J. Exp. Med.* **184,** 2025–2030.
76. Pelanda, R., Schaal, S., Torres, R. M., and Rajewsky, K. (1996) A prematurely expressed Igκ transgene, but not a $V_κJ_κ$ gene segment targeted into the Igκ locus, can rescue B cell development in λ5–deficient mice. *Immunity* **5,** 229–239.
77. Alt, F. W., Yancoupoulos, G. D., Blackwell, T. K., Wood, C., Thomas, E., Boss, M., Coffman, R., Rosenberg, N., Tonegawa, S., and Baltimore, D. (1984) Ordered rearrangement of immunoglobulin heavy chain variable region segments. *EMBO J.* **3,** 1209–1219.
78. Weaver, D., Constantini, F., Imanishi–Kari, T., and Baltimore, D. (1985) A transgenic immunoglobulin μ gene prevents rearrangement of endogenous genes. *Cell* **42,** 117–127.
79. Kitamura, D. and Rajewsky, K. (1992) Targeted disruption of μ–chain membrane exon causes loss of heavy–chain allelic exclusion. *Nature* **356,** 154–156.

80. Constantinescu, A. and Schlissel, M. S. (1997) Changes in Locus–specific V(D)J recombinase activity induced by immunoglobulin gene products during B cell development. *J. Exp. Med.* **185,** 609–620.
81. Lin, W.–C. and Desiderio, S. (1994) Cell cycle regulation of V(D)J recombination–activating protein RAG–2. *Proc. Natl. Acad. Sci. USA* **91,** 2733–2737.
82. Lin, W.–C. and Desiderio, S. (1993) Regulation of V(D)J recombination activator protein RAG–2 by phosphorylation. *Science* **260,** 953–959.
83. Alt, F. W., Oltz, E. M., Young, F., Gorman, J., Taccioli, G., and Chen, J. (1992) VDJ recombination. *Immunol. Today* **13,** 306–314.
84. Stanhope–Baker, P., Hudson, K. M., Shaffer, A. L., Constantinescu, A., and Schlissel, M. S. (1996) Cell type–specific chromatin structure determines the targeting of V(D)J recombinase activity in vitro. *Cell* **85,** 887–897.
85. Löffert, D., Ehlich, A., Müller, W., and Rajewsky, K. (1996) Surrogate light chain expression is required to establish immunoglobulin heavy chain allelic exclusion during early B cell development. *Immunity* **4,** 133–144.
86. Sonoda, E., Pewzner–Jung, J., Schwers, S., Taki, S., Jung, S., Eilat, D., and Rajewsky, K. (1997) B cell development under the condition of allelic inclusion. *Immunity* **6,** 225–233.
87. Wabl, M. and Steinberg, C. (1982) A theory of allelic and isotypic exclusion for immunoglobulin genes. *Proc. Natl. Acad. Sci. USA* **79,** 6976–6978.
88. Freitas, A. A., Andrade, L., Lembezat, M. P., and Coutinho, A. (1990) Selection of VH gene repertoires: differentiating B cells of adult bone marrow mimic fetal development. *Int. Immunol.* **2,** 15–23.
89. Gu, H., Tarlinton, D., Müller, W., Rajewsky, K., and Förster, I. (1991) Most peripheral B cells in mice are ligand–selected. *J. Exp. Med.* **173,** 1357–1371.
90. Malynn, B. A., Yancopoulos, G. D., Barth, J. E., Bona, C. A., and Alt, F. W. (1990) Biased expression of Jh–proximal VH genes occurs in the newly generated repertoire of neonatal and adult mice. *J. Exp. Med.* **171,** 843–859.
91. Decker, D. J., Boyle, N. E., and Klinman, N. R. (1991) Predominance of nonproductive rearrangements of VH81X gene segments evidences a dependence of B cell clonal maturation on the structure of nascent H chains. *J. Immunol.* **147,** 1406–1411.
92. Huetz, F., Carlsson, L., Tornberg, U. C., and Holmberg, D. (1993) V–region directed selection in differentiating B lymphocytes. *EMBO J.* **12,** 1819–1826.
93. Yancopoulos, G. D., Desiderio, S. V., Paskind, M., Kearney, J. F., Baltimore, D., and Alt, F. W. (1984) Preferential utilization of the most DH–proximal VH gene segments in pre–B cell lines. *Nature* **311,** 727–733.
94. Carlsson, L., Övermo, C., and Holmberg, D. (1992) Developmentally controlled selection of antibody genes, characterization of individual VH7183 genes and evidence for stage–specific somatic diversification. *Eur. J. Immunol.* **22,** 71–78.
95. Marshall, A. J., Wu, G. E., and Paige, C. J. (1996) Frequency of VH81X usage during B cell development. *J. Immunol.* **156,** 2077–2084.
96. Martin, F., Chen, X., and Kearney, J. F. (1997) Development of VH81X transgene–bearing B cells in fetus and adult, site for expansion and deletion in conventional and CD5/B1 cells. *Int. Immunol.* **9,** 493–505.
97. Ye, J., McCray, S. K., and Clarke, S. H. (1996) The transition of preB–I to preB–II cells is dependent on the VH structure of the μ/surrogate L chain receptor. *EMBO J.* **15,** 1524–1533.
98. Chen, J., Ma, A., Young, F., and Alt, F. W. (1994) IL–2 receptor a chain expression during early B lymphocyte differentiation. *Int. Immunol.* **6,** 1265–1268.
99. Grawunder, U., Rolink, A., and Melchers, F. (1995) Induction of sterile transcription from the kappa L chain gene locus in V(D)J recombinase–deficient progenitor B cells. *Int. Immunol.* **7,** 1915–1925.
100. Papavasiliou, F., Jancovic, M., Suh, H., and Nussenzweig, M. C. (1995) The cytoplasmic domains of immunoglobulin (Ig) alpha and Ig beta can independently induce the precursor B cell transition and allelic exclusion. *J. Exp. Med.* **182,** 1389–1394.
101. Papavasiliou, F., Misulovin, Z., Suh, H., and Nussenzweig, M. C. (1995) The role of Ig beta in precursor B cell transition and allelic exclusion. *Science* **268,** 408–411.
102. Torres, R. M., Flaswinkel, H., Reth, M., and Rajewsky, K. (1996) Aberrant B cell development and immune response in mice with a compromised BCR complex. *Science* **272,** 1804–1808.
103. Reth, M. (1989) Antigen receptor tail clue. *Nature* **338,** 383–384.

104. Satterwaite, A. and Witte, O. (1996) Genetic analysis of tyrosine kinase function in B cell development. *Ann. Rev. Immunol.* **14,** 131–154.
105. Cheng, A. M., Rowley, B., Pao, W., Hayday, A., Bolen, J. B., and Pawson, T. (1995) Syk tyrosine kinase required for mouse viability and B–cell development. *Nature* **378,** 303–306.
106. Turner, M., Mee, P. J., Costello, P. S., Williams, O., Price, A. A., Duddy, L. P., Furlong, M. T., Geahlen, R. L., and Tybulewicz, V. L. (1995) Perinatal lethality and blocked B–cell development in mice lacking the tyrosine kinase Syk. *Nature* **378,** 298–302.
107. Hirabayashi, Y., Lecerf, J. M., Dong, Z., and Stollar, B. D. (1995) Kinetic analysis of the interactions of recombinant human VpreB and Ig V domains. *J. Immunol.* **155,** 1218–1228.
108. Fehling, H. J. and von Boehmer, H. (1997) Early αβ T cell development in the thymus of normal and genetically altered mice. *Curr. Opin. Immunol.* **9,** 263–275.
109. Padlan, E. A. (1977) Structural basis for the specificity of antibody–antigen reactions and structural mechanisms for the diversification of antigen–binding specificities. *Q. Rev. Biophys.* **10,** 35–65.
110. Klein, J. (1990) Immunology. Blackwell Scientific, Oxford, pp. 136.

Chapter 21

Molecular Mechanisms Regulating Negative Selection in Immature-Stage B-Cells

Leslie B. King, Peter Sandel, Richard A. Sater, and John G. Monroe

1. Introduction

Although the tremendous clonal diversity expressed in the B-cell receptor (BCR) repertoire is beneficial for mounting immune responses to foreign antigens, it is simultaneously detrimental in that it may include a multitude of BCRs capable of recognizing self antigens. Therefore, mechanisms must exist to functionally silence these self-reactive B-cells. Negative selection of autoreactive cells has been proposed to occur by clonal elimination or abortion (deletion), clonal silencing (anergy), and clonal alteration (receptor editing). Although there has been a significant advance in our understanding of these various modes of tolerance in recent years, the biochemical mechanisms regulating tolerance remain largely unknown. Rather than present a comprehensive review of the findings in this area, the authors will concentrate on the role of clonal deletion in the tolerization of immature B-cells. In particular, the following questions will be addressed:

1. Which target cell populations are sensitive to deletion?
2. What are the molecular mechanisms responsible for rendering these target populations tolerance sensitive? and
3. Is clonal deletion necessary for the maintenance of B-cell tolerance?

Although definitive answers will not be provided, the authors hope to present the most current experimental data addressing these issues as well as to point out controversial aspects of B-cell negative selection that await resolution.

From: *Molecular Biology of B-Cell and T-Cell Development*
Edited by: J. G. Monroe and E. V. Rothenberg © Humana Press Inc., Totowa, NJ

2. Historical Basis For Negative Selection

Given the enormous diversity of specificities displayed by surface immunoglobulin (sIg) on B-cells and the consequent potential for the generation of autoreactive B-cells, it became apparent that preservation of immunologic self-tolerance required a mechanism for eliminating or inactivating autoreactive B-cells. It was first hypothesized that such regulation would occur during neonatal development *(1)*. Hypotheses on the sensitivity of immature B-cells to tolerogenic signals were formalized in the clonal selection theory of Burnet *(2)* which predicted that:

1. Developing cells should be more sensitive to tolerance induction than mature cells.
2. Immature cells should be sensitive to a wide range of antigen concentrations and structures.
3. Immune tolerance should be exquisitely specific such that autoreactive clones are eliminated without jeopardizing the organism's ability to respond to foreign antigens.

Despite the lack of scientific evidence to support such views at the time, these basic tenets still hold true today.

Although B-cell tolerance was first speculated to occur only during the neonatal period, it was soon appreciated that a continued ability to negatively select newly developing autoreactive B-cells would be required throughout the lifetime of the animal. It was therefore hypothesized that the maturational status of the B-cell, rather than the age of the animal, would dictate immune responsiveness. Newly developing B-cells that had just begun to express specific antigen receptors were proposed to be the target of negative selection. This hypothesis was supported by the seminal studies of Metcalf and Klinman *(3,4)* and Nossal and Pike *(5,6)*, which demonstrated that exposure of immature B-cells from either neonatal spleen or adult bone marrow to low doses of antigen rendered them nonresponsive to subsequent antigenic stimulation. In these same studies, mature B-cells were not tolerized, emphasizing the dichotomy in inherent immunologic responsiveness of immature and mature B-cells. Similar results were obtained in in vitro assays using anti-immunoglobulin (anti-Ig) as a polyclonal stimulant *(7,8)*.

The studies described above suggested that stimulation through the BCR complex elicits distinct functional responses at the immature and mature stages of B-cell development. Using "knockout" mice deficient in various BCR components (reviewed in ref. *9*), differential developmentally regulated responses to pre-BCR/BCR stimulation have been shown to play a critical role in the developmental progression of B lymphocytes at several maturational stages (Fig. 1). For instance, signaling through the pre-BCR may provide a positive signal by enhancing proliferation and/or survival during the pro-B to pre-B transition *(10)*. Similarly, BCR engagement of mature B-cells leads to proliferation and differentiation into antibody secreting cells. In this chapter, the authors will focus on the extreme sensitivity of immature B-cells to negative selection following antigenic stimulation and the potential molecular mechanisms that may differentiate a tolerogenic response from the BCR-induced activation response observed in mature B-cells.

The extremely low frequency of B-cells specific for any one particular antigen makes following the fate of a particular specificity of autoreactive cell in vivo technically challenging, and thus makes it difficult to address the mechanisms responsible for B-cell tolerance. In the late 1980s, the advent of transgenic mice expressing BCRs of defined specificities represented a significant technical advancement for future analysis of the mechanisms responsible for B-cell tolerance *(11,12)*. Using these systems, three types of tolerance could be distinguished: clonal abortion or deletion, clonal anergy, and clonal

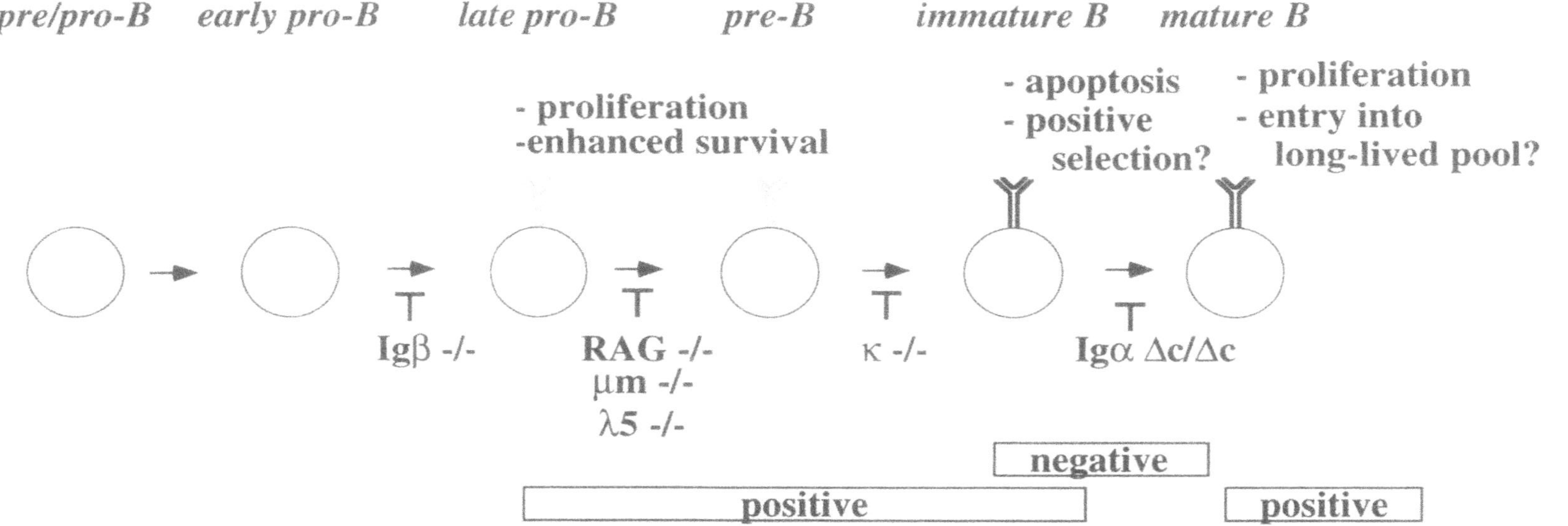

Fig. 1. BCR-induced signal transduction influences B-cell development. This schematic depicts the developmental stages during which BCR-induced signal transduction can influence B-cell maturation. Such signals can be either positive in that they induce survival and/or proliferation (indicated by the stippled bar) or negative in that they induce apoptosis (indicated by the open bar). Transitions between developmental stages that are affected by "knockout" mice deficient in the indicated genes are indicated under the T bars. The black Y indicates the BCR while the gray Y indicates the pre-BCR.

alteration (receptor editing). All three mechanisms appear to be utilized in vivo, and the ultimate fate of the immature B-cell likely depends upon the valency and concentration of the antigen, the maturational stage of the B-cell and the anatomic site in which antigen is first encountered, and the presence of T_h cells.

3. Clonal Abortion or Deletion of Autoreactive B-Cells

The physical elimination of autoreactive B-cells would appear to be the most fail-safe mechanism for silencing autoreactive B-cells. The ability of immature B-cells to be clonally deleted in response to BCR engagement was suggested in experiments in which treatment of neonatal mice or chickens with anti-immunoglobulin (Ig) resulted in the elimination of all peripheral B-cells *(13,14)*. These early observations were substantiated by work in transgenic mouse systems: reduced numbers of transgene-expressing B-cells were found in the bone marrow and spleen of mice expressing a BCR specific for the MHC class I molecule H-2K^k when expressed on the selecting H-2^k background *(12)*, and deletion of DNA-specific B-cells was observed in transgenic mice expressing an anti-DNA specific BCR *(15)*. Finally, antigen–specific B-cells were not observed in the periphery of double–transgenic mice expressing both an anti-hen egg lysozyme (HEL) Ig transgene and a membrane bound HEL transgene *(16)*. In this system, the clonal deletion of autoreactive B-cells could be dissociated into two distinct and potentially differentially regulated events: developmental arrest and cell death *(17)*. Continuous binding of antigen by immature B-cells in the bone marrow led to an arrest in their development that was followed by clonal deletion after one to three days. Although overexpression of the anti-apoptotic molecule Bcl-2 could rescue the cells from cell death, the developmental arrest was still apparent. Importantly, removal of antigen could reverse the developmental arrest, suggesting that immature B-cells have a window of opportunity after antigenic exposure during which they can be rescued, either by removal of antigen or by receptor editing (*see* Subheading 9.3.).

4. Targets of Negative Selection

A large body of literature indicates that immature B-cells in adult bone marrow and neonatal spleen are the target of negative selection *(3–5,18,19)*. However, the recent description of tolerance-sensitive, late immature, or transitional B-cells in the spleen *(20–22)* suggests that clonal deletion may also occur in the periphery. Therefore, the question remains—which subset of immature B-cells is the most physiologically relevant tolerance-sensitive target cell population in vivo?

4.1. Immature B-Cells in the Bone Marrow

The sensitivity of bone-marrow–derived immature B-cells to negative selection makes intuitive sense, since immature B-cells in the bone marrow are in contact with autoantigens but are largely protected from exposure to foreign antigens. Negative selection in this environment would therefore promote the elimination of unwanted autoreactive specificities while simultaneously preserving immature B-cells reactive with foreign antigens. Although it is clear that immature B-cells can bind antigen in the bone marrow *(23)*, the evidence that immature autoreactive B-cells receive a signal in the bone marrow that will result in deletion is somewhat indirect. In transgenic systems in which clonal deletion appears operational, immature B-cells expressing autoreactive specificities are often present in the bone marrow, albeit in some cases at reduced frequencies, but mature B-cells are absent in the periphery *(12,17,24,25)*. Phenotypic analysis of bone marrow B-cells from transgenic mice expressing BCRs specific for anti-double stranded DNA clearly indicates the presence of pre-B-cells, but the absence of subsequent stages of B-cell development, suggesting that immature B-cells expressing newly acquired sIg are the likely targets for negative selection *(25)*. In all of these systems, disappearance is equated with deletion, despite the inability to detect large numbers of dying immature B-cells *(17)*. Thus, although it is possible that immature B-cells are triggered to die in the bone marrow, it is also conceivable that BCR engagement on immature B-cells promotes exit from the bone marrow and that antigenic exposure in the periphery leads to cell death (*see* Subheading 4.2.). Although BCR-signaling of immature B-cells in the bone marrow can result in a developmental arrest, this signal does not necessitate death *(17)*. Indeed, it has been suggested that the bone marrow may provide a protective environment for immature B-cells, preventing them from being deleted following antigenic exposure *(22)*, (P.S. and J.G.M., unpublished observation) and perhaps allowing them sufficient time to receptor edit *(26)*. Thus, the microenvironment in which immature B-cells first encounter antigen may dramatically affect their subsequent functional response.

4.2. Late Immature or Transitional B-Cells in the Periphery

Although autoreactive immature B-cells can be negatively selected by autoantigens present in the bone marrow, autoreactive B-cells specific for peripheral autoantigens would escape such a selection process. Therefore, mechanisms must exist to functionally silence such cells once they reach the periphery. The recent description of late immature or transitional B-cells that share many of the phenotypic characteristics of bone marrow-derived immature B-cells ($IgM^{hi}IgD^{lo}HSA^{hi}$), but which have recently emigrated from the bone marrow to the spleen *(20–22)* suggests that these cells might also be tolerance-sensitive. Indeed further studies revealed that this population of cells is sensitive to negative selection in vitro *(27)* and in vivo *(22)*. The susceptibility of immature B-cells to clonal deletion in the peripheral lymphoid organs has been confirmed in other systems *(28)*, suggesting that antigen-induced negative selection is certainly not confined to the bone marrow. However, it remains to be seen whether the bulk of immature B-cells are eliminated in the bone marrow, or whether newly emigrating transitional B-cells that have escaped the potentially protective bone marrow microenvironment account for the majority of autoreactive B-cells actively undergoing clonal deletion.

5. Mechanisms Regulating Clonal Deletion

It has long been known that thymocytes undergoing negative selection die by apoptosis or programmed cell death *(29)*. The ability of immature B-cells to undergo apoptosis in response to BCR ligation was directly tested using immature B-cells isolated from adult bone marrow *(30)*, or late immature/transitional B-cells *(27)* and anti-Ig as a polyclonal activator. In contrast to mature B-cells, immature B-cells are exquisitely sensitive to BCR-induced apoptosis in vitro. These results support the clonal deletion model of negative selection and further demonstrate that deletion can occur via an apoptotic mechanism. Interestingly, the clonal deletion of immature B-cells appears to be preceded by an abortive attempt to enter the cell cycle. Although immature B-cells leave G_0 and enter the cell cycle in response to anti-Ig, they fail to make the G_1/S transition. This is apparently because of an inability to generate functional cyclin E/cdk2 complexes *(31)*. It is not yet clear at this time if the cell-cycle arrest and the induction of apoptosis are functionally related or are the consequence of two separate and distinct signaling events. Current investigation centers on the mechanism responsible for the enhanced sensitivity of immature B-cells to BCR-induced apoptosis and begs the Talmudic question—why are these B-cells different from all other B-cells?

5.1. The Potential Role of IgD as a Protective Signaling Mechanism

Immature B-cells (IgM^{hi} IgD^{lo}) progressively acquire more IgD as they develop into mature B-cells (IgM^{lo} IgD^{hi}). Associated with this progression is a shift from a tolerance-sensitive phenotype to a tolerance-insensitive one. These observations suggested that signaling through the IgD surface receptor could result in either a protective or a proliferative signal, whereas signaling through the IgM receptor would result in a tolerogenic signal (reviewed in ref. *32*). Evidence that IgD could provide a protective signal to developing immature B-cells was provided in a transgenic mouse system in which an anti-TNP Ig transgene was expressed as either an IgM alone or as IgM and IgD *(24)*. In this system, multivalent TNP led to the efficient deletion of immature B-cells in the IgM-only expressing mice, but deletion was partially blocked in the mice expressing both IgM and IgD. However, this putative protective effect of IgD is not universally observed; transgenic mice expressing an anti-HEL Ig transgene constructed to express both IgM and IgD, IgM alone, or IgD alone indicate that IgM and IgD are virtually indistinguishable in their ability to induce deletion, anergy, or proliferation *(33)*. In addition, the authors have recently shown that stimulation of late immature B-cells with either anti-IgD or anti-IgM leads to apoptosis *(27)*, and, importantly, anti-IgD does not protect immature B-cells from anti–IgM-induced apoptosis. Finally, IgD-deficient mice are capable of responding to both T-dependent and T-independent antigens *(34,35)*, indicating that the presence of IgD is not required for either the prevention of tolerance or the induction of proliferation in mature B-cells.

5.2. The Role of T-Cell Help in B-Cell Tolerance

According to the original model of Bretscher and Cohn, B lymphocytes stimulated through their antigen receptor (signal 1) in the absence of T-cell help (signal 2) would be tolerized *(36)*. The relative lack of T-cells in the bone marrow that could provide a "second signal" to immature B-cells exposed to self antigen suggested that the negative selection of immature B-cells occurred because of a lack of T-cell help. However, despite a lack of T-cell help, highly purified populations of mature B-cells proliferate in response to anti-Ig stimulation in vitro. In contrast, immature B-cells undergo apoptosis under identical conditions *(27,30)*. If signal 1 (anti-Ig) in the absence of signal 2 (T-cell help) were solely responsible for inducing tolerance, then both immature and mature B-cells should be tolerized in this assay. Thus, these results suggest that an intrinsic developmentally regulated difference in BCR-induced signal transduction is responsible for the functional dichotomy between antigen-stimulated immature and mature B-cells.

Although the experiments described above suggest that B-cell tolerance is not a direct consequence of inadequate T-cell help, T-cell help can have a profound influence on the induction of immature B-cell tolerance *(3,4)*. In particular, ligation of the B-cell surface antigen CD40 by CD40L expressed on activated T-cells, or the T_h lymphokine, IL-4, can efficiently rescue immature B-cells from anti-Ig-induced apoptosis in vitro *(18,30,37)* and activated T_h cells can prevent tolerance induction in vivo *(28)*.

Table 1
Comparison of Immature- and Mature-Stage B-Cells

	Immature	Mature
Functional Aspects		
Sensitivity to tolerance induction	Sensitive	Resistant
Stimulation with anti-IgM or IgD	Apoptosis	Proliferation
Stimulation with LPS	Proliferation	Proliferation
Stimulation with anti-Ig + IL-4 or anti-CD40	Rescue from apoptosis	Enhanced proliferation
BCR-induced Ca^{2+} flux[a]	"Normal"	"Normal"
BCR-induced PIP_2 hydrolysis[a]	Reduced	"Normal"
Molecular aspects		
Fgr expression[a]	Reduced	"Normal"
Bcl-2 and Bcl-x expression[a]	Reduced	"Normal"
BCR-induced *c-myc* expression[a]	Reduced	"Normal"
CD45 expression	Intermediate	High
CD22 expression	Dull to intermediate	High
CD19 expression	Intermediate	High

[a]Relative levels or activity when compared with those of mature B-cells.

5.3. Developmentally Regulated Signaling Differences in Immature and Mature B-Cells

In general, naive mature B-cells proliferate in response to BCR engagement and are resistant to BCR-induced apoptosis, whereas immature B-cells are unable to proliferate and instead undergo apoptosis in response to BCR crosslinking in vitro *(27,30)*. In addition, immature B-cells appear to be much more sensitive to antigenic stimulation, undergoing apoptosis at approximately 100-fold lower concentration of anti-Ig than is required for the induction of mature B-cell proliferation (R. A. Sater and J. G. Monroe, unpublished observation). Such observations suggest that either quantitative or qualitative differences in BCR-induced signal transduction events will dictate the negative response of immature B-cells and activation response of mature B-cells. What then are the molecular mechanisms that distinguish the induction of tolerance from the initiation of activation events?

6. Qualitative vs Quantitative Differences in the Induction of B-Cell Negative Selection

The induction of apoptosis in immature B-cells and activation in mature B-cells following anti-Ig stimulation in vitro suggests that an intrinsic developmentally regulated difference in BCR-induced signal transduction may be responsible for their apparent functional dichotomy. This hypothesis is supported by the authors' observation that although mature B-cells increase intracellular Ca^{2+} and hydrolyze phosphatidylinositol 4,5-*bis* phosphate (PIP_2) in response to BCR crosslinking, immature B-cells increase intracellular Ca^{2+} levels in the relative absence of PIP_2 hydrolysis *(19)* (Table 1). Since PIP_2 hydrolysis results in the generation of inositol triphosphate (IP_3) and diacylglycerol (DAG), an activator of protein kinase C (PKC), these results suggest that an unbalanced signal consisting of increased intracellular Ca^{2+} levels in the absence of PKC activation could potentially result in apoptosis. This hypothesis is supported by the findings that pharmacologic activation of PKC is capable of rescuing immature B-cells from anti–Ig-induced apoptosis and that PKC-depleted mature B-cells are rendered sensitive to this type of tolerance (King et al., submitted manuscript). It, therefore, appears that a developmentally regulated, functional coupling of PKC to BCR induced signaling is essential for an activating response.

The inability of immature B-cells to hydrolyze PIP_2 in response to anti-Ig stimulation suggested that the tyrosine kinase pathway involved in the activation of phospholipase C_γ (PLC_γ), the enzyme responsible for PIP_2 hydrolysis, may be differentially regulated in immature and mature B-cells. Although the increase in tyrosine kinase activity observed in BCR-induced mature B-cells is grossly intact in immature B-cells, analysis of the expression of *src* family kinases revealed a deficiency in the expression of two kinases, *fyn* and *fgr*, in immature B-cells obtained from neonatal spleen *(38)*. However, although these results are provocative, they cannot totally account for the signaling defect responsible for negative signaling in immature B-cells since late immature/transitional B-cells, which are also sensitive to BCR-induced apoptosis, express both *fyn* and *fgr (39)* and mature B lymphocytes from *fyn* -deficient mice proliferate in response to anti-Ig *(40)*. The molecular mechanisms underlying the uncoupling of the BCR from PIP_2 hydrolysis and the apoptotic pathway activated by this imbalance in signal transduction remain unclear, but are actively being pursued in the author's laboratory.

The role of tyrosine kinases in the induction of immature B-cell apoptosis has been extensively analyzed in tumor models (WEHI-231, DT40, Ramos) thought to represent immature-stage B-cells. Increased tyrosine kinase activity following BCR engagement suggested that a tyrosine kinase-activated apoptotic pathway may be operative in these cell lines. In these systems, activation of Btk and PLCγ appeared to be required for the induction of BCR-induced apoptosis *(41,42)* but Lyn appeared unlikely to play an active role in this process *(41,43)*. However, distinct BCR-induced signaling differences have been observed between WEHI-231 cells and primary immature B lymphocytes *(19,44)*, suggesting that different apoptotic mechanisms may be utilized by each. Therefore, although data obtained in cell lines representing immature B-cells may provide insights into the mechanisms responsible for apoptosis in general, such data may not be indicative of mechanisms utilized during the negative selection of immature B-cells in vivo.

The induction of tyrosine kinase activity following BCR engagement in immature B-cells suggests that tyrosine phosphorylation of a substrate linked to the "death pathway" could be involved in the induction of apoptosis. An analysis of substrates in the WEHI-231 cell line revealed that a potentially relevant apoptosis-related substrate could be HS-1, a protein with a C-terminal SH3 domain capable of binding proline rich regions of proteins, and an N-terminal region characteristic of helix-loop-helix proteins *(45)*. Although lymphoid development appears relatively normal in HS-1-deficient mice, both B1 and B2 peritoneal B-cells appear resistant to anti–Ig-induced apoptosis *(46)*. Although it is not clear what functional role HS-1 may play in the induction of apoptosis, its inducible nuclear localization and homology to helix-loop-helix transcription factors suggest that it may act to regulate the expression of apoptosis-related gene products.

Based upon the authors' hypothesis that an unbalanced signal of increased intracellular Ca^{2+} in the absence of an increase in PKC activation is responsible for the BCR-induced apoptosis of immature B-cells, they believe that PKC is likely to play an active role in determining whether a B-cell is activated or undergoes apoptosis in response to receptor crosslinking. The recent generation of mutant mice that are deficient in PKC-β suggests that PKC-β plays an important role in the activation responses of mature B-cells *(47)*. PKC-β deficient mice respond poorly to anti-Ig *in vitro*, although it remains to be seen whether this is because of an inadequate proliferative signal or to the induction of apoptosis, as would be predicted by the authors' hypothesis. Other PKC isoenzymes appear unable to compensate for the deficiency in PKC-β, suggesting that PKC-β is either uniquely regulated following BCR crosslinking or has a distinct substrate specificity. Interestingly, the phenotype of PKC-β deficient mice resembles that observed in the Btk $^{-/-}$ mouse *(48,49)*. Since the pleckstrin homology domain of Btk binds PKC *(50)*, it is possible that these molecules are intimately associated during BCR-induced signal transduction and B-cell activation.

In contrast to PKC-β, a recently identified isoenzyme of PKC, PKC-μ, appears to function as a negative regulator of BCR activation *(51)*. PKC-μ is found associated with the resting BCR, and its activity is upregulated by BCR crosslinking. PKC-μ also associates with Syk and PLCγ, and it has been shown that both of these molecules are potential substrates for this serine/threonine kinase. Interestingly, PKC-μ activation appears to inhibit the tyrosine-kinase activity of Syk, a kinase thought to be involved in PLCγ activation *(52,53)*. Therefore, it is possible that developmentally regulated alterations in the regulation of PKC-μ activity could affect the ability of immature B-cells to hydrolyze PIP_2 following BCR ligation.

Although the molecular mechanisms regulating the negative selection of B-cells remain largely undefined, several signaling pathways known to modulate apoptotic processes are activated following BCR engagement. For instance, BCR crosslinking in mature B-cells activates the Ras pathway *(54)*, as well as phosphoinositide 3-kinase (PI-3K) *(55)*. Ras activation ultimately results in the activation of the mitogen activated protein kinases (MAPKs), the extracellular signal-regulated kinases (ERKs), and the c-Jun N-terminal kinase (JNKs) (reviewed in ref. *56*). A dynamic balance between JNK and ERK activation has been shown to be critical for the regulation of apoptosis in some cell systems *(57)*. Although ERK/JNK regulation of apoptosis in immature B-cells has not been directly assessed, anti-Ig stimulation upregulates ERK activity in WEHI-231, a cell line sensitive to BCR-induced apoptosis, whereas stimulation with anti-CD40 rescues WEHI-231 from BCR-induced death *(58)* and leads to JNK activation *(59)*. PI-3K may play a role in the regulation of apoptotic vs activation signals by decreasing the levels of PLCγ substrate, PIP_2, and through the generation of novel phospholipid second messengers. One product of PI-3K, phosphatidylinositol 3,4 bisphosphate, has recently been shown to be responsible for the activation of another serine/threonine kinase, Akt *(60)*, recently shown to function as an antiapoptotic effector molecule *(61,62)*. However, as yet there is no direct evidence that any of these signaling pathways plays a role in the intrinsic difference in signaling observed between immature and mature B-cells.

Although it is thought that clonal deletion of immature B-cells requires *de novo* gene expression *(63)*, the transcription factors involved in this process remain largely unknown. The protooncogene c-Myc has been shown to play a role in the BCR-induced apoptosis of WEHI-231 cells (reviewed in ref. *64*). Treatment of WEHI-231 cells with agents that lead to an elevation in the NF-κB inhibitor, I-κB, resulted in a decrease in c-*myc* expression and the subsequent induction of cell death, an effect that could be reversed by the ectopic expression of c-*myc (65,66)*. Of note, unlike mature B-cells, immature B-cells do not upregulate c-*myc* expression after BCR engagement *(31)*, suggesting that an inability to upregulate Myc expression following BCR engagement may play a role in the induction of apoptosis in primary immature B-cells as well. The identity and role of other transcription factors involved in the induction of immature B-cell apoptosis, as well as the gene products that they regulate, remain to be elucidated.

7. B-Cell Coreceptors

In addition to the intrinsic signal delivered to the B-cell through direct BCR occupancy, ligation of other cell surface molecules have been shown to modulate BCR-induced responses. For instance, coreceptors such as CD19 (reviewed in ref. *67*) and CD45 are thought to positively regulate BCR-induced responses *(68)* although, in contrast, CD22 appears to negatively regulate BCR-induced signals (reviewed in ref. *69*). Since engagement of these coreceptors can influence the threshold of BCR-induced signal transduction, it is possible that the relative level of expression of these coreceptors may influence the induction of B-cell tolerance and/or activation. Indeed, the differential expression of these coreceptors on immature and mature B-cells (Table 1) suggests that they could indeed play a role in developmentally regulated differences in signal transduction. However, it is unclear whether these coreceptors could qualitatively affect signal transduction (i.e., convert a tolerogenic signal to a proliferative one) or alternatively quantitatively alter the signal by regulating the threshold at which B-cell tolerance or activation is achieved.

The CD19 coreceptor has been hypothesized to play a positive role in regulating BCR-induced activation signals; co-crosslinking of the CD19/CD21 complex and the BCR results in a synergistic response *(70,71)*, perhaps because of the ability of CD19 to bind PI3-K *(67)*. The threshold for mature B-cell stimulation is clearly influenced by levels of CD19: CD19-deficient mice exhibit decreased responses to anti-Ig stimulation *(72,73)*, whereas CD19-overexpressing transgenic mice are hyperresponsive *(72,74)*. If signaling in immature B-cells was similarly affected, a deficiency in CD19 expression might allow for less efficient negative selection of immature B-cells and, conversely, overexpression of CD19 could potentially lead to the increased deletion of immature B-cells. However, an analysis of B-cell development in CD19 $^{-/-}$ mice suggested that negative selection is not dramatically altered *(72)*. In contrast, CD19-overexpressing mice exhibited significant defects in the development of bone marrow B-cell compartments in that the number of immature and mature B-cells were significantly reduced *(72)*. Thus it appears that the hyperresponsiveness of B-cells from CD19-overexpressing mice could result in the stimulation of immature B-cells expressing BCRs with an avidity that in normal mice would be below the threshold for negative selection, resulting in their clonal elimination and a consequent reduction in B-cell numbers. Together, these results suggest that CD19 levels can affect the threshold at which immature B-cell negative selection and mature B-cell activation take place, but cannot qualitatively convert an activation signal to a deletional signal or vice versa.

CD22 was originally proposed to augment BCR-induced proliferative signaling *(69)*, but a negative modulatory role for CD22 was suggested by experiments in which CD22 sequestration away from the BCR complex augmented BCR-induced responses *(75)*. The existence of immunoreceptor tyrosine-based activation motifs (ITAM) capable of binding positive regulators of signal transduction, *(76)* as well as negative regulatory ITIM motifs capable of binding SHP-1 *(75,77–79)* in the cytoplasmic domain of CD22 supports a dual role for CD22 in signal transduction. The tyrosine phosphatase, SHP-1, recently found to be mutated in motheaten (*me*) and motheaten viable (*me^{v}*) mice *(80,81)*, has been hypothesized to function as a negative regulator of BCR-induced signaling *(82)*, potentially regulating the threshold at which negative selection of immature B-cells occurs *(83)*.

CD22 is expressed at very low levels on pre- B-cells and is upregulated as B-cells mature *(84,85)*. As expected, early B-cell development in CD22-deficient mice progresses normally. However, mature B-cells appear hyperresponsive to receptor signaling in that BCR-induced Ca^{2+} fluxes are increased and achieved at lower doses of anti-Ig *(85–88)*. Although mature B-cells appear in relatively normal numbers, there is a shift in phenotype resulting in a depletion of $IgM^{hi}IgD^{lo}$ and an enrichment of $IgM^{lo}IgD^{hi}$ cells *(86–88)*, a phenotype reminiscent of the chronically stimulated B-cells found in anti-HEL Ig/soluble HEL transgenic mice. The apparent chronic activation of $CD22^{-/-}$ B-cells, coupled with the similarity in phenotype to B-cells from SHP-1-deficient me^v/me^v mice *(83)*, suggested that CD22 negatively regulates BCR signaling, perhaps via binding of SHP-1. In the absence of CD22, the BCR may be spontaneously activated or the activation threshold may be lowered sufficiently so that it is stimulated following exposure to endogenous antigens. In contrast to their apparent chronic activation, in most cases, CD22-deficient B-cells exhibit a reduced proliferative responses to anti-Ig *in vitro (85,87,88)*. While reduced proliferation could reflect the apparent anergic status of the cells, B-cells from CD22-deficient mice appear unable to desensitize their BCR *(88)*, suggesting that CD22 may normally play a positive role in BCR-induced activation. Alternatively, the decrease in proliferation observed in B-cells from $CD22^{-/-}$ mice has been proposed to occur as a result of enhanced apoptosis, consistent with the reduced life span of mature B-cells in these animals *(85,87)*. Although these results were far from dramatic, they suggest that, in the absence of CD22, an activation signal may be converted to an apoptotic one, perhaps because of, in part, the substantial increases in intracellular calcium observed in stimulated cells. Thus it appears that the developmentally regulated expression of CD22 (lower in immature B-cells) may contribute to their susceptibility to BCR-induced negative selection

In B-cells, CD45 expression appears to act as a positive regulator of B-cell activation, critical for ras activation *(89,90)*, Ca^{2+} mobilization *(68)*, and recruitment of Lyn to the BCR complex *(91)*. Analysis of signal transduction events in B-cells from CD45-deficient mice reveal that although Ig-α and PLCγ2 were phosphorylated following BCR crosslinking, there appeared to be an abrogation in the influx of calcium from extracellular stores *(92)*. Phenotypically and functionally, B-cells from CD45-deficient mice resemble late immature or transitional B-cells from nontransgenic mice, exhibiting a reduced ability to proliferate in response to anti-Ig *(92–94)*. However, in contrast to traditional immature B-cells, they do not undergo apoptosis *(94)*. The “immature” phenotype of CD45-deficient B-cells is a B-cell intrinsic phenomenon; mixed bone marrow chimeras containing $CD45^{+/+}$ T-cells do not rescue B-cell development *(92)*. CD45 has recently been suggested to play a role in setting the threshold between negative and positive selection of immature B-cells into the long-lived B-cell pool *(95)*. Somewhat surprisingly, exposure of CD45-deficient anti-HEL Ig expressing immature B-cells to soluble HEL in vivo led to an increased recovery of IgD^+ B-cells. These results suggest that in the absence of CD45, a normally tolerogenic signal is converted to a positively selecting one, and further suggest that a BCR-induced response of very low affinity may be required for efficient entry of B-cells into the long-lived pool (*see* Subheading 9.1.).

8. Modulators of the Apoptotic Response

8.1. Bcl-2 Family Members

Bcl-2 is a 25–26 kDa protein predominantly located in the membranes of mitochondria, the endoplasmic reticulum, and the nuclear envelope *(96)*. Bcl-2 forms either homodimers or heterodimers with an ever-expanding family of Bcl-2 family members including, but not limited to, pro-apoptotic members such as Bax *(97)*, Bcl-x_s *(98)*, and Bad *(99)* as well as anti-apoptotic molecules such as Bcl-x_L *(98)* and A1 *(100)*. It has been theorized that the relative expression of these family members functions as a rheostat mechanism, setting the threshold for determining whether a cell lives or dies when exposed to potentially lethal stimuli *(101)*.

The expression patterns of Bcl-2 and Bcl-x have been evaluated throughout B-cell development, and indicate that the different family members are likely to play unique roles in the prevention of apoptosis at distinct stages of B-cell development. For instance, Bcl-2 is highly expressed at the pro-B-cell and mature B-cell stage, but is down-regulated at the pre-B and immature B-cell stage *(102,103)*. In contrast, Bcl-x_L is highly expressed at the pre-B-cell stage and in activated mature B-cells *(104)* ; it is somewhat controversial whether immature-stage B-cells also express Bcl-x_L *(105)*. Based upon these results, it was hypothesized that expression of Bcl-2 may be responsible for the continued survival of mature B-cells. Furthermore, pre-BCR-induced Bcl-x_L expression in pre-B-cells may extend cell survival and thereby promote the pre-B to immature B-cell transition, whereas BCR-induced Bcl-x_L expression in activated B-cells may similarly promote entry into the long-lived B-cell pool. Importantly, the relative inability of immature B-cells to express high levels of either Bcl-2 or Bcl-x_L may render them particularly sensitive to stimuli that would induce apoptosis, thus correlating with their tolerance sensitivity.

The role of Bcl-2, Bcl-x_L, and Bax in B-cell negative selection have been addressed in "knockout" mice, as well as in transgenic mice overexpressing these molecules. Normal B-cell development is not dependent upon expression of Bcl-2 since this process occurs normally in Bcl-$2^{-/-}$ mice up until 3–4 weeks of age, at which time massive lymphoid apoptosis occurs *(106,107)*. In contrast, the absence of Bcl-x_L appears to result in a reduced survival of pre-B-cells *(108)*, suggesting that upregulation of Bcl-x_L by engagement of the pre-BCR may play an important role in B-cell development. In contrast, mice deficient in the pro-apoptotic family member, Bax, displayed an increased number of B-cells with a mature B-cell phenotype, suggesting that a proportion of B-cells may be eliminated through a Bax-dependent mechanism *(109)*, perhaps during negative selection.

In most cases, overexpression of a Bcl-2 transgene in the B-cell lineage does not prevent the negative selection of immature B-cells *(110)*, nor does it promote entry of tolerized B-cells into the long-lived pool *(111)*. However, Bcl-2 overexpressing mice do have increased numbers of peripheral mature B-cells, presumably because of the increased life span of these cells *(112)*. Although Bcl-2 overexpressing mice exhibit autoimmune symptoms late in life, it is not clear whether this break in tolerance is because of a defect in central tolerance or whether peripheral tolerance is compromised by a reduced ability to delete autoreactive mature B-cells. Similarly, overexpression of Bcl-x_L in the B-cell compartment of transgenic mice can lead to an accumulation of pre-B, immature and mature B-cells. However, in this case, it appears that the increase in the number of mature B-cells reflects an increased survival of pre-B-cells rather than a lack of negative selection, since B-cell depletion in response to anti-IgD in vivo was relatively normal *(104)*. Thus overexpression of antiapoptotic members of the Bcl-2 family can certainly lead to increased numbers of B-lineage cells, presumably as a consequence of a prolongation of the time in which they can receive signals for developmental progression and/or entry into the long-lived B-cell pool. Despite this, there is little direct evidence to suggest that Bcl-2/Bcl-x_L overexpression can prevent the negative selection of immature B-cells or that the lack of Bcl-2 or Bcl-x_L is directly responsible for the tolerance-sensitivity of immature B-cells.

8.2. Fas/FasL Family Members

The tumor necrosis factor (TNF)/TNF receptor families are ever-expanding gene superfamilies encoding receptor/ligand pairs that influence the life and death decisions of lymphocytes (reviewed in ref. *113*). Fas, a member of the TNF receptor family, is capable of inducing apoptosis by virtue of a "death domain" in its intracytoplasmic tail. The expression of both Fas and Fas ligand (FasL) in activated lymphocytes *(114,115)* suggested that Fas could normally be involved in the deletion of autoreactive lymphocytes. Consistent with this, deletion of activated peripheral T-cells in vivo appears to occur via a Fas-dependent pathway *(116)*. Fas is expressed, at least at low levels, on B-cells representing all stages of B-cell development *(117)*. However, B-cell development in the bone marrow appears normal in Fas-deficient mice *(118)*, suggesting that, as with thymocytes, development and central deletion of immature B lymphocytes occurs via a relatively Fas-independent pathway *(119,120)*. This is not to say that Fas has no role in the regulation of self-tolerance. As in the T-cell system, Fas appears to play a role in maintaining peripheral tolerance and may function to eliminate both activated *(121)* and anergized *(122)* B-cells during collaborative T-B-cell interactions.

CD40 is a multifaceted member of the TNFR family. Signaling through CD40 is capable of inducing B-cell proliferation as well as synergizing with anti-Ig to stimulate B-cell growth *(123)*, inducing Fas expression on B-cells to render them sensitive to Fas-mediated apoptosis *(121)*, and antagonizing BCR-induced death *(58)*. CD40 can actively prevent apoptosis by altering the expression of molecules such as myc and Bcl-x, thought to be involved in regulating apoptosis *(104,124–126)*. Despite the ability of activated, CD40L-expressing T-cells to abrogate tolerance induction in immature B-cells, there is little evidence to suggest that a lack of CD40 signaling is directly responsible for the tolerance sensitivity of immature B-cells. Consistently, although there are subtle abnormalities in the phenotype of mature B-cells in CD40-deficient mice, these cells are not tolerized by antigenic stimulation *(127)*.

In summary, the sensitivity of immature B-cells to BCR-induced apoptosis suggests that antigen-driven, programmed cell death contributes to the negative selection of autoreactive, immature B-cells in vivo. It is likely that developmentally regulated differences in BCR-induced signal transduction events play a role in distinguishing an apoptotic response in immature B-cells from an activation response in mature B-cells. In addition, there are suggestions that modulation of BCR-induced signal transduction by co-receptors can either quantitatively or qualitatively alter B-cell responses. Finally, developmentally regulated alterations in the expression of both pro- and antiapoptotic modulators could potentially regulate the negative selection of immature B-cells in vivo. Although progress is being made, an analysis of the molecular mechanisms regulating immature B-cell apoptosis is in its infancy and clearly deserves more intensive investigation before firm conclusions can be drawn. However, the relative importance of such an analysis presupposes that clonal deletion of immature B-cells represents a key fate decision during B-cell development—a concept that will be discussed more thoroughly in the next section.

9. To Die or Not to Die—Is That the Question?

While it is clear that clonal deletion can play a role in central B-cell tolerance in transgenic mice, its relative importance in the negative selection of autoreactive B-cells in normal mice remains unknown. The rate of generation of immature B-cells in the bone marrow (1.5×10^7 cells/day) *(128)*, greatly exceeds the number of mature B-cells entering the periphery *(129)*, suggesting that there is a substantial loss of cells during this transition. However, the frequency of dying cells is difficult to determine *in situ* because cells undergoing apoptosis are rapidly scavenged by resident macrophages *(130)*. Despite this, it is possible to detect low frequencies of apoptotic cells that have an immature B-cell phenotype in the bone marrow of normal mice *(131)*. Although apoptotic cells are present, it is not yet clear if these are autoreactive B-cells dying as a consequence of negative selection. It is possible that immature B-cells enter a default death pathway unless they either join the mature B-cell pool stochastically or are positively selected (Fig. 2). Immature B-cells may also die as a consequence of anergy, since anergic B-cells have been shown to have a shortened half-life (*see* Subheading 9.2.). Thus, by an assortment of mechanisms, immature B-cells seem to be at a pivotal stage in their development and must decide—to die or not to die?

9.1. Death by a Lack of Positive Selection

The hypothesis that B-cells undergo a positive selection step to progress from the immature to the mature stage is not universally held. Although the "requirement" for positive selection during thymocyte development can easily be explained by their obligate need to recognize peptide in the context of self MHC molecules, B-cells are under no such restriction. However, antigen-driven positive selection could provide a mechanism for "testing" for a functional BCR on immature B-cells. Failure to be positively selected could then lead to the elimination of immature B-cells that either fail to express sIg or that express functionally compromised sIg. Death of these cells could contribute to the substantial number of dying cells observed during the immature to mature B-cell transition.

Based upon the repertoire skewing of long-lived conventional B-cells relative to the repertoire observed in pre-B-cells, it has been suggested that all mature B-cells must undergo a positive selection step during the immature to mature B-cell transition *(132)*. Alternatively, this skewing could reflect expansion of B-cell clones reactive to environmental and gut-associated antigens. An intact, signaling-competent BCR appears to be required for the efficient progression of immature B-cells to a mature, long-lived B-cell population *(133)* (Fig. 1), suggesting that a BCR-induced signal is necessary for this positive selection step. Furthermore, in a CD45-deficient/ anti-HEL Ig transgenic mouse system it was observed that, in the absence of CD45, a tolerizing signal normally induced by BCR engagement was converted into a positively selecting one, resulting in the accumulation of IgD^+ B-cells *(95)*. These results suggest that although moderate avidity antigen/BCR interactions result in a tolerization signal, a lowering of the signal transduction capacity of this interaction by the removal of CD45 (effectively lowering the sensitivity) can transform this signal to a positively selecting one. Additionally, *syk*-deficient mice appear to be defective in the immature to mature B-cell transition, suggesting that a *syk*-dependent (and perhaps BCR-inducible) signaling event is required *(134)*. Importantly, however, it is not clear at this time if a BCR-induced signal would be required to drive the immature to mature B-cell transition, or instead may be required to promote entry into the long-lived B-cell pool. Additionally, it remains to be determined whether entry into the long-lived pool is a necessary consequence of transition to the mature B-cell stage or rather reflects antigen-induced activation of clonally-selected mature B-cells.

9.2. Anergy

Clonal deletion of autoreactive B-cells provides the most fail-safe method for preventing self-reactive B-cells from entering or being activated in the periphery. However,

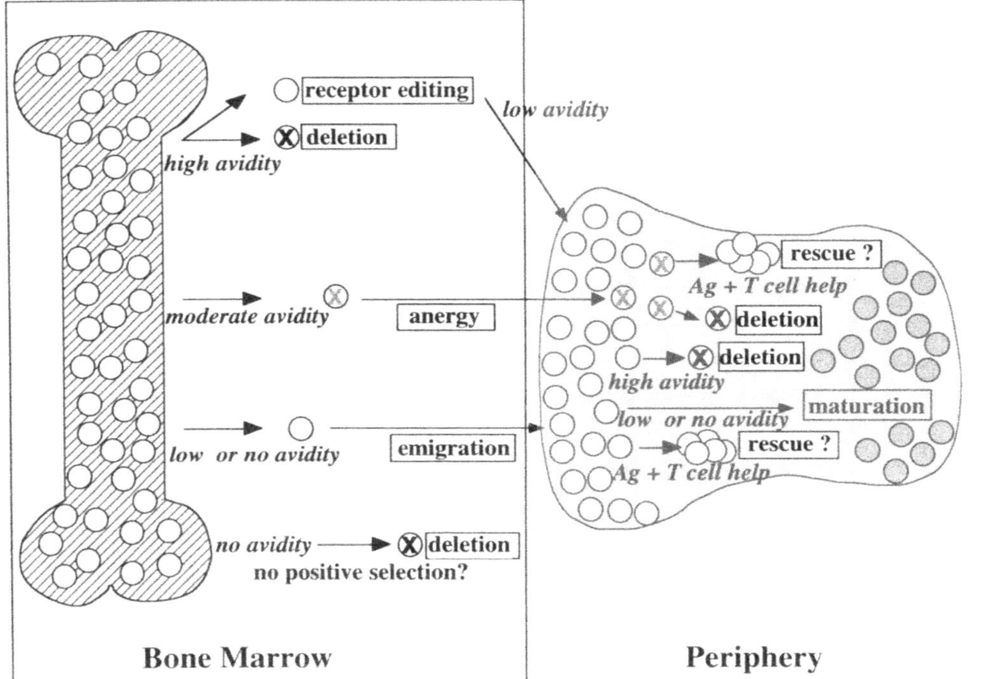

Figure 2. Potential outcomes of BCR-signaling in immature B-cells in the bone marrow and late immature/transitional B-cells in the periphery. In this schematic, the outcomes of engagement of the BCR on immature B-cells with antigens of different avidity are indicated. Immature B-cells in the bone marrow as well as late immature/transitional B-cells in the periphery are subject to negative selection. However, immature B-cells in the bone marrow may be protected from BCR-induced apoptosis by bone marrow-derived stromal cells, potentially allowing for receptor editing. Similarly, late immature/transitional B-cells in the periphery may be protected from negative selection by T-cell help. Anergized B-cells may undergo a delayed form of death, perhaps by follicular exclusion. In the absence of BCR-induced signal transduction, B-cells may undergo death by neglect. Open circles represent live, immature B-cells (both immature and late immature/transitional), gray circles represent live, mature B-cells, circles with a black X represent apoptotic cells, and circles with a gray X represent anergized B-cells.

another form of B-cell tolerance, clonal inactivation or anergy, can be induced in both nontransgenic *(135)*, as well as BCR transgenic mice *(11,15,136)*. Anergic B-cells express a unique surface phenotype in that they express reduced sIgM (presumably because of receptor modulation following chronic antigenic exposure), normal IgD levels *(11)* and are desensitized to further receptor-induced signal transduction *(137,138)*. The "choice" of an immature B-cells to undergo either clonal deletion or clonal anergy is mainly determined by the concentration and valency of the interacting antigen. In general, highly expressed membrane-bound antigen or antigens with multiple repeating epitopes that promote extensive BCR crosslinking induce deletion *(12,15,16,139)*, whereas anergy is induced by soluble, paucivalent antigens *(11,136)*. Importantly, even in cases where the identical anti-HEL Ig transgene was utilized, membrane bound HEL induced deletion whereas soluble HEL induced anergy *(11,16,136)*, indicating that receptor affinity plays a relatively minor role in this decision.

Although it appears that clonal deletion and clonal anergy represent distinct mechanisms of B-cell tolerance, the ultimate fate of the tolerized B-cell may be similar in both cases. Anergic cells exhibit a shortened half-life in the periphery *(140)*, suggesting that anergy may simply represent an intermediate stage in the functional elimination of weakly autoreactive B-cells. The shortened life span of anergic B-cells correlates with an inability to enter lymphoid follicles, although the mechanism responsible for the follicular exclusion of anergic B-cells remains controversial *(28,111,141)*. Upon binding antigen, anergic B-cells accumulate in the T-cell rich zone, the periarteriolar lymphoid sheath (PALS). Anergic B-cells have a limited life span in the PALS in which they can potentially receive T-cell help: addition of preactivated T_h cells prevents the induction of anergy and allows the HEL-specific B-cells to enter the follicle *(28)*. Anergized B-cells are unable to be rescued by naive T-cells, presumably because of their inability to upregulate costimulatory molecules *(141)*. In either case, autoreactive B-cells that have bound self-antigen are unable to enter the follicle. Follicular exclusion appears to result in the physical elimination of the anergized B-cells, thus preventing their subsequent entry into the long-lived B-cell pool.

9.3. Clonal Alteration or Receptor Editing

In addition to the tolerance mechanisms described above, a nondeletional mechanism termed receptor editing, has been recently described. During receptor editing, immature B-cells appear to escape clonal deletion by altering their BCRs so that they are no longer autoreactive. Molecular analysis of the surviving B-cells revealed that they had rearranged their endogenous light chains in an apparent attempt to alter their autoreactive specificity *(142,143)*, and that these endogenous light chains could effectively compete for heavy chain association *(144)*. Subsequent analysis with "knock-in" mice revealed that B-cells can rearrange both heavy *(145)* and light *(146)* chains in an attempt to avoid expressing an autoreactive antigen receptor and that receptor editing is antigen driven *(26,147)*.

It is not clear whether receptor editing can rescue large numbers of immature autoreactive B-cells from BCR-induced apoptosis. Such a possibility is not unwarranted since the ability of immature B-cells to undergo a reversible developmental arrest in the bone marrow prior to clonal deletion *(17)* would provide them with a "window of opportunity" in which receptor editing could take place. However, the universal role of receptor editing in the negative selection of normal, autoreactive B-cells has not been formally demonstrated. B-cells from nontransgenic mice do appear capable of undergoing receptor editing *(26)*, and it is possible that the bone marrow may provide them with a protective environment in which cell death can be delayed long enough for a new, functional, autoreactive BCR to be expressed. However, the high frequency of unrearranged κ and λ alleles in κ-expressing B-cells suggests that the potential rescue of autoreactive cells from autoantigen-induced negative selection is a relatively rare event *(148)*. During receptor editing, autoreactive BCRs are replaced with potentially functionally competent nonautoreactive specificity BCRs; B-cells without new productive rearrangements are thought not to survive *(149)*. These results implicitly suggest that a positive selection step may be occurring during B-cell development, and that a BCR-induced signal may be required for B-cell survival. Immature B-cells that are still autoreactive upon emerging from the receptor-edited pool would be subject to deletional (apoptotic) processes of negative selection.

10. Is B-Cell Negative Selection Necessary?

Activation of mature B-cells in response to protein antigens requires cognate T-cell help. As T-cells are generally rendered tolerant at much lower antigen concentrations than are B-cells *(136,150,151)*, negative selection of these B-cells might at first appear an unnecessary redundancy since autoreactive B-cells should not be activated in the absence of autoreactive T-cells. However, autoreactive B-cells specific for DNA or polysaccharides, molecules that are not readily recognized by T-cells, are often activated in the apparent absence of T-cell help. Moreover, proteins may exist that contain both "self" epitopes as well as epitopes shared by foreign proteins. Selective uptake of the protein by self-reactive B-cells by virtue of its BCR could lead to the presentation of foreign-peptide epitopes to T-cells, providing T-cell help to the autoreactive B-cell and leading to their activation *(152)*. Therefore, the ability of both T and B lymphocyte populations to be tolerized enables redundant controls to negatively regulate autoantibody production and prevent inappropriate activation of autoreactive B-cells.

10.1. Central vs Peripheral B-Cell Tolerance

Although central tolerance appears to be the most efficient way to eliminate newly emerging autoreactive B-cells, not all autoantigens are present in the bone marrow. Furthermore, autoreactive B-cells may be generated during the process of somatic hypermutation in germinal centers. Clearly, mechanisms of tolerance in the periphery must exist. Although mature, peripheral B-cells are generally thought to be relatively resistant to sIg-mediated deletion in vitro *(7,30,32,153)*, under conditions of extreme BCR-crosslinking, such cells do undergo apoptosis *(154,155)*. Moreover, in vivo, mature B-cells are deleted following exposure to anti-IgD *(156)* and mature B-cells from anti-H-2^k Ig-expressing transgenic mice appear to be deleted following exposure to antigen in the periphery *(157)*. Furthermore, peripheral B-cells exposed to antigen in the absence of T-cell help are capable of being anergized *(136)* and are follicularly excluded *(141)*, suggesting that multiple peripheral tolerance mechanisms may exist. The recent discovery of the transitional immature B-cell subset may extend the window of opportunity for immature autoreactive B-cells to be deleted in the periphery *(20,21)* (Fig. 2). Therefore, it is possible that all B-cells that have not yet entered the long-lived B-cell pool may be tolerance sensitive in the absence of T-cell help.

10.2. The Physiologic Relevance of Maintaining Central Tolerance

The important physiologic role in maintaining self-tolerance is underscored by the immunopathology resulting from natural or transgenic interruption of this process such as observed in the Fas-deficient MRL *lpr/lpr* strain *(158)* and Bcl-2 overexpressing transgenic mice *(112)*. However, in many cases, central deletion appears relatively intact. For instance, crossing anti-HEL transgenic mice onto the *lpr/lpr* background did not appreciably affect the clonal deletion of autoreactive B-cells in response to membrane bound HEL or induction of anergy of B-cells following interaction with soluble HEL in young mice *(119)*. Similarly, the ability to tolerize in the anti-H-2^k/H-2^k system was not adversely affected by a deficiency in Fas expression *(120)*. In both cases, however, tolerance to the designated autoantigen, as well as to endogenous autoantigens was compromised in a subset of older mice. This suggests that B-cell tolerance may break down with age in Fas-deficient mice, perhaps because of the accumulation of autoreactive T-cells capable of either breaking tolerance or reactivating tolerized peripheral B-cells. Similarly, Bcl-2 overexpressing transgenic mice appear to have a functional central deletion mechanism *(17,112)*, but develop an autoimmune syndrome relatively late in life, perhaps as a consequence of an inability to delete activated, autoreactive peripheral B-cells *(112)*. In contrast, it appears that the central deletion of anti-DNA expressing B-cells (particularly the antihomogeneous nuclear specific subtype) may be defective in Fas-deficient mice *(159,160)*. However, these conclusions were based on the ability to generate anti–DNA-specific hybridomas from peripheral B-cells of older mice, therefore, it is still possible that the observed accumulation of anti–DNA-specific B-cells in *lpr/lpr* mice was the result of a breakdown in peripheral tolerance.

Together, these data suggest that autoimmune syndromes generally result from a breakdown in peripheral tolerance. It is possible that defects in central tolerance may also exist, but that they are not observed in systems in which peripheral tolerance is intact. For instance, although high affinity BCRs for rheumatoid factor are centrally deleted or receptor-edited, low-to-moderate avidity receptors are commonly found in the periphery *(161,162)*. In the absence of a breakdown in peripheral T-cell tolerance or aberrant B-cell activation, peripheral B-cell tolerance appears sufficient to avert autoimmune reactions. Alternatively, aberrancies in central deletion may not be commonly observed, if such deficiencies are severely detrimental to the host and result in early lethality.

10.3. Is the Determination of Self vs Nonself Necessary for Negative Selection?

Using the perspective that the immune system is more concerned with the perception of danger, in the form of tissue destruction, than with the discrimination of self and nonself, an alternative hypothesis of tolerance induction has been proposed *(152)*. In this model, both B- and T-cells will die after receiving a primary signal through their antigen receptors unless a second signal is also received. In the case of B-cells, signal 2 must come from "experienced" T-cells and central deletion of immature B-cells would occur following antigen stimulation because of the absence of appropriate T-cell help in the bone marrow. However, several observed aspects of both B- and T-cell development are inconsistent with this model. For instance, receptor editing is not compatible with the "Danger" hypothesis since any engagement with immature B-cells should lead to deletion, not a change in BCR specificity. Similarly, under this scenario, positive selection cannot occur. Therefore, it is unlikely that the "Danger hypothesis" predicts B-cell negative selection better than the conventional self/nonself discrimination model. Furthermore, with either hypothesis, the exquisite sensitivity of immature B-cells to tolerization signals remains enigmatic and awaits further resolution.

Acknowledgments

The authors wish to thank all of the members of the Monroe laboratory, past and present, for the data and ideas utilized in the preparation of this manuscript. The authors also thank Dr. Michael S. Marks for critical review of the manuscript. This work was supported in part by grants AI23568 and AI32592 from the National Institutes of Health and from the Lucille Markey Trust.

References

1. Lederberg, J. (1959) Genes and antibodies: Do antigens bear instructions for antibody specificity or do they select cell lines that arise by mutation? *Science* **129,** 1649–1653.
2. Burnet, F.M. (1959) Clonal Selection Theory of Acquired Immunity. Vanderbilt University, Nashville, TN.
3. Metcalf, E. S. and Klinman, N. R. (1976) *In vitro* tolerance induction of neonatal murine B cells. *J. Exp. Med.* **143,** 1327–1340.
4. Metcalf, E. S. and Klinman, N. R. (1977) In vitro tolerance induction of bone marrow cells: a marker for B cell maturation. *J. Immunol.* **118,** 2111–2116.
5. Nossal, G. J. V. and Pike, B. L. (1975) Evidence for the clonal abortion theory of B-lymphocyte tolerance. *J. Exp. Med.* **141,** 904–917.
6. Pike, B. L., Kay, T. W., and Nossal., G. J. V. (1980) Relative sensitivity of fetal and newborn mice to induction of hapten-specific B cell tolerance. *J. Exp. Med.* **152,** 1407–1412.
7. Raff, M. C., Owen, J. J. T., Cooper, M. D., Lawton, A. D., Megson, M., and Gathings, W. E. (1975) Differences in susceptibility of mature and immature mouse B lymphocytes to anti-immunoglobulin-induced immunoglobulin suppression in vitro: possible implications for B cell tolerance to self. *J. Exp. Med.* **142,** 1052–1064.
8. Sidman, C. L. and Unanue, E. R. (1975) Receptor-mediated inactivation of early B lymphocytes. *Nature* **257,** 149–151.
9. Roth, P. E. and DeFranco, A. L. (1996) Receptor tails unlock developmental checkpoints for B lymphocytes. *Science* **272,** 1752–1754.
10. Rajewsky, K. (1996) Clonal selection and learning in the antibody system. *Nature* **381,** 751–758.
11. Goodnow, C. C., Crosbie, J., Adelstein, S., Lavoie, T. B., Smith-Gill, S. J., Brink, R. A., Pritchard-Briscoe, H., Wotherspoon, J. S., Loblay, K. Raphael, R. H., Trent, R. J. and Basten, A. (1988) Altered immunoglobulin expression and functional silencing of self-reactive B lymphocytes in transgenic mice. *Science* **334,** 676–682.
12. Nemazee, D. A. and Burki, K. (1989) Clonal deletion of B lymphocytes in a transgenic mouse bearing anti-MHC class I antibody genes. *Nature* **337,** 562–566.
13. Kincade, P. W. and Cooper, M. D. (1971) Development and distribution of immunoglobulin-containing cells in the chicken. An immunofluorescent analysis using purified antibodies to mu, gamma and light chains. *J. Immunol.* **106,** 371–382.
14. Waldschmidt, T. J. and Vitetta, E. S. (1985) The use of haptenated-immunoglobulin molecules to induce tolerance in B cells from neonatal mice. *J. Immunol.* **134,** 1436–1441.
15. Erikson, J., Radic, M. Z., Camper, S. A., Hardy, R. R., Carmack, C., and Weigert, M. (1991) Expression of anti-DNA immunoglobulin trangenes in non-autoimmune mice. *Nature* **349,** 331–334.
16. Hartley, S. S., Crosbie, J., Brink, R., Kantor, A. B., Basten, A., and Goodnow, C. C. (1991) Elimination from peripheral lymphoid tissues of self-reactive B lymphocytes recognizing membrane-bound antigens. *Nature* **353,** 765–769.
17. Hartley, S. B., Cooke, M. P., Fulcher, D. A., Harris, A. W., Cory, S., Basten, A., and Goodnow, C. C. (1993) Elimination of self-reactive B lymphocytes proceeds in two stages: arrested development and cell death. *Cell* **72,** 325–335.
18. Chang, T.-L., Capraro, G., Kleinman, R. E., and Abbas, A. K. (1991) Anergy in immature B lymphocytes. Differential responses to receptor-mediated stimulation and helper T lymphocytes. *J. Immunol.* **147,** 750–756.
19. Yellen, A. J., Glenn, W., Sukhatme, V. P., Cao, X., and Monroe, J. G. (1991) Signaling through surface IgM in tolerance- susceptible immature murine B lymphocytes. *J. Immunol.* **146,** 1446–1454.

20. Allman, D. M., Ferguson, S. E., and Cancro, M. P. (1992) Peripheral B cell maturation. I. Immature peripheral B cells in adults are heat-stable antigen^{hi} and exhibit unique signaling characteristics. *J. Immunol.* **149,** 2533–2540.
21. Allman, D. M., Ferguson, S. E., Lentz, V. M., and Cancro, M. P. (1993) Peripheral B cell maturation. II. Heat-stable antigen hi splenic B cells are an immature developmental intermediate in the production of long-lived marrow-derived B cells. *J. Immunol.* **151,** 4431–4444.
22. Carsetti, R., Kohler, M. P., and Lamers, M. C. (1995) Transitional B cells are the target of negative selection in the B cell compartment. *J. Exp. Med.* **181,** 2129–2140.
23. Mason, D. Y., Jones, M., and Goodnow, C. C. (1992) Development and follicular localization of tolerant B lymphocytes in lysozyme/anti-lysozyme IgM/IgD transgenic mice. *Int. Immunol.* **4,** 163–175.
24. Carsetti, R., Kohler, G., and Lamers, M. C. (1993) A role for immunoglobulin D: interference with tolerance induction. *Eur. J. Immunol.* **23,** 168–178.
25. Chen, C., Nagy, Z., Radic, M. Z., Hardy, R. R., Huszar, D., Camper, S. A., and Weigert, M. (1995) The site and stage of anti-DNA B-cell deletion. *Nature* **373,** 252–255.
26. Hertz, M. and Nemazee, D. (1997) BCR ligation induces receptor editing in IgM^+IgD^- bone marrow cells in vitro. *Immunity* **6,** 429–436.
27. Norvell, A. and Monroe, J. G. (1996) Acquisition of surface IgD fails to protect from tolerance-induction. Both surface IgM- and surface IgD-mediated signals induce apoptosis of immature murine B lymphocytes. *J. Immunol.* **156,** 1328–1332.
28. Fulcher, D. A., Lyons, A. B., Korn, S. L., Cook, M. C., Koleda, C., Parish, C., Groth, B. F. D. S., and Basten, A. (1996) The fate of self-reactive B cells depends primarily on the degree of antigen receptor engagement and availability of T cell help. *J. Exp. Med.* **183,** 2313–2328.
29. Smith, C. A., Williams, G. T., Kingston, R., Jenkinson, E. J., and Owen, J. J. T. (1989) Antibodies to CD3/T-cell receptor complex induce death by apoptosis in immature T cells in thymic cultures. *Nature* **337,** 181–184.
30. Norvell, A., L. Mandik and J. G. Monroe. (1995) Engagement of the antigen-receptor on immature murine B lymphocytes results in death by apoptosis. *J. Immunol.* **154,** 4404–4413.
31. Carman, J. A., Wechsler-Reya, R. J., and Monroe, J. G. (1996) Immature stage B cells enter but do not progress beyond the early G1 phase of the cell cycle in response to antigen receptor signaling. *J. Immunol.* **156,** 4562–4569.
32. Monroe, J. G. (1996) Tolerance sensitivity of immature stage B cells: can developmentally regulated B cell antigen receptor (BCR) signal transduction play a role? *J. Immunol.* **156,** 2657–2660.
33. Brink, R., Goodnow, C. C., Crosbie, J., Adams, E., Eris, J., Mason, D. Y., Hartley, S. B., and Basten, A. (1992) Immunoglobulin M and D antigen receptors are both capable of mediating B lymphocyte activation, deletion, or anergy after interaction with specific antigen. *J. Exp. Med.* **176,** 991–1005.
34. Nitschke, L., Kosco, M. H., Kohler, G., and Lamers, M. C. (1993) Immunoglobulin D-deficient mice can mount normal immune responses to thymus-independent and -dependent antigens. *Proc. Natl. Acad. Sci. USA* **90,** 1887–1891.
35. Roes, J. and Rajewsky, K. (1993) Immunoglobulin D (IgD)-deficient mice reveal an auxiliary receptor function for IgD in antigen-mediated recruitment of B cells. *J. Exp. Med.* **177,** 45–55.
36. Bretscher, P. A. and Cohn, M. (1968) Minimal model for the mechanism of antibody induction and paralysis by antigen. *Nature* **220,** 444–448.
37. Brines, R. D. and Klaus, G. G. B. (1992) Inhibition of lipopolysaccharide-induced activation of immature B cells by anti-μ and anti-δ antibodies and its modulation by interleukin-4. *Int. Immunol.* **4,** 765–771.
38. Wechsler, R. J. and Monroe., J. G. (1995) Immature B lymphocytes are deficient in expression of the *src*-family kinases $p59^{fyn}$ and $p55^{fgr}$. *J. Immunol.* **154,** 1919–1929.
39. Norvell, A., Birkeland, M. L., Carman, J., Sillman, A. L., Wechsler-Reya, R., and Monroe, J. G. (1996) Use of isolated immature-stage B cells to understand negative selection and tolerance induction at the molecular level. *Immunol. Res.* **15,** 191–207.
40. Sillman, A. L. and Monroe, J. G. (1994) Surface IgM-stimulated proliferation, inositol phospholipid hydrolysis, Ca^{2+} flux, and tyrosine phosphorylation are not altered in B cells from $p59^{fyn-/-}$ mice. *J. Leuk. Biol.* **56,** 812–816.
41. Takata, M., Homma, Y. and Kurosaki, T. (1995) Requirement of phospholipase C-γ2 activation in surface immunoglobulin M-induced B cell apoptosis. *J. Exp. Med.* **182,** 907–914.

42. Uckun, F. M., Waddick, K. G., Mahajan, S., Jun, X., Takata, M., Bolen, J., and Kurosaki, T. (1996) BTK as a mediator of radiation-induced apoptosis in DT-40 lymphoma B cells. *Science* **273,** 1096–1100.
43. Scheuermann, R. H., Racila, E., Tucker, T., Yefenof, E., Street, N. E., Vitetta, E. S., Picker, L. J., and Uhr., J. W. (1994) Lyn tyrosine kinase signals cell cycle arrest but not apoptosis in B-lineage lymphoma cells. *Proc. Natl. Acad. Sci. USA* **91,** 4048–4052.
44. Monroe, J. G., Seyfert, V. L., Owen, C. S., and Sykes, N. (1989) Isolation and characterization of a B lymphocyte mutant with altered signal transduction through its antigen receptor. *J. Exp. Med.* **169,** 1059–1070.
45. Fukuda, T., Kitamura, D., Taniuchi, I., Maekawa, Y., Benhamou, L. E., Sarthou, P., and Watanabe, T. (1995) Restoration of surface IgM-mediated apoptosis in an anti-IgM-resistant variant of WEHI-231 lymphoma cells by HS1, a protein-tyrosine kinase substrate. *Proc. Nat. Acad. Sci. USA* **92,** 7302–7306.
46. Taniuchi, I., Kitamura, D., Maekawa, Y., Fukuda, T., Kishi, H., and Watanabe, T. (1995) Antigen-receptor induced clonal expansion and deletion of lymphocytes are impaired in mice lacking HS1 protein, a substrate of the antigen-receptor-coupled tyrosine kinases. *EMBO J.* **14,** 3664–3678.
47. Leitges, M., Schmedt, C., Guinamard, R., Davoust, J., Schaal, S., Stabel, S., and Tarakhovsky, A. (1996) Immunodeficiency in protein kinase c β-deficient mice. *Science* **273,** 788–791.
48. Kerner, J. D., Appleby, M. W., Mohr, R. N., Chien, S., Rawlings, D. J., Maliszewski, C. R., Witte, O. N., and Perlmutter, R. M. (1995) Impaired expansion of mouse B cell progenitors lacking Btk. *Immunity* **3,** 301–312.
49. Khan, W. N., Alt, F. W., Gerstein, R. M., Malynn, B. A., Larsson, I., Rathbun, G., Davidson, L., Muller, S., Kantor, A. B., Herzenberg, L. A., Rosen, F.S., and Sideras, P. (1995) Defective B cell development and function in Btk-deficient mice. *Immunity* **3,** 283–299.
50. Yao, L., Kawakami, Y., and Kawakami, T. (1994) The pleckstrin homology domain of Bruton tyrosine kinase interacts with protein kinase C. *Proc. Natl. Acad. Sci. USA* **91,** 9175–9179.
51. Sidorenko, S. P., Law, C.-L., Klaus, S. J., Chandran, K. A., Takata, M., Kurosaki, T., and Clark, E. A. (1996) Protein kinase C mu (PKC μ) associates with the B cell antigen receptor complex and regulates lymphocyte signaling. *Immunity* **5,** 353–363.
52. Law, C. L., Chandran, K. A., Sidorenko, S. P., and Clark, E. A. (1996) Phospholipase C-gamma1 interacts with conserved phosphotyrosyl residues in the linker region of Syk and is a substrate for Syk. *Mol. Cell. Biol.* **16,** 1305–1315.
53. Sillman, A. L. and Monroe, J. G. (1995) Association of p72syk with the src homology-2 (SH2) domains of PLCγ1 in B lymphocytes. *J. Biol. Chem.* **270,** 11,806–11,811.
54. Gold, M. R., Crowley, M. T., Martin, G. A., McCormick, F., and DeFranco, A. L. (1993) Targets of B lymphocyte antigen receptor signal transduction include the p21ras GTPase-activating protein (GAP) and two GAP-associated proteins. *J. Immunol.* **150,** 377–386.
55. Gold, M. R., Chan, V. W. F., Turck, C. W., and DeFranco, A. L. (1992) Membrane Ig cross-linking regulates phosphatidylinositol 3 kinase in B lymphocytes. *J. Immunol.* **148,** 2012–2022.
56. Marshall, C. J. (1995) Specificity of receptor tyrosine kinase signaling: transient versus sustained extracellular signal-regulated kinase activation. *Cell* **80,** 179–185.
57. Xia, Z., Dickens, M., Raingeaud, J., Davis, R. J., and Greenberg, M. E. (1995) Opposing effects of ERK and JNK-p38 MAP kinases on apoptosis. *Science* **270,** 1326–1331.
58. Tsubata, T., Wu, J., and Honjo, T. (1993) B-cell apoptosis induced by antigen receptor crosslinking is blocked by a T-cell signal through CD40. *Nature* **364,** 645–648.
59. Sutherland, C. L., Heath, A. W., Pelech, S. L., Young, P. R., and Gold, M. E. (1996) Differential activation of the ERK, JNK, and p38 mitogen-activated protein kinases by CD40 and the B cell antigen receptor. *J. Immunol.* **157,** 3381–3390.
60. Franke, T. F., Kaplan, D. R., Cantley, L. C., and Toker, A. (1997) Direct regulation of the Akt proto-oncogene product by phosphatidylinositol-3,4-bisphosphate. *Science* **275,** 665–668.
61. Kauffmann-Zeh, A., Rodriguez-Viciana, P., Ulrich, E., Gilbert, C., Coffer, P., Downward, J., and Evan, G. (1997) Suppression of c-Myc-induced apoptosis by Ras signalling through PI(3)K and PKB. *Nature* **385,** 544–548.
62. Kennedy, S. G., Wagner, A. J., Conzen, S. D., Jordan, J., Bellacosa, A., Tsichlis, P. N., and Hay, N. (1997) The PI 3-kinase/Akt signaling pathway delivers an anti-apoptotic signal. *Genes Dev.* **11,** 701–713.
63. Teale, J. M. and Klinman, N. R. (1984) Membrane and metabolic requirements for tolerance induction of neonatal B cells. *J. Immunol.* **133,** 1811–1817.

64. Sonenshein, G. E. (1997) Down-modulation of c-myc expression induces apoptosis of B lymphocyte models of tolerance via clonal deletion. *J. Immunol.* **158,** 1994–1997.
65. Wu, M., Arsura, M., Bellas, R. E., FitzGerald, M. J., Lee, H., Schauer, S. L., Sherr, D. H. and Sonenshein, G. E. (1996) Inhibition of c-myc expression induces apoptosis of WEHI 231 murine B cells. *Mol. Cell. Biol.* **16,** 5015–5025.
66. Wu, M., Lee, H., Bellas, R. E., Schauer, S. L., Arsura, M., Katz, D., FitzGerald, M. J., Rothstein, T. L., Sherr, D. H., and Sonenshein, G. E. (1996) Inhibition of NF-kappaB/Rel induces apoptosis of murine B cells. *EMBO J.* **15,** 4682–4690.
67. Fearon, D. T. and Carter, R. H. (1995) The CD19/CR2/TAPA-1 complex of B lymphocytes: linking natural to acquired immunity. *Ann. Rev. Immunol.* **13,** 127–149.
68. Justement, L. B., Campbell, K. S., Chien, N., and Cambier, J. C. (1991) Regulation of B cell antigen receptor signal transduction and phosphorylation by CD45. *Science* **252,** 1839–1842.
69. Tedder, T. F., Tuscano, J., Sato, S., and Kehrl, J. H. (1997) CD22, a B lymphocyte-specific adhesion molecule that regulates antigen receptor signaling. *Ann. Rev. Immunol.* **15,** 481–504.
70. Carter, R. H. and Fearon., D. T. (1992) CD19, lowering the threshold for antigen receptor stimulation of B lymphocytes. *Science* **256,** 105–107.
71. Dempsey, P. W., Allison, M. E. D., Akkaraju, S., Goodnow, C. C., and Fearon, D. T. (1996) C3d of complement as a molecular adjuvant: bridging innate and acquired immunity. *Science* **271,** 348–350.
72. Engel, P., Zhou, L. J., Ord, D. C., Sato, S., Koller, B., and Tedder, T. F. (1995) Abnormal B lymphocyte development, activation, and differentiation in mice that lack or overexpress the CD19 signal transduction molecule. *Immunity* **3,** 39–50.
73. Rickert, R. C., Rajewsky, K., and Roes, J. (1995) Impairment of T-cell-dependent B-cell responses and B-1 cell development in CD19-deficient mice. *Nature* **376,** 352–355.
74. Sato, S., Steeber, D. A., and Tedder, T. F. (1995) The CD19 signal transduction molecule is a response regulator of B-lymphocyte differentiation. *Proc. Natl. Acad. Sci. USA* **92,** 11,558–11,562.
75. Doody, G. M., Justement, L. B., Delibrias, C. C., Matthews, R. J., Lin, J., Thomas, M. L., and Fearon, D. T. (1995) A role in B cell activation for CD22 and the protein tyrosine phosphatase SHP. *Science* **269,** 242–244.
76. Tuscano, J. M., Engel, P., Tedder, T. F., Agarwal, A., and Kehrl, J. H. (1996) Involvement of p72syk kinase, p53/56lyn kinase and phosphatidyl inositol-3 kinase in signal transduction via the human B lymphocyte antigen CD22. *Eur. J. Immunol.* **26,** 1246–1252.
77. Campbell, M. A. and Klinman, N. R. (1995) Phosphotyrosine-dependent association between CD22 and protein tyrosine phosphatase 1C. *Eur. J. Immunol.* **25,** 1573–1579.
78. Lankester, A. C., van Schijndel, G. M., and van Lier, R. A. (1995) Hematopoietic cell phosphatase is recruited to CD22 following B cell antigen receptor ligation. *J. Biol. Chem.* **270,** 20,305–20,308.
79. Law, C. L., Sidorenko, S. P., Chandran, K. A., Zhao, A., Shen, S. H., Fischer, E. H., and Clark, E. A. (1996) CD22 associates with protein tyrosine phosphatase 1C, Syk, and phospholipase C-γ1 upon B cell activation. *J. Exp. Med.* **183,** 547–560.
80. Shultz, L. D., Schweitzer, P. A., Rajan, T. V., Yi, T., Ihle, J. N., Matthews, R. J., Thomas, M. L., and Beier, D. R. (1993) Mutations at the murine motheaten locus are within the hematopoietic cell protein-tyrosine phosphatase (Hcph) gene. *Cell* **73,** 1445–1454.
81. Tsui, H. W., Siminovitch, K. A., de Souza, L., and Tsui, F. W. (1993) Motheaten and viable motheaten mice have mutations in the haematopoietic cell phosphatase gene. *Nat. Gen.* **4,** 124–129.
82. Pani, G., Kozlowski, M., Cambier, J. C., Mills, G. B., and Siminovitch, K. A. (1995) Identification of the tyrosine phosphatase PTP1C as a B cell antigen receptor-associated protein involved in the regulation of B cell signaling. *J. Exp. Med.* **181,** 2077–2084.
83. Cyster, J. G. and Goodnow, C. C. (1995) Protein tyrosine phosphatase 1C negatively regulates antigen receptor signaling in B lymphocytes and determines thresholds for negative selection. *Immunity* **2,** 13–24.
84. Erickson, L. D., Tygrett, L. T., Bhatia, S. K., Grabstein, K. H., and Waldschmidt, T. J. (1996) Differential expression of CD22 (Lyb8) on murine B cells. *Int. Immunol.* **8,** 1121–1129.
85. Nitschke, L., Carsetti, R., Ocker, B., Kohler, G., and Lamers, M. C. (1997) CD22 is a negative regulator of B-cell receptor signalling. *Curr. Biol.* **7,** 133–143.
86. O'Keefe, T. L., Williams, G. T., Davies, S. L., and Neuberger, M. S. (1996) Hyperresponsive B cells in CD22-deficient mice. *Science* **274,** 798–801.

87. Otipoby, K. L., Andersson, K. B., Draves, K. E., Klaus, S. J., Farr, A. G., Kerner, J. D., Perlmutter, R. M., Law, C. L., and Clark, E. A. (1996) CD22 regulates thymus-independent responses and the lifespan of B cells. *Nature* **384,** 634–637.
88. Sato, S., Miller, A. S., Inaoki, M., Bock, C. B., Jansen, P. J., Tang, M. L., and Tedder, T. F. (1996) CD22 is both a positive and negative regulator of B lymphocyte antigen receptor signal transduction: altered signaling in CD22-deficient mice. *Immunity* **5,** 551–562.
89. Kawauchi, K., Lazarus, A. H., Rapoport, M. J., Harwood, A., Cambier, J. C., and Delovitch, T. L. (1994) Tyrosine kinase and CD45 tyrosine phosphatase activity mediate p21ras activation in B cells stimulated through the antigen receptor. *J. Immunol.* **152,** 3306–3316.
90. Pao, L. I., Bedzyk, W. D., Persin, C., and Cambier, J. C. (1997) Molecular targets of CD45 in B cell antigen receptor signal transduction. *J. Immunol.* **158,** 1116–1124.
91. Pao, L. I. and Cambier, J. C. (1997) Syk, but not Lyn, recruitment to B cell antigen receptor and activation following stimulation of CD45- B cells. *J. Immunol.* **158,** 2663–2669.
92. Benatar, T., Carsetti, R., Furlonger, C., Kamalia, N., Mak, T., and Paige, C. J. (1996) Immunoglobulin-mediated signal transduction in B cells from CD45-deficient mice. *J. Exp. Med.* **183,** 329–334.
93. Blyth, K. F., Conroy, L. A., Howlett, S., Smith, A. J. H., May, J., Alexander, D. R., and Holmes, N. (1996) CD45-null transgenic mice reveal a positive regulatory role for CD45 in early thymocyte development, in the selection of $CD4^+CD8^+$ thymocytes, and in B cell maturation. *J. Exp. Med.* **183,** 1707–1718.
94. Kong, Y.-Y., Kishihara, K., Sumichika, H., Nakamura, T., Kaneko, M., and Nomoto, K. (1995) Differential requirements of CD45 for lymphocyte development and function. *Eur. J. Immunol.* **25,** 3431–3436.
95. Cyster, J. G., Healy, J. I., Kishihara, K., Mak, T. W., Thomas, M. L., and Goodnow, C. C. (1996) Regulation of B-lymphocyte negative and positive selection by tyrosine phosphatase CD45. *Nature* **381,** 325–328.
96. Hockenbery, D., Nunez, G., Milliman, C., Schreiber, R. D., and Korsmeyer, S. J. (1990) Bcl-2 is an inner mitochondrial membrane protein that blocks programmed cell death. *Nature* **348,** 334–336.
97. Oltvai, Z. N., Milliman, C. L., and Korsmeyer, S. J. (1993) Bcl-2 heterodimerizes in vivo with a conserved homolog, Bax, that accelerates programmed cell death. *Cell* **74,** 609–619.
98. Boise, L. H., Gonzalez-Garcia, M., Postema, C. E., Ding, L., Lindsten, T., Turka, L. A., Mao, X., Nunez, G., and Thompson, C. B. (1993) *bcl-x,* a bcl-2-related gene that functions as a dominant regulator of apoptotic cell death. *Cell* **74,** 597–608.
99. Yang, E., Zha, J., Jockel, J., Boise, L. H., Thompson, C. B., and Korsmeyer, S. J. (1995) Bad, a heterodimeric partner for Bcl-XL and Bcl-2, displaces Bax and promotes cell death. *Cell* **80,** 285–291.
100. Lin, E. Y., Orlofsky, A., Berger, M. S., and Prystowsky, M. B. (1993) Characterization of A1, a novel hemopoietic-specific early-response gene with sequence similarity to bcl-2. *J. Immunol.* **151,** (1979–1988.
101. Oltvai, Z. N. and Korsmeyer, S. J. (1994) Checkpoints of dueling dimers foil death wishes. *Cell* **79,** 189–191.
102. Li, Y.-S., Hayakawa, K., and Hardy, R. R. (1993) The regulated expression of B lineage associated genes during B cell differentiation in bone marrow and fetal liver. *J. Exp. Med.* **178,** 951–960.
103. Merino, R., Ding, L., Veis, D. J., Korsmeyer, S. J., and Nunez, G. (1994) Developmental regulation of the Bcl-2 protein and susceptiblity to cell death in B lymphocytes. *EMBO J.* **13,** 683–691.
104. Grillot, D. A. M., Merino, R., Pena, J. C., Fanslow, W. C., Finkelman, F. D., Thompson, C. B., and Nunez, G. (1996) bcl-x exhibits regulated expression during B cell development and activation and modulates lymphocyte survival in transgenic mice. *J. Exp. Med.* **183,** 381–391.
105. Choi, M. S., Holmann, M., Atkins, C. J., and Klaus, G. G. (1996) Expression of bcl-x during mouse B cell differentiation and following activation by various stimuli. *Eur. J. Immunol.* **26,** 676–682.
106. Nakayama, K., Nakayama, K., Negishi, I., Kuida, K., Shinkai, Y., Louie, M. C., Fields, L. E., Lucas, P. J., Stewart, V., Alt, F. W., and Loh, D. Y. (1993) Disappearance of the lymphoid system in Bcl-2 homozygous mutant chimeric mice. *Science* **261,** 1584–1588.

107. Veis, D. J., Sorenson, C. M., Shutter, J. R., and Korsmeyer, S. J. (1993) Bcl-2-deficient mice demonstrate fulminant lymphoid apoptosis, polycystic kidneys, and hypopigmented hair. *Cell* **75,** 229–240.
108. Motoyama, N., Wang, F., Roth, K. A., Sawa, H., Nakayama, K., Nakayama, K., Negishi, I., Senju, S., Zhang, Q., Fujii, S., and Loh, D. Y. (1995) Massive cell death of immature hematopoietic cells and neurons in Bcl-x-deficient mice. *Science* **267,** 1506–1510.
109. Knudson, C. M., Tung, K. S., Tourtellotte, W. G., Brown, G. A., and Korsmeyer, S. J. (1995) Bax-deficient mice with lymphoid hyperplasia and male germ cell death. *Science* **270,** 96–99.
110. Nisitani, S., Tsubata, T., Murakami, M., Okamoto, M., and Honjo, T. (1993) The bcl-2 gene product inhibits clonal deletion of self-reactive B lymphocytes in the periphery but not in the bone marrow. *J. Exp. Med.* **178,** 1247–1254.
111. Cyster, J. G., Hartley, S. B., and Goodnow, C. C. (1994) Competition for follicular niches excludes self-reactive cells from the recirculating B cell repertoire. *Nature* **371,** 389–395.
112. Strasser, A., Whittingham, S., Vaux, D. L., Bath, M. L., Adams, J. M., Cory, S., and Harris, A. W. (1991) Enforced BCL2 expression in B-lymphoid cells prolongs antibody responses and elicits autoimmune disease. *Proc. Natl. Acad. Sci. USA* **88,** 8661–8665.
113. Smith, C. A., Farrah, T., and Goodwin, R. G. (1994) The TNF receptor superfamily of cellular and viral proteins: activation, costimulation, and death. *Cell* **76,** 959–962.
114. Itoh, N., Yonehara, S., Ishii, A., Yonehara, M., Mizushima, S., Sameshima, M., Hase, A., Seto, Y., and Nagata, S. (1991) The polypeptide encoded by the cDNA for human cell surface antigen Fas can mediate apoptosis. *Cell* **66,** 233–243.
115. Suda, T., Takahashi, T., Golstein, P., and Nagata, S. (1993) Molecular cloning and expression of the Fas ligand, a novel member of the tumor necrosis factor family. *Cell* **75,** 1169–1178.
116. Singer, G. G. and Abbas, A. K. (1994) The fas antigen is involved in peripheral but not thymic deletion of T lymphocytes in T cell receptor transgenic mice. *Immunity* **1,** 365–371.
117. Mandik, L., Nguyen, K.-A. T., and Erikson, J. (1995) Fas receptor expression on B-lineage cells. *Eur. J. Immunol.* **25,** 3148–3154.
118. Adachi, M., Suematsu, S., Suda, T., Watanabe, D., Fukuyama, H., Ogasawara, J., Tanaka, T., Yoshida, N., and Nagata, S. (1996) Enhanced and accelerated lymphoproliferation in Fas-null mice. *Proc. Nat. Acad. Sci. USA* **93,** 2131–2136.
119. Rathmell, J. C. and Goodnow, C. C. (1994) Effects of the lpr mutation on elimination and inactivation of self-reactive B cells. *J. Immunol.* **153,** 2831–2842.
120. Rubio, C. F., Kench, J., Russell, D. M., Yawger, R., and Nemazee, D. (1996) Analysis of central B cell tolerance in autoimmune-prone MRL/lpr mice bearing autoantibody transgenes. *J. Immunol.* **157,** 65–71.
121. Rothstein, T. L., Wang, J. K. M., Panka, D. J., Foote, L. C., Wang, Z., Stanger, B., Cul, H., Ju, S.-T., and Marshak-Rothstein, A. (1995) Protection against Fas-dependent Th1-mediated apoptosis by antigen receptor engagement in B cells. *Nature* **374,** 163–165.
122. Rathmell, J. C., Cooke, M. P., Ho, W. Y., Grein, J., Townsend, S. E., Davis, M. M., and Goodnow, C. C. (1995) CD95 (Fas)-dependent elimination of self-reactive B cells upon interaction with $CD4^+$ T cells. *Nature* **376,** 181–184.
123. Clark, E. A. and Ledbetter, J. A. (1994) How B and T cells talk to each other. *Nature* 367, 425–428.
124. Choi, M. S., Boise, L. H., Gottschalk, A. R., Quintans, J., Thompson, C. B., and Klaus, G. G. (1995) The role of bcl-XL in CD40-mediated rescue from anti-mu-induced apoptosis in WEHI-231 B lymphoma cells. *Eur. J. Immunol.* **25,** 1352–1357.
125. Schauer, S. L., Wang, Z., Sonenshein, G. E., and Rothstein, T. L. (1996) Maintenance of nuclear factor-kappa B/Rel and c-myc expression during CD40 ligand rescue of WEHI 231 early B cells from receptor-mediated apoptosis through modulation of I kappa B proteins. *J. Immunol.* **157,** 81–86.
126. Wang, Z., Karras, J. G., Howard, R. G., and Rothstein, T. L. (1995) Induction of bcl-x by CD40 engagement rescues sIg-induced apoptosis in murine B cells. *J. Immunol.* **155,** 3722–3725.
127. Kawabe, T., Naka, T., Yoshida, K., Tanaka, T., Fujiwara, H., Suematsu, S., Yoshida, N., Kishimoto, T., and Kikutani, H. (1994) The immune responses in CD40-deficient mice: impaired immunoglobulin class switching and germinal center formation. *Immunity* **1,** 167–178.
128. Opstelten, D. and Osmond, D. G. (1983) Pre-B cells in mouse bone marrow: immunofluorescence stathmokinetic studies of the proliferation of cytoplasmic mu-chain-bearing cells in normal mice. *J. Immunol.* **131,** 2635–2640.

129. Osmond, D. G. (1986) Population dynamics of bone marrow B lymphocytes. *Immunol. Rev.* **93,** 103–124.
130. Ellis, R. E., Yuan, J. Y., and Horvitz, H. R. (1991) Mechanisms and functions of cell death. *Ann. Rev. Cell Biol.* **7,** 663–698.
131. Lu, L. and Osmond, D. G. (1997) Apoptosis during B lymphopoiesis in mouse bone marrow. *J. Immunol.* **158,** 5136–5145.
132. Gu, H., Tarlinton, D., Muller, W., Rajewsky, K., and Forster, I. (1991) Most peripheral B cells in mice are ligand selected. *J. Exp. Med.* **173,** 1357–1371.
133. Torres, R. M., Flaswinkel, H., Reth, M., and Rajewsky, K. (1996) Aberrant B cell development and immune response in mice with a compromised BCR complex. *Science* **272,** 1804–1808.
134. Turner, M., Mee, P. J., Costello, P. S., Williams, O., Price, A. A., Duddy, L. P., Furlong, M. T., Geahlen, R. L., and Tybulewicz, V. L. (1995) Perinatal lethality and blocked B-cell development in mice lacking the tyrosine kinase Syk. *Nature* **378,** 298–302.
135. Pike, B. L., Boyd, A. W., and Nossal, G. J. V. (1982) Clonal anergy: The universally anergic B lymphocyte. *Proc. Natl. Acad. Sci. USA* **79,** 2013–2017.
136. Goodnow, C. C., Crosbie, J., Jorgensen, H., Brink, R. A., and Basten, A. (1989) Induction of self-tolerance in mature peripheral B lymphocytes. *Nature* **342,** 385–391.
137. Cooke, M. P., Heath, A. W., Shokat, K. M., Zeng, Y., Finkelman, F. D., Linsley, P. S., Howard, M., and Goodnow, C. C. (1994) Immunoglobulin signal transduction guides the specificity of B cell-T cell interactions and is blocked in tolerant self-reactive B cells. *J. Exp. Med.* **179,** 425–438.
138. Healy, J. I., Dolmetsch, R. E., Timmerman, L. A., Cyster, J. G., Thomas, M. L., Crabtree, G. R., Lewis, R. S., and Goodnow, C. C. (1997) Different nuclear signals are activated by the B cell receptor during positive versus negative signaling. *Immunity* **6,** 419–428.
139. Murakami, M., Tsubata, T., Okamoto, M., Shimizu, A., Kumagai, S., Imura, H., and Honjo, T. (1992) Antigen-induced apoptotic death of Ly-1 B cells responsible for autoimmune disease in transgenic mice. *Nature* **357,** 77–80.
140. Fulcher, D. A. and Basten, A. (1994) Reduced life span of anergic self-reactive B cells in a double-transgenic model. *J. Exp. Med.* **179,** 125–134.
141. Cyster, J. G. and Goodnow, C. C. (1995) Antigen-induced exclusion from follicles and anergy are separate and complementary processes that influence peripheral B cell fate. *Immunity* **3,** 691–701.
142. Radic, M. Z., Erikson, J., Litwin, S., and Weigert, M. (1993) B lymphocytes may escape tolerance by revising their antigen receptors. *J. Exp. Med.* **177,** 1165–1173.
143. Tiegs, S. L., Russell, D. M., and Nemazee, D. (1993) Receptor editing in self-reactive bone marrow B cells. *J. Exp. Med.* **177,** 1009–1020.
144. Gay, D., Saunders, T., Camper, S., and Weigert, M. (1993) Receptor editing: an approach by autoreactive B cells to escape tolerance. *J. Exp. Med.* **177,** 999–1008.
145. Chen, C., Nagy, Z., Prak, E. L., and Weigert, M. (1995) Immunoglobulin heavy chain gene replacement: a mechanism of receptor editing. *Immunity* **3,** 747–755.
146. Prak, E. L. and Weigert, M. (1995) Light chain replacement: a new model for antibody gene rearrangement. *J. Exp. Med.* **182,** 541–548.
147. Chen, C., Prak, E. L., and Weigert, M. (1997) Editing disease-associated autoantibodies. *Immunity* **6,** 97–105.
148. Coleclough, C. (1992) Is expression of the B-cell antigen receptor repertoire chaotic? *Res.Immunol.* **143,** 824–830.
149. Andersson, J., F. Melchers and Rolink, A. (1995) Stimulation by T cell independent antigens can relieve the arrest of differentiation of immature auto-reactive B cells in the bone marrow. *Scand. J. Immunol.***42,** 21–33.
150. Adelstein, S., Pritchard-Briscoe, H., Anderson, T. A., Crosbie, J., Gammon, G., Loblay, R. H., Basten, A., and Goodnow, C. C. (1991) Induction of self-tolerance in T cells but not B cells of transgenic mice expressing little self antigen. *Science* **251,** 1223–1225.
151. Chiller, J. M., Habicht, G. S., and Weigle, W. O. (1971) Kinetic differences in unresponsiveness of thymus and bone marrow cells. *Science* **171,** 813–815.
152. Matzinger, P. (1994) Tolerance, danger and the extended family. *Annu. Rev. Immunol.* **12,** 991–1045.
153. Yellen-Shaw, A. and Monroe, J. G. (1992) Differential responsiveness of immature- and mature-stage murine B cells to anti-IgM reflects both FcR-dependent and -independent mechanisms. *Cell. Immunol.* **145,** 339–350.

154. Parry, S. L., Hasbold, J., Holman, M., and Klaus, G. G. (1994) Hypercross-linking surface IgM or IgD receptors on mature B cells induces apoptosis that is reversed by costimulation with IL-4 and anti-CD40. *J. Immunol.* **152,** 2821–2829.
155. Parry, S. L., Holman, M. J., Hasbold, J., and Klaus, G. G. B. (1994) Plastic-immobilized anti-m or anti-d antibodies induce apoptosis in mature murine B lymphocytes. *Eur. J. Immunol.* **24,** 974–979.
156. Finkelman, F. D., Holmes, J. M., Dukhanina, O. I., and Morris, S. C. (1995) Cross-linking of membrane IgD, in the absence of T cell help, kills mature B cells in vivo. *J. Exp. Med.* **181,** 515–525.
157. Russell, D. M., Dembic, Z., Morahan, G.J. F., Miller, A. P., Burki, K., and Nemazee, D. (1991) Peripheral deletion of self-reactive B cells. *Nature* **354,** 308–311.
158. Watanabe-Fukunaga, R., C. I. Brannan, N. G. Copeland, J. N. A. Jenkins and S. Nagata. (1992) Lymphoproliferative disorder in mice explained by defects in Fas antigen that mediated apoptosis. *Nature* **356,** 314–317.
159. Roark, J. H., Kuntz, C. L., Nguyen, K.-A., Caton, A. J., and Erikson, J. (1995) Breakdown of B cell tolerance in a mouse model of systemic lupus erythematosus. *J. Exp. Med.* **181,** 1157–1167.
160. Roark, J. H., Kuntz, C. L., Nguyen, K. A., Mandik, L., Cattermole, M., and Erikson, J. (1995) B cell selection and allelic exclusion of an anti-DNA Ig transgene in MRL-lpr/lpr mice. *J. Immunol.* **154,** 4444–4455.
161. Wang, H. and Shlomchik, M. J. (1997) High affinity rheumatoid factor transgenic B cells are eliminated in normal mice. *J. Immunol.* **159,** 1125–1134.
162. Hannum, L. G., Ni, D., Haberman, A. M., Weigert, M. G., and Shlomchik, M. J. (1996) A disease-related rheumatoid factor autoantibody is not tolerized in a normal mouse: implications for the origins of autoantibodies in autoimmune disease. *J. Exp. Med.* **184,** 1269–1278.

Part VI

Selection Processes Operating During T-Lymphocyte Development

Chapter 22

How Essential is the Pre-T-Cell Receptor?

Jan Buer and Harald von Boehmer

1. Introduction

The immune system has the capacity to distinguish and respond specifically to a large variety of antigens. This function is performed mostly by the lymphocytes that form two major cell lineages: the B-cells and T-cells. Cells of the two lymphoid lineages express distinct, but related cell-surface antigen receptors, and thereby recognize different types of antigens. Although the diverse immunoglobulin (Ig) receptors on different B lymphocytes generally can bind to a large variety of different substances, the T-cell receptor (TCR) for antigen is built in such a way that it binds preferentially to major histocompatibility complex (MHC) encoded molecules that present various peptides, which are degradation products of either cell exogenous or cell endogenous proteins. TCR-peptide–MHC recognition regulates immune responses including graft and tumor rejection, antiviral cytolysis, and the recruitment and control of other immune cells such as antibody-producing B-cells. Lymphocyte antigen receptors are composed of two variable glycoprotein subunits: the Ig heavy (IgH) and light chains (IgL) on B-cells and the TCRα and β, or γ and δ chains on T-cells. The genes coding for Ig and TCR chains are formed through somatic rearrangement of V, D, and J gene segments *(1,2)*. During V-D-J recombination, coding gene segments are generally subjected to varying degrees of base deletion, addition, or both *(3)*. As a consequence, V-D-J joining could result either in productive rearrangements that maintain an "open reading frame" throughout the gene or in "out-of-frame," nonproductive rearrangements. Rearrangement of both TCR and Ig genes requires the expression of recombination activating genes (RAG1 and RAG2) *(4,5)*. Given its diploid nature, a lymphocyte could theoretically express up to four distinct combinations of antigen receptor chains on its surface. However, each B-cell has only one antibody receptor specificity, a phenomenon referred to as allelic exclusion. In thymocytes developing along the TCRαβ lineage, the situation is different; although virtually all T lymphocytes of the αβ lineage express only one particular TCRβ chain, a significant proportion of T-cells can express two different α chains at the cell surface *(6,7)*.

From: *Molecular Biology of B-Cell and T-Cell Development*
Edited by: J. G. Monroe and E. V. Rothenberg © Humana Press Inc., Totowa, NJ

The diverse lineages of the hematopoietic system including both B and T lymphocytes are derived from a single progenitor, the pluripotent bone marrow stem cell. Unlike B-cells, T-cells do not differentiate in the bone marrow; rather, they are derived from bone marrow progenitors that mature within the thymus. Although the thymus is the predominant site of maturation of T lymphocytes found in the peripheral lymphoid tissues, some subsets of T-cells, especially those present in gut-epithelia, mature outside the thymus *(8)*. Understanding how functionally different lineages of T-cells develop from multipotential hematopoietic stem cells is a great challenge. The generation of transgenic and gene-deficient knockout mice has greatly contributed to our present views on T-cell development. Thymocyte development depends on receptor-mediated signals that confer survival as well as differentiation. In the absence of these signals, developing T-cells die by apoptosis. Several checkpoints have been identified at which developing T-cells have to make a particular type of receptor in order to proceed to the next developmental stage. One such checkpoint for the development of αβ T-cells depends on the binding of the T-cell receptor to thymic MHC molecules, which can rescue immature αβ T-cells from programmed cell death *(9)*. At this stage, TCRα expression begins, and TCRαβ-mediated recognition of peptide-MHC ligands expressed on thymic stromal cells selects some double positive (DP, $CD4^+8^+$) cells to mature into $CD4^+8^-$ or $CD4^-8^+$ single positive cells. Another important checkpoint occurs earlier in development and ensures that only thymocytes with a functional TCRβ gene rearrangement will survive, and continue to mature from the double negative (DN, $CD4^-8^-$) to the double positive stage. The transition of thymocytes from a population of cells undergoing TCRβ chain rearrangement, to a population enriched in cells with productively rearranged TCRβ chain genes, is known as β-selection. This developmental event is regulated by the pre-TCR complex consisting of a conventional TCRβ chain disulfide-linked to a novel transmembrane protein termed pre-TCRα (pTα) in noncovalent association with components of the CD3 complex *(10)*. The cloning and gene-targeting of the pre-TCRα gene in mice demonstrated the crucial role of the pTα in early T-cell development *(11,12)*.

This chapter summarizes our current understanding of the pre-TCR in early thymocyte development. Pre-TCR independent pathways from the double negative to the double positive stage will be discussed further. Finally, recent data indicating that signaling from the pre-TCR inhibits further V-D-J recombination and establishes allelic exclusion at the TCRβ locus will be examined.

2. Early T-Cell Development

Throughout life, precursors of T lymphocytes leave the bone marrow, enter the blood stream, and seed the thymus. In the thymus, the immature T-cells proliferate and differentiate, passing through a series of discrete phenotypic stages that can be identified by distinct patterns of expression of various cell-surface molecules. The programmed series of events that lead to the generation of a mature T-cell population with a diverse TCR repertoire may be divided into an early phase, in which the development of thymocytes proceeds in the absence of a mature TCR, and a late phase, in which further maturation of developing thymocytes critically depends on the cell-surface expression of a functional αβ TCR. Precursor cells entering the thymus carry their TCR loci in germline configuration and may develop along the γδ or αβ lineages. These thymic lymphoid progenitors express high levels of CD44, CD117 (c-kit), low levels of Thy-1, CD4 and heat-stable antigen (HSA), and are not yet committed exclusively to the T-cell lineage *(13,14)*. Following adoptive transfer they can give rise not only to γδ and αβ T-cells, but also to B-cells *(15)*, natural killer (NK) cells *(15,16)*, and dendritic cells *(17)*. In the absence of single cell assays, it remains to be established whether or not these precursors are really pluripotent *(18)*. During the initial step of maturation, these $CD4^{low}$ precursors upregulate Thy1 and HSA and lose CD4 to become triple negative (TN) cells ($CD4^-8^-3^-$).

Early TN cells express CD44, do not yet express the low affinity chain of the IL-2 receptor (CD25), and retain the ability to home to the thymus ($CD44^+25^-c\text{-}kit^+$). Intermediate TN cells express higher levels of HSA and upregulate CD25. They have lost expression of CD44 and downregulate c-kit ($CD44^-25^+c\text{-}kit^-$/low). Late triple negative cells are $CD44^-25^-$ and can progress to the $CD4^+8^+$ stage via intermediates which express either CD8 or CD4 in the absence of mature αβ TCR. These immature $CD4^+8^-$ or $CD4^-8^+$ cells are probably the result of variations in the order in which CD4 and CD8 genes are activated in individual thymocytes. Such cells differentiate rapidly both in vivo and in vitro into DP cells.

Rearrangement of TCRβ,γ and δ chain genes begins at the $CD44^{low/-}25^+$ TN stage and generally precedes rearrangements at the TCRα locus. Developmental control points appear to ensure that T-cells do not complete their intrathymic differentiation program in the absence of productive TCR gene rearrangements, and in the case of expression of the TCRαβ, do not mature with receptors displaying inappropriate specificities. If the γ and δ genes are rearranged productively, the cells express the TCRγδ receptor at the surface and subsequently follow the γδ lineage. If the γδ genes are not rearranged productively, then the cells can go on and attempt to enter the αβ lineage *(19–21)*. Although successful rearrangement of either β or γδ TCR genes may influence the lineage decision, the mechanisms by which thymocytes choose between the αβ and γδ lineage remain unknown. It appears that the decision to become a γδ T-cell is not strictly determined by the type of receptor that is expressed, but rather by the timing of receptor expression *(22)*. More recently, Notch, originally identified in the fruit fly *Drosophila*, has been suggested to act together with the newly formed TCR to direct differentiation along the αβ lineage *(23)*.

Cells that enter the αβ lineage express the TCRβ chain that covalently binds to the pTα chain *(11,24)* and form the pre-TCR that rescues from programmed cell death $CD44^{low/-}25^+$ TN cells that have succeeded in TCRβ rearrangement. Based on a recent study, the $CD44^{low/-}25^+$ TN population can be sorted into two subsets representing small cells not yet TCRβ-selected (denoted E for "expected size") and large cells (denoted L for "large size") that contain TCRβ selected cells *(25)*. Cells that have passed β-selection differ from the preceding cells by several criteria, including hyperphosphorylation of the retinoblastoma protein (Rb), increased expression of cyclins A and B, increased cyclin-dependant protein kinase activity (Cdk2 and Cdc2), downregulation of p27 (a Cdk inhibitor), and progression through DNA synthesis. Consistent with these changes being attributable to productive TCRβ chain rearrangement the identified β-selected subset is not detected in mutant mice that cannot assemble a functional pre-TCR. These findings clearly demonstrate that productive TCRβ rearrangement is tightly associated with the induction of massive cellular proliferation. The selected cells assume the $CD4^-8^-44^-25^-$ phenotype *(14)* and eventually become $CD4^+8^+$ cells that bear the αβ TCR on the cell surface; expression of the pTα is terminated at this point *(12,26)*. Cells that fail β-selection, because both alleles are rearranged in a nonproductive way, remain quiescent, and eventually die, unless they have the potential to develop into γδ lineage cells *(27)*. In $pT\alpha^{-/-}$ mice, the increase in the absolute number of γδ cells suggests that the pre-TCR terminates γδ lineage commitment and initiates development along the αβ pathway *(26)*.

Although the presence of a productively rearranged TCRβ chain gene prevents further rearrangement *(28)*, both alleles of the α chain gene rearrange until a productive TCRαβ is formed *(29–32)*. The $CD4^{+}8^{+}$ expressing cells are programmed to die unless the αβ TCR binds to thymic MHC molecules, and cells are rescued from cell death once more and eventually become mature T-cells that leave the thymus *(29,32a)*. Thymocytes whose TCRs recognize MHC class I expressed on thymic epithelial cells as a rule develop as CD8 cells, whereas thymocytes whose antigen receptor recognize MHC Class II proteins develop as CD4 cells *(33)*. Although it is clear that MHC recognition influences the choice between the CD4 and CD8 lineage, the mechanistic basis for this influence is not known; again Notch has been implicated as a participant in the CD4 versus CD8 lineage decision *(34)*.

3. Molecular Characteristics of the Pre-T-Cell Receptor

The pre-T-cell receptor contains the TCRβ chain disulfide linked to a 33kDa transmembrane glycoprotein termed pTα, as well as components of CD3 *(10,11,24)*. Although CD3ε, CD3δ, CD3γ and CD3ζ have been found to be associated with the pre-TCR complex expressed in pre–T-cell lines, in early thymocytes CD3ζ and CD3δ have been more difficult to detect and may therefore be only loosely or not all associated with the pre-TCR *(35)*. Under physiological conditions, the pre-TCR complex is likely to signal via its CD3 subunits *(36–40)*.

Analysis of the murine and human pTα cDNA shows the existence of conserved and nonconserved regions in the protein that may be related to its function. The deduced amino acid sequence has revealed a type I transmembrane protein that belongs to the Ig superfamily. Alignment of the extracellular regions of the mouse and human pTα shows that they are identical in length with 77% homology at the amino acid level *(41)*. This would be consistent with the possibility that a conserved extracellular ligand is needed for pre-TCR function, as this extent of conservation is not required for pairing with TCRβ. As for the IgH chain/surrogate light chain complex (VpreB) on immature B-cells, little is known about the nature of the putative ligand(s) for the pre-TCR. CD81 has been proposed as a potential ligand for the pre-TCR as interactions between immature thymocytes and stromal cells expressing CD81 are required, and may be sufficient to induce early events associated with T-cell development *(42)*. However, CD81 knockout mice appear to undergo normal thymic development and produce normal numbers of mature T-cells *(43)*. In addition, the association of signal transducing CD3 molecules with the pre-TCR heterodimer may be sufficient for signaling in the absence of a putative ligand. The pTα-TCRβ heterodimer has an asymmetrical structure, because the TCRβ has two, and the pTα only one extracellular Ig-like domain *(11,26)*. This could suggest that an additional small protein may be part of the pre-TCR much like the VpreB is part of the pre-BCR. Such a protein might be essential for proper assembly, glycosylation, and transport of the pre-TCR complex to the cell surface as cotransfection of TCRβ and pTα into a mature T-cell line, which lacks TCRα protein, does not lead to efficient cell-surface expression of the pre-TCR complex *(11)*.

The cytoplasmic tail of the murine pTα chain is about 31 residues long and contains two potential serine and threonine phosphorylation sites, as well as SH3 binding sites. In contrast, the 127 amino acids that are predicted to compose the human cytoplasmic region do not show any significant identity with the 31 residues found in the mouse cytoplasmic tail. The lack of homology between the cytoplasmic tail of mouse and human pTα and recent functional data obtained in pTα-deficient mice, which express a tailless pTα transgene under the control of the proximal lck promoter *(44)*, suggest that the cytoplasmic portion of the pTα is not required for signal transduction. Both the pre-TCR and the αβ TCR associate with signal transducing CD3 molecules and may signal through activation of src kinases like $p56^{lck}$ and fyn *(24,45,46)*.

Lck was the first protein tyrosine kinase clearly implicated in signaling through the pre-TCR. The targeted disruption of the lck gene or the overexpression of a catalytically inactive lck transgene results in a substantial reduction of double positive cells *(47,48)*. The ability of TCRβ transgenes, but not CD3 crosslinking to restore normal double positive thymocyte development in $RAG1^{-/-}$ or $RAG2^{-/-}$ mice, requires Lck activity *(49)* (A. Weiss, et al., unpublished data). Overexpression of a constitutively active lck transgene promotes the development of double positive cells in the absence of TCRβ expression *(49)*, suggesting that Lck functions downstream of the pre-TCR complex. In addition, Lck signals regulate allelic exclusion of the TCRβ locus in double negative cells *(45)*. However, T-cell development is only partially compromised in Lck-deficient mice, suggesting that other kinases may also transduce TCR and pre-TCR signals. Recent data support the notion that also fyn may promote the transition from double negative to double positive cells under conditions in which lck is limiting or absent *(46,50)*. Activation of lck or fyn is likely to involve phosphorylation of the immune receptor tyrosine-based activation motifs (ITAM) of CD3 proteins and recruitment of ZAP-70, syk, or both into the phosphorylated ITAMs of the pre-TCR *(40,51)*. Further experiments are necessary to determine how pre-TCR signals are directed via these kinases. In addition, p21 (Ras) protein and the MAP kinase cascade have been implicated in the pre-TCR signal transduction pathway *(52,53)*.

3.1. Expression of the pTα Gene

Expression of the pTα gene is developmentally regulated in that it is found in immature thymocytes prior to rearrangement, but it is switched off in mature single positive cells *(11,54)*. pTα gene expression has been analyzed by RT-PCR in cells from various anatomical sites to investigate the lineage specificity of pTα mRNA, as well as its presence in early precursors in and outside the thymus *(54)*. In addition to the expression of pTα in immature thymocytes, pTα mRNA can be detected in the gut and the liver, which are well known as extra-thymic sites of T-cell development, and in adult bone marrow, as well as in a T-lineage-committed precursor population from fetal blood. Pluripotent stem cells are pTα negative. Consistently, pTα mRNA could not be detected in human B-cells, NK cells, myeloid, and dendritic cells *(55)*. More recently, the expression of the pTα gene has been used to identify a potential human T-cell precursor in the peripheral blood of adult donors *(56)*.

4. Pre-T-Cell Receptor Independent Pathways from the Double Negative to the Double Positive Stage

Recent evidence suggests that the survival, as well as differentiation of early thymocytes, depends critically on molecular signals such as those generated by the pre-TCR. Most thymocytes require the TCRβ protein in association with the pTα chain to receive a signal to survive (rescue from programmed cell death), proliferate, and further differentiate. Likewise, the pre–B-cell receptor, composed of membrane-bound μ heavy chain (μ_m), surrogate light chain, Igα and Igβ, has been postulated to play critical roles during the early stages of B-cell development *(57)*.

The important role of the TCRβ chain in thymic development has been described first by studies that involved the reconstitution of rearrangement-deficient severe combined immunodeficient (SCID) mice with a functionally rearranged TCRβ transgene *(10,29,58)*. The TCRβ transgene was sufficient to induce expansion and differentiation of double negative cells into double positive cells. Likewise, in mice lacking recombination activating genes (RAG1 or RAG2) *(4,5)*, TCRβ *(59)*, pre-TCRα *(12)*, or CD3ε *(35)*, development of double positive thymocytes from double negative progenitors is diminished or completely abrogated, reducing thymic cellularity 10–100-fold. Thus, expression of the pre-TCR complex regulates this critical checkpoint. Consistent with this notion, productively rearranged TCRβ-transgenes *(32,58,59)* or anti-CD3ε treatment *(36,38,39)* restores thymic cellularity and the development of double positive thymocytes in SCID or RAG1- or RAG2-deficient mice. In contrast with TCRβ-deficient mice, the thymus of TCRα-deficient mice contains normal numbers of double positive cells, excluding a role for the TCRα chain in early thymic differentiation *(59,60)*.

Experiments in pre-TCR deficient $TCR\beta^{-/-}$ or $pT\alpha^{-/-}$ mice have shown that the pre-TCR, although having an important function in generating large numbers of $CD4^+8^+$ cells from $CD4^-8^-$ precursors, was likely not to be the only TCR able to mediate these events, since both types of mutant mice still contained significant, though, reduced numbers of $CD4^+8^+$ thymocytes *(12,59)*. In fact, the origin of $CD4^+8^+$ cells in $TCR\beta^{-/-}$ mice was obscure, and the possibility was discussed that they may belong to the γδ lineage *(59)*. In $pT\alpha^{-/-}$ mice, however, some of the $CD4^+8^+$ cells expressed αβ TCRs on the cell surface and could undergo positive selection to become mature T-cells, (i.e., they belonged to the αβ lineage). Accordingly, it was important to define alternative rescue pathways that could avoid a total deficiency of αβ T-cells in pTα defective mice.

Therefore, it was determined whether either the γδ or the αβ TCR could be responsible for the production of $CD4^+8^+$ T-cells in $pT\alpha^{-/-}$ mice by analyzing the cellular composition of thymuses from either $pT\alpha^{-/-}$ $TCR\alpha^{-/-}$ or $pT\alpha^{-/-}$ $TCR\delta^{-/-}$ double mutant mice that can only produce the γδ and the αβ TCR, respectively (Fig. 1). Both types of double mutant mice contained $CD4^+8^+$ T-cells. In wild-type mice, the vast majority of $CD4^+8^+$ cells contained TCRβ chains in their cytoplasm because of TCRβ selection by the pre-TCR. In $pT\alpha^{-/-}$ mice, only 39% of the $CD4^+8^+$ cells were TCRβ positive. The expression of cytoplasmic TCRδ chains was restricted to the $CD4^-8^-$ cells. In $pT\alpha^{-/-}$ $TCR\alpha^{-/-}$ mice the proportion of $TCR\beta^+CD4^+8^+$ cells was even further reduced (15%). By contrast, in $pT\alpha^{-/-}$ $TCR\delta^{-/-}$ mice all of the $CD4^+8^+$ cells are TCRβ positive, (i.e., are generated through a mechanism that involves TCRβ selection). Thus, not only the pre-TCR, but both the γγ TCR, as well as the αβTCR can further the differentiation of $CD4^-8^-25^+$ pre-T-cells, albeit by distinct mechanisms. Although the γδ TCR affects $CD4^-8^-$ precursor cells irrespective of their rearrangement status by intercellular mechanisms, both the pre-TCR and the αβ TCR select only cells with productive TCRβ genes for expansion and maturation *(61)*. The latter results suggest that the αβ TCR could assume much of the function of the pre-TCR, and that the low numbers of $TCR\beta^+CD4^+8^+$ cells in $TCR\beta^{-/-}$ $\delta^{-/-}$ mice are because of the fact that TCRα chains are only poorly expressed in early precursors that undergo TCRβ rearrangement. This hypothesis was tested in TCRαβ transgenic $pT\alpha^{-/-}$ mice that express TCRα chains earlier than nontransgenic mice. Indeed, the early expression of TCRα chains in these mice could largely overcome the developmental block that is seen in both $pT\alpha^{-/-}$ as well as TCRβ transgenic $pT\alpha^{-/-}$ mice *(61)*.

The notion of intercellular communication by γδ T-cells is consistent with experiments that involved transfer of γδ T-cells into thymuses of rearrangement-deficient mice

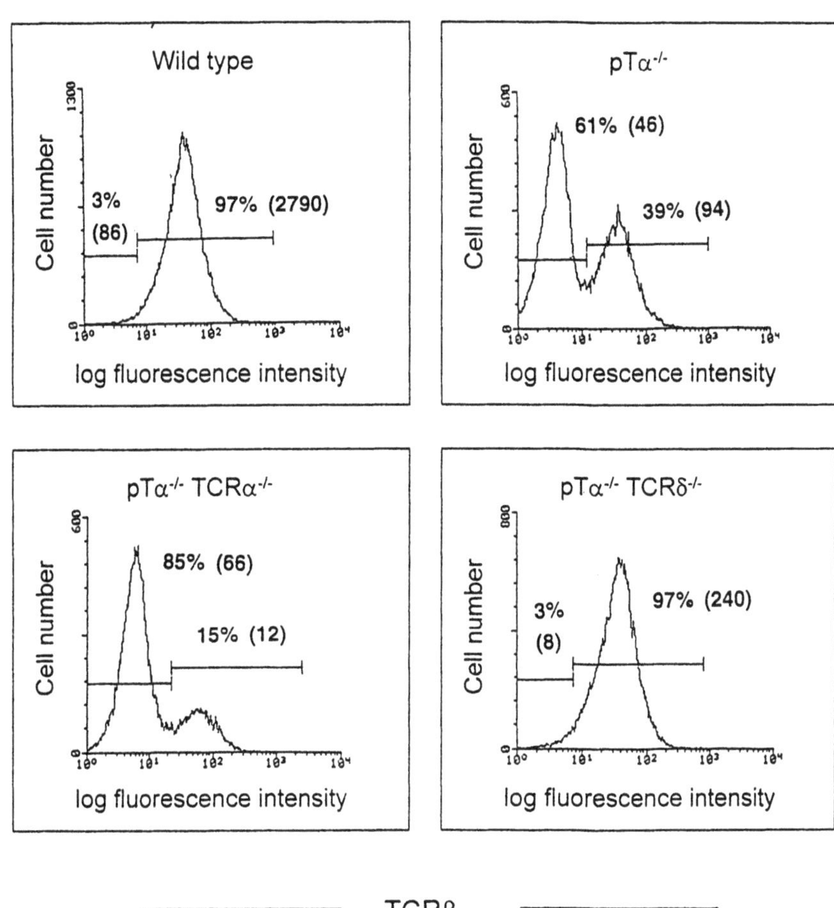

Fig. 1. Intracytoplasmic staining for TCRβ ($TCR\beta_{IC}$) within the double positive ($CD4^+8^+$) compartment from C57BL/6 (wild-type), $pT\alpha^{-/-}$, $pT\alpha^{-/-}$ $TCR\alpha^{-/-}$, and $pT\alpha^{-/-}$ $TCR\delta^{-/-}$ mice. The percentages of cells and absolute numbers ($\times 10^4$) (in brackets) are indicated.

that resulted in generation of $CD4^+8^+$ cells of host origin *(62)* and also with earlier data by Shores and colleagues *(63)*. The αβ TCR appears to be much less effective than the pre-TCR, because of the paucity of TCRα proteins in TCRβ positive precursors, since an early expressed transgenic αβ TCR can largely substitute for the pre-TCR. Thus, the αβ TCR can assume a role not only in the rescue from programmed cell death of $CD4^+8^+$, but also of $CD4^-8^-$ thymocytes. A schematic overview of various gene-deficient mice and the corresponding defects in T-cell development is given in Fig. 2.

5. Allelic Exclusion in the Absence of the Pre-T-Cell Receptor?

The variable region genes of the TCRα and β chains are assembled by somatic recombination of Vβ, Dβ, and Jβ segments at the TCRβ loci and of Vα and Jα elements at the TCRα loci *(2)*. At the TCRβ locus, D-J rearrangements precede V-D-J rearrangements. During thymocyte development, gene rearrangements display both an ordered progres-

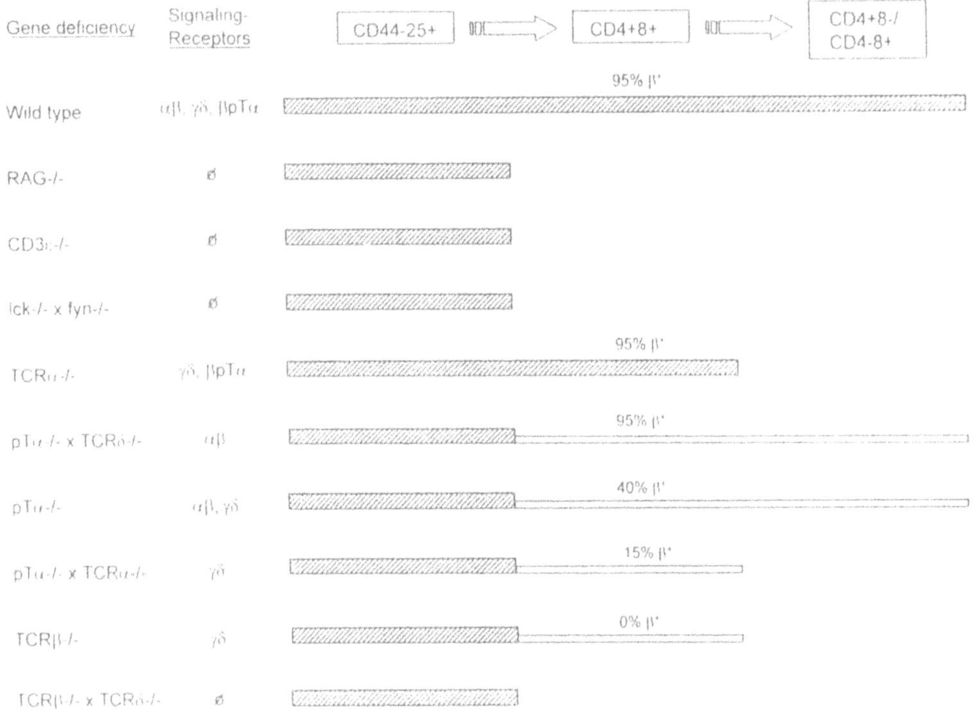

Fig. 2. Overview of various gene-deficient mice and the corresponding defects in T cell development. Percentages given indicate the proportion of cells which stain positive for intracellular TCRβ protein. The thickness of the bars is meant to correlate with the numbers of cells within the different subsets.

sion, with β chain formation preceding α chain, and allelic exclusion, with each TCRβ selected cell containing only a single functional β chain rearrangement. Whereas TCRβ genes are subject to allelic exclusion, TCRα genes are generally not allelically excluded and TCRα rearrangement is terminated only by signals that result in positive selection *(29–32)*.

The phenomenon of allelic exclusion has been extensively analyzed in transgenic mice. Thymocytes from mice bearing a functionally rearranged TCRβ transgene manifest a profound suppression of rearrangement of endogenous Vβ gene segments associated with nearly uniform surface expression of the Vβ transgene *(28)*. Suppression of endogenous Vβ gene rearrangement requires the TCRβ protein, since introduction of a frame shift mutation abolishes suppression of endogenous Vβ rearrangement *(64)*. This phenomenon has been widely interpreted to provide evidence supporting the regulation of allelic exclusion via a feedback mechanism, first proposed for allelic exclusion at the IgH locus *(65)*. Transgenes encoding a functional membrane-bound μ-chain (μ_m) prevent or profoundly impede rearrangements at the endogenous IgH loci, suggesting that the μ_m may be involved in feedback control of allelic exclusion at the IgH locus *(66,67)*. In contrast, mutants expressing only the secreted form of the μ-chain from one chromosome generate allelically" included" double producing cells *(68)*. It has been proposed that the μ_m chain exert its effect on allelic exclusion through the pre-BCR *(69,70)*. In analogy, the discovery of pre-TCR has provided a likely candidate mediating allelic exclusion at the TCRβ locus.

The role of the pTα chain in allelic exclusion at the TCRβ locus was recently analyzed by introduction of a functionally rearranged TCRβ transgene into pTα$^{-/-}$ and

$pT\alpha^{+/-}$ embryonic stem cells, which were subsequently assayed by RAG2 deficient blastocyst complementation. In the absence of pTα, expression of the TCRβ transgene inhibited rearrangement of the TCRβ locus to an extent similar to that seen in normal TCRβ transgenic mice *(65)*. When these results were repeated in pTα knockout mice, staining of CD3 positive thymocytes and lymph node cells with a Vβ6 and a Vβ8 specific antibody, vs a pool of other Vβ-specific antibodies, did not reveal any violation of allelic exclusion at the level of surface staining *(71)*. Moreover, expression of endogenous TCRβ chains could not be detected on the surface of T-cells from $pT\alpha^{-/-}$ mice expressing a functionally rearranged TCRβ transgene. However, PCR analysis of endogenous Vβ rearrangement in both total thymocytes and sorted $CD25^{+}$ cells from these TCRβ transgenic, $pT\alpha^{-/-}$ mice revealed that the TCRβ transgene was not able to fully inhibit endogenous TCRβ rearrangements in the absence of pTα. However, the extent of Vβ rearrangement in TCRβ transgenic $pT\alpha^{-/-}$ mice was much less pronounced than that seen in normal mice, indicating that the transgene exhibited most of its function in the absence of the pre-TCR. These results clearly indicate an involvement of the pre-TCR in the feedback inhibition of TCRβ rearrangements, but at least in TCRβ transgenic mice, pTα is not absolutely required. This may represent a transgenic artifact because of unphysiological amounts and forms of transgene expression *(10,12)* which may generate signals that cause allelic exclusion. Although this may explain allelic exclusion of TCRβ in TCRα negative cells, recent data indicate that also TCRα chains can partially substitute for pTα, since they induce the generation of almost normal numbers of thymocytes in pTα-deficient mice, when expressed at a relatively early developmental stage *(61)*. The fact that an early expressed αβ TCR can account for the transition of a few double negative cells to double positive cells in $pT\alpha^{-/-}$ mice could suggest an additional role of the αβ TCR in allelic exclusion of the TCRβ locus, which takes place at an early developmental stage. Moreover, in $CD3^{-/-}$ mice, TCRβ rearrangement appears essentially complete, and there is a total lack of allelic exclusion (B. Malissen, personal communication).

In order to analyze whether under physiological condition the pre-TCR has an essential role in allelic exclusion of cells that do not express TCRα chain at an early stage of development, one needs to analyze allelic exclusion in single cells in $pT\alpha^{+}$ and $pT\alpha^{-/-}$ mice. Recently such analysis has been conducted in the author's laboratory and indicates that under physiological conditions the pre-TCR is the only receptor to terminate Vβ gene rearrangement in cells that carry already a single productive TCRβ gene *(72)*.

6. Conclusion

Experiments in pTα gene deficient mice have shown that the pre-TCR has a crucial role in maturation, as well as allelic exclusion of αβ T-cells, but is not required for the development of γδ expressing cells *(12,26,61)*.

The pre-TCR, composed of the TCRβ chain, pTα chain, and CD3 molecules, rescues from programmed cell death $CD4^{-}8^{-}25^{+}$ thymocytes that have successfully rearranged the TCRβ chain. The assembly of the pre-TCR therefore establishes a key checkpoint in early thymocyte differentiation at which developing T-cells undergo "β-selection." As a result, TCRβ positive $CD4^{-}8^{-}25^{+}$ cells not only are rescued from programmed cell death, but also stimulated to proliferate, downregulate CD25, and express CD4 and CD8 molecules to become double positive cells (Fig. 3).

The molecular characterization of the pre-TCR complex has provided a fundamental insight into regulation at this early developmental checkpoint. The pre-TCR appears to

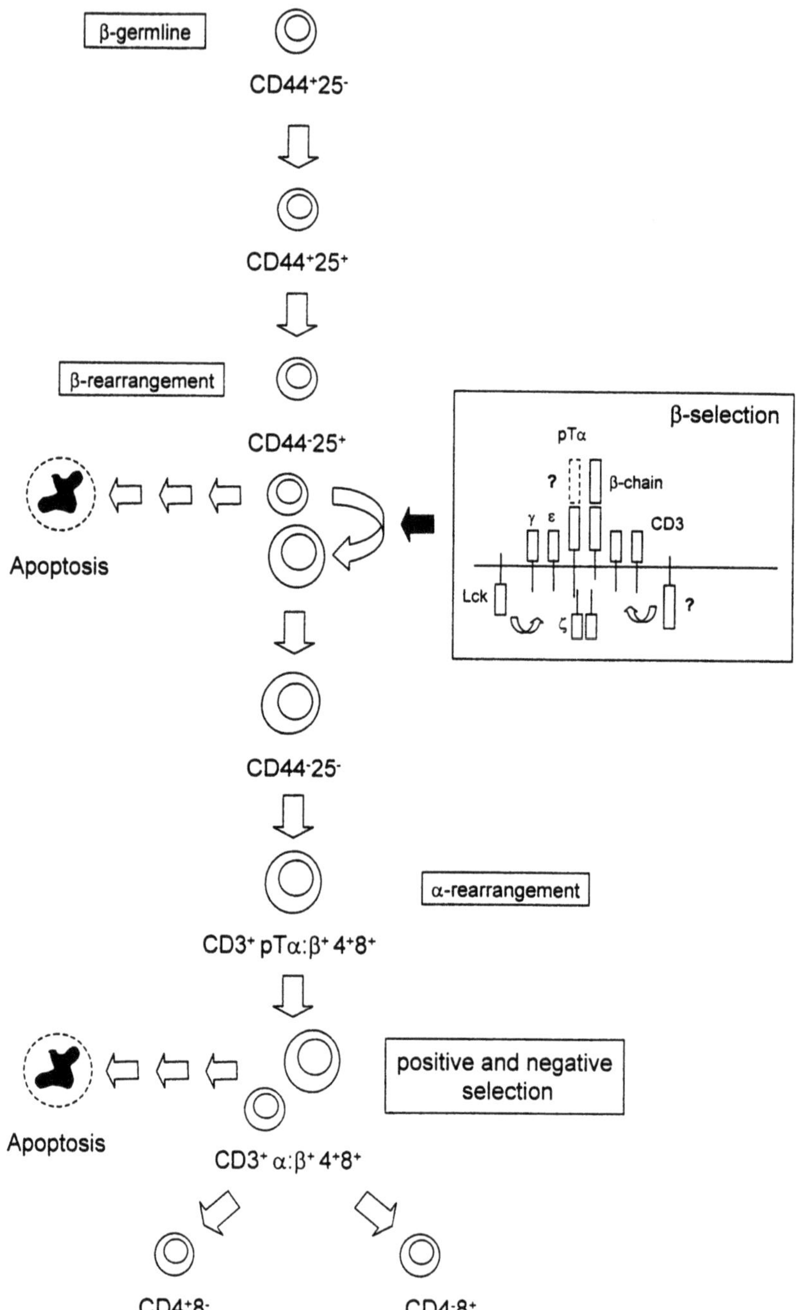

Fig. 3. Control points in early αβ T-cell development. The pre-TCR that consists of the TCRβ chain, the pTα chain, and perhaps other proteins in association with signal transducing CD3 proteins has the function to rescue from programmed cell death (apoptosis) $CD4^-8^-44^-25^+$ thymocytes that have successfully rearranged the TCRβ chain. The pre-TCR induces expansion and differentiation of these cells such that they become TCRαβ bearing double positive ($CD4^+8^+$) thymocytes, which express only a single TCRβ chain (i.e., the cells are allelically excluded). A second round of selection takes place during the double positive stage. At this stage, TCRα gene rearrangement begins and thymocytes are subsequently subjected to repertoire selection based on the specificity of the mature αβ TCR (positive and negative selection). The relative size of the thymocyte symbols indicates their proliferative status.

work as a surface receptor that employs both CD3 proteins and src family protein kinases. It remains to be established how protein kinases are recruited by the pre-TCR. The origin of the pre-TCR signals is likewise unclear. They may spontaneously arise as a result of receptor assembly, or the pre-TCR may engage a specific ligand on thymocytes or stromal cells.

The results and observations obtained using pTα knockout mice demonstrate that signaling by the pre-TCR inhibits further V-D-J recombination and establishes allelic exclusion at the TCRβ locus. Allelic exclusion may initially be achieved by the temporary downregulation of recombination activating genes and may later be secured by making the loci inaccessible to the recombinase.

In addition to its role, in αβ lineage T-cell development, recent results show that the pre-TCR can significantly influence the γδ versus αβ lineage decision. However, not much is known about the molecular mechanisms that trigger commitment to either the αβ or the γδ T-cell lineage.

Finally, data on the extrathymic expression of the pTα argue that this protein also plays a role in T-cell precursors that may either seed the thymus or develop outside the thymus.

In the absence of the pre-TCR, the development of early T-cell progenitors can be mediated, albeit inefficiently, by the αβ TCR, and to some extent, also by the γδ TCR. Although the γδ TCR affects $CD4^{-}8^{-}$ cells irrespective of their TCRβ rearrangement status by mechanisms not involving TCRβ selection, the αβ TCR only selects cells with a functional TCRβ chain for expansion and maturation. Thus, the early expressed αβ TCR avoids a severe immunodeficiency by enabling the formation of a significant number of mature T-cells bearing αβ TCRs. The fact that the αβ TCR promotes T-cell development much in the same way as the pre-TCR, i.e., by cell-autonomous signaling and thereby β-selection, suggests that T-cell development may have proceeded in this way before the event of the pTα chain in evolution. Thus the pre-TCR has a major role in inducing allelic exclusion and maturation in pre-T-cells that have not yet succeeded in TCRα rearrangement, and is thereby responsible for the generation of a large number of TCRβ allelically excluded T-cell precursors, which can now efficiently "test" several TCRα chains to form a TCR αβ that permits positive selection.

Acknowledgments

The authors are grateful to Hans Jörg Fehling, Bernard Malissen, Iannis Aifantis, and Orly Azogui for unpublished communications. This work was supported in part by the Institut National de la Santé et Recherche Medicale, Paris. J. B. is a recipient of a research grant from the Deutsche Forschungsgemeinschaft. H. v. B. is supported by the Institut Universitaire de France and by the Körber Foundation.

References

1. Tonegawa, S. (1983) Somatic generation of antibody diversity. *Nature* **302,** 575–581.
2. Davis, M. M., and Bjorkman, P. J. (1988) T-cell antigen receptor genes and T-cell recognition. *Nature* **334,** 395–402.
3. Lewis, S. M. (1994) The mechanisms of V(D)J joining: lessons from molecular, immunological, and comparative analyses. *Adv. Immunol.* **56,** 27–150.
4 Mombaerts, P., Iacomoni, J., Johnson, R. S., Herrup, K., Tonegawa, S., and Papioannou, V. E. (1992a) RAG-1 deficient mice have no mature B and T lymphocytes. *Cell* **68,** 869–877.
5. Shinkai, Y., Rathbun, G., Lam, K. P., Oltz, E. M., Steward, V., Mendelsohn, M., Charron, J., Datta, M., Young, F., Stall, A. M., and Alt, F. (1992) RAG-2 deficient mice lack mature lymphocytes owing to inability to initiate V(D)J rearrangement. *Cell* **68,** 855–867.

6. Padovan, E., Casorati, G., Dellabona, P., Meyer, S., Brockhaus, M., and Lanzavecchia, A. (1993) Expression of two T cell receptor α chains: dual receptor T cells. *Science* **262,** 422–424.
7. Heath, W. R., Carbone, F. R., Bertolino, P., Kelly, J., Cose, S., and Miller, J. F. A. P. (1995) Expression of two α chains on the surface of T cells in T cell receptor transgenic mice. *J. Exp. Med.* **178,** 1807–1811.
8. Rocha, B., Vassalli, P., and Guy-Grand, D. (1991) The Vβ repertoire of mouse gut homodimeric $\alpha CD8^+$ intraepithelial T cell receptor $\alpha\beta^+$ lymphocytes reveals a major extrathymic pathway of T cell differentiation. *J. Exp. Med.* **173,** 483–486.
9. von Boehmer, H. (1994) Positive selection of lymphocytes. *Cell* **76,** 219–228.
10. Groettrup. M., Baron, A., Griffiths, R., Palacios, R., and von Boehmenr, H. (1992) T-cell receptor (TCR) β chain homodimers on the surface of immature but not mature α, γ, δ chain deficient T-cell lines. *EMBO J.* **11,** 2735–2746.
11. Saint-Ruf, C., Ungewiss, K., Groettrup, M., Bruno, L., Fehling, H. J., and von Boehmer, H. (1994) Analysis and expression of a pre-T cell receptor gene. *Science* **266,** 1208–1212.
12. Fehling, H. J., Krotkova, A., Saint-Ruf, C., and von Boehmer, H. (1995) Crucial role of the pre-T-cell receptor alpha in development of alpha/beta but not gamma/delta T cells. *Nature* **375,** 795–798.
13. Wu, L., Scollay, R., Egerton, M., Pearse, M., Spangrude, G. J., and Shortman, K. (1991) CD4 expressed on earliest T-lineage precursor cells in adult murine thymus. *Nature* **349,** 71–74.
14. Godfrey, D. I., Kennedy, J., Suda, T., and Zlotnik, A. (1993) A developmental pathway involving four phenotypically and functionally distinct subsets of CD3-CD4-CD8- triple-negative adult mouse thymocytes defined by CD44 and CD25 expression. *J. Immunol.* **150,** 4244–4252.
15. Matsuzaki, Y., Gyotoku, J., Ogawa, M., Nishikawa, S., Katsura, Y., Gachelin, G., and Nakauchi, H. (1993) Characterization of c-kit positive intrathymic stem cells that are restricted to lymphoid differentiation. *J. Exp. Med.* **178,** 1283–1292.
16. Rodewald, H. R., Moingeon, P., Lucich, J. L., Dosiou, C., Lopez, P., and Reinherz, L. E. (1992) A population of early fetal thymocytes expressing FcγRII/III contains precursors of T lymphocytes and NK cells. *Cell* **69,** 139–150.
17. Ardavin, C., Wu, L., Li, C. L., and Shortman, K. (1993) Thymic dendritic cells and T cells develop simultaneously in the thymus from a common precursor population. *Nature* **362,** 761–763.
18. Kisielow, P., and von Boehmer, H. (1995) Development and selection of T cells, facts and puzzles. *Adv. Immunol.* **58,** 87–209.
19. Livak, F., Petrie, H. T., Crispe, I. N., and Schatz, D. G. (1995) In-frame TCRδ rearrangements play a critical role in the αβ/γδ lineage decision. *Immunity* **2,** 617–627.
20. Dudley, E., Girardi, M., Owen, M., and Hayday, A. (1995) Alpha beta and gamma delta T cells can share a late common precursor. *Curr. Biol.* **5,** 659–669.
21. Kang, J., Baker, J., and Raulet, D. (1995) Evidence that productive rearrangements of TCR gamma genes influence the commitment of progenitor cells differentiate into alpha beta or gamma delta T cells. *Eur. J. Immunol.* **9,** 2706–2709.
22. Bruno, L., Fehling, H. J., and von Boehmer, H. (1996) The alpha/beta T cell receptor can replace the gamma/delta receptor in the development of the gamma/delta lineage cells. *Immunity* **5,** 343–352.
23. Washburn, T., Schweighoffer, E., Gridley, T., Chang, D., Fowlkes, B. J., Cado, D., and Robey, E. (1997) Notch activity influences the αβ vs. γδ T cell lineage decision. *Cell* **88,** 833–843.
24. Groettrup, M., Ungewiss, K., Azogui, O., Palacios, R., Owen, M. J., Hayday, A. C., and von Boehmer, H. (1993a) A novel disulfide-linked heterodimer on pre-T cells consists of the T cell receptor beta chain and a 33 kd glycoprotein. *Cell* **75,** 283–94.
25. Hoffman, E. S., Passoni, L., Crompton, T., Leu, T. M., Schatz, D. G., Koff, A., Owen, M. J., and Hayday, A. C. (1996) Productive T-cell receptor beta-chain gene rearrangement: coincident regulation of cell cycle and clonality during development in vivo. *Genes Dev.* **10,** 948–962.
26. von Boehmer, H. and Fehling, H. J. (1997) Structure and function of the pre-T cell receptor. *Annu. Rev. Immunol.* **15,** 433–452.
27. Penit, C., Lucas, B., and Vasseur, F. (1995) Cell expansion and growth arrest phases during the transition from precursor ($CD4^-8^-$) to immature ($CD4^+8^+$) thymocytes in normal and genetically modified mice. *J. Immunol.* **154,** 5103–5105.

28. Uematsu, Y., Ryser, S., Dembic, S. Z., Borgulya, P., Krimpenfort, P., Berns, A., von Boehmer, H., and Steinmetz, M. (1988) In transgenic mice the introduced functional T cell receptor β gene prevents expression of endogenous β genes. *Cell* **52,** 831–841.
29. von Boehmer, H. 1990. Developmental biology of T cells in T-cell receptor transgenic mice. *Annu. Rev. Immunol.* **8,** 531–556.
30. Casanova, J. L., Romero, P., Widman, C., Kourilsky, P., and Maryanski, J. L. (1991) T cell receptor genes in a series of class I major histocompatibility complex-restricted cytotoxic T lymphocyte clones specific for a Plasmodium berghei nonapeptide: implications for T cell allelic exclusion and antigen-specific repertoire. *J. Exp. Med.* **174,** 1371–1383.
31. Borgulya, P., Kishi, H., Uematsu, Y., and von Behmer, H. (1992) Exclusion and inclusion of α and β T cell receptor alleles. *Cell* **69,** 529–537.
32. Malissen, M., Trucy, J., Jouvin-Marche, E., Cazenave, P. A., Scollay, R., and Malissen, B. (1992) Regulation of TCRa and b gene allelic exclusion during T cell development. *Immunol. Today* **13,** 315–322.
32a. Shinkai, Y., Koyasu, S., Nakayama, K. I., Murphy, K. M., Loh, D. Y., Reinherz, E. L., and Alt, F. W. (1993) Restoration of T cell development in RAG-2 deficient mice by functional TCR transgenes. *Science* **259,** 822–825.
33. Teh, H. S., Kisielow, P., Scott, B., Kishi, H., Uematsu, Y., Bluethmann, H., and von Boehmer, H. (1988) Thymic major histocompatibility complex antigens and the specificity of the αβ T cell receptor determine the CD4/CD8 phenotype of T cells. *Nature* **335,** 229–233.
34. Robey, E., Chang, D., Itano, A., Cado, D., Alexander, H., Lans, D., Weinmaster, G., and Salmon, P. (1996) An activated form of Notch influences the choice be tween CD4 and CD8 T cell lineages. *Cell* **87,** 483–492.
35. Malissen, M., Gillet, A., Ardouin, L., Bouvier, G., Trucy, J., Ferrier, P., Vivier, E., and Malissen, B. (1995) Altered T cell development in mice with a targeted mutation of the CD3epsilon gene. *EMBO J.* **14,** 4641–4653.
36. Levelt, C. N., Mombaerts, P., Iglesias, A., Tonegawa, S., and Eichmann, K. (1993) Restoration of early thymocyte differentiation in T-cell receptor β-chain-deficient mutant mice by transmembrane signaling through CD3ε. *Proc. Natl. Acad. Sci. USA* **90,** 11,401–11,405.
37. Levelt, C. N., Mombaerts, P., Wang, B., Kohler, H., Tonegawa, S., Eichmann, K., and Terhorst, C. (1993) Regulation of thymocyte development through CD3, functional dissociation between $p56^{lck}$ and CD3ζ in eraly thymic selection. *Immunity* **3,** 215–222.
38. Jacobs, H., Vandeputte, D., Tolkamp, L., de Vries, E., Borst, J., and Berns, A. (1994) CD3 components at the surface of pro-T cells can mediate pre-T cell development in vivo. *Eur. J. Immunol.* **24,** 934–939.
39. Shinkai, Y., and Alt, F. W. (1994) CD3ε-mediated signals rescue the development of $CD4^+8^+$ thymocytes in $RAG2^{-/-}$ mice in the absence of TCRβ chain expression. *Int. Immunol.* **6,** 995–1001.
40. van Oers, N. S. C., von Boehmer, H., and Weiss, A. (1995) The pre-T cell receptor (TCR) complex is functionally coupled to the TCR-ζ subunit. *J. Exp. Med.* **182,** 1585–1590.
41. Del Porto, P., Bruno, L., Mattei, M. G., von Boehmer, H., and Saint-Ruf, C. (1995) Cloning and comparitive analysis of the human pre-T cell receptor α-chain gene. *Proc. Natl. Acad. Sci. USA* **92,** 12105–12109.
42. Boismenu, R., Rhein, M., Fischer, W. H., and Havran, W. L. (1996) A role for CD81 in early T cell development. *Science* **271,** 198–200.
43. Maecker, H. T. and Levy, S. (1997) Normal lymphocyte development but delayed humoral immune response in CD81-null mice. *J. Exp. Med.* **185,** 1505–1510.
44. Fehling, H. J., Iritani, B. M., Krotkova, A., Forbush, K. A., Laplace, C., Perlmutter, R. M., and von Boehmer, H. (1997) Restoration of early T cell development in pTα-deficient mice by anti-CD3e antibody treatment or with transgenes encoding activated lck or tailless pTα. *Immunity* **6,** 703–714.
45. Anderson, S. J., Levin, S. D., and Perlmutter, R. M. (1994) Involvement of the protein tyrosine kinase $p56^{lck}$ in T cell signaling and thymocyte development. *Adv. Immunol.* **56,** 151–178.
46. van Oers, N. S. C., Lowin-Kropf, B., Finlay, D., Connolly, K., and Weiss, A. (1996) Alpha/beta T cell development is abolished in mice lacking both lck and fyn protein tyrosine kinases. *Immunity* **5,** 429–436.
47. Molina, T. J., Kishihara, K., Siderovski, D. P., van Ewijk, W., Narendran, A., Timms, E., Wakeham, A., Paige, C. J., Hartmann, K. U., Veillette, A., Davidson, D., and Mak, T. W. (1992) Profound block in thymocyte development in mice lacking p56lck. *Nature* **357,** 161-164.

48. Levin, S., Anderson, S., Forbush, K., and Perlmutter, R. (1993) A dominant-negative transgene defines a role for $p56^{lck}$ in thymopoiesis. *EMBO J.* **12,** 1671–1680.
49. Mombaerts, P., Anderson, S. J., Perlmutter, R. M., Mak, T. W., and Tonegawa, S. (1994) An activated lck transgene promotes thymocyte development in RAG-1 mutant mice. *Immunity* **1,** 261–267.
50. Groves, T., Smiley, P., Cooke, M. P., Forbush, K., Perlmutter, R. M., and Guidos, C. J. (1996) Fyn can partially substitute for lck in T lymphocyte development. *Immunity* **5,** 417–428.
51. Weiss, A. and Littman, D. R. (1994) Signal transduction by lymphocyte antigen receptors. *Cell* **76,** 263–274.
52. Swat, W., Shinkai, Y., Cheng, H. L., Davidson, L., and Alt, F. W. (1996) Activated ras signals differentiation and expansion of $CD4^+8^+$ thymocytes. *Proc. Natl. Acad. Sci. USA* **93,** 4683–4687.
53. Crompton, T., Gilmour, K. C., and Owen, M. J. (1996) The MAP kinase pathway controls differentiation from double-negative to double-positive thymocytes. *Cell* **86,** 243–251.
54. Bruno, L., Rocha, B., Rolink, A., von Boehmer, H., and Rodewald, H. R. (1995) Intra- and extra-thymic expression of the pre-T cell receptor a gene. *Eur. J. Immunol.* **25,** 1877–1882.
55. Ramiro, A. R., Trigueros, C., Marquez, C., San Millan, J. L., and Toribio, M. L. (1996) Regulation of pre-T cell receptor (pTα-TCRβ) gene expression during human thymic development. *J. Exp. Med.* **184,** 519–530.
56. Bruno, L., Res, P., Dessing, M., Cella, M., and Spits, H. (1997) Identification of a committed T cell precursor population in adult human peripheral blood. *J. Exp. Med.* **185,** 875–884.
57. Rajewsky, K. (1996) Clonal selection and learning in the antibody system. *Nature* **381,** 751–758.
58. Kishi, H., Borgulya, P., Scott, B., Karjalainen, K., Traunecker, A., Kaufman, J., and von Boehmer, H. (1991) Surface expression of the β T cell receptor (TCR) chain in the absence of other TCR or CD3 proteins on immature T cells. *EMBO J.* **10,** 93–100.
59. Mombaerts, P., Clark, A. R., Rudnicki, M. A., Iacomini, J., Itohara, S., Lafaille, J. J., Wang, L., Ichikawa, Y., Jaenisch, R., Hooper, M. L., and Tonegawa, S. (1992b) Mutations in T-cell antigen receptor genes alpha and beta block thymocyte development at different stages. *Nature* **360,** 225–231.
60. Philpott, K. L., Viney, J. L., Kay, G., Rastan, S., Gardiner, E. M., Chae, S., Hayday, A. C., and Owen, M. J. (1992) Lymphoid development in mice lacking T cell receptor alpha/beta-expressing cells. *Science* **256,** 1448–1452.
61. Buer, J., Aifantis, I., DiSanto, J. P., Fehling, H. J., and von Boehmer, H. (1997) Role of different T cell receptors in the development of pre-T cells. *J. Exp. Med.* **185,** 1541–1547.
62. Lynch, F. and Shevach, E. M. (1993) Gamma/delta T cells promote CD4 and CD8 expression of SCID thymocytes. *Int. Immunol.* **8,** 991–995.
63. Shores, E. W., Sharrow, S. O., Uppenkamp, I., and Singer, A. (1990) T cell receptor negative thymocytes from SCID mice can be induced to enter the CD4/CD8 differentiation pathway. *Eur. J. Immunol.* **20,** 69–77.
64. Krimpenfort, P., Ossendrop, F., Borst, J., Melief, C., and Berns, A. 1989. T cell depletion in transgenic mice carrying a mutant gene for TCRβ. *Nature* **341,** 742–746.
65. Xu, Y., Davidson, L., Alt, F. W., and Baltimore, D. (1996) Function of the pre-T-cell receptor a chain in T-cell development and allelic exclusion at the T-cell receptor β locus. *Proc. Natl. Acad. Sci. USA* **93,** 2169–2137.
66. Storb, U., Pinkert, C., Arp, B., Engler, P., Gollanhon, K., Manz, J., Brady, W., and Brinster, R. L. (1986) Transgenic mice with mu and kappa genes encoding antiphosphorylcholine antibodies. *J. Exp. Med.* **164,** 627–652.
67. Nussenzweig, M., Shaw, A., Sinn, E., Danner, D. B., Holmes, K. L., Morse, H. C., and Leder, P. (1988) Allelic exclusion in transgenic mice that express the membrane form of immunoglobulin μ. *Science* **236,** 816–819.
68. Kitamura, D. and Rajewsky, K. (1992) Targeted disruption of mμ chain membrane exon cuases loss of heavy-chain allelic exclusion. *Nature* **356,** 154–156.
69. Karasuyama, H., Rolink, A., Shinkai, Y., Young, F., Alt, F. W., and Melchers, F. (1993) The expression of $V_{pre}B/\lambda5$ surrogate light chain in early bone marrow precursor B cells of normal and B-cell deficient mice. *Cell* **77,** 133–143.

70. Loeffert, D., Ehrlich, A., Mueller, W., and Rajewsky, K. (1996) Surrogate light chain expression is equired to establish immunoglobulin heavy chain allelic exclusion during early B cell development. *Immunity* **4,** 133–144.
71. Krotkova, A., von Boehmer, H., and Fehling, H. J. (1997) Allelic exclusion in pTα-deficient mice: no evidence for cell surface expression of two T cell receptor (TCR)-β chains, but less efficient inhibition of endogenous Vβ→(D)Jβ rearrangements in the presence of a functional TCR-β transgene. *J. Exp. Med.* **186,** 767–775.
72. Aifandis, I., Buer, J., von Boehmer, H., and Azogui, O. (1997) Essential role of the pre-T-cell receptor in allelic exclusion of the T-cell receptor β locus. *Immunity J.* **7,** 601–607.

Chapter 23

Developmental Stage-Specific Responses to Ligation of CD3-Containing Complexes

Christiaan N. Levelt

1. Introduction

The vast repertoire of T-cell receptor specificities is accomplished by somatic assembly of V, D, and J gene segments into genes encoding the T-cell receptor (TCR) -α and -β chains. Because chances are that this partially random process does not produce a useful TCR, several selection events are imposed on developing T-cells. These selection events are all controlled by signals transduced through TCR-CD3 complexes. The composition of the TCR-CD3 complex, the signals transduced by it, and the responses of the thymocytes differ at distinct stages of development. This chapter describes the molecular composition of the CD3-containing complexes, as well as the signals and maturation events that are inducible upon ligation with antibodies.

2. Stages of T-Cell Development

Extensive research efforts over the last 20 years have provided us with detailed knowledge of stage-specific properties of developing T-cells in the thymus. An overview of these maturational stages is depicted in Fig. 1. The earliest T-cell precursors that enter the thymus are characterized by expression of c-kit, Pgp-1, and low levels of CD4 *(1)*. The TCR genes of these cells are all in germline configuration *(2)*. Already at this stage, mRNAs encoding components of the CD3 complex can be detected. CD3ε and γ are expressed first, followed by CD3δ and CD3ζ *(3)*. Within a day or so after entry into the thymus, these cells downregulate CD4 and express the IL-2Rα chain to become IL-2Rα$^+$Pgp-1$^+$c-kit$^+$ pro-T-cells (IL-2Rα = CD25; Pgp–1 = CD44). Many of these cells are in an apparently activated state and proliferate. The major signal for this proliferation and the continued maturation into IL-2Rα$^+$Pgp-1$^-$c-kit$^-$ pre-T-cells is probably provided by the cytokines c-kit ligand and IL-7 produced by thymic epithelial cells *(4–9)*.

From: *Molecular Biology of B-Cell and T-Cell Development*
Edited by: J. G. Monroe and E. V. Rothenberg © Humana Press Inc., Totowa, NJ

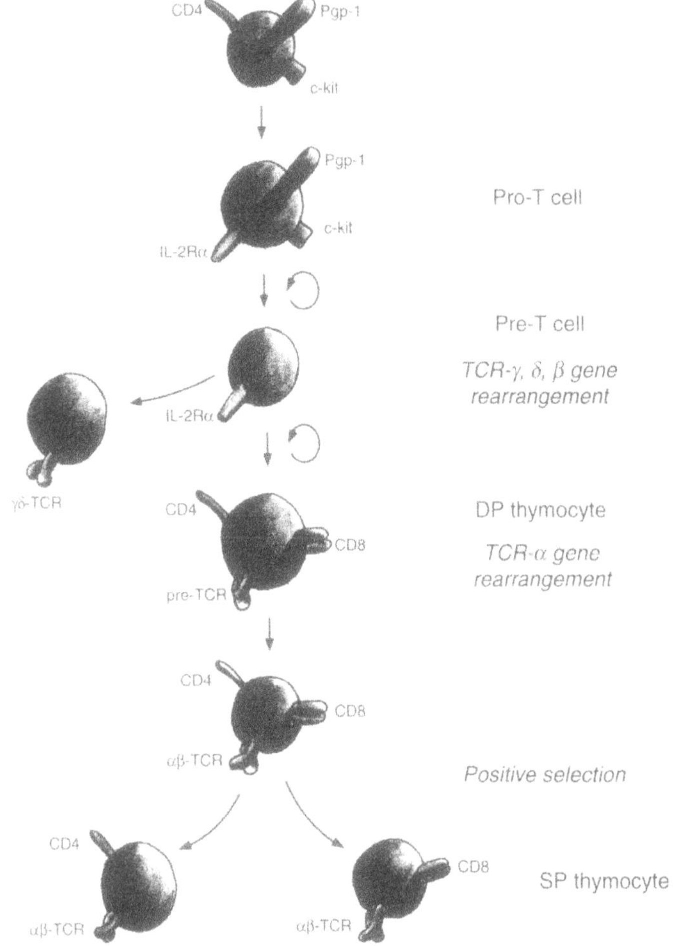

Fig. 1. Stages of T-cell development in the thymus. Surface markers characterizing each maturation stage are indicated. Circular arrows represent maturation events accompanied by proliferation.

IL-2Rα$^+$Pgp-1$^-$c-kit$^-$ pre-T-cells are fully committed to the T-cell lineage, but may still develop into γδ or αβ lineage T-cells *(10)*. How the branching into the two classes is regulated is not clear. Recent experiments suggest that the successful rearrangement of the TCR-γ and δ loci and signaling by Notch may be involved *(10–14)*. Early during the pre-T-cell stage, rearrangement of the TCR-γ, -δ, and -β loci is initiated. Transcription of the Rag-1 and -2 genes can already be detected in the earliest thymic precursors, indicating that other factors are responsible for the onset of rearrangement *(15–17)*. If recombination of the TCR-β locus is in frame, a pre–T-cell receptor (pre-TCR) containing the TCR-β chain is expressed on the cell surface *(18,19)*, inducing the thymocytes to undergo a second burst of proliferation, down regulate IL-2Rα, and express CD4 and CD8. Progression to the CD4$^+$CD8$^+$ double positive (DP) stage is accompanied by rearrangements of TCR-α genes *(17,20,21)*. Once a complete TCR is synthesized and expressed on the cell surface, cells are selected based on the specificity of their TCR *(22)*. Only a minority of thymocytes fulfills the stringent criteria for positive selection and escaping negative selection. These thymocytes upregulate the level of TCR expression,

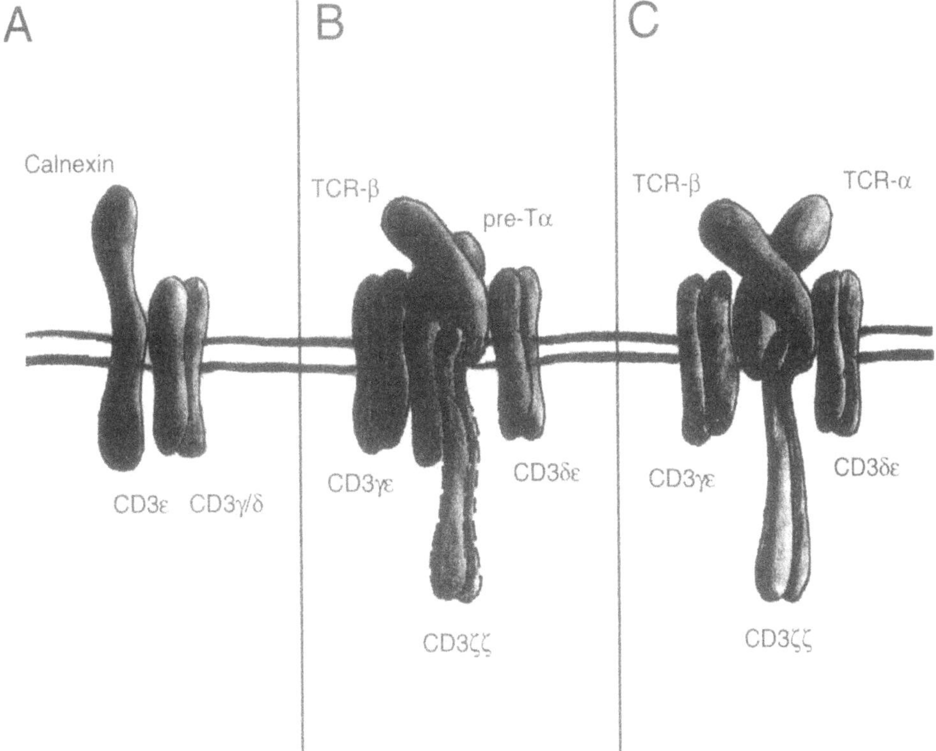

Fig. 2. Composition of CD3-containing complexes at progressing stages of T-cell development. **(A)** Before in frame rearrangement of the TCR-β locus, pre-T-cells express CD3γε or δε dimers associated with calnexin on the surface. **(B)** Upon production of the TCR-β chain, the pre-TCR is assembled. **(C)** The complete TCR-CD3 complex as found on mature T-cells.

and mature into $CD4^+$ or $CD8^+$ single positive (SP) T-cells, depending on the MHC restriction of their TCR.

3. Stage-Specific Composition of the CD3-Containing Complexes

T-cell development is regulated by signals originating from CD3-containing complexes, which vary with regard to density at the cell surface and composition (*see* Fig. 2). The variation in composition results from differences in intracellular sorting and from the differential availability of some of the components.

The TCR found on mature T-cells is a multi-unit complex, consisting of the variable TCR-α and -β chains, and the invariant CD3γ, δ, ε, and ζ/η chains. The α- and β- chains are responsible for antigen recognition, whereas the CD3 chains transfer signals into the cell upon ligation of the TCR.

The TCR chains are members of the immunoglobulin superfamily, and consist of a variable and a constant domain that are linked by a joining region. The TCR-α and -β chain constant domains are anchored in the cell membrane and are linked by disulfide bridges. They contain short cytoplasmic regions that are not involved in signal transduction but in the regulation of transport from the endoplasmic reticulum (ER) to the cell surface. The transmembrane regions of the TCR-α and -β chains are positively charged, and interact with the negatively charged transmembrane regions of the CD3 complex. The variable N-terminal regions form the antigen recognition domain, which can interact with MHC-peptide ligands.

The CD3γ,δ and ε chains are also members of the immunoglobulin superfamily *(23)*. In contrast to the TCR chains, the extracellular regions consist of a single immunoglobulin domain and are not known to have any specific ligand. The cytoplasmic tails comprise one immunoreceptor tyrosine-based activation motif (ITAM), containing tyrosines that can be phosphorylated. The cytoplasmic tails also embody ER retention sequences, preventing the export of incomplete TCR-CD3 complexes out of the ER *(24)*.

The CD3-ζ and -η chains do not belong to the Ig superfamily and are products of alternatively spliced mRNAs from the same gene *(25,26)*. The extracellular domains consist of only a few amino acids. The cytoplasmic tails have three ITAMs, giving it a robust signaling capacity. Like the other CD3 chains, the cytoplasmic tails of the CD3ζ/η chains contain ER retention sequences.

The TCR-CD3 complex is assembled in the ER. The core element of the complex is the CD3ε chain. It forms a dimer with a CD3-γ or -δ chain and subsequently associates with a TCR-α or -β chain *(27)*. Such partial complexes are targeted for destruction and need to associate with each other to form a stable hexameric complex which consists of one TCR αβ heterodimer, one CD3γε, and one CD3δε dimer *(27a)*. Such complexes can exit the ER, and are capable of signal transduction, but addition of a CD3-ζζ, -ζη, or -ηη dimer greatly facilitates these processes *(28–33)*. Nearly all TCR's found on the cell surface of mature T-cells are associated with a complete set of CD3 chains.

In the last few years, it was recognized that the situation in immature thymocytes is quite different. As mentioned in Subheading 2., maturation of pre-T-cells to the DP stage depends on the surface expression of the pre-TCR. This immature TCR complex is similar to the mature TCR complex in that it contains the TCR-β chain and CD3 chains. At this stage, the TCR-α chain is not yet available, and instead, the pre-TCR utilizes a pre-Tα chain *(18,19)*. The pre-Tα chain is also a member of the Ig superfamily and contains a single Ig domain and a 31-residue cytoplasmic tail. In contrast to the mature TCR complex, there is no evidence that CD3ζ is stably associated with the pre-TCR complex. However, functional data show that the CD3ζ chain does play a role in signal transduction through the pre-TCR complex *(30–34)*.

Surprisingly, CD3 complexes are also expressed on the cell surface of pre-T-cells in the absence of the TCR-β chain. This was recognized by the observation that thymocytes already respond to anti-CD3 antibodies before successful rearrangement of the TCR-β locus *(35,36)*. Such immature CD3 complexes consist of CD3γε or CD3δε heterodimers, associated with the ER resident molecular chaperone calnexin *(37–39)*. This finding was unexpected, because CD3 chains contain ER retention sequences, and mature T-cells are unable to express partial CD3 complexes on the cell surface. Recent experiments have shown that the CD3 chains are not the only calnexin associated molecules found on the surface of pre-T-cells *(40)*. Possibly, certain types of ER retention receptors are absent in pre-T-cells, allowing certain molecular chaperones to escape ER retention, thus providing a mechanism for surface expression of the pre-TCR. Consistent with this idea is that the pre-T-cell receptor is only expressed on the surface of immature, but not of mature T-cell lines that were transfected with a rearranged TCR-β chain gene and a pre-Tα gene *(19)*. The observed surface expression of CD3 dimers in the absence of TCR-β and pre-Tα chains probably has no specific role in T-cell development, but may simply reflect the absence of certain ER retention receptors. Indeed, T-cell maturation is normal until the pre-T-cell stage in mice that are deficient for the CD3γ, δ, and ε chains *(41)*. As will be discussed in Subheading 4. 2., the presence of these partial CD3 complexes has been useful in exploring the role of the pre-TCR in early T-cell development.

4. CD3-Mediated Responses of Pre-T-Cells

4.1. Regulation of Early T-Cell Development

The important role of the TCR-β chain in driving maturation of pre-T-cells to the DP stage is evident by analyzing thymocyte development in mice that cannot produce the TCR-β chain, such as rearrangement deficient (Rag-1$^-$, Rag-2$^-$, or severe combined immunodeficient [SCID]) or TCR-β deficient mice *(42–45)*. In such mice, thymocyte development does not proceed efficiently beyond the pre–T-cell stage. However, introduction of a functionally rearranged TCR-β transgene in these mice fully restores maturation of DP thymocytes *(43,46)*. Evidence for the importance of the other components of the pre-TCR also comes from gene-targeting experiments. In mice deficient for pre-Tα, CD3γ, δ, and ε, or CD3ζ, the DP population is absent or significantly decreased *(30–33,41,47,48)*.

The reason for regulation of T-cell development by the pre-TCR is the need to verify in frame rearrangement of the TCR-β locus. During the pre–T-cell stage, the TCR-β gene is formed by recombination of V (variable), D (diversity), J (joining), and C (constant) gene segments *(49)*. Initially, a D gene segment is brought into proximity of one of the J gene segments. Subsequently, a V gene segment is fused to the newly rearranged D-J region. During these recombination events, random nucleotides are inserted by the action of terminal deoxyribonucleotidyl transferase in order to increase diversification. Chances that this process leads to an in frame TCR-β gene are one out of three. T-cells are diploid cells, and contain two TCR-β loci. Therefore, the probability that a pre-T-cell produces an inframe TCR-β gene is one minus the probability of two failures: $1-(2/3)^2 = 5/9$. However, analysis of expression of the TCR-β chain by intracellular stainings reveals that 95% of all DP thymocytes have functionally rearranged the TCR-β locus *(50)*. Also, 75% of all TCR-β loci of DP thymocytes are in frame, in contrast to 33% expected in the absence of selection for functional TCR-β gene rearrangements *(51)*. Taken together, these experiments show that pre-T-cells are selected on the basis of in frame rearrangement of the TCR-β locus. Maturation events mediated by the pre-TCR are collectively called β-selection.

In addition to spurring pre-T-cells that successfully rearranged the TCR-β locus to continue maturation, the pre-TCR mediated selection event also functions as part of a feedback mechanism for controlling rearrangement of the TCR-β locus. In order to avoid the production of T-cells expressing two different TCR-β chains, V to D rearrangement on the second allele is inhibited upon production of the TCR-β chain *(52)*. This process is referred to as allelic exclusion.

Once the pre-TCR is expressed on the cell surface, it proclaims its presence by signal transduction through components of the CD3 complex. Crosslinking of CD3 complexes on pre-T-cells in fetal thymic organ cultures (FTOC) from mice incapable of producing the TCR-β chain (such as severe combined immunodeficiency [SCID] mice, or mice deficient for Rag-1, or TCR-β) fully restores development of DP thymocytes *(36–48)*. This shows that signals mediated by CD3 regulate this maturation step. Addition of anti-CD3 MAb to FTOC from wild-type mice before successful TCR-β gene rearrangement leads to the production of DP thymocytes that have both TCR-β loci in D-J configuration *(21,35)*. This indicates that the same CD3 mediated signal also inhibits V to D rearrangement of the TCR-β locus, and thus regulates allelic exclusion. How the signal through the pre-TCR is initiated is not clear. It is conceivable that a ligand for the pre-TCR is present on cortical epithelium, but no evidence for this exists yet.

4.2. Signaling Events in β-Selection

The tyrosine kinase p56[lck] (lck) plays a crucial role in signaling through the pre-TCR (*see* Fig. 3 for an overview of signaling pathways in T-cells). In mice in which the function of lck is disrupted by gene targeting or by introducing a dominant negative lck mutant, maturation of DP thymocytes is hampered *(20,53)*. Moreover, in mice transgenic for a constitutively active form of lck, V-D rearrangement of the TCR-β locus is inhibited *(54)* , as it is in anti-CD3ε-treated mice *(21)*. If the active lck transgene is introduced in Rag-1 deficient mice, maturation and expansion of DP thymocytes is fully restored *(55)*.

Some confusion arose with regard to the exact role of lck in β-selection, because of phenotypic differences between lck deficient mice and transgenic mice expressing a dominant negative lck mutant. The dominant negative mutant fully inhibits allelic exclusion of the TCR-β locus and development of DP thymocytes *(20,56)*. In lck deficient mice, however, some DP thymocytes develop, and allelic exclusion of the TCR-β locus is 85% complete *(53,57)*. What explains this discrepancy? Recently, it has been shown that the tyrosine kinase p59[fyn] (fyn) can partially substitute for lck in driving β-selection. In mice doubly deficient for fyn and lck, no DP thymocytes develop *(58,59)*. Therefore, it is likely that the dominant negative form of lck is capable of blocking the activities of both lck and fyn.

What remains surprising is the finding that in lck deficient mice, allelic exclusion is much less affected than the accumulation of DP thymocytes. A similar phenotype is observed in pre-Tα deficient mice *(48)*. A possible explanation is that early responses such as allelic exclusion, CD69 expression and downregulation of IL-2Rα depend on different signals than the proliferative response of DP thymocytes. However, there is no evidence for such differential signaling. In Rag-1 and lck double deficient mice, for example, anti-CD3 treatment did neither efficiently induce early responses nor the expansion of the DP pool *(60)*. An alternative explanation may be that allelic exclusion depends on a single signal, whereas proliferation of DP thymocytes depends on a continued signal through the pre-TCR. Thus, as long as some signal is mediated, allelic exclusion may still operate satisfactorily. The need for a sustained signal in driving proliferation of DP thymocytes is supported by the finding that restoring the deficient signaling capacity of the pre-TCR in CD3ζ-deficient mice by crosslinking with anti-CD3 antibodies results in enhanced proliferation of pre-existing DP thymocytes *(60)*.

Whatever the precise mechanisms of β-selection are, it is clear that signal transduction through CD3 components and activation of lck are involved. What is the contribution of each of the CD3 chains? It seems that CD3ε and CD3ζ are both important in signaling through the pre-TCR. Although it could not be shown that the CD3ζ chain is stably associated with the pre-TCR, several lines of evidence substantiate its engagement during β-selection. In CD3ζ deficient mice, DP thymocytes develop, but their number is 10–20-fold reduced *(30–33)*. Furthermore, crosslinking of the pre-TCR on pre–T-cell lines results in the phosphorylation of CD3ζ *(34)*. The CD3ζ mediated signal is not specific, though, as anti-CD3 treatment of Rag-1/CD3ζ double deficient mice fully restores maturation of DP thymocytes *(60)*. Furthermore, rearrangement of the TCR-β locus is effectively inhibited by crosslinking of CD3ε-containing complexes on thymocytes of CD3ζ-deficient mice *(61)*. Interestingly, the signal through CD3ε does not seem to be any more specific than that mediated by CD3ζ. This was shown by blastocyst reconstitution experiments. Rag-2 deficient ES cell lines were transfected with a transgene encoding the transmembrane and extracellular domains of the IL-2Rα chain

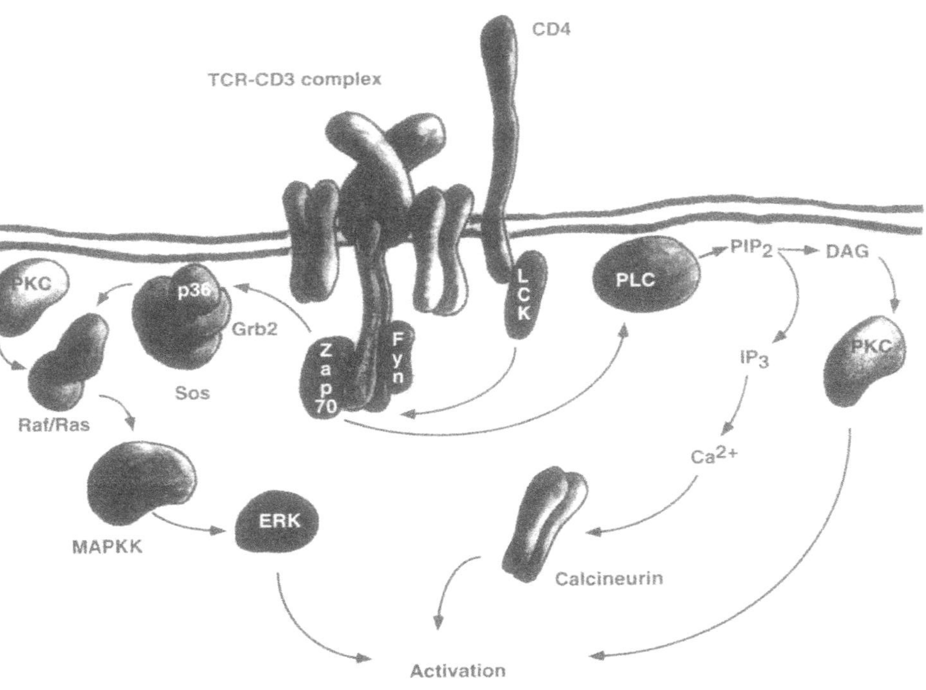

Fig. 3. The major signaling cascades regulating T-cell activation.

fused to the cytoplasmic domain of either CD3ε or CD3ζ. Pre-T-cells that developed from either of these ES cell lines could be induced to mature to the DP stage equally well by crosslinking with anti-IL-2Rα antibodies *(62)*. The role that the different CD3 proteins play in early T-cell development may be summarized as follows: The CD3ζ chain facilitates surface expression of the pre-TCR and amplifies its signaling capacity through its multiple ITAM's. The CD3ε chain is essential for the surface expression of the pre-TCR. This is not the case for the CD3δ chain, which is not required for the maturation of pre-T-cells *(63)*.

The downstream signals initiated by the CD3 chains of the pre-TCR complex remain elusive. What is clear though, is that maturation of DP thymocytes is independent of Zap-70, as Zap-70 deficient animals show no defect in T-cell development at this developmental stage *(64)*. Mobilization of extracellular Ca^{2+} is also not required for β-selection. In Rag-1 deficient, or CD3ζ deficient thymocytes, anti-CD3 crosslinking does not result in detectable Ca^{2+} influx, but does stimulate maturation to the DP stage *(36,60)*. Therefore, it is no surprise that inhibition of the Ca^{2+} dependent phosphatase calcineurin by CsA or FK506 has no effect on early thymocyte maturation *(61)*.

Although several signaling pathways can be ruled out, identification of second messengers that do regulate early thymocyte development remains problematic. In particular, experiments addressing the involvement of the $p21^{ras}$ (ras) signaling pathway in this process have produced conflicting results. In mice expressing dominant negative forms of MAP kinase kinase 1 (MAPKK1), ras, or both ras and MAPKK1, the appearance of DP thymocytes is not affected *(65–67)*. However, other experiments do support the involvement of MAPKK1 in β-selection. Infection of FTOCs with a retroviral vector expressing a dominant negative form of MAPKK1 has an inhibitory effect on anti-CD3 induced development of Rag-1 deficient thymocytes to the DP stage *(63)*. However, infection of Rag-1 deficient FTOCs with constitutively active forms of MAPKK1 or ras did not result in the production of DP thymocytes. To further complicate the picture, in Rag-2 deficient blastocyst reconstitution experiments, an active form of ras was described to stimulate production of DP thymocytes *(69)*. These results may be conflicting because of differences in the assays used, or in the inhibitory potential of the various dominant negative members of the ras signaling pathway. The elucidation of the role of the ras pathway in β-selection needs more extensive research, probably involving T-cell specific gene targeting experiments.

5. CD3-Mediated Responses of DP Thymocytes

5.1. Selection Events Imposed on DP Thymocytes

Once thymocytes have matured to the DP stage and successfully rearranged the TCR-α locus, they are subjected to repertoire selection. In order to create a T-cell repertoire that is self tolerant and capable of MHC-restricted antigen recognition, thymocytes are selected according the specificity of their receptor for allelic forms of MHC (Class I or Class II) and endogenous peptides associated with these molecules *(70,71)*. Thymocytes that have a TCR that interacts weakly with self-MHC/peptide complexes that are positively selected, as they are self-MHC-restricted and may be capable of recognizing foreign peptides with high affinity. Thymocytes that receive a strong signal through their TCR upon encountering self-MHC/peptide are negatively selected, as they would develop into potentially dangerous self-reactive T-cells *(72,73)*. Most thymocytes receive no signal at all, because their TCRs do not interact with self-MHC/peptide complexes. These cells continue rearrangement of the TCR-α genes and are subjected to selection if they generate a useful receptor within the three to four day life-span of the cell *(74)*.

Positively selected cells not only receive a signal for survival but also shut off the expression of one of the coreceptors, CD4 or CD8. Initially it was thought that depending on the engagement of the TCR and one of the coreceptors with Class I or Class II MHC, signals transmitted by the cytoplasmic tails of CD4 or CD8 instruct the cell which maturational pathway to follow *(75–77)*. Other studies suggested that the decision between development into $CD4^+$ or $CD8^+$ lineage T-cells is stochastic and that a second selection event is necessary for survival of thymocytes that retained the coreceptor matching the MHC restriction of the TCR *(78–80)*. Over the last few years, evidence has accumulated suggesting that the pathways are not symmetrical. Development into the $CD4^+$ pathway may be default, and maturation of $CD8^+$ cells may depend on second signals possibly provided by the cytoplasmic tail of CD8 *(81,92)*. A recent study suggests that a second signal driving the development of $CD8^+$ cells is mediated by the Notch 1 protein *(83)*. It is not known if the Notch signal correlates with an instructive signal or with a signal for survival of cells committed to the $CD8^+$ lineage.

It is not clear how differences in TCR ligand interactions result in different signals. Probably the number of TCRs that are engaged per time unit is crucial *(72)*. When this number is low, positive selection occurs, and when it is high, negative selection takes place. Some evidence exists that the longevity of the engagement between the TCR and MHC/peptide is an important factor influencing the outcome of T-cell selection *(84)*. This may explain why very high affinity ligands are not very efficient in mediating positive selection *(85)*.

Whatever the mechanisms of positive and negative selection are, it is clear that the signals involved are finely tuned, and depend on delicate differences in the type of TCR/MHC-peptide interactions. Consequently, only limited information can be obtained from studies involving ligation of TCR/CD3 complexes using antibodies. The current models of positive and negative selection have been derived predominantly from in vivo and in vitro studies using genetically engineered mice expressing a single TCR, a single TCR ligand, or both *(10–14,70–73,85–89)*. Nonetheless, antibody crosslinking studies have been useful to dissect the roles of the TCR and the coreceptors CD4 and CD8 to study consequences of different modes of TCR engagement and to analyze signal transduction pathways involved in T-cell selection.

5.2. Negative Selection

The first evidence that clonal deletion is mediated by death through apoptosis was obtained by addition of anti-CD3 antibodies to FTOCs *(90)*. It was shown that engaging the CD3/TCR complex on DP thymocytes with anti-CD3 antibodies produced cell death and DNA fragmentation typical of apoptosis. Similar results were obtained when examining thymuses from mice treated with anti-CD3 antibodies. The role of the coreceptors CD4 and CD8 in negative selection was also assessed using antibodies *(91)*. It was demonstrated that anti-CD3 or anti-TCR-β mediated negative selection is strongly enhanced when antibodies to CD4 or CD8 are also added to FTOCs. Some evidence implicating potential roles for costimulatory molecules in negative selection was obtained using a similar approach. For example, anti-CD3 induced apoptosis in FTOC can be enhanced by anti-CD28 antibodies *(92)* and inhibited by antibodies to LFA-1 *(93)* or Sca-2 (TSA-1) *(94)*. The implications of these studies are controversial, as mice deficient for CD28 or LFA-1 *(95,96)* show no alterations in negative selection. It is conceivable that the presence of multiple costimulatory molecules masks the function of each individually. But this is not supported by the finding that negative selection or anti-CD3 induced apoptosis are clearly affected in mice deficient of other costimulatory ligands such as CD30 *(97)* or CD40L *(98)*.

5.3. Positive Selection

Although antibodies to components of the TCR-CD3 complex have been used extensively for examining negative selection, only a few studies have provided evidence that positive selection can also be induced using antibodies. For example, hybrid antibodies with dual specificity for thymic epithelium and TCR-β have been shown to drive the maturation of $CD4^+$ SP thymocytes in FTOC, even in the complete absence of MHC class II molecules *(99)*. More recent experiments show that TCR engagement induces positive selection in FTOC when antibodies are used that cannot mediate TCR aggregation *(100)*. Crosslinking of such antibodies with protein A or using antibodies that do result in TCR aggregation lead to negative selection. An interpretation for this finding is that when thymocytes encounter low avidity ligands mediating positive selection, TCR aggregation does not occur because of the paucity of the ligand or the fast dissociation of the TCR-ligand interaction. In contrast, high avidity ligands are expected to mediate TCR aggregation resulting in negative selection. It is noteworthy that antibody-mediated positive selection always drives development into the $CD4^+$ pathway, supporting the notion that this may be the default pathway for T-cell maturation.

In another recent study, it was demonstrated that maturation of DP thymocytes into $CD4^+$ SP thymocytes could be driven by antibody mediated TCR engagement and ligation of costimulatory molecules such as CD2, CD5, CD24, CD28, CD49d, CD81, and TSA-1 in the complete absence of thymic stroma *(101)*. This type of experiments that employ antibodies as artificial mediation of selection, may help to identify signaling pathways that are involved in positive selection.

5.4. Signaling Pathways Involved in Positive and Negative Selection

Since anti-CD3 antibodies induce Ca^{2+} influx in immature T-cells and mediate negative selection when added to FTOCs, initial experiments focused on the role of Ca^{2+} mobilization in clonal deletion. It was demonstrated that the calcium ionophore ionomycin induces apoptosis in DP thymocytes *(90,102)*. Moreover, when anti-CD3 antibodies were added to DP thymocytes together with a calcium chelator, induction of programmed cell death is reduced to background levels. Therefore, it seems that mobilization of extracellular Ca^{2+} is essential for the induction of negative selection. In thymuses from mice transgenic for a self-reactive TCR, representing a more physiological model of negative selection, a large number of DP thymocytes with increased levels of intracellular Ca^{2+} are detected *(103)*. At the same time, Ca^{2+} influx by itself is not always sufficient, and although addition of Conavalin A to FTOC also results in Ca^{2+} mobilization, it does not induce apoptosis *(104)*. Therefore, negative selection must be controlled by the strength or duration of the calcium signal and/or additional signaling pathways *(105)*. The same conclusions were reached from studies on the role of phosphatidyl inositol triphosphate hydrolysis, an upstream event of Ca^{2+} mobilization *(5,16)*. When thymocyte responses to anti-CD3, Conavalin A and other mitogenic substances are measured in thymic organ cultures from newborn mice (NTOC), it is observed that like Ca^{2+} mobilization, phosphatidyl inositol triphosphate hydrolysis is essential, but not sufficient, for mediating apoptosis.

The calcium-dependent phosphatase calcineurin is an important signal transduction intermediate in the activation of mature T-cells. Therefore, calcineurin has been suspected to also play a role in downstream events mediating negative selection. However, ablation of calcineurin activity using CsA or FK506 does not inhibit anti-CD3 or peptide-ligand induced apoptosis of DP thymocytes *(61)*. These findings suggest that other calcium-dependent enzymes mediate negative selection. Since the calcineurin inhibitor FK506 does hinder positive selection, it must be assumed that different calcium-dependent signal transduction pathways distinguish positive from negative selection.

Recently, the ras pathway has received attention for its differential role in positive and negative selection. Mice expressing dominant negative forms of kinases of the Ras pathway such as raf, ras, and MAPKK1 show defects in positive selection, whereas negative selection is not affected *(65–67,106)*. These exciting results have to be interpreted with some caution, because the inhibitory effect of these dominant negative molecules may not be complete. It is thus conceivable that weak signals involved in positive selection are more severely affected than strong signals resulting in negative selection. But an important role for the ras pathway in inducing positive selection is also supported by experiments analyzing T-cell selection events in response to the phorbol ester PMA, which activates the ras pathway independently of TCR signaling by activating Protein Kinase C (PKC). It was found that when added at low concentrations together with ionomycin, PMA mediates the maturation of $CD4^+$ SP T-cells in FTOC or suspension cultures *(108,109)*.

What are the events upstream of ras activation or phosphatidyl inositol triphosphate hydrolysis? The main players are the tyrosine kinases fyn, lck, and Zap-70 (*110*; for review, *see* ref. *38*). Lck associates with CD4 or CD8 and upon crosslinking of the TCR, phosphorylates the tyrosines in the ITAMs of CD3 chains. Fyn has a similar specificity to lck, but may have a preference for the CD3ζ chain *(111)*. Phosphorylation of the CD3 chains leads to recruitment of Zap-70 through its SH2 domains. When Zap-70 is brought in proximity of the TCR complex, it may become activated by lck or fyn mediated phosphorylation. Active Zap-70 subsequently phosphorylates p36, which in turn associates with adaptor molecules and guanine exchange proteins. These complexes mediate activation of ras and inositol phopholipid metabolism. In lck deficient mice, very few T-cells develop *(53)*. This is partially because of defective development of DP cells, but positive selection and expansion of peripheral T-cells are also impaired. Injection of anti-CD3ε MAb into lck deficient mice does not result in the deletion of DP thymocytes. At first glance this may seem to imply that negative selection is lck dependent. But as lck deficient DP thymocytes are also resistant to (lck independent) dexamethasone induced apoptosis, it is more likely that the DP thymocytes in these mice do not effectively reach an apoptosis sensitive stage *(60)*. Fyn's role in T-cell selection is less significant. Although thymocytes from fyn deficient mice show inhibition of Ca^{2+} mobilization upon TCR crosslinking, positive and negative selection events are not severely affected *(112,113)*.

Mice in which the Zap-70 gene is disrupted by homologous recombination show a different phenotype. In these mice, positive selection is completely blocked, and no single positive thymocytes or mature T-cells are detected. Negative selection is similarly perturbed, and neither anti-CD3 nor MHC-peptide ligands can induce apoptosis of DP thymocytes *(64)*. In contrast to lck-deficient mice, DP thymocytes are present in normal numbers and are sensitive to dexamethasone induced apoptosis, suggesting that maturation events that occur before positive or negative selection are unaffected in the absence of Zap-70.

Recently, it was demonstrated that in immature thymocytes, the phosphorylation of Zap-70 upon TCR crosslinking is inefficient because of the sequestration of lck by CD4. Only when CD4 or CD8 are coaggregated, bringing coreceptor associated lck in the proximity of the TCR complex, phosphorylation of Zap-70 is observed *(114)*. However, in other experiments mentioned in Subheading 5.3., antibody mediated engagement of TCR's resulted in positive or negative selection even in the absence of coreceptor engagement *(100)*. Hence, the extent of the inefficiency of Zap-70 phosphorylation in immature thymocytes and the implications for thymic selection are not clear.

Anti-CD3 antibodies do not only have direct effects on thymocytes, but may also influence T-cell development via the induction of cytokines *(115)*. Crosslinking of TCRs on DP thymocytes induces the production of lymphokines such as IL-4, GM-CSF, TNF-α, and IFN-γ. These factors activate macrophages, dendritic cells, and thymic epithelium to upregulate the expression of cell surface proteins such as MHC molecules and cytokine receptors and to produce other cytokines including IL-1 and Mig. Cytokines may influence T-cell selection, for example by sustaining the TCR mediated apoptosis signal and may be required for the clearance of apoptotic thymocytes by macrophages.

6. Extrathymic T-Cell Development

Most studies exploring the effects of ligation of CD3-containing complexes on T-cell development have focused on intrathymic selection events. But anti-CD3 antibodies also mediate phenotypic changes of CD3-containing cells in the gut, spleen, and lymph nodes of Rag-1 or -2 deficient mice. In the spleen and lymph nodes of Rag-1 deficient mice, small numbers of cells are found that express Thy1.2, Pgp-1, Rag-2, intracellular CD3ε, and probably pre-Tα. Crosslinking of CD3ε results in their proliferation, downregulation of Pgp-1, and, in some cells, upregulation of CD4 and CD8 *(116)*. These cells are thymus-dependent, as anti-CD3 induced expansion of this population is strongly reduced one month after thymectomy. The physiological significance of this finding is not clear. It is possible that some immature T-cells leave the thymus and home to peripheral lymphoid organs. Such cells may follow an alternative developmental pathway, as has been shown for intestinal epithelial lymphocytes, which complete maturation in the gut. Alternatively, the thymus may provide endocrine factors, which are required for the survival of immature cells in the periphery. Recently it was shown that full T-cell maturation can occur in lymph nodes from mice transgenic for oncostatin M (OM), or upon treatment of wild type mice with this cytokine *(117)*. It is conceivable that the pro–T-cell like cells found in the secondary lymphoid organs of Rag-1 deficient mice are identical to the precursor cells that give rise to mature T-cells in OM-transgenic animals. In contrast to anti-CD3 induced responses, peripheral T-cell development in OM transgenic mice is thymus independent. Possibly, the transgene encoded OM overcomes the need for OM or other endocrine factors produced by the thymus.

Phenotypic changes in T-cell lineage cells are also seen in the gut of Rag-2 deficient mice after injection of anti-CD3 antibodies. In the gut, three major T-cell types of intra epithelial lymphocytes (IEL) are recognized: CD8$\alpha^+\beta^+$TCR$\alpha\beta^+$, CD8$\alpha^+\beta^-$TCR$\alpha\beta^+$, and CD8$\alpha^+\beta^-$TCR$\gamma\delta^+$ T-cells. A subset of the CD8$\alpha^+\beta^-$ T-cells expresses B220 and FcγRIII. These cells can replace the CD3ζ chain of the TCR-CD3 complex with the FcεRIγ chain, which is part of the FcγRIII complex. In the intestine of Rag-2 deficient mice, CD8$\alpha^+\beta^+$ IELs do not mature, but CD8$\alpha^+\beta^-$FcγRIII$^+$B220$^+$ IELs (obviously not expressing TCR-$\alpha\beta$ or -$\gamma\delta$ chains) are present. Treatment of Rag-2 deficient mice with anti-CD3 antibodies results in the downregulation of B220 and FcγRIII on these cells *(116)*. This finding indicates that CD8$\alpha^+\beta^-$FcγRIII$^+$B220$^+$ IELs are precursors of CD8$\alpha^+\beta^-$FcγRIII$^-$B220$^-$ IELs, and that their maturation depends on signaling through CD3. This idea is supported by the observation that CD8$\alpha^+\beta^-$FcγRIII$^+$B220$^+$ IELs from wild-type mice develop into CD8$\alpha^+\beta^-$FcγRIII$^-$B220$^-$ IELs when transferred to Rag-2 deficient recipients.

7. Future Directions

Many of the principles governing T-cell selection events have been extensively researched and are understood in great detail. Yet, some important questions remain unanswered. For example, it is unclear if the signal through the pre-TCR is initiated by interaction with a specific ligand or if the pre-TCR is capable of signaling autonomously. The downstream signaling events regulating β-selection will need further analysis, as recent studies have produced conflicting results. Furthermore, it remains unknown how allelic exclusion of the TCR-β locus is regulated at the molecular level. And last, it is still not fully understood how the TCR is capable of transducing signals regulating entirely different developmental programs depending on the nature of its ligand and on the involvement of various costimulatory molecules. Resolving this question has proved a tour de force but is of major importance for our understanding of the formation of the T-cell repertoire and maintaining tolerance.

Acknowledgments

The author is grateful to Drs. Werner Haas, David Gerber, and Johannes Huppa for the critical reading of the manuscript. The author is supported by the Cancer Research Institute.

References

1. Wu, L., Scollay, R., Egerton, M., Pearse, M., Spangrude, G. J., and Shortman, K. (1991. CD4 expressed on earliest T-lineage precursor cells in the adult murine thymus. *Nature* **349,** 71–74.
2. Shortman, K. and Wu, L. (1996) Early T lymphocyte progenitors. *Annu. Rev. Immunol.* 14, 29–47.
3. Wilson, A. and MacDonald, H. R. (1995) Expression of genes encoding the pre-TCR and CD3 complex during thymus development. *Int. Immunol.* **7,** 1659–1664.
4. Hozumi, K., Kondo, M., Nozaki, H., Kobori, A., Nishimura, T., Nishikawa, S., Sugamura, K., and Habu, S. (1994) Implication of the common gamma chain of the IL-7 receptor in intrathymic development of pro-T cells. *Int. Immunol.* **6,** 1451–1454.
5. Peschon, J. J., Morrissey, P. J., Grabstein, K. H., Ramsdell, F. J., Maraskovsky, E., Gliniak, B. C., Park, L. S., Ziegler, S. F., Williams, D. E., Ware, C. B., et al. (1994) Early lymphocyte expansion is severely impaired in interleukin 7 receptor-deficient mice. *J. Exp. Med.* **180,** 1955–1960.
6. Rodewald, H. R., Kretzschmar, K., Swat, K., and Takeda, S. (1995) Intrathymically expressed c-kit ligand (stem cell factor) is a major factor driving expansion of very immature thymocytes in vivo. *Immunity* **3,** 313–319.
7. von Freeden-Jeffry, U., Vieira, P., Lucian, L. A., McNeil, T., Burdach, S. E., and Murray, R. (1995) Lymphopenia in interleukin (IL)-7 gene-deleted mice identifies IL-7 as a nonredundant cytokine. *J. Exp. Med.* **181,** 1519–1526.
8. Oosterwegel, M. A., Haks, M. C., Jeffry, U., Murray, R., and Kruisbeek, A. M. (1997) Induction of TCR gene rearrangements in uncommitted stem cells by a subset of IL-7 producing, MHC class-II-expressing thymic stromal cells. *Immunity* **6,** 351–360.
9. Rodewald, H. R., Ogawa, M., Haller, C., Waskow, C., and DiSanto, J. P. (1997) Pro-thymocyte expansion by c-kit and the common cytokine receptor gamma chain is essential for repertoire formation. *Immunity* **6,** 265–272.
10. Dudley, E. C., Girardi, M., Owen, M. J., and Hayday, A. C. (1995) Alpha beta and gamma delta T cells can share a late common precursor. *Curr. Biol.* **5,** 659–669.

11. Kang, J., Baker, J., and Raulet, D. H. (1995) Evidence that productive rearrangements of TCR gamma genes influence the commitment of progenitor cells to differentiate into alpha beta or gamma delta T cells. *Eur. J. Immunol.* **25,** 2706–2709.
12. Livak, F., Petrie, H. T., Crispe, I. N., and Schatz, D. G. (1995) In-frame TCR delta gene rearrangements play a critical role in the alpha beta/gamma delta T cell lineage decision. *Immunity* **2,** 617–627.
13. Wilson, A., J. P. de Villartay and MacDonald, H. R. (1996) T cell receptor delta gene rearrangement and T early alpha (TEA) expression in immature alpha beta lineage thymocytes: implications for alpha beta/gamma delta lineage commitment. *Immunity* **4,** 37–45.
14. Washburn, T., Schweighoffer, E., Gridley, T., Chang, D., Fowlkes, B. J., Cado, D., and Robey, E. (1997) Notch activity influences the αβ versus γδ T cell lineage decision. *Cell* **88,** 833–843.
15. Godfrey, D. I., Kenney, J., Mombaerts, P., Tonegawa, S., and Zlotnik, A. (1994) Onset of TCR-beta rearrangement and role of TCR-beta expression during CD3-CD4-CD8- thymocyte differentiation. *J. Immunol.* **152,** 4783–4792.
16. Hozumi, K., Kobori, A., Sato, T., Nozaki, H., Nishikawa, S., Nishimura, T., and Habu, S. (1994) Pro-T cells in fetal thymus express c-kit and RAG-2 but do not rearrange the gene encoding the T cell receptor beta chain. *Eur. J. Immunol.* **24,** 1339–1344.
17. Wilson, A., Held, W., and MacDonald, H. R. (1994) Two waves of recombinase gene expression in developing thymocytes. *J. Exp. Med.* **179,** 1355–1360.
18. Groettrup, M., U. K., Azogui, O., Palacios, R., Owen, M. J., Hayday, A. C., and von Boehmer, H. (1993) A novel disulfide-linked heterodimer on pre-T cells consists of the T cell receptor beta chain and a 33 kd glycoprotein. *Cell* **75,** 283–294.
19. Saint-Ruf, C., Ungewiss, K., Groettrup, M., Bruno, L., Fehling, H. J., and von Boehmer, H. (1994) Analysis and expression of a cloned pre-T cell receptor gene. *Science* **266,** 1208–1212.
20. Levin, S. D., Anderson, S. J., Forbush, K. A., and Perlmutter, R. M. (1993) A dominant-negative transgene defines a role for p56lck in thymopoiesis. *EMBO J.* **12,** 1671–1680.
21. Levelt, C. N., Wang, B., Ehrfeld, A., Terhorst, C., and Eichmann, K. (1995) Regulation of T cell receptor (TCR)-beta locus allelic exclusion and initiation of TCR-alpha locus rearrangement in immature thymocytes by signaling through the CD3 complex. *Eur. J. Immunol.* **25,** 1257–1261.
22. Kisielow, P., Teh, H. S., Bluthmann, H., and von Boehmer, H. (1988) Positive selection of antigen-specific T cells in thymus by restricting MHC molecules. *Nature* **335,** 730–733.
23. Gold, D. P., Clevers, H., Alarcon, B., Dunlap, S., Novotny, J., Williams, A. F., and Terhorst, C. (1987) Evolutionary relationship between the T3 chains of the T-cell receptor complex and the immunoglobulin supergene family. *Proc. Natl. Acad. Sci. USA* **84,** 7649-7653.
24. Mallabiabarrena, A., Fresno, M., and Alarcon, B. (1992) An endoplasmic reticulum retention signal in the CD3 epsilon chain of the T-cell receptor. *Nature* **357,** 593–596.
25. Weissman, A. M., Hou, D., Orloff, D. G., Modi, W. S., Seuanez, H., O'Brien, S. J., and Klausner, R. D. (1988) Molecular cloning and chromosomal localization of the human T-cell receptor zeta chain: distinction from the molecular CD3 complex. *Proc. Natl. Acad. Sci. USA* **85,** 9709–9713.
26. Kuster, H., Thompson, H., and Kinet, J. P. (1990) Characterization and expression of the gene for the human Fc receptor gamma subunit. Definition of a new gene family. *J. Biol. Chem.* **265,** 6448–6452.
27. Kearse, K. P., Roberts, J. L., and Singer, A. (1995) TCR alpha-CD3 delta epsilon association is the initial step in αβ dimer formation in murine T cells and is limiting in immature $CD4^+$ $CD8^+$ thymocytes. *Immunity* **2,** 391–399.
27a. Punt, J. A., Roberts, J. L., Kearse, K. P. and Singer, A. (1994) Stoichiometry of the T cell antigen receptor (TCR) complex: each TCR/CD3 complex contains one TCR alpha, one TCR beta, and two CD3 epsilon chains. *J. Exp. Med.* **180,** 587–593.
28. Sussman, J. J., Bonifacino, J. S., Lippincott-Schwartz, J., Weissman, A. M., Saito, T., Klausner, R. D., and Ashwell, J. D. (1988) Failure to synthesize the T cell CD3-zeta chain, structure and function of a partial T cell receptor complex. *Cell* **52,** 85–95.
29. Wegener, A. M., Letourneur, F., Hoeveler, A., Brocker, T., Luton, F., and Malissen, B. (1992) The T cell receptor/CD3 complex is composed of at least two autonomous transduction modules. *Cell* **68,** 83–95.
30. Liu, C. P., Ueda, R., She, J., Sancho, J., Wang, B., Weddell, G., Loring, J., Kurahara, C., Dudley, E. C., Hayday, A., et al. (1993) Abnormal T cell development in CD3-$zeta^{-/-}$ mutant mice and identification of a novel T cell population in the intestine. *EMBO J.* **12,** 4863–4875.

31. Love, P. E., Shores, E. W., Johnson, M. D., Tremblay, M. L., Lee, E. J., Grinberg, A., Huang, S. P., Singer, A., and Westphal, H. (1993) T cell development in mice that lack the zeta chain of the T cell antigen receptor complex. *Science* **261,** 918–921.
32. Malissen, M., Gillet, A., Rocha, B., Trucy, J., Vivier, E., Boyer, C., Kontgen, F., Brun, N., Mazza, G., Spanopoulou, E., et al. (1993) T cell development in mice lacking the CD3-zeta/eta gene. *EMBO J.* **12,** 4347-4355.
33. Ohno, H., Goto, S., Taki, S., Shirasawa, T., Nakano, H., Miyatake, S., Aoe, T., Ishida, Y., Maeda, H., Shirai, T. et al. (1994) Targeted disruption of the CD3 eta locus causes high lethality in mice: modulation of Oct-1 transcription on the opposite strand. *EMBO J.* **13,** 1157–1165.
34. van Oers, N. S., von Boehmer, H., and Weiss, A. (1995) The pre-T cell receptor (TCR) complex is functionally coupled to the TCR-zeta subunit. *J. Exp. Med.* **182,** 1585–1590.
35. Levelt, C. N., Ehrfeld, A., and Eichmann, K. (1993) Regulation of thymocyte development through CD3. I. Timepoint of ligation of CD3 epsilon determines clonal deletion or induction of developmental program. *J. Exp. Med.* **177,** 707–716.
36. Levelt, C. N., Mombaerts, P., Iglesias, A., Tonegawa, S., and Eichmann, K. (1993) Restoration of early thymocyte differentiation in T-cell receptor beta- chain-deficient mutant mice by transmembrane signaling through CD3 epsilon. *Proc. Natl. Acad. Sci. USA* **90,** 11,401–11,405.
37. Jacobs, H., Vandeputte, D., Tolkamp, L., de, V. E., Borst, J., and Berns, A. (1994) CD3 components at the surface of pro-T cells can mediate pre-T cell development in vivo. *Eur. J. Immunol.* **24,** 934–939.
38. Shinkai, Y. and Alt, F. W. (1994) CD3 epsilon-mediated signals rescue the development of $CD4^+CD8^+$ thymocytes in RAG-$2^{-/-}$ mice in the absence of TCR beta chain expression. *Int. Immunol.* **6,** 995–1001.
39. Wiest, D. L., Kearse, K. P., Shores, E. W. and Singer, A. (1994) Developmentally regulated expression of CD3 components independent of clonotypic T cell antigen receptor complexes on immature thymocytes. *J. Exp. Med.* **180,** 1375–1382.
40. Wiest, D. L., Bhandoola, A., Punt, J., Kreibich, G., McKean, D., and Singer, A. (1997) Incomplete endoplasmic reticulum (ER) retention in immature thymocytes as revealed by surface expression of "ER-resident" molecular chaperones. *Proc. Natl. Acad. Sci. USA* **94,** 1884–1889.
41. Malissen, M., Gillet, A., Ardouin, L., Bouvier, G., Trucy, J., Ferrier, P., Vivier, E., and Malissen, B. (1995) Altered T cell development in mice with a targeted mutation of the CD3- epsilon gene. *EMBO J.* **14,** 4641–4653.
42. Bosma, M. J. and Carroll, A. M. (1991) The Scid mouse mutant: definition, characterization and potential uses. *Annu. Rev. Immunol.* **9,** 323–335.
43. Mombaerts, P., Clarke, A. R., Rudnicki, M. A., Iacomini, J., Itohara, S., Lafaille, J. J., Wang, L., Ichikawa, Y., Jaenisch, R., Hooper, M. L., et al. (1992) Mutations in T-cell antigen receptor genes alpha and beta block thymocyte development at different stages. *Nature* **360,** 225–231.
44. Mombaerts, P., Iacomini, J., Johnson, R. S., Herrup, K., Tonegawa, S., and Papaioannou, V. E. (1992) RAG-1-deficient mice have no mature B and T lymphocytes. *Cell* 68, 869–877.
45. Shinkai, Y., G. Rathbun, K. P. Lam, E. M. Oltz, V. Stewart, M. Mendelsohn, J. Charron, M. Datta, F. Young, A. M. Stall et al. (1992. RAG-2-deficient mice lack mature lymphocytes owing to inability to initiate V(D)J rearrangement. *Cell* **68,** 855–867.
46. Shinkai, Y., Koyasu, S., Nakayama, K., Murphy, K. M., Loh, D. Y., Reinherz, E. L., and Alt, F. W. (1993) Restoration of T cell development in RAG-2-deficient mice by functional TCR transgenes. *Science* **259,** 822–825.
47. Fehling, H. J., Krotkova, A., Saint-Ruf, C., and von Boehmer, H. (1995) Crucial role of the pre-T-cell receptor alpha gene in development of alpha beta but not gamma delta T cells. *Nature* **375,** 795–798.
48. Xu, Y., Davidson, L., Alt, F. W., and Baltimore, D. (1996) Function of the pre-T-cell receptor alpha chain in T-cell development and allelic exclusion at the T-cell receptor beta locus. *Proc Natl. Acad. Sci. USA* **93,** 2169–2173.
49. Prosser, H. M. and Tonegawa, S. (1995) T cell receptor V(D)J recombination: mechanisms and developmental regulation, in *T Cell Receptors* (Bell, J. I., Owen, M. J., and Simpson, E., eds.) Oxford, Oxford University Press, pp. 326–351.
50. Levelt, C. N., Carsetti, R., and Eichmann, K. (1993) Regulation of thymocyte development through CD3. II. Expression of T cell receptor beta CD3 epsilon and maturation to the $CD4^+8^+$ stage are highly correlated in individual thymocytes. *J. Exp. Med.* **178,** 1867–1875.

51. Mallick, C. A., Dudley, E. C., Viney, J. L., Owen, M. J., and Hayday, A. C. (1993) Rearrangement and diversity of T cell receptor beta chain genes in thymocytes: a critical role for the beta chain in development. *Cell* **73,** 513–519.
52. Borgulya, P., Kishi, H., Uematsu, Y., and von Boehmer, H. (1992) Exclusion and inclusion of alpha and beta T cell receptor alleles. *Cell* **69,** 529–536.
53. Molina, T. J., Kishihara, K., Siderovski, D. P., van Ewijk, W., Narendran, A., Timms, E., Wakeham, A., Paige, C. J., Hartmann, K. U., Veillette, A., et al. (1992) Profound block in thymocyte development in mice lacking $p56^{lck}$. *Nature* **357,** 161–164.
54. Anderson, S. J., Abraham, K. M., Nakayama, T., Singer, A., and Perlmutter, R. M. (1992) Inhibition of T-cell receptor beta-chain gene rearrangement by overexpression of the non-receptor protein tyrosine kinase $p56^{lck}$. *EMBO J.* B 4877–4886.
55. Mombaerts, P., Anderson, S. J., Perlmutter, R. M., Mak, T. W., and Tonegawa, S. (1994) An activated lck transgene promotes thymocyte development in RAG-1 mutant mice. *Immunity* **1,** 261–267.
56. Anderson, S. J., Levin, S. D., and Perlmutter, R. M. (1993) Protein tyrosine kinase p56lck controls allelic exclusion of T-cell receptor beta-chain genes. *Nature* **365,** 552–554.
57. Wallace, V. A., Kawai, K., Levelt, C. N., Kishihara, K., Molina, T., Timms, E., Pircher, H., Penninger, J., Ohashi, P. S., Eichmann, K., et al. (1995) T lymphocyte development in $p56^{lck}$ deficient mice: allelic exclusion of the TCR beta locus is incomplete but thymocyte development is not restored by TCR beta or TCR alpha beta transgenes. *Eur. J. Immunol.* **25,** 1312–1318.
58. Groves, T., Smiley, P., Cooke, M. P., Forbush, K., Perlmutter, R. M., and Guidos, C. J. (1996) Fyn can partially substitute for Lck in T lymphocyte development. *Immunity* **5,** 417–428.
59. van Oers, N. S., Lowin, K. B., Finlay, D., Connolly, K., and Weiss, A. (1996) alpha beta T cell development is abolished in mice lacking both Lck and Fyn protein tyrosine kinases. *Immunity* **5,** 429–436.
60. Levelt, C. N., Mombaerts, P., Wang, B., Kohler, H., Tonegawa, S., Eichmann, K., and Terhorst, C. (1995) Regulation of thymocyte development through CD3, functional dissociation between p56lck and CD3 sigma in early thymic selection. *Immunity* **3,** 215–222.
61. Wang, C. R., Hashimoto, K., Kubo, S., Yokochi, T., Kubo, M., Suzuki, M., Suzuki, K., Tada, T., and Nakayama, T. (1995) T cell receptor-mediated signaling events in $CD4^+CD8^+$ thymocytes undergoing thymic selection: requirement of calcineurin activation for thymic positive selection but not negative selection. *J. Exp. Med.* **181,** 927–941.
62. Shinkai, Y., Ma, A., Cheng, H. L., and Alt, F. W. (1995) CD3 epsilon and CD3 zeta cytoplasmic domains can independently generate signals for T cell development and function. *Immunity* **2,** 401–411.
63. Dave, V. P., Cao, Z., Browne, C., Alarcon, B., Fernandez-Miguel, G., Lafaille, J., de la Hera, A., Tonegawa, S., and Kappes, D. J. (1997) CD3delta deficiency arrests development of the alpha beta but not the gamma delta T cell lineage. *EMBO J.* **16,** 1360–1370.
64. Negishi, I., Motoyama, N., Nakayama, K., Nakayama, K., Senju, S., Hatakeyama, S., Zhang, Q., Chan, A. C., and Loh, D. Y. (1995) Essential role for ZAP-70 in both positive and negative selection of thymocytes. *Nature* **376,** 435–438.
65. Alberola-Ila, J., Forbush, K. A., Seger, R., Krebs, E. G., and Perlmutter, R. M. (1995) Selective requirement for MAP kinase activation in thymocyte differentiation. *Nature* **373,** 620–623.
66. Alberola-Ila, J., K. A. Hogquist, K. A. Swan, M. J. Bevan and R. M. Perlmutter. (1996) Positive and negative selection invoke distinct signaling pathways. *J. Exp. Med.* **184,** 9–18.
67. Swan, K. A., Alberola-Ila, J., Gross, J. A., Appleby, M. W., Forbush, K. A., Thomas, J. F. and Perlmutter, R. M. (1995) Involvement of p21ras distinguishes positive and negative selection in thymocytes. *EMBO J.* **14,** 276–285.
68. Crompton, T., Gilmour, K. C., and Owen, M. J. (1996) The MAP kinase pathway controls differentiation from double-negative to double-positive thymocyte. *Cell* **86,** 243–251.
69 Swat, W., Shinkai, Y., Cheng, H. L., Davidson, L. and Alt, F. W. (1996) Activated Ras signals differentiation and expansion of $CD4^+8^+$ thymocytes. *Proc. Natl. Acad. Sci. USA* **93,** 4683–4687.
70. Benoist, B. and Mathis, D. (1997) Positive selection of T cells: fastidious or promiscuous? *Curr. Opin. Immunol.* **9,** 245–249.
71. Marrack, P. and Kappler, J. (1997) Positive selection of thymocytes bearing $\alpha\beta$ T cell receptors. *Curr. Opin. Immunol.* **9,** 250–255.
72. Ashton-Rickardt, P., Bandeira, A., Delaney, J. R., van Kaer, L., Pircher, H. P., Zinkernagel, R. M. and Tonegawa, S. (1994) Evidence for a differential avidity model of T cell selection in the thymus. *Cell* **76,** 651–663.

73. Hogquist, K. A., Jameson, S. C., Heath, W. R., Howard, J. L., Bevan, M. J. and Carbone, F. R. (1994) T cell receptor antagonist peptides induce positive selection. *Cell* **76,** 17–27.
74. Petrie, H. T., Livak, F., Schatz, D. G., Strasser, A., Crispe, I. N. and Shortman, K. (1993) Multiple rearrangements in T cell receptor alpha chain genes maximize the production of useful thymocytes. *J. Exp. Med.* **178,** 615–622.
75. Robey, E. A., Fowlkes, B. J., Gordon, J. W., Kioussis, D., von, B. H., Ramsdell, F., and Axel, R. (1991) Thymic selection in CD8 transgenic mice supports an instructive model for commitment to a CD4 or CD8 lineage. *Cell* **64,** 99–107.
76. Itano, A., Cado, D., Chan, F. K., and Robey, E. (1994) A role for the cytoplasmic tail of the beta chain of CD8 in thymic selection. *Immunity* **1,** 287–290.
77. Itano, A., Salmon, P., Kioussis, D., Tolaini, M., Corbella, P. and Robey, E. (1996) The cytoplasmic domain of CD4 promotes the development of CD4 lineage T cells. *J. Exp. Med.* **183,** 731–741.
78. Chan, S. H., Cosgrove, D., Waltzinger, C., Benoist, C., and Mathis, D. (1993) Another view of the selective model of thymocyte selection. *Cell* **73,** 225–236.
79. Crump, A. L., Grusby, M. J., Glimcher, L. H., and Cantor, H. (1993) Thymocyte development in major histocompatibility complex-deficient mice: evidence for stochastic commitment to the CD4 and CD8 lineages. *Proc. Natl. Acad. Sci. USA* **90,** 10739–10743.
80. Davis, C. B., Killeen, N., Crooks, M. E., Raulet, D., and Littman, D. R. (1993) Evidence for a stochastic mechanism in the differentiation of mature subsets of T lymphocytes. *Cell* **73,** 237–247.
81. Punt, J. A., Suzuki, H., Granger, L. G., Sharrow, S. O., and Singer, A. (1996) Lineage commitment in the thymus: only the most differentiated ($TCR^{hi}bcl\text{-}2^{hi}$) subset of $CD4^+CD8^+$ thymocytes has selectively terminated CD4 or CD8 synthesis. *J. Exp. Med.* **184,** 2091–2099.
82. Suzuki, H., Punt, J. A., Granger, L. G., and Singer, A. (1995) Asymmetric signaling requirements for thymocyte commitment to the $CD4^+$ versus $CD8^+$ T cell lineages: a new perspective on thymic commitment and selection. *Immunity* **2,** 413–425.
83. Robey, E., Chang, D., Itano, A., Cado, D., Alexander, H., Lans, D., Weinmaster, G., and Salmon, P. (1996) An activated form of Notch influences the choice between CD4 and CD8 T cell lineages. *Cell* **87,** 483–492.
84. Alam, S. M., Travers, P. J., Wung, J. L., Nasholds, W., Redpath, S., Jameson, S. C., and Gascoigne, N. R. (1996) T-cell-receptor affinity and thymocyte positive selection. *Nature* **381,** 616–620.
85. Hogquist, K. A., Jameson, S. C., and Bevan, M. J. (1995) Strong agonist ligands for the T cell receptor do not mediate positive selection of functional $CD8^+$ T cells. *Immunity* **3,** 79–86.
86. Fung, L. W., Surh, C. D., Liljedahl, M., Pang, J., Leturcq, D., Peterson, P. A., Webb, S. R., and Karlsson, L. (1996) Antigen presentation and T cell development in H2-M-deficient mice. *Science* **271,** 1278–1281.
87. Ignatowicz, L., Kappler, J., and Marrack, P. (1996) The repertoire of T cells shaped by a single MHC/peptide ligand. *Cell* **84,** 521–529.
88. Martin, W. D., Hicks, G. G., Mendiratta, S. K., Leva, H. I., Ruley, H. E., and Van, K. L. (1996) H2-M mutant mice are defective in the peptide loading of class II molecules, antigen presentation, and T cell repertoire selection. *Cell* **84,** 543–550.
89. Miyazaki, T., Wolf, P., Tourne, S., Waltzinger, C., Dierich, A., Barois, N., Ploegh, H., Benoist, C., and Mathis, D. (1996) Mice lacking H2-M complexes, enigmatic elements of the MHC class II peptide-loading pathway. *Cell* **84,** 531–541.
90. Smith, C. A., Williams, G. T., Kingston, R., Jenkinson, E. J., and Owen, J. J. (1989) Antibodies to CD3/T-cell receptor complex induce death by apoptosis in immature T cells in thymic cultures. *Nature* **337,** 181–184.
91. McConkey, D. J., Fosdick, L., D'Adamio, L., Jondal, M., and Orrenius, S. (1994) Co-receptor (CD4/CD8) engagement enhances CD3-induced apoptosis in thymocytes. Implications for negative selection. *J. Immunol.* **153,** 2436–2443.
92. Punt, J. A., Osborne, B. A., Takahama, Y., Sharrow, S. O., and Singer, A. (1994) Negative selection of CD4+CD8+ thymocytes by T cell receptor-induced apoptosis requires a costimulatory signal that can be provided by CD28. *J. Exp. Med.* **179,** 709–713.
93. Zhao, Y. and Iwata, M. (1995) Cross-linking of the TCR-CD3 complex with CD4, CD8 or LFA-1 induces an anti-apoptotic signal in thymocytes: the signal is canceled by FK506. *Int. Immunol.* **7,** 1387–1396.
94. Noda, S., Kosugi, A., Saitoh, S., Narumiya, S., and Hamaoka, T. (1996) Protection from anti-TCR/CD3-induced apoptosis in immature thymocytes by a signal through thymic shared antigen-1/stem cell antigen-2. *J. Exp. Med.* **183,** 2355–2360.

95. Shahinian, A., Pfeffer, K., Lee, K. P., Kundig, T. M., Kishihara, K., Wakeham, A., Kawai, K., Ohashi, P. S., Thompson, C. B., and Mak, T. W. (1993) Differential T cell costimulatory requirements in CD28-deficient mice. *Science* **261,** 609–612.
96. Shier, P., Otulakowski, G., Ngo, K., Panakos, J., Chourmouzis, E., Christjansen, L., Lau, C. Y., and Fung, L. W. (1996) Impaired immune responses toward alloantigens and tumor cells but normal thymic selection in mice deficient in the beta2 integrin leukocyte function-associated antigen-1. *J. Immunol.* **157,** 5375–5386.
97. Amakawa, R., Hakem, A., Kundig, T. M., Matsuyama, T., Simard, J. J., Timms, E., Wakeham, A., Mittruecker, H. W., Griesser, H., Takimoto, H., et al. (1996) Impaired negative selection of T cells in Hodgkin's disease antigen CD30-deficient mice. *Cell* **84,** 551–562.
98. Foy, T. M., Page, D. M., Waldschmidt, T. J., Schoneveld, A., Laman, J. D., Masters, S. R., Tygrett, L., Ledbetter, J. A., Aruffo, A., Claassen, E., et al. (1995) An essential role for gp39, the ligand for CD40, in thymic selection. *J. Exp. Med.* **182,** 1377–1388.
99. Muller, K. P. and Kyewski, B. A. (1993) T cell receptor targeting to thymic cortical epithelial cells in vivo induces survival, activation and differentiation of immature thymocytes. *Eur. J. Immunol.* **23,** 1661–1670.
100. Takahama, Y., Suzuki, H., Katz, K. S., Grusby, M. J., and Singer, A. (1994) Positive selection of $CD4^+$ T cells by TCR ligation without aggregation even in the absence of MHC. *Nature* **371,** 67–70.
101. Cibotti, R., Punt, J. A., Dash, K. S., Sharrow, S. O. and Singer, A. (1997) Surface molecules that drive T cell development in vitro in the absence of thymic epithelium and in the absence of lineage–specific signals. *Immunity* **6,** 245–255.
102. McConkey, D. J., Hartzell, P., Orrenius, S., and Jondal, M. (1989) Calcium-dependent killing of immature thymocytes by stimulation via the CD3/T cell receptor complex. *J. Immunol.* **143,** 1801–1806.
103. Nakayama, T., Ueda, Y., Yamada, H., Shores, E. W., Singer, A., and June, C. H. (1992. In vivo calcium elevations in thymocytes with T cell receptors that are specific for self ligands. *Science* **257,** 96–99.
104. Vasquez, N. J., Kane, L. P., and Hedrick, S. M. (1994) Intracellular signals that mediate thymic negative selection. *Immunity* 1, 45–56.
105. Anderson, K. L., Anderson, G., Michell, R. H., Jenkinson, E. J., and Owen, J. J. (1996) Intracellular signaling pathways involved in the induction of apoptosis in immature thymic T lymphocytes. *J. Immunol.* **156,** 4083–4091.
106. Conroy, L. A., Jenkinson, E. J., Owen, J. J., and Michell, R. H. (1995) Phosphatidylinositol 4,5-bisphosphate hydrolysis accompanies T cell receptor-induced apoptosis of murine thymocytes within the thymus. *Eur. J. Immunol.* **25,** 1828–1835.
107. O'Shea, C. C., Crompton, T., Rosewell, I. R., Hayday, A. C., and Owen, M. J. (1996) Raf regulates positive selection. *Eur. J. Immunol.* **26,** 2350–2355.
108. Ohoka, Y., Kuwata, T., Tozawa, Y., Zhao, Y., Mukai, M., Motegi, Y., Suzuki, R., Yokoyama, M., and Iwata, M. (1996) In vitro differentiation and commitment of $CD4^+$ $CD8^+$ thymocytes to the CD4 lineage, without TCR engagement. *Int. Immunol.* **8,** 297–306.
109. Takahama, Y. and Nakauchi, H. (1996) Phorbol ester and calcium ionophore can replace TCR signals that induce positive selection of CD4 T cells. *J. Immunol.* **157,** 1508–1513.
110. Izquirdo-Pastor, M., Reif, K., and Cantrell, D. (1995) The regulation and function of $p21^{ras}$ during T-cell activation and growth. *Immunol. Today* **16,** 159–164.
111. Hall, C. G., Sancho, J., and Terhorst, C. (1993) Reconstitution of T cell receptor zeta-mediated calcium mobilization in nonlymphoid cells. *Science* **261,** 915–918.
112. Appleby, M. W., Gross, J. A., Cooke, M. P., Levin, S. D., Qian, X., and Perlmutter, R. M. (1992) Defective T cell receptor signaling in mice lacking the thymic isoform of $p59^{fyn}$. *Cell* **70,** 751–763.
113. Stein, P. L., Lee, H. M., Rich, S., and Soriano, P. (1992) $pp59^{fyn}$ mutant mice display differential signaling in thymocytes and peripheral T cells. *Cell* **70,** 741–750.
114. Wiest, D. L., Ashe, J. M., Abe, R., Bolen, J. B., and Singer, A. (1996) TCR activation of ZAP70 is impaired in $CD4^+CD8^+$ thymocytes as a consequence of intrathymic interactions that diminish available p56lck. *Immunity* **4,** 495–504.
115. Lerner, A., Clayton, L. K., Mizoguchi, E., Ghendler, Y., van Ewijk, W., Koyasu, S., Bhan, A. K., and Reinherz, E. L. (1996) Cross-linking of T-cell receptors on double-positive thymocytes

induces a cytokine-mediated stromal activation process linked to cell death. *EMBO J.* **15,** 5876–5887.

116. Falk, I., Potocnik, A. J., Barthlott, T., Levelt, C. N., and Eichmann, K. (1996) Immature T cells in peripheral lymphoid organs of recombinase- activating gene-1/-2-deficient mice. Thymus dependence and responsiveness to anti-CD3 epsilon antibody. *J. Immunol.* **156,** 1362–1368.
117. Clegg, C. H., Rulffes, J. T., Wallace, P. M., and Haugen, H. S. (1996) Regulation of an extrathymic T-cell development pathway by oncostatin M. *Nature* **384,** 261–263.
118. She, J., Simpson, S. J., Gupta, A., Hollaender, G., Levelt, C., Liu, C. P., Allen, D., van Houten, N., Wang, B., and Terhorst, C. (1997) CD16-Expressing CD8α/α^+ T lymphocytes in the intestinal epithelium: Possible precursors of FcγR$^-$CD8α/α^+ T cells. *J. Immunol.* **158,** 4678–4687.

Chapter 24

The Molecular Basis of Thymocyte Positive Selection and CD4/CD8 Lineage Commitment

Cynthia J. Guidos

1. Introduction

It has been 20 years since it was first postulated that developing T-cells undergo a positive selection process that ensures that only those bearing self-MHC restricted TCRαβ mature and exit the thymus to form the peripheral T-cell pool *(1,2)*. It is now clear that positive selection operates on a pool of immature $TCR\alpha\beta^+$ thymocytes that express high levels of CD4 and CD8. These coreceptors recognize MHC Class II or Class I molecules, respectively, and function both to stabilize TCRαβ interactions with MHC/peptide ligands, as well to recruit the Lck protein tyrosine kinase to the TCRαβ/CD3 complex, thus facilitating TCR-mediated signal transduction. In response to low avidity interactions between TCRαβ and MHC/peptide ligands expressed in the thymic cortex, DP thymocytes bearing potentially useful, self MHC-restricted TCRαβ are positively selected to survive and to mature into MHC II-restricted $CD4^+$ helper, or MHC I-restricted $CD8^+$ cytotoxic T-cells. Thus, positively selected DP thymocytes are rescued from programmed cell death, the fate of most DP cells, and become committed to the CD4 or CD8 single positive (SP) lineage. However, high avidity TCR-ligand interactions preferentially mediate clonal deletion of potentially autoreactive precursors, usually before the DP→SP transition is complete.

Despite this progress in achieving a clearer understanding of the repertoire selection process during αβ T-cell development, several fundamental questions remain unanswered. Two distinct mechanisms have been proposed to explain how the process of CD4/CD8 lineage commitment ensures that DP precursors bearing class II MHC-specific TCRαβ will retain expression of CD4, whereas those bearing class I MHC-specific TCR will retain expression of CD8, but no clear consensus has been reached. Indeed, recent

From: *Molecular Biology of B-Cell and T-Cell Development*
Edited by: J. G. Monroe and E. V. Rothenberg © Humana Press Inc., Totowa, NJ

data suggest that the process of CD4 or CD8 downregulation during the DP→SP transition involves a complex series of transitional intermediate steps, rather than a simple loss of either CD4 or CD8. Emerging studies on transcriptional regulation of CD4 and CD8 reinforce the notion that this developmental decision is mechanistically complex. This article will review recent observations relevant to each of these areas, highlighting areas of consensus and controversy.

2. Transitional Intermediate Stages During Positive Selection of DP Thymocytes

During positive selection, DP thymocytes increase expression of TCR, CD5, CD69, and Bcl-2, and decrease expression of RAG-1 and RAG-2, before beginning to downregulate expression of CD4 or CD8 (reviewed in ref. *3*). These maturational events can be elicited by in vitro engagement of the TCR on purified DP thymocytes *(4–6)*, and require intact TCR-mediated signaling pathways in vivo *(7,8)*. $TCR^{int}/CD69^{+}$ DP thymocytes develop into SP thymocytes faster than their $TCR^{lo}/CD69^{-}$ counterparts, suggesting that they have begun to undergo positive selection *(9,10)*. Some $TCR^{int}/CD69^{+}$ DP thymocytes appear to already be CD4 or CD8-committed in a coreceptor re-expression assay *(11)*, but the DP cells were not stringently purified and were probably contaminated with small numbers of SP thymocytes. Thus, TCR-dependent maturation events temporally precede changes in coreceptor expression and evidence of CD4/CD8 lineage commitment during the DP→SP transition.

Coreceptor downregulation first becomes apparent two to three days following intrathymic transfer of DP thymocytes, with CD8 downregulation being apparent before CD4 downregulation *(12,13)*. Thymocytes with incompletely downregulated expression of either CD4 or CD8 represent transitional intermediates that arise during the DP→SP transition *(14)*. The fact that $CD4^{+}CD8^{int/lo}$ thymocytes or $CD4^{int/lo}CD8^{+}$ thymocytes are $CD69^{+}$ suggests that TCR engagement has recently occurred *(15)*. TCR expression on $CD4^{+}CD8^{int/lo}$ thymocytes is unimodal, and is 5–10× greater than that on DP thymocytes, but 3–5× less (on average) than that on CD4 SP thymocytes or peripheral T-cells *(14)*. In contrast, TCR expression is bimodally distributed on $CD4^{int/lo}CD8^{+}$ thymocytes, with the TCR^{int} subset expressing 3× more, and the TCR^{hi} subset 12–15× more, TCR than DP thymocytes *(14,16,17)*. Thus, upregulation of TCR levels begins at the DP stage, but the pattern of upregulation is different among cells losing CD4 vs CD8.

Originally, $CD4^{+}CD8^{int/lo}$ thymocytes were postulated to represent CD4-committed cells, whereas $CD4^{int/lo}CD8^{+}$ thymocytes were thought to represent CD8-committed cells *(14)*. Studies of the developmental potential of these transitional subsets in vivo or in vitro confirmed the presence of CD8-committed cells in the TCR^{hi} $CD4^{int/lo}CD8^{+}$ subset *(16,17)*. Unexpectedly, however, $TCR^{int/hi}$ $CD4^{+}CD8^{int/lo}$ thymocytes were shown to contain both CD4-committed and CD8-committed cells *(18–21)*. These studies identified a possible asymmetry in the development of CD4 versus CD8 SP, in that CD8-committed cells appear to transiently downregulate CD8, whereas CD4-committed cells appear to maintain constant expression of CD4.

More recent work suggests that both coreceptors are transiently downregulated as a consequence of TCR-mediated signaling early in the positive selection process. In addition to the maturational events described above, TCR engagement of DP thymocytes in vitro induces partial downregulation of both CD4 and CD8 *(4,5)*. Because some of the resulting $CD4^{lo}CD8^{lo}$ cells are apoptotic *(22)*, coreceptor downregulation has become a widely used assay for negative selection in vivo. However, when the analysis of

$CD4^{lo}CD8^{lo}$ cells is limited to those with intact plasma membranes, excluding cells that have already died and thus stain nonspecifically, very few apoptotic cells are detected *(4)*. The adult steady-state thymus contains small numbers of $CD4^{lo}CD8^{lo}$ cells that express levels of TCR and CD69 intermediate between those on DP thymocytes and $CD4^{+}CD8^{int/lo}$ or $CD4^{int/lo}CD8^{+}$ thymocytes *(19)*. Although some of these cells may be apoptotic *(23)*, $CD4^{lo}CD8^{lo}$ thymocytes can mature into CD4 and CD8 SP cells in vivo and in vitro *(4,19,24)*. When $CD4^{lo}CD8^{lo}$ cells are pronase-treated to proteolytically strip the cell surface and then cultured, re-expression of CD4 occurs significantly faster than re-expression of CD8, potentially explaining the apparent asymmetry in the commitment status of $CD4^{+}CD8^{int/lo}$ vs $CD4^{int/lo}CD8^{+}$ thymocytes *(19)*.

3. Signaling Pathways that Regulate CD4/CD8 Lineage Commitment

Lineage commitment is operationally determined to have taken place when a particular cell fate is autonomously maintained, irrespective of the cellular environment. Two general models have been proposed to explain how binary cell fate decisions are made. The instruction model posits that alternative fates are instructively promoted by different environmental signals. The instructionist view of CD4/CD8 lineage commitment proposes that TCR/CD4 signaling of MHC II-restricted DP thymocytes will promote CD4 commitment and loss of CD8, whereas TCR/CD8 signaling of MHC I-restricted DP thymocytes will cause CD8 commitment and loss of CD4. Stochastic models attest that all cell fate decisions are made randomly, but that survival of progenitors committed to alternative lineages requires particular environmental signals. In a stochastic model, DP cells would randomly commit to CD4 or CD8 expression without regard to TCR MHC specficity. If the MHC specificity of the retained coreceptor happens to match that of the TCR, committed precursors will be selected for survival and complete maturation by coengagement of a cognate MHC/peptide ligand. Thus, an individual precursor will choose the wrong cell fate 50% of the time. In contrast to the instructional model, the stochastic model views lineage commitment and positive selection as distinct events. As it is clear that TCR-ligand interactions are essential for development of CD4 and CD8 SP cells, the key to understanding the mechanism of CD4/CD8 lineage commitment lies in determining whether TCR/coreceptor signals are necessary for commitment per se, or only for survival of committed progenitors.

3.1. TCR/Coreceptor Signals in CD4/CD8 Lineage Commitment

An instructional mechanism would be supported if CD4/CD8 lineage commitment could be demonstrated to depend on the transmission of distinct signals through TCR/CD4 vs TCR/CD8. Signaling through both CD4 and CD8 is Lck-dependent, and to date, little evidence supports the notion that CD4 signaling is qualitatively distinct from CD8 signaling *(25)*. However, the cytoplasmic tail of CD4 binds considerably more Lck than that of CD8α, and in thymocytes, this inherent bias is accentuated by the abundant expression of CD8α', a cytoplasmically truncated isoform that can't bind Lck *(26)*. Thus, TCR/CD4 signaling is inherently more efficient than TCR/CD8 signaling in DP thymocytes *(27)*. This observation has lead to a quantitative instructional model which suggests that CD4 commitment is instructed by strong (CD4-mediated) Lck signals, whereas CD8 commitment is instructed by weak (CD8-mediated) signals.

Quantitative instruction is supported by studies in which chimeric CD8/CD4 transgenes, encoding the extracellular domain of CD8α fused to the cytoplasmic domain of CD4, switch the fate of DP cells expressing transgenic MHC I-restricted TCR from the CD8 to the CD4 lineage *(28,29)*. However, expression of endogenous TCRα chains, which occurs frequently in TCRαβ transgenic mice *(30,31)*, could have allowed generation of MHC II-specific endogenous TCR that were selected using CD4. Matechak et al. also argued in favor of a quantitative instructional model, based on their finding that DP thymocytes expressing a transgenic MHC II-restricted TCR choose the CD8 fate when CD4 is absent *(32)*. Interestingly, this choice is MHC I-dependent, though not allele-specific. Similarly, Kirberg et al. observed MHC I-dependent selection of an MHC II-specific transgenic TCR into the CD8 lineage, even in the presence of CD4 *(33)*. In the latter two studies, selection based on endogenous TCRα chains was ruled out.

These observations make some sense when considered in the context of the finding that $CD4^{lo}CD8^{lo}$ thymocytes re-express CD4 more rapidly than CD8 *(19)*. Although the mechanistic basis of this kinetic asymmetry has not been defined, it could ensure that all thymocytes first have the opportunity to be selected by MHC II. Only those that fail to receive survival signals mediated by TCR/CD4-MHC II interactions would subsequently lose CD4 and attempt to be selected as $CD4^{int/lo}CD8^{+}$ thymocytes. Accordingly, cells with MHC II-specific, but weakly MHC I crossreactive TCR would usually develop into the CD4 lineage; however, they could sometimes develop as CD8 cells. It would be predicted that such cells would be more likely to choose the CD8 over the CD4 fate when the selecting MHC II ligand is limiting, or when CD4 is absent.

A variant of the instruction model suggests that only one fate is determined by extracellular signaling, and that the alternative fate will occur by default in the absence of the instructive signal. Two groups have recently proposed that lineage commitment is mechanistically asymmetric, in that CD4 commitment occurs by default, and CD8 commitment is instructed *(20,21)*. Suzuki et al. evaluated lineage commitment using a novel assay in which transitional intermediate subsets are sorted, proteolytically stripped of surface CD4/CD8 (and other molecules) by pronase treatment, and then recultured to determine which coreceptors are still being actively synthesized. As mentioned in Subheading 2., CD8-committed cells were identified among both $CD4^{+}CD8^{int/lo}$ and $CD4^{int/lo}$ $CD8^{+}$ thymocytes, but only when these cells were isolated from MHC I^{+} mice. In contrast, CD4-committed cells were detected among $CD4^{+}CD8^{int/lo}$ thymocytes from normal and MHC II-deficient mice. However, a minor subset of $CD4^{+}$ MHC I-restricted NKT lineage cells has been identified, and these are the only CD4 lineage cells that can be detected in MHC II-deficient mice *(34–37)*. Therefore, it cannot be assumed that the CD4 committed cells detected by Suzuki et al. are bonafide MHC II-restricted CD4 lineage cells. Moreover, using the same coreceptor re-expression assay, Lucas et al. did not detect significant numbers of CD4-committed cells among $CD4^{+}CD8^{int/lo}$ thymocytes isolated from MHC II-deficient mice *(19)*. Rather, these investigators observed that detection of CD4 or CD8-committed cells in the coreceptor re-expression assay is strictly dependent on engagement of MHC II or MHC I, respectively, prior to cell purification, arguing that commitment to both lineages is instructed. However, this assay can only detect committed cells that survive in overnight culture, and it is possible that it is survival, rather than commitment *per se*, which requires TCR/coreceptor signals.

In summary, there is little, if any, unambiguous experimental support for an instructive model of CD4/CD8 lineage commitment. The recent demonstration that coengagement of either TCR/CD4 or TCR/CD8 induces development of CD4 SP in fetal thymus organ culture argues strongly against coreceptor-dependent instructional lineage commitment *(38)*. In addition, positive selection of some MHC I-restricted transgenic TCR (and CD8 commitment) can occur in the complete absence of CD8 *(39,40)*, so CD8 signals do not play a requisite instructional role in CD8 commitment. Although it is formally possible that the TCR itself can transduce distinct signals upon recognition of MHC I vs MHC II, this has never been observed experimentally. In contrast, the observation that the CD4/CD8 lineage choice is not perfectly correlated with TCR specificity *(32,33)* fulfils a major prediction of the stochastic model. The MHC I-dependence of the "inappropriate" lineage choice may indicate that CD8-MHC I adhesive interactions can sometimes stabilize TCR-MHC II interactions when CD4 is genetically absent or has been stochastically downregulated.

3.2. CD4/CD8 Lineage Commitment is TCR-Independent

Some studies support the notion that TCR/CD3 signals are required to induce lineage commitment stochastically, without regard for TCR specificity. This was first suggested because $CD4^{+}CD8^{int/lo}$ or $CD4^{int/lo}CD8^{+}$ thymocytes arise in mice lacking MHC II or MHC I, respectively, and are $TCR^{int/hi}$ and $CD69^{+}$, suggesting that TCR signaling has taken place *(16,41,42)*. Additionally, simultaneous engagement of TCR with either CD2, CD5, CD24, or CD28 generates CD4 SP from DP thymocytes in suspension culture *(43)*. Although this finding is provocative and suggests that CD4-independent TCR signaling can induce CD4 commitment, further studies are needed to show that the CD4 SP generated in vitro represent TCR^{hi} functionally mature helper T-cells rather than immature transitional cells.

Studies of mice with TCR signaling defects argue that the decision to downregulate CD4 or CD8 can be made without TCR signals. DP thymocytes from Vav-deficient mice are not responsive to TCR/coreceptor engagement in vitro, and very few SP thymocytes are produced. Nonetheless, $CD4^{+}CD8^{int/lo}$ or $CD4^{int/lo}CD8^{+}$ thymocytes are readily detected in these animals, but they are largely TCR^{lo} and $CD69^{-}$, arguing that they arose independently of TCR-signaling *(7)*. Studies of Lck-deficient or CD45-deficient mice confirm that the generation of thymocytes with CD4/CD8 transitional phenotypes can be uncoupled from TCR signaling (G. Cheng, P. Smiley, T. Groves, and C. Guidos, unpublished observations) *(8)*. Contrary to these findings, the generation $CD4^{+}CD8^{int/lo}$ thymocytes from $TCR^{-}/CD3^{+}$ RAG-deficient DP thymocytes was reported to depend on prior CD3 signals *(44)*. However, we have found that $CD4^{+}CD8^{int/lo}$ thymocytes develop readily from $TCR^{-}/CD3^{+}$ DP thymocytes independently of CD3 signals (Fig. 1). Of course, these cells do not survive to complete the maturation process because they are incapable of receiving TCR-mediated rescue signals. Similarly, $TCR^{lo}/CD69^{-}$ $CD4^{+}CD8^{int/lo}$ or $CD4^{int/lo}CD8^{+}$ thymocytes are present in MHC I/II double mutant mice *(19,45)*, although their reduced numbers relative to mice lacking only MHC I or MHC II would suggest that their survival is enhanced by TCR engagement. Studies demonstrating that antibody-mediated TCR signals can restore development of CD4 SP in fetal thymus organ culture of MHC I/II-deficient thymus lobes are consistent with the idea that stochastically CD4-committed precursors survive if they receive TCR signals *(46,47)*. Generation of mature CD8 SP in these cultures was not evaluated.

3.3. Thymic Epithelium Provides Unique Signals for Positive Selection

Multiple lines of evidence suggest that thymic epithelium provides specialized functions in positive selection. This was first hinted at when Poirier et al. observed that a clonal DP cell line could generate CD4 SP cells when cultured with MHC II^{+} thymic epithelial cells, but not when cultured with MHC II^{+} bone marrow-derived cells *(48)*. Two groups confirmed this finding using a novel reaggregate thymus organ culture system, in which purified thymic stomal cell populations will reaggregate with thymic progenitor subsets to form intact thymic lobes *(49)*. In this system, production of CD4

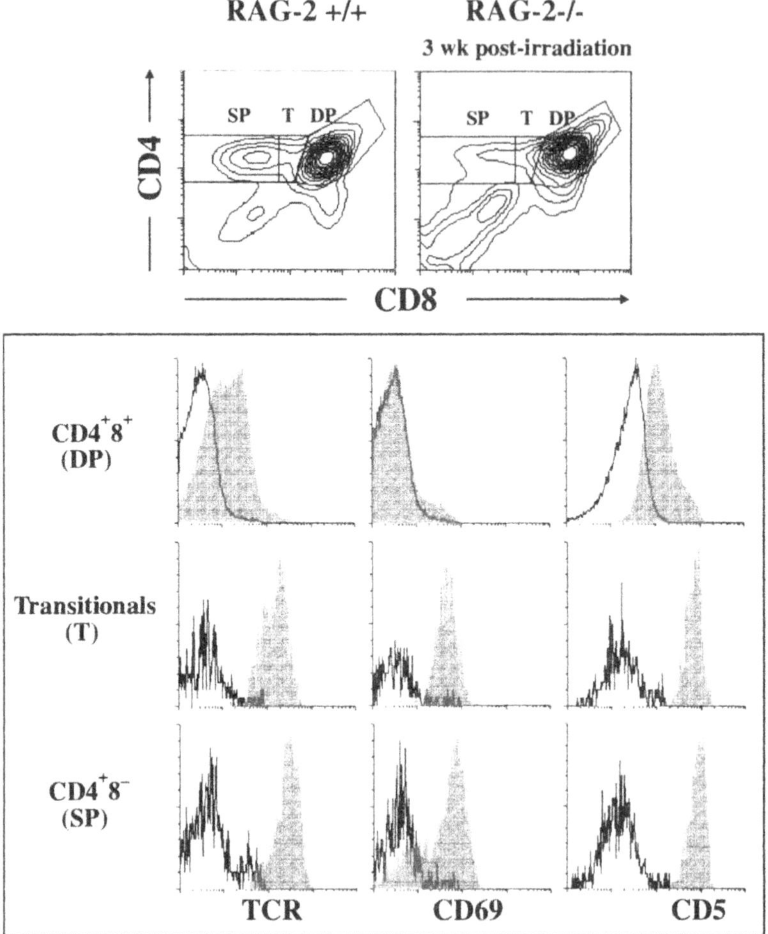

Fig. 1. $CD4^+CD8^{int/lo}$ thymocytes develop from $TCR\alpha\beta^-$ DP thymocytes without CD3-mediated signals. Thymocytes were isolated from untreated $RAG\text{-}2^{+/+}$ mice, or from $RAG\text{-}2^{-/-}$ mice three weeks following irradiation with 700 cGy, and stained with antibodies specific for CD4, CD8, and either TCR, CD69, or CD5, and analyzed by 3-color flow cytometry as previously described *(108)*. For each thymus, TCR, CD69, and CD5 expression was evaluated on DP, transitional, and CD4 SP thymocytes from $RAG\text{-}2^{+/+}$ (shaded histograms) or $RAG\text{-}2^{-/-}$ (clear histograms) mice. Note that $CD4^+CD8^{int/lo}$ thymocytes develop from DP thymocytes in irradiated $RAG\text{-}2^{-/-}$ mice, but, in contrast to their wild-type counterparts, these cells do not express significant levels of TCR, CD69, or CD5, indicating the absence of TCR/CD3-mediated signals.

and CD8 SP thymocytes was observed when DP precursors were reaggregated with MHC II^+ thymic cortical epithelial cells, but failed to be produced with nonthymic MHC II^+ epithelial or bone marrow-derived cells *(50,51)*. Similarly, Tanaka et al. observed positive selection of MHC I-specific TCR transgenic thymocytes in reaggregate cultures with an immortalized thymic epithelial clone, but not a kidney epithelial clone *(52)*. A potential role for MHC-independent thymic epithelium-derived signals is also consistent with the finding that bispecific hybrid antibodies, engineered to simultaneously bind TCR and cortical epithelial cells, rescue CD4 SP development in MHC II-deficient mice much more efficiently than bivalent TCR antibodies not specifically targeted to epithelium *(53,54)*. Interestingly, fibroblasts have been reported to positively select T-cells restricted to the fibroblast MHC type following intrathymic injection *(55)*, arguing that, at least in some circumstances, the MHC need not be expressed by thymic epithelium to mediate positive selection. Taken together, these data argue that the role of thymic epithelium in positive selection is not limited to presentation of a selecting MHC/peptide ligand. Rather, these data indicate that thymic epithelium also provides specialized, MHC-independent signals for positive selection. Recent work has identified Notch receptor-ligand interactions as a candidate for providing such MHC-independent signals during positive selection.

3.4. Notch Signals in CD4/CD8 Lineage Commitment

Notch is a transmembrane receptor first identified in Drosophila as an important regulator of cell fate decisions in several tissues (reviewed in ref. *64*). Upon interaction of Notch with its ligands, the Delta or Serrate proteins, the cytoplasmic domain is translocated to the nucleus. The Suppressor of Hairless (RBPJκ/CBF-1) transcription factor normally acts as a transcriptional repressor, but in association with the Notch cytoplasmic domain, it activates transcription of N-box basic helix-loop-helix (bHLH) proteins in the *Enhancer of Split* (E[spl]) gene complex *(56,57)*. These E(spl) proteins then repress transcription of E-box bHLH proteins required for neurogenesis. Mammalian homologues of Notch (mNotch), Delta/Serrate, RBPJκ/CBF-1, and E(spl) have been identified and shown to regulate neurogenesis and myogenesis by a very similar pathway to that described for Drosophila Notch *(58–61)*.

Recently, Robey and colleagues have implicated Notch signaling in CD4/CD8 lineage commitment *(62)*. mNotch-1 is expressed in murine thymocytes, with the highest protein levels being found in the most immature DN thymocytes, and much lower levels in the major DP thymocyte population *(63)*. In Drosophila, truncated Notch proteins retaining only the cytoplasmic domain function as dominant gain-of-function alleles *(64)*. Therefore, Robey et al. evaluated the effect of transgenic overexpression of the mNotch-1 cytoplasmic domain on T-cell development *(62)*. Transgenic, but otherwise wild-type, mice dramatically overproduced CD8 SP thymocytes. This bias toward the CD8 lineage did not require thymic expression of MHC 1, since it was seen in MHC I-deficient mice. However, downregulation of HSA on CD8 SP thymocytes was incomplete in Notch transgenic, MHC I-negative mice, suggesting that MHC I recognition facilitates maturation of CD8-committed cells. Strikingly, however, activated Notch could not restore CD8 SP T-cell development in mice lacking both MHC I and MHC II. Based on this finding, the authors suggest that TCR-mediated MHC signaling may be required to allow the survival of thymocytes induced to undergo CD8 commitment in response to Notch signaling.

These data provide novel insights into the molecular control of CD4/CD8 lineage commitment. However, in keeping with the multifunctional nature of Notch in Drosophila, mNotch is likely to play multiple roles in T-cell development. mNotch-1 was first identified as by virtue of its oncogenic activation in humans with acute lymphoblastic leukemia *(65)*. Subsequent studies have demonstrated that activated mNotch-1 is a powerful, T-cell–specific oncogene *(66–68)*, revealing that it can have profound effects on thymocyte proliferation and/or survival. This is consistent with the fact that the highest mNotch-1-expressing thymocytes are $CD25^+$ DN thymocytes poised to undergo a proliferative burst in response to pre-TCR signaling *(63)*. Indeed, activated mNotch-1 can also influence the TCRαβ vs TCRγδ lineage decision, which occurs precisely at this time *(69)*.

Although enhanced thymocyte proliferation was not demonstrable in the mNotch-1 transgenic mice, they ultimately succumbed to thymic lymphoma. Thus, it will be important to determine whether mNotch-1 is acting exclusively to effect the CD4/CD8 lineage decision, or whether it functions to regulate the survival of lineage-committed progenitors. A survival gene would not be expected to discriminate between CD4-committed and CD8-committed cells, as mNotch-1 apparently does. However, similar to activated mNotch-1, transgenic overexpression of the Bcl-2 survival gene rescues the development of CD8 lineage cells in the absence of MHC I, but does not rescue production of CD4 lineage cells in the absence of MHC II *(70)*. Moreover, Bcl-2-mediated rescue of CD8 SP thymocytes in MHC I-negative mice is MHC II-dependent. Thus, Bcl-2 and mNotch-1 have similar, if not identical, effects on T-cell development in MHC-deficient mice. Clearly, sifting apart the diverse roles played by Notch in T-cell development presents a significant challenge for the future.

3.5. Postcommitment Events in Positive Selection

Considerable evidence points to the existence of important developmental events that occur after CD4/CD8 lineage commitment has taken place. Acquisition of a completely mature phenotype, characterized by low HSA expression, does not occur until many days after SP thymocytes are produced *(71)*, and recent data suggest that positively selected thymocytes reside in the thymic medulla for up to one week before migrating to the periphery *(72)*. Although positive selection and CD4/CD8 lineage commitment can occur in the complete absence of proliferation *(73)*, some SP thymocytes undergo a proliferative burst several days after they were first generated, perhaps to expand successfully selected cells *(74)*. Surprisingly, newly generated SP thymocytes survive in Bcl-2-deficient mice, but the long-term survival of selected cells in the periphery is Bcl-2-dependent *(75)*. One particulary important postcommitment event is the functional specialization of CD4 helper T-cells into TH1 versus TH2 cells that regulate cellular and humoral immunity, respectively *(76)*.

Several lines of evidence indicate that even once cells are positively selected, they require continuing TCR engagements for long-term survival in the periphery. For example, transgenic expression of activated Fyn under control of the Lck proximal promoter can rescue the production of phenotypically mature SP thymocytes in Lck-deficient mice, but it does not restore peripheral T-cell homeostasis, presumably because this promoter is relatively inactive in mature T-cells *(8)*. Similarly, intrathymic expression of MHC II restores CD4 SP thymocyte development in MHC II-negative mice, but long-term survival of these cells is compromised in the absence of peripheral MHC II expression *(72,76)*. Finally, transgenic expression of CD45RO or CD45ABC restores development of CD4 and CD8 SP thymocytes in CD45-deficient mice, but peripheral T-cells only accumulate in the lymph node, and are absent from the spleen and skin *(77)*. Thus, particular CD45 isoforms may be required for the homing and/or survival of T-cells in distinct peripheral microenvironments.

4. Transcriptional Regulation of CD4 and CD8 in Developing and Mature T-Cells

CD4/CD8 lineage commitment is likely effected through changes in transcription of the CD4 vs CD8 genes *(78,79)*. One relatively simple possibility is that CD4 expression is extinguished in CD8-committed cells by negative regulation of CD4 enhancer-specific trans-acting factors. Thus, selective changes in coreceptor expression could be accomplished by modulation of CD4 vs CD8-specific enhancer activity as DP precursors mature into SP cells. However, data accumulated over the last few years suggests that lineage-restricted expression of CD4 is effected by a complex interplay between transcriptional enhancers and silencers, and recent studies suggest that CD8 expression may be regulated by similar mechanisms. A final resolution to the instruction/selection debate will require a complete understanding of the *cis*- and trans-acting factors responsible for transcriptional regulation of CD4 and CD8 expression, as well as the identification of signaling pathways emanating from the cell surface that control transcription factor expression and repression. Immediately below is a summary of current knowledge in these areas, followed by a discussion of how these observations fit into instructionist versus selectionist views of CD4/CD8 lineage commitment.

4.1. The CD4 Promoter

For both human and murine CD4 (hCD4 and mCD4), the core promoter region extends 40–100 bp upstream of the transcriptional start site and lacks a classical TATA box *(80,81)*. However, the promoter contains binding sites for Myb and Ets transcription factors that are critical for its function in transient transfection assays *(80–82)*. Interestingly, the core promoter functions only in T-cells in transient assays, and is much more active in CD4 SP than in DN, DP or CD8 SP T-cells *(80,81)*. Expression of dominant negative or constitutively active Myb alleles in transgenic mice inhibits or promotes, respectively, the development of CD4 T-cells, suggesting that Myb could regulate CD4 expression in vivo *(83,84)*. Nonetheless, since Myb is expressed in many hematopoietic cells types, the relative CD4 SP specificity of this promoter region is not explained by Myb activity alone. Rather, CD4 specificity may reflect cooperation between Myb and Ets proteins, given the greater abundance of Ets-1 and Ets-2 in CD4 relative to CD8 T-cells. Moreover, as described below, transcription from the CD4 promoter is also subject to regulation by at least two enhancers, which can override the apparent CD4 lineage preference of the core promoter.

4.2. CD4 Enhancers

Using transient transfection assays, two distinct CD4 enhancers have been identified that are localized within DNase I hypersensitive sites upstream of the mCD4 gene. Sawada and Littman identified a 339 bp minimal enhancer region 13 kb 5' of the transcription initiation site for mCD4 *(85)*, and a similar enhancer exists 6.5 kb 5' of the hCD4 gene *(86)*. This enhancer motif, in conjunction with either the mCD4 promoter or a heterologous promoter, did not activate reporter gene expression in non-T-cell lines, but it functioned equally well in DP, CD4, and CD8 SP T-cell lines *(85,87)*. Thus, this particular mCD4 enhancer is T-cell–specific, but its function is not restricted to a particular developmental stage or T-cell lineage. An E-box site (CAGNTG) within the CD4-3 region of the enhancer binds E12 and HEB, a complex of bHLH transcription factors, and appears crucial for T-cell-specific CD4 enhancer function *(88)*.

Siu and Hedrick identified a second CD4 enhancer 24 kb upstream of the mCD4 gene *(89)*. In transient assays, this distal enhancer worked well in CD4 SP T-cells with a heterologous promoter, and synergized with the mCD4 core promoter, but did not function in non-T-cells. However, it differs from the more proximal enhancer described by Sawada and Littman, in that it does not function in immature DP T-cell lines, nor in CD8 SP or DN T-cell lines *(85)*. Thus, the distal enhancer appears to be functional only in mature CD4 lineage T-cells. The distal enhancer includes putative binding sites for AP-1, Sp1, GATA, and Ets transcription factors, but mutational analysis implicated only the Ets site as being essential for enhancer function *(89)*.

Several groups have reported that the murine or human proximal CD4 enhancer can direct expression of hCD4 reporter gene constructs to immature DP thymocytes and mature CD4 SP T-cells in transgenic mice *(86,90–92)*. In contrast, Salmon et al. found that the murine proximal enhancer was incapable of driving expression of a hCD4 transgene in murine DP thymocytes *(93)*. Similarly, Siu and colleagues found that the proximal and distal mCD4 enhancers did not allow expression of an HLA-B7 reporter transgene in DP thymocytes *(94)*. Instead, these investigators found that expression of the reporter gene in DP thymocytes was dependent on sequences that coincide with DNase I hypersensitive sites found at least 10 kb 3' of the last CD4 exon *(95)*. Subtle differences between the transgenic constructs used in the various studies may account for these discrepancies. For example, the hCD4 reporter mini-gene constructed by Salmon et al. *(93)* contained no hCD4 intronic sequences, whereas those made by the other groups minimally had sequences derived from introns 1–3. Sequences within introns 1 and 2 of hCD4 appear incapable of supporting reporter gene expression in immature DP thymocytes *(91)*. However, transgenes containing the proximal enhancer together with intron 1 plus the 5' part of intron 3 from hCD4 are expressed in DP thymocytes *(86,96)*. Thus, a DP enhancer appears to reside within these intronic sequences of hCD4, but not within the same region of mCD4 *(95)*.

Interestingly, transgenic constructs containing the CD4 enhancer and promoter, but lacking the putative DP enhancer, were only expressed in a subset of CD4 SP thymocytes *(93,95,96)*. Reporter gene-positive CD4 SP thymocytes expressed higher levels of TCR/CD3 and H-2K, and lower levels of HSA and CD69, than the reporter gene-negative subset *(93,95,96)*. Moreover, $CD4^{+}CD8^{int}$ transitional thymocytes included approximately equal proportions of reporter gene negative and reporter gene positive cells *(96)*. Since $CD4^{+}CD8^{int}$ $CD3^{int}$ HSA^{hi} $CD69^{hi}$ thymocytes are more immature than $CD4^{+}CD8^{-}$ $CD3^{hi}$ HSA^{lo} $CD69^{lo}$ thymocytes *(14,17,19,20,41,97)*, these phenotypic distinctions between CD4 SP subsets suggest that the CD4 enhancer/promoter becomes functional only after cells have completed positive selection. Thus, although CD4 expression is maintained at relatively constant levels throughout the DP $\rightarrow$ CD4 SP transition, distinct transcriptional control elements regulate mCD4 expression in immature DP vs mature CD4 T-cells.

4.3. The CD4 Silencer

Although the distal CD4 enhancer alone could be responsible for lineage-restricted CD4 expression in vivo, recent studies have identified a transcriptional silencer in murine and hCD4 that extinguishes CD4 expression in CD8 lineage T-cells *(79,87,98)*. Human CD2, CD4, or HLA-B7 reporter transgenic constructs containing the CD4 distal and/or proximal enhancers and promoter without intron 1 were expressed in both CD4 and CD8 T-cells *(79,87,93,98)*. In contrast, intron 1-derived sequences in conjunction with the CD4 enhancer/promoter confers expression of reporter genes exclusively to the CD4 SP lineage in transgenic mice *(79,86,87,90–93,98)*. Although the hCD4 silencer may also be active in CD4-committed thymocytes *(96)*, studies of the murine silencer do not support this conclusion *(79,87,94,95)*. Enhancer-containing transgenes lacking the silencer were also expressed in immature DN thymocytes and in B-cells and macrophages, revealing that CD4 expression is also actively silenced in very immature T-cells and non-T-cells *(79,95)*.

A minimal CD4 silencer consisting of 428 or 484 bp from intron 1 of mCD4 or hCD4, respectively, is able to limit CD4 enhancer and promoter activity to CD4 lineage cells in transient assays and in transgenic mice *(87,98)*. This murine element could also silence reporter transgene expression from a heterologous T-cell-specific promoter/enhancer *(87)*. DNase I footprinting and gel mobility shift assays identified sites binding sites for three different nuclear factors within the mCD4 silencer *(94)*. Sites I and II were bound by T-cell-specific factors, whereas site III was bound by a ubiquitously expressed protein. Deletional studies indicate that site II, in conjunction with either site I or III, are required for silencer function. Further analyses suggested that site II binds an E-box bHLH protein complex very similar, if not identical, to the CD4 proximal enhancer-binding E12/HEB heterodimer. Interestingly, site I has a consensus binding site (CACNAG) for N-box bHLH proteins, which are induced by Notch-mediated signal transduction and often act as transcriptional repressors (*see* Subheading 3.4.). In light of a potential role for Notch signaling in CD8 lineage commitment, it is intriguing to speculate that Notch-regulated induction of mammalian N-box-binding bHLH genes, such as HES-1 or HES-3 *(99)*, might be important for transcriptional repression of CD4 in CD8 lineage cells.

4.4. Transcriptional Regulation of CD8 Expression

Thymically-derived CD8 SP T-cells of the TCRαβ lineage express a heterodimer consisting of two unrelated proteins, CD8α and CD8β, encoded by closely linked genes. CD8β cannot be expressed on the T-cell surface without CD8α, but some NK cells and IEL express CD8αα homodimers (reviewed in ref. *100*). Although both MHC class I recognition and Lck-mediated signal transduction can be accomplished by CD8αα homodimers, CD8β can influence MHC specificity and its function is essential for positive selection of CD8 lineage T-cells (reviewed in ref. *26*). Thus, it is important to understand how expression of both CD8α and CD8β are regulated as DP thymocytes commit to the CD8 lineage.

Transcriptional elements regulating lineage-specific CD8 expression are not as well defined as those that regulate CD4 transcription. Studies by Kavathas and colleagues have shown that the core promoter region for hCD8α contains cyclic AMP response elements, but its function is not T-cell–specific *(101)*. However, a T-cell–specific enhancer is associated with a DNase I hypersensitive site in the last hCD8α intron *(102)*. This enhancer bears some resemblance to the CD4 enhancers in that it contains consensus binding sites for Ets, TCF-1/Lef-1, GATA, and bHLH transcription factors. It also contains a putative silencer, but in contrast to the CD4 silencer, its negative regulatory function is position-dependent, most likely because its self-complementarity allows formation of DNA cruciforms, which structurally impede CD8α transcription *(103)*. A transgene construct including the hCD8α intronic enhancer does not direct reporter gene expression to CD8 SP T-cells, but is important for CD8α expression in NK cells *(104)*.

Very recent studies have begun to identify *cis*-acting DNA elements that regulate mCD8α expression during T-cell development in vivo. Hostert et al. made transgenic mice using a very large genomic construct containing both mCD8β and mCD8α, the 36 kb in between, as well as 6.5 kb of 5' and 25 kb of 3' flanking sequence *(78)*. Transgenic mCD8α was expressed in DP and CD8 SP thymocytes, but not in DN or CD4 SP thymocytes or other cell lineages, suggesting that this construct contains all sequences necessary for developmental stage- and lineage-specific CD8 expression. Importantly, two groups have recently identified DNA elements, located in between mCD8β and mCD8α, that direct expression of reporter transgenes exclusively to mature CD8 SP T-cells and IEL *(105,106)*. This regulatory region may also contain a CD8 silencer, since reporter gene expression was not observed in mature CD4 SP thymocytes in these studies *(105,106)*. Although a CD8 silencer was not positively identified in these studies, appropriate lineage-specific expression of mCD8α requires negative regulatory elements, located outside the mCD8α gene and its immediate flanking regions, to prevent its expression in CD4 lineage cells *(78)*. Some evidence suggests that posttranscriptional mechanisms may also contribute to subset-specific regulation of CD8α and CD8β expression *(78,107)*.

4.5. CD4 and CD8 Transcription and Lineage Commitment

These advances in elucidating developmental stage- and lineage-specific transcriptional regulation of CD4/CD8 expression, combined with a more complete description of transitional intermediate stages in the DP → SP transition, have begun to provide fundamental insights into mechanisms of CD4/CD8 lineage commitment. Why should thymocytes proceed through a $CD4^{lo}CD8^{lo}$ intermediate stage before committing to the CD4 or CD8 lineage? The answer awaits further study, but the fact that distinct transcriptional control elements regulate CD4 and CD8 expression in DP vs SP thymocytes may provide an important clue. Transient downregulation of CD4 and CD8 could be necessary to prepare cells to transcriptionally reprogram expression from the mature enhancers. Thus, CD4 commitment would require at least three events:

1. Cessation of CD4 transcription from the DP enhancer,
2. Activation of the CD4 enhancer, and
3. Silencing of CD8 expression by transcriptional or posttranscriptional means.

It is striking that there is a significant temporal separation between steps 1 and 2. CD4 enhancer activity is only detected in a subset of $CD4^{+}CD8^{int/lo}$ and the most mature, HSA^{lo} $H\text{-}2K^{hi}$ CD4 SP thymocytes. BUdR labeling studies demonstrate that significant numbers of TCR^{hi} CD4 SP are generated by three days after cell division ceases, but these cells do not acquire a completely mature phenotype (HSA^{lo}, $H\text{-}2K^{hi}$, $Qa\text{-}2^{hi}$) until five to nine days after cell division ceases *(71)*. If activation of the CD4 enhancer occurs as a consequence of CD4 commitment, why would instructional activation of CD4 enhancer activity occur so long after acquisition of the CD4 SP phenotype? It seems more likely that activation of the CD4 enhancer occurs when stochastically CD4-committed cells are positively selected. Similar considerations apply to the CD8 commitment process. Whether or not the switch in enhancer usage is a cause or a consequence of CD4/8 lineage commitment, these findings minimally reveal that commitment is a mechanistically complex process in which there are multiple steps, each potentially subject to regulation by inputs from different signaling pathways.

5. Conclusions

The past several years have yielded many important advances towards understanding the molecular basis of thymocyte positive selection and CD4/CD8 lineage commitment. The lack of a clear consensus with regard to the mechanisms underlying this process attests to the difficulties of observing cell lineage decisions in rare thymocyte subsets, most of which are destined to die, and to the tremendous complexity of these events. Moreover, it has proven to be particularly difficult to devise experimental strategies and perturbations that can unambiguously distinguish between commitment per se, and survival of committed progenitors. Additional progress in understanding transcriptional regulation of CD4 and CD8 is likely to be made, although not rapidly, given the necessity of using a transgenic approach. It will be particulary informative to learn whether a CD8 silencer exists. Finally, further studies of Notch, or other molecules, such homeobox and polycomb group genes, which play fundamental roles in regulating many cell fate decisions, as potential regulators of CD4/CD8 lineage commitment are likely to yield important insights. These issues all represent significant challenges for the future.

Acknowledgments

The author is supported by operating grants from the Medical Research Council of Canada, the National Cancer Institute of Canada, and also holds an MRC Scientist award. The author wishes to acknowledge Dr. Tim Groves for providing Fig. 1.

References

1. Fink, P. J. and Bevan, M. J. (1978) H-2 antigens of the thymus determine lymphocyte specificity. *J. Exp. Med.* **148,** 766–775.
2. Zinkernagel, R. M., Callahan, G. N., Althage, A., Cooper, S., Klein, P. A., and Klein, J. (1978) On the thymus in the differentiation of "H-2 self-recognition" by T-cells: Evidence for dual recognition? *J. Exp. Med.* **147,** 882–896.
3. Guidos, C. J. (1996) Positive selection of $CD4^+$ and $CD8^+$ T cells. *Curr. Opin. Immunol.* **8,** 225–232.
4. Groves, T., Parsons, M., Miyamoto, N., and Guidos, C. J. (1997) TCR engagement of $CD4^+CD8^+$ thymocytes in vitro induces early aspects of positive selection, but not apoptosis. *J. Immunol.* **158,** 65–75.
5. Kearse, K., Takahama, Y., Punt, J., Sharrow, S., and Singer, A. (1995) Early molecular events induced by TCR signaling in immature $CD4^+CD8^+$ thymocytes. *J. Exp. Med.* **181,** 193–202.
6. Turka, L. A., Schatz, D. G., Oettinger, M. A., Chun, J., Gorka, C., Lee, K., McCormack, W. T., and Thompson, C. B. (1991) Thymocyte expression of RAG-1 and RAG-2: Termination by T cell receptor cross-linking. *Science* **253,** 778–781.
7. Fischer, K.-D., Zmuidzinas, A., Gardner, S. , Barbacid, M., Bernstein, A., and Guidos, C. (1995) Defective T-cell receptor signaling and positive selection of Vav-deficient $CD4^+CD8^+$ thymocytes. *Nature* **374,** 474–477.
8 Groves, T., Smiley, P., Cooke, M. P., Forbush, K., Perlmutter, R. M., and Guidos, C. J. (1996) Fyn can partially substitute for Lck in T lymphocyte development. *Immunity* **5,** 417–428.
9. Petrie, H. T., Strasser, A., Harris, A. W., Hugo, P., and Shortman, K. (1993) $CD4^+8^-$ and $CD4^-8^+$ mature thymocytes require different post-selection processing for final development. *J. Immunol.* **151,** 1273–1279.
10. Wilkinson, R. W., Anderson, G., Owen, J. J. T., and Jenkinson, E. J. (1995) Positive selection of thymocytes involves sustained interactions with the thymic microenvironment. *J. Immunol.* **155,** 5234–5240.
11. Punt, J. A., Suzuki, H., Granger, L. G., Sharrow, S. O., and Singer, A. (1996) Lineage commitment in the thymus: only the most differentiated ($TCR^{hi}bcl\text{-}2^{hi}$) subset of $CD4^+CD8^+$ thymocytes has selectively terminated CD4 or CD8 synthesis. *J. Exp. Med.* **184,** 2091–2099.
12. Guidos, C. J. and Weissman, I. L. (1993) Sequential occurrence of positive and negative selection during T lymphocyte maturation, in *Molecular Mechanisms of Immunological Self-Recognition* (Alt, F., and Vogel, H. J., eds.) Academic, San Diego, CA, 137–147.
13. Guidos, C. J., Weissman, I. L., and Adkins, B. (1989) Intrathymic maturation of murine T lymphocytes from $CD8^+$ precursors. *Proc. Natl. Acad. Sci. USA* **86,** 7542–7546.
14. Guidos, C. J., Danska, J. S., Fathman, C. G., and Weissman, I. L. (1990) T cell receptor-mediated negative selection of autoreactive T lymphocyte precursors occurs after commitment to the CD4 or CD8 lineages. *J. Exp. Med.* **172,** 835–845.
15. Bendelac, A., Matzinger, P., Seder, R. A., Paul, W. E., and Schwartz, R. H. (1992) Activation events during thymic selection. *J. Exp. Med.* **175,** 731–742.
16. van Meerwijk, J. P. M. and Germain, R. N. (1993) Development of mature $CD8^+$ thymocytes: selection rather than instruction? *Science* **261,** 911–915.
17. van Meerwijk, J. P. M., O'Connell, E. M., and Germain, R. N. (1995) Evidence for lineage commitment and initiation of positive selection by thymocytes with intermediate surface phenotypes. *J. Immunol.* **154,** 6314–6323.
18. Benveniste, P., Knowles, G., and Cohen, A. (1996) CD8/CD4 lineage commitment occurs by an instructional/default process followed by positive selection. *Eur. J. Immunol.* **26,** 461–471.

19. Lucas, B., and Germain, R. N. (1996) Unexpectedly complex regulation of CD4/CD8 coreceptor expression supports a revised model for $CD4^+CD8^+$ thymocyte differentiation. *Immunity* **5,** 461–477.
20. Lundberg, K., Heath, W., Köntgen, F., Carbone, F. R., and Shortman, K. (1995) Intermediate steps in positive selection: differentiation of $CD4^+8^{int}TCR^{int}$ thymocytes into $CD4^-8^+TCR^{hi}$ thymocytes. *J. Exp. Med.* **181,** 1643–1651.
21. Suzuki, H., Punt, J., Granger, L., and Singer, A. (1995) Asymmetric signaling requirements for thymocyte commitment to the $CD4^+$ versus $CD8^+$ T cell lineages: a new perspective on thymic commitment and selection. *Immunity* **2,** 413–425.
22. Swat, W., Ignatowicz, L., von Boehmer, H., and Kisielow, P. (1991) Clonal deletion of immature $CD4^+8^+$ thymocytes in suspension culture by extrathymic antigen-presenting cells. *Nature* **351,** 150–153.
23. Kersh, G. J., and Hedrick, S. M. (1995) Role of TCR specificity in CD4 versus CD8 lineage commitment. *J. Immunol.* **154,** 1057–1068.
24. Akashi, K., and Weissman, I. L. (1996) The c-kit^+ maturation pathway in mouse thymic T cell development, lineages and selection. *Immunity* **5,** 147–161.
25. Weiss, A., and Littman, D. R. (1994) Signal transduction by lymphocyte antigen receptors. *Cell* **76,** 263–274.
26. Zamoyska, R. (1994) The CD8 coreceptor revisited: one chain good, two chains better. *Immunity* **1,** 243–246.
27. Wiest, D. L., Yuan, L., Jefferson, J., Benveniste, P., Tsokos, M., Klausner, R. D., Glimcher, L. H., Samelson, E., and Singer, A. (1993) Regulation of T cell receptor expression in immature $CD4^+CD8^+$ thymocytes by $p56^{lck}$ tyrosine kinase: Basis for differential signaling by CD4 and CD8 in immature thymocytes expressing both coreceptor molecules. *J. Exp. Med.* **178,** 1701–1712.
28. Itano, A., Salmon, P.,Kioussis, D., Tolaini, M., Corbella, P., and Robey, E. (1996) The cytoplasmic domain of CD4 promotes the development of CD4 lineage T cells. *J. Exp. Med.* **183,** 731–741.
29. Seong, R. H., Chamberlain, J. W., and Parnes, J. R. (1992) Signal for T-cell differentiation to a CD4 cell lineage is delivered by CD4 transmembrane region and/or cytoplasmic tail. *Nature* **356,** 718–720.
30. Borgulya, P., Kishi, H., Uematsu, Y., and von Boehmer, H. (1992) Exclusion and inclusion of α and β T cell receptor alleles. *Cell* **69,** 529–537.
31. Petrie, H. T., Livak, F., Schatz, D. G., Strasser, A., Crispe, I. N., and Shortman, K. (1993) Multiple rearrangements in TCRα chain genes maximize the production of useful thymocytes. *J. Exp. Med.* **178,** 615–622.
32. Matechak, E. O., Killeen, N., Hedrick, S. M., and Fowlkes, B. J. (1996) MHC class II-specific T cells can develop in the CD8 lineage when CD4 is absent. *Immunity* **4,** 337–347.
33. Kirberg, J., Baron, A., Jakob, S., Rolink, A., Karjalainen, K., and von Boehmer, H. (1994) Thymic selection of $CD8^+$ single positive cells with a class II major histocompatibility complex-restricted receptor. *J. Exp. Med.* **180,** 25–34.
34. Bendelac, A. (1995) Positive selection of mouse $NK1^+$ T cells by CD1-expressing cortical thymocytes. *J. Exp. Med.* **182,** 2091–2096.
35. Bendelac, A., Killeen, N., Littman, D. R., and Schwartz, R. H. (1994) A subset of $CD4^+$ thymocytes selected by MHC class I molecules. *Science* **263,** 1774–1778.
36. Coles, M. C. and Raulet, D. H. (1994) Class I dependence of the development of $CD4^+CD8^-$ $NK1.1^+$ thymocytes. *J. Exp. Med.* **180,** 395–399.
37. Cosgrove, D., Gray, D., Dierich, A., Kaufman, J., Lemeur, M., Benoist, C., and Mathis, C. C. (1991) Mice lacking MHC class II molecules. *Cell* **66,** 1051–1066.
38. Bommhardt, U., Cole, M. S., Tso, J. Y., and Zamoyska, R. (1997) Signals through CD8 or CD4 can induce commitment to the CD4 lineage in the thymus. *Eur. J. Immunol.* **27,** 1152–1163.
39. Goldrath, A. W., Hogquist, K. A., and Bevan, M. J. (1997) CD8 lineage commitment in the absence of CD8. *Immunity* **6,** 633–642.
40. Sebzda, E., Choi, M., Fung-Leung, W. P., T. Mak, W., and Ohashi, P. S. (1997) Peptide-induced positive selection of TCR transgenic thymocytes in a coreceptor-independent manner. *Immunity* **6,** 643–653.
41. Chan, S. H., Cosgrove, D., Waltzinger, C., Benoist, C., and Mathis, D. (1993) Another view of the selective model of thymocyte selection. *Cell* **73,** 225–236.

42. Davis, C. B., Killeen, N., Crooks, M. E. C., Raulet, D., and Littman, D. R. (1993) Evidence for a stochastic mechanism in the differentiation of mature subsets of T lymphocytes. *Cell* **73,** 237–247.
43. Cibotti, R., Punt, J. A., Dash, K. S., Sharrow, S. O., and Singer, A. (1997) Surface molecules that drive T cell development in vitro in the absence of thymic epithelium and in the absence of lineage-specific signals. *Immunity* **6,** 245–255.
44. Suzuki, H., Shinkai, Y., Granger, L. G., Alt, F. W., Love, P. E., and Singer, A. (1997) Commitment of immature $CD4^+CD8^+$ thymocytes to the CD4 lineage requires CD3 signaling but does not require expression of clonotypic T cell receptor (TCR) chains. *J. Exp. Med.* **186,** 17–23.
45. Crump, A. L., Grusby M. J., Glimcher, L. H., and Cantor, H. (1993) Thymocyte development in major histocompatibility complex-deficient mice: Evidence for stochastic commitment to the CD4 and CD8 lineages. *Proc. Natl. Acad. Sci. USA* **90,** 10739–10743.
46. Takahama, Y., Suzuki, H., Katz, K. S., Grusby, M. J., and Singer, A. (1994) Positive selection of $CD4^+$ T cells by TCR ligation without aggregation even in the absence of MHC. *Nature* **371,** 67–70.
47. Zerrahn, J., Held, W., and Raulet, D. H. (1997) The MHC reactivity of the T cell repertoire prior to positive and negative selection. *Cell* **88,** 627–636.
48. Poirier, G., Lo, D., Reilly, C. R., and Kaye, J. (1994) Discrimination between thymic epithelial cells and peripheral antigen-presenting cells in the induction of immature T cell differentiation. *Immunity* **1,** 385–391.
49. Anderson, G., Jenkinson, E. J., Moore, N. C., and Owen, J. J. T. (1993) MHC class II-positive epithelium and mesenchyme cells are both required for T-cell development in the thymus. *Nature* **362,** 70–73.
50. Anderson, G., Owen, J. J. T., Moore, N. C., and Jenkinson, E. J. (1994) Thymic epithelial cells provide unique signals for positive selection of $CD4^+CD8^+$ thymocytes in vitro. *J. Exp. Med.* **179,** 2027–2031.
51. Ernst, B. B., Surh, C. D., and Sprent, J. (1996) Bone marrow-derived cells fail to induce positive selection in thymus reaggregation cultures. *J. Exp. Med.* **183,** 1235–1240.
52. Tanaka, Y., Williams, O., Tarazona, R., Wack, A., Norton, T., and Kioussis, D. (1996) In vitro positive selection of αβ TCR transgenic thymocytes by a conditionally immortalized cortical epithelial clone. *Int. Immunol.* **9,** 381–393.
53. Muller, K. P. and Kyewski, B. A. (1993) T cell receptor targeting to thymic cortical epithelial cells in vivo induces survival, activation and differentiation of immature thymocytes. *Eur. J. Immunol.* **23,** 1661–1670.
54. Muller, K. P. and Kyewski, B. A. (1995) Intrathymic T cell receptor (TCR) targeting in mice lacking CD4 or major histocompatibility complex (MHC) class II, rescue of CD4 T cell lineage without co-engagement of TCR/CD4 by MHC class II. *Eur. J. Immunol.* **25,** 896–902.
55. Pawlowski, T., Elliott, J. D., Loh, D. Y., and Staerz, U. D. (1993) Positive selection of T lymphocytes on fibroblasts. *Nature* **364,** 642–645.
56. Bailey, A. M., and Posakony, J. W. (1995) Suppressor of hairless directly activates transcription of enhancer of split complex genes in response to Notch receptor activity. *Genes Dev.* **9,** 2609–2622.
57. Fortini, M. E. and Artavanis-Tsakonas, S. (1994) The suppressor of hairless protein participates in Notch receptor signaling. *Cell* **79,** 273–282.
58. Hsieh, J. J., Henkel, T., Salmon, P., Robey, E., Peterson, M. G., and Hayward, S. D. (1996) Truncated mammalian Notch1 activates CBF1/RBPJk-repressed genes by a mechanism resembling that of Epstein-Barr virus EBNA2. *Mol. Cell. Biol.* **16,** 952–959.
59. Ishibashi, M., Ang, S. L., Shiota, K., Nakanishi, S., Kageyama, R., and Guillemot, F. (1995) Targeted disruption of mammalian hairy and Enhancer of split homolog-1 (HES-1) leads to up-regulation of neural helix-loop-helix factors, premature neurogenesis, and severe neural tube defects. *Genes Dev.* **9,** 3136–3148.
60. Jarriault, S., Brou, C., Logeat, F., Schroeter, E. H., Kopan, R., and Israel, A. (1995) Signalling downstream of activated mammalian Notch. *Nature* **377,** 355–358.
61. Tomita, K., Ishibashi, M., Nakahara, K., Ang, S. L., Nakanishi, S., Guillemot, F., and Kageyama, R. (1996) Mammalian hairy and Enhancer of split homolog 1 regulates differentiation of retinal neurons and is essential for eye morphogenesis. *Neuron* **16,** 723–734.
62. Robey, E., Chang, D., Itano, A., Cado, D., Alexander, H., Lans, D., Weinmaster, G., and Salmon, P. (1996) An activated form of Notch influences the choice between CD4 and CD8 T cell lineages. *Cell* **87,** 483–492.

63. Hasserjian, R. P., Aster, J. C., Davi, F., Weinberg, D. S., and Sklar, J. (1996) Modulated expression of Notch1 during thymocyte development. *Blood* **88,** 970–976.
64. Artavanis-Tsakonas, S., Matsuno, K., and Fortini, M. E. (1995) Notch signaling. *Science* **268,** 225–232.
65. Ellisen, L. W., Bird, J., West, D. C., Soreng, A. L., Reynolds, T. C., Smith, S. D., and Sklar, J. (1991) TAN-1, the human homolog of the Drosophila Notch gene, is broken by chromosomal translocations in T lymphoblastic neoplasms. *Cell* **66,** 649–661.
66. Aster, J. C., Robertson, E. S., Hasserjian, R. P., Turner, J. R., Kieff, E., and Sklar, J. (1997) Oncogenic forms of NOTCH1 lacking either the primary binding site for RBP-Jκ or nuclear localization sequences retain the ability to associate with RBP-Jκ and activate transcription. *J. Biol. Chem.* **272,** 11336–11343.
67. Girard, L., Hanna, Z., Beaulieu, N., Hoemann, C. D., Simard, C., Kozak, C. A., and Jolicoeur, P. (1996) Frequent provirus insertional mutagenesis of Notch1 in thymomas of MMTVD/myc transgenic mice suggests a collaboration of c-myc and Notch1 for oncogenesis. *Genes Dev.* **10,** 1930–1944.
68. Pear, W. S., Aster, J. C., Scott, M. L., Hasserjian, R. P., Soffer, B., Sklar, J., and Baltimore, D. (1996) Exclusive development of T cell neoplasms in mice transplanted with bone marrow expressing activated Notch alleles. *J. Exp. Med.* **183,** 2283–2291.
69. Washburn, T., Schweighoffer, E., Gridley, T., Chang, D., Fowlkes, B. J., Cado, D., and Robey, E. (1997) Notch activity influences the αβ versus γδ T cell lineage decision. *Cell* **88,** 833–843.
70. Linette, G. P., Grusby, M. J., Hedrick, S. M., Hansen, T. H., Glimcher, L. H., and Korsmeyer, S. J. (1994) *Bcl-2* is upregulated at the $CD4^+CD8^+$ stage during positive selection and promotes thymocyte differentiation at several control points. *Immunity* **1,** 197–205.
71. Lucas, B., Vasseur, F., and Penit, C. (1994) Production, selection, and maturation of thymocytes with high surface density of TCR. *J. Immunol.* **153,** 53–62.
72. Rooke, R., Waltzinger, C., Benoist, C., and Mathis, D. (1997) Targeted complementation of MHC class II deficiency by intrathymic delivery of recombinant adenoviruses. *Immunity* **7,** 123–134.
73. Huesmann, M., Scott, B., Kisielow, P., and von Boehmer, H. (1991) Kinetics and efficiency of positive selection in the thymus of normal and T cell receptor transgenic mice. *Cell* **66,** 533–540.
74. Ernst, B., Surh, C. D., and Sprent, J. (1995) Thymic selection and cell division. *J. Exp. Med.* **182,** 961–971.
75. Nakayama, K.-I., Nakayama, K., Negishi, I., Kuida, K., Shinkai, Y., Louie, M., Fields, I. E., Lucas, P. J., Stewart, V., Alt, F. W., and Loh, D. Y. (1993) Disappearance of the lymphoid system in Bcl-2 homozygous mutant chimeric mice. *Science* **261,** 1584–1588.
76. Abbas, A. K., Murphy, K. M., and Sher, A. (1996) Functional diversity of helper T lymphocytes. *Nature* **383,** 787–793.
76a. Takeda, S., Rodewald, H. R., Arakawa, H., Bluethmann, H., and Shimizu, T. (1996) MHC class II molecules are not required for survival of newly generated $CD4^+$ T cells, but affect their long-term life span. *Immunity* **5,** 217–228.
77. Kozieradzki, I., Kundig, T., Kishihara, K., Ong, C. J., Chiu, D., Wallace, V. A., Kawai, V. A., Timms, E., J. Ionescu, J., Ohashi, P., Marth, J. D., Mak, T. W., and Penninger, J. M. (1997) T cell development in mice expressing splice variants of the protein tyrosine phosphatase CD45. *J. Immunol.* **158,** 3130–3139.
78. Hostert, A., Tolaini, M., Festenstein, R., McNeill, L., Malissen, B., Williams, O., Zamoyska, R., and Kioussis, D. (1997) A CD8 genomic fragment that directs subset-specific expression of CD8 in transgenic mice. *J. Immunol.* **158,** 4270–4281.
79. Siu, G., Wurster, A. L., Duncan, D. D., Soliman, T. M., and Hedrick, S. M. (1994) A transcriptional silencer controls the developmental expression of the CD4 gene. *EMBO J.* **13,** 3570–3579.
80. Salmon, P., Giovane, A., Wasylyk, B., and Klatzmann, D. (1993) Characterization of the human CD4 gene promoter: transcription from the CD4 gene core promoter is tissue-specific and is activated by Ets proteins. *Proc. Natl. Acad. Sci. USA* **90,** 7739–7743.
81. Siu, G., Wurster, A. L., Lipsick, J. S., and Hedrick, S. M. (1992) Expression of the CD4 gene requires a Myb transcription factor. *Mol. Cell. Biol.* **12,** 1592–1604.
82. Duncan, D. D., Stupakoff, A., Hedrick, S. M., Marcu, K. B., and Siu, G. (1995) A Myc-associated zinc finger protein binding site is one of four important functional regions in the CD4 promoter. *Mol. Cell. Biol.* **15,** 3179–3186.

83. Badiani, P., Corbella, P., Kioussis, D., Marvel, J., and Weston, K. (1994) Dominant interfering alleles define a role for c-Myb in T-cell development. *Genes Dev.* **8,** 770–782.
84. Badiani, P. A., Kioussis, D., Swirsky, D. M., Lampert, I. A., and Weston, K. (1996) T-cell lymphomas in v-Myb transgenic mice. *Oncogene* **13,** 2205–2212.
85. Sawada, S. and Littman, D. R. (1991) Identification and characterization of a T-cell-specific enhancer adjacent to the murine CD4 gene. *Mol. Cell. Biol.* **11,** 5506–5515.
86. Blum, M. D., Wong, G. T., Higgins, K. M., Sunshine, M. J., and Lacy, E. (1993) Reconstitution of the subclass-specific expression of CD4 in thymocytes and peripheral T cells of transgenic mice: identification of a human CD4 enhancer. *J. Exp. Med.* **177,** 1343–1358.
87. Sawada, S., Scarborough, J. D., Killeen, N., and Littman, D. R. (1994) A lineage-specific transcriptional silencer regulates CD4 gene expression during T lymphocyte development. *Cell* **77,** 917–929.
88. Sawada, S. and Littman, D. R. (1993) A heterodimer of HEB and an E12-related protein interacts with the CD4 enhancer and regulates its activity in T-cell lines. *Mol. Cell. Biol.* **13,** 5620–5628.
89. Wurster, A. L., Siu, G., Leiden, J. M., and Hedrick, S. M. (1994) Elf-1 binds to a critical element in a second CD4 enhancer [published erratum appears in Mol Cell Biol 1994 Dec;14(12),8493]. *Mol. Cell. Biol.* **14,** 6452–6463.
90. Gillespie, F. P., Doros, L., Vitale, J., Blackwell, C., Gosselin, J., Snyder, B. W., and Wadsworth, S. C. (1993) Tissue-specific expression of human CD4 in transgenic mice. *Mol. Cell. Biol.* **13,** 2952–2958.
91. Hanna, Z., Simard, C., Laperriere, A., and Jolicoeur, P. (1994) Specific expression of the human CD4 gene in mature $CD4^+$ $CD8^-$ and immature $CD4^+$ $CD8^+$ T cells and in macrophages of transgenic mice. *Mol. Cell. Biol.* **14,** 1084–1094.
92. Killeen, N., Sawada, S., and Littman, D. R. (1993) Regulated expression of human CD4 rescues helper T cell development in mice lacking expression of endogenous CD4. *EMBO J.* **12,** 1547–1553.
93. Salmon, P., Boyer, O., Lores, P., Jami, J., and Klatzmann, D. (1996) Characterization of an intronless CD4 minigene expressed in mature CD4 and CD8 T cells, but not expressed in immature thymocytes. *J. Immunol.* **156,** 1873–1879.
94. Duncan, D. D., Adlam, M., and Siu, G. (1996) Asymmetric redundancy in CD4 silencer function. *Immunity* **4,** 301–311.
95. Adlam, M., Duncan, D. D., Ng, D. K., and Siu, G. (1997) Positive selection induces CD4 promoter and enhancer function. *Int. Immunol.* **9,** 877–887.
96. Uematsu, Y., Donda, A., and De Libero, G. (1997) Thymocytes control the CD4 gene differently from mature T lymphocytes. *Int. Immunol.* **9,** 179–187.
97. Kydd, R., Lundberg, K., Vremec, D., Harris, A. W., and Shortman, K. (1995) Intermediate steps in thymic positive selection. Generation of $CD4^-8^+$ T cells in culture from $CD4^+8^+$, $CD4^{int}8^+$, and $CD4^+8^{int}$ thymocytes with up-regulated levels of TCR-CD3. *J. Immunol.* **155,** 3806–3814.
98. Donda, A., Schulz, M., Burki, K., De Libero, G., and Uematsu, Y. (1996) Identification and characterization of a human CD4 silencer. *Eur. J. Immunol.* **26,** 493–500.
99. Sasai, Y., Kageyama, R., Tagawa, Y., Shigemoto, R., and Nakanishi, S. (1992) Two mammalian helix-loop-helix factors structurally related to Drosophila hairy and Enhancer of split. *Genes Dev.* **6,** 2620–2634.
100. Poussier, P. and Julius, M. (1994) Thymus independent T cell development and selection in the intestinal epithelium. *Ann. Rev. Immunol.* **12,** 521–553.
101. Gao, M. H. and Kavathas, P. B. (1993) Functional importance of the cyclic AMP response element-like decamer motif in the CD8 alpha promoter. *J. Immunol.* **150,** 4376–4385.
102. Hambor, J. E., Mennone, J., Coon, M. E., Hanke, J. H., and Kavathas, P. (1993) Identification and characterization of an Alu-containing, T-cell-specific enhancer located in the last intron of the human CD8 alpha gene. *Mol. Cell. Biol.* **13,** 7056–7070.
103. Hanke, J. H., Hambor, J. E., and Kavathas, P. (1995) Repetitive Alu elements form a cruciform structure that regulates the function of the human CD8 alpha T cell-specific enhancer. *J. Mol. Biol.* **246,** 63–73.
104. Kieffer, L. J., Bennett, J. A., Cunningham, A. C., Gladue, R. P., McNeish, J., Kavathas, P. B., and Hanke, J. H. (1996) Human CD8 alpha expression in NK cells but not cytotoxic T cells of transgenic mice. *Int. Immunol.* **8,** 1617–1626.

105. Hostert, A., Tolaini, M., Roderick, K., Harker, N., Norton, T., and Kioussis, D. (1997) A region in the CD8 gene locus that directs expression to the mature CD8 T cell subset in transgenic mice. *Immunity* **7,** 525–536.
106. Ellmeier, W., Sunshine, M. J., Losos, K., Hatam, F., and Littman, D. R. (1997) An enhancer that directs lineage-specific expression of CD8 in positively selected thymocytes and mature T cells. *Immunity* **7,** 537–547.
107. Gao, M. H., Walz, M., and Kavathas, P. B. (1996) Post-transcriptional regulation associated with control of human CD8α expression of $CD4^+$ T cells. *Immunogenetics* **45,** 130–135.
108. Guidos, C. J., Williams, C. J., Wu, G. E., Paige, C. J., and Danska, J. S. (1995) Development of $CD4^+CD8^+$ thymocytes in RAG-deficient mice through a T cell receptor β chain-independent pathway. *J. Exp. Med.* **181,** 1187–1195.

Part VII

Clinical Applications of Hematolymphoid Development

Chapter 25

Stem Cell Transplants for Hematopoietic Malignancies

Susan C. Guba and Bart Barlogie

1. Introduction

The purpose of this chapter is to identify clinical models or approaches that can be exploited to improve the curability of hematopoietic malignancies. The chapter begins by identifying tumor and host factors that the clinician must consider when identifying a specific clinical approach for a specific patient that ultimately will determine the curability of that particular tumor. The remaining sections in the chapter focus on strategies to approach hematopoietic malignancies, particularly those that may be either palliated or cured as a result of their inherent responsiveness to at least high-dose chemotherapy. These approaches include the goals, limitations, and timing of dose-intensive therapy, which are utilized to maximize tumor response and which may be required to provide curative therapy. Subsequently, there is a discussion of strategies to decrease the incidence of relapse. Such strategies include both ex vivo and in vivo mechanisms to eliminate minimal residual disease (e.g., autograft manipulation by purging or positive selection of normal stem cells; graft-vs-tumor effects, tumor vaccines, cytokine modulation). The authors hope that this chapter will suggest that early intensive therapy for patients with potentially curable malignancies should be a new paradigm for future clinical trials.

2. Tumor and Host Factors Influencing Response to Cancer Therapy

A plethora of intrinsic tumor and host factors contribute to the clinical behavior of a hematopoietic malignancy in an individual patient. A cartoon of these relationships is shown in Fig. 1. The presence or absence, and the nature of these factors, influence the therapeutic approach, determines clinical outcome and, especially, curability.

From: *Molecular Biology of B-Cell and T-Cell Development*
Edited by: J. G. Monroe and E. V. Rothenberg © Humana Press Inc., Totowa, NJ

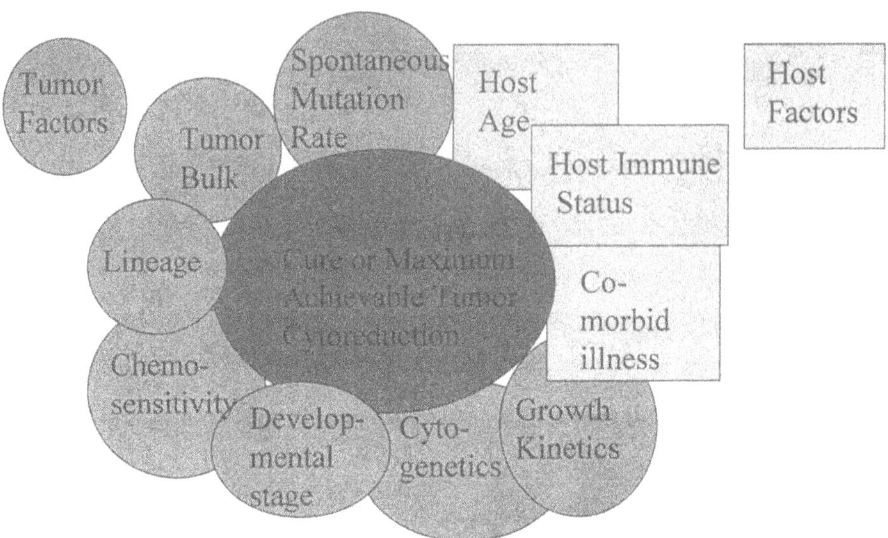

Fig. 1. The interaction between intrinsic tumor and host-specific factors affects the clinical behavior and curability of a tumor, treatment approach and outcome for a patient. For example, tumor bulk is a function of growth kinetics, the immune status of the patient, and response to prior therapy. In part, response to prior therapy relates to the host's comorbid illnesses and performance status. These host and tumor factors may predict for good or poor prognosis and may change spontaneously or in response to treatment (e.g., karyotype, minimal residual disease [MRD]).

2.1. Tumor Factors

2.1.1. Lineage

The lineage of a hematopoietic malignancy is important for selecting appropriate chemotherapeutic agents for treatment of the malignancy, or for selecting an appropriate conditioning regimen pretransplantation. However, lineage by itself is a poor determinant for predicting outcome; instead, the clinician must rely on other tumor characteristics to predict clinical behavior.

2.1.2. Developmental Stages

Developmental stages for both benign and malignant cells may be divided into self-renewal and differentiated compartments. These different compartments can be defined phenotypically and cytogenetically. Differentiation antigens may be selectively targeted so that the renewal compartment and hence, a tumor's ability to self-perpetuate, is eliminated. Tumor self-antigens may also be used to develop specific idiotype antibodies. These antibodies may be used to purge autologous marrow. Alternatively, antibodies may be used to develop idiotype vaccines to induce an idiotype specific immunological response of the humoral or cell-mediated type.

2.1.3. Genetic Alterations

Genetic alterations, present in all tumor cells, result in activation of oncogenes, inactivation of tumor suppressor genes, or development of fusion genes. Such genetic alterations result in changes of normal cellular functions, that often predict prognosis (Table 1). In AML, younger patients (< 60 years) more often have specific chromosomal translocations *(1,2)* identified in leukemic progenitors at a more mature stage of differentiation

Table 1
Tumor Cytogenetics and Prognosis

Malignancy	Genetic alteration	Fusion gene or oncogene	Prognosis	Transplant timing
AML *(de novo)*	t(8;21)	ETO/AML 1	Good	All good to intermediate prognosis AML:
AML *(de novo)*	inv(16)	AML 1, CBFβ/MYH11	Good	1. allogeneic transplants established in 2nd or greater CR;
AML *(de novo)*	t(15;17)	PML-RARα	Good-intermediate	2. purged autologous transplants established in 2nd CR if patients has no donor or is too old for allo transplant;
AML *(de novo)*	Normal		Good-intermediate	3. worthy of investigation by cytogenetic groups in first CR
ALL, CML, AML	t(9;22)	bcr-abl	Poor	Established or under investigation in 1st CR; worthy of investigation as primary therapy
MDS, t-ANLL	–5, –5q, –7, +8		Poor	Worthy of investigation in 1st CR
Follicular lymphoma	t(14;18)	bcl-2	Good	Autotransplantation under investigation in 2nd-3rd CR
Large cell lymphoma	t(3;14), t(3;22)	bcl-6	Good	Autotransplantation established in 1st relapse 2nd CR, especially in high-risk patients
Burkitt's lymphoma	t(8;14)	c-myc	Poor (50%) Good (50%)	Established in 1st relapse in poor prognosis group; autoBMT under investigation in 1st CR
Mantle cell lymphoma	t(11;14)	Ig heavy chain/bcl-1 (PRAD1)	Good	Worthy of investigation in 2nd CR

Data from refs. *1, 3, 59–75*. CR, complete remission.

Table 2
Prognostic Factors Associated with Tumor Relapse

Bulky disease
Advanced clinical stage
Bone marrow or CNS involvement
Elevated serum markers (LDH or b2M)
Poor prognosis cytogenetics
Chemorefractoriness
Other antiapoptotic mechanisms, e.g., bcl-2, IL-6

and a superior outcome. In contradistinction, older patients more commonly present with numerical abnormalities in less mature undifferentiated leukemia cells.

2.1.4. Mutation Rate

The spontaneous mutation rate of the tumor contributes to tumor heterogeneity and increases the potential for drug resistance.

2.1.5. Growth Kinetics

The net growth kinetics of a tumor are determined by several factors including cell-cycle kinetics, the differentiation rate of the cells, and the rate of cell death or apoptosis. These factors combine to determine tumor doubling time.

2.1.6. Tumor Bulk

Tumor bulk, usually at 10^{12} cells at the time of clinical presentation, can often be approximated by imaging studies to assess clinical stage of disease or, indirectly, by tumor secretory products (e.g., LDH or β_2M). Increased tumor bulk usually correlates with poor prognosis, because advanced tumor mass reflects a longer subclinical course with higher mutation rates of one mutation per 10^6–10^9 tumor cells. Such mutations account for resistance to chemotherapy, even without prior chemotherapy, or are further enhanced as a result of ineffective cell-kill where surviving cells display multiple antiapoptotic devices. Large tumor bulk also implies that the tumor is poorly modulated by the host's immune system, implying either poor tumor immunogenicity, host immunosuppression, or both.

2.1.7. Chemosensitivity

Chemosensitivity, clinically discernible only by response to therapy, is the single most important indicator of curability. Complete remission (CR) following initial therapy signals potential cure with standard therapy. However, early relapse or the persistence of minimal residual disease signals the need for additional therapy. Such additional therapy for tumors that remain chemosensitive at relapse should include myeloablative therapy at a time when apoptotic mechanisms, as a result of cytotoxic or immunologic intervention, are still operative. Relapsed tumors that are resistant to standard-dose therapy may respond to high-dose therapy and can be potentially overcome sufficiently by dose-escalation to result in cures. However, complete response rates and disease-free survival for patients with resistant tumors are less than for patients with preserved chemosensitivity. The resistance of tumors that have never responded to standard-dose chemotherapy (primary unresponsive disease) can generally not be overcome sufficiently by dose-escalation to result in cures *(3)*.

2.2. Host Factors

Host factors important in predicting outcome include the following:

2.2.1. Age

Increasing host age has been associated in some hematological malignancies with worse prognosis. However, differences in outcome between patients of different ages are not a function of age per se, but of inherent differences in the disease (e.g., manifested by cytogenetic differences) or differences in the host (e.g., the presence of serious comorbid illness), both of which should influence treatment approaches. For example, host age should not by itself exclude otherwise eligible patients from high-dose therapy with stem cell support. The authors have recently reported on patients over the age of 60 who have undergone double autologous bone marrow or PBSC transplantation for multiple myeloma *(4)*. No age-related differences in the number of CD34 cells collected or infused were observed. In addition, the rate of hematopoietic recovery following both the first and second transplant was not affected by patient age, when corrected for the amount of prior therapy. Although age of 60 years or greater was associated with increased treatment-related mortality compared to younger patients (0% vs 9%); overall survival was not significantly different between age groups. The important determining factor in the success of these transplants was the underlying health of the stem cells pretransplantation. In this chapter, patients of all ages who had received extensive prior therapy were found to have prolonged time to engraftment and time to count recovery compared to minimally pretreated patients.

2.2.2. Impaired Immune Response

An impaired host immune response occurs when tumor products, such as cytokines or cytokine receptors, or abnormalities in tumor ligands, paralyze the host immune system.

2.2.3. Comorbid Illnesses

Comorbid illnesses result in increased treatment-associated morbidity and, if sufficiently severe, may preclude treatment entirely.

The complexity of these interrelationships suggests that a treatment strategy should be based upon the anticipated long-term behavior of a particular disease in a particular patient and should include transplantation in potentially treatable diseases. The goals and timing of transplantation as well as the role of posttransplant modulation are examined in the remainder of the chapter.

3. Dose-Intensive Cancer Therapy

The role of dose-intensive or high-dose therapy with stem cell support in the treatment of malignancy was first established in patients with advanced poor-prognosis disease (Table 2). Once high-dose therapy was determined to be tolerated by the host, the use of high-dose therapy was expanded to include patients with less advanced disease and with better prognosis. The discussion on dose intensity that follows will include only a discussion of high-dose therapy with autologous stem cell support. Autologous transplantation provides a better model of dose-intensive therapy than allogeneic transplantation, because the ability of dose-intensive therapy to eradicate tumor in the autologous setting is not complicated by immunological modulating factors such as a graft-vs-leukemia effect present in an allogeneic transplant.

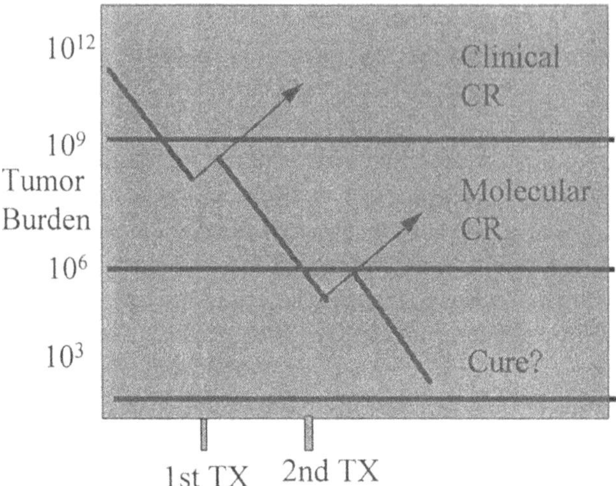

Fig. 2. The limits of a clinical complete remission are a tumor burden of $<10^9$ cells, whereas molecular techniques may detect tumor cells to a level of one tumor cell per 10^6 cells. Induction therapy, followed by transplant (TX) therapy, strives to reduce the tumor burden below the limits of molecular detection in an attempt to provide curative therapy. Between courses of therapy, or because of the development of chemorefractory cells, tumor cells may regrow and the tumor may escape remission.

3.1. Goals and Limitations of High-Dose Therapy

The putative goal of high-dose therapy is to improve response rates, particularly in tumor cells resistant to standard-dose therapy and, by achieving both a clinical and molecular complete remission, improve cure rates (Fig. 2). Cytoreduction to submolecular detection levels also theoretically diminishes the chance of developing spontaneous (endogenous) or treatment–induced resistance mutations, and hence, enhances the probability that a tumor will remain chemosensitive. At present, the data for improved survival as a result of high-dose therapy with autologous stem cell support have been most convincing for multiple myeloma and intermediate and high-grade lymphomas *(5,6)*. In addition, for those hematological malignancies in which clinical trials have shown a benefit for high-dose therapy, such therapy is likely to be the "best" therapy, whether that therapy is given for cure or palliation.

Two important corollaries follow. First, because first-order kinetics are followed, a single course of therapy will not eradicate all tumor cells even in the setting of high-dose therapy. Second, even though chemosensitive tumors will always demonstrate the best response to therapy, high-dose therapy is expected to improve response in relatively chemoresistant tumors, since some "resistant" tumors exhibit a threshold effect and are relatively chemosensitive at sufficiently high doses of chemotherapy. The key in overcoming such tumor resistance is the choice of the conditioning regimen. Optimally, such regimens deliver a sufficiently high cytotoxic dose to tumor cells to surpass the threshold necessary to overcome resistance. Thus, the conditioning regimen should be designed to shift the survival curve to the right, thereby improving survival or serving as high-quality palliative therapy.

High-dose therapy for hematological malignancies is designed to be myeloablative; high-dose therapy is limited by the ability to spare other end organs. Within a tolerable toxicity range, a variety of different conditioning regimens have been shown to be, apparently, equally efficacious. For example, most clinical trials of high-dose therapy in non-Hodgkin's lymphoma and CML suggest that combination TBI/chemotherapy regimens are comparable to chemotherapy alone with respect to efficacy of the regimen *(7–13)*. For malignancies in which an efficacious conditioning regimen is not well defined, therapeutic strategies can be borrowed from diseases with similar biology. For example, treatment approaches for Waldenstrom's macroglobulinemia may be modeled after approaches for multiple myeloma.

3.2. Efficacy of Timing of Dose-Intensive Therapy in Hematological Malignancies

High-dose therapy with autologous stem cell support has been shown to be efficacious in non-Hodgkin's lymphoma and in multiple myeloma *(5,6)*. Ongoing and future clinical trials will determine whether high-dose therapy with stem cell support is efficacious for other hematological malignancies and under what circumstances (e.g., stage, remission, conditioning regimen). In part, efficacy is determined by the timing of the high-dose therapy. Dose-intensive therapy should be utilized early in the course of a disease before stem cell damage has occurred from chronic or repetitive use of standard-dose chemotherapy. Such damage limits the number of stem cells that can be procured for transplant, impairs engraftment of those stem cells, and leads to treatment-related myelodysplasias (MDS) and leukemias. Vincristine, adriamycin, dexamethasone (VAD) exemplifies a stem cell-sparing standard therapy used in multiple myeloma, because it limits stem cell damage by minimizing alkylator exposure *(14,15)*. The importance of minimizing stem cell damage was demonstrated by Govindarajan et al. *(16)* who studied 188 patients with multiple myeloma; 71 of whom had no more than one prior regimen of chemotherapy (median duration of chemotherapy exposure 7.6 months), whereas 117 patients had more prolonged conventional chemotherapy (median duration of chemotherapy exposure 24 months). Following autologous transplantation, seven patients developed MDS; all seven patients were from the more extensively pretreated group ($p = 0.02$), suggesting that prolonged alkylator therapy pretransplantation, rather than early myeloablative therapy, is associated with development of MDS. Moreover, exposure to chemotherapy, even to <6 months of alkylator therapy, is associated with delayed hematopoietic recovery posttransplantation *(17)*. Thus, early high-dose therapy, even in the setting of palliation, strives to maintain hematopoietic integrity following therapy by minimizing treatment-related stem cell damage.

The efficacy of dose-intensive therapy is also improved with increasing chemosensitivity of the malignant cells. The prognostic impact of chemotherapy-sensitive disease on clinical outcome with autotransplants is exemplified by data by Philip et al. from relapsed non-Hodgkin's lymphomas: the CR rate is highest and three year disease-free survival longest in sensitive disease (91%, 36%), intermediate for resistant relapse (45%, 14%), and lowest for unresponsive lymphoma (26%, 0%) *(3,12,18)*. These results underscore that dose intensification even to the myeloablative range, at least in large cell lymphoma, can induce a response in patients in resistant relapse, but cannot overcome primary drug resistance sufficiently to effect cure.

The efficacy of dose-intensive therapy early in the treatment of newly diagnosed multiple myeloma patients was demonstrated by a total therapy regimen by Barlogie et al. *(19,20)*. This program utilized a series of noncross-resistant induction regimens followed by double transplantation. This protocol exploited the advantages of treating

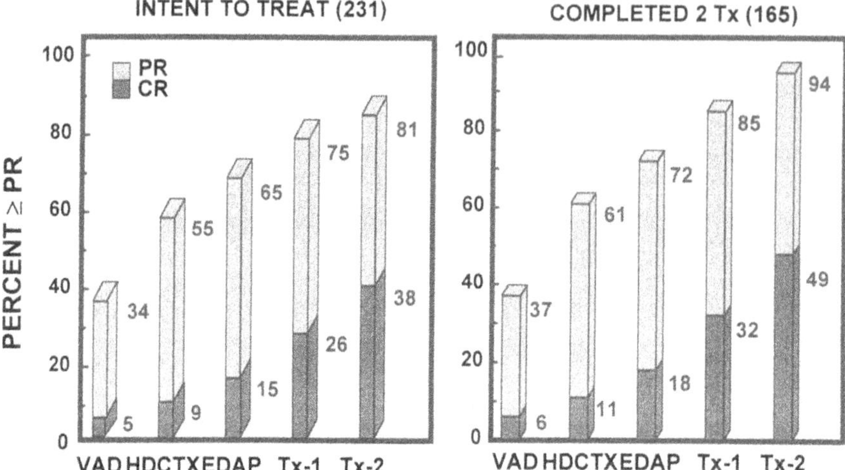

Fig. 3. The response to the Total Therapy Multiple Myeloma Regimen demonstrates a marked increase in the incidence of partial remission (PR) and complete remission (CR) as patients proceed through the different phases of the protocol consisting of remission induction with mutually non-cross-resistant therapy (vincristine, doxorubicin, dexamethasone; high-dose cyclophosphamide; etoposide, dexamethasone, ara-C, cisplatin and two transplants (Tx-1, Tx-2). *See* refs. *19* and *20* for details.

patients early in the course of their disease when they were still chemosensitive, and their stem cells were minimally affected by prior chemotherapy. Utilizing this regimen, 84% of patients completed one transplant and 72% of patients completed two transplants. This study demonstrates the importance of dose intensification: analysis on an intent to treat basis shows that 15% of 231 patients achieved CR at the end of induction whereas 26 and 38% achieved complete remission at the end of first and second transplants (Fig. 3). When only the 164 patients who completed two transplants are considered, 18, 32, and 49% achieved a CR following induction, first transplant, and second transplant, respectively. Double transplantion does require greater hematopoietic reserve than single transplantation. Since hematopoietic reserve is a function of extent of prior therapy, double transplantation requires early referral of patients to a transplant center.

Third, the efficacy of dose-intensive therapy is improved when such therapy is delivered at a time of greatest host tolerance. This typically occurs early in the course of disease, before end-organ damage has occurred as the result of prior standard therapy and at a time when host performance status is optimized. For example, non-Hodgkin's lymphoma patients who have received prior radiation therapy who subsequently undergo autologous bone marrow transplantation have an increased risk to develop pulmonary complications when treated with TBI-containing regimens. Thus, especially for high-risk patients, standard therapies should be chosen to minimize complications should dose-intensive therapy be required *(11,12)*.

4. Implications and Management of Minimal Residual Disease

For hematological malignancies, minimal residual disease (MRD) may be defined as disease undetectable by standard methods and suspected when relapse occurs. For example, standard immunohistochemistry can detect malignant cells to a level of 5%; if a marrow contains less than 5% malignant cells they are not detectable by standard techniques and represent minimal residual disease *(21)*. MRD is detectable by molecular techniques to a level of 10^{-6} cells; molecular techniques to detect fusion gene products or immunoglobulin gene rearrangements include PCR or Southern blot.

Does MRD in the patient or the autograft contribute to relapse? This question has been the focus of several important studies, and available data suggest that MRD in either source may contribute to relapse. Gribben et al. have utilized PCR to detect the bcl-2 translocation t(14; 18) to establish the presence of MRD in the bone marrow of B-cell lymphoma patients following purged autologous bone marrow transplantation. In those patients in whom the translocation was known to be present at the time of transplantation, detection of the bcl-2 translocation in serial bone marrow samples following transplantation was associated with a decreased disease-free survival compared to those patients in whom the translocation could not be identified following transplantation ($p < 0.00001$) *(22)*. In another study by Gribben et al., patients with follicular lymphoma underwent induction therapy with CHOP followed by anti–B-cell monoclonal antibody purged autologous bone marrow transplantation. In this study, freedom from relapse was significantly longer in those patients whose bone marrow was PCR-negative following purging ($p = 0.0006$). In addition, the continued inability to detect the t(14;18) translocation by PCR in the bone marrow following transplantation correlated with continued complete remission *(22,23)*. Bone marrow, rather than peripheral blood, was found in a subsequent study to be more informative in predicting relapse *(24)*. These studies suggest that autograft purging, particularly in chemosensitive malignancies, presumably eradicated by high-dose therapy, may be critical to improve disease-free and overall survival *(22–24)*.

Putatively, to be most efficacious, purging must distinguish between malignant progenitors and benign progenitors. Elimination of the malignant self-renewal compartment is crucial to eradication of the malignant clone. Such purging might be achieved with an antibody cocktail, if the malignant progenitor cells express differentiation antigens that are distinct from those expressed by normal progenitor cells. In an early differentiation phenotype, such as early leukemias, differentiation antigens may not be expressed on the malignant cells in the self-renewal compartment, precluding elimination of these progenitor leukemia cells by purging. Gorin, who has shown improved leukemia-free survival in first remission acute myelogenous leukenia (AML) patients following mafosfamide purged autologous bone marrow transplantation (ABMT) compared to those who received unpurged marrow *(25)*, has also shown an alternative approach by purging with the combination of mafosfamide and protective agents providing for selective toxicity to malignant cells and protection to benign progenitor cells. This work has shown that pretreatment of bone marrow with amifostine protected normal progenitor cells so that a higher LD95 of mafosfamide could be used for ex vivo purging. Conversely, the amifostine increased the toxicity of the mafosfamide on the leukemic progenitors *(26)*.

Brenner et al. have reported on a series of patients who underwent autologous bone marrow transplantation for AML and neuroblastoma *(27–29)*. Autologous marrow was transduced with the neomycin-resistance gene so that at the time of relapse, the source of the malignant relapse could be tracked. Results demonstrated the presence of the marker gene in 6/8 relapsed marrows. These important studies document that residual malignant cells in the autograft may directly contribute to relapse, although the presence of residual disease in the marrow may be a surrogate marker of residual tumor bulk in the patient. Moreover, these studies raise the possibility that for patients without other residual disease at the time of transplant, the presence of malignant cells in the autograft may be the only potential source of relapse.

Rather than selection of tumor cells to eliminate minimal residual disease, positive selection of benign stem cells may select for a purified autograft. In chronic myelogenous leukemia (CML), Philadelphia chromosome negative stem cells may be selected by in vitro depletion of the malignant clone by selectively expanding normal benign hematopoietic stem cells *(30–32)*.These studies illustrate an important issue: the self-renewal compartment for benign hematopoiesis is distinct from the transformed compartment. If markers such as t(9;22) can be identified to distinguish the two compartments, the difference can be exploited to separate benign and malignant cells and to re-establish normal hematopoiesis.

Tricot et al. have reported the selection of $CD34^{+}Lin^{-}Thy1$- hematopoietic progenitor cells free of clonal myeloma cells. In this report, the progenitor cells were separated mechanically, first by centifugal elutriation and chemical lysis, and subsequently by high-speed cell sorting. Although this method provided viable, purified progenitor cells, delayed engraftment, and decreased viability of stored progenitor cells have resulted in early closing of this study. Nonetheless, this study demonstrates that benign stem cells can be selected, although mechanisms to maintain the integrity of stem cells following manipulation remain to be developed *(33,34)*.

5. Tumor Immunomodulation

Despite efforts to eliminate malignant cells, minimal residual disease may persist, and immunomodulation may be an important mechanism for tumor eradication. Tumor immunomodulation may result from a graft-vs-leukemia (tumor) [GVL] effect, particularly in allogeneic or cord blood transplants, or from the use of immunotherapy. GVL and GVHD are distinct clinical entities, mediated apparently by different immune cell types and occurring at different times following transplantation. Nonetheless, in clinical practice, development of GVL is known to decrease the relapse rate in several hematological malignancies, and can often be best predicted by development of acute GVHD. The magnitude of the importance of GVL is demonstrated by lymphoma data comparing the rate of relapse following allogeneic and autologous bone marrow transplantation. In a prospective study reported by Ratanatharathorn et al. *(35)*, 66 consecutive patients with intermediate or high-grade lymphoma with relapsed or primary refractory disease were treated with either allogeneic bone marrow transplant (BMT) (age <55 and appropriate sibling donor) or with autologous BMT (all others). At a median follow-up of 14 months, progression-free survival was not significantly different between the two groups (24% [auto] vs 47% [allo], $p = 0.21$). However, the probability of disease progression was significantly different (69% [auto] vs 10% [allo], $p = 0.001$). This difference, at least in part, is attributed to the graft vs lymphoma effect.

The immune mechanisms involved in GVHD involve activated T-cells. Some data indicate that these T-cells belong phenotypically to the Th2-like T-cell subset. Takai et al. *(36)* have demonstrated that in mice injected with hybrid spleen cells, subsequent GVHD was characterized by immunologic features, including the presence of autoantibodies, immune complex nephritis, hepatosplenomegaly, and increased IgE levels. Indeed, IgE levels were found to correlate strongly with the histologic stage of graft-vs-host liver disease. Autoantibodies were found to be of the IgG1 subclass. Both IgG1 and IgE represent immunoglobulin class switching consistent with a Th2 phenotype.

When the mice were concurrently injected with monoclonal anti–IL-4 antibody, IgE, and IgG1 levels were markedly reduced and graft-vs-host associated liver disease was markedly reduced. In similar murine studies, Ushiyama et al. reported *(37)* induction of GVHD in (BALB/c X C57BL/6)F_1 mice with bone marrow and spleen cells of BALB/c mice. The GVHD was characterized by liver disease, splenomegaly, hypergammopathy, and IgE and IgG1 levels correlated with the extent of liver disease. Treatment with anti–IL-4 antibody eliminated the liver disease and splenomegaly. These data suggest a critical role for IL-4 in the development of graft-vs-host disease. Since IL-4 is critical in inducing the Th2 phenotype, the importance of the Th2 like T-cell in graft-vs-host disease is further suggested. Other murine studies by Weiss et al. *(38)* have shown that a Graft-vs-Leukemia effect can be induced, which is independent of graft-vs-host disease. In this study, C57BL/6 → BALB/c chimeras, free of GVHD, were inoculated three months after T-cell-depleted allogeneic BMT with murine B-cell leukemia (BCL 1). None of these mice developed leukemia, whereas control mice all developed leukemia and died. These data demonstrate that in this murine model, GVL may develop even in the absence of immunocompetent donor T-cells.

Other evidence that suggests that GVL and GVHD may be mediated, at least in part, by different immune cells or mechanisms was demonstrated by Horowitz et al. *(39)*. In this analysis of the International BMT Registry, patients with first CR ALL and AML, or first chronic phase CML following allogeneic transplantation, could be divided into three groups based upon risk of leukemic relapse. Patients with the highest risk of relapse received syngeneic or T-cell depleted transplants, and developed no GVHD. The second and third groups received non–T-cell depleted allogeneic transplants. The intermediate group developed neither acute nor chronic GVHD, but presumably in the transplant received some "immune cells." Patients who developed either acute or chronic GVHD, or both, had the lowest relapse rates. Because the patients in the intermediate group presumably derived some benefit from immune cells that did not mediate GVHD, the data suggest that the mechanism of GVL is, at least in part, distinct from that of GVHD, and that GVL may occur in the absence of GVHD.

Kolb has also reported a GVL effect, which is apparently distinct from GVHD, following donor lymphocyte transfusions *(40)*. In this study, patients with CML, AML, ALL, myelodysplastic syndrome (MDS), or polycythemia vera with osteomyelofibrosis received donor lymphocyte transfusions after relapse following allogeneic BMT. Interestingly, the patients with ALL did not respond to the adoptive immunotherapy, whereas patients with chronic phase CML had an 87% three-year probability of remission. Following donor lymphocyte transfusions, most CML patients studied developed GVHD, myelosuppression, or both (46/75); however, 29/75 developed neither. Of these, 91% in the former group and 45% in the latter group demonstrated disease response following transfusion, presumably because of a GVL effect. These data suggest that GVL is associated with, or can be predicted by, GVHD, but that GVL may occur independently of GVHD. Moreover, the difference in response between ALL and CML patients to donor lymphocyte transfusions may be explained by the difference between leukemia-specific antigens expressed on ALL vs CML leukemia progenitors. Expression of different antigens may enhance or diminish interaction with minor histocompatibility antigens on donor lymphocytes, hence, induce or suppress a GVL reaction *(40)*.

An alternative mechanism to achieve GVL with little or no GVHD is by the use of cord blood as the donor source. Data recently reported by the Eurocord Transplant Group and the European Blood and Marrow Transplantation Group shows that 78 recipients of cord blood from related donors for different hematological disorders experienced timely engraftment and an estimated 63% one-year survival, whereas 65 patients who received unrelated-donor cord blood transplants experienced a 29% estimated one-year survival *(41)*. For the patients who received related-donor cord blood transplants, the incidence of acute GVHD (Grade 2 or higher) was 9% for HLA-matched and 50% for HLA-mismatched transplants *(41)*. Following unrelated cord blood transplantation, the New York Blood Center Program also reported a low incidence of acute or chronic GVHD even with multiple HLA-mismatches *(42)*. If a patient has significant tumor involvement in their marrow, cord blood offers the advantage of an uncontaminated allograft. Banked cord blood may also provide the advantage of serving as an available source of stem cells for patients who otherwise might not have a matched donor. Cord blood is composed of immature lymphocytes, which cannot exert mature T-cell functions, and thus induce GVHD.

The most important asset of cord blood transplants is the difference in immunogenicity between cord blood and standard allogeneic bone marrow. Because of intrinsic defects in mature T-cell function, the incidence of both acute and chronic GVHD is very low following cord blood transplantation *(41,42)*. In contradistinction, GVL activity has been demonstrated because of activation of NK cells (which become LAK cells) and expansion of $CD8^+$ T-cells with nonspecific lytic function. The ability of these cells to lyse tumor cells in vitro was enhanced by the presence of IL-2, however, lytic activity occurred even in the absence of added IL-2. In an in vivo model, cord blood was also able to cure tumors in SCID mice *(43–45)*. Thus, cord blood offers an important alternative for patients who would benefit from allogeneic transplantation and GVL effect. These data further support that GVHD and GVL are distinct immunological entities.

IL-2 has been reported to have a GVL-like effect in mice receiving IL-2 activated syngeneic marrow followed by IL-2 therapy. Both survival and cure were superior to syngenic marrow alone, suggesting IL-2 induction of a GVL-like effect *(46)*. One possible mechanism for this GVL-like effect may be related to IL-2 dependent cytokine induction of lymphocytes following autologous transplantation. Heslop et al. have reported *(47)* that increased IFN-γ and TNF are detectable in the serum and from lymphocytes of multiple myeloma or AML patients after IL-2 infusion. Increased IFN-γ may directly antagonize IL-4, and the IL-4 mediated Th2 or GVHD effects. These data taken together suggest that GVL effect may be mediated by Th-1 like cytokines and cytotoxic NK and CD8 T-cells, whereas GVHD is mediated by Th2-like T-cells.

Other potential mechanisms to eradicate minimal residual disease by immunomodulation include specific idiotype antibodies and idiotype vaccines. The vaccine can induce idiotype specific immunologic responses of the humoral or cell-mediated type targeted to tumor specific antigen. As previously discussed, these specific antigens would optimally be present on tumor cells in the self-renewal compartment. Potentially, such antigens could be transduced into progenitor tumor cells to either increase immunogenicity or specificity.

Other immunomodulation therapy requires an understanding of cytokines, cytokine receptors, or tumor ligands in hematological malignancies. For example, hairy cell leukemia cells secrete soluble IL-2R *(48,49)*; this soluble cytokine receptor may impair T-cell function by binding available IL-2 and may contribute to the immunoparesis observed in hairy cell leukemia patients. Reduction in the sIL-2R levels occurs following response to therapy. In CML, leukemic progenitor cells have decreased or absent expression of the LFA-3 (CD58) molecule, the natural ligand to the CD2 T-cell receptor. The result is loss of generation of autoregulatory T-cells, and unregulated proliferation of the leukemic clone *(50)*. Interferon-α up-regulates expression of LFA-3 (CD58) on CML progenitor cells, thereby restoring the normal regulatory proliferative control of autoregulatory T-cells over CML progenitor cells *(50)*. Immunoregulation of CML progenitor cells also occurs by an interferon-α induced increase of Fas-receptor expression on CML progenitor cells *(51)*. The combination of interferon-α and Fas-receptor antibody suppressed proliferation of CML progenitor cells more strongly than normal progenitor cells; the hematopoietic suppression was because of induction of apoptosis *(51)*. Fas-receptor/Fas-ligand activity has also been reported in multiple myeloma. Anti-Fas antibody has been shown to induce apoptosis in multiple myeloma cells; this activity is mitigated by IL-6, a myeloma growth factor *(52)*. Conversely, Fas ligand production by myeloma cells has recently been implicated in T- and B-cell immunoparesis associated with this disease *(52)*.

6. Future Directions of Stem Cell Transplants in Hematopoietic Malignancies

Improved understanding of the importance of early high-dose therapy with stem cell support to exploit dose-response in relatively chemosensitive tumors, although minimizing damage to the normal hematopoietic stem cell compartment, requires continued clinical trials of dose-intensive therapy in hematopoietic malignancies. Since end-organ toxicity limits dose-intensive therapy, new mechanisms to decrease extramedullary toxicities need to be developed, such as the use of protective cytokines (e.g., TGF-β3) capable of protecting epithelial cells and hematopoietic cells by arresting cells in the G1 phase, thus protecting them against cytotoxic agents preferentially active in cycling cells *(53)*.

Another future challenge in the treatment of hematological malignancies is to restore immunocompetence to the patient, lost both as a result of the malignancy and the treatment applied. This might be achieved by developing methods of autologous stem cell procurement, which, because of decreased manipulation of the stem cells, render the stem cell more immunocompetent. Alternatively, with allografts, a graft vs tumor effect, which may be achieved when T-cells are transduced with a suicide gene such as the TK gene *(54–57)* may more effectively eliminate residual disease and thereby restore immunocompetence. Alternatively, restoration of immunocompetence may be achieved by partial mismatched related donors recently shown to establish partial chimerism *(58)*. Eradicating residual disease may require additional immunologic approaches such as radio-labeled antibodies to specific tumor antigens that serve to delivery localized radiation to the site of residual tumor cells. Further understanding of mechanisms to eliminate tumor resistance, eliminate minimal residual disease and minimize toxicity to the host will all be important avenues to explore in future clinical trials.

References

1. Dastugue, N., Lafage-Pochitaloff, M., Leroux, D., Payen, C., Bernard, P., Huguet-Rigal, F., Stoppa, A., Marit, G., Molina, L., Michallet, M., et al. (1995) Prognostic significance of karyotype in de novo adult acute myeloid leukemia. The BGMT Group *Leukemia* **9,** 1491–1498.
2. Mrozek, K., Heinonen, K., de la Chapelle, A., and Bloomfield, C. (1997) Clinical significance of cytogenetics in acute myeloid leukemia. *Sem. Oncol.* **24,** 17–31.
3. Armitage, J. (1997) The development of bone marrow transplantation as a treatment for patients with lymphoma-Twentieth Richard and Hinda Rosenthal Foundation Award Lecture. *Clin. Cancer Res.* **3,** 829–836.
4. Guba, S., Vesole, D., Jagannath, S., Bracy, D., Barlogie, B., and Tricot, G. (1997) Peripheral stem cell mobilization and engraftment in patients over age 60. *Bone Marrow Transplant* **20,** 1–3.

5. Savarese, D., Hsieh, C.-C., and Steward, F. (1997) Clinical impact of chemotherapy dose escalation in patients with hematologic malignancies and solid tumors. *J. Clin. Oncol.* **15,** 2981–2995.
6. Siu, L. and Tannock, I. (1997) Chemotherapy dose escalation: case unproven. *J. Clin. Oncol.* **15,** 2765–2768.
7. Biggs, J., Szer, J., Crilley, P., Atkinson, K., Downs, K., Dodds, A., Concannon, A., Avalos, B., Tutschka, P., Kapoor, N., Brodsky, I., Topolsky, D., Bulova, S., and Copelan, E. (1992) Treatment of chronic myeloid leukemia with allogeneic bone marrow transplantation after preparation with BuCy2. *Blood* **80,** 1352–1357.
8. Buckner, C., Clift, R., Appelbaum, F., and Thomas, E. (1992) A randomized study comparing two transplant regimens for CML in chronic phase. *Blood* **80,** 72a.
9. Copeland, E., Grever, M., Kapoor, N., and Tutschka, P. (1989) Marrow transplantation following busulfan and cyclophosphamide for chronic myelogenous leukemia in accelerated or blastic phase. *Br. J. Haematol.* **71,** 487–491.
10. Santos, G. (1993) Busulfan and cyclophosphamide versus cyclophosphamide and total body irradiation for marrow transplantation in chronic myelogenous leukemia-a review. *Leuk. Lymphoma* **11,** 201–204.
11. Petersen, F., Appelbaum, F., Hill, R., Fisher, L., Bigelow, C., Sanders, J., Sullivan, K., Bensinger, W., Witherspoon, R., Storb, R., Clift, R., Fefer, A., Priss, O., Weiden, P., Singer, J., Thomas, E., and Buckner, C. (1990) Autologous marrow transplantation for malignant lymphoma: a report of 101 cases from Seattle. *J. Clin. Oncol.* **8,** 638–647.
12. Philip, T., Armitage, J., Spitzer, G., Chauvin, F., Jagannath, S., Cahn, J., Colombat, P., Goldstone, A., Gorin, N., Flesh, M., Laporte, J.-P., Maraninchi, D., Pico, J., Bosly, A., Anderson, C., Schots, R., Bion, P., Cabanillas, F., and Dicke, K. (1987) High-dose therapy and autologous bone marrow transplantation after failure of conventional chemotherapy in adults with intermediate-grade or high-grade non-Hodgkin's lymphoma. *N. Engl. J. Med.* **316,** 1493–1498.
13. Vose, J., Armitage, J., Bierman, P., Weisenburger, D., Hutchins, M., Dowling, M., Moravec, D., Sorensen, S., Okerbloom, J., Bascom, G., Howe, D., Johnson, P., Langdon, R., Mailliard, J., Pevnick, W., Westberg, M., and Kessinger, A. (1989) Salvage therapy for relapsed or refractory non-Hodgkin's lymphoma utilizing autologous bone marrow transplantation. *Am. J. Med.* **87,** 285–288.
14. Jagannath, S., Vesole, D., Glenn, L., Crowley, J., and Barlogie, B. (1992) Low-risk intensive therapy for multiple myeloma with combined autologous bone marrow and blood stem cell support. *Blood* **80,** 1666–1672.
15. Tricot, G., Jagannath, S., Vesole, D., Crowley, J., and Barlogie, B. (1995) Relapse of multiple myeloma after autologous transplantation: survival outcome after salvage. *Bone Marrow Transplant* **16,** 7–11.
16. Govindarajan, R., Jagannath, S., Flick, J., Vesole, D., Sawyer, J., Barlogie, B., and Tricot, G. (1996) Preceding standard therapy is the likely cause of MDS after autotransplants for multiple myeloma. *Br. J. Haematol.* **95,** 349–353.
17. Tricot, G., Jagannath, S., Vesole, D., Nelson, J., Tindle, S., Miller, L., Cheson, B., Crowley, J., and Barlogie, B. (1995) Peripheral blood stem cell transplants for multiple myeloma: identification of favorable variables for rapid engraftment of 225 patients. *Blood* **85,** 588–596.
18. Philip, T., Guglielmi, C., Hagenbeek, A., Somers, R., Van deer Lelie, H., Bron, D., Sonneveld, P., Gisselbrecht, C., Cahn, J., Harousseau, J., Coiffier, B., Biron, P., Mandelli, F., and Chauvin, F. (1995) Autologous bone marrow transplantation as compared with salvage chemotherapy in relapses of chemotherapy-sensitive non-Hodgkin's lymphoma. *N. Engl. J. Med.* **333,** 1540–1545.
19. Barlogie, B., Jagannath, S., and Tricot, G. (1998) Advances in the treatment of multiple myeloma, in *Advances in Internal Medicine*, vol. 43 (Schrier, R., Abboud, F., Baxter, J., and Fauci, A., eds.), Mosby, St. Louis, MO, 279–320.
20. Barlogie, B., Jagannath, S., Vesole, D., Naucke, S., Cheson, B., Mattox, S., Bracy, D., Salmon, S., Jacobson, J., Crowley, J., and Tricot, G. (1997) Superiority of tandem autologous transplantation over standard therapy for previously untreated multiple myeloma. *Blood* **89,** 789–793.
21. Gribben, J. and Nadler, L. (1993) Monitoring minimal residual disease. *Sem. Oncol.* **20,** 143–155.
22. Gribben, J., Neuberg, D., Freedman, A., Gimmi, C., Pesek, K., Barber, M., Saporito, L., Woo, S., Coral, F., Spector, N., Rabinowe, S., Grossbard, M., Ritz, J., and Nadler, L. (1993) Detection of polymerase chain reaction of residual cells with the bcl-2 translocation is associated with

increased risk of relapse after autologous bone marrow transplantation for B-cell lymphoma. *Blood* **81,** 3449–3457.
23. Freedman, A., Gribben, J., Neuberg, D., Mauch, P., Soiffer, R., Anderson, K., Pandite, L., Robertson, M., Kroon, M., Ritz, J., and Nadler, L. (1996) High-dose therapy and autologous bone marrow transplantation in patients with follicular lymphoma during first remission. *Blood* **88,** 2780–2786.
24. Gribben, J., Neuberg, D., Barber, M., Moore, J., Pesek, K., Freedman, A., and Nadler, L. (1994) Detection of residual lymphoma cells by polymerase chain reaction in peripheral blood is significantly less predictive for relapse than detection in bone marrow. *Blood* **83,** 3800–3807.
25. Gorin, N., Aegerter, P., Auvert, B., Meloni, G., Goldstone, A., Burnett, A., Carella, A., Korbling, M., Herve, P., Maraninchi, D., Lowenberg, R., Verdonck, L., de Planque, M, Hermans, J., Helbig, W., Porcellini, A., Rizzoli, V., Alesandrino, E., Franklin, I., Reiffers, J., Colleselli, P., and Goldman, J. (1990) Autologous bone marrow transplantation for acute myelocytic leukemia in first remission: a European survey of the role of marrow purging. *Blood* **75,** 1606–1614.
26. Douay, L., Hu, C., Giarratana, M., Bouchet, S., Conlon, J., Capizzi, R., and Gorin, N. (1995) Amifostine improves the antileukemic therapeutic index of mafosfamide: implications for bone marrow purging. *Blood* **86,** 2849–2855.
27. Brenner, M., Rill, D., Moen, R., Krance, R., Heslop, H., Mirro, J. J., Anderson, W., and Ihle, J. (1994) Gene marking and autologous bone marrow transplantation [Review]. *Ann. NY Acad. Sci.* **716,** 204–214.
28. Brenner, M., Rill, D., Moen, R., Krance, R., Mirro, J. J., Anderson, W., and Ihle, J. (1993) Gene-marking to trace origin of relapse after autologous bone-marrow transplantation. *Lancet* **341,** 85,86.
29. Heslop, H., Rooney, C., Rill, D., Krance, R., and Brenner, M. (1996) Use of gene marking in bone marrow transplantation. *Cancer Detect. Prev.* **20,** 108–113.
30. Barnett, M., Eaves, C., Phillips, G., Kalousek, D., Klingemann, K., Landsdorp, P., Reece, D., Shepherd, J., Shaw, G., and Eaves, A. (1989) Successful autografting in chronic myeloid leukemia after maintenance of marrow in culture. *Bone Marrow Transplant* **4,** 345–351.
31. Coulombel, L., Kalousek, D., Eaves, C., Gupta, C., and Eaves, A. (1983) Long-term marrow culture reveals chromosomally normal hematopoietic progenitor cells in patients with Philadelphia chromosome-positive chronic myelogenous leukemia. *N. Engl. J. Med.* **308,** 1493–1498.
32. Udomsakdi, C., Eaves, C., Swolin, B., Reid, D., Barnett, M., and Eaves, A. (1992) Rapid decline of chronic myeloid leukemic cells in long-term culture due to a defect at the leukemic stem cell level. *Proc. Natl. Acad. Sci. USA* **89,** 6192–6196.
33. Gazitt, Y., Reading, C., Hoffman, R., Wickrema, A., Vesole, D., Jagannath, S., Condino, J., Lee, B., Barlogie, B., and Tricot, G. (1995) Purified $CD34^+$ Lin-Thy^+ stem cells do not contain clonal myeloma cells. *Blood* **86,** 381–389.
34. Tricot, G. (1997) Multiparameter cell sorting of PBSC. VI International Workshop on Multiple Myeloma, Boston.
35. Ratanatharathorn, V., Uberti, J., Karanes, C., Abella, E., Lum, L., Momin, F., Cummings, G., and Sensenbrenner, L. (1994) Prospective comparative trial of autologous versus allogeneic bone marrow transplantation in patients with non-Hodgkin's lymphoma. *Blood* **84,** 1050–1055.
36. Takai, S., Tateno, M., Hirano, T., Kondo, N., Hirose, S., and Yoshiki, T. (1993) Increased IgE level as a marker of host-versus-graft disease: inhibition of this HVGD with a monoclonal antibody to IL-4. *Cell. Immunol.* **149,** 1–10.
37. Ushiyama, C., Hirano, T., Miyajima, H., Okumura, K., Ovary, Z., and Hashimoto, H. (1995) Anti-IL-4 antibody prevents graft-versus-host disease in mice after bone marrow transplantation. *J. Immunol.* **154,** 2687–2696.
38. Weiss, L., Lubin, I., Factorowich, I., Lapidot, Z., Reich, S., Reisner, Y., and Slavin, S. (1994) Effective graft-versus-leukemia effects independent of graft-versus-host disease after T cell-depleted allogeneic bone marrow transplantation in a murine model of B cell leukemia/lymphoma. *J. Immunol.* **153,** 2562–2567.
39. Horowitz, M., Gale, R., Sondel, P., Goldman, J., Kersey, J., Kolb, H.-J., Rimm, A., Ringden, O., Rozman, C., Speck, B., Truitt, R., Zwaan, F., and Bortin, M. (1990) Graft-versus-leukemia reactions after bone marrow transplantation. *Blood* **75,** 555–562.
40. Kolb, H.-J., Schattenberg, A., Goldman, J., Hertenstein, B., Jacobsen, N., Arcese, W., Ljungman, P., Ferrant, A., Verdonck, L., Niederwieser, D., van Rhee, F., Mittermueller, J., de Witte, T., Holler, E., and Ansari, H. for the European Group for Blood and Marrow Transplantation

Working Party Chronic Leukemia. (1995) Graft-versus-leukemia effect of donor lymphocyte transfusions in marrow grafted patients. *Blood* **86,** 2041–2050.

41. Gluckman, E., Rocha, V., Boyer-Chammard, A., Locatelli, F., Arcese, W., Pasquini, R., Ortega, J., Souillet, G., Ferreira, E., Laporte, J.-P., Fernandez, M., and Chastang, C. (1997) Outcome of cord-blood transplantation from related and unrelated donors. *N. Engl. J. Med.* **337,** 373–381.
42. Rubinstein, P., Carrier, C., Adamson, J., Migliaccio, A., Berkowitz, R., Kurtzberg, J., Scaradavou, A., and Stevens, C. (1996) New York Blood Center's Program for unrelated placental/umbilical cord blood (PCB) transplantation: 243 transplants in the first 3 years. *Blood* **88,** 142a.
43. Harris, D. (1994) Cord blood transplantation: implications for graft vs. host disease and graft vs. leukemia. *Blood Cells* **20,** 560–565.
44. Harris, D. (1995) In vitro and in vivo assessment of the graft-versus-leukemia activity of cord blood. *Bone Marrow Transplant* **15,** 17–23.
45. Keever, C., Abu-Hajir, M., Graf, W., McFadden, P., Prichard, P., O'Brien, J., and Flomberg, N. (1995) Characterization of the alloreactivity and anti-leukemia reactivity of cord blood mononuclear cells. *Bone Marrow Transplant* **15,** 407–419.
46. Charak, B., Brynes, R., Groshen, S., Chen, S.-C., and Mazumder, A. (1990) Bone marrow transplantation with interleukin-2 activated bone marrow followed by interleukin-2 therapy for acute myeloid leukemia in mice. *Blood* **76,** 2187–2190.
47. Heslop, H., Gottlieb, D., Bianchi, A., Meager, A., Prentice, H., Mehta, A., Hoffbrand, A., and Brenner, M. (1989) In vivo induction of gamma interferon and tumor necrosis factor by interleukin-2 infusion following intensive chemotherapy or autologous marrow transplantation. *Blood* **74,** 1374–1380.
48. Chrobak, L., Podzimek, K., Pliskova, L., Kerekes, Z., Zak, P., Voglova, J., Spacek, J., and Palicka, V. (1996) Serum soluble IL-2 receptor as a reliable and noninvasive marker of disease activity in patients with hairy cell leukemia. *Neoplasm* **43,** 321–325.
49. Srivastava, M., Srivastava, A., and Srivastava, B. (1994) Soluble interleukin-2 receptor, soluble CD8 and soluble intercellular adhesion molecule-1 levels in hematologic malignancies. *Leukemia Lymphoma* **12,** 241–251.
50. Upadhyaya, G., Guba, S., Sih, S., Feinberg, A., Talpaz, M., Kantarjian, H., Deisseroth, A., and Emerson, S. (1991) Interferon-alpha restores the deficient expression of the cytoadhesion molecule lymphocyte function antigen-3 by chronic myelogenous leukemia progenitor cells. *J. Clin. Invest.* **88,** 2131–2136.
51. Selleri, C., Sato, T., Del Vecchio, L., Luciano, L., Barrett, A., Rotoli, B., Young, N., and Maciejewski, J. (1997) Involvement of Fas-mediated apoptosis in the inhibitory effects of interferon-α in chronic myelogenous leukemia. *Blood* **89,** 957–964.
52. Chauhan, D., Kharbanda, S., Ogata, A., Urashima, M., Teoh, G., Robertson, M., Kufe, D., and Anderson, K. (1997) Interleukin-6 inhibits Fas-induced apoptosis and stress-activated protein kinase activation in multiple myeloma cells. *Blood* **89,** 227–234.
53. McCormack, E., Borzillo, G., Ambrosino, C., Mak, G., Hamablet, L., Qu, G., and Haley, J. (1997) Transforming growth factor-beta3 protection of epithelial cells from cycle-selective chemotherapy in vitro. *Biochem. Pharmacol.* **53,** 1149–1159.
54. Bonini, C., Ferrari, G., Verzeletti, S., Servida, P., Zappone, E., Ruggieri, L., Ponzoni, S., Mavilio, F., Traversari, C., and Bordignon, C. (1997) HSV-TK gene transfer into donor lymphocytes for control of allogeneic graft-versus-leukemia. *Science* **276,** 1719–1724.
55. Cohen, J., Boyer, O., Salomon, B., Onclercq, R., Charlotte, F., Bruel, S., Boisserie, G., and Klatzmann, D. (1997) Prevention of graft-versus-host disease in mice using a suicide gene expressed in T lymphocytes. *Blood* **89,** 4636–4645.
56. Munshi, N., Govindarajan, R., Drake, R., Ding, L., Iyer, R., Saylors, R., Kornbluth, J., Marcus, S., Chiang, Y., Ennist, D., Kwak, L., Reynolds, C., Tricot, G., and Barlogie, B. (1997) Thymidine kinase (TK) gene-transduced human lymphocytes can be highly purified, remain fully functional, and are killed efficiently with ganciclovir. *Blood* **89,** 1334–1340.
57. Munshi, N., Jagannath, S., Vesole, D., Desikan, K., Barlogie, B., and Tricot, G. (1996) Graft vs. myeloma effect: Thymidine kinase (TK) gene transduced lymphocyte infusion following allogeneic transplantation in myeloma. *Blood* **88,** 244a.
58. Henslee-Downey, P., Abhyankar, S., Parrish, R., Pati, A., Goddar, K., Neglia, W., et al. (1997) Use of partially mismatched donors extends access to allogeneic marrow transplant. *Blood* **89,** 3864–3872.

59. Bloomfield, C., Lawrence, D., Arthur, D., Berg, D., Schiffer, C., and Mayer, R. (1994) Curative impact of intensification with high-dose cytarabine (HiDAC) in acute myeloid leukemia (AML) varies by cytogenetic group. *Blood* **84,** 111a.
60. Cattoretti, G., Chang, C.-C., Cechova, K., Zhang, J., Ye, B., Falini, B., Louie, D., Offit, K., Chaganti, R., and Dalla-Favera, R. (1995) BCL-6 protein is expressed in germinal-center B cells. *Blood* **86,** 45–53.
61. Clark, S., Mclaughlin, J., Crist, W., Changlin. R., and Witte, O. (1987) Unique forms of the abl tyrosine kinase distinguish Ph-positive CML from Ph-positive ALL. *Science* **235,** 85–88.
62. deThe, H., Lavau, C., Marchio, A., Chomienne, C., Degos, L., and Dejean, A. (1991) The PML/RARa fusion mRNA generated by the t(15;17) translocation in acute promyelocytic leukemia encodes a functionally altered RAR. *Cell* **66,** 675–684.
63. Erickson, P., Gao, J., Chang, K.-S., Look, T., Whisenant, E., Raimondi, S., Lasher, R., Trujillo, H., Rowley, H., and Drabkin, H. (1992) Identification of breakpoints in t(8;21) acute myelogenous leukemia and isolation of a fusion transcript, AML1/ETO, with similarity to Drosophila segmentation gene, runt. *Blood* **80,** 1825–1831.
64. Haioun, C., Lepage, E., Gisselbrecht, C., Bastion, Y., Coiffier, B., Brice, P., Bosly, A., Dupriez, B., Nouvel, C., Tilly, H., Lederlin, P., Biron, P., Briere, J., Gaulard, P., and Reyes, F., for the Groupe d'Etudes des Lymphomes de l'Adulte. (1997) Benefit of autologous bone marrow transplantation over sequential chemotherapy in poor-risk aggressive non-Hodgkin's lymphoma: updated results of the prospective study LNH87-2. *J. Clin. Oncol.* **15,** 1131–1137.
65. Kakizuka, A., Miller, W., Umesono, K., Warrel, R., Frankel, S., Murty, V., Dmitrovsky, E., and Evans, R. (1991) Chromosomal translocation t(15;17) in human acute promyelocytic leukemia fuses RARa with a novel putative transcription factor, PML. *Cell* **66,** 663–674.
66. Keating, M., Cork, A., Broach, Y., Smith, T., Walters, R., McCredie, K., Trujillo, J., and Freireich, E. (1987) Toward a clinically relevant cytogenetic classification of acute myelogenous leukemia. *Leukemia Res.* **11,** 119–133.
67. Kelliher, M., Knott, A., Mclaughlin, J., Witte, O., and Rosenberg, N. (1991) Differences in oncogenic potency but not target cell specificity distinguish the two forms of the BCR/ABL oncogene. *Mol. Cell. Biol.* **11,** 4710–4716.
68. Levine, E., Arthur, D., Frizzera, G., Peterson, B., Hurd, D., and Bloomfield, C. (1985) There are differences in cytogenetic abnormalities among histologic subtypes of the non-Hodgkin's lymphomas. *Blood* **66,** 1414–1422.
69. Liu, P., Tarle, S., Hajra, A., Claxton, D., Marlton, P., Freedman, M., Siciliano, M., and Collins, F. (1993) Fusion between transcription factor CBFβ/PEBP2β and myosin heavy chain in acute myeloid leukemia. *Science* **261,** 1041–1044.
70. Marosi, C., Koller, U., Koller-Weber, E., Schwarzinger, I., Schneider, B., Jager, U., Vahls, P., Nowotny, H., Pirc-Danoewinata, H., Steger, G., Kreiner, G., Wagner, B., Lechner, K., Lutz, D., Bettelheim, P., and Haas, O. (1992) Prognostic impact of karyotype and immunologic phenotype in 125 adult patients with de novo AML. *Cancer Genet. Cytogenet.* **61,** 14–25.
71. Meyers, S., Downing, J., and Hiebert, S. (1993) Identification of AML-1 and the (8;21) translocation protein (AML-1/ETO) as sequence specific DNA binding proteins: the runt homology domain is required for DNA binding and protein-protein interactions. *Mol. Cell. Biol.* **13,** 6336–6345.
72. Miyoshi, H., Shimizu, K., Kozu, T., Maseki, N., Kaneko, Y., and Ohki, M. (1991) t(8;21) breakpoints on chromosome 21 in acute myeloid leukemia are clustered within a limited region of a single gene, AML1. *Proc. Natl. Acad. Sci. USA* **88,** 10,431–10,434.
73. Offit, K., Wong, G., Filippa, D., Tao, Y., and Chaganti, R. (1991) Cytogenetic analysis of 434 consecutively ascertained specimens of non-Hodgkin's lymphoma: clinical correlations. *Blood* **77,** 1508–1515.
74. Rimokh, R., Berger, F., Delsol, G., Digonnet, I., Rouault, J., Tigaud, J., Gadoux, M., Coiffier, B., Bryon, C. B, P., and Magaud, J. (1994) Detection of the chromosomal translocation t(11;14) by polymerase chain reaction in mantle cell lymphomas. *Blood* **83,** 1871–1875.
75. Swansbury, G., Lawler, S., Alimena, G., Arthur, D., Berger, R., Van Den Berghe, H., Bloomfield, C., de la Chappelle, A., Dewald, G., Garson, O., Hagemeijer, A., Mitelman, F., Rowley, J., and Sakurai, M. (1994) Long-term survival in acute myelogenous leukemia: a second follow-up of the fourth international workshop on chromosomes in leukemia. *Cancer Genet. Cytogenet.* **73,** 1–7.

Chapter 26

Placental Blood

Immunology, Transplantation, and Gene Therapy

Anne F. Eder and Leslie E. Silberstein

1. Introduction

Placental blood is an alternative to bone marrow for hematopoietic transplantation, and repositories of cryopreserved placental blood will be a valuable adjunct to bone marrow donor registries *(1–4)*. Although thousands have benefitted from bone marrow transplantation since its introduction 25 year ago, only one third of patients requiring this treatment have an HLA-genotypically matched sibling *(5)*. For those remaining, the probability of finding an HLA-identical unrelated match in a database of more than 2.6 million volunteers registered with the National Marrow Donor Program is influenced by race. The registry identifies HLA-A, -B, and -DR identical matches for approx 70% of Caucasian patients, but only for approx 34% of African American patients *(6)*. This discrepancy is because of under representation of African Americans in the registry and increased HLA heterogeneity among African Americans compared to Caucasians. Unfortunately, even if an appropriate match is identified, some donors in the registry refuse or are medically unable to undergo the donation procedure, which requires hospitalization and anesthesia. Finally, the three to six months required to obtain bone marrow through the registry (NBMDR, personal communication) is problematic for some acutely ill patients with advancing disease or ensuing secondary complications.

For these reasons, additional sources of hematopoietic progenitor cells have been investigated, such as peripheral blood, fetal liver, and placental blood (umbilical cord blood, cord blood) *(7)*. Placental blood collected from the umbilical cord shortly after the delivery of an infant contains progenitor cells capable of reconstituting the human hematopoietic system *(8–10)*. Practical advantages of placental blood compared to bone marrow include the ease of procurement, cryopreservation and long-term storage, immediate accessibility, elimination of donor attrition, and expansion of the donor pool. Moreover, biological advantages associated with placental blood have emerged from clinical transplantation trials. In addition to the rich content of stem cells, placental blood

From: *Molecular Biology of B-Cell and T-Cell Development*
Edited by: J. G. Monroe and E. V. Rothenberg © Humana Press Inc., Totowa, NJ

is less likely to provoke a severe immune response in recipients, even in the face of 1-3 HLA antigen mismatches *(8–11)*.

The first placental blood transplant in 1988 proved effective treatment for a child with Fanconi's anemia, a disease associated with complete bone marrow failure *(12)*. To date, placental blood transplantation has been performed for more than 350 patients, the vast majority of whom are children, suffering from various diseases including hematologic cancers, such as acute lymphocytic leukemia, bone marrow failure syndromes such as Fanconi's anemia, immunodeficiency disorders such as severe combined immunodeficiency, and genetic metabolic diseases such as mucopolysaccharidoses *(8–20)*. Finally, placental blood may facilitate gene therapy protocols. Recently, the gene required to correct a metabolic defect was introduced into hematopoietic progenitor cells from autologous placental blood and delivered to three affected infants *(21,22)*. This chapter reviews the hematopoietic potential and immunologic properties of placental blood compared to adult bone marrow and summarizes results from clinical transplantation and gene therapy protocols utilizing hematopoietic progenitor cells from placental blood.

2. Hematopoietic Potential and Immunologic Properties of Placental Blood

2.1. Placental Blood Progenitor Cell Content and Characteristics

Comparison of the content and functional properties of stem and hematopoietic progenitors in bone marrow, peripheral blood, and placental blood have revealed differences in the quality and quantity of these multipotent cells *(1,23)*. Because there is no quantitative assay for the stem cell subset that has long-term marrow repopulating capacity in humans, surrogate assays for the presence of progenitor cells in vitro are performed and correlated with clinical outcome of transplantation trials. The assays evaluate the ability of lineage-committed progenitor cells to form differentiated colonies on semi-solid media (CFU or colony forming assay) or the capacity of early progenitors to self renew. Colony forming units-granulocyte macrophage (CFU-GM) and blast forming units-erythrocyte (BFU-E) reflect committed progenitors; whereas, colony forming units-granulocyte, erythrocyte, monocyte, macrophage (CFU-GEMM or CFU-Mix) reflect earlier multipotent progenitors. The ability of an individual progenitor cell colony to form additional generations of colonies after replating in vitro has been used as an indicator of the self-renewal potential of that progenitor cell. Additional clonogenic assays for subsets of cells with the capacity for self-renewal include high proliferative potential-colony forming cells (HPP-CFC) and long-term culture initiating cells (LTC-ICs). The LTC-IC assay identifies cells with the ability to sustain prolonged hematopoiesis and progenitor cell generation when inoculated onto preformed irradiated marrow stroma and represents the earliest stem cell compartment that can be evaluated in vitro *(24)*. Alternatively, flow cytometry is used to detect expression of the CD34 cell surface antigen characteristic of immature hematopoietic cells *(25)*. Murine and ovine models have also been developed as assay systems for human placental blood progenitor cell engraftment *(26,27)*. Recently, Larochelle et al. identified a novel human hematopoietic cell more primitive than most LTC-ICs in placental blood and bone marrow, capable of multilineage repopulation of the bone marrow of severe combined immunodeficiency disease (SCID) mice *(28)*. However, broad interpretation of these assays is limited because none is a direct assay for the earliest subset of hematopoietic stem cells with long-term marrow engrafting capacity in humans.

Regardless, these assays serve as the foundation to evaluate the quantity and quality of stem and progenitor cells in hematopoietic transplants. For example, engraftment and recovery after myeloablative therapy and bone marrow transplantation has been shown to correlate with CFU-GM content and $CD34^+$ cell dose *(29,30)*. Several groups have shown that the quantity of stem and progenitor cells present in placental blood are at least comparable to the numbers found in adult bone marrow, and greater than the numbers found in adult peripheral blood *(23,31–35)*. Broxmeyer et al. demonstrated that placental blood donations contained a mean (SD) total of 1.9 (1.5) $\times 10^6$ CFU-GM *(31)*. Consequently, a placental blood collection would be sufficient for bone marrow reconstitution for a recipient weighing as much as 70 kg, because its CFU-GM content compares favorably to the mean CFU-GM per kilogram of recipient body weight associated with successful engraftment in adults receiving bone marrow allografts ($4.3 \pm 4.1 \times 10^4$ CFU-GM/kg) *(36)*. Moreover, the CFU-GM content of placental blood would be above the threshold ($>10^3$ CFU-GM/kg) associated with favorable recovery kinetics for hematopoiesis in adults receiving bone marrow autografts *(37)*. The significant interlaboratory variability associated with the CFU-GM assay weakens the validity of this prediction. However, direct comparison of placental blood and adult bone marrow confirmed comparable numbers of CFU-GM in placental blood and adult bone marrow *(32)*. Although CFU-GM reflects the content of committed progenitors in the graft and correlates with time to early engraftment in bone marrow transplantation trials, long-term culture is a measure of more primitive progenitor cells and is more likely to relate to the potential for sustained engraftment. Direct comparison of LTC-IC suggest that the incidence of hematopoietic stem cells is at least equivalent or greater in placental blood compared to adult bone marrow *(34)*, or to adult bone marrow and peripheral blood leukoapheresis collections *(35)*. Immunophenotypic data also suggest placental blood is enriched for more immature progenitors *(33,38)*.

In several studies, early hematopoietic cells in placental blood differed qualitatively as well as quantitatively from their counterparts in adult bone marrow. The CD34 cell surface antigen is expressed at low density on committed hematopoietic progenitor cells and at high density on earlier precursors *(25)*. The phenotype of $CD34^+$ stem cells in both placental blood and bone marrow has been characterized as $CD34^{bright}$ *(39)*, $CD45RA^{lo}$, $CD71^{lo}$ *(40)*, $CD38^-$ *(33)*, $Thy1^+$ *(41)*, and $CD45RO^+$ *(38,42)*. Differences are apparent at the HLA-DR locus; these $CD34^+$ cells in bone marrow are $HLA\text{-}DR^{lo}$ or $HLA\text{-}DR^-$, those in placental blood are $HLA\text{-}DR^+$ *(43)*.

Functional as well as phenotypic differences exist between hematopoietic progenitor cells in placental blood and adult bone marrow. First, the hematopoietic progenitor cells in placental blood demonstrate high proliferative and replating potential compared with their counterparts in adult bone marrow *(7,42,44)*. For example, Carow et al. demonstrated that both placental blood and adult bone marrow CFU-GEMM have the capacity to be replated (self-renew) and generate secondary CFU-GEMM when cultured with stem cell factor or cord blood plasma *(44)*. Replating single placental blood CFU-GEMM resulted in up to 1000 secondary colonies, many of multiple lineages such as CFU-GEMM, whereas replating adult bone marrow CFU-GEMM gave rise to a maximum of 50 secondary colonies, most of which were lineage-restricted colonies such as CFU-GM and BFU-E *(44)*. Lansdorp et al. found that placental blood $CD34^+$ cells demonstrated a more active proliferative response to cytokines in culture and generated significantly more $CD34^+$ progeny than adult bone marrow $CD34^+$ cells *(42)*. Several studies confirmed that placental blood contains progenitor cells that are more responsive to the proliferative effects of cytokines, such as stem-cell factor and IL-3, than their counterparts in adult bone marrow or peripheral blood *(23,32,45)*. Finally, placental blood long-term culture initiating cells were maintained in vitro for significantly longer periods of time than adult bone marrow long-term culture initiating cells *(34)*. The proliferative potential of a cell may be regulated by telomere length, because the total number of cellular divisions is correlated with sequential loss of telomeric sequences *(46)*. Interestingly, shorter telomeric regions have been found in $CD34^+$ cells from adult bone marrow compared to those from placental blood (*47*; *see* also Chapter 2).

These data suggest that placental blood is enriched for progenitor cells possessing greater proliferative potential than their counterparts in adult bone marrow. In addition to inherent qualitative differences in stem-cell populations, placental blood may contain a subset of stem cells representing an earlier developmental stage not found in adult bone marrow. Evidence for differences in growth factors and cytokines in plasma from placental blood compared to adult blood have also been described. For example, placental plasma, but not adult plasma, enhanced the replating capacity of both placental blood and bone marrow CFU-GEMM *(44)*. The differences observed in the clonogenic in vitro assays could translate into a clinical advantage, if the minimum cell numbers of stem and progenitor cells required for durable hematopoietic engraftment is lower, and the potential for ex vivo expansion of immature stem cells is greater for placental blood than for adult bone marrow.

2.2. Lymphocyte Populations— Graft vs Host Disease and Graft vs Leukemia Effect

In a broader context, the unique immunological status of placental blood compared to adult bone marrow may also prove beneficial in clinical transplantation trials. A dire complication of bone marrow transplantation is severe graft-vs-host disease (GVHD) in which T lymphocytes contained in the graft mount a reaction against the recipient's tissues because of antigenic disparities in histocompatibility antigen (HLA) expression *(48)*. Clinical manifestations of GVHD include maculopapular skin rash, liver function abnormalities, and gastrointestinal dysfunction. An acute form of GVHD may develop around the time of hematopoietic engraftment or a chronic form of the disease may develop more than 100 days after transplantation. Cellular mediators of GVHD include $CD8^+$ cytotoxic lymphocytes directed against histocompatibility antigens, nonspecific effector systems such as NK cells, and $CD4^+$ T lymphocytes. Cytokines, such as IL-1, IL-2, TNF-α, and IFN-γ, that are produced by T lymphocytes and other mononuclear cells are also implicated in the pathogenesis of GVHD *(49)*. The graft-vs-leukemia effect is related to GVHD, except that the allogeneic reaction of the donor T lymphocytes is directed against residual leukemia in the host. Bone marrow grafts depleted of T lymphocytes are associated with less severe and less frequent GVHD; however, they are also associated with increased rate of graft rejection and leukemic relapse *(50)*. Delineation of the T lymphocyte populations mediating GVHD and graft vs leukemia effect and separation of these two entities has been an elusive goal in clinical bone marrow transplantation. Observations from the first two placental blood transplantations for Fanconi's anemia suggested that GVHD was less severe in patients who received placental blood from HLA-identical siblings than in those patients who received HLA-identical bone marrow *(12,51)*. This preliminary finding supported the hypothesis that placental hematopoietic cells differed immunologically from adult hematopoietic cells.

Functional differences between placental blood and adult peripheral blood have been observed with respect to cellular and humoral immunity, as well as to natural host defenses such as macrophage activation. The neonatal immune system is functionally less mature at birth and, under the influence of both genetic programming and environmental stimulation, undergoes a complex process of development. The total leukocyte and absolute lymphocyte counts are highest at birth and decline with age *(52,53)*. Because of the increased number of lymphocytes in placental blood, the absolute number of cells within virtually every lymphocyte population is significantly higher in placental blood than in adult peripheral blood *(54–57)*. Placental blood contains a lower percentage of T-cells ($CD3^+$) and a higher percentage of B-cells ($CD19^+$) than adult peripheral blood. Despite the decline in absolute counts, the relative proportions of T lymphocyte subsets, including both $CD4^+$ and $CD8^+$ subsets, generally increase with age *(54,55,58)*.

2.2.1. T-Lymphocyte Subpopulations in Placental Blood

Placental blood contains T lymphocytes that are phenotypically immature. Approximately 90% of T lymphocytes from placental blood express the CD45RA antigen compared to 40–50% of T-cells from adult peripheral blood *(2,55,56,58–60)*. The reciprocal trend is observed for CD45RO expression on placental blood and adult blood lymphocytes *(54,56)*. Higher expression of CD38 and lower expression of CD29 within T lymphocyte populations in placental blood compared to those in adult peripheral blood also likely represents their naïve status *(54,57–59)*. The percentage of T lymphocytes expressing activation markers, such as IL-2R and HLA-DR, is low in neonatal blood and increases with age *(54,55,57)*. Evidence for phenotypic immaturity and antigenic naiveté of placental T lymphocytes compared to their adult counterparts also includes the lower density expression of CD3, of cellular adhesion molecules such as CD11a (LFA-1), CD18 and CD58 (LFA-3), and of activation markers such as HLA class II antigen *(59,61,62)*.

The major immunoregulatory function for the predominant T lymphocyte subsets, both within the $CD4^+$ and within the $CD8^+$ populations, in placental blood has been speculated to involve suppression of immune responses *(56,63)*. For example, the majority of cord $CD4^+$ lymphocytes express the phenotype $CD4^+CD45RA^+$ which is associated with the induction of suppressor activity by $CD8^+$ T-cells *(64)*. Similarly, within the $CD8^+$ T lymphocyte population in placental blood, a predominance of $CD11a^{dim}$ cells, a phenotype associated with suppressor function, compared to $CD11a^{bright}$ cells, a phenotype associated with killer-effector function, could contribute to the immune suppression associated with placental blood *(56,65)*. In summary, the "suppressor activity" of placental blood may be a result of the overrepresentation of subsets of $CD4^+$ and $CD8^+$ cells that express the suppressor inducer and suppressor phenotypes, respectively. This model predicts that the suppressor-type cells in placental blood modulate the activation of transplanted lymphocytes and NK cells to minimize the risk of GVHD.

Although the vast majority of data support a predominant population of immature, unactivated T lymphocytes in placental blood, consensus has not been reached regarding the frequency of other T lymphocyte populations within placental blood. For example, increased *(2,56,58,59)*, decreased *(65)* and equivalent *(55)* $CD4^+/CD8^+$ (helper/suppressor) ratios have been found in placental blood compared to adult blood. Similarly, the mean proportion of NK cells ($CD3^-CD16^+/CD56^+$) in placental blood ranges from 5%, lower than the mean proportion in adult peripheral blood, to 25%, greater than the mean proportion in adult peripheral blood *(54,55,57,66,67)*. Variance among studies likely reflects a number of factors including sample size, antibody panel, and technique of lymphocyte preparation. In addition, variation in placental blood populations has been reported between sexes and among races *(58,68)*. Finally, factors related to obstetric history, such as glucocorticoid exposure, may influence lymphocyte subsets and surface phenotype *(55,69)*.

2.2.2. Alloreactivity of T-Cells in Placental Blood

Although phenotypic analysis permits these correlations between maturation and function of T-cell populations, experimental evaluation of proliferative and cytotoxic responses of placental blood T lymphocytes following allogeneic stimulation provides the most direct estimation of their functional status in the unrelated donor transplantation setting. Induction of cytotoxic responses is a balance between the interaction of different T lymphocyte subsets. Although often contradictory, most studies demonstrate T-cells in placental blood are deficient in a variety of functional assays when compared to their counterparts in adult peripheral blood *(59,62,70–74)*. For example, the generation of specific cytotoxicity after primary, secondary, and tertiary allogeneic stimulation of placental blood T lymphocytes in bulk assay is minimal compared to adult T lymphocytes *(70,73)*. Some groups, but not others, have reported lower frequencies of cytotoxic T-cell precursors and alloreactive T-cell precursors in placental blood than adult peripheral blood by limiting dilution analysis *(59,70,75)*. Several investigators extrapolated from their results that the probability of GVHD after transplantation would be lower with placental blood than with adult bone marrow *(70–73)*. However, predictions to the contrary were also proffered *(75,76)*.

The most likely source of this controversy lies in the variability inherent to cellular immunological assays such as the mixed lymphocyte reaction (MLR) and mixed lymphocyte culture (MLC). The MLR is an estimate of the proliferative response of T-cells after allogeneic stimulation. The MLC generates cytotoxic lymphocytes upon allogeneic stimulation in culture, which are evaluated for their ability to lyse various allogeneic cellular targets. The purification of the responder T-cells, the source of the stimulator cells (allogeneic tumor cell lines or primary peripheral blood mononuclear cells), and the experimental conditions (stimulation with phytohemagglutinin or cytokines, source of serum) are all variables that influence the results and consequently the interpretation of the experiment. In conclusion, the alloresponsiveness of placental blood T lymphocytes may differ from that of peripheral blood T lymphocytes because of differences in the precursor frequencies of alloreactive and cytotoxic T lymphocytes, impaired activation of $CD8^+$ effectors, more stringent lymphocyte activation requirements or the unique cytokine and cytokine receptor profile of placental blood lymphocytes.

A narrow spectrum of cytokines is produced by placental blood T lymphocytes on primary activation as predicted by the cells' naïve phenotype *(77,78)*. Following allogeneic stimulation, placental blood T-cells produce IL-2, but significantly less IFN-γ, IL-4, and other cytokines compared to adult peripheral blood T lymphocytes *(70,73,74)*. Receptors for virtually all cytokines are expressed on the surface of placental blood T-cells, albeit at lower cell surface density than observed on adult blood T-cells *(79)*. Decreased expression of the IL-2 receptor gamma chain that is shared with receptors for IL-4, IL-7, IL-9, IL-15, as well as IL-2 in placental blood lymphocytes compared to adult blood lymphocytes, could contribute to these differences *(80)*. T lymphocytes in placental blood do not express the receptor for IL-1 *(56)*. Since dysregulated production of cytokines such as IL-1, IL-2, and TNFα may contribute to GVHD, the cytokine and cytokine receptor profile on placental blood T-cells may modulate the activation of placental blood lymphocytes and their ability to mediate GVHD.

2.2.3. NK and LAK Activity

Placental blood contains a comparable or increased proportion and an increased absolute number of cells expressing natural killer (NK) markers ($CD3^-$, $CD16^+$, $CD56^+$)

than adult peripheral blood *(55,59,61,67)*. However, NK cytotoxicity is barely detectable in fresh placental blood *(62,81)*. Incubation of placental blood cells in IL-2 alone, IL-2, and mitogens, or IL-12, induces lytic ability *(62,81,82)*. Limiting dilution analysis revealed a higher frequency of lymphokine-activated killer (LAK) precursors and a more rapid expansion of NK cells in response to stimulation with IL-2 in placental blood, compared to adult peripheral blood *(59)*. These differences may be related to a unique population of $CD34^-CD7^+$ lineage-negative cells that are precursors to NK cells and are activated in response to IL-2 in placental blood *(81)*. The lack of NK cytotoxicity in fresh preparations of NK cells from placental blood may be a result of inhibition by soluble HLA class I antigen in placental blood *(83)*. Because activation of nonspecific effector systems such as NK cells during GVHD in bone marrow allografts has been implicated in the graft vs leukemia response, a similar mechanism may occur in umbilical cord grafts *(84)*. Interestingly, a prominent population of NK cells emerges within weeks following placental blood transplantation *(11)*. Moreover, IL-2 activated placental blood LAK cells were capable of lysing a variety of noncultured leukemia targets in vitro and placental blood demonstrated significant graft vs leukemia capacity in an animal model in vivo *(59,85)*.

2.3. Humoral Immunity and Accessory Cell Function

Despite the increased numbers of B lymphocytes in placental blood, newborns are deficient in their ability to mount humoral immune responses. The neonatal immune system is incapable of producing significant levels of immunoglobulins other than IgM in response to antigens. The B lymphocytes ($CD19^+/CD20^+$) in placental blood express a unique phenotype with the majority demonstrating CD5 and an increased proportion demonstrating CD10 (CALLA) on their cellular surface *(55,58,62)*. Although functionally naïve, neonatal B lymphocytes are intrinsically capable of isotype switching, if provided with appropriate signals *(86,87)*. Placental blood T lymphocytes suppress immunoglobulin production, and the defect in isotype switching has been attributed to ineffective T-cell help because of deficient CD40 ligand expression *(86,87)*, and other mechanisms such as deficient cytokine production by T-cells and delayed maturation of antigen presenting cells *(88,89)*. Independently from T-cell help, neonatal B lymphocytes produce polyreactive autoantibodies spontaneously, which may play role in regulation of immune responses or in non-specific host defenses *(90)*.

Deficits in macrophage and accessory cell function have also been demonstrated in placental blood *(91–93)*. For example, neonatal T lymphocytes produce less IFN-γ than adult T lymphocytes. Because T lymphocytes acquire the ability to produce IL-4 and IFN-γ after exposure to exogenous activation, reduced expression of IL-4 and IFN-γ by neonatal T lymphocytes may reflect, in part, their antigenically naïve status *(77,78)*. However, placental T lymphocytes produced IFN-γ only in the presence of adult macrophages, whereas adult T lymphocytes produced minimal IFN-γ in the presence of placental macrophages. Consequently, dysfunctional macrophage function may contribute to impaired IFN-γ production in placental blood. Another mechanism for deficient T lymphocyte function in placental blood compared to adult bone marrow is defective dendritic cell function. Because the predominant T lymphocyte population expresses the CD45RA antigen characteristic of naïve T-cells, their activation likely requires presentation of antigen by dendritic cells. Dendritic cells have been isolated or propagated from placental blood; however, they perform poorly as accessory cells for T-lymphocyte mitogenic responses *(91)*. Moreover, placental blood dendritic cells were associated with significantly less stimulation in MLR than adult dendritic cells. This effect was observed when either adult or placental blood mononuclear cells or T lymphocytes were used as responder cells. In contrast, placental blood T lymphocytes and mononuclear cells responded vigorously to allogeneic adult dendritic cells. The impaired function of the placental blood dendritic cells correlated with lower cell surface expression of cell adhesion and MHC molecules. Thus, deficient dendritic cell activity may contribute to the functional immaturity of placental blood.

3. Placental Blood Transplantation

The first placental blood transplant was performed in 1988 to treat a child with Fanconi's anemia *(12)*. More than seven years after transplantation, the child is hematologically normal and healthy *(14)*. Following additional preliminary successes with placental blood transplantation from sibling donors, placental blood banks were established in the United States and Europe *(4,94)*. Placental blood transplantation has been used for over 350 patients with high-risk or recurrent hematological malignancies, bone marrow failure, and selected hereditary immunodeficiency syndromes, hemoglobinopathies, and metabolic disorders *(8–20)*. There are few contraindications for collecting blood from the umbilical cord following delivery of the placenta. Indeed, the umbilical cord is usually clamped without consideration to the elapsed time after delivery of the infant, and the placenta discarded. There is no measurable detriment to infants whose umbilical cord is clamped within 30 seconds of delivery to allow optimal collection of blood from the placenta *(95,96)*. In rare instances, delayed clamping of the umbilical cord may be advocated to benefit the newborn. In other settings, placental blood can be used for laboratory testing to decrease iatrogenic blood loss in the neonatal period or can be used for red cell transfusion to the neonate to decrease the risk of exposure to transfusion transmitted infectious diseases *(97)*. If fetal distress, intrauterine infection, or congenital abnormalities are suspected, evaluation of the placenta for pathological changes will preclude blood collection. However, in the vast majority of cases, placental blood can be collected, cryopreserved, and used for hematopoietic transplantation *(4)*.

3.1. Clinical Efficacy of Placental Blood Transplantation

The safety and efficacy of placental blood transplantation utilizing sibling or unrelated donors has been evaluated in clinical trials *(8–10)*. Several key properties of the placental blood used in these trials are summarized in Table 1. Most patients weighed less than 50 kg and received less than 100 mL of placental blood containing the hematopoietic progenitor cells that repopulated the bone marrow and generated differentiated peripheral blood cells in 3–12 wk. The smallest dose associated with successful engraftment in these studies was 0.7×10^7 nucleated cells/kg *(8)*. The probability of engraftment was 85–100% and the probability of survival at six months after transplantation was approx 65%. Although follow-up intervals are short, late graft failure was not reported for any of the patients. Causes of death were similar to the experience with bone marrow transplantation and included early fungal sepsis, chemotherapy related toxicity/multi-organ failure, and leukemic relapse. Grade IV GVHD was reported as the cause of death for two patients *(9,10)*.

3.2. Engraftment of Placental Blood vs Adult Bone Marrow

The number of nucleated cells infused per kilogram of body weight correlated with the rate of myeloid engraftment in recipients of placental blood from unrelated donors in a study performed at a single medical center, but not in recipients of placental blood

Table 1
Placental Blood Transplantation: Experience with Sibling and Unrelated Donors[a]

Reference	Kurtzberg et al. (Unrelated)	Wagner et al. (Unrelated)	Wagner et al. (Sibling)
Patient and placental blood characteristics			
Number of patients	25	18	44
Median patient weight (kg)	19.4	15.4	20
HLA compatibility of patient and product			
No. identical	1	7	34
No. discordant (1–3 Ags)	24	11	10
Median NC/kg ($\times 10^{-7}$)	3.0	4.1	5.2
Median CFU-GM/kg ($\times 10^{-4}$)	3.6	N.R.	2.4
$CD34^+$/kg ($\times 10^{-6}$)	1.43	N.R.	N.R.
Median vol collected (mL)	68	83.1	100
Clinical outcome measures			
Median recovery (days)			
PMN > 500/µL	22	24	22
Plts > 50,000/µL	56	54	49
Engraftment (no./no. evaluable)	23/25	13/13	33/39
GVHD grade III, IV acute	2/21	2/13	1/34
Chronic	2/21	N.R.	2/34
Survival	64%[b]	65%[c]	62%[d]

[a]Abbreviations: kg, kilogram; CFU-GM, colony forming unit-granulocyte, macrophage; NC, nucleated cells; vol, volume; PMN, polymorphonuclear cells; Plts, platelets; GVHD, graft-vs-host disease; N.R., not reported.

[b]Median follow-up 12.5 months, 100 day survival.

[c]Median follow-up 6 months, 6 month survival.

[d]Median follow-up 1.6 years.

from related or unrelated donors in two other multicenter studies *(8–10)*. This difference could reflect differences among protocols at different study sites. Regardless, the time to myeloid recovery did not correlate with CFU-GM or $CD34^+$ content of the umbilical cord grafts in contrast to clinical results from bone marrow and mobilized peripheral blood transplantation trials *(29,30,36,37)*. These observations suggest differences between these early progenitor cell compartments in placental blood compared to adult bone marrow. Development of additional assays directed at detecting the earliest stem cells may correlate more closely with engraftment kinetics following placental blood transplantation than the currently available assays.

The time to neutrophil recovery following placental blood transplantation is comparable to that observed following bone marrow transplantation. Neutrophil recovery has been expedited following autologous bone marrow and peripheral blood transplantation by administration of hematopoietic growth factors such as GM-CSF (Neupogen) *(98,99)*. The role for such growth factors after placental blood transplantation has not been clearly established. The time to neutrophil recovery in a group receiving growth factors compared to a group not receiving growth factors was slightly improved in one study but unaffected in another *(9,10)*. In all studies performed to date, the average rate of platelet recovery is remarkably delayed following placental blood transplantation (50 d) as compared to that following bone marrow (30 d), or peripheral blood stem cell transplantation (14 d). Strategies to accelerate platelet recovery following hematopoietic transplantation, such as the use of thrombopoietin and its derivative megakaryocyte growth and differentiation factor (MGDF), are currently being evaluated in clinical trials *(100)*.

3.3. Risk of GVHD

The first case reports of successful umbilical cord transplantation suggested a lower risk of severe graft vs host disease than typically observed following bone marrow transplantation *(11,12,51)*. Kurtzberg et al. demonstrated that despite significant HLA incompatibility, acute graft vs host disease (grade I-III) affected 52% overall but was mild (<grade II) in all but two out of 25 recipients of placental blood transplants *(8)*. Chronic graft vs host disease occurred in only two of 25 recipients, and no deaths resulted from graft vs host disease in this series. Wagner et al. reported the incidence of grade II-IV GVHD was approx 50% among patients receiving HLA mismatched grafts *(10)*. However, most of these individuals had limited disease that responded to steroid treatment, and only two patients developed grade III-IV GVHD. One of these patients, despite clinical manifestations, had no evidence of pathologic changes in the skin and lower GI tract, and responded promptly to steroid therapy. The other individual did not respond to steroids or various other immunosuppressive agents and ultimately died from complications of acute GVHD. Consequently, the probability of grade III-IV acute graft vs host disease at 100 days was 11% in this series. The statistics from these two series compares favorably to estimates of the risk of acute and chronic GVHD following bone marrow transplantation. In pediatric (<18 year old) recipients of HLA-matched unrelated donor marrow, the incidence of grade III or IV acute GVHD is 30–37%, and the incidence of chronic GVHD is 60% *(101,102)*. In young recipients of HLA-mismatched unrelated donor bone marrow, the incidence of grade III-IV acute GVHD was 62% and the incidence of chronic graft vs host disease was 69% *(101)*. In conclusion, placental blood lymphocytes are capable of inducing graft-vs-host pathology. Placental blood transplantation, however, is associated with a low risk of severe refractory acute graft vs host disease. The duration of follow-up is not sufficient to evaluate the risk of leukemic relapse or the graft vs leukemia activity associated with placental blood transplantation compared to adult bone marrow transplantation.

The risk of GVHD may be minimized in sibling transplantations by matching the paternal HLA alleles of the donor and recipient *(103)*. For example, several recipients of placental blood from donors who shared a paternal haplotype, but differed at the maternal one, did not develop GVHD or developed low grade and limited disease, despite HLA disparities *(9,104)*. Conversely, two patients with grade II and grade III acute GVHD had donors who differed with respect to the paternal haplotype *(9)*. These observations may be explained by the partial tolerance to noninherited maternal alleles that develops during gestation *(105,106)*. This suggests that placental blood T lymphocytes will be tolerant to the disparate maternal haplotype and will be less likely to initiate GVHD.

Another consideration in evaluating the risk of GVHD associated with placental blood transplantation is the potential for contaminating maternal T lymphocytes in grafts to initiate host tissue damage *(76)*. Maternal lymphocytes may be introduced into the placental circulation either during gestation and parturition by transplacental passage or during collection. Cellular traffic across the placenta results in the presence of maternal lymphocytes in more than 25% of neonates with severe combined immunodeficiency *(4)*. The frequency of this phenomenon in healthy neonates has not been reported. Contamination with maternal blood during the collection procedure is minimized by utilizing a closed system, such as a whole blood collection bag after aseptic venipuncture of the umbilical cord, rather than an open system in which blood is collected by gravity into bottles or tubes *(107)*. Estimates of maternal cell contamination in samples of placental blood have varied with respect to both the frequency of maternal cells within a unit and the proportion of units containing maternal cells. Several groups were unable to detect maternal cells in placental blood from sibling donors utilizing restriction fragment length polymorphism, karyotypic analysis or HLA Class II typing *(4,11,20,108)*. Socie et al. reported only one sample in 47 (2%) had a positive PCR signal for maternal minisatellite sequences, and estimated the frequency of maternal cells as 0.1–1% in the whole blood and lymphocyte fraction of placental blood samples *(109)*. Hall et al. utilized fluorescence *in situ* hybridization to identify X and Y chromosomes and reported maternal cells were found in 7 of the 49 (14%) placental blood samples collected from male infants, at levels ranging 0.04–1.0% in the mononuclear or the lymphocyte fractions *(110)*. Scaradavou et al., utilizing a sensitive PCR-hybridization technique capable of detecting 1 maternal cell in 10^5 fetal cells, reported small numbers of maternal cells (less than 1%) in 38% of the 213 placental blood samples *(107)*. In conclusion, a low level of maternal cell contamination (less than 1%) may be present in as many as 38% of CB samples.

Although these estimates are within the range of cell doses capable of inducing GVHD after HLA-identical BM transplantation *(111)*, the low frequency and severity of GVHD in recent clinical trials suggest that maternal T-cell contamination is not key contributing factor to graft-vs-host disease pathogenesis. Kurtzberg et al. reported that maternal cells from the donor unit were not found in the tissue-biopsy specimens from any patient with GVHD *(8)*. Moreover, a recent successful transplant performed with a sample of placental blood containing significant maternal cell contamination suggests that the likelihood of GVHD even in this setting is unlikely *(104)*. This observation may reflect the ability of placental blood T-cells to suppress the proliferation of maternal T lymphocytes *(103)*. Moreover, maternal NK activity is depressed at the time of birth. Maternal lymphocytes in this context may not be predisposed to generate graft-vs-host disease. A systematic evaluation of the ability of maternal cells to mediate graft-vs-host disease in recipients of placental blood transplants is warranted.

3.4. Applicability of Placental Blood Transplantation for Adults

Clinical experience with umbilical cord transplantation in adults is much less extensive than in children (Table 2). Laporte et al. reported the successful engraftment of placental blood from an unrelated donor in a 26-year-old woman with chronic myelogenous leukemia *(17)*. She weighed 55 kg and received the relatively low dose of 10 million nucleated cells per kilogram. In Kurtzberg's series, a 24-year-old woman with leukemia weighing 44 kg and two adolescent subjects with leukemia weighing 53 and 79 kg also demonstrated successful engraftment and significant event free survival *(8)*. Wagner et al. included two patients weighing more than 50 kg in whom hematopoietic reconstitution was accomplished with $1.4–1.7 \times 10^7$ nucleated cells/kg of placental blood: a 15-year-old with AML weighing 78.8 kg, and a 21-year-old with adrenoleukodystrophy weighing 53.6 kg *(10)*. Placental blood may achieve hematopoietic reconstitution with fewer stem and progenitor cells than adult bone marrow because of its enhanced proliferative potential and self-renewal capacity. The minimum dose required for adequate engraftment and bone marrow repopulation is not clearly defined. Additional follow-up is necessary to establish the durability of the graft in these patients. These preliminary results, however, indicate placental blood transplantation may be a suitable alternative to bone marrow transplantation for adults as well as children.

3.5. Issues in Establishing an Placental Blood Bank

Many blood banks already collect and process bone marrow and peripheral blood stem cells for use in transplantation and possess experience that is directly applicable to

Table 2
Placental Blood Transplantation:
Published Experience with Recipients Weighing more than 50 kg

Weight (kg)	Age (years)	Vol. CB (mL)	NC/kg ($\times 10^{-7}$)	CFU-GM/kg ($\times 10^{-4}$)	Engraftment	Reported survival/ cause of death	Reference
55.0	26.0	79	1.0	1.40	Yes	8 months	*(17)*
53.0	11.9	122	3.8	0.23	Yes	469 days	*(8)*
79.0	15.1	98	1.1	1.48	Yes	103 days/adenovirus	*(8)*
78.8	14.9	88	1.4	N.R.	Yes	85 days	*(10)*
53.6	21.3	83	1.7	N.R.	Yes	88 days/grade IV GVHD	*(10)*

handling and preserving hematopoietic progenitor cells in placental blood *(112)*. Standards for stem cell programs have been detailed by the Foundation for the Accreditation of Hematopoietic Cell Therapy (FAHCT) and the American Association of Blood Banks. The FDA currently requires an Investigational New Drug (IND) application from those collecting and storing placental blood for allogeneic human transplantation. These agencies ensure appropriate standards to protect the safety of both the donor and recipient, to maintain donor confidentiality, and to provide a source of viable hematopoietic stem cells effective for transplantation. Their guidelines address the issues of informed consent, donor selection and deferral, product evaluation, and quality assurance and provide the basis for further refinement of standard operating procedures. Ethical issues such as the ramifications of results of infectious disease and genetic testing for the newborn are still open topics of discussion *(113)*.

The New York Blood Center, leading the effort in this country to establish a publicly accessible bank, has collected more than 5000 placental blood specimens *(4)*. The National Heart Lung and Blood Institute of the NIH has invested approx 38 million dollars to support a network of placental blood banks and experimental transplant centers as a public resource similar to the current blood banks. At least four commercial placental blood banks currently exist. Public, government-funded allogeneic placental blood banks view placental blood that would otherwise be discarded as a commonly owned good, which should be collected and distributed to whomever medically needs it. To date, all umbilical cord transplantations have been performed for sibling or unrelated donors. The potential for autologous umbilical cord transplantation is being advocated by investigators, but the cost benefit ratio for autologous storage of placental blood is not clear. Commercial placental blood banks charge a processing fee and yearly payments adding up to several thousand dollars to collect and store placental blood for later use only by the infant donor or a designated relative. Several concerns regarding this commercial endeavor have been raised. The probability a child will develop leukemia and require hematopoietic transplantation has been estimated as 1:200,000, a statistic seldomly included in advertisements from private companies. In addition, should a child with leukemia require hematopoietic transplantation, an autologous product may not be an appropriate option because it may already harbor the malignant cells. The degree of HLA disparity that has been tolerated in trials of unrelated placental blood transplantation may also diminish the advantage of autologous placental blood. Finally, the effect of long-term storage on the viability of placental blood hematopoietic stem and progenitor cells has not been clearly defined and potentially could limit utility of autologous storage. To address these concerns regarding the viability of the immature hematopoietic progenitor cells in cryopreserved placental blood, Broxmeyer et al. demonstrated that recovery after 10 year without loss of viability is possible *(14)*. Despite the controversy, autologous umbilical cord transplantation offers clinical benefit in specific scenarios and has been utilized in a gene therapy protocol *(21,22)*.

4. Placental Blood as a Vehicle for Gene Therapy

Gene therapy holds the ultimate promise to cure various inherited disorders *(114,115)*. Hematopoietic stem and progenitor cells in placental blood present an attractive target for introducing candidate genes because of their proliferative potential and capacity for self renewal. Goals of effective gene therapy include efficient gene transfer into hematopoietic cells, sufficient expression of introduced genetic sequences to complement the genetic deficiency, and persistence of the transduced cells for the lifetime of the host

(22). In primate models, long-term and stable expression of the introduced sequences after bone marrow reconstitution has been achieved *(116,118)*. However, low efficiency of gene transfer into pluripotent hematopoietic stem cells resulted in only 0.1–2% of circulating peripheral blood cells demonstrating the transduced sequence after transplantation *(116,117)*.

4.1. Efficiency of Gene Transfer into Placental Blood

A significant challenge has been to improve the efficiency of gene transfer into human hematopoietic stem cells responsible for long-term reconstitution. Efficient transduction and expression of foreign genes in committed and early progenitor cells in placental blood has been accomplished with retrovirus derived vectors in vitro. When CFU and LTC-IC assays are used as the endpoint, gene transfer into human progenitor cells occurs with 30–50% efficiency *(119,120)*. Placental blood cells were more efficiently transduced via retroviral-mediated gene transfer as compared with adult bone marrow cells *(121)*. Stable expression of an introduced adenosine deaminase gene was demonstrated in the progeny of infected LTC-ICs after five weeks in long-term marrow cultures. Moreover, expression of the introduced ADA cDNA was higher than the endogenous human ADA gene in the LTC-IC-derived colonies. Lu et al. reported the efficient retroviral-mediated gene transduction of single, isolated $CD34^+$ placental blood cells, which retained extensive replating capacity *(122)*. These results demonstrate early hematopoietic progenitor cells with high proliferative potential and replating capacity are transduced with high efficiency as assessed by clonogenic and long-term culture assays in vitro.

This population likely contains the subset of stem cells responsible for long-term marrow repopulation and suggests this subset may be amenable to gene transfer. However, the low efficiency of gene transfer observed in canine and primate models and in human gene therapy trials suggests that the transduction efficiency into the reconstituting stem cell may not be accurately assessed by in vitro assays, even those assays for more primitive cells. Recently, a primitive human hematopoietic cell capable of repopulating SCID mice was described *(28)*. Several features of this SCID repopulating cell (SRC) suggest that it represents a more primitive and distinct cell population than those detected in LTC-IC and CFU assays. Whereas CFUs and LTC-ICs were efficiently transduced, SRCs were rarely transduced with retroviruses. The SRC assay more accurately predicts the low levels of gene marking in human trials and may serve as a model to improve transduction methods.

The efficiency of retroviral gene transfer into hematopoietic stem and progenitor cells in placental blood is enhanced by cytokines, growth factors, and culture conditions. Growth stimulation is required for retroviral gene transduction, because the vector only infects cells in the cell cycle, not those in G0. Combinations of SLF, IL-3, and IL-6 exert a positive effect, whereas IL-12 exerts a negative effect on transduction efficiency *(122,123)*. Higher transduction efficiency has been obtained in cocultivation infection protocols compared to supernatant infection protocols, because direct contact is provided between hematopoietic cells and viral packaging cell lines or other sources of stroma. However, cocultivation on producer cell lines is not applicable to human gene therapy trials because of the risks associated with contamination of the graft with allogeneic stromal cells. Interaction between hematopoietic stem and progenitor cells and purified fragments of bone marrow extracellular matrix molecules has also been associated with improved retroviral-mediated gene transfer *(124)*. The improved efficiency may result from colocalization of retrovirus and target hematopoietic cells, with a resultant increase in the local viral titer presented to the cells.

Development of additional gene transfer vectors may improve efficiency and overcome potential shortcomings of retroviral-based protocols. For example, the requirement for growth factor stimulation for optimal transduction by retroviral vectors could potentially lead to differentiation of these cells and decrease their utility in the transplantation setting. Moreover, the potential for insertional oncogenesis with retroviruses, although reduced by utilizing replication defective vectors, cannot be eliminated. Adeno-associated virus 2 (AAV) is a single-stranded DNA parvovirus that demonstrates several advantages compared to retrovirus-derived vectors for gene therapy. AAV, unlike retroviruses, has not been associated with any known human disease. In addition, AAV-derived vectors demonstrate high stability, high titer, and high transduction efficiency, and may possess the ability to transduce slowly cycling or resting cells *(125)*. High efficiency transduction of $CD34^+$ cells from human placental blood cells with AAV occurred in the absence of cytokine stimulation as assessed by the presence of the marker gene in clonogenic assays in vitro. The utility of recombinant adeno-associated viruses has been demonstrated by its ability to complement the genetic defect in a cell line derived from patients with Fanconi anemia *(126)*. The safety and efficacy of recombinant adeno-associated viruses is being evaluated in human gene therapy trials.

4.2. Clinical Trial of Genetically Corrected Placental Blood

The first use of autologous placental blood cells for clinical gene therapy was for the treatment of severe combined immunodeficiency (SCID) caused by inherited deficiency of adenosine deaminase (ADA) *(21,22)*. A rare autosomal recessive disorder, ADA-deficiency results in accumulation of deoxyadenosine triphosphate to levels that are toxic to T lymphocytes. SCID ensues and is characterized by defective cell mediated and humoral immune responses. Conventional therapy for ADA-deficiency is bone marrow transplantation or enzyme replacement with ADA complexed with polyethylene glycol (PEG-ADA). Three infants with SCID were recently treated with autologous transplantation of gene modified $CD34^+$ hematopoietic progenitors from placental blood *(21)*. Gene transfer of the cDNA for ADA into $CD34^+$ hematopoietic progenitors from placental blood was mediated by a retrovirus. The transduced cells were introduced into the infants who did not receive prior myeloablative therapy. Even without this preconditioning, the frequency of vector-containing cells in the peripheral blood and bone marrow mononuclear cells fractions was 0.001–0.03% after transplantation. Because the infants were maintained on ADA enzyme replacement therapy, expression of the transduced ADA protein could not be evaluated. However, mRNA for the transduced ADA gene was detected in vivo, and enzymatically active ADA was detected in cultured transduced progenitor cells in vitro. Expression of the ADA gene in leukocytes from bone marrow and peripheral blood persisted for the 18 month follow-up period.

This preliminary clinical study establishes the feasibility of genetic modification of placental blood and engraftment in neonates for gene therapy. Clinical benefit of this intervention has not yet been demonstrated. However, SCID patients are likely to benefit even from the small fraction of genetically corrected hematopoietic stem cells for two reasons *(22)*. First, relatively low levels of ADA enzyme are associated with clinical improvement. Second, the progeny of the genetically corrected hematopoietic stem cells may have a survival advantage over the progeny of the endogenous ADA deficient stem cells. In this clinical trial, the infants simultaneously received enzyme replacement that would blunt any selective advantage afforded to transduced T lymphocyte precursors by detoxifying deoxyadenosine metabolites. When the dosage of PEG-ADA was decreased by 50%, the frequency of T lymphocytes containing the ADA gene was selectively increased 30–100 fold in each patient *(22)*. These patients may tolerate further dosage reduction. Wider application of gene therapy, such as correction of hemoglobinopathies and lysosomal storage diseases awaits improved protocols to allow for a greater fraction of transduced hematopoietic stem cells in the transplanted recipient.

5. Conclusions and Future Prospects

Human placental blood is a unique source of hematopoietic stem and progenitor cells for scientific analysis and clinical protocols. Hematopoietic progenitors in placental blood possess extensive proliferative potential and capacity for self renewal. T lymphocytes, B lymphocytes, and other accessory cell populations in placental blood are immature compared to their counterparts in adult bone marrow and peripheral blood. T lymphocytes in placental blood are deficient in a variety of functional assays with respect to proliferative and cytotoxic responses after allogeneic stimulation. The deficiency of B lymphocyte responses in placental blood is primarily due to defective T lymphocyte function. T lymphocytes produce a more narrow spectrum of cytokines and relatively low levels of cytokine receptors. NK activity is also depressed compared to that in adults, but can be activated with IL-2 and other stimuli. The immunologic status of placental blood as assessed in vitro likely underlies observations made in the initial clinical studies: placental blood is more tolerogenic and less alloreactive, permitting significant HLA disparity between donor and recipient and less frequently inducing severe GVHD than adult bone marrow. Future advances such as a more direct assay for the long-term marrow repopulating cell and further delineation of the lymphocyte subsets that mediate GVHD and graft vs leukemia effect will aid in characterization of early hematopoietic stem cell populations and alloreactive potential of placental blood.

In the clinical realm, placental blood is a suitable alternative to bone marrow for hematopoietic transplantation and gene therapy. Advantages of placental blood compared to bone marrow for hematopoietic transplantation include immediate availability, absence of risk to the donor during collection, absence of donor attrition, and lower risk of severe refractory GVHD. In addition, infants are less likely than adults to be infected with latent viruses such as EBV and CMV, important pathogens in immunosuppressed transplant recipients. The feasibility of placental blood transplantation in adults is supported by several studies, but clinical experience is still limited. In addition, the durability of engraftment, the rate of leukemic relapse in placental blood transplants compared to bone marrow transplants, the contribution of maternal lymphocytes to GVHD following placental blood transplantation, and the clinical utility of ex vivo expansion of placental blood require closer scrutiny and continued surveillance. Finally, improved transduction efficiency of early hematopoietic stem cells, physiologic regulation of gene expression, and reduced immunogenicity of viral vectors and expressed transgenes are necessary before gene therapy fulfills its clinical potential.

Note Added in Proof

Recently, Gluckman et al. reported the results of 143 placental blood transplants performed at 45 centers *(127)*. Seventy-eight patients received cord blood from related donors, and 65 patients received cord blood from unrelated donors. The Kaplan-Meier estimate of survival at one year was greater for recipients of cord blood from related donors (63%) compared to that from unrelated donors (29%). Among recipients of cord blood from related donors, younger age, lower weight, HLA-identity with the donor, and cytomegalovirus-negative serologic status was associated with a more favorable prognosis. Severe acute graft versus host disease (grades III, IV) occurred in 4 recipients in the related groups and 12 recipients in the unrelated group. Chronic graft versus host disease, evaluated in those who survived more than 100 days, occurred in 8 of 56 patients in the related group and 0 of 23 in the unrelated group.

References

1. Broxmeyer, H. E. (1995) Questions to be answered regarding umbilical cord blood hematopoietic stem and progenitor cells and their use in transplantation. *Transfusion* **35,** 694–702.
2. Flomenberg, N. and Keever, C. A. (1992) Cord blood transplants: potential utility and potential limitations. *Bone Marrow Transplant* **10,** 115–120.
3. Kurtzberg, J. (1996) Umbilical cord blood: a novel alternative source of hematopoietic stem cells for bone marrow transplantation. *J. Hematother.* **5,** 95,96.
4. Rubinstein, P., Rosenfield, R. E., Adamson, J. W., and Stevens, C. E. (1993) Stored placental blood for unrelated bone marrow reconstitution. *Blood* **81,** 1679–1690.
5. Beatty, P. G., Kollman, C., and Howe, C. W. S. (1995) Unrelated-donor marrow transplants: The experience of the National Marrow Donor Program, *in Clinical Transplants 1995* (Cecka and Terasaki, eds.), UCLA Tissue Typing Laboratory, Los Angeles, CA, pp. 271–277.
6. Beatty, P. D., Mori, M., and Milford, E. (1995) Impact of racial genetic polymorphism on the probability of finding an HLA-matched donor. *Transplantation* **60,** 778–783.
7. Lu, L., Shen, R. N., and Broxmeyer, H. E. (1996) Stem cells from bone marrow, umbilical cord blood and peripheral blood for clinical application: current status and future application. *Crit. Rev. Oncol.-Hematol.* **22,** 61–78.
8. Kurtzberg, J., Laughlin, M., Graham, M. L., et al. (1996) Placental blood as a source of hematopoietic stem cells for transplantation into unrelated recipients. *N. Engl. J. Med.* **335,** 157–166.
9. Wagner, J. E., Kernan, N. A., Steinbuch, M., Broxmeyer, H. E., and Gluckman, E. (1995) Allogeneic sibling umbilical-cord-blood transplantation in children with malignant and non-malignant disease. *Lancet* **346,** 214–219.
10. Wagner, J. E., Rosenthal, J., Sweetman, R., et al. (1996) Successful transplantation of HLA-matched and HLA-mismatched umbilical cord blood from unrelated donors: Analysis of engraftment and acute graft-versus-host disease. *Blood* **88,** 795–802.
11. Vilmer, E., Sterkers, G., Rahimy, C., et al. (1992) HLA-mismatched cord blood transplantation in a patient with advanced leukemia. *Transplantation* **53,** 1155–1157.
12. Gluckman, E., Broxmeyer, H. E., Auerbach, A. D., et al. (1989) Hematopoietic reconstitution in a patient with Fanconi's anemia by means of umbilical cord blood from an HLA-identical sibling. *N. Engl. J. Med.* **321,** 1174–1178.
13. Bogdanic, V., Nemet, D., Kastelan, A., et al. (1993) Umbilical cord blood transplantation in a patient with Philadelphia chromosome-positive chronic myeloid leukemia. *Transplantation* **56,** 477–479.
14. Broxmeyer, H. E. and Cooper, S. (1997) High efficiency recovery of immature haematopoietic progenitor cells with extensive proliferative capacity from human cord blood cryopreserved for 10 years. *Clin. Exp. Immunol.* **107,** 45–53.
15. Issaragrisil, S., Visuthisakchai, S., Suvatte, V., et al. (1995) Brief report: transplantation of cord-blood stem cells into a patient with severe thalassemia. *N. Engl. J. Med.* **332,** 367–369.
16. Kohli-Kumar, M., Shahidi, T., Broxmeyer, H. E., et al. (1993) Haemopoietic stem/progenitor cell transplant in Fanconi anaemia using HLA-matched sibling umbilical cord blood cells. *Br. J. Haematol.* **85,** 419–422.
17. Laporte, J.-P., Gorin, N.-C., Rubinstein, P., et al. (1996) Cord-blood transplantation from an unrelated donor in an adult with chronic myelogenous leukemia. *N. Engl. J. Med.* **335,** 167–170.
18. Miniero, R., Busca, A., Roncarolo, M. G., et al. (1995) HLA-haploidentical umbilical cord blood stem cell transplantation in a patient with advanced leukemia: clinical outcome and analysis of hematopoietic recovery. *Bone Marrow Transplant* **16,** 229–240.

19. Vowels, M. R., Lam-Po-Tang, R., Berdoukas, V., et al. (1993) Brief report: correction of X-linked lymphoproliferative disease by transplantation of cord-blood stem cells. *N. Engl. J. Med.* **329,** 1623–1625.
20. Wagner, J. E., Broxmeyer, H. E., Byrd, R. L., et al. (1992) Transplantation of umbilical cord blood after myeloablative therapy: Analysis of engraftment. *Blood* **79,** 1874–1881.
21. Kohn, D. B., Weinberg, K. I., Nolta, J. A., et al. (1995) Engraftment of gene-modified umbilical cord blood cells in neonates with adenosine deaminase deficiency. *Nature Med.* **1,** 1017–1023.
22. Kohn, D. B. (1997) Gene therapy for hematopoietic and lymphoid disorders. *Clin. Exp. Immunol.* **107,** 54–57.
23. Migliaccio, G., Baiocchi, M., Hamel, N., et al. (1996) Circulating progenitor cells in human ontogenesis: Response to growth factors and replating potential. *J. Hematother.* **5,** 161–170.
24. Sutherland, H. J., Eaves, C. J., Eaves, A. C., Dragouwska, W., and Lansdorp, P. (1989) Characterization and partial purification of human marrow cells capable of initiating long-term hematopoiesis *in vitro*. *Blood* **74,** 1563–1570.
25. Krause, D. S., Fackler, M. J., Civin, C. I., and May, W. S. (1996) CD34: structure, biology and clinical utility. *Blood* **87,** 1–13.
26. Vormoor, J., Lapidot, T., Pflumio, F., et al. (1994) Immature human cord blood progenitors engraft and proliferate to high levels in severe combined immunodeficient mice. *Blood* **83,** 2489–2497.
27. Zanjani, E. D., Silva, M. R. G., and Flake, A. W. (1994) Retention and multilineage expression of human hematopoietic stem cells in human-sheep chimera. *Blood Cells* **20,** 331–340.
28. Larochelle, A., Vormoor, J., Hanenberg, H., et al. (1996) Identification of primitive human hematopoietic capable of repopulating NOD/SCID mouse bone marrow: implications for gene therapy. *Nature Med.* **2,** 1329–1337
29. Mavroudis, D., Read, E., Cottler-Fox, M., et al. (1996) $CD34^+$ cell dose predicts survival, posttransplant morbidity and rate of hematologic recovery after allogeneic marrow transplants for hematologic malignancies. *Blood* **88,** 3223–3229.
30. Spitzer, G., Verma, D. S., Zander, A., et al. (1980) The myeloid progenitor cell-its value in predicting hematopoietic recovery after autologous bone marrow transplantation. *Blood* **55,** 317–323.
31. Broxmeyer, H. E., Douglas, G. W., Hangoc, G., et al. (1989) Human umbilical cord blood as a potential source of transplantable hematopoietic stem/progenitor cells. *Proc. Natl. Acad. Sci. USA* **86,** 3828–3832.
32. Broxmeyer, H. E., Hangoc, G., Cooper, S., et al. (1992) Growth characteristics and expansion of human umbilical cord blood and estimation of its potential for transplantation in adults. *Proc. Natl. Acad. Sci. USA* **89,** 4109–4113.
33. Cardoso, A. A., Li, M. L., Batard, P., et al. (1993) Release from quiescence of $CD34^+CD38^-$ human umbilical cord blood cells reveals their potentiality to engraft adults. *Proc. Natl. Acad. Sci. USA* **90,** 8707–8711.
34. Hows, J. M., Bradley, B. A., Marsh, J. C., et al. (1992) Growth of human umbilical-cord blood in long-term haematopoietic cultures. *Lancet* **340,** 73–76.
35. Pettengell, R., Luft, T., Henschler, R., et al. (1994) Direct comparison by limiting dilution analysis of long-term culture-initiating cells in human bone marrow, umbilical cord blood and blood stem cells. *Blood* **84,** 3653–3659.
36. Ma, D. D. F., Varga, D. E., and Biggs, J. C. (1987) Donor marrow progenitors (CFU-Mix, BFU-E and CFU-GM) and hematopoietic engraftment following HLA matched sibling bone marrow transplantation. *Leukaemia Res.* **11,** 141–147.
37. Douay, L., Gorin, N. C., Jean-Yves, M., et al. (1986) Recovery of CFU-GM from cryopreserved marrow and in vivo evaluation after autologous bone marrow transplantation are predictive of engraftment. *Exper. Hematol.* **14,** 358–365.
38. Kinniburgh, D. and Russell, N. H. (1993) Comparative study of CD34-positive cells and subpopulations of human umbilical cord blood and bone marrow. *Bone Marrow Transplant* **12,** 489–494.
39. Lu, L., Xiao, M., Shen, R. N., Grigsby, S., and Broxmeyer, H. E. (1993) Enrichment, characterization an responsiveness of single primitive CD34 human umbilical cord blood hematopoietic progenitors with high proliferative and replating potential. *Blood* **81,** 41–48.

40. Lansdorp, P. M., Sutherland, H. J., and Eaves, C. J. (1990) Selective expression of CD45 isoforms on functional subpopulations of $CD34^+$ hematopoietic cells from human bone marrow. *J. Exp. Med.* **172,** 363–366.
41. Mayani, H. and Lansdorp, P. M. (1994) Thy1 expression is linked to functional properties of primitive hematopoietic progenitor cells from human umbilical cord blood. *Blood* **83,** 2410–2417.
42. Lansdorp, P. M., Droagowska, W., and Mayani, H. (1993) Ontogeny-related changes in proliferative potential of human hematopoietic cells. *J. Exp. Med.* **178,** 787–791.
43. Traycoff, C. M., Abboud, M. R., Laver, J., et al. (1994) Evaluation of the in vitro behavior of phenotypically defined populations of umbilical cord blood hematopoietic progenitor cells. *Exp. Hematol.* **22,** 215–222.
44. Carow, C. E., Hangoc, G., and Broxmeyer, H. E. (1993) Human multipotential progenitor cells (CFU-GEMM) have extensive replating capacity for secondary CFU-GEMM: an effect enhanced by cord blood plasma. *Blood* **81,** 942–949.
45. Traycoff, C. M., Abboud, M. R., Laver, J., et al. (1994) Human umbilical cord blood hematopoietic progenitor cells: Are they the same as their adult bone marrow counterparts? *Blood Cells* **20,** 382–391.
46. Goldstein, S. (1990) Replicative senescence: the human fibroblast comes of age. *Science* **249,** 1129.
47. Vaziri, H., Dragowska, W., Allsopp, R. C., et al. (1994) Evidence for a mitotic clock in human hematopoietic stem cells: loss of telomeric DNA with age. *Proc. Natl. Acad. Sci. USA* **91,** 9857–9860.
48. Chao, N. J. and Schlegel, P. G. (1995) Prevention and treatment of graft-versus-host disease. *Bone Marrow Transplant NY Acad. Sci.* **770,** 130–141.
49. Antin, J. H. and Ferrara, J. L. M. (1992) Cytokine dysregulation and acute graft-versus-host disease. *Blood* **80,** 2964–2968.
50. Champlin, R. (1990) T cell depletion to prevent graft-versus-host disease after bone marrow transplantation. *Hematol. Oncol. Clin. North Amer.* **4,** 687–698.
51. Auerbach, A. D., Liu, Q., Ghosh, R., Pollack, M. S., Douglas, G. W., and Broxmeyer, H. E. (1990) Prenatal identification of potential donors for umbilical cord blood transplantation for Fanconi anemia. *Transfusion* **30,** 682–687.
52. Campbell, A. C., Waller, C., Wood, J., Aynsley-Green, A., and Yu, V. (1974) Lymphocyte subpopulations in the blood of newborn infants. *Clin. Exp. Immunol.* **18,** 469–482.
53. Kato I. (1935) Leukocytes in infancy and childhood. *J. Pediatr.* **7,** 7–15.
54. Beck, R. and Lam-Po-Tang, P. R. (1994) Comparison of cord blood and adult blood lymphocyte normal ranges: a possible explanation for decreased severity of graft versus host disease after cord blood transplantation. *Immunol. Cell. Biol.* **72,** 440–444.
55. Erkeller-Yuksel, F. M., Deneys, V., Yuksel, B., et al. (1992) Age-related changes in human blood lymphocyte subpopulations. *J. Pediatr.* **120,** 216–222.
56. Han, P., Hodge, G., Story, C., and Xu, X. (1995) Phenotypic analysis of functional T-lymphocyte subtypes and natural killer cells in human cord blood: relevance to umbilical cord blood transplantation. *J. Haematol.* **89,** 733–740.
57. Rabian-Herzog, C., Lesage, S., Gluckman, E., and Charron, D. (1993) Characterization of lymphocyte subpopulations in cord blood. *J. Hematother.* **2,** 255–257.
58. Motley, D., Meyer, M. P., King, R. A., and Naus, G. J. (1996) Determination of lymphocyte immunophenotypic values for normal full-term cord blood. *Am. J. Clin. Pathol.* **105,** 38–43.
59. Keever, C. A., Abu-Hajir, M., Graf, W., et al. (1995) Characterization of the alloreactivity and anti-leukemia reactivity of cord blood mononuclear cells. *Bone Marrow Transplant* **15,** 407–419.
60. Amlot, P. L., Tahami, F., Chinn, D., and Rawlings, E. (1996) Activation antigen expression on human T cells. I. Analysis by two-colour flow cytometry of umbilical cord blood, adult blood and lymphoid tissue. *Clin. Exper. Immunol.* **105,** 176–182.
61. Harris, D. T., Schumacher, M. J., LoCascio, J., et al. (1992) Phenotypic and functional immaturity of human umbilical cord blood T lymphocytes. *Proc. Natl. Acad. Sci. USA* **89,** 10,006–10,010.

62. Clement, L. T. (1992) Isoforms of the CD45 common leukocyte antigen family: markers for human T-cell differentiation. *J. Clin. Immunol.* **12,** 1–10.
63. Morimoto, C., Letvin, N. L., Distasco, J. A., Aldrich, W. R., and Schlossman, S. F. (1985) The isolation and characterisation of the human suppressor inducer T cell subset. *J. Immunol.* **134,** 1508–1513.
64. Morimoto, C., Rudd, C. E., Letvin, N. L., and Schlossman, S. F. (1987) A novel epitope of the LFA-1 antigen which can distinguish killer effector and suppressor cells in human CD8 cells. *Nature* **330,** 479–482.
65. Griffiths-Chu, S., Patterson, J. A. K., Berger, C. L., et al. (1984) Characterization of immature T cell subpopulations in neonatal blood. *Blood* **64,** 296–300.
66. Kotylo, P. K., Baenzinger, J. C., Yoder, M. C., et al. (1990) Rapid analysis of lymphocyte subsets in cord blood. *Am. J. Clin. Pathol.* **93,** 263–266.
67. Milosevits, J., Pocsik, E., Schmidt, B., et al. (1995) Immunophenotypic and functional characteristics of haemopoietic cells from human cord blood. *Scand. J. Immunol.* **42,** 493–500.
68. Lee, B.-W., Yap, H.-K., Chew, F.-T., et al. (1996) Age- and sex-related changes in lymphocyte subpopulations of healthy Asian subjects: from birth to adulthood. *Cytometry* **26,** 8–15.
69. Lim, F. T., van Winsen, L., Willemze, R., et al. (1994) Influence of delivery on numbers of leukocytes, leukocyte subpopulations, and hematopoietic progenitor cells in human umbilical cord blood. *Blood Cells* **20,** 547,558.
70. Harris, D. T., LoCascio, J., and Besencon, F. J. (1994) Analysis of the alloreactive capacity of human umbilical cord blood: implications for graft-versus-host disease. *Bone Marrow Transplant* **14,** 545–553.
71. Risdon, G., Gaddy, J., and Broxmeyer, H. E. (1994) Allogeneic responses of human umbilical cord blood. *Blood Cells* **20,** 566–572.
72. Risdon, G., Gaddy, J., Horie, M., and Broxmeyer, H. E. (1995) Alloantigen priming induces a state of unresponsiveness in human cord blood T cells. *Proc. Natl. Acad. Sci. USA* **92,** 2413–2417.
73. Risdon, G., Gaddy, J., Stehman, F. B., and Broxmeyer, H. E. (1994) Proliferative and cytotoxic responses of human cord blood T lymphocytes following allogeneic stimulation. *Cell. Immunol.* **154,** 14–24.
74. Roncarolo, M. G., Bigler, M., Martino, S., et al. (1996) Immune functions of cord blood cells before and after transplantation. *J. Hematother.* **5,** 157–160.
75. Deacock, S. J., Schwarer, A. P., Bridge, J., et al. (1992) Evidence that umbilical cord blood contains a higher frequency of HLA class II-specific alloreactive T cells than adult peripheral blood. A limiting dilution analysis. *Transplantation* **53,** 1128–1134.
76. Linch, D. C. and Brent, L. (1989) Can cord blood be used? *Nature* **340,** 676.
77. Ehlers, S. and Smith, K. A. (1991) Differentiation of T cell lymphokine gene expression: the in vitro acquisition of T cell memory. *J. Exp. Med.* **173,** 25–36.
78. Lewis, D. B., Yu, C. C., Meyer, J., et al. (1991) Cellular and molecular mechanisms for reduced interleukin 4 and interferon-γ production by neonatal T cells. *J. Clin. Invest.* **87,** 194–202.
79. Zola, H., Fusco, M., Macardle, P. J., et al. (1995) Expression of cytokine receptors by human cord blood lymphocytes: comparison with adult blood lymphocytes. *Pediatr. Res.* **38,** 397–403.
80. Saito, S., Morii, T., and Umekage, H. (1996) Expression of the interleukin-2 receptor gamma chain on cord blood mononuclear cells. *Blood* **87,** 3344–3350.
81. Cicuttini, F. M., Martin, M., Petrie, H. T., and Boyd, A. W. (1993) A novel population of natural killer progenitor cells isolated from human umbilical cord blood. *J. Immunol.* **151,** 29–37.
82. Gaddy, J., Risdon, G., and Broxmeyer, H. E. (1995) Cord blood natural killer cells are functionally and phenotypically immature but readily respond to interleukin-2 and interleukin-12. *Interferon Cytokine Res.* **15,** 527–536.
83. Webb, B. J., Bochan, M. R., Montel, A., et al. (1994) The lack of NK cytotoxicity associated with fresh HUCB may be due to the presence of soluble HLA in the serum. *Cell. Immunol.* **159,** 246–261.
84. Hauch, M., Gazzola, M. V., Small, T., et al. (1990) Anti-leukemia potential of interleukin-2 activated natural killer cells after bone marrow transplantation for chronic myelogenous leukemia. *Blood* **75,** 2250–2262.

85. Harris, D. T. (1995) *In vitro* and *in vivo* assessment of the graft-versus-leukemia activity of cord blood. *Bone Marrow Transplant* **15,** 17–23.
86. Brugnoni, D., Airo, P., Graf, D., et al. (1994) Ineffective expression of CD40 ligand on cord blood T cells may contribute to poor immunoglobulin production in the newborn. *Eur. J. Immunol.* **24,** 1919–1924.
87. Fuleihan, R., Ahern, D., and Geha, R. S. (1994) Decreased expression of the ligand for CD40 in newborn lymphocytes. *Eur. J. Immunol.* **24,** 1925–1928.
88. Servet-Delprat, C., Bridon, J.-M., Djossou, O., et al. (1996) Delayed IgG2 humoral response in infants is not due to intrinsic T or B cell defects. *Int. Immunol.* **8,** 1495–1502.
89. Splawski, J., Nishioka, J., Nishioka, Y., and Lipsky, P. E. (1996) CD40 ligand is expressed and functional on activated neonatal T cells. *J. Immunol.* **156,** 119–127.
90. Barbouche, R., Forveille, M., Fischer, A., et al. (1992) Spontaneous IgM autoantibody production *in vitro* by B lymphocytes of normal human neonates. *Scand. J. Immunol.* **35,** 659–667.
91. Hunt, D. W., Huppertz, H. I., Jiang, H. J., and Petty, R. E. (1994) Studies of human cord blood dendritic cells: evidence for functional immaturity. *Blood* **84,** 4333–4343.
92. Marodi, L., Kaposzta, R., Campbell, D. E., et al. (1994) Candidacidal mechanisms in the human neonate. Impaired IFN-γ activation of macrophages in newborn infants. *J. Immunol.* **153,** 5643–5649.
93. Taylor, S. and Bryson, Y. J. (1985) Impaired production of γ-interferon by newborn cells in vitro is due to a functionally immature macrophage. *J. Immunol.* **134,** 1493–1497.
94. Gluckman, E., Wagner, J., Hows, J., Kernan, N., Bradley, B., and Broxmeyer, H. E. (1993) Cord blood banking for haematopoietic stem cell transplantation: an international cord blood transplant registry. *Bone Marrow Transplant* **11,** 199,200.
95. Bertolini, F., Battaglia, M., De Iulio, C., and Sirchia, G. (1995) Placental blood collection: effects on newborns. *Blood* **85,** 3361,3362.
96. Kinmond, S., Aitchison, T. C., Holland, B. M., et al. (1993) Umbilical cord clamping and preterm infants: a randomised trial. *Br. Med. J.* **306,** 172–175.
97. Ballin, A., Arbel, E., Kenet, G., et al. (1995) Autologous umbilical cord blood transfusion. *Archives Disease Childhood* **73,** F181–183.
98. Brandt, S. J., Peters, W. P., Atwater, S. K., et al. (1988) Effect of recombinant human granulocyte-macrophage colony-stimulating factor on hematopoietic reconstitution after high-dose chemotherapy and autologous bone marrow transplantation. *N. Engl. J. Med.* **318,** 869–876.
99. Neumunaitis, J., Singer, J. W., Buckner, C. K., et al. (1988) Use of recombinant human granulocyte-macrophage colony-stimulating factor in autologous marrow transplantation for lymphoid malignancies. *Blood* **72,** 834–836.
100. Levin, J. (1997) Thrombopoietin; clinically realized? *N. Engl. J. Med.* **336,** 434–436.
101. Balduzzi, A., Gooley, T., Anasetti, C., et al. (1995) Unrelated donor bone marrow transplantation in children. *Blood* **86,** 3247–3256.
102. Kernan, N. A., Bartsch, G., Ash, R. C., et al. (1993) Analysis of 462 transplantations from unrelated donors facilitated by the National Marrow Donor Program. *N. Engl. J. Med.* **328,** 593–602.
103. Harris, D. T., Schumacher, M. J., LoCascio, J., et al. (1994) Immunoreactivity of umbilical cord blood and post-partum maternal peripheral blood with regard to HLA-haploidentical transplantation. *Bone Marrow Transplant* **14,** 63–68.
104. Abecasis, M. M., Machado, A. M., Boavida, G., et al. (1996) Case report: Haploidentical cord blood transplant contaminated with maternal T cells in a patient with advanced leukaemias. *Bone Marrow Transplant* **17,** 891–895.
105. Claas, F. H. J., Gijbels, Y., van der Velden-de Munch, J., and van Rood, J. J. (1988) Induction of B cell unresponsiveness to noninherited maternal HLA antigens during fetal life. *Science* **241,** 1815–1817.
106. van Rood, J. J. and Claas, F. H. J. (1990) The influence of allogeneic cells on the human T and B cell repertoire. *Science* **248,** 1388–1393.

107. Scaradavou, A., Carrier, C., Mollen, N., et al. (1996) Detection of maternal DNA in placental/umbilical cord blood by locus specific amplification of the noninherited maternal HLA gene. *Blood* **4,** 1494–1500.
108. Broxmeyer, H. E., Kurtzberg, J., Gluckman, E., et al. (1991) Umbilical cord blood hematopoietic stem and repopulating cells in human clinical transplantation. *Blood Cells* **17,** 313–329.
109. Socie, G., Gluckman, E., Carosella, E., et al. (1994) Search for maternal cells in human umbilical cord blood by polymerase chain reaction amplification of two minisatellite sequences. *Blood* **83,** 340–344.
110. Hall, J., Lingenfelter, P., Adams, S., et al. (1995) Detection of maternal T-cells in human umbilical cord blood using fluorescence in situ hybridization. *Blood* **86,** 2829–2832.
111. Kernan, N. A., Collin, N. H., Juliano, L., et al. (1986) Clonable T lymphocytes in T cell-depleted bone marrow transplants correlate with development of graft-v-host disease. *Blood* **68,** 770–773.
112. McCullough, J., Clay, M. E., Fautsch, S., et al. (1994) Proposed policies and procedures for the establishment of a cord blood bank. *Blood Cells* **20,** 609–626.
113. Sugarman, J., Reisner, E. G., and Kurtzberg, J., (1995) Ethical aspects of banking placental blood for transplantation. *JAMA* **274,** 1783–1785.
114. Anderson, W. F. (1992) Human gene therapy. *Science* **256,** 808–813.
115. Miller, A. D. (1992) Human gene therapy comes of age. *Nature* **357,** 455–460.
116. Bodine, D. M., Moritz, T., Donahue, R. E., et al. (1993) Long term in vivo expression of a murine adenosine deaminase gene in rhesus multilineage haematopoietic cells following retroviral mediated gene transfer into $CD34^+$ bone marrow cells. *Blood* **82,** 1975–1980.
117. van Beusechem, V. W., Kukler, A., Heidt, P. J., and Valerio, D. (1992) Long-term expression of human adenosine deaminase in rhesus monkeys transplanted with retrovirus-infected bone marrow cells. *Proc. Natl. Acad. Sci. USA* **89,** 7640–7644.
118. Williams, D. A. and Moritz, T. (1994) Umbilical cord blood stem cells as targets for genetic modification: New therapeutic approaches to somatic gene therapy. *Blood Cells* **20,** 504–516.
119. Hanley, M. E., Nollta, J. A., Parkman, R., and Kohn, D. (1994) Umbilical cord blood cell transduction by retroviral vectors: Preclinical studies to optimize gene transfer. *Blood Cells* **20,** 539–546.
120. Shi, Y.-J., Shen, R.-N., Lu, L., and Broxmeyer, H. E. (1994) Comparative analysis of retroviral-mediated gene transduction into $CD34^+$ cord blood hematopoietic progenitors in the presence and absence of growth factors. *Blood Cells* **20,** 517–524.
121. Moritz, T., Keller, D. C., and Williams, D. A. (1993) Human cord blood cells as targets for gene transfer: potential use in genetic therapies of severe combined immunodeficiency disease. *J. Exp. Med.* **178,** 529–536.
122. Lu, L., Xiao, M., Clapp, D. W., et al. (1993) High efficiency retroviral mediated gene transduction into single isolated immature and replatable CD34+ hematopoietic stem/progenitor cells from human umbilical cord blood. *J. Exp. Med.* **178,** 2089–2096.
123. Xiao, M., Li, Z.-H., McMahel, J., et al. (1996) Inhibitory effects of interleukin 12 on retroviral gene transduction into $CD34^{+++}$ cord blood myeloid progenitors mediated by induction of tumor necrosis factor-α. *J. Hematother.* **5,** 171–177.
124. Moritz, T., Dutt, P., Xiao, X., et al. (1996) Fibronectin improves transduction of reconstituting hematopoietic stem cells by retroviral vectors: evidence of direct viral binding to chymotryptic carboxy-terminal fragments. *Blood* **88,** 855–862.
125. Zhou, S. Z., Cooper, S., Kang, L. Y., et al. (1994) Adeno-associated virus 2-mediated high efficiency gene transfer into immature and mature subsets of hematopoietic progenitor cells in human umbilical cord blood. *J. Exp. Med.* **179,** 1867–1875.
126. Walsh, C. E., Nienhuis, A. W., Samulski, R. J., et al. (1994) Phenotypic correction of Fanconi anemia in human hematopoietic cells with a recombinant Adeno-associated virus vector. *J. Clin. Invest.* **94,** 1440–1448.
127. Gluckman, E., Rocha, V., Boyer-Chammard, A., Locatelli, F., Arcese, W., Pasquini, Ortega, J., Souillet, G., Ferreira, E., Laporte, J-P., Fernandez, M., and Chastang, C., for the Eurocord Transplant Groups and the European Blood and Marrow Transplantation Group (1997) Outcome of cord-blood transplantation from related and unrelated donors. *N. Eng. J. Med.* **337,** 373–381.

Chapter 27

Human Hematopoietic Stem Cells, Progenitors, and Peripheral Blood Lymphocytes as Targets for the Correction of Immune System Disorders via Gene Therapy

Karen E. Pollok and David A. Williams

1. Introduction

As genetic defects responsible for congenital disorders are delineated at the DNA level, it is possible to design strategies to express the corrected gene in autologous-derived cells *(1–3)*. A large number of gene therapy clinical trials encompassing a broad spectrum of human diseases are in progress *(4,5)*. Therapies to prevent and treat human immunodeficiency virus (HIV) *(6)*, adenosine deaminase deficiency associated with severe combined immunodeficiency disease (ADA^- SCID) *(7–11)*; lysosomal storage diseases *(12,13)*, autoimmune diseases *(3,14)*, as well as a variety of cancers *(15)*, are ongoing. In this chapter, the authors will review the current status on gene transfer technology and discuss current findings on treatment of ADA^- SCID by gene therapy. In addition, five primary immunodeficiency diseases that affect the B- and T-cell lineages at various stages of differentiation will be highlighted, and the potential treatment of these diseases by gene therapy will be discussed.

The ethical dilemma of introducing new genetic information into humans has received much attention in the medical field as well as in the media. Is it worthwhile to pursue this avenue, and if it is, how can clinical trials be designed to ascertain the efficacy of gene therapy? Furthermore, to what extent should concurrent treatment deemed efficacious be reduced or stopped? There is a growing consensus that gene therapy may provide, in the future, a worthwhile alternative to current therapies in terms of both efficiency and cost-effectiveness. For example, ADA^- SCID patients ineligible for bone marrow trans-

From: *Molecular Biology of B-Cell and T-Cell Development*
Edited by: J. G. Monroe and E. V. Rothenberg © Humana Press Inc., Totowa, NJ

plantation may receive regular injections of bovine adenosine deaminase conjugated to polyethylene glycol (PEG-ADA) as an enzyme replacement therapy. Such therapy is estimated to cost over a $100,000 per year *(16)*, whereas bone marrow transplantation costs range $200,000–$1,000,000 *(13)*.

2. Vectors Used For Gene Transfer

A variety of gene transfer vehicles and liposomal reagents are currently being evaluated in preclinical studies *(17,18)*. At present, the best candidates for gene transfer in the clinical setting are replication-defective retroviral-, adenoviral- or adeno-associated viral-vectors. The advantages and disadvantages of each are discussed in the following sections.

2.1. Adenovirus

Adenoviruses can carry large fragments of DNA and will infect nondividing cells such as $CD34^+$ bone marrow progenitor cells *(19,20)*. Replication-defective adenoviral vectors were generated by deletions in the E1 and E2 genes *(21)*. Although high level expression can be obtained in target cells *(21)*, adenoviral vectors do not integrate, and long-term expression is not likely. Presently, it cannot be guaranteed that high-titer recombinant adenoviral stocks are free of wild-type helper virus; this could be problematic, since wild-type adenovirus infection could lead to a productive infection with or without the recombinant vector. In addition, much work has been done to decrease the immunogenicity of these vectors, yet this remains a major obstacle for their use in the clinic *(22)*.

2.2. Adeno-Associated Virus

Adeno-Associated Virus (AAV) is a potential candidate as a vehicle for gene delivery since it integrates into the host chromosomal DNA in a site-specific fashion *(23)*, and is able to infect a variety of cell types *(24)*. Studies have indicated that AAV will infect noncycling cells quite efficiently *(24,25)*; one study reported, however, that proliferating human fibroblasts, were preferentially infected with AAV vector compared to nondividing fibroblasts *(26)*. Additionally, AAV-based vectors are attractive from a safety standpoint, since wild-type AAV is not associated with any known human disease. The ability to use a vector that would integrate in a site-specific fashion in the genome is attractive, since this would decrease the likelihood of insertional mutagenesis or activation of a putative oncogene. Although wild-type AAV undergoes site-specific integration on chromosome 19q *(23)*, recent studies indicate that recombinant AAV vectors may not integrate in the same site because of the absence of the *rep* protein, which is responsible for DNA replication. However, the presence of *rep* could confer enhanced immunogenicity to the vector, although this has not been formally proven. AAV packaging protocols require transfection of the vector plasmid with plasmid providing the rep and cap proteins (virion proteins) into helper-virus infected cells. After 48–72 hours, recombinant vectors are harvested by cell lysis, and subsequently heated to inactivate helper virus. Further purification is performed on cesium chloride gradients *(24)*. Unfortunately, long-term reconstitution studies to date have demonstrated that integration and expression of AAV-introduced genes are low *(27)*.

2.3. Retroviruses

Retroviral-mediated gene transfer (RMGT) is a well-studied choice of vector technology, since integration into the host DNA occurs and long-term expression in vivo is possible *(28)*. For long-term correction of immunodeficiency disease, the introduced gene must integrate into the target cell in such a way that all progeny derived from this cell will contain a copy of the sequence. Moloney murine leukemia virus (MoMuLV)-based vectors are probably not immunogenic, but these vectors require that the target cells undergo an additional cell division for proviral integration to occur *(29)*. This has proven problematic since hematopoietic stem cells cycle infrequently. On the other hand, prestimulation of hematopoietic cells to increase their cycling could alter the capacity of the cells to engraft and function appropriately in the recipient *(30,31)*. Another concern with the MoMuLV-based retroviruses is that such viruses and vectors derived from these viruses integrate relatively randomly throughout the genome. Concerns about the probability of insertional mutagenesis or activation of transforming genes have not to date been realized using replication-defective viruses. However, one study involving primates documented serendipitously the consequence of infecting target hematopoietic cells with replication-competent retrovirus. In this study, there was an increase in the number of viral integrations in the peripheral blood, indicative of viral spread, and 3/8 of the animals developed a thymic lymphoma *(32)*. By screening for the presence of helper-free virus prior to transduction, the likelihood of disrupting the genome should be greatly diminished.

Since retroviruses are being used in a wide variety of gene-therapy clinical trials, the next section will discuss the state of the art in terms of designing and generating retroviruses and retrovirus packaging lines. In addition, methodologies for optimizing the efficiency of gene transfer into hematopoietic stem cells, progenitors, and peripheral blood lymphocytes will be discussed.

2.3.1. Gene Transfer Utilizing Replication-Defective Retroviruses

2.3.1.1. Design of Retroviral Packaging Lines. A prerequisite for safe gene therapy is the use of retroviral vectors that are replication-defective *(33)*. These viruses infect the target cell and if integrated, the provirus will be replicated along with the host DNA. Most significantly, the integrated provirus will be incapable of producing infectious virions since it lacks sequences encoding essential viral packaging proteins (Fig. 1). Retroviruses utilized at present in preclinical and clinical studies are based on the MoMuLV backbone. The genome of this retrovirus contains *gag*, *pol*, and *env* genes. The *gag*-encoded proteins are responsible for encapsidation and assembly of the viral particle. The *pol*-encoded proteins reverse transcribe viral RNA into proviral DNA, which can then integrate into the host genome. The *env*-encoded proteins are present in the viral envelope and mediate attachment to receptors on the target cells. To generate replication-defective retroviruses, these gene products are provided *in trans* by packaging lines usually derived from fibroblasts. However, the defective retroviruses must carry the viral-encoded *pol* protein, sequences (ψ) required *in cis* for packaging of the RNA genome, and sequences responsible for directing the integration of the provirus into the DNA of the host. These sequences are located in the long terminal repeats (LTR) of the provirus and in the areas just flanking the LTR. Deletion of the *gag*, *pol*, and *env* sequences allows insertion of up to 8 kb of foreign DNA.

Once the retroviral vector plasmid is transfected into the packaging line, its RNA is packaged, and once virions are assembled, they bud off from the plasma membrane into the medium. Clones selected from the transfected pool are subsequently screened for the titer of virus particles and the fidelity of the packaged virus. Packaging lines have been constructed that confer an ecotropic, xenotropic, or amphotropic host range. Retroviruses produced in ecotropic lines have a narrow host range and are only able to infect mouse

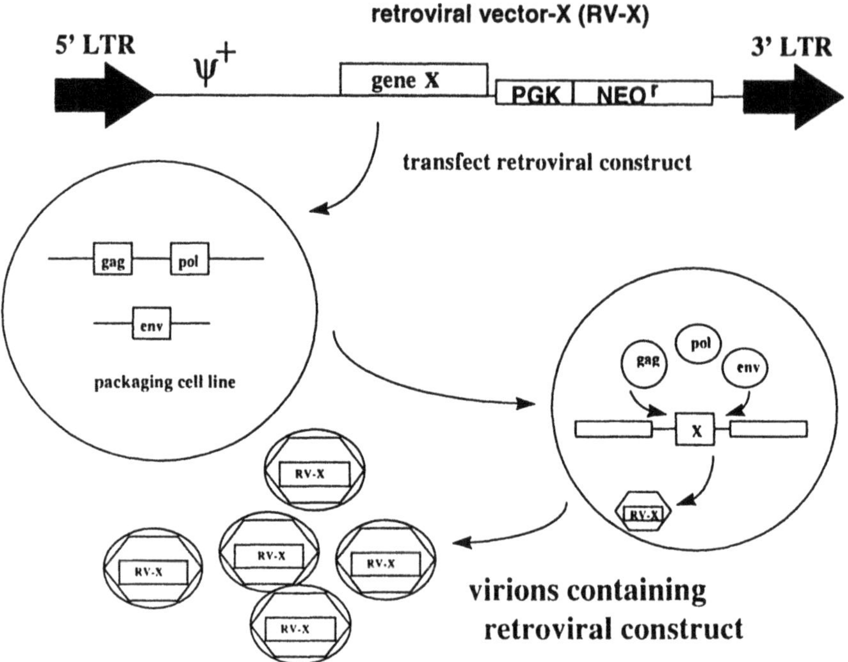

Fig. 1. Generation of a prototypical retroviral-packaging line producing replication-defective retroviruses. In this example, gene X expression is under the control of the viral 5' LTR, whereas expression of the selectable marker gene, neomycin phosphotransferase (Neo^r), is under the control of the human phosphoglycerate kinase promoter (PGK). The retroviral construct is transfected into the packaging cell line and stable transfectants are selected for by incubation with the neomycin analogue, G418. The *gag*, *pol*, and *env* proteins are constitutively expressed in the packaging cells (*see* text). The placement of the *gag* and *pol* genes on one plasmid and the *env* gene on a separate plasmid decreases the probability of recombination events which could generate helper-free virus. Supernatants from producer clones are then analyzed for production of high-titer replication-defective virus (RV-X).

and rat cells, whereas those packaged in amphotropic lines are capable of infecting a variety of mammalian cells, including human cells. One of the initial problems with the first generation of producer lines was the ability of the retroviral vector to undergo homologous recombination with the *gag*, *pol*, and *env* genes resulting in the generation of replication-competent virus. The risk of this potentially serious problem has been reduced by further deletions in the regions of homology between the vector and the helper genome *(33,34)* and by separation of DNA sequences within the genome encoding *gag* and *pol* and the *env* gene products *(34)*. Thus, newer generation producer lines now require at least three recombination events for the generation of replication-competent virus.

2.3.2. Influence of Promoter Elements on Retroviral-Encoded Gene Expression

Extensive efforts have been focused on developing a retroviral vector, which meets the needs of a variety of circumstances. However, retroviral technology is still an inexact science. Many different vector designs have been tested to determine optimal *cis*-regulatory elements needed for high level and stable expression. In most vectors, the gene of interest is either expressed alone (so-called "simplified vectors") or in association with a dominant selectable marker (Fig. 1). Gene expression is controlled by the retroviral promoter located in the LTR or by an internal promoter. This internal transcription unit has been used successfully in the same or opposite orientation of transcription as the viral LTR *(1)*. Replication-defective retroviruses generated to date contain one to two genes under the control of the viral promoter in the 5' LTR or by alternative promoters cloned into the vector *(1)*. A few examples of vectors encoding three gene products or fusion genes have been published *(35–40)*. More recently, vectors have been developed that contain an internal ribosome entry sequence (IRES), which allows for two independent translational units *(41–44)*. IRES elements are 500–600 bp sequences that are characteristic of 5' untranslated regions of picornaviruses and form tertiary structures that facilitate cap-independent translation of virus proteins. These elements may prevent RNA processing steps which affect the expression of multiple genes.

In studies designed to examine expression of the human adenosine deaminase gene, vectors were constructed that contained the ADA gene under the transcriptional control of the promoter/enhancers of MoMuLV, the simian virus 40 early region, the cytomegalovirus immediate-early gene, the lymphotropic papovavirus, and the human beta-globin gene *(45)*. In the hematopoietic cell lines, DHL-9 and K562, vectors containing ADA regulated by MoMuLV or the cytomegalovirus promoters expressed ADA at the highest level. A comparative analysis of promoters derived from hematopoietic-specific genes, CD11b, CD18, and CD34, vs viral promoters, such as MoMuLV, CMV immediate early gene or the SV40 early region, indicated that expression of a reporter gene in undifferentiated and differentiated hematopoietic cell lines varied, depending on the promoter used *(46)*. For example, in undifferentiated HL60 cells, the MoMuLV promoter yielded the highest expression of the reporter gene, whereas in HL60 cells induced to differentiate into the monocyte/macrophage lineage, the CD11b promoter resulted in highest expression levels. This study suggested that it may be feasible to regulate expression of retrovirally introduced sequences by using promoters of a specific cell lineage. This has been intensively studied with respect to the expression of globin genes via retroviral constructs *(47–50)*. However, it is also clear that transcriptional activities of retroviral vectors in cell lines do not predict the usefulness of the same regulatory elements in primary hematopoietic cells, especially in vivo *(50–55)*.

Vectors derived from the lentiviridae (HIV 1,2) *(56)* and spumaviridae (foamy virus) *(56,57)* are two alternatives for gene transfer currently under study. A replication-defective HIV-based vector has been constructed that was capable of infecting growth arrested-HeLa cells or -rat 208F fibroblasts *(56)*. In this vector, key virion determinants known to interact with the nuclear import machinery and drive the active transport of the HIV preintegration complex through the nucleopore were included. This approach, if successful, could be very useful for gene transfer into rarely dividing cells such as hematopoietic stem cells. The foamy viral-based vectors can potentially infect a broader host range than the lentiviral vectors, but integration is dependent on cell cycling *(57)*.

The maintenance of long-term ADA expression in hematopoietic cells in vivo has been studied extensively *(1,36,51,59–68)*. A prerequisite for clinical applicability is to evaluate vector expression in vivo following bone marrow transplantation and long-term reconstitution. Studies utilizing retroviral vectors expressing human ADA and a selectable marker have indicated that expression of ADA in hematopoietic cells is possible *(55,69–71)*; other studies documented that vectors containing dominant selectable markers may be problematic *(1)*. In vectors expressing a dominant selectable marker, expression of the second gene of interest was either markedly reduced or completely silenced in vivo in primary hematopoietic cells *(51–55)*. These same vectors, however, expressed both genes efficiently in hematopoietic cell lines in vitro *(51,52)*. In vectors in which ADA is expressed off the MoMuLV-based LTR, serial bone marrow transplantation of transduced stem cells into lethally irradiated mice demonstrated a correlation between increased methylation of the retroviral LTR and decreased gene expression in vivo *(72)*. In hematopoietic cells, the highest expression levels of the ADA cDNA in vivo have generally been from vectors that contain the ADA cDNA but no selectable marker gene *(55,64,67,73)*. Successful gene transfer into stem cells has been accomplished in rhesus monkeys *(60,62,74)* and dogs *(61)*, where vector sequences were detected more than one year after transplant. Gene transfer efficiencies were low, however, with only 0.1–3.0% gene-marked cells detected in the peripheral blood and bone marrow. In some primate experiments, ADA cDNA sequences have been detected up to four years after transplant (D. Bodine and D. A. Williams, unpublished results).

In addition to downregulation of sequences at the transcriptional level, the expression of bacterial-derived, dominant selectable marker genes such as neomycin phosphotransferase may also confer immunogenicity to the target cell. Studies in humans by Riddell and colleagues *(75)* reported that HIV-specific T-cell clones transduced with a retrovirus encoding for a hygromycin phosphotransferase (Hy) and the herpes simplex thymidine kinase fusion protein persisted in vivo after the first two infusions but were cleared during the third and fourth infusions. In vitro analysis of peripheral blood from these patients indicated that in five out of six patients, $CD8^+$ cytotoxic T-cells recognizing Hy-TK were detected and presumably responsible for the clearance of the infused lymphocytes. The inclusion of a selectable marker gene in a retroviral vector allows for easy selection and titering in vitro. Likewise, selection in vivo, whether positive or negative, could be beneficial in some clinical settings. However, it is clear from the above studies, that problems associated with gene expression and potential immunogenicity of selectable markers in vivo raise valid concerns about the inclusion of such sequences in vectors destined for in vivo studies.

2.4. Factors Influencing the Efficiency of RMGT

2.4.1. Titer of Producer Lines

Several studies have reported the half life of MoMuLV-derived retroviruses in culture medium at 37°C to be three to eight hours *(76–78)*. This short half-life may be a limiting factor in gene-transfer efficiency. Stability of retroviral particles is increased when supernatant is harvested at 32°C in contrast to 37°C *(79)*. Polycations, such as polybrene, are used in many infection protocols and are thought to assist in the binding of viruses to the cell surface by neutralizing electrostatic repulsion *(80)*. One recent study indicated that gene transfer efficiency was dependent on the relative amounts of calf serum in the retroviral supernatant *(81)*. Increasing amounts of serum required increasingly higher amounts of polybrene to achieve maximal gene transfer efficiency. Unique characteristics of each producer clone may also contribute to efficiency of gene transfer *(82)*. For example, the level of transduction of primary human $CD34^+$ progenitors has been shown to vary with the level of TGF-β made by the retroviral producer line *(83)*; TGF-β is known to be a negative regulator of hematopoiesis and may inhibit cells from entering the cell cycle, thereby lowering infection efficiency *(84)*.

2.4.2. Retroviral Receptors

In some cases, titer may not necessarily correlate with the efficiency of gene transfer. A factor influencing gene transfer efficiency in these cases may relate to the absolute number of receptors on the target cell. Eight classes of retroviral receptors used for viral entry have been identified thus far *(85,86)*. Murine ecotropic retroviruses bind to the *Rec1* receptor, a basic amino acid transporter, whereas murine amphotropic retroviruses bind to *Ram1*, a phosphate transporter. Delineation of growth factors and medium conditions, which simultaneously maintain the functional integrity of the target cells and increase receptor expression, may increase gene transfer efficiency. Other improvements in producer lines and in retroviral constructs may also result in significantly increasing gene transfer efficiency. The development of alternative packaging lines such as PG13 cells derived from the gibbon ape leukemia virus (GALV) envelope has led to increased gene transfer rates in human and primate PBLs *(87,88)*. An optimized protocol used PG13-derived retroviral supernatant, metabolic induction of GALV receptor by phosphate depletion, low-temperature incubation and centrifugation to increase gene transfer efficiency. At 72 hours posttransduction, >50% lymphocyte transduction using PG13-packaged vectors and >25% transduction efficiency with amphotropic-packaged retroviral vectors was observed. In other studies, a retroviral vector pseudotyped with vesicular stomatitis G glycoprotein (VSV-G) envelope was used to enhance gene transfer *(37)*. Theoretical advantages of this vector include the fact that receptors for VSV-G may be widely expressed in mammalian cells and that pseudotyped retroviruses could be concentrated to high titers. A gene transfer efficiency of 16–32% was observed at 48–72 hours posttransduction in activated human peripheral blood lymphocytes (PBLs).

Other targeting strategies have included modification of the retroviral glycoprotein envelope as a means of delivering genes in a highly specific manner *(89,90)*. Valsesia-Wittman et al. *(91)* generated chimeric MoMuLV-derived envelopes targeted to the *Ram-1* phosphate transporter. While all recombinant virions bound to *Ram-1*, optimal interdomain spacing between the *Ram-1*-binding domain and the MoMuLV surface proteins correlated with the highest gene transfer. Schwarzenberger et al. *(92)* reported a novel gene transfer system containing the growth factor, stem cell factor (SCF), which is a ligand for the receptor tyrosine kinase, c-kit. Specific targeting of c-kit$^+$ hematopoietic cell lines was demonstrated. This receptor-mediated gene-transfer protocol could be potentially useful for the specific targeting of a wide array of cell types.

It is likely that a wide array of gene-transfer vehicles will ultimately be available for therapeutic use *(18)*. As gene-transfer technology continues to develop, ongoing efforts to understand the basic principles of hematopoiesis will be instrumental in selecting the optimal gene-transfer vehicle to be used for a particular target cell.

2.4.3. Modes of Retroviral Transduction

The most common method of transducing target cells is incubation with retroviral supernatant in the presence of a polycation, such as polybrene (Fig. 2). Cocultivation of target cells with irradiated or mitomycin C-treated producer cells *(93–98)* or a stromal cell layer *(98–100)*, leads to increased gene transfer compared to transduction with supernatant and polybrene only. Mortiz et al. *(98)* compared gene transfer efficiencies of cord blood progenitors utilizing retroviral supernatant and polybrene versus cocultivation with the producer line, retroviral supernatant with stromal lines expressing human membrane-bound SCF, or retroviral supernatant and bone marrow stroma. Gene transfer efficiency was the greatest using cocultivation.

In terms of enhancing retroviral-mediated gene transfer, the authors have developed gene transfer strategies for transduction of murine and human bone marrow cells, as well as human peripheral blood T-cells that result in high levels of gene transfer (*30,96–98,101,* Pollok et al. submitted). These transduction strategies arose from the authors'

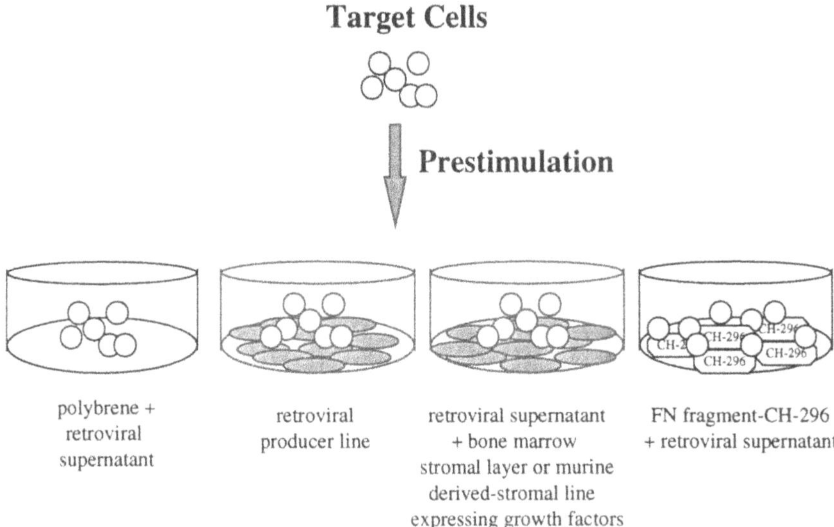

Fig. 2. Enhancement of retroviral-mediated gene-transfer efficiency utilizing alternative transduction strategies. Schematically shown are supernatant infection in the presence of polybrene, cocultivation of target cells with irradiated or mitomycin C-treated producer cells *(93–97)* infection on stromal cell layer *(98–100)* and the use of chimeric FN fragment CH-296 (*see* text) *(96)*.

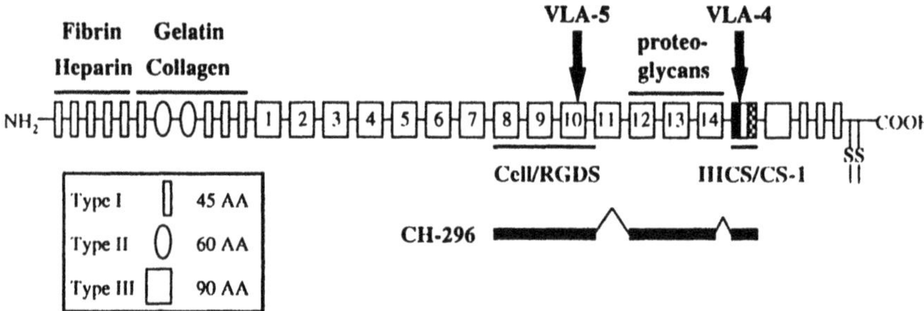

Fig. 3. Diagram of the A chain of fibronectin and the recombinant FN peptide, CH-296. The A chain of FN contains multiple binding sites for extracellular matrix components such as fibrin, heparin, gelatin, and collagen. In addition, it contains sequences involved in cell adhesion via the integrins, VLA-4 and VLA-5. The FN type I, II, III repeats are indicated and the type III repeats numbered 1-14. Mammalian cells expressing the integrin, VLA-4, bind to the CS-1 sequence located in the alternatively spliced IIICS region; cells expressing VLA-5 can bind to the tetrapeptide Arg-Gly-Asp-Ser (RGDS) in the cell binding domain (Cell) of FN. Cell surface proteoglycan molecules bind to another heparin binding domain contained within the type III repeats 12–14. The recombinant FN fragment, CH-296, contains sequences involved in cell adhesion via the integrins, VLA-4 and VLA-5 separated by a heparin binding domain.

interest in interactions of the hematopoietic cells with the hematopoietic microenvironment *(102)*. Fibronectin (FN) contains multiple sites important for interaction with cells (Fig. 3) *(102,103)*. The authors originally demonstrated that bone marrow stem and progenitor cells express VLA-4 and bind to the extracellular matrix component, FN *(104)*. They then reported an improvement in the efficiency of retrovirus-mediated gene

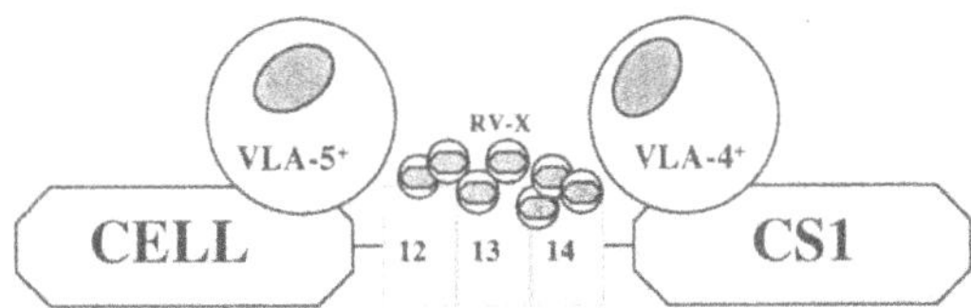

Fig. 4. Facilitation of retroviral-mediated gene transfer utilizing the recombinant fibronectin fragment, CH-296. The close proximity of target cells and retrovirus leads to a local increase in viral titer, resulting in increased gene transfer efficiency. Target cells expressing VLA-5 bind to the CELL binding domain, while cells expressing VLA-4 bind to the CS-1 region; retroviral particles (RV-X) bind to the type III repeats 12–14 via proteoglycan molecules.

transfer of human hematopoietic progenitors utilizing a carboxy terminal chymotryptic fragment of FN, 30/35, derived from human plasma *(97,98)* (Fig. 3). Mammalian cells expressing the integrin, very late antigen (VLA)-4, adhere to the CS-1 sequence located in the alternatively spliced IIICS region within the A chain of FN; cells expressing VLA-5 adhere to the tetrapeptide Arg-Gly-Asp-Ser (RGDS) in the central cell binding domain of FN. Cells expressing proteoglycan molecules adhere to heparin binding sequences contained within the type III repeats 12-14 of FN. Recently, the authors have utilized a recombinant chimeric FN fragment, CH-296 (Figs. 3,4), which contains CS-1, RGDS, and type III repeats 12–14 *(105)* and demonstrated that the colocalization of retrovirus and target cells on the CH-296 fragment resulted in enhanced gene transfer into human and murine hematopoietic stem and progenitors cells *(96)*. Routinely, the authors have observed 60–80% transduction of human CD34$^+$-derived progenitors after a short prestimulation period in cytokines followed by transduction using cell-free retrovirus supernatant on CH-296 *(96,101)*.

Since T-cells are potential targets in some gene therapy protocols *(59,106,107)*, they have also assessed the effect of transducing primary-culture T lymphocytes with retroviruses on CH-296–coated plates. Although resting T-cells express both VLA-4 and VLA-5, activation of T-cells results in a rapid increase in the binding affinity of VLA-4 and VLA-5 to FN molecules *(108–110)*. Using a retroviral vector that expresses the cell surface murine B7-1 molecule as an indicator of gene transfer efficiency, activated T-cells transduced with cell-free supernatant on CH-296 resulted in gene transfer efficiencies approaching 100%. Since lymphocytes have been used as targets for gene therapy of adenosine deaminase deficiency, we have also transduced normal and ADA-deficient PBLs on CH-296 with the PGK-mADA retrovirus, which expresses murine adenosine deaminase. At 12 days post-transduction, the level of mADA expression from this patient was two to three fold higher than endogenous human ADA expression observed in normal human lymphocytes (K. Pollok and D. A. Williams, submitted). This gene transfer protocol provides a simple and reliable method of delivering genes at high efficiency to human PBLs and may be useful in a wide variety of gene therapy protocols designed to target T lymphocytes.

Although direct cocultivation of amphotropic-packaging lines with target cells yields high levels of gene transfer in murine and human studies, concerns about the safety, reproducibility, and quality control of cocultivation make it a less than desirable avenue for human gene therapy protocols. The gene transfer strategy summarized above using recombinant FN molecules results in levels of gene transfer comparable to those cultures using the cocultivation method. Utilization of supernatant infection on recombinant FN fragments represents a highly reproducible and efficacious way to achieve high levels of gene transfer using low titer retroviruses. The safety of this approach is currently being evaluated in human trials.

An important question still being addressed is whether the ex vivo manipulation required for gene transfer of hematopoietic cells, such as stem cells, affects the functional capacity of these target cells. Several xenogeneic transplant models to assess human hematopoietic stem cell function have been developed *(30,111–117)*. However, it is not yet clear to what degree these models assay a human long-term repopulating stem cell. Interestingly, in the NOD/SCID model, transplants of human hematopoietic cells have revealed a primitive cell that engrafts in these mice that appears distinct from primitive cells defined by in vitro assays *(30)*. In these experiments, NOD/SCID mice were transplanted with large numbers of retroviral-transduced progenitors, including long-term culture-initiating cells (LTC-IC). Strikingly, the majority of engrafted cells, in contrast to in vitro colony forming and LTC-IC cells, were not transduced, indicating that progenitors assayed in vitro did not contribute significantly to the graft. This transplant model may be utilized to design strategies that lead to sufficient engraftment of transduced cells.

3. Primary Immunodeficiency Diseases to be Approached by Gene Transfer Technology

3.1. Adenosine Deaminase Deficiency Associated with Severe Combined Immunodeficiency

Severe combined immunodeficiency (SCID) caused by adenosine deaminase deficiency is associated with 30% of SCIDs and the feasibility of using gene therapy as a treatment of this rare disorder has been evaluated *(4,8,9,11)*. ADA^- SCID is a fatal condition secondary to mutations in the ADA gene *(118)*. In particular, lymphocytes are sensitive to the build up of toxic ADA substrates resulting in lymphopenia with impairment of both cell-mediated and humoral immunity. Although ADA historically has been considered to be an intracellular enzyme, a recent study indicates that a proportion of the ADA pool in T-cells directly associates on the cell surface with the costimulator molecule CD26 *(119)*. Cell surface ADA is functional and can detoxify medium containing high levels of adenosine, which would normally be toxic to T-cells. Current therapy is limited to either allogeneic bone marrow transplantation *(120)* or enzyme replacement with polyethylene-glycol modified ADA (PEG-ADA) *(10,16,121)*, both of which restore immune competence.

The feasibility of gene therapy utilizing ADA-transduced autologous T-cells as an alternative to marrow transplantation or supplementary to PEG-ADA therapy has been reported *(9,35,36,59,69,106,122)*. Prior to these trials, in vitro studies indicated that ADA-deficient T lymphocytes could be genetically corrected when transduced with retroviruses encoding for human ADA *(8,36,59,98,122)*. Analysis of ADA-transduced T lymphocytes transferred into immunodeficient mice *(89,106,123)* or rhesus monkeys *(62,70)* indicated that these cells continued to express ADA and persisted for long periods of time. These preclinical data suggested that the genetic correction of ADA-deficient T lymphocytes in vitro followed by adoptive transfer may be a beneficial therapy in patients receiving PEG-ADA. The ADA^- SCID clinical trials utilizing ADA-transduced PBLs *(8,9)* demonstrated that these cells were long-lived and their existence correlated with improved immune function even as the PEG-ADA dose was lowered. In vitro studies also had indicated that ADA-transduced and expressing cells may have a growth advantage compared to nontransduced populations. These data would imply that even though gene transfer efficiency may be low in these populations, a selective growth advantage in vivo may contribute to their persistence. However, this hypothesized selective growth advantage may not adequately compensate for low gene transfer efficiency. Blaese et al. *(9)* performed multiple infections on activated T-cells using cell-free retroviral supernatant. Transduced PBLs from one patient showed an in vitro transduction efficiency of 1–10% whereas PBLs from a second patient were transduced in the range 0.1–1.0%. In the second year of the protocol, in which no transduced-cell infusions were given, vector sequences were detected in the peripheral blood of both patients by PCR. However, the level detected in the second patient was equivalent to that detected in the first patient in spite of the low gene transfer documented in vitro.

Bordignon et al. *(8)* transduced PBLs or BM cells following T-cell depletion from ADA^- SCID patients with either multiple exposure to cell-free viral supernatant or by cocultivation with irradiated packaging cells. Gene transfer efficiency increased from 1–2.5% using cell-free retroviral supernatant up to 40% by cocultivation. Gene transfer efficiency into colony forming units-granulocyte/macrophage (CFU-GM) and burst forming units-erythroid (BFU-E) hematopoietic progenitors averaged 30–40%. In Bordignon's study *(8)*, the contribution of PBLs, BM stem, and progenitor cells were evaluated by transducing them with two similar, but molecularly distinguishable retroviral vectors. It was shown in vivo that the transduced PBLs comprised 0.8–8.5% of the circulating PBLs and provided an immediate reserve of immunocompetent lymphocytes prior to the maturation of BM-derived lymphocytes. However, contribution of these PBL-derived transduced cells was not long-lived. Kohn et al. *(7)* transduced CD34-enriched cord blood cells from three ADA^- SCID neonates with three infection cycles resulting in gene transfer efficiencies of 12–21%. In the absence of cytoablative therapy, 0.03–0.001% of peripheral blood leukocytes contained vector-derived sequences at 18 months posttransplant.

Gene transfer strategies mentioned previously in this chapter, which significantly enhance the efficiency of genetic transduction, may be utilized in future ADA^- SCID gene therapy trials. With the development of protocols yielding high efficiency gene transfer, it may be reasonable to design a gene therapy protocol whereby enzyme replacement with PEG-ADA, is lowered or stopped for a period of time, to assess the biological contribution of ADA-transduced cells in maintaining lower levels of adenosine and deoxyadenosine in the circulation.

3.2. X-linked Severe Combined Immunodeficiency

The most common form of X-linked SCID is inherited as an X-linked genetic defect, referred to as SCIDX1 *(124)*. Affected males show a pronounced impairment of both humoral and cell-mediated immunity. These individuals usually die of infection at an early age unless treated by bone marrow transplantation. The number of T-cells in SCIDX1 patients are low, whereas B-cell numbers are normal or even elevated. However, circulating B-cells may be dysfunctional, since antibody production is deficient. The SCIDX1 disease locus has been mapped to Xq13.1 *(125)*. Cloning of the common γ chain gene (γ_c) of the interleukin-2 (IL-2) receptor indicated that this gene mapped to the SCIDX1 region and subsequent studies indicated that the γ_c gene was defective in

SCIDX1 patients *(124,126–128)*. Analysis of γ_c mutations from multiple patients indicated a broad array of genetic lesions scattered throughout each exon of the γ_c cDNA. These mutations have been recently catalogued in a data base by Puck et al. *(125)*.

The IL-2 receptor plays a pivotal role in activation and differentiation of T-cells into effector cells. It was initially puzzling to investigators that genetic lesions in the γ_c could cause such a severe impairment of immunity in these patients. These observations were clarified when it was discovered that the γ_c chain is also a component of receptors for interleukin-4 (IL-4) *(129,130)*, interleukin-7 (IL-7) *(131,132)*, interleukin-9 (IL-9) *(133)*, and interleukin-15 (IL-15) *(134)*. T-cell development and differentiation are dependent on IL-7-mediated signals *(135,136)*, so a lack of this signaling pathway may be responsible for low T-cell numbers in the periphery. Likewise, the initiation of a T-cell–mediated immune response is regulated by γ_c expression. Several studies have shown that signals delivered through γ_c in T-cell clones were necessary for the prevention of clonal anergy *(137)*.

Since the γ_c chain is intricately involved in normal hematopoiesis (*see* below) *(135,136)*, treatment of X-linked SCID by gene therapy would presumably need to be done at the level of the hematopoietic stem cell. Correction of SCIDX1 by gene therapy may be possible. In vitro studies utilizing EBV-transformed B-cells from X-SCID patients have shown that gene transfer using γ_c retroviruses could correct the lack of γ_c-mediated signal transduction *(42,138,139)* in these cell lines. After gene transfer of γ_c cDNA into X-SCID B-cell lines, high affinity IL-2 receptors *(139)* were reconstituted, and the phosphorylation of the Janus family tyrosine kinases, JAK1 and JAK3, was restored *(42,140)*. In addition, expression of the γ_c gene in SCIDX1 B-cells may promote a selective growth advantage in vitro *(139)*. Hacein-Bey et al. demonstrated that the percentage of SCIDX1 B-cells transduced with the MFG(B2)-γ_c cDNA-retroviral vector increased over time in culture *(139)*. Other studies have shown that human $CD34^+$ and murine bone marrow cells could be transduced with a γ_c retroviral vector *(141)*. Murine bone marrow transduced with the γ_c retroviral vector and transplanted into syngeneic Balb/c mice, yielded vector-marked donor cells for at least three months posttransplant.

The availability of γ_c-deficient animals will assist in evaluating the feasibility of gene therapy for treatment of SCIDX1 *(142–144)*. In mice, targeted deletion of the γ_c gene has confirmed that γ_c expression was essential for normal lymphoid development. Mature splenic B- and T-cells were decreased in $\gamma_c^{-/-}$ animals 10-fold, and natural killer (NK) cells were undetectable. The presence of gut-associated intraepithelial lymphocytes was reduced and Peyer's patches were absent. T-cell responses to γ_c-dependent signaling were defective and mitogenic stimulation of thymocytes was impaired. In the B-cell compartment, IL-4-mediated immunoglobulin class switching did not occur. Since some SCIDX1 patients express a mutant γ_c chain on the cell surface, it will also be useful to develop mouse models to study the feasibility of performing gene therapy in patients expressing a defective γ_c protein. These animals could be used to address whether expression of a corrected γ_c gene will sufficiently reconstitute functional cytokine receptors in the presence of defective molecules, which in some instances, may still bind IL-2 and initiate some level of signal transduction. To approach this issue, Ohbo et al. *(145)* used homologous recombination of the γ_c gene to create a mouse, which expresses a mutant gene encoding for a truncated γ_c protein; the mutant protein was expressed on the cell surface, could bind IL-2, but was not capable of signal transduction. In these mice, the number of lymphocytes was decreased, whereas the number of monocytes was increased; no NK cells were present. Although B-cell numbers were decreased, the levels of IgM in serum of eight-week-old mice was higher than control littermates.

Interestingly, CD34$^+$, c-kit$^+$, Sca-1$^+$ cells were significantly increased, and measurements of colony forming cells indicated that mutant mice had 15-fold increase in hematopoietic progenitor cells compared to controls. This study revealed that γ_c expression plays an intricate role at multiple levels during hematopoiesis.

A canine model for SCIDX1 has also been described *(146,147)*. These dogs exhibit a severe impairment of immunity similar to that observed in SCIDX1 patients. As SCIDX1 dogs age, the percentage of T-cells increases *(147)*. Flow cytometric analysis of PBLs from these dogs, indicated that at less than three weeks of age, there was increased B-cell numbers and low to nonexistent levels of T-cells. However, by five weeks of age, T-cells were present in about 50% of the SCIDX1 dogs, whereas the absolute numbers of T-cells were still only 30% of normal. These data suggest that some thymic maturation and lymphocyte migration and, hence, peripheral expansion of T-cells can occur in these mutant animals *(147)*. In contrast, the appearance of T-cells in the periphery is not normally observed in patients with SCIDX1; this could be because of the fact that SCIDX1 is usually lethal at an early age in the absence of bone marrow transplantation *(148)*.

These animal models for SCIDX1 provide invaluable tools for the analysis of gene therapy strategies designed to correct the defective γ_c gene. By transplanting autologous bone marrow transduced with a γ_c retrovirus, it will be possible to assess whether the constitutive expression of γ_c can correct the severe immunodeficiency seen in these animals at both the developmental and functional level, and whether such constitutive expression has deleterious consequences. Constitutive γ_c expression may be sufficient for some aspects of hematolymphopoiesis. In one report *(149)*, SCIDX1 CD34-enriched cells were transduced with a γ_c-retrovirus. In the presence of SCF, IL-2, and IL-7, or in the presence of SCF and IL-15, NK-cell development occurred; these cells expressed the γ_c transgene, and were capable of NK-mediated target-cell lysis. It will also be informative to study the effects of constitutive γ_c expression on the thymic-maturation of bone-marrow-derived T-cell precursors. In the future, the construction of retroviruses capable of regulated γ_c expression may be optimal. In this regard, the recent characterization of the γ_c promoter may provide useful information for construction of constructs conferring regulated expression *(142)*.

Future correction of SCIDX1 by gene transfer may offer additional advantages over BMT. Successful BMT routinely corrects the T-cell defect in the majority of SCIDX1 patients, but it is common for B-cell engraftment not to occur. Because of a persistent defect in the B-cell compartment, the administration of gamma globulin is often necessary. Although successful retroviral-mediated gene- transfer of primary-culture murine B-cells has been reported, gene transfer of primary-culture human B-cells has not been documented *(150)*, however, transduction of hematopoietic stem cells should yield correction of both T- and B-cell lineages.

3.3. Hyper-IgM Syndrome

Another exciting example of basic research successfully delineating the cause of an immunodeficiency disease, are observations linking the CD40-CD40 ligand (CD40L) and X-linked Hyper- IgM Syndrome (HIGMX-1) *(151,152)*. HIGMX-1 patients show normal to increased serum IgM, very low IgG, and nondetectable serum levels of IgA and IgE *(152–158)*. These patients are prone to recurrent bacterial infections, autoimmune, and lymphoproliferative diseases. Without gamma globulin therapy, these patients are highly susceptible to opportunistic infections. Although B-cell numbers are within the normal range in these patients, the B-cells are exclusively IgM/IgD-positive with no cells expressing other isotypes. The CD40 receptor is expressed on immature and mature

B-cells, interdigitating cells, follicular dendritic, and thymic epithelial cells, as well as some carcinomas *(158)*. Previous reports have shown that CD40 is instrumental in regulating B-cell proliferation, and differentiation. For example, treatment of B-cells with anti-CD40 MAbs in the presence of IL-4 is associated with B-cell proliferation, which can be maintained for weeks in culture *(159,160)*. During B-cell differentiation, signals generated via CD40 block apoptosis possibly by upregulating *bcl-2 (161)*. CD40 plays a pivotal role in isotype switching. During the progression of a humoral immune response, B lymphocytes can express different heavy chain isotypes, but retain the same VDJ region. In the case of human B-cells, two signals are required for effective class switching to IgE. One signal is provided by IL-4 and the second signal is provided by direct T-cell contact *(162–165)*. This T-cell component can be replaced by anti-CD40 antibodies, which suggests that a potential ligand for CD40 may exist on T-cells *(162)*. A CD40L has been cloned from both murine and human cDNA libraries generated from activated T-cells *(166,167)*. The gene encoding CD40L was mapped to chromosome Xq26 *(168)*. EBV-transformed B-cell lines transfected with CD40L were able to induce IgE switching in both murine and human B-cells in the presence of IL-4, providing direct evidence for the role of CD40-CD40L interactions in isotype switching *(166)*. Although alternative pathways exist for isotype switching, this pathway appears to be the most pivotal one described to date. Most strikingly, it has been shown that CD40L expression is absent on T-cells from patients with HIGMX-1 *(153–157)* and T-cell-dependent IgE synthesis is absent in HIGM-X1 B-cells, and can be restored by anti-CD40 antibodies and IL-4 *(157)*. Cloning of CD40L from HIGMX-1 patient cells has demonstrated point mutations, deletions, and insertions throughout the entire coding region *(168)*.

Although T-cells from these patients are defective in CD40L expression, T-cell numbers are within the normal range. A detailed analysis of normal expression patterns may ultimately be informative in determining which hematopoietic cells need to be targeted for correction of a particular genetic defect. For instance, CD40L expression is tightly controlled. It is not expressed on resting immature double positive ($CD4^+/CD8^+$) or resting mature single positive ($CD4^+/CD8^-$ or $CD4^-/CD8^+$) thymocytes *(151)*. Immature thymocytes fail to express CD40L after stimulation with phorbol ester and ionophore, but stimulated $CD4^+/CD8^-$ thymocytes do express CD40L. These data predict that CD40L expression is required late in thymocyte development. Although resting mature T-cells do not express CD40L, time course studies of CD40L expression demonstrate maximal surface expression at 16–18 hours postactivation *(169)*.

Since genetic lesions in CD40L do not cause any gross defects in T-cell development, and HIGMX-1 patients have normal T-cell counts in the periphery, these cells may be excellent targets for gene therapy. Activated T-cells are infectible with retroviral vectors and gene transfer of the CD40L cDNA could potentially reconstitute the ability of CD4 T-cells to direct isotype switching in B lymphocytes. This hypothesis can be formally tested in CD40L-deficient animals. CD40L-deficient mice have been generated by gene targeting and exhibit decreased IgM response to thymus-dependent antigens and completely lack an antigen-specific IgG1 response *(170)*. These mice do not develop germinal centers in response to immunization with thymus-dependent antigens implying that memory B-cell responses are abrogated. In contrast to HIGMX-1 observed in humans, CD40L knock-out mice do not show elevated IgM in their serum. Likewise, in CD40-deficient mice, immune responses to thymus-dependent antigens resulted in IgM but no IgG, IgA, or IgE production *(171)*. In addition, a group of patients with Hyper-IgM Syndrome and normal CD40L expression have also been identified *(172)*. A lesion in the

CD40-mediated signaling cascade may be the cause of defective Ig class switching in these patients.

3.4. Wiskott-Aldrich Syndrome and X-linked Agammaglobulinemia

The Wiskott-Aldrich Syndrome (WAS) represents another X-linked immunodeficiency disease which maps to Xp11.23, and has been characterized by thrombocytopenia, increased risk of bacterial and viral infections, autoimmune disease, and malignancies *(152,173)*. Many abnormalities in both the T-cell and B-cell compartment have been observed in WAS patients. For instance, the relative number of CD4 and CD8 T lymphocytes expressing CD45RA is increased in WAS patients, suggesting involvement of the WAS protein in memory cell differentiation *(174)*. CD8 molecules predominantly exist as α/α homodimers in the thymus and as T-cell differentiation progresses, there is a switch to α/β heterodimers. In WAS patients, however, the majority of peripheral CD8 T-cells continue to express the α/α homodimer *(174,175)*. The WAS protein (WASP) contains proline-rich motifs including the PxxP binding consensus for src homology-3 domains (SH3) domains *(176,177)*. The function of WASP is unclear, but recent reports suggest it plays a role in lymphoid signaling *(178)*. The WASP has been shown to interact with the *Cdc42*, a member of the *Rho* family of GTPases *(179)*. The *Cdc42* protein plays a pivotal role in regulating cytoskeletal elements and reorganization of the cytoskeleton is important during B- and T-cell interactions *(180)*. Cory et al. *(178)* reported recently that WASP bound to the SH3 domains of Grb2 and phospholipase C-γ as well as the *Tec* family of cytoplasmic tyrosine kinases (*Btk*, *Itk*, and *Tec*). Interestingly, this observation suggests a functional connection between WAS and X-linked agammaglobulinemia (XLA), since the defective gene in XLA is the Bruton's tyrosine kinase (*Btk*). The *Btk* gene is located on the X chromosome at Xq21.3-Xq22 *(181,182)*. Btk is expressed early in B-cell development but is not expressed in T-cells or plasma cells *(183,184)*. Abnormalities in Btk lead to an absence of peripheral B lymphocytes, but do not affect the appearance of pro-B-cells and pre-B-cells in the bone marrow *(185)*. Similarly, in *Btk*-deficient mice, B-cell development is abrogated *(186)*; these mice may provide a clinically relevant model to study gene therapy of *Btk*-deficient B-cell progenitors.

3.5. ZAP-70 Kinase Deficiency

One autosomal recessive form of SCID is caused by defects in the ZAP-70 protein tyrosine kinase *(187–189)*. ZAP-70 is selectively expressed in thymocytes, T-cells, and NK cells *(190)*. There is a complete absence of $CD8^+$ T-cells and normal to high levels of $CD4^+$ T-cells in the peripheral blood of patients with ZAP-70 kinase deficiency. However, the $CD4^+$ cells present are incapable of delivering signals through the T-cell receptor complex. Retroviruses expressing ZAP-70 have been used to transduce human T-cell leukemia virus type I (HTLV I)-transformed $CD4^+$ T-cells from ZAP-70-deficient patients *(191)*. After transduction, ZAP-70 was expressed at levels observed in normal cells, and upon TCR crosslinking, was phosphorylated on tyrosine residues. Calcium mobilization was normal after TCR crosslinking. In ZAP-70 kinase-deficient mice, T-cell development was blocked, because mature CD4- or CD8-single-positive cells were not apparent *(192)*. These deficient mice can be used to design gene therapy strategies suitable for correction of this defect. By transducing bone marrow from these animals with a ZAP-70 kinase retroviral vector, the effect of constitutive expression during hematopoiesis can be determined. It will be informative to determine whether constitutive expression is sufficient for correction of this defect or if regulated expression of the ZAP-70 kinase is more desirable.

In gene therapy protocols for ZAP-70-deficient patients, the specific targeting of T-cell progenitors could be beneficial since the ZAP-70 kinase is exclusively expressed in the NK/T-cell lineages and ex vivo expansion of T-cell progenitors may be feasible. For instance, studies *(193)* using rhesus monkey and human thymic stroma have indicated that these stromal layers can promote normal T lymphopoiesis of human or rhesus $CD34^+$ progenitor cells into both double positive ($CD4^+/CD8^+$) and single positive cells ($CD4^+$ or $CD8^+$). The T-cell populations generated contained a polyclonal TCR repertoire.

4. Conclusions

With continued improvements in gene transfer technology, and ex vivo expansion of hematopoietic progenitor cells and lymphoid precursor cells *(194)*, somatic gene therapy may become a viable therapeutic option in the future. The generation of gene-knock out mice will make it possible to prove the feasibility of gene therapy for a broad variety of diseases. For example, a gene-knock out mouse model for X-linked chronic granulomatous disease (X-CGD) has been developed in which the gp91phox gene was disrupted *(195)*. In healthy individuals, the gp91phox protein is an integral component of the respiratory burst oxidase pathway. In a landmark study by Bjorgvinsdottir et al. *(196)*, bone marrow from X-CGD mice was transduced with a retrovirus expressing gp91phox and transplanted into these immunodeficient animals. Deficient mice transplanted with transduced bone marrow did not develop lung disease after respiratory challenge with *Aspergillus fumigatus*, a phenotypic correction directly applicable to human X-CGD patients. Strikingly, gp91phox-deficient mice transplanted with mixtures of wild-type and gp91phox-deficient bone marrow only required approximately 5% wild-type neutrophils to protect against *Aspergillus fumigatus* challenge. This study suggested that a very low percentage of corrected cells was sufficient for survival of these mice. Whether low levels of corrected cells in humans will be sufficient for maintenance of immunity awaits further study.

In conclusion, the issues surrounding gene-transfer efficiency, although still a major obstacle to gene therapy, may be circumvented in some cases of immune deficiency diseases by targeting more differentiated progenitors of the lymphoid compartment. The major challenge for the future is to determine in humans, strategies to optimize ex vivo gene transfer that lead to phenotypic correction of specific diseases while not compromising engraftment capabilities.

Acknowledgments

The authors especially thank Dr. Arthur Baluyut for his support and critical evaluation of this chapter. They also thank him for his assistance with computer graphics. The authors also thank Wendy Schroeder for her critical review of this chapter. A special thanks to Dana Waddell for her expert assistance with preparation of this chapter. This work was supported by the National Heart, Lung and Blood Institute (PO1 HL 53586). The Herman B Wells Center for Pediatric Research is a Center of Excellence in Molecular Hematology funded by the National Institute of Diabetes and Digestive and Kidney Diseases (P50 DK 49218).

References

1. Williams, D. A. (1990) Expression of introduced genetic sequences in hematopoietic cells following retroviral-mediated gene transfer. *Hum. Gene Ther.* **1**, 229–239.

2. Brenner, M. K. (1996) Gene transfer to hematopoietic cells. *Mol. Med.* **335,** 337–339.
3. Blau, H. M. and Springer, M. L. (1995) Gene therapy; a novel form of drug delivery. *Mol. Med.* **333,** 1204–1207.
4. Kohn, D. B. (1997) Gene therapy for haematopoietic and lymphoid disorders. *Clin. Exp. Immunol.* **107,** 54–57.
5. Rosenberg, S. A., Blaese, R. M., Brenner, M. K., Deisseroth, A. B., Ledley, F. D., Lotze, M. T., Wilson, J. M., Nabel, G. J., Cornetta, K., Economou, J. S., Freeman, S. M., Riddell, S. R., Oldfield, E., Gansbacher, B., Dunbar, C., Walker, R. E., Schuening, F. G., Roth, J. A., Crystal, R. G., Welsh, M. J., Culver, K., Heslop, H. E., Simons, J., Wilmott, R. W., and Aevischer, P., et al. Human gene marker/therapy clinical protocols. *Hum. Gene Ther.* 7, 1621–1647.
6. Lisziewicz, J. (1996) Tar decoys and trans-dominant gag mutant for HIV-1 gene therapy. *Antibiot. Chemother.* **48,** 192–197.
7. Kohn, D. B., Weinberg, K. I., Nolta, J. A., Heiss, L. N., Lenarsky, C., Crooks, G. M., Hanley, M. E., Annett, G., Brooks, J. S., El-Khoureiy, A., Lawrence, K., Wells, S., Moen, R. C., Bastian, J., Williams-Herman, M. Elder, D. E., Wara, D., Bowen, T., Hershfield, M. S., Mullen, C. A., Blaese, R. M., and Parkman, R. (1995) Engraftment of gene-modified umbilical cord blood cells in neonates with adenosine deaminase deficiency. *Nat. Med.* **1,** 1–10.
8. Bordignon, C., Notarangelo, L. D., Nobili, N., Ferrari, G., Casorati, G., Panina, P., Mazzolari, E., Maggioni, D., Rossi, C., Servida, P., Ugazio, A. G., and Mavilio, F. (1995) Gene therapy in peripheral blood lymphocytes and bone marrow for ADA^- Immunodeficient patients. *Science* **270,** 470–474.
9. Blaese, R. M., Culver, K. W., Miller, A. D., Carter, C. S., Fleisher, T., Clerici, M., Shearer, G., Chang, L., Chiang, Y., Tolstoshev, P., Greenblatt, J. J., Rosenberg, S. A., Klein, H., Berger, M., Mullen, C. A., Ramsey, W. J., Muul, L., Morgan, R. A., and Anderson, W. F. (1995) T-lymphocyte-directed gene therapy for ADA^- SCID, Initial trial results after 4 years. *Science* **270,** 475–480.
10. Hershfield, M. S., Chaffee, S., and Sorensen, R. U. (1993) Enzyme replacement therapy with polyethylene glycol-adenosine deaminase in adenosine deaminase deficiency: overview and case reports of three patients including two now receiving gene therapy. *Ped. Res.* **33,** S42–S47.
11. Hoogerbrugge, P. M., van Beusechem, V. W., Fischer, A., Debree, M., le Deist, F., Perignon, J. L., Morgan, G., Gaspar, B., Fairbanks, L. D., Skeoch, C. H., Moseley, A., Harvey, M., Levinsky, R. J., and Valerio, D. (1996) Bone marrow gene transfer in three patients with adenosine deaminase deficiency. *Gene Ther.* **3,** 179–183.
12. Dunbar, C. and Kohn, D. (1996) Retroviral mediated transfer of the cDNA for human glucocerebrosidase into hematopoietic stem cells of patients with Gaucher disease: a Phase I study. *Hum. Gene Ther.* **7,** 231–253.
13. Whitley C. B. (1996) Retroviral mediated gene transfer of the Iduronate-2-Sulfatase gene into lymphocytes for treatment of mild Hunter Syndrome (Mucopolysaccharidosis type II). *Hum. Gene Ther.* **7,** 537–549.
14. Evans, C. H. and Robbins, P. D. (1995) Progress toward the treatment of arthritis by gene therapy. *Annals of Med.* **27,** 543–546.
15. Roth, J. A. and Cristiano, R. J. (1997) Gene therapy for cancer: what have we done and where are we going? *JNCI.* **89,** 21–39.
16. Hershfield, M. S. (1995) PEG-ADA Replacement therapy for adenosine deaminase deficiency: an update after 8.5 years. Clin. Immunol. Immunopath. 76, S228–S232.
17. Mulligan, R. C. (1993) The basic science of gene therapy. *Science* **260,** 926–932.
18. Dunbar, C. E. (1996) Gene transfer to hematopoietic stem cells: implications for gene therapy of human disease. *Annu. Rev. Med.* **47,** 11–20.
19. Watanabe, T., Kuszynski, C., Ino, K., Heimann, D. G., Shepard, H. M., Yasui, Y., Maneval, D. C., and Talmadge, J. E. (1996) Gene transfer into human bone marrow hematopoietic cells mediated by adenovirus vectors. *Blood* **87,** 5032–5039.
20. Descamps, V., Duffour, M. T., Mathieu, M. C., Fernandez, N., Cordier, L., Abina, M. A., Kremer, E., Perricaudet, M., and Haddada, H. (1996) Strategies for cancer gene therapy using adenoviral vectors. *J. Molec. Med.* **74,** 183–189.

21. Trapnell, B. C. and Gorziglia, M. (1994) Gene therapy using adenoviral vectors. *Curr. Opin. Biotechnol.* **5,** 617–625.
22. Hardy, S., Kitamura, M., Harris-Stansil, T., Dai, Y., and Phipps, M. L. (1997) Construction of adenovirus vectors through cre-lox recombination. *J. Virol.* **71,** 1842–1849.
23. Samulski, R. J., Zhu, X., Xiao, X., and Brook, J. D. (1991) Targeted integration of adeno-associated virus (AAV) into human chromosome 19. *EMBO J.* **10,** 3941–3950.
24. Chatterjee, S. and Wong, K. K., Jr. (1996) Adeno-associated virus vectors for gene therapy of the hematopoietic system. *Curr. Top. Micro. Immunol.* **218,** 61–71.
25. Podsakoff G., Wong, K. K., Jr., and Chatterjee, S. (1994) Stable and efficient gene transfer into non-dividing cells by adeno-associated virus (AAV)-based vectors. *J. Virol.* **68,** 656–666.
26. Russell, D. W., Miller, A. D., and Alexander, I. E. (1994) Adeno-associated virus vectors preferentially transduce cells in S phase. *Proc. Natl. Acad. Sci. USA* **91,** 8915–8919.
27. Podsakoff, G., Shaughnessy, E. A., Lu, D., Wong, K. K. Jr., and Chatterjee, S. (1994) Long term in vivo reconstitution with murine marrow cells transduced with an adeno-associated virus vector. *Blood* **84,** (S) 256a.
28. Einerhand, M. P. W. and Valero, D. (1992) Gene transfer into hematopoietic stem cells: prospects for human gene therapy. *Curr. Top. Microbiol. Immunol.* **177,** 217–231.
29. Miller, D. G., Adam, M. A., and Miller, A. D. (1990) Gene transfer by retrovirus vectors occurs only in cells that are actively replicating at the time of infection. *Mol. Cell. Biol.* **10,** 4239–4242.
30. Larochelle, A., Vormoor, J., Hanenberg, H., Wang, J. C. Y., Bhatia, M., Lapidot, T., Moritz, T., Murdoch, B., Xiao, X. L., Kato, I., Williams, D. A., and Dick, J. E. (1996) Identification of primitive human hematopoietic cells capable of repopulating NOD/SCID mouse bone marrow: implications for gene therapy. *Nat. Med.* **2,** 1329–1337.
31. Luskey, B. D., Rosenblatt, M., Zsebo, K., and Williams, D. A. (1992) Stem cell factor, interleukin-3, and interleukin-6 promote retroviral-mediated gene transfer into murine hematopoietic stem cells. *Blood* **80,** 396–402.
32. Donahue, R. E., Kessler, S. W., Bodine, D., McDonagh, K., Dunbar, C., Goodman, S., Agricola, B., Byrne, E., Raffeld, M., Moen, R., et al. (1992) Helper virus induced T cell lymphoma in nonhuman primates after retroviral mediated gene transfer. *J. Exp. Med.* **176,** 1125–1135.
33. Miller , A. D. (1990) Retrovirus Packaging Cells. *Hum. Gene Ther.* **1,** 5–14.
34. Markowitz, M., Goff, S., and Bank, A. (1988) A safe packaging line for gene transfer: separating viral genes on two different plasmids. *J. Virol.* **62,** 1120–1124.
35. Mavilio, F., Ferrari, G., Rossini, S., Nobili, N., Conini, C., Casorati, G., Traversari, C., and Bordignon, C. (1994) Peripheral blood lymphocytes as target cells of retroviral vector-mediated gene transfer. *Blood* **83,** 1988–1997.
36. Ferrari, G., Rossini, S., Nobili, N., Maggioni, D., Garofalo, A., Giavazzi, R., Mavilio, F., and Bordignon, C. (1992) Transfer of the ADA gene into human ADA-deficient T lymphocytes reconstitutes specific immune functions. *Blood* **80,** 1120–1124.
37. Sharma, S., Cantwell, M., Kipps, T. J., and Friedmann, T. (1996) Efficient infection of a human T-cell line and of human primary peripheral blood leukocytes with a pseudotyped retrovirus vector. *Proc. Natl. Acad. Sci. USA* **93,** 11842–11847.
38. Schumann, G., Qin, L., Rein, A., Natsoulis, G., Boeke, J. D. (1996) Therapeutic effect of gag-nuclease fusion protein on retrovirus-infected cell cultures. *J. Virol.* **70,** 4329–4337.
39. Rogulski, K. R., Kim, J. H., Kim, S. H. and Freytag, S. O. (1997) Glioma cells transduced with an *Escherichia coli* CD/HSV-1 TK fusion gene exhibit enhanced metabolite suicide and radiosensitivity. *Hum. Gene Ther.* **8,** 73–85.
40. Gervaix, A., Li, X., Kraus, G., and Wong-Staal, F. (1997) Multigene antiviral vectors inhibit diverse human immunodeficiency virus type 1 clades. *J. Virol.* **71,** 3048–3053.
41. Ghattas, I. R., Sanes, J. R., and Majors, J. E. (1991) The encephalomyocarditis virus internal ribosome entry sites allows efficient coexpression of two genes from a recombinant provirus in cultured cells and in embryos. *Mol. Cell. Biol.* **11,** 5848–5859.
42. Candotti, F., Johnston, J. A., Puck, J. M., Sugamura, K., O'Shea, J. J., and Blaese, R. M. (1996) Retroviral-mediated gene correction for X-linked severed combined immunodeficiency. *Blood* **87,** 3097–3102.

43. Medin, J. A., Makoto, M., Pawliuk, R., Jacobson, S., Amiri, M., Kluepfel-Stahl, S., Brady, R. O., Humphries, R. K., and Karlsson, S. (1996) A bicistronic therapeutic retroviral vector enables sorting of transduced CD34$^+$ cells and corrects the enzyme deficiency in cells from Gaucher patients. *Blood* **87,** 1754–1762.
44. Sokolic, R. A., Sekhsaria, S., Sugimoto, Y., Whiting-Theobald, N., Linton, G. F., Li, F., Gottesman, M. M., and Malech, H. L. (1996) A bicistronic retrovirus vector containing a picornavirus internal ribosome entry site allows for correction of X-linked CGD by selection for MDR1 expression. *Blood* **87,** 42–50.
45. Hock, R. A., Miller, A. D., and Osborne, W. R. (1989) Expression of human adenosine deaminase from various strong promoters after gene transfer into human hematopoietic cell lines. *Blood* **74,** 876–881.
46. Malik, P., Krall, W. J., Yu, X. J., Zhou, C., and Kohn, D. B. (1995) Retroviral-mediated gene expression in human myelomonocytic cells: a comparison of hematopoietic cell promoters to viral promoters. *Blood* **86,** 2993–3005.
47. Li, C. L., Dwarki, V. J., and Verma, I. M. (1990) Expression of human α-globin and mouse/human hybrid β-globin genes in murine hemopoietic stem cells transduced by recombinant retroviruses. *Proc. Natl. Acad. Sci. USA* **87,** 4349–4353
48. Rixon, M. W., Harris, E. A. S., and Gelinas, R. E. (1990) Expression of the human γ-globin gene after retroviral transfer to transformed erythroid cells. *Biochemistry* **29,** 4393–4400.
49. Bender, M. A., Miller, A. D., and Gelinas, R. E. (1988) Expression of the human β-globin gene after retroviral transfer into murine erythroleukaemia cells and human BFU-E cells. *Mol. Cell. Biol.* **8,** 1725–1735.
50. Novak, U., Harri, E. A. S., Forrester, W., Groudine, M., and Gelinas, R. (1990) High-level β-globin expression after retroviral transfer of locus activation region-containing human β-globin gene derivatives into murine erythroleukemia cells. *Proc. Natl. Acad. Sci. USA* **87,** 3386–3390.
51. Williams, D. A., Orkin, S. H., and Mulligan, R. C. (1986) Retrovirus-mediated gene transfer of human adensoine deaminase gene sequences into cells in culture and into murine hematopoietic cells in vivo. *Proc. Natl. Acad. Sci. USA* **83,** 2566–2570.
52. Williams, D. A., Lim, B., Spooner, E., Longtine, J., and Dexter, T. M. (1988) Restriction of expression of an integrated recombinant retrovirus in primary but not immortalized murine hematopoietic stem cells. *Blood* **71,** 1738–1743.
53. Kantoff, P. W., Gillio, A, McLachlin, J. R., Flake, A. W. Eglitis, M. A., Moen, R., Karlsson, S., Kohn, D. B., Karson, E., Zwiebel, J. A., Bordignon, C., Hutton, J. J., Harrison, M. R., Blaese, R. M., Nienhuis, A., Gilboa, E., Zanjani, E. D., O'Reilly, R., and Anderson, W. F. (1986) Retroviral-mediated gene transfer into hematopoietic cells. *Trans. Assoc. Amer. Phys.* **99,** 92–102.
54. McIvor, R. S., Johnson, M. J., Miller, A. D., Pitts, S., Williams, S. R., Valerio, D., Martin, D. W., Jr., and Verma, I. R. (1987) Human purine nucleoside phosphorylase and adenosine deaminase: gene transfer into cultured cells and murine hematopoietic stem cells by using a recombinant amphotropic retrovirus. *Mol. Cell. Biol.* **7,** 383–846.
55. Belmont, J. W., Macgregor, G. R., Wagner-Smith, K., Fletcher, F. A., Moore, K. A., Hawking, D., Villalon, D., Chang, S. M. W., and Caskey, C. T. (1988) Expression of human adenosine deaminase in murine hematopoietic cells. *Mol. Cell. Biol.* **8,** 5116–5125.
56. Naldini, L., Blomer, U., Gallay, P., Ory, D., Mulligan, R., Gage, F. H., Verma, I. M., and Trono, D. (1996) *In vivo* gene delivery and stable transduction of nondividing cells by a lentiviral vector. *Science* **272,** 263–267.
57. Bieniasz, P. D., Weiss, R. A., and McClure, M. O. (1995) Cell cycle dependence of foamy retrovirus infection. *J. Virol.* **69,** 7295–7299.
58. Russell, D. W. and Miller, A. D. (1996) Foamy virus vectors. *J. Virol.* **70,** 217–222.
59. Culver, K. W., Anderson, W. F., and Blaese, R. M. (1991) Lymphocyte gene therapy. *Hum. Gene Ther.* **2,** 107–109.
60. van Beusechem, V. W. and Valerio, D. (1996) Gene transfer into hematopoietic stem cells of nonhuman primates. *Hum. Gene Ther.* **7,** 1649–1668.
61. Kiem, H. -P., Darovsky, B., von Kalle, C., Goehle, S., Graham, T., Miller, A. D., Storb, R., and Schuening, F. G. (1995) Long-term persistence of canine hematopoietic cells genetically marked by retrovirus vectors. *Hum. Gene Ther.* **7,** 89–96.

62. Bodine, D. M., Moritz, T., Donahue, R. E., Luskey, B. D., Kessler, S. W., Martin, D. I. K., Orkin, S. H., and Nienhuis, A. W., and Williams, D. A. (1993) Long-term in vivo expression of a murine adenosine deaminase gene in rhesus monkey hematopoietic cells of multiple lineages after retroviral mediated gene transfer into $CD34^+$ bone marrow cells. *Blood* **82,** 1975–1980.
63. Kaleko, M., Garcia, J. V., Osborne, W. R. A., and Miller, A. D. (1990) Expression of human adenosine deaminase in mice after transplantation of genetically-modified bone marrow. *Blood* **75,** 1733–1741.
64. Lim, B., D. A. Williams, and Orkin, S. H. (1987) Retrovirus-mediated gene transfer of human adenosine deaminase: expression of functional enzyme in murine hematopoietic stem cells in vivo. *Mol. Cell. Biol.* **7,** 3459–3465.
65. Moore, K. A., Fletcher, F. A., Villalon, D. K., Utter, A. E., and Belmont, J. W. (1990) Human adenosine deaminase expression in mice. *Blood* **75,** 2085–2092.
66. Osborne, W. R. A., Hock, R. A., Kaleko, M., and Miller, A. D. (1990) Long-term expression of human adenosine deaminase in mice after transplantation of bone marrow infected with amphotropic retroviral vectors. *Hum. Gene Ther.* **1,** 31–41.
67. Lim, B., Apperly, J. F., Orkin, S. H., and Williams, D. A. (1989) Long-term expression of human adenosine deaminase in mice transplanted with retrovirus-infected hematopoietic stem cells. *Proc. Natl. Acad. Sci. USA* **86,** 8892–8896.
68. Correll, P. H., Colilla, S., and Karlsson, S. (1994) Retroviral vector design for long-term expression in murine hematopoietic cells in vivo. *Blood* **84,** 1812–1822.
69. Mullen, C. A., Snitzer, K., Culver, K. W., Morgan, R. A., Anderson, W. F., and Blaese, R. M. (1996) Molecular analysis of T lymphocyte-directed gene therapy for adenosine deaminase deficiency: long-term expression in vivo of genes introduced with a retroviral vector. *Hum. Gene Ther.* **7,** 1123–1129.
70. Culver, K. W., Morgan, R. A., Osborne, W. R. A., Lee, R. T., Lenschow, D., Able, C., Cornetta, K., Anderson, W. F., and Blaese, R. M. (1990) In vivo expression and survival of gene-modified T lymphocytes in rhesus monkeys. *Hum. Gene Ther.* **1,** 399–410.
71. Kantoff, P. W., Kohn, D. B., Mitsuya, H., Armentano, D., Sieberg, M., Zwiebel, J. A., Eglitis, M. A., McLachlin, J. R., Wiginto, D. A., Hutton, J. J., Horowitz, S. D., Gilboa, E., Blaese, R. M., and Anderson, W. F. (1986) Correction of adenosine deaminase deficiency in cultured human T and B cells by retrovirus-mediated gene transfer. *Proc. Natl. Acad. Sci. USA* **83,** 6563–6567.
72. Challita, P. and Kohn, D. B. (1994) Lack of expression from a retroviral vector after transduction of murine hematopoietic stem cells is associated with methylation in vivo. *Proc. Natl. Acad. Sci. USA* **91,** 2567–2571.
73. Wilson, J. M., Danos, O., Grossman, M., Raulet, D. H., and Mulligan, R. C. (1990) Expression of human adenosine deaminase in mice reconstituted with retrovirus-transduced hematopoietic stem cells. *Blood* **71,** 1738–1743.
74. van Beusechem, V., Kukler, A., Heidt, P. J., and Valerio, D. (1992) Long-term expression of human adenosine deaminase in rhesus monkeys transplanted with retrovirus-infected bone-marrow cells. *Proc. Natl. Acad. Sci. USA.* **89,** 7640–7644.
75. Riddell, S. R., Elliott, M., Lewinsohn, D. A., Gilbert, M. J., Wilson, L., Manley, S. A., Lupton, S. D., Overll, R. W., Reynolds, T. C., Corey, L., and Greenberg, P. D. (1996) T-cell mediated rejection of gene-modified HIV-specific cytotoxic T lymphocytes in HIV-infected patients. *Nat. Med.* **2,** 216–223.
76. Sanes J., Rubenstein, J., and Nicolas, J. (1986) Use of a recombinant retrovirus to study post implantation cell lineage in mouse embryos. *EMBO J.* **5,** 3133–3142.
77. Paul R., Morris, D., Hess, B., Dunn, J., and Overell, R. (1993) Increased viral titer through concentration of viral harvests from retroviral packaging cell lines. *Hum. Gene Ther.* **4,** 609–615.
78. Chuck, A. and Palsson, B. (1996a) Consistent and high rates of gene transfer can be obtained using the flow through transduction over a wide range of retroviral titers. *Hum. Gene Ther.* **7,** 743–750.
79. Kotani, H., Newton, P. B., Zhang, S., Chiang, Y., Otto, E., Weaver, L. Blaese, R. M., Anderson, W. F., and McGarrity, G. J. (1994) Improved methods of retroviral vector transduction and production for gene therapy. *Hum. Gene Ther.* **5,** 19–28.

80. Coelen, R., Jose, D., and May, J. (1983) The effect of hexadimethrine bromide (polybrene) on the infection of primate retroviruses SSV1/SSAV1 and BaEV. *Arch. Virol.* **75,** 307–311.
81. Andreadis, S. and Palsson, B. O. (1997) Coupled effects of polybrene and calf serum on the efficiency of retroviral transduction and the stability of retroviral vectors. *Hum. Gene Ther.* **8,** 285–291.
82. Bagnis, C., Cischportich, C., Imbert, A., Van den Broeke, A., Cornet, V., and Mannoni, P. (1997) Efficiency of retroviral transduction into hematopoietic cells by cocultivation procedure does not correlate with viral titer. *Cancer Gene Ther.* **4,** 5–8.
83. Xu, L. C., Young, H. A., Blanco, M., Kessler, S., Roberts, A. B., and Karlsson, S. (1994) Poor transduction efficiency of human hematopoietic progenitor cells by high titer amphotropic retrovirus producer cell clones. *J. Virol.* **68,** 7634–7636.
84. Mayani, H., Little, M. T., Dragowska, W., et al. (1995) Differential effects of the hematopoietic inhibitors MIP1-α, TGF-β, and TNF-α on cytokine-induced proliferation of subpopulations of $CD34^+$ cells purified from cord blood and from liver. *Exp. Hemat.* **23,** 422–427.
85. Miller, A. D. (1996) Cell-surface receptors for retroviruses and implications for gene transfer. *Proc. Natl. Acad. Sci. USA* **93,** 11407–11413.
86. Weiss, R. A., and Tailor, C. S. (1995) Retrovirus receptors. *Cell* **82,** 531–533.
87. Miller A. D., Garcia, J. V., von Suhr, N., Lynch, C. M., Wilson, C., and Eiden, M. V. (1991) Construction and properties of retrovirus packaging cells based on gibbon ape leukemia virus. *J. Virol.* **65,** 2220–2224.
88. Bunnel, B. A., Muul, L. M., Donahue, R. E., Blaese, R. M., and Morgan, R. A. (1995) High-efficiency retroviral-mediated gene transfer into human and nonhuman primate peripheral blood lymphocytes. *Proc. Natl. Acad. Sci. USA.* **92,** 7739–7743.
89. Cosset, F. L., and Russell, S. J. (1996) Targeting retrovirus entry. *Gene Ther.* **3,** 946–956.
90. Kasahara N., Dozy, A. M., Kan, Y. W. (1994) Tissue-specific targeting of retroviral vectors through ligand-receptor interactions. *Science* **266,** 1373–1376.
91. Valsesia-Wittmann, S., Morling, F. J., Nilson, B. H., Takeuchi, Y., Russell, S. J., and Cosset, F. L. (1996) Improvement of retroviral retargeting by using amino acid spacers between an additional binding domain and the N terminus of Moloney murine leukemia virus SU. *J. Virol.* **70,** 2059–2064.
92. Schwarzenberger, P., Spence, S. E., Gooya, J. M., Michiel, D., Curiel, D. T., Ruscetti, F. W., and Keller, J. R. (1996) Targeted gene transfer to human hematopoietic progenitor cell lines through the c-kit receptor. *Blood* **87,** 472–478.
93. Williams, D. A., Lenischka, I. R., Nathan, D. G., and Mulligan, R. C. (1984) Introduction of new genetic material into pluripotent stem cells of the mouse. *Nature* **310,** 476–480.
94. Dick, J. E., Magli, M. C., Huszar, D., Phillips, R. A., and Bernstein, A. (1985) Introduction of a selectable gene in primitive stem cells capable of long-term reconstitution of the hematopoietic system of w/wv mice. *Cell* **42,** 71–79.
95. Lemischka, I. R., Raulet, D. H., and Mulligan, R. C. (1986) Developmental potential and dynamic behavior of hematopoietic stem cells. *Cell* **45,** 917–927.
96. Hanenberg, H., Xiao, X. L., Dilloo, D., Hashino, K., Kato, I., and Williams, D. A. (1996) Colocalization of retrovirus and target cells on specific fibronectin fragments increases genetic transduction of mammalian cells. *Nat. Med.* **2,** 876–882.
97. Moritz, T., Dutt, P., Xiao, X., Carstanjen, D., Vik, T., Hanenberg, H., and Williams, D. A. (1996) Fibronectin improves transduction of reconstituting hematopoietic stem cells by retroviral vectors: evidence of direct viral binding to chymotryptic carboxy-terminal fragments. *Blood* **88,** 855–862.
98. Moritz, T., Keller, D. C., and Williams, D. A. (1993) Human cord blood cells as targets for gene transfer: potential use in genetic therapies of severe combined immunodeficiency disease. *J. Exp. Med.* **178,** 529–536.
99. Moore, K. A., Deisseroth, A. B., Reading, C. L., Williams, D. E., and Belmont, J. W. (1992) Stromal support enhances cell-free retroviral vector transduction of human bone-marrow long-term culture-initiating cells. *Blood* **79,** 1393–1399.
100. Toksoz, D., Zsebo, K. M., Smith, K. A., Hu, S., Brankow, D., Suggs, S. V., Martin, F. H., and Williams, D. A. (1992) Support of human hematopoiesis in long-term bone marrow cultures by

murine stromal cells selectively expressing the membrane-bound and secreted forms of the human homolog of the steel gene product, stem cell factor. *Proc. Natl. Acad. Sci.* **89,** 7350–7354.
101. Hanenberg, H., Hashino, K., Konishi, H., Hock, R. A., Kato, I., and Williams, D. A. (1997) Optimization of fibronectin-assisted retroviral gene transfer into human CD34⁺ hematopoietic cells. *Human Gene Ther.* **8,** 2193–2206.
102. Yoder, M. C. and Williams, D. A. (1995) Matrix molecule interactions with hematopoietic stem cells. *Exp. Hematol.* **23,** 961–967.
103. Ruoslahti, E. (1988) Fibronectin and its receptors. *Ann. Rev. Biochem.* **57,** 375–413.
104. Williams, D. A., Rios, M., Stephens, C., and Patel, V. P. (1991) Fibronectin and VLA-4 in hemotopoietic stem-cell-microenvironment interactions. *Nature* **352,** 438–441.
105. Kimizuka, F., Taguchi, Y., Ohdate, Y., Kawase, Y., Shimojo, T., Hashino, K., Kato, I., Sekiguchi, K., and Titani, K. (1991) Production and characterization of functional domains of human fibronectin expressed in Escherichia coli. *J. Biochem.* **110,** 284–291.
106. Culver, K., Cornetta, K., Morgan, R., Morecki, S., Aebersold, P., Kasid, A., Lotze, M., Rosenberg, S. A., Anderson, W. F., and Blaese, R. M. (1991) Lymphocytes as cellular vehicles for gene therapy in mouse and man. *Proc. Natl. Acad. Sci. USA* **88,** 3155–3159.
107. Hege, K. M. and Roberts, M. R. (1996) T-cell gene therapy. *Curr. Opin. Biotech.* **7,** 629–634.
108. Shimizu, Y., van Seventer, G. A., Ennis, E., Newman, W., Horgan, K. J., and Shaw, S. (1992) Crosslinking of the T cell-specific accessory molecules CD7 and CD28 modulates T cell adhesion. *J. Exp Med.* **175,** 577–582.
109. Shimizu, Y., van Seventer, G. A., Horgan, K. J., and Shaw, S. (1990) Regulated expression and binding of three VLA (β1) integrin receptors on T cells. *Nature* **345,** 250–253.
110. Turcovski-Corrales, S. M., Fenton, R. G., Peltz, G., and Traub, D. D. (1995) CD28:B7 interactions promote T cell adhesion. *Eur. J. Immunol.* **25,** 3087–3093.
111. Bock, T. A., Orlic, D., Dunbar, C. E., Broxmeyer, H. E., and Bodine, D. M. (1995) Improved engraftment of human hematopoietic cells in severe combined immunodeficient (SCID) mice carrying human cytokine transgenes. *J. Exp. Med.* **182,** 2037–2043.
112. Lubin, I., Segall, H., Marcus, H., David, M., Kulova, L., Steinitz, M., Erlich, P., Gan, J., and Reisner, Y. (1994) Engraftment of human peripheral blood lymphocytes in normal strains of mice. *Blood* **83,** 2368–2381.
113. Nolta, J., Dao, M., Wells, S., Smogorzewska, E., and Kohn, D. (1996) Transduction of pluripotent human hematopoietic stem cells demonstrated by clonal analysis after engraftment in immune deficient mice. *Proc. Natl. Acad. Sci. USA.* **93,** 2414–2419.
114. Champsiex, C., Marechal, V., Khazaal, I., Schwartz, O., Fournier, S., Schlegel, N., Dranoff, G., Danos, O., Blot, P., Vilmer, E., Heard, J. M., Peault, B., and Lehn, P. (1996) A cell surface marker gene transferred with a retroviral vector into CD34⁺ cord blood cells is expressed by their T-cell progeny in the SCID-hu thymus. *Blood* **88,** 107–113.
115. Tary-Lehmann, M., Lehmann, P. V., Schols, D., Roncarolo, M. G., and Saxon, A. (1994) Anti-SCID mouse reactivity shapes the human CD4⁺ T cell repertoire in hu-PBL-SCID chimeras. *J. Exp. Med.* **180,** 1817–1827.
116. Srour, E. F., Zanjani, E. D., Cornetta, K., Traycoff, C. M., Flake, A. W., Hedrick, M., Brandt, J. E., Leemhuis, T., Hoffman, R. (1993) Persistence of human multilineage, self-renewing lymphohematopoietic stem cells in chimeric sheep. *Blood* **82,** 3333–3342.
117. Zanjani, E. D., Srour, E. F., and Hoffman, R. (1995) Retention of long-term repopulating ability of xenogeneic transplanted purified adult human bone marrow hematopoietic stem cells in sheep. *J. Lab. Clin. Med.* **126,** 24–28.
118. Hirschhorn, R. (1995) Adenosine deaminase deficiency: molecular basis and recent developments. *Clin. Immun. Immunopath.* **76,** S219–S227.
119. Dong, R., Kameoka, J., Hegen, M., Tanaka, T., Xu, Y., Schlossman, S. F., and Morimoto, C. (1996) Characterization of adenosine deaminase binding to human CD26 on T cells and its biologic role in immune response. *J. Immunol.* **156,** 1349–1355.
120. Parkman, R. (1986) The application of bone marrow transplantation to the treatment of genetic diseases. *Science* **232,** 1373–1378.

121. Fairbanks, L. D., Simmonds, A. A., Hoogerbrugge, P. M., van Beusechem, V. W., Valerio, D., Moseley, A., Levinsky, R. J., Gaspar, H. B., and Morgan, G. (1995) Biochemical and immunological status following gene therapy and PEG-ADA therapy for adenosine deaminase (ADA) deficiency, in *Purine and Pyrimidine Metabolism in Man* VIII. (Sahota, A. and Taylor, M., eds.), Plenum Press, New York.
122. Braakman, E., van Beusechem, V. W., van Krimpen, B. A., Fischer, A., Bolhuis, R. L. H., and Valerio, D. (1992) Genetic correction of cultured T cells from an adenosine deaminase-deficient patient: characteristic of non-transduced and transduced T cells. *Eur. J. Immunol.* **22,** 63–69.
123. Ferrari, G., Rossini, S., Giavazzi, R., Maggioni, D., Nobili, N., Soldati, M., Ungers, G., Mavilio, F., Gilboa, E., and Bordignon, C. (1991) An in vivo model of somatic cell gene therapy for human severe combined immunodeficiency. *Science* **251,** 1363–1366.
124. Leonard, W. J. (1996) The molecular basis of X-linked severe combined immunodeficiency: defective cytokine receptor signaling. *Annu. Rev. Med.* **47,** 229–239.
125. Puck, J. M., de Saint Basile, G., Schwarz, K., Fugmann, S., and Fischer, R. E. (1996) IL2RGbase: a database of γ_c-chain defects causing human X-SCID. *Immunol. Today* **17,**
126. Leonard, W. J., Noguchi, M., Russell, S. M., and McBride, O. W. (1994) The molecular basis of X-linked severe combined immunodeficiency: the role of the interleukin-2 receptor γ chain as a common γ chain, γ_c. *Immunol. Rev.* **138,** 61–86.
127. Noguchi, M., Yi, H., Rosenblatt, H. M., Filipovich, A. H., Adelstein, A., Modl, W. S., McBride, O. W., and Leonard, W. J. (1993) Interleukin-2 receptor γ chain mutation results in X-linked severe combined immunodeficiency in humans. *Cell* **73,** 147–157.
128. Puck, J. M., Deschenes, S. M., Porter, J. C., Dutra, A. S., Brown, C. J., Willard, H. F., and Henthorn, P. S. (1993) The interleukin-2 receptor γ chain maps to Xq13. 1 and is mutated in X-linked severe combined immunodeficiency, SCIDX1. *Hum. Mol. Gen.* **2,** 1099–1104.
129. Russell, S. M., Keegan, A. D., Harada, N., Nakamura, Y., Noguchi, M., Leland, P., Friedmann, M. C., Miyajima, A., Puri, R. K., Paul, W. E., and Leonard, W. J. (1993) Interleukin-2 receptor γ chain: a functional component of the interleukin-4 receptor. *Science* **262,** 1880–1883.
130. Kondo, M., Takeshita, T., Ishii, N., Nakamura, M., Watanabe, S., Arai, K., and Sugamura, K. (1993) Sharing of the interleukin-2 (IL-2) receptor γ chain between receptors for IL-2 and IL-4. *Science* **262,** 1874–1876.
131. Noguchi, M., Nakamura, Y., Russell, S. M., Ziegler, S. F., Tsang, M., Cao, X. G., and Leonard, W. J. (1993) Interleukin-2 receptor γ chain: a functional component of the interleukin-7 receptor. *Science* **262,** 1877–1880.
132. Kondo, M., Takeshita, T., Higuchi, M., Nakamura, M., Sudo, T., Nishikawa, S., and Sugamura, K. (1994) Functional participation of the IL-2 receptor γ chain in IL-7 receptor complexes. *Science* **364,** 1453–1454.
133. Russell, S. M., Johnston, J. A., Noguchi, M., Kawamura, M., Bacon, C. M., Friedmann, M., Berg, M., McVicar, D. W., Witthuhn, B. A., Silvennoinen, O., Goldman, A. S., Schmalstieg, F. C., Ihle, J. N., O'Shea, J. J., and Leonard, W. J. (1994) Interaction of IL-2Rβ and γ_c chains with Jak1 and Jak3: implications for XSCID and XCID. *Science* **266,** 1042–1045.
134. Giri, J. G., Ahdieh, M., Eisenman, J., Shanebeck, K., Grabstein, K., Kumaki, S., Namen, A., Park, L. S., Cosman, D., and Anderson, D. (1994) Utilization of the β and γ chains of the IL-2 receptor by the novel cytokine IL-15. *EMBO J.* **13,** 2822–2830.
135. Peschon J., Morrissey, P. J., Grabstein, K. H., Ramsdell, F. J., Maraskovsky, E., Gliniak, B. C., Park, L. S., Ziegler, S. F., Williams, D. E., Ware, C. B., Meyer, J. D., and Davison, B. L. (1994) Early lymphocyte expansion is severely impaired in interleukin 7 receptor-deficient mice. *J. Exp. Med.* **180,** 1955–1960.
136. Grabstein, K. H., Waldschmidt, T. J., Finkelman, F. D., Hess, B. W., Alpert, A. R., Boiani, N. E., Namen, A. E., and Morrissey, P. J. (1993) Inhibition of murine B and T lymphopoiesis in vivo by an anti-interleukin 7 monoclonal antibody. *J. Exp Med.* **178,** 257–264.
137. Boussiotis, V. A., Barber, D. L., Nakarai, T., Freeman, G. J., Gribben, J. G., Bernstein, G. M., D'Andrea, A. D., Ritz, J., and Nadler, L. M. (1994) Prevention of T cell anergy by signaling through the γ_c chain of the IL-2 receptor. *Science* **266,** 1039–1050.

138. Taylor, N, Uribe, L., Smith, S., Jahn, T., Kohn, D. B., and Weinberg, K. (1996) Correction of interleukin-2 receptor function in X-SCID lymphoblastoid cells by retrovirally mediated transfer of the γ_c gene. *Blood* **87,** 3103–3107.
139. Hacein-Bey, B., Cavazzana-Calvo, M., Le Deist, F., Dautry-Varsat, A., Hivroz, C., Riviere, I., Danos, O., Heard, J. M., Sugamura, K., Fischer, A., and De Saint Basile, G. (1996) γ_c gene transfer into SCID X1 patients' B-cell lines restores normal high-affinity interleukin-2 receptor expression and function. *Blood* **87,** 3108–3116.
140. Miyazaki, T., Kawahara, A., Fujii, H., Nakagawa, Y., Minami, Y., Liu, Z. -J., Oishi, I., Silvennoinen, O., Witthuhn, B. A., Ihle, J. N., and Taniguchi, T. (1994) Functional activation of Jak1 and Jak3 by selective association with IL-2 receptor subunits. *Science* **266,** 1045–1047.
141. Qazilbash, M. H., Walsh, C. E., Russell, S. M., Noguchi, M., Mann, M. M., Leonard, W. J., and Liu, J. M. (1995) Retroviral vector for gene therapy of X-linked severe combined immunodeficiency syndrome. *J. Hematother.* **4,** 91–98.
142. Ohbo, K., Takasawa, N., Ishii, N., Tanaka, N., Nakamura, M., and Sugamura, K. (1995) Functional analysis of the human interleukin-2 receptor γ chain gene promoter. *J. Biol. Chem.* **270,** 7479–7486.
143. Cao, X., Shores, E. W., Hu-Li, J., Anver, M. R., Keisall, B. L., Russell, S. M., Drago, J., Noguchi, M., Grinberg, A., Bloom, E. T., Paul, W. E., Katz, S. I., Love, P. E., and Leonard, W. J. (1995) Defective lymphoid development in mice lacking expression of the common cytokine receptor γ chain. *Immunity* **2,** 223–238.
144. DiSanto, J. P., Muller, W., Guy-Grand, D., Fischer, A., and Rajewsky, K. (1995) Lymphoid development in mice with a targeted deletion of the interleukin 2 receptor γ chain. *Proc. Natl. Acad. Sci. USA* **92,** 377–381.
145. Ohbo, K., Suda, T., Haashiyama, M., Mantani, A., Ikebe, M., Miyakawa, K., Moriyama, M., Nakamura, M., Katsuki, M., Takahashi, K., Yamamura, K., and Sugamura, K. (1996) Modulation of hematopoiesis in mice with a truncated mutant of the interleukin-2 receptor γ chain. *Blood* **3,** 956–967.
146. Henthorn, P. S., Somberg, R. L., Fimiani, V. M., Puck, J. M., Patterson, D. F., and Felsburg, P. J. (1994) IL-2Rγ gene microdeletion demonstrates that canine X-linked severe combined immunodeficiency is a homologue of the human disease. *Genomics* **23,** 69–74.
147. Somberg, R. L., Tipold, A., Hartnett, B. J., Moore, P. F., Henthorn, P. S., and Felsburg, P. J. (1996) Postnatal development of T cells in dogs with X-linked severe combined immunodeficiency. *J. Immunol.* **156,** 1431–1435.
148. Buckley, R. H., Schiff, S. E., Roberts, J. L., Markert, M. L., Peters, W., Williams, L. W., and Ward, E. (1993) Haploidentical bone marrow stem cell tranplantation in human severe combined immunodeficiency. *Semin. Hematol.* **30,** 92–101.
149. Cavazzana-Calvo, M., Hacein-Bey, S., de Saint Basile, G., De Coene, C., Self, F., Le Deist, F., and Fischer, A. (1996) Role of interleukin-2 (IL-2), IL-7, and IL-15 in natural killer cell differentiation from cord blood hematopoietic progenitor cells and from γ_c transduced severe combined immunodeficiency X1 bone marrow cells. *Blood* **88,** 3901–3909.
150. Sutkowski, N., Kuo, M., Varela-Echavarria, A., Dougherty, J. P., and Ron, Y. (1994) A murine model for B-lymphocyte somatic cell gene therapy. *Proc. Natl. Acad. Sci. USA* **91,** 8875–8879.
151. Noelle, R. J. (1995) The role of gp39 (CD40L) in immunity. *Clin. Immunol. Immunopath.* **76,** S203–S207.
152. Rosen F. S., Cooper, M. D., and Wedgwood, R. J. P. (1995) The primary immunodeficiencies. *NEJM* **333,** 431–440.
153. Allen, R., Armitage, R. J., Conley, M. E., Rosenblatt, H., Jenkis, N. A., Copeland, N. G., Bedell, M. A., Edilhoff, S., Desteche, C. M., Simoneaux, D. K., Fanslow, W. C., Belmont, J., and Spriggs, M. K. (1993) CD40 ligand gene defects responsible for X-linked hyper IgM syndrome. *Science* **259,** 990–993.
154. Aruffo, A., Farrington, M., Hollenbaugh, D., Xu, L., Milatovich, A., Nonoyama, S., Bejorath, J., Grosmaire, L. S., Stenkamp, R., Neubauer, M., Roberts, R. L., Noelle, R. J., Ledbetter, J. A., Francke, U., and Ochs, H. D. (1993) The CD40 ligand, gp39, is defective in activated T cells from patients with X-linked Hyper-IgM Syndrome. *Cell* **72,** 291–300.

155. Korthauer, U., Graf, D., Mages, H. W., Briere, F., Padayachee, M., Malcolm, S., Ugazio, A. G., Notarangelo, L. D., and Kroczek, R. A. (1993) Defective expression of T cell CD40 ligand causes X-linked immunodeficiency with hyper IgM. *Nature* **361,** 539–541.
156. DiSanto, J. P., Bonnefoy, J. Y., Gauchat, J. F., Fischer, A., and de Saint Basile, G. (1993) CD40 ligand mutations in the X-linked form of hyper -IgM syndrome. *Nature* **361,** 541–543.
157. Fuleihan, R., Ramesu, N., Loh, R., Jabara, H., Rosen, F. S., Chatila, T., Fu, S. M., Stamenkovic, I., and Geha, R. S. (1993) Defective expression of the CD40-ligand in X chromosome-linked immunoglobulin deficiency with normal or elevated IgM. *Proc. Natl. Acad. Sci. USA* **90,** 2170–2173.
158. Banchereau, J., Bazan, F., Blanchard, D., Briere, F., Galizzi, J. P., van Kooten, C., Liu, Y. J., Rousset, F., and Saeland, S. (1994) The CD40 antigen and its ligand. *Annu. Rev. Immunol.* **12,** 881–922.
159. Banchereau, J., de Paoli, P., Valle, A., Garcia, E., and Rousset, F. (1991) Long term human B cell lines dependent on interleukin 4 and antibody to CD40. *Science* **291,** 70–72.
160. Rousset, F., Garcia, E., and Banchereau, J. (1991) Cytokine-induced proliferation and immunoglobulin production of human B lymphocytes triggered through their CD40 antigen. *J. Exp. Med.* **173,** 671–682.
161. Kehry, M. R. (1996) CD40-mediated signaling in B cells. *J. Immunol.* **156,** 2345–2348.
162. Foy, T. M., Shepherd, D. M., Durie, F. H., Aruffo, A., Ledbetter, J. A., and Noelle, R. J. (1993) In vivo CD40-gp39 interactions are essential for thymus-dependent humoral immunity. II. Prolonged suppression of the humoral immune response by an antibody to the ligand for CD40, gp39. *J. Exp. Med.* **178,** 1567–1575.
163. Shapira, S., Vercelli, D., Jabara, H., Fu, S. M., and Geha, R. (1992) Molecular analysis of the induction of IgE synthesis in human B cells by IL-4 and engagement of CD40 antigen. *J. Exp. Med.* **175,** 289–292.
164. Vercelli, D., Jabara, H. H., Arai, K., and Geha, R. S. (1989) Induction of human IgE synthesis requires interleukin-4 and T/B cell interactions involving the T cell receptor/CD3 complex and MHC class II antigens. *J. Exp. Med.* **169,** 1295–1307.
165. Vercelli, D. and Geha, R. S. (1991) Regulation of IgE synthesis in humans: a tale of two signals. *J. Allergy Clin. Immunol.* **88,** 285–295.
166. Armitage, R. J., Fanslow, W. C., Stockbine, L., Sato, T. A., Clifford, K. N., Macduff, B. M., Anderson, D. M., Glimpel, S. D., Davis-Smith, T., Maliszewski, C. R., Clark, E. A., Smith, C. A., Grabstein, K. H., Cosman, D., and Spriggs, M. K. (1992) Molecular and biological characterization of a murine ligand for CD40. *Nature* **357,** 80–82.
167. Hollenbaugh, D., Gosmaire, L., Kullas, C. D., Chalupny, N. J., Noelle, R. J., Stamenkovic, I., Ledvetter, J. A., and Aruffo, A. (1992) The human T cell antigen gp39, a member of the TNF gene family, is a ligand for the CD40 receptor: expression of a soluble form of gp39 with B cell co-stimulatory activity. *EMBO J.* **11,** 4313–4321.
168. Notarangelo, L. D., et al. (1996) CD40Lbase, a database of CD40L gene mutations causing X-linked hyper-IgM syndrome. *Immuol. Today* **17,** 511–516.
169. Ramesh, N., Morio, T., Fuleihan, R., Worm, M., Horner, A., Tsitsikov, E., Castigli, E., and Geha, R. S. (1995) CD40-CD40 ligand (CD40L) interactions and X-linked HyperIgM Syndrome (HIGMX-1). *Clin. Immunol. Immunopath.* **76,** S208–S213.
170. Xu, J., Foy, T. M., Laman, J. D., Elliott, E. A., Dunn, J. J., Waldschmidt, T. J., Elsemore, J., Noelle, R. J., and Flavell, R. A. (1994) Mice deficient for the CD40 ligand. *Immunity* **1,** 423–431.
171. Kawabe, T., Naka, T., Yoshida, K., Tanaka, T., Fujiwara, H., Suematsu, S., Yoshida, N., Kishimoto, T., and Kikutani, H. (1994) The immune responses in CD40-deficient mice: impaired immunoglobulin class switching and germinal center formation. *Immunity* **1,** 167–178.
172. Durandy, A., Hivroz, C., Mazerolles, F., Schiff, C., Bernard, F., Jouanguy, E., Revy, P., DiSanto, J. P., Gauchat, J. F., Gauchat, J. Y., Bonnefoy, J. Y., Casanova, J. L., and Fischer, A. (1997) Abnormal CD40-mediated activation pathway in B lymphocytes from patients with Hyper-IgM Syndrome and normal CD40 ligand expression. *J. Immunol.* **158,** 2576–2584.

173. Schwarz, K., Nonoyama, S., Peitsch, M. C., de Saint Basile, G., Espanol, T., Fasth, A., Fischer, A., Freitag, K., Friedrich, W., Fugmann, S., Hossle, H., Jones, A., Kinnon, C., Meindl, A., Notarangelo, L. D., Weschsler, A., Weiss, M., and Ochs, H. D. (1996) WASPbase: a database of WAS- and XLT-causing mutations. *Immunol. Today* **17,** 496–502.
174. Gerwin, N., Friedrich, C., Perez-Atayde, A., Rosen, F. S., and Gutierrez-Ramos, J. C. (1996) Multiple antigens are altered on T and B lymphocytes from peripheral blood and spleen of patients with Wiskott-Aldrich syndrome. *Clin. Exp. Immunol.* **106,** 208–217.
175. Kawabata, K., Nagasawa, M., Morio, T., Okawa, H., and Yata, J. (1996) Decreased alpha/beta heterodimer among CD8 molecules of peripheral blood T cells in Wiskott-Aldrich syndrome. *Clin. Immunol. Immunopath.* **81,** 129–135.
176. Kwan, S. -P., Hagemann, T. L., Radtke, B. E., Blaese, R. M., and Rosen, F. S. (1995) Identifications of mutations in the Wiskott-Aldrich syndrome gene and characterization of a polymorphic dinucleotide repeat at DXS6940, adjacent to the disease gene. *Proc. Natl. Acad. Sci. USA* **92,** 4706–4710.
177. Symons, M., Derry, J. M. J., Karlak, B., Jiang, S., Lemahieu, V., McCormick, F., Francke, U., and Abo, A. (1996) Wiskott-Aldrich syndrome protein, a novel effector for the GTPase CDC42Hs, is implicated in actin polymerization. *Cell* **84,** 723–734.
178. Cory, G. O. C., MacCarthy-Morrogh, L., Banin, S., Gout, I., Brickell, P. M., Levinsky, R. J., Kinnon, C., and Lovering, R. C. (1996) Evidence that the Wiskott-Aldrich Syndrome protein may be involved in lymphoid cell signaling pathways. *J. Immunol.* **157,** 3791–3795.
179. Kolluri, R., Tolias, K. F., Carpenter, C. L., Rosen, F. S., and Kirchhausen, T. (1996) Direct interaction of the Wiskott-Aldrich syndrome protein with the GTPase Cdc42. *Proc. Natl. Acad. Sci. USA* **93,** 5615–5618.
180. Stowers L., Yelon, D., Berg, L. J., and Chant, J. (1995) Regulation of the polarization of T cells toward antigen-presenting cells by Ras-related GTPase CDC42. *Proc. Natl. Acad. Sci. USA* **92,** 5027–5031.
181. Sideras, P. and Smith, C. I. (1995) Molecular and cellular aspects of X-linked agammaglobulinemia. *Adv. Immunol.* **59,** 135–233.
182. Vetrie, D., Vorechovsky, I., Sideras, P., Holland, J., Davies, A., Flinter, F., Hammarstrom, L., Kinnon, C., Levinsky, R., Bobrow, M., Smith, C. I. E., and Bentley, D. R. (1993) The gene involved in X-linked agammaglobulinaemia is a member of the *src* family of protein tyrosine kinases. *Nature* **361,** 226–233.
183. Smith, C. I., Baskin, B., Humire-Greiff, P., Zhou, J. N., Olsson, P. G., Maniar, H. S., Kjellen, P., Lambris, J. D., Christensson, B., Hammarstrom, L., Bentley, D., Vetrie, D., Islam, K. B., Vorechovsky, I., and Sideras, P. (1994) Expression of Bruton's agammaglobulinemia tyrosine kinase gene, BTK, is selectively down-regulated in T lymphocytes and plasma cells. *J. Immunol.* **152,** 557–565.
184. de Weers, M., Verschuren, M. C., Kraakman, M. E., Mensink, R. G., Schuurman, R. K., van Dongen, J. J., and Hendriks, R. W. (1993) The Bruton's tyrosine kinase gene is expressed throughout B cell differentiation, from early precursor B cell stages preceding immunoglobulin gene rearrangement up to mature B cell stages. *Eur. J. Immunol.* **23,** 3109–3114.
185. Conley, M. E. (1985) B cells in patients with X-linked aggammaglobulinemia. *J. Immunol.* **134,** 3070–3074.
186. Kerner, J. D., Appleby, M. W., Mohr, R. N., Chien, S., Rawlings, D. J., Maliszewski, C. R., Witte, O. N., and Perlmutter, R. M. (1995) Impaired expansion of mouse B cell progenitors lacking Btk. *Immunity* **3,** 301–312.
187. Arpaia, E., Shahar, M., Dadi, H., Cohen, A., and Roifman, C. M. (1994) Defective T cell receptor signaling and $CD8^+$ thymic selection in humans lacking ZAP kinase. *Cell* **76,** 947–958.
188. Elder, M. E., Lin, D., Clever, J., Chan, A. C., Hope, T. J., Weiss, A., and Parslow, T. G. (1994) Human severe immunodeficiency due to a defect in ZAP-70, a T cell tyrosinase kinase. *Science* **264,** 1596–1601.
189. Chan, A. C., Kadlecek, T., Elder, M., Filipovich, A., Grey, J., Iwashima, M., Parslow, T., and Weiss, A. (1994) ZAP–70 protein tyrosine kinase deficiency in an autosomal recessive form of severe combined immunodeficiency. *Science* **264,** 1599–1601.

190. Chan, A. C., van Oers, N. S. C., Tran, A., Turka, L., Law, C. L., Ryan, J. C., Clark, E. A., and Weiss, A. (1994) Differential expression of ZAP-70 and Syk protein tyrosine kinases, and the role of this family of protein tyrosine kinases in TCR signaling. *J. Immunol.* **152,** 4758–4766.
191. Taylor, N., Bacon, K. B., Smith, S., Jahn, T., Kadlecek, T. A., Uribe, L., Kohn, D. B., Gelfand, E. W., Weiss, A., and Weinberg, K. (1996) Reconstitution of T cell receptor signaling in ZAP-70-deficient cells by retroviral transduction of the ZAP-70 gene. *J. Exp. Med.* **184,** 2031–2036.
192. Negishi, I., Motoyams, N., Nakayama, K. -I., Nakayama, K., Senju, S., Hatakeyama, S., Zhang, Q., Chan, A. C., and Loh, D. Y. (1995) Essential role for ZAP-70 in both positive and negative selection of thymocytes. *Nature* **376,** 435–438.
193. Rosenzweig, M., Marks, D. F., Zhu, H., Hempel, D., Mansfield, K. G., Sehgal, P. K., Kalams, S., Scadden, D. T., and Johnson, R. P. *In vitro* T lymphopoiesis of Human and Rhesus CD34$^+$ progenitor cells. *Blood* **87,** 4040–4048.
194. Emerson, S. G. (1996) *Ex vivo* expansion of hematopoietic precursors, progenitors, and stem cells: the next generation of cellular therapeutics. *Blood* **87,** 3082–3088.
195. Pollock, J. D., Williams, D. A., Gifford, M. A., Li, L. L., Du, X., Fisherman, J., Orkin, S. H., Doerschuk, C. M., and Dinauer, M. C. (1996) Mouse model of X-linked chronic granulomatous disease, an inherited defect in phagocyte superoxide production. *Nat. Gen.* **9,** 202–209.
196. Bjorgvinsdottir, H., Ding, C., Pech, N., Gifford, M. A., Li, L. L., and Dinauer, M. C. (1997) Retroviral-mediated gene transfer of gp91phox into bone marrow cells rescues defect in host defense against Aspergillus fumigatus in murine X-linked chronic granulomatous disease. *Blood* **89,** 41–48.

Index

www.ingramcontent.com/pod-product-compliance
Ingram Content Group UK Ltd.
Pitfield, Milton Keynes, MK11 3LW, UK
UKHW051131260726
13967UKWH00010B/2989